Orthotics and Prosthetics in Rehabilitation

Orthotics and Prosthetics in Rehabilitation

FIFTH EDITION

Kevin K. Chui, PT, DPT, PhD, GCS, OCS, CEEAA, FAAOMPT
Endowed Chair and Professor, Department of Physical Therapy, Waldron College of Health and Human Services, Radford University, Roanoke, Virginia

Sheng-Che Yen, PT, PhD
Clinical Professor, Department of Physical Therapy, Movement and Rehabilitation Sciences, Bouvé College of Health Professions, Northeastern University, Boston, Massachusetts

Daniele Piscitelli, PT, MSc, PhD, OMPT
Assistant Professor, Doctor of Physical Therapy Program, Department of Kinesiology, University of Connecticut, Storrs, Connecticut

Inga Wang, PhD, OTR/L
Professor, Programs in Occupational Therapy, Science, Technology & Rehabilitation, School of Rehabilitation Sciences & Technology, Milwaukee, Wisconsin

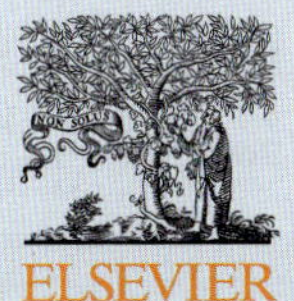
ELSEVIER

ELSEVIER
3251 Riverport Lane
St. Louis, Missouri 63043

ORTHOTICS AND PROSTHETICS IN REHABILITATION, FIFTH EDITION ISBN: 978-0-443-11369-7

Executive Content Strategist: Lauren Willis
Content Development Manager: Ranjana Sharma
Content Development Specialist: Vaishali Singh
Publishing Services Manager: Deepthi Unni
Senior Project Manager: Kamatchi Madhavan
Book Designer: Ryan Cook

Printed in India

Last digit is the print number: 9 8 7 6 5 4 3 2 1

Contributors

Kelly Allegro, PT, DPT, NCS
Assistant Professor and Co-Director of Clinical Education
School of Physical Therapy and Rehabilitation Sciences
University of South Florida
Tampa, Florida

Katherine Bendix, PT, ATP
Therapy Team Leader
Clinical Services
Encompass Health Rehabilitation Hospital of Braintree
Braintree, Massachusetts
Part-Time Lecturer
Bouvé College of Health Sciences
Northeastern University
Boston, Massachusetts

Anna Berardi, OT, PhD
Researcher
Human Neurosciences
Sapienza University of Rome
Rome, Italy

Donna M. Bowers, PT, DPT, MPH, PCS
Clinical Professor
Department of Physical Therapy and Human Movement Science
Sacred Heart University
Fairfield, Connecticut

Luke L. Brisbin, PT, DPT, OCS
Assistant Clinical Professor
Department of Physical Therapy, Movement and Rehabilitation Sciences
Northeastern University
Boston, Massachusetts
Physical Therapist
Rehabilitation Department
Boston Medical Center
Boston, Massachusetts

Steven Brown, CPO
Clinical Assistant Professor and Residency Director
OU Health Orthotics & Prosthetics
Oklahoma City, Oklahoma

Kevin M. Carroll, MS, CP, FAAOP(D)
Vice President of Prosthetics
Lower Limb Prosthetics
Hanger Clinic
Orlando, Florida

Michael K. Carroll, PhD, CPO, FAAOP(D)
National Program Manager, Orthotist-Prosthetist
Orthotic, Prosthetic & Pedorthic Clinical Services
U.S. Department of Veterans Affairs
Washington, District of Columbia
Assistant Professor
Medical Education, College of Medicine
University of Central Florida
Orlando, Florida

Heidi Cheerman, PT, MS, DPT, NCS
Assistant Professor
Department of Physical Therapy, Movement and Rehabilitation Sciences
Northeastern University
Boston, Massachusetts

Kevin K. Chui, PT, DPT, PhD, GCS, OCS, CEEAA, FAAOMPT
Endowed Chair and Professor
Department of Physical Therapy
Waldron College of Health and Human Services
Radford University
Roanoke, Virginia

Matteo Cioeta, PT, OMPT
Clinical Researcher
Research Area in Neuromotor and Robotic Rehabilitation
Department of Neurological and Rehabilitation Sciences
IRCCS San Raffaele
Rome, Italy

Marie B. Corkery, PT, DPT, MHS, FAAOMPT
Clinical Professor
Department of Physical Therapy, Movement and Rehabilitation Sciences
Northeastern University
Boston, Massachusetts

Michelle G. Criss, PT, DPT, PhD, GCS
Associate Professor
Physical Therapy Program
Chatham University
Pittsburgh, Pennsylvania

Jonathan Day, PhD, CPO
Clinical Associate Professor
Orthopedic Surgery and Rehabilitation
The University of Oklahoma Health Sciences Center
Oklahoma City, Oklahoma

Marika Demers, OT, PhD
Assistant Professor
School of Rehabilitation
Université de Montréal
Montréal, Quebec, Canada
Researcher
Institut universitaire sur la réadaptation en déficience physique de Montréal
Centre for Interdisciplinary Research in Rehabilitation of Greater Montreal, CIUSSS du Centre-Sud-de-l'Île-de-Montréal
Montreal, Quebec, Canada

Todd DeWees, MHA, CPO
Manager—Prosthetist Orthotists
POPS
Shriner's Hospital for Children
Portland, Oregon

Jamie Dyson, PT, DPT
Assistant Clinical Professor
Department of Physical Therapy
Graceland University
Independence, Missouri

Duffy Felmlee, MSPO, CPO, FAAOP(D)
Associate Professor
Rehabilitation Sciences
University of Hartford
West Hartford, Connecticut

Eric Folmar, PT, DPT, OCS
Associate Clinical Professor and Associate Department Chair
Department of Physical Therapy, Movement, and Rehabilitation Sciences
Northeastern University
Boston, Massachusetts

Marco Franceschini, MD
Professor Emeritus of Physical and Rehabilitation Medicine
Head of the Research Area in Neuromotor and Robotic Rehabilitation
Department of Neurological and Rehabilitation Sciences
IRCCS San Raffaele
Rome, Italy

Giovanni Galeoto, PT, PhD
Professor
Human Neurosciences
Sapienza University of Rome
Rome, Italy

Michela Goffredo, PhD
Biomedical Engineer
Professor in Physical Medicine and Rehabilitation
Department of Neurological and Rehabilitation Sciences
IRCCS San Raffaele
Rome, Italy
Department of Human Sciences and Promotion of Quality of Life, San Raffaele Open University, Rome, Italy

Tamara N. Gravano, PT, DPT, MSPT, EdD, GCS
Director and Associate Professor
Physical Therapy Program
Temple University
Philadelphia, Pennsylvania

Patrick D. Grimm, MD
Attending Orthopaedic Surgeon
Department of Orthopaedic Surgery
Eisenhower Army Medical Center
Fort Eisenhower, Georgia
Clinical Associate Professor
Department of Orthopaedic Surgery
WellStar MCG Health
Augusta, Georgia

William Holbrook, CP, LP
Senior Clinical Coordinator
Prosthetics
Fourroux Prosthetics
Duluth, Georgia

Renée M. Huth, PhD, DPT
Director of Clinical Education and Assistant Professor
Department of Physical Therapy
Radford University
Roanoke, Virginia

Kent E. Irwin, PT, DHS, MS, GCS
Professor
Physical Therapy Program
Midwestern University
Downers Grove, Illinois

Heather Jennings, PT, DPT
Service Line Manager, Physical Therapist
Physical Medicine and Rehabilitation
Department of Veterans Affairs Hospital
West Roxbury, Massachusetts

Milagros "Millee" Jorge, PT, MA, EdD
Professor Emerita
School of Physical Therapy
Langston University
Langston, Oklahoma

Amanda Knowles, MPO, CPO
Medical Director
OU Health Orthotics & Prosthetics Clinic
Department of Orthopedic Surgery & Rehabilitation
OU Health
Oklahoma City, Oklahoma

Theresa E. Leahy, PT, PhD, MHS
Assistant Professor
School of Physical Therapy
Langston University
Langston, Oklahoma

Daniel J. Lee, PT, DPT, PhD, GCS, OCS, COMT
Chair and Clinical Associate Professor
Department of Physical Therapy
Stony Brook University
Stony Brook, New York

Edward Mahoney, PT, DPT, EdD, CWS
Associate Professor and Program Director
Physical Therapy Program
Louisiana State University Health Sciences Center Shreveport
Shreveport, Louisiana

Jessica M. Marengo, PT, DPT, SM
Visiting Assistant Clinical Professor
Department of Physical Therapy, Movement and Rehabilitation Sciences
Northeastern University
Boston, Massachusetts
Adjunct Assistant Professor
Department of Physical Therapy
University of Pittsburgh
Pittsburgh, Pennsylvania
Physical Therapist
Inpatient Rehabilitations
Beth Israel Deaconess Medical Center
Boston, Massachusetts

Brendan McNulty, PT, DPT, CSCS, CDNS
Physical Therapist
Outpatient Clinic
Ivy Rehab
Palmyra, Virginia

Carol Ann Miller, PT, PhD, GCS
Professor
Department of Physical Therapy
Philadelphia College of Osteopathic Medicine—Georgia
Suwanee, Georgia

Daniel G. Miner, PT, DPT, CCS, NCS
Associate Professor
Department of Physical Therapy
Radford University
Roanoke, Virginia

Kelly J. Negley, PT, DPT, EdD, NCS
Associate Professor
Physical Therapy Program
Marymount University
Arlington, Virginia
Physical Therapist
Rehabilitation
Virginia Hospital Center
Arlington, Virginia

Arco P. Paul, PT, PhD, PGDM, NCS, CSRS
Associate Professor
Department of Physical Therapy
Radford University
Roanoke, Virginia
Physical Therapist
Inpatient Rehabilitation Unit
Lewis Gale Medical Center
Salem, Virginia

Daniele Piscitelli, PT, MSc, PhD, OMPT
Assistant Professor
Doctor of Physical Therapy Program
Department of Kinesiology
University of Connecticut
Storrs, Connecticut

Elicia Pollard, PT, PhD, MEd
Dean
School of Physical Therapy
Langston University
Langston, Oklahoma

Benjamin K. Potter, MD, FAAOS, FAOA, FACS
Norman M. Rich Professor and Chair
Walter Reed Department of Surgery
Uniformed Services University
Bethesda, Maryland

Sanaz Pournajaf, MSc, DPT
Senior Clinical Researcher
Research Area in Neuromotor and Robotic Rehabilitation
Department of Neurological and Rehabilitation Sciences
IRCCS San Raffaele
Rome, Italy
Lecturer in Rehabilitation Methodology
Department of Medical and Surgical Sciences and Translational Medicine—Faculty of Medicine and Psychology
Sapienza Università di Roma
Rome, Italy

John Rheinstein, CP, FAAOP(D)
Upper and Lower Limb Prosthetic Specialist
Metro New York
Hanger Clinic
New York, New York

Julie D. Ries, PT, PhD
Professor
Physical Therapy Program
Marymount University
Arlington, Virginia

S. Tyler Shultz, PT, DPT, OCS
Associate Professor
Department of Physical Therapy
Wingate University
Wingate, North Carolina

Stanislaw Solnik, PT, PhD
Associate Professor
Department of Physical Therapy
University of North Georgia
Dahlonega, Georgia

Donna Sylvester, PT, DPT
Assistant Professor
School of Physical Therapy
Langston University
Langston, Oklahoma

Susan Hallenborg Ventura, PT, MEd, PhD
Associate Clinical Professor (Retired)
Department of Physical Therapy, Movement, and Rehabilitation Sciences
Northeastern University
Boston, Massachusetts

Inga Wang, PhD, OTR/L
Professor
Programs in Occupational Therapy, Science, Technology & Rehabilitation
School of Rehabilitation Sciences & Technology
Milwaukee, Wisconsin

Mariana Wingood, PT, DPT, PhD, MPH, GCS, CEEAA
Assistant Professor
Department of Implementation Science
Department of Internal Medicine/Section of Gerontology and Geriatric Medicine
Wake Forest University School of Medicine
Winston Salem, North Carolina

Christopher K. Wong, PT, PhD, OCS
Orthopedic Clinical Residency Curriculum Director
Department of Physical Therapy
Columbia University Irving Medical Center
New York, New York
Professor
Department of Rehabilitation & Regenerative Medicine
Columbia University Irving Medical Center
New York, New York

Pei-Tzu Wu, PT, PhD, CCS
Professor
Physical Therapy Program
Southern California University of Health Sciences
Whittier, California

Sheng-Che Yen, PT, PhD
Clinical Professor
Department of Physical Therapy, Movement and Rehabilitation Sciences
Bouvé College of Health Professions
Northeastern University
Boston, Massachusetts

Preface

The roots of *Orthotics and Prosthetics in Rehabilitation* can be traced to a novice faculty member haunting what was then known as "publisher's row" in multiple exhibit halls in successive years of the American Physical Therapy Association's Combined Sections and Annual Conference, searching for resources to use in the course content she had been assigned to teach at University of Connecticut. Eventually one of the publisher's representatives challenged her: "Well, if you can't find what you want, why don't you write it? Hmm... Perhaps an edited text? Having recently survived the dissertation process, how much more difficult could it be to assemble a team to prepare one chapter in their area of expertise?

Caroline Nielsen, Director of a Master's program for orthotists and prosthetists, and I, a physical therapist who recently transitioned from clinic to academics, colleagues at the University of Connecticut, put our heads together to develop a plan of action. Our edited text should emphasize an interdisciplinary and collaborative perspective, present "best evidence" to guide practice, recognize the person rather than the illness or disability they are living with, include foundational knowledge about development and aging (i.e., take a lifespan approach), and include principles of motor control and motor learning since using orthoses or prostheses requires skill development. We decided to organize chapters into three components: foundational content such as gait analysis, materials, and footwear; content related to the use of orthoses in rehabilitation; and finally content relevant to prosthetic rehabilitation. We tapped our professional networks, twisted a few arms, and assembled a wonderful team of prosthetists and orthotists, physical and occupational therapists, physicians and surgeons, epidemiologists, and psychologists willing to share their expertise. Our goal was to create a resource useful for students during their professional education, as well as for practicing clinicians actively involved in the rehabilitation of persons with mobility issues needing orthoses and those at risk of and experiencing amputation.

We had to develop strong editorial skills to ensure the tone and flow of content were consistent across chapters. We became quite familiar with the process of securing permission to reprint or adapt existing figures and tables and create new art or photos to meet our needs. We could transform references into AMA format in our sleep! Although the project required a few more years than expected to complete, we were so very proud of the text when the first edition was published in 2000! Feedback from academic colleagues in physical therapy (PT) and the orthotics and prosthetics (O&P) world was incredibly positive, and students in the problem-based learning program at Sacred Heart University (where I now teach) found the text to be a readable and reliable resource for their tutorial preparation.

We were rather surprised at how quickly the request to prepare a second edition arrived! There was an abundance of feedback that the organization of the text into foundational, orthotic-related, and prosthetic-related sections was effective to navigate. We had to address improvements in technology and materials, as well as change within the healthcare delivery and reimbursement system; both created new opportunity and constraining challenges to the rehabilitation process for those needing an orthosis or prosthesis. Many of our original contributors (thankfully) took on the challenge of updating their chapters. We developed action-oriented learning objectives to direct readers as they reviewed each chapter. With the development of the *Guide to Physical Therapist Practice*, we incorporated the patient/client management system framework, and the World Health Organization's International Classification of Functioning, Disability and Health into chapter content as well as the case reports we created for the second edition. We saw it published in 2007!

When the request for third edition came along, Caroline had retired, and I was not sure about taking on the task alone! Milagros (Millie) Jorge was adamant that the text should not be lost and signed on to organize the process with me. Millie's network stretched to the west coast; this gave us the opportunity to engage contributors from across the country. We also included new educators needing opportunity to write to document their scholarship, several of whom were graduates of Sacred Heart's PT program! Caroline's historical contribution to this book was acknowledged by including her as editor emeritus. This edition found its way to print in 2013.

I was honored the text was successful enough for Elsevier to request a fourth edition be developed! I had retired myself by that time and no longer had convenient access to the resources used for earlier editions. I turned to my colleague and research partner, Kevin K. Chui, to ask if he might be willing to take the revision on with Millie, and, thankfully, he was. He brought Sheng-Che Yen into the project as well, and together they organized a wonderful cadre of former and new contributors to face the healthcare system challenges and technical advances in the O&P world. Their efforts both updated content and improved "flow" of the text, making it much more reader friendly. That they included me as editor emeritus was wonderful as well, acknowledging the effort that I contributed to previous editions. This one appeared on PT and O&P bookshelves in 2020.

As I write this, the fifth edition is nearing production under Kevin's watchful eyes. I could not have imagined, when Caroline and I started planning the text in 1995, the longevity of our work. Over the years, the text has introduced me to many wonderful professionals from many different fields from whom I have learned much. It has provided opportunity to help shape the way developing professionals coming through my classroom examine, evaluate, and choose interventions to assist those with amputation or other mobility issues regain function, activity, and the ability to participate. It has been a vehicle to mentor developing academics and researchers, a role that I treasured. Preparing each edition has honed the skills, editorial and organizational, necessary to manage a professional journal. It has been a vehicle with which to truly contribute to my beloved profession. I am so very grateful that *Orthotics and Prosthetics in Rehabilitation* will continue.

Now, as an "elder" in rehabilitation, what words of wisdom can I offer to the students, clinicians, and future academics who might use this text during their careers? First, it is truly a privilege, as well as a responsibility to "see possibility for" rather than disability in the individuals and families we care for: we often interact with those whose situation clouds their ability to see a positive future. How wonderful to be part of the team that helps them regain their feet! Second, seek mentorship when you need it, no matter where you are along your professional path; there is always something to learn or a new perspective to consider. Be willing to mentor a colleague when the opportunity presents itself; this text would not have come into being, or continued quite as long as it has, without the support, advice, and questioning of my mentors; and being a mentor is one of the most fulfilling professional role one can take on. Finally, embrace opportunity when one comes your way, even if you wonder if you have the skills or ability that the opportunity might require. We all learn as we go!

There are many individuals who made substantive contributions to this text. I would like to acknowledge a mentor and friend in the O&P world who we lost to COVID-19. When we started the project in 1995, Joan Edelstein, PT, MA, FISPO, CPed, was recognized as a leading expert in prosthetics, primarily working with children with limb deficiency. She had authored many of the manuals and texts available at that time. Rather than viewing *Orthotics and Prosthetics in Rehabilitation* as competition, she enthusiastically welcomed our efforts, reviewed and edited many first edition chapters, contributed an excellent chapter of her own, and wrote the forward. A generous colleague who was a true lifelong learner, and she is much missed by her former students and colleagues. I will always be grateful for her guidance and assistance. I am sure Joan would be pleased that her legacy is, in one way, continuing in the fifth edition of this text.

Thank you for taking the time to read my thoughts. What a wonderful *Orthotics and Prosthetics in Rehabilitation* journey it has been.

Michelle M. Lusardi, PT, DPT, PhD, FAPTA
Professor Emerita
Department of Physical Therapy and
Human Movement Science
Sacred Heart University
Fairfield, Connecticut

Acknowledgments

To my family, for their endless support. To Dr. Michelle Lusardi, PT, DPT, PhD, FAPTA, for her friendship and mentorship. To our returning editor Dr. Sheng-Che Yen, PT, PhD, and our new editors Drs Daniele Piscitelli, PT, MSc, PhD, OMPT, and Inga Wang, OTR/L, PhD, for their commitment to the fifth edition. To all of our colleagues who contributed to the textbook, for their willingness to share their expertise to advance practice. And to my Dean, Dr. Kenneth M. Cox, AuD, MPH, CCC-A, for his guidance.

Kevin K. Chui

To my beloved wife Sara, you have been the support and inspiration behind all my research developments. To my daughters, Diletta A. and Dafne R., you bring joy and wonder into my life every day, reminding me of what truly matters. To my family your sacrifices have allowed me to become the person I am today. To my friends and mentors, Drs. Mindy F. Levin, PT, PhD; Anatol G. Feldman, PhD, DSc; and Mark L. Latash, PhD, you have shown me the path to becoming a scientist. To Dr. Kevin K. Chui, PT, DPT, PhD, GCS, OCS, CEEAA, FAAOMPT, for believing in me for this project.

Daniele Piscitelli

To my beloved wife, Shao-Jen Cheng, and our wonderful sons, you all have been my source of inspiration and interest for all of my scholarly works. To my parents, for your endless support in my life. To my students, it has been a privilege working with you, and you do not know how much I have learned from you.

Sheng-Che Yen

To my beloved partner, Gary Felts, for his unwavering support throughout this journey. I would like to express my deepest gratitude to Dr. Kevin K. Chui, PT, DPT, PhD, GCS, OCS, CEEAA, FAAOMPT, and Dr. Sheng-Che Yen, PT, PhD, for giving me the incredible opportunity to contribute to such a meaningful project. To my students at the University of Wisconsin-Milwaukee (UWM), it has been a privilege to work with you, and your curiosity and innovative ideas continue to inspire me. I would also like to thank the College of Health Professions & Sciences at UWM for providing a supportive environment and the resources necessary to make this possible.

Inga Wang

Acknowledgments

Contents

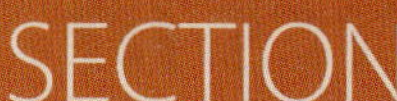

I

Building Baseline Knowledge

1 Orthotics and Prosthetics in Rehabilitation: Multidisciplinary Approach

PEI-TZU WU AND DUFFY FELMLEE

LEARNING OBJECTIVES

On completion of this chapter, the reader will be able to do the following:

1. Describe the role of the orthotist, prosthetist, physical therapist, and other professionals in the rehabilitation of persons with movement dysfunction.
2. Discuss the history and development of physical rehabilitation professions associated with the practice of orthotics and prosthetics in healthcare.
3. Identify contemporary critical factors that continue to influence the need for the use of orthotics and prosthetics in rehabilitation.
4. Apply the use of disablement frameworks in physical rehabilitation.
5. Discuss the role of health professionals in multidisciplinary and interdisciplinary rehabilitation teams.
6. Determine key attributes and attitudes that health professionals should possess to be successful members of interdisciplinary rehabilitation teams.

Health professionals work in healthcare settings to meet the physical rehabilitation needs of diverse patient populations. The current healthcare environment strives to be patient centered and advocates the use of best-practice models that maximize patient outcomes and contain costs. The use of evidence-based treatment approaches, clinical practice guidelines, and standardized outcome measures provides a foundation for evaluating and determining efficacy in healthcare across disciplines and health conditions. The World Health Organization (WHO) International Classification of Functioning, Disability and Health (ICF)[1] provides a disablement framework that enables health professionals to maximize patient/client participation and function while minimizing disability. The current complex environment of healthcare and evolving patterns of healthcare delivery require a focus on multidisciplinary and interdisciplinary approaches to the total care of the patient.

For a healthcare team to function effectively, each member of the healthcare team must develop a positive attitude toward multidisciplinary and interdisciplinary collaboration. The collaborating health professional must understand the functional roles of each healthcare discipline within the team and must respect and value each discipline's input in the decision-making process of the healthcare team. Rehabilitation, particularly when related to orthotics and prosthetics, requires an interdisciplinary approach and lends itself well to collaboration among the various health professionals involved in the management of providing physical rehabilitation. Persons with orthopedic and neurologic impairments caused by a variety of health conditions require a wide range of expert knowledge and technical skills. The physician, prosthetist, orthotist, physical therapist, occupational therapist, nurse, and social worker are important participants in the rehabilitation team who will provide the knowledge and skills necessary for effective patient management. Understanding the roles and professional responsibilities of each of these disciplines maximizes the ability of the rehabilitation team members to function effectively to provide comprehensive care for the patient.

According to disability data from the American Community Survey 2019,[2] 12.7% of noninstitutionalized populations, male or female, of all ages and races regardless of ethnicity, reported having a disability. Among six types of functional disability, mobility disability is the second most common disability type (12.1%) after cognition disability (12.8%), followed by independent living, hearing, vision, and self-care. Nearly 30% of noninstitutionalized civilian veterans aged 21 to 64 years report having a Veterans Administration (VA) service-connected disability.[3]

The continued rise in persons with obesity has increased the number of people with diabetes. The Centers for Disease Control and Prevention 2019 National Diabetes Statistics Report indicates 37.3 million Americans (11.3% of the US population) have diabetes; 96 million Americans (38% of the adult US population) have prediabetes (Box 1.1).[4] Persons with diabetes are at risk for vascular disease, such as peripheral arterial disease (PAD),[5] which often results in musculoskeletal and neuromuscular impairments to the lower extremities. Ischemic disease can cause peripheral neuropathy, loss of sensation, poor skin care and wound formation, trophic ulceration, osteomyelitis, and gangrene, which can result in the need for limb amputation.

Persons coping with illness, injury, disease, impairments, and disability often require rehabilitation inclusive of special orthotic and prosthetic devices to help with mobility, stability, pain relief, and skin and joint protection. Appropriate prescription, fabrication, instruction, and

Box 1.1 Fast Facts on Diabetes

37.3 Million Americans have diabetes (11.3% of the US population)
Diagnosed: 28.7 million people
Undiagnosed: 8.5 million people
96 Million Americans have prediabetes (38.0% of the adult US population)

Centers for Disease Control and Prevention. *National Diabetes Statistics Report*. https://www.cdc.gov/diabetes/data/statistics-report/index.html

application of orthotic and prosthetic devices help persons to engage in activities of daily living as independently as possible. Orthotists and prosthetists are healthcare professionals who custom fabricate and fit orthoses and prostheses. Along with other healthcare professionals, including nurses, physical therapists, and occupational therapists, orthotists and prosthetists are integral members of the multidisciplinary and interdisciplinary rehabilitation teams responsible for returning patients to productive and meaningful lives.

The WHO ICF[1] is a common framework to understand and describe functioning and disability. The use of the WHO ICF disablement framework enables health professionals from across healthcare disciplines to endorse a more inclusive model that uses expertise within the many sectors in rehabilitative care. A multidisciplinary approach to patient care in rehabilitation is the current standard when addressing the needs of persons with physical impairments, limitations, and disabilities. The 2016 American Heart Association (AHA)/American College of Cardiology (ACC) clinical guideline supports an interdisciplinary approach to the management of persons with PAD.[6] The AHA/ACC clinical guideline identifies a team of professionals representing different disciplines to assist in the evaluation and management of patients with PAD. This chapter discusses the developmental history of the art and science of orthotics, prosthetics, and physical therapy as professions dedicated to rehabilitating persons with injury, impairment, and disability.

Orthotists and Prosthetists

Orthotists provide care to persons with neuromuscular and musculoskeletal impairments that contribute to functional limitation and disability by designing, fabricating, and fitting orthoses or custom-made braces. The orthotist is responsible for evaluating the patient's functional and cosmetic needs, designing the orthosis, selecting appropriate components, and fabricating, fitting, and aligning the orthosis. The orthotist educates the patient and the care providers on the appropriate use of the orthosis, care of the orthosis, and how to assess the continued appropriateness of the orthosis (Figs. 1.1 and 1.2).

Prosthetists provide care to patients with partial or total absence of limbs by designing, fabricating, and fitting prostheses or artificial limbs. The prosthetist creates the design to fit the individual's particular functional and cosmetic needs, selects the appropriate materials and components; makes all necessary casts, measurements, and modifications

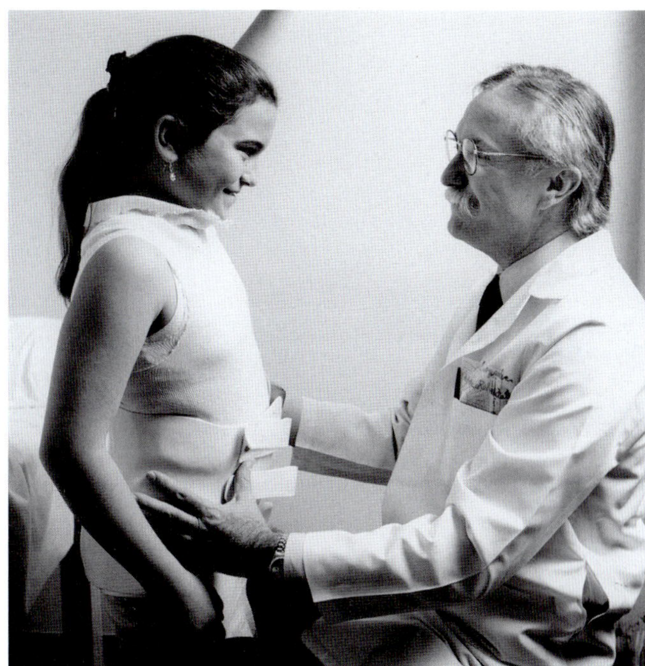

Fig. 1.1 Orthotist is evaluating the proper fit of a spinal orthosis to determine whether it meets the prescriptive goals and can be worn comfortably during functional activities or whether modifications need to be made.

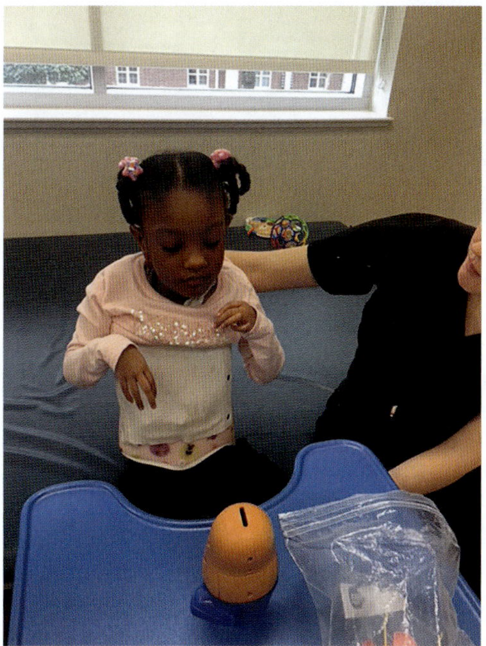

Fig. 1.2 Child is wearing a spinal orthosis during a physical therapy session. Orthotist is observing the child as she is engaged in therapeutic play to assess the child's level of support and comfort while wearing the orthosis.

(including static and dynamic alignment); evaluates the fit and function of the prosthesis on the patient; and teaches the patient how to care for the prosthesis (Figs. 1.3 and 1.4).

According to the US Department of Labor, Bureau of Labor Statistics, in 2023 there were an estimated 8820 orthotists and/or prosthetists practicing in the United

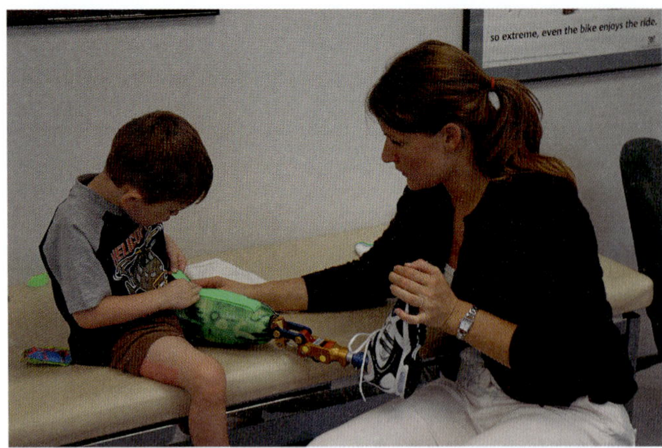

Fig. 1.3 Prosthetist is assisting the child in donning prosthetic limb. Prosthetist will check the prosthesis for alignment, fit, and comfort.

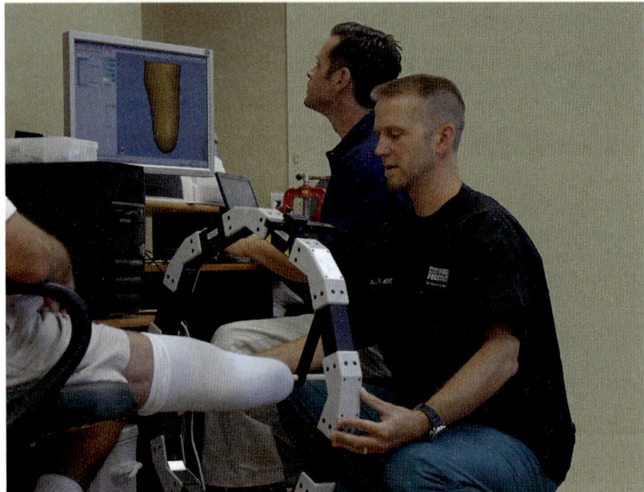

Fig. 1.4 Prosthetist using computer-aided design in fabricating a lower-extremity prosthesis.

States.[7] Individuals who enter the fields of orthotics and prosthetics must complete advanced education (beyond an undergraduate degree) and a residency program before becoming eligible for certification. Registered assistants and technicians in orthotics or prosthetics assist the certified practitioner with patient care and fabrication of orthotic and prosthetic devices.

History

The emergence of orthotics and prosthetics as healthcare professions has followed a course similar to the profession of physical therapy. The development of all three professions is closely related to three significant events in world history: World War I, World War II, and the onset and spread of polio in the 1950s. Unfortunately it has taken war and disease to provide the major impetus for research and development in these key areas of rehabilitation.

Although the profession of physical therapy has its roots in the early history of medicine, World War I was a major impetus to its development. During the war, female "physical educators" volunteered in physicians' offices and Army hospitals to instruct patients in corrective exercises. After the war ended, a group of these "reconstruction aides" joined together to form the American Women's Physical Therapy Association. In 1922 the association changed its name to the American Physiotherapy Association and opened membership to males and aligned itself closely with the medical profession. In the late 1940s the Association had once again changed its name to the American Physical Therapy Association , as it remains at present.[8]

Until World War II, the practice of prosthetics depended on the skills of individual craftsmen. The roots of prosthetics can be traced to early blacksmiths, armor makers, other skilled artisans, and even individuals with amputations, who fashioned makeshift replacement limbs from materials at hand. During the Civil War, more than 30,000 amputations were performed on Union soldiers injured in battle; at least as many occurred among injured Confederate troops. At that time, most prostheses consisted of carved or milled wooden sockets and feet. Many were procured by mail order from companies in New York or other manufacturing centers at a cost of US$75 to US$100 each.[9] Before World War II, prosthetic practice required much hands-on work and craftsman's skill. D.A. McKeever, a prosthetist who practiced in the 1930s, described the process: "You went to [the person with an amputation's] house, took measurements and then carved a block of wood, covered it with rawhide and glue, and sanded it." During his training, McKeever spent 3 years in a shop carving wood: "You pulled out the inside, shaped the outside, and sanded it with a sandbelt."[10]

The development of the profession of orthotics mirrors the field of prosthetics. Early "bracemakers" were also artisans such as blacksmiths, armor makers, and patients who used many of the same materials as the prosthetist: metal, leather, and wood. By the 18th and 19th centuries splints and braces were also mass produced and sold through catalogs. These bracemakers were also frequently known as "bonesetters" until surgery replaced manipulation and bracing in the practice of orthopedics. "Bracemaker" then became a profession with a particular role distinct from that of the physician.[9]

World War II and the period following were times of significant growth for the professions of physical therapy, prosthetics, and orthotics. During the war many more physical therapists were needed to treat the wounded and rehabilitate those who were left with functional impairments and disabilities. The Army became the major resource for physical therapy training programs, and the number of physical therapists serving in the armed services increased more than sixfold.[11] The number of soldiers who required braces or artificial limbs during and after the war increased the demand for prosthetists and orthotists as well.

After World War II, a coordinated program for persons with amputations was developed. In 1945 a conference of surgeons, prosthetists, and scientists organized by the National Academy of Sciences revealed that little scientific effort had been devoted to the development of artificial limbs. A "crash" research program was initiated, funded by the US Department of Veterans Affairs Office of Scientific Research and Development, and continued by the VA. A direct result of this effort was the development of the patellar tendon-bearing prosthesis for individuals with transtibial (below-knee) amputation and the quadrilateral socket design for those with transfemoral (above-knee) amputation. This program also included educating prosthetists, physicians, and physical therapists in the skills of fitting and training of patients with these new prosthetic designs.[11]

The needs of soldiers injured in the military conflicts in Korea and Vietnam ensured continuing research, further refinements, and the development of new materials. The development of myoelectrically controlled upper extremity prostheses and the advent of modular endoskeletal lower-extremity prostheses occurred in the post-Vietnam conflict era. The US Department of Defense reports data on the casualties from military engagements in Iraq and Afghanistan, including Operation Freedom's Sentinel, Operation Inherent Resolve, Operation New Dawn, Operation Iraqi Freedom, and Operation Enduring Freedom. Based on the 2015 Congressional Research Service report on the military casualties of war, 327,299 servicemen and servicewomen sustained traumatic brain injury (TBI) and 1645 sustained major limb amputations.[12]

The use of orthotics and prosthetics to support individuals with TBI and amputation is critical when seeking to reduce impairments and enhance functional abilities. The Veterans Health Administration Research Development is committed to exploring the use of new technology such as robotics, tissue engineering, and nanotechnology to design and build lighter, more functional orthoses and prostheses.[13]

The current term *orthotics* emerged in the late 1940s and was officially adopted by American orthotists and prosthetists when the American Orthotic and Prosthetic Association was formed to replace its professional predecessor, the Artificial Limb Manufacturers' Association. *Orthosis* is a more inclusive term than *brace* and reflects the development of devices and materials for dynamic control in addition to stabilization of the body. In 1948 the American Board for Certification in Orthotics and Prosthetics[14] was formed to establish and promote high professional standards.

Although the polio epidemic of the 1950s played a role in the further development of the physical therapy profession, this epidemic had the greatest effect on the development of orthotics. By 1970 many new techniques and materials, some adapted from industrial techniques, were being used to assist patients in coping with the effects of polio and other neuromuscular disorders. The scope of practice in the field of orthotics is extensive, including working with children with muscular dystrophy, cerebral palsy, and spina bifida; patients of all ages recovering from severe burns or fractures; adolescents with scoliosis; athletes recovering from surgery or injury; and older adults with diabetes, cerebrovascular accident, severe arthritis, and other disabling conditions.

Like physical therapists, orthotists and prosthetists practice in a variety of settings. The largest employers of orthotists and prosthetists are medical equipment and supplies manufacturing, which account for 32% of the jobs in 2021.[15] Many large institutions, such as hospitals, rehabilitation centers, and research institutes, have departments of orthotics and prosthetics with on-site staff to provide services to patients. The prosthetist or orthotist may also be a supplier or fabrication manager in a central production laboratory. In addition, orthotists and prosthetists serve as full-time faculty in orthotic and prosthetic professional education programs. Orthotists and prosthetists also serve as residency directors and clinical educators in a variety of facilities for the year-long residency program required before the certification examination.

Prosthetic and Orthotic Professional Roles and Responsibilities

With rapid advances in technology and healthcare, the roles of the prosthetist and orthotist have expanded from a technological focus to a more inclusive focus on being a member of the rehabilitation team. Patient examination, evaluation, education, and treatment are currently significant responsibilities of prosthetic and orthotic practitioners. Many technical tasks are completed by technicians who work alongside the practitioner in the practice or at a separate central fabrication facility. The advent and availability of modifiable prefabrication systems has reduced the amount of custom fabricated prostheses and especially orthoses provided to patients. Orthotists and prosthetists are vital members of the rehabilitation team to assess the patient's needs for prosthetics and orthotic intervention. They are uniquely qualified to determine if a custom or prefabrication intervention is most appropriate to meet the patient's needs. Current educational requirements reflect these changes in orthotic and prosthetic practice. Entry into professional training programs requires completion of a bachelor's degree from an accredited college or university, with a strong emphasis on prerequisite courses in the sciences. Professional education in orthotics or prosthetics requires an accredited master's degree. Along with the specific orthotics and prosthetic courses, students study research methodology, kinesiology and biomechanics, material science, musculoskeletal and neuromuscular pathology, communication and education, and current healthcare issues. Orthotics and prosthetics programs may be based within academic health centers or in colleges or universities with hospital affiliations. On completion of the educational and experiential requirements, the student must complete an accredited residency in each discipline before being eligible to take the certification and licensure examinations. To address the rehabilitation needs of individuals who require prosthetic and orthotic intervention, physical therapists, orthotists, prosthetists, occupational therapists, and other members of the healthcare team must have discreet knowledge and skills in the management of persons with a variety of health conditions across the life span. Working as a rehabilitation team, physicians, nurses, prosthetists, orthotists, physical therapists, occupational therapists, social workers, patients, and family members seek to alleviate disease, injury, impairments, and disability by maximizing function.

Disablement Frameworks

Historically disability was described using a theoretical medical model of disease and pathology. Over time, various conceptual frameworks have been developed to organize information about the process and effects of disability.[16] Disablement frameworks in the past have been used to understand the relationship of disease and pathology to human function and disability.[16–19] The need to understand the impact that acute injury or illness and chronic health conditions have on the functioning of specific body systems, human performance in general, and the typical activities of daily living from both the individual and a societal perspective has been central to the development of the disablement models. The biomedical model of pathology and dysfunction provided the conceptual framework for understanding human function, disability, and handicap as a consequence of pathological and disease processes.

The Nagi model was among the first to challenge the appropriateness of the traditional biomedical model of disability.[17] Nagi developed a model that looked at the individual in relationship to the pathologic condition, functional limitations, and the role that the environment and society or the social environment played. The four major elements of Nagi's theoretical formulation included active pathology (interference with normal processes at the level of the cell), impairment (anatomic, physiologic, mental, or emotional abnormalities or loss at the level of body systems), functional limitation (limitation in performance at the level of the individual), and disability. Nagi defined disability as "an expression of physical or mental limitation in a social context."[17] The Nagi model was the first theoretical construct on disability that considered the interaction between the individual and the environment from a sociologic perspective rather than a purely biomedical perspective. Despite the innovation of the Nagi model in the 1960s, the biomedical model of disability persisted.

In 1980 the WHO developed the International Classification of Impairments, Disabilities, and Handicaps (ICIDH) to provide a conceptual framework for disability which is described in three dimensions: Impairment, Disability, and Handicap (Fig. 1.5).[20] The ICIDH focused on the effects of pathologic processes on the individual's activity level. Disability was viewed as a result of an impairment and considered a lack of ability to perform an activity in a normal manner.

The Institute of Medicine enlarged Nagi's original concept in 1991 to include the individual's social and physical environment (Fig. 1.6). This revised model describes the environment as "including the natural environment, the built environment, the culture, the economic system, the political system, and psychological factors." In this model disability is not viewed as a pathologic condition residing in a person but instead is a function of the interaction of the person with the environment.[21]

In 1993 the WHO began a revision of the ICIDH disablement framework. The new factors in the ICIDH-2: International Classification of Functioning and Disability include a dimension for participation in social activities and a listing of environmental factors that are important for understanding the complexity of disability. In addition, the revised ICIDH-2 attempts to use neutral terminology that gave rise to the concept that a person's handicap was less related to the health condition that created a disadvantage for completing the necessary life roles but rather to the level of participation that the person with the health condition was able to engage in within the environment.

In 2001 the World Health Assembly endorsed International Classification of Functioning, Disability and Health (ICF) for international use.[22,23] The ICF is the successor of the ICIDH and is the final result of a long-lasting revision process. The ICF provides a standard language for the description of health and health-related states from different perspectives: the perspective of the body (classification of body functions and body structures) and the perspective of the individual and the society (classification of activities and participation). The ICF model helps in the description of changes in body function and structure, what people with particular health conditions can do in standard environments (their level of capacity), and what they actually do in their usual environments (their level of performance). One of the major innovations of the ICF model is the presence of an environmental factor classification that considers the role of environmental barriers and facilitators in the performance of tasks of daily living. The ICF model emphasizes health and functioning rather than disability. The ICF model provides a radical departure from emphasizing a person's disability to focusing on the level of health and facilitating an individual's participation to whatever extent is possible within that level of health. In the ICF disability and functioning are viewed as outcomes of interactions between health conditions (diseases, disorders, and injuries) and contextual factors (Fig. 1.7).

As stated on the ICF website,[24] "To make the ICF more applicable for everyday use, WHO and the ICF Research Branch created a process for developing core sets of ICF categories, or 'ICF Core Sets'."[25] ICF Core Sets facilitate the description of functioning, for example, in clinical practice by providing lists of essential categories that are relevant for specific health conditions and healthcare contexts. These ICF categories were selected from the entire ICF following a scientific process based on preparatory studies and the involvement of a multidisciplinary group of experts.

The evolution of disablement frameworks from the biomedical models to the newer, contemporary models that include the biopsychosocial domains provides theoretical constructs that guide the rehabilitation professional in clinical practice. The development of the ICF Core Sets derived from input from members of the rehabilitation team is essential for clinical decision-making that addresses pathologic conditions or disease processes, impairments, functional limitations, and disabilities. Interrelationships among all four of these elements are the focus of the rehabilitation team. The physical therapist, orthotist, prosthetist, and other team members work together to create the most effective outcome for the patient by identifying and addressing pathologic processes, functional limitations, impairments, and disability. The ICF Core Sets and ICF

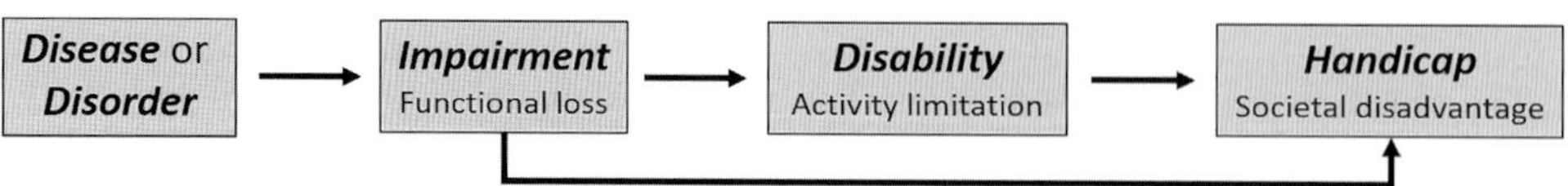

Fig. 1.5 **World Health Organization International Classification of Impairments, Disabilities, and Handicaps Framework.** (Modified from World Health Organization. International classification of impairments, disabilities, and handicaps: a manual of classification relating to the consequences of disease, published in accordance with resolution WHA29.35 of the Twenty-ninth World Health Assembly, May 1976. World Health Organization.)

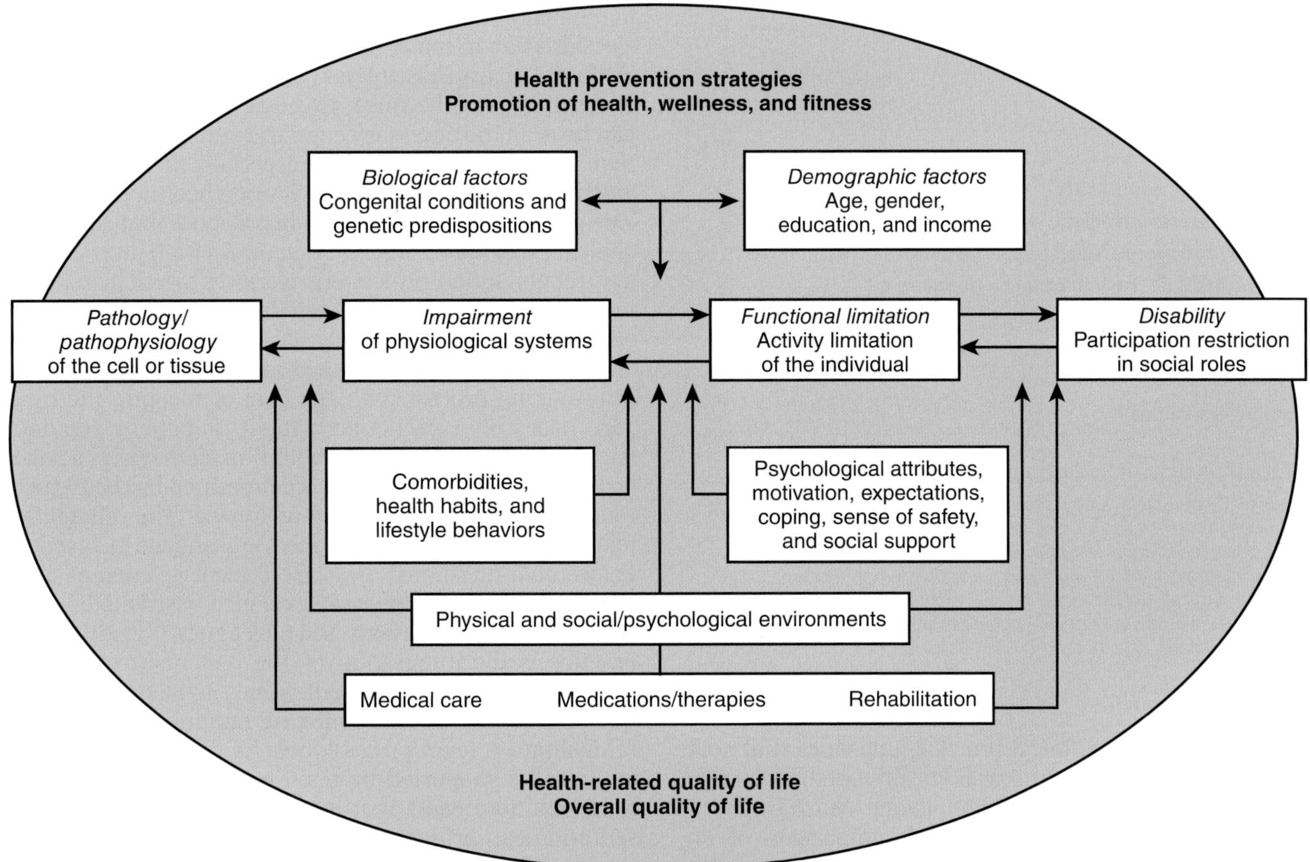

Fig. 1.6 The revised Institute of Medicine/Nagi model of the disablement process considers the impact of pathologic conditions and impairment, as well as intraindividual and extraindividual factors, that may influence functional limitation and disability affecting health-related and overall quality of life. (Modified from Guccione AA. Arthritis and the process of disablement. *Phys Ther.* 1994;74(5):410.)

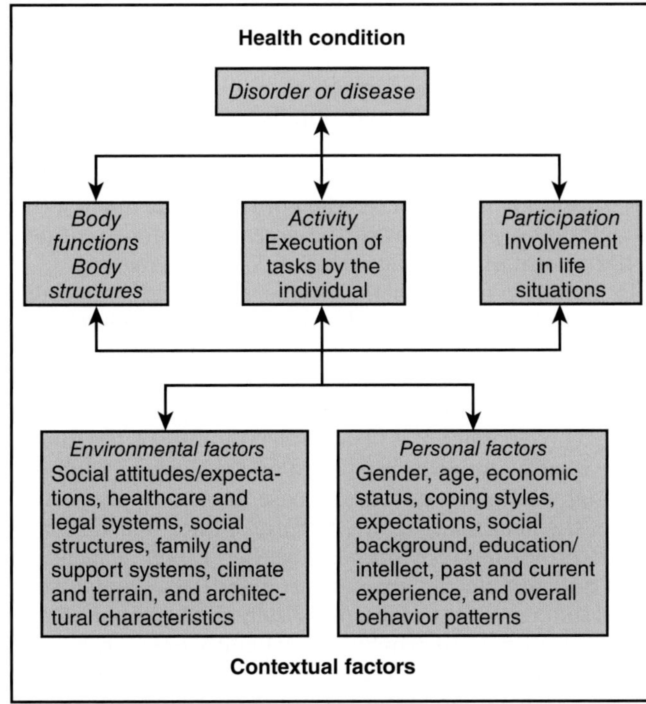

Fig. 1.7 World Health Organization International Classification of Functioning, Disability and Health Framework. (Modified from World Health Organization. *Towards a Common Language for Functioning, Disability and Health.* World Health Organization; 2002:9–10.)

Documentation System[26] allow for data collection that can be useful in research leading to improved patient interventions, assessment of patient outcomes, and development of health and social policies.

Characteristics of Rehabilitation HealthCare Teams

The complexity of the healthcare arena and the level of care required by individuals in rehabilitation care settings require the collaboration of many healthcare practitioners with varied professional skills who can form multidisciplinary, interdisciplinary, and transdisciplinary teams as needed.[27–30] The multidisciplinary rehabilitation team is composed of different health professionals such as the physician, nurse, physical therapist, occupational therapist, prosthetist, orthotist, and social worker. Each professional operates with an area of specialization and expertise. The members of the multidisciplinary teamwork parallel to one another, and the medical record is the collecting source for the information gleaned and shared. Interdisciplinary teams also include representatives of a variety of health disciplines, but there is interdependence among the professionals. In the interdisciplinary team process there is structure and organization that promotes program planning to support patient-centered care through effective communication and effective

Table 1.1 AHA/ACC Clinical Guidelines for Management of Patients With Lower-Extremity Peripheral Artery Disease

- Nurses
- Orthopedic surgeons and podiatrists
- Endocrinologists
- Internal medicine specialists
- Infectious disease specialists
- Radiology and vascular imaging specialists
- Physical medicine and rehabilitation clinicians
- Orthotics and prosthetics specialists
- Social workers or exercise physiologists
- Physical and occupational therapists
- Nutritionists/dietitians

From Gerhard-Herman MD, et al. 2016 AHA/ACC Lower Extremity PAD Guideline. 2016 AHA/ACC guideline on the management of patients with lower extremity peripheral artery disease. A report of the American College of Cardiology/American Heart Association Task Force on clinical practice guidelines. *J Am Coll Cardiol*. 2017;69(11):1465–1508.
Recommendations for interdisciplinary care team members include vascular medical and surgical specialists (i.e., vascular medicine, vascular surgery, interventional radiology, and interventional cardiology). *ACC*, American College of Cardiology; *AHA*, American Heart Association.

clinical management. Clinical practice guidelines that seek to promote best practices for specific health conditions often include information on the interdisciplinary team.[6] Table 1.1 provides an example of the suggested composition of an interdisciplinary team for the management of patients with PAD. The interdisciplinary team members work to establish goals for the team that drive the rehabilitation process for the patient. Interdisciplinary teams traditionally follow a patient-centered approach to goal setting. Establishing the patient as the focus of the work for the team, the interdisciplinary team members collaborate to execute the goals and meet the desired outcomes. Most team processes in rehabilitation centers strive for an interdisciplinary team approach that promotes patient-centered care.[29] Each discipline works within its scope of practice to optimize care through coordinated efforts.

Transdisciplinary teams comprise the same professional members identified in the multidisciplinary and interdisciplinary teams; however, the team members in the transdisciplinary model function differently in that they share clinical responsibilities and overlap in duties and responsibilities. In the transdisciplinary model of team building the professional roles and responsibilities are so familiar to the team members that there is an interchange of tasks and functions.[30] Transdisciplinary teams engage in the release of professional roles typical to the discipline in an effort to have the patient receive the interventions needed within a context that is supportive of the learning and the practice. The transdisciplinary model is operational in the management of infants and toddlers who receive early intervention rehabilitation services and have an Individualized Family Service Plan (IFSP).[31]

Two major issues emerging in healthcare that affect healthcare professionals include (1) the need for healthcare professionals with advanced education and training in specialty and subspecialty areas and (2) the need for collaboration among health practitioners to ensure efficiency of patient management that results in best practice and improves patient outcomes. The information explosion in healthcare, particularly in rehabilitation, has led to increasing specialization and subspecialization in many fields. The multidisciplinary, interdisciplinary, or transdisciplinary healthcare team concept has evolved, in part, because no single individual or discipline can have all the necessary expertise and specialty knowledge required for high-quality care, especially the care of patients with complex disorders. Rehabilitation healthcare teams provide patient care management approaches that capitalize on clinical expertise by engaging members from diverse medical and rehabilitation professions working together, collaborating, and communicating closely to optimize patient care and clinical outcomes.[32,33]

Collaboration is defined as a joint communication and decision-making process with the goal of meeting the healthcare needs of a particular patient or patient population. Each participant on the rehabilitation team brings a particular expertise, and leadership is determined by the particular rehabilitation situation being addressed. The rehabilitation team has the opportunity to meet and engage in "asking the answerable questions" that are critical in current clinical practice when engaging in an evidence-based model of practice. According to Strauss and colleagues,[34] evidence-based practice is the integration of the best research evidence, clinical expertise, and patient values. Evidence-based practice and clinical decision-making enhance the role of the rehabilitation team professionals as they share their clinical insights supported by historical and current evidence. Rehabilitation teams that are diverse in professional representation can bring a wide perspective of expertise on particular rehabilitation issues. With this perspective, clinical decision-making becomes a more inclusive process.

The role of the healthcare professional on a rehabilitation team begins during professional education. Rehabilitation sciences health professionals must work at understanding, evaluating, and analyzing the many facets of healthcare that require specialized professionals who will work to meet the goals and objectives of the specialty and healthcare delivery on the whole. The formation of a rehabilitation team provides a cohort of professionals who individually and collectively strive for effective and efficient management of patients. The team process allows for a deeper understanding of and appreciation for the contributions of the other rehabilitation disciplines in the assessment and treatment of the patient and management of patient problems.

In addition to discipline-specific skills and knowledge, health professionals must be aware of the interrelationships among healthcare workers. One of the major barriers to effective team functioning is a lack of understanding or misconception of the roles of different disciplines in the care of the whole patient.[32] A clear understanding of the totality of the healthcare delivery system and the role of each professional within the system increase the potential effectiveness of the healthcare team. A group of informed, dedicated health professionals working together to set appropriate goals and initiate patient care to meet these goals uses a model that exceeds the sum of its individual components.

Almost all current rehabilitation healthcare is provided in a team setting using a patient-centered approach. This integrated approach facilitates appreciation of the patient as a person with individual strengths and needs rather than as a dehumanized diagnosis or problem. The diverse perspectives and knowledge that are brought to the rehabilitation

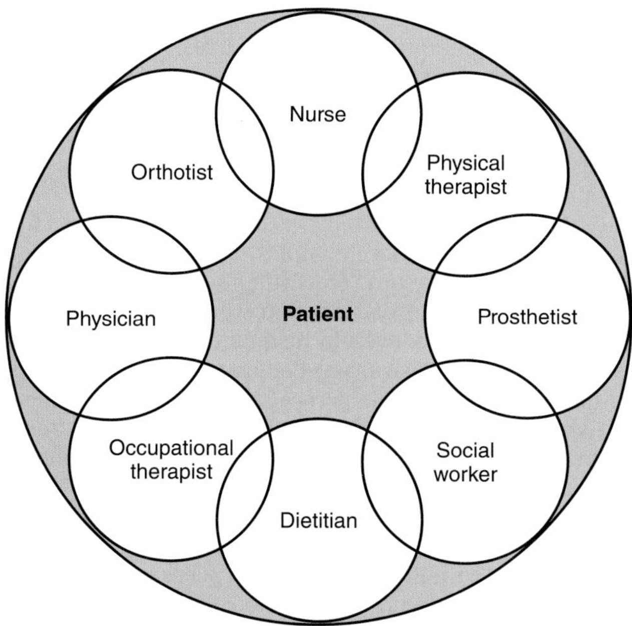

Fig. 1.8 Patient-centered rehabilitation teams. Key components of a successful healthcare team are a clear understanding of the role, responsibilities, and unique skills and knowledge of each member of the rehabilitation team, combined with open and effective communication.

process by the members of the interdisciplinary team provide insight into all aspects of the patient's concerns (Fig. 1.8). Conceptually all members of the healthcare team contribute equally to patient care. The contribution of each is important and valuable; otherwise, the quality of patient care and efficacy of intervention would be diminished. Although one member of the team may take an organization or management role, decision-making occurs through consensus building and critical discussion. Professionals with different skills function together with mutual support, sharing the responsibility of patient care. The multidisciplinary team then develops and implements an integrated and individualized treatment plan for each patient.

VALUES AND BEHAVIORS

Some of the factors that tend to limit the effectiveness of a work group are large group size, poor decision-making practices, lack of fit between group members' skills and task demands, and poor leadership.[35–37] Other factors that influence team dynamics are classified as formal (tangible or visible) and informal (submerged). Formal factors include the policies and objectives of the group or its parent organization, the systems of communication available to the group, and the job descriptions of its members. Informal factors, which are often less obvious but equally influential on the group process, include working relationships among team members; power networks within and external to the group; and the values, beliefs, and goals of individuals within the group. Team-building initiatives are often focused on the formal, or visible, areas, but informal communication, values, and norms play key roles in the functioning of the healthcare team.

A variety of characteristics and considerations also enhance the effectiveness of the interdisciplinary healthcare team. In addition to having strong professional backgrounds and appropriate skills, team members must appreciate the diversity within the group, taking into account age and status differences and the dynamics of individual professional subgroups.[36] The size of the team is also important: the most capable and effective teams tend to have no more than 12 members. Team members who know each other and are aware of and value each other's skills and interests are often better able to set and achieve goals. Clearly defined goals and objectives about the group's purpose and primary task, combined with a shared understanding of each member's roles and skills, increase the likelihood of effective communication.

Values and behaviors that facilitate the collaborative team care model include the following:

- Trust among members that develops over time as members become more familiar with each other.
- Knowledge or expertise necessary for the development of trust.
- Shared responsibility for joint decision-making regarding patient outcomes.
- Mutual respect for all members of the team.
- Two-way communication that facilitates the sharing of patient information and knowledge.
- Cooperation and coordination to promote the use of skills of all team members.
- Optimism that the team is indeed the most effective means of delivering quality care.

In the early stages of development, it is essential that the team spend time developing goals, tasks, roles, leadership, decision-making processes, and communication methods. In other words, the team needs to know where it is going, what it wants to do, who is going to do it, and how it will get done. One of the most important characteristics of an effective healthcare team is the ability to accommodate personal and professional differences among members and to use these differences as a source of strength. A well-functioning team often becomes a means of support, growth, and increased effectiveness and professional satisfaction for the physical therapist and other health professionals who wish to maximize their strengths as individuals while participating in professional responsibilities.

REHABILITATION TEAMS

The interdisciplinary healthcare team has become essential in the rehabilitation of patients whose body function and level of participation in the tasks of daily living could be enhanced by assistive technology such as an orthosis or prosthesis. The complexity of the rehabilitation process and the multidimensional needs of patients frequently require the expertise of many different professional disciplines. The rehabilitation team is often shaped by the typical needs and characteristics of the patient population that it is designed to serve. The individuals most often represented on the rehabilitation team include one or more physicians with specialties in rehabilitation medicine, orthopedics, vascular surgery, or neurology; nurses; prosthetists and/or orthotists; physical therapists; occupational therapists; dietitians; social workers; and vocational rehabilitation counselors, as well as patients and caregivers (Fig. 1.8). Each member of the interdisciplinary team has an important role to play in the rehabilitation of the patient. Patient education is often one of the primary concerns of the team. Imparting information regarding the health condition, etiology, treatment, progression, management, and prognosis helps patients become active partners in the rehabilitation process rather than passive recipients of care. Patient education addresses prevention and treatment strategies; patients and their families are able to identify their needs and concerns and communicate them to the team members. Each member of the team has the responsibility for contributing to patient education so that patients have the information needed for an effective partnership and positive outcome of rehabilitation efforts.

Caring for patients with diabetic foot is complicated by a nexus of comorbidities including diabetes, vascular disease, neuroarthropathy, and peripheral neuropathy that cross the boundaries of usual medical care. These comorbidities, coupled with secondary infection and care gaps, further increase the risk of major amputation.[38] Studies have recommended a multidisciplinary team approach, defined as clinicians from at least two different disciplines working together, to optimally address these comorbidities in a coordinated manner and reduce major amputations.[39–41] A recent systemic review revealed that despite a variety of multidisciplinary team composition across all included studies, multidisciplinary teams are found to be associated with significant reductions in major amputations for patients with diabetic foot ulcers.[39]

The Department of Veterans Affairs has instituted a system of care for US veterans with limb amputations, using outcome measures. The Amputation System of Care (ASoC) was introduced in 2008 with a goal of providing "lifelong care for service members with combat-related amputations from military conflicts in Iraq and Afghanistan and for veterans with amputations from diseases such as diabetes and peripheral vascular disease." The ASoC provides coordinated care that enables persons with amputation to receive the prosthetic technology and rehabilitation management that will maximize function and independence.[42]

Coordinated patient-centered care by an interdisciplinary rehabilitation team is just as essential for the effective rehabilitation of children as it is for adults. For children with myelomeningocele or cerebral palsy the broad knowledge base available through team interaction provides a stronger foundation for tailoring interventions to the ever-changing developmental needs of the child and family. Initially, the optimal delivery of care for children is best provided in a comprehensive healthcare setting in which the various specialists can provide a truly collaborative approach. Orthopedic surgeons, neurologists, orthotists, prosthetists, physical therapists, occupational therapists, nurses, dietitians, social workers, psychologists, and special education professionals may all be involved in setting goals and formulating and carrying out plans for intervention and outcomes assessment.

The concept of a multidisciplinary pediatric clinic team was formulated as World War II came to an end.[43] This structure has evolved further over the years and is particularly effective for the more complex orthotic and prosthetic challenges. A "mini-team" consisting of the patient's physician, a physical therapist, and a prosthetist or orthotist can usually be assembled, even in a small town with few facilities. Regardless of its size, an effective team views the child and family from a holistic perspective, with the input from each specialty being of equal value. Under these circumstances the setting of treatment priorities, such as whether prosthetic fitting or training in single-handed tasks is most appropriate at a child's current age or developmental level, is made on the basis of the particular needs of the individual. Children with orthotic and prosthetic needs are followed in the community and within the school setting. As appropriate, a child may receive rehabilitation or habilitation services under the Individuals with Disabilities Education Act.[44] The rehabilitation/educational team is a diverse group of healthcare professionals, educators, family, and caregivers, each with essential skills necessary to address the needs of the child that encourage maximum participation in tasks of daily living. Each member of the team works in a collaborative manner with the family and caregivers and with the child's teachers and other health professionals to ensure that the goals of the IFSP or the Individualized Education Plan are addressed and met. Clear and frequent communication is essential for the team to function effectively and to achieve the desired outcomes for the child.

While evidence supports that multidisciplinary team care is an effective strategy for optimizing patient care and clinical outcomes, a tiered approach is also suggested to care based on symptom severity and appropriate triage. Relatively straightforward cases can be managed with collaboration between primary care and certain specialties, and highly specialized multidisciplinary teams should be reserved for patients with severe or complicated symptoms.[41] In addition, clear and effective referral pathways to provide timely, comprehensive care is an essential element of a successful multidisciplinary team model.[45] Future research should focus on how to best identify the threshold for initiating these resource-intense, multidisciplinary teams.

Case Example 1.1 **Interdisciplinary Teams**

P.G. is a 23-year-old male admitted to a level 3 trauma center 2 weeks ago after sustaining severe crush injuries to both lower extremities and a closed-head injury in an accident involving a motorcycle and a sport utility vehicle. Initially unconscious with a Glasgow Coma Scale score of 8, P.G. was placed on life support in the emergency department. Radiographs revealed a severely comminuted fracture of the distal right femur and displaced fractures of the left tibia and fibula at midshaft. Examination revealed partial-thickness "road burn" abrasions on the left anterior thorax and thigh; these were thoroughly cleaned and covered with semipermeable dressings.

A computed tomography scan of his cranium and brain revealed a subdural hematoma over the left sylvian fissure and moderate contusion of the anterior pole and undersides of the frontal lobes. Arteriography indicated a rupture of the right femoral artery 4 inches above the knee. Given the extent of the crush injuries, the trauma team determined P.G. was not a candidate for reconstructive surgery to salvage his right limb.

P.G. was taken to the operating room, where a standard-length transfemoral amputation was performed on the right lower extremity. Simultaneously, orthopedic surgeons performed an open-reduction internal fixation with an intramedullary rod in the tibia and used surgical plates and screws to repair the fibula. Neurosurgeons drained the subdural hematoma through

Case Example 1.1 Interdisciplinary Teams (Continued)

a burr hole in his skull. P.G. was started on high-dose broad-spectrum antibiotics in the operating room. He was transferred to the surgical intensive care unit for postoperative care.

P.G. was weaned from the ventilator and is now functioning at a Rancho Los Amigos Scale level of 7. He is able to follow one- and two-step commands but becomes easily confused and angry in complex environments and when fatigued. His postoperative pain is currently being managed with Tylenol No. 3 as needed. His right lower extremity has been managed with soft dressings and elastic bandages; his residual limb is moderately bulbous, with resolving ecchymosis from the accident and surgery. Moderate serosanguineous drainage continues from the medial one-third of the suture line. Although most of the skin abrasions show signs of regranulation, one area on his left thigh is red and hot, with yellowish drainage. When transferred (maximum assist of two) into a bedside recliner, P.G. tolerates 30 minutes in a 45- to 60-degree reclined position. He becomes lightheaded and has significant pain when sitting upright with his left lower extremity dependent. He has been referred to physical therapy for evaluation of rehabilitation potential and initiation of mobility activities.

Before his accident, P.G. was a graduate student in physics at a nearby university. He lived in a third-floor walk-up apartment with his fiancé and his golden retriever. Besides his motorcycle, his interests and hobbies included long-distance running and mountain climbing. His mother and father have traveled to be with him during the acute hospital stay.

QUESTIONS TO CONSIDER

- Who are the clinical specialists and health professionals needed to address the medical needs of the patient?
- What are the priorities, specific roles, and responsibilities for each potential member of the team? What team structure do you envision?
- How are the roles and responsibilities similar or different across the team?
- What external influences will affect team formation and functioning in a busy level 3 trauma center?
- What factors might facilitate team development?
- What factors might challenge the effectiveness of the team?
- As P.G. recovers from his injuries, how might the roles and responsibilities of the various team members change or evolve?
- When and how would you apply the International Classification of Functioning (ICF) disablement model for P.G.?
- Is there an ICF Core Set that applies to this clinical situation?
- Are there recommended clinical practice guidelines that apply to the management of this patient?

Case Example 1.2 Interdisciplinary Teams

E.L. is a 73-year-old female with a 10-year history of type 2 diabetes mellitus. She is insulin dependent. Two weeks before her most recent hospitalization, she and her husband (who is in the early stages of Alzheimer disease) moved from their home of 50 years to an assisted-living complex in a neighboring town. Although the furniture is set up and functional, they have not had the chance to fully unpack and make the apartment their own.

Over the past 3 years, E.L. has been monitored by her team of physicians for progressive polyneuropathy of diabetes and for moderate peripheral vascular disease. She had a transmetatarsal amputation of her right forefoot 8 months ago because of nonhealing recurrent neuropathic ulcer. Despite wearing custom-molded shoes and accommodative orthoses, another ulcer of her first metatarsal head developed on the left foot 2 months ago. This new ulcer did not heal with conservative care and progressed to osteomyelitis 2 weeks ago. When vascular studies suggested inadequate circulation to heal the ulcer, she received arterial revascularization intervention, but the ischemia persisted and E.L. underwent an elective transtibial amputation of her left lower extremity. Despite a short bout of postoperative delirium thought to be related to pain management with morphine, E.L. (5 days postoperatively) was adamant about returning to her new assisted-living apartment, using a wheelchair for mobility, and receiving home care until her residual limb is healed and ready for prosthetic fitting.

Currently she is able to ambulate two lengths of 15-foot-long parallel bars before needing to rest and has begun gait training with a "hop-to" gait pattern with a standard walker. She is able to transfer from sitting on a firm seating surface with armrests to standing with standby guarding and verbal cueing and needs minimal assistance from low and soft seats without armrests. She believes that she and her husband will be able to manage at home because her bathroom has grab bars on the toilet, and a tub seat and handheld shower head are available from the "loaner closet" at her assisted-living facility.

At discharge, the suture line had one small area of continued moderate drainage, requiring frequent dressing changes. She is unable to move her residual limb into a position for effective visual self-inspection of the healing surgical wound without significant discomfort. Her husband, although attentive, becomes confused with the routine of wound care. E.L.'s postoperative limb volume and edema are being managed with a total contact cast, which she is able to don and doff independently. She had one late evening fall, when she awoke from a sound sleep having to go to the bathroom and was surprised when her left limb "wasn't really there" to stand on when she tried to get out of bed.

Since her amputation, E.L.'s insulin dosages have had to be adjusted frequently because of unpredictable changes in her serum glucose levels. She has lost 20 pounds (half of which can be attributed to her amputation) since admission.

QUESTIONS TO CONSIDER

- Who are the healthcare professionals likely to be involved in her care?
- Which team approach is most desirable for patient-centered care: multidisciplinary, interdisciplinary, or transdisciplinary? Why?
- What are the major challenges facing the team of care providers involved in the postoperative, preprosthetic care of E.L. and her husband? How are these similar to or different from challenges and issues the trauma center team considered before her amputation?
- What strategies are currently in place or must be developed to ensure that E.L.'s care at home is comprehensive and coordinated?
- How will the roles and responsibilities of the team members evolve and change as she recovers from her surgery and is ready to begin prosthetic use?
- When and how would you apply the International Classification of Functioning (ICF) disablement model for E.L.?
- Is there an ICF Core Set that applies to this clinical situation?
- Are there recommended clinical practice guidelines that apply to the management of this patient?

Case Example 1.3 **Interdisciplinary Teams**

M.S. is a 12-year-old girl with myelomeningocele (spina bifida) who uses a wheelchair for mobility. In the past year, she has developed significant thoracolumbar scoliosis believed to be associated with a growth spurt. Concerned about the rate of increase in her S-shaped thoracolumbar curve, her parents sought the advice of an orthopedic surgeon who has been involved as a consultant in her care since birth. The surgeon recommends surgical stabilization of M.S.'s spine with Harrington rods and bony fusion to (1) prevent further progression of the curve and rib hump so that secondary impairment of the respiratory system will be minimized as she grows and (2) provide more efficient upright sitting posture for wheelchair propulsion in the years ahead.

M.S. currently attends classes in her neighborhood middle school where she receives related health services including physical therapy. Until 2 years ago, she ambulated for exercise by using a reciprocal gait orthosis during gym periods at school, but with recent spurts in growth the use of a manual wheelchair is more efficient for mobility (to keep up with her classmates). She is also followed up on a regular basis by a neurologist who monitors the operation of her ventriculoperitoneal shunt (commonly used in the management of hydrocephalus associated with myelomeningocele).

In addition to their concerns about the risk of the surgical procedure, M.S.'s parents are quite concerned about how the anticipated 4-month postoperative immobilization in a thoracolumbosacral orthosis will affect her capacity for self-care and independent wheelchair mobility. They are also concerned about how the surgery and postoperative period will potentially interrupt the effective bowel and bladder management routine for which M.S. has just begun to assume responsibility. As witnesses to their daughter's deconditioning and loss of stamina over the past 6 months, they are concerned that she might not be "physically ready" for the surgery and postoperative rehabilitation. They are also asking questions about whether this spinal surgery will ultimately improve the prognosis of a successful return to ambulation with her reciprocal gait orthosis.

QUESTIONS TO CONSIDER

- Who are the members of the rehabilitation team?
- What is the structure of the team that will best address the needs of the patient?
- What are the priorities, roles, and responsibilities of the health professionals involved in the care of this child and her family?
- How is the composition of M.S.'s rehabilitation team similar to or different from that of P.G.'s and E.L.'s teams?
- How will the health and education professionals support M.S. and her family through the postoperative recovery process?
- When and how would you apply the International Classification of Functioning disablement model to M.S.?

Summary

Patient-centered care, whether in tertiary care medical centers, in-patient rehabilitation facilities, skilled nursing facilities, or ambulatory community settings, currently relies on interdisciplinary rehabilitation teams that function to address patient goals and maximize patient outcomes. The use of rehabilitation teams has evolved in part because no one person or discipline has the expertise in all the areas of specialty knowledge required for the established standards of care. The success of the rehabilitation team process requires health professionals to work together in a collaborative and cooperative manner. The rehabilitation team professional must demonstrate attitudes and attributes that foster collaboration, including:

1. Openness and receptivity to the ideas of others.
2. An understanding of, value of, and respect for the roles and expertise of other professionals on the team.
3. Value interdependence and acceptance of a common commitment to comprehensive patient-centered care.
4. Willingness to share ideas openly and take responsibility.

This chapter introduces the topic of orthotics and prosthetics in rehabilitation and advocates for a multidisciplinary and interdisciplinary approach to patient-centered care. There is a burgeoning demand for the use of orthotics and prosthetics, based on several varying health concerns for the population, including limb loss associated with US servicemen and servicewomen military duties; traumatic injuries sustained by US servicemen and servicewomen involved in military conflicts; and on the projected rise in the number of persons with chronic health conditions such as obesity, type 2 diabetes, and vascular disease. The overarching goal is to rehabilitate persons to the highest level of functional independence, which is possible for the individual. The WHO ICF is the current disablement framework endorsed by 191 countries. Rehabilitation professionals including orthotists, prosthetists, and physical and occupational therapists will apply the ICF disablement model to maximize strategies for patient participation in the tasks of daily living through enhancement of environmental factors such as providing appropriate, cost-effective assistive technology including orthoses and prostheses. A rehabilitation model of patient-centered care that uses a multidisciplinary or interdisciplinary team approach to enhance communication, address goals and objectives, apply best practice, and improve patient outcomes is the current standard of care for persons in rehabilitation settings. Collaboration, mutual respect, and an understanding of the roles and responsibilities of colleagues engender productive teamwork and improved outcomes for the rehabilitation patient.

References

The complete listing of the References are available in the accompanying enhanced eBook version included with the print purchase of this textbook. Visit Elsevier eBooks+ (eBooks.Health.Elsevier.com) to access this content.

2 Aging and Activity Tolerance: Implications for Orthotic and Prosthetic Rehabilitation

KENT E. IRWIN, MICHELLE G. CRISS, KEVIN K. CHUI, AND MARIANA WINGOOD

LEARNING OBJECTIVES

On completion of this chapter, the reader will be able to do the following:

1. Describe the role of the cardiopulmonary and cardiovascular systems as "effectors" for goal-driven functional motor activity.
2. Define the key components of the cardiopulmonary and cardiovascular systems as they relate to energy expenditure during functional activity.
3. Describe the functional consequences of age-related change in cardiopulmonary and cardiovascular structures, especially with respect to the effect on exercise and activity tolerance.
4. Apply principles of cardiopulmonary and cardiovascular conditioning to rehabilitation interventions for older and/or deconditioned individuals who will be using a prosthesis or an orthosis.
5. Weigh the benefits and limitations with respect to energy cost and facilitation of daily function in selecting an appropriate orthosis or prosthesis for an older or deconditioned individual.
6. Appreciate technological advances in prosthetics and orthotics and their role in activity tolerance.

Many individuals who rely on orthotic or prosthetic devices to accomplish functional tasks (e.g., walking, transfers, and standing activities) have impairments of the musculoskeletal or neuromuscular systems that limit movement efficiency and increase daily energy costs. Physiologic aging causes changes in numerous systems that have the potential to impact movement.[1] The prevalence of chronic conditions, such as cardiovascular disease, chronic obstructive pulmonary disease, or diabetes, is on the rise and presents as a significant healthcare burden.[2] Physical inactivity is far too common as almost all (91%) older adults do not meet the recommended levels of physical activity.[3,4] The cumulative effects of aging, inactivity, and chronic conditions place individuals at increased risk for further functional decline, additional chronic disease development, poor tolerance of activity in general, and more specifically after limb loss.

Consider this example: a 79-year-old female with insulin-controlled type 2 diabetes has been referred for physical therapy evaluation after transfemoral amputation (TFA) following a failed femoral-popliteal bypass graft due to peripheral arterial disease. She has been on bed rest for two weeks because of her multiple surgeries. The physical effort required in undergoing rehabilitation and prosthetic training may initially feel overwhelming to this female. Taken together, this patient's inactivity, diabetes, and recent amputation combined with normal aging changes have the potential to accelerate her decline and increase her risk for loss of independence.[5] In her deconditioned state, preprosthetic ambulation with a walker is likely to increase her heart rate (HR) close to the upper limits of a safe-target HR for aerobic training. Considering the cumulative effects of her multiple conditions, what is her prognosis for functional use of a prosthesis? What are the most important issues to address in her plan of care? What intensity of intervention is most appropriate given her deconditioned state? In what setting and for how long will care be provided? These questions have no simple answers.

Rehabilitation professionals must recognize factors that can be successfully modified to enhance performance and activity tolerance when decisions about prescription and intervention strategies are being made. Aerobic fitness should be a key component of the rehabilitation program for those who will be using a prosthesis or orthosis for the first time. Rehabilitation professionals must also recognize and respond to the warning signs of significant cardiopulmonary or cardiovascular dysfunction during treatment encounters.

Although the anatomic and physiologic changes in the aging cardiopulmonary system are important to our discussion, our focus is on the contribution of cellular and tissue-level changes to the performance of the cardiopulmonary and cardiovascular systems and, consequently, on the individual's ability to function. During the rehabilitation process, clinicians should consider the following questions:

- Can the individual complete functional activities to enable full life participation?
- What impact does the use of an orthosis or prosthesis have on energy use and cost during functional activities for this person?
- Is it possible for this individual to become more efficient during functional activities?

Oxygen Transport System

The foundation for the functional view of the cardiopulmonary system is the equation for the oxygen transport system (Fig. 2.1). Aerobic capacity (VO_{2max}) is the body's ability to deliver and use oxygen (maximum rate of oxygen consumption) to support the energy needs of demanding physical activity. VO_{2max} is influenced by three factors: the efficiency of ventilation and oxygenation in the lungs, how much oxygen-rich blood can be delivered from the heart (cardiac output, or CO) to active peripheral tissues, and how well oxygen

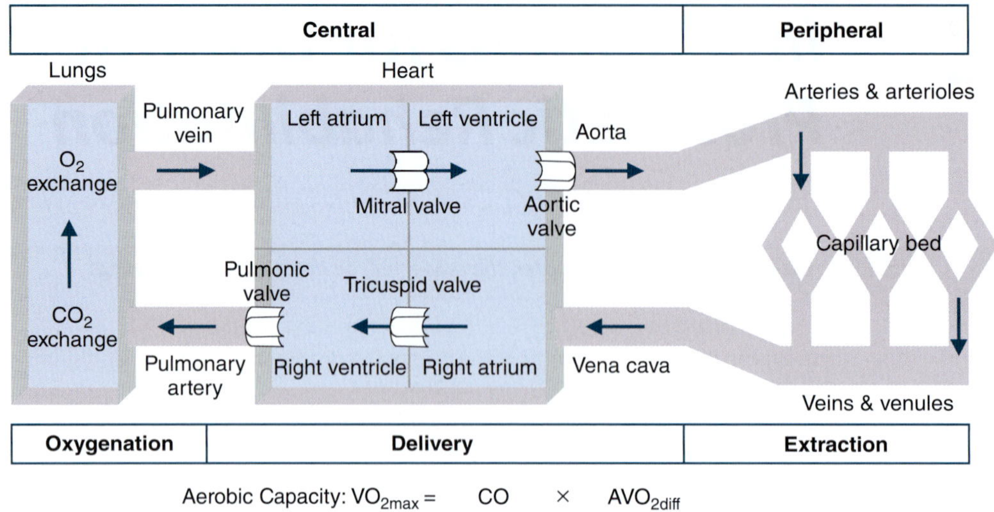

Fig. 2.1 Functional anatomy and physiology of the cardiopulmonary system. After blood has been oxygenated in the lungs, the left side of the heart contracts to deliver the blood, through the aorta and its branches (arteries and arterioles), to active tissues in the periphery. Oxygen must be effectively extracted from blood by peripheral tissues to support their activity. Deoxygenated blood, high in carbon dioxide, returns from venules and veins through the vena cava to the right side of the heart, which pumps it to the lungs for reoxygenation. Aerobic capacity (VO_{2max}) is the product of how well oxygen is delivered to active tissues (cardiac output [CO]) and extracted from the blood to support active tissues (arteriovenous oxygen difference [AVO_{2diff}]). *HR*, Heart rate; *SV*, stroke volume.

is extracted from the blood to support muscle contraction and other peripheral tissues during activity (arteriovenous oxygen difference, or AVO_{2diff}).[6–9] Aerobic capacity can be represented by the following formula:

$$VO_{2max} = CO \times AVO_{2diff}$$

The energy cost of doing work is based on the amount of oxygen consumed for the activity, regardless of whether the activity is supported by aerobic (with oxygen) or anaerobic (without oxygen) metabolic mechanisms for producing energy. VO_{2max} provides an indication of the maximum amount of work that can be supported.[6–9]

CO is the product of two elements. The first is the HR, the number of times the heart contracts (or beats) per minute. The second is stroke volume (SV), the amount of blood pumped from the left ventricle with each beat (measured in milliliters or liters). CO is expressed by the following formula (measured in milliliters or liters per minute):

$$CO = HR \times SV$$

As a product of HR and SV, CO is influenced by four factors: (1) the amount of blood returned from the periphery through the vena cava, (2) the ability of the heart to match its rate of contraction to physiologic demand, (3) the efficiency or forcefulness of the heart's contraction, and (4) the ability of the aorta to deliver blood to peripheral vessels. The delivery of oxygen to the body tissues to be used to produce energy for work is, ultimately, a function of the central components of the cardiopulmonary system.[6–9]

The second determinant of aerobic capacity, the AVO_{2diff}, reflects the extraction of oxygen from the capillary bed by the surrounding tissues. The AVO_{2diff} is determined by subtracting the oxygen concentration on the venous (postextraction) side of the capillary bed (CvO_2) from that of the arteriole (preextraction) side of the capillary bed (CaO_2), according to the formula:

$$AVO_{2diff} = CaO_2 - CvO_2$$

The smaller vessels and capillaries of the cardiovascular system are involved in the process of extraction of oxygen from the blood by the active tissues. Extraction of oxygen from the blood to be used to produce energy for the work of the active tissues is a function of the peripheral components of the cardiopulmonary system.[6–9]

During exercise or a physically demanding activity, CO must increase to meet the need for additional oxygen in the more active peripheral tissues. This increased CO is the result of a more rapid HR and a greater SV. As the return of blood to the heart increases, the heart contracts more forcefully and a larger volume of blood is pumped into the aorta by the left ventricle. Chemical and hormonal changes that accompany exercise enhance the peripheral shunting of blood to the active muscles, and oxygen depletion in muscle assists transfer of oxygen from the capillary blood to the tissue at work.[7,9,10]

The efficiency of central components, primarily of CO, accounts for as much as 75% of VO_{2max}. Peripheral oxygen extraction (AVO_{2diff}) contributes the remaining 25% to the process of making oxygen available to support tissue work.[11] In healthy adults under most conditions, more oxygen is delivered to active tissues (muscle mass) than is necessary.[9,11] During exercise in healthy adults, CO may increase five times, allowing for oxygen to be available to working muscles.[7]

For those who are significantly deconditioned or who have cardiopulmonary or cardiovascular disease, the ability to deliver oxygen efficiently to the periphery as physical activity increases may be compromised. With normal aging, there are age-related physiologic changes in the heart that limit maximum attainable HR. Because of these changes, clinicians must assess whether and to what degree SV can be increased safely and effectively if rehabilitation interventions are to be successful.

Age-Related Changes to the Heart

The ability to plan an appropriate intervention to address cardiovascular endurance and conditioning in older adults who may need to use a prosthesis or orthosis is founded on an understanding of "typical" age-related changes in cardiovascular structure and physiology as well as on the functional consequences of these changes.

CARDIOVASCULAR STRUCTURE

Age-related structural changes in the cardiovascular system occur in five areas: myocardium, cardiac valves, coronary arteries, conduction system, and coronary vasculature (i.e., arteries) (Table 2.1).[12–16] Despite these cellular and tissue-level changes, a healthy older heart can meet energy demands of daily and recreational activities. Cardiovascular disease and a habitually sedentary lifestyle, both of which increase in later life, can significantly compromise activity tolerance.[17–20]

Myocardium

With age, cells of the myocardium show microscopic signs of degeneration, including increases in myocardial fat content (i.e., storage of triglyceride droplets within cardiomyocytes); however, the relationship between the quantity of fat and disease severity remains unclear.[21] Unlike aging skeletal muscle cells, there is minimal atrophy of cardiac smooth muscle cells. More typically, there is hypertrophy of the left ventricular myocardium, increasing the diameter of the left atrium.[19,22–24] These changes have been attributed to cardiac tissue responses to an increased systolic blood pressure (SBP) and reduced compliance of the left ventricle; they are associated with an increase in the weight and size of the heart.[22,24–27]

Valves

The four valves (i.e., mitral, aortic, tricuspid, and pulmonic) of the aged heart often become fibrous and thickened at their margins as well as somewhat calcified.[28] Calcification of the aorta at the base of the cusps of the aortic valve (aortic stenosis) is clinically associated with the slowed exit of blood from the left ventricle into the aorta.[29] Such aortic stenosis contributes to a functional reduction in CO. A baroreflex-mediated increase in SBP attempts to compensate for this reduced CO.[30,31] Over time, the larger residual of blood in the left ventricle after each beat (increased end-systolic volume, or ESV) begins to weaken the left ventricular muscle.[32] This muscle must work harder to pump the blood out of the ventricle into a more resistant peripheral vascular system.[33,34]

Calcification of the annulus of the mitral valve can restrict blood flow from the left atrium into the left ventricle during diastole. As a result, end-diastolic volume (EDV) of blood in the left ventricle is decreased because the left atrium is not completely empty. Over time, this residual blood in the left atrium elongates the muscle of the atrial walls and increases the diameter of the atrium of the heart.[33–35]

Coronary Arteries

Age-related changes of the coronary arteries are similar to those in any aged arterial vessel: an increase in the thickness of the vessel walls and tortuosity of the vessel's path.[36] These changes tend to occur earlier in the left coronary artery than in the right.[37] When coupled with atherosclerosis, these changes may compromise the muscular contraction and pumping efficiency and effectiveness of the left ventricle during exercise or any activity of high physiologic demand.[9,38,39]

Conduction System

Age-related changes in the heart's conduction system can have a substantial impact on cardiac function. On average, a 75-year-old person has less than 10% of the original number of pacemaker cells of the sinoatrial node.[40,41] Fibrous tissue builds within the internodal tracts as well as within the atrioventricular node, including the bundle of His and its main bundle branches.[40,41] As a consequence, the ability of the heart to coordinate the actions of all four chambers

Table 2.1 Age-Related Changes in the Cardiovascular System

Structure	Change	Functional Consequences
Heart	Deposition of lipids, lipofuscin, and amyloid within cardiac smooth muscle	Less excitability
	Increased connective tissue and fibrosity	Diminished cardiac output
	Hypertrophy of left ventricle	Diminished venous return
	Increased diameter of atria	Susceptibility to dysrhythmia
	Stiffening and calcification of valves	Reduction in maximal attainable heart rate
	Fewer pacemaker cells in sinoatrial and atrioventricular nodes	Less efficient dilation of cardiac arteries during activity
	Fewer conduction fibers in bundle of His and branches	Less efficient left ventricular filling in early diastole, leading to reduced stroke volume
	Less sensitivity to extrinsic (autonomic) innervation	
	Slower rate of tension development during contraction	Increased afterload, leading to weakening of heart muscle
Blood vessels	Altered ratio of smooth muscle to connective tissue and elastin in vessel walls	Less efficient delivery of oxygenated blood to muscle and organs
	Decreased baroreceptor responsiveness	Diminished cardiac output
	Susceptibility to plaque formation within vessel	Less efficient venous return
	Rigidity and calcification of large arteries, especially the aorta	Susceptibility to venous thrombosis
	Dilation and increased tortuosity of veins	Susceptibility to orthostatic hypotension
	Vascular inflammation	

may be compromised.[40] Arrhythmias are pathologic conduction system conditions that become more common in later life. Emerging consumer smartwatch technology has been reported to identify potential arrhythmias in individuals 55 years and older.[42,43] Arrhythmias are managed pharmacologically or with the implantation of a pacemaker/defibrillator.[44,45] Rehabilitation professionals must be aware of the impact of medications or pacemaker settings on an individual's ability to physiologically respond to exercise and to adapt to the intervention accordingly.[46]

Arterial Vascular Tree

Age-related changes in the arterial vascular tree, demonstrated most notably by the thoracic aorta and eventually the more distal vessels, can disrupt the smooth or streamlined flow (i.e., laminar flow) of blood from the heart toward the periphery.[47,48] Altered alignment of endothelial cells of the intima creates rough or turbulence flow (i.e., nonlaminar flow), which increases the likelihood of deposition of collagen and lipid.[49] Fragmentation of elastic fibers in the intima and media of larger arterioles and arteries further compromises the functionally important "rebound" characteristic of arterial vessels.[50] Rebound normally assists directional blood flow through the system, preventing the backward reflection of fluid pressure waves of blood. This loss of elasticity increases vulnerability of the aorta, which, distended and stiffened, cannot effectively resist the tensile force of left ventricular ejection. Not surprisingly, the incidence of abdominal aortic aneurysms rises sharply among older adults, and stiffness (distensibility) of the ascending aorta is associated with the severity of coronary artery disease.[51,52]

CARDIOVASCULAR PHYSIOLOGY

Although the physiologic changes in the cardiovascular system are few, their impact on the performance of the older adult can be substantial. The healthy aging heart continues to be an effective pump, maintaining its ability to develop enough myocardial contraction to support daily activity. The response of cardiac muscle to calcium (Ca^{2+}) is preserved, and its force-generating capacity is maintained.[53] Two aspects of myocardial contractility do, however, change with aging: the rate of tension development in the myocardium slows, and the duration of contraction and relaxation becomes prolonged.[54,55]

Sensitivity to β-Adrenergic Stimulation

One of the most marked age-related changes in cardiovascular function is the reduced sensitivity of the heart to sympathetic stimulation, specifically to the stimulation of β-adrenergic receptors.[55,56] Age-related reduction in β-adrenergic sensitivity includes a decreased response to norepinephrine and epinephrine released from sympathetic nerve endings in the heart as well as a decreased sensitivity to any of these catecholamines circulating in the blood.[56,57] Normally, norepinephrine and epinephrine are potent stimulators of ventricular contraction.

An important functional consequence of the change in receptor sensitivity is less efficient cardioacceleratory response, which leads to a lower HR at submaximal and maximal levels of exercise or activity.[40,58] The time for HR rise to the peak rate is prolonged, so more time is necessary to reach the appropriate HR level for physically demanding activities. A further consequence of this reduced β-adrenergic sensitivity is less than optimal vasodilation of the coronary arteries with increasing activity.[56,59] In peripheral arterial vessels β-adrenergic receptors do not appear to play a primary role in mediating vasodilation in the working muscles.[60]

Baroreceptor Reflex

Age-related change in the cardiovascular baroreceptor reflex also contributes to prolongation of cardiovascular response time in the face of an increase in activity (physiologic demand).[55] The baroreceptors in the proximal aorta appear to become less sensitive to changes in blood volume (pressure) within the vessel. Normally any drop in proximal aortic pressure triggers the hypothalamus to begin a sequence of events that leads to increased sympathetic stimulation of the heart. Decreased baroreceptor responsiveness may increase individuals' susceptibility to orthostatic (postural) and postprandial (after eating) hypotension or may compromise their tolerance of the physiologic stress of a Valsalva maneuver associated with breath holding during strenuous activity.[61–64] Clinically, this is evidenced by lightheadedness when rising from a lying or sitting position, especially after a meal, or if one tends to hold one's breath during effortful activity.

The effects of age-related physiologic changes on the cardiovascular system can often be managed satisfactorily. If the older adult presents with decreased baroreceptor responsiveness or orthostatic hypotension, then use simple lower extremity warmup exercises before position changes. Several repetitions of ankle and knee exercises before standing up, especially after a prolonged time sitting (including for meals) or lying down (after a night's rest), help maximize blood return to the heart (preload), assisting cardiovascular function for the upcoming physical activity. In addition, taking a bit more time in initiating activities and progressing their difficulty may help the slowed cardiovascular response time reach an effective level of performance. Scheduling physical therapy or physical activity at a reasonable time after a meal might also be beneficial for older adults who are particularly vulnerable to postprandial hypotension. Fortunately, many of the aging effects on the cardiovascular system can be minimized or reversed with exercise training.[7,65]

FUNCTIONAL CONSEQUENCES OF CARDIOVASCULAR AGING

What are the functional consequences of cardiovascular aging for those participating in exercise or rehabilitation activities? This question can best be answered by focusing on factors that affect CO changes (Fig. 2.2). The age-related structural and physiologic changes in the cardiovascular system give rise to two loading conditions that influence CO: cardiac filling (preload) and vascular impedance (afterload).[9,31]

Preload

Cardiac filling (preload) determines the volume of blood in the left ventricle at the end of diastole. The most effective ventricular filling occurs when pressure is low within the

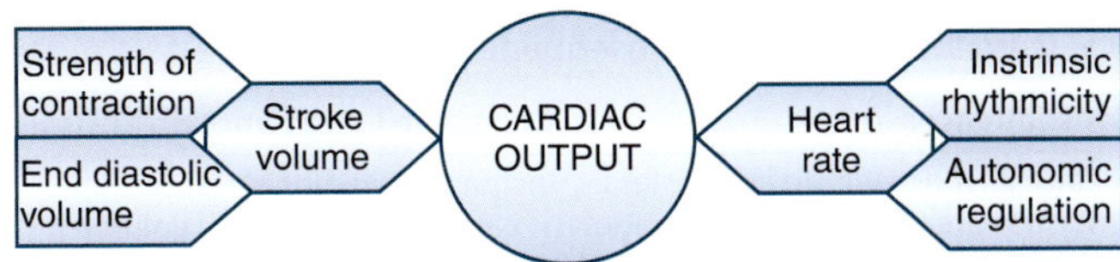

Fig. 2.2 Factors affecting cardiac output are influenced by the aging process. If strength of contraction decreases and end-diastolic volume increases, stroke volume is reduced. Coupled with alterations in heart rate response to increasing workload, activities that were submaximal in intensity at a younger age may become more physiologically demanding in later life.

heart and relaxation of the muscular walls of the ventricle is maximized.[6,7,11] Mitral valve calcification, decreased left ventricle compliance, and prolonged relaxation of myocardial contraction can contribute to less effective filling of the left ventricle in early diastole.[66] Doppler studies of the flow of blood into the left ventricle in aging adults demonstrate decreased rates of early filling, an increased rate of late atrial filling, and an overall decrease in the peak filling rate.[11,32,66] When compared with healthy 45- to 50-year-old adults, the early diastolic filling of a healthy 65- to 80-year-old is 50% less.[11,32,67] This reduced volume of blood in the ventricle at the end of diastole does not effectively stretch the ventricular muscle of the heart, thus compromising the Frank-Starling mechanism and the myocontractility of the left ventricle.[68] The functional outcome of decreased early diastolic filling and the reduced EDV is a proportional decrease in SV, one of the determinants of CO and, consequently, aerobic capacity (VO_{2max}).[11,30,55]

Afterload

High vascular impedance and increased afterload disrupt the flow of blood as it leaves the heart and moves toward the peripheral vasculature. Increased afterload is partly a function of age-related stiffness of the proximal aorta, an increase in systemic vascular resistance (elevation of SBP, hypertension), or a combination of both.[55,69] Ventricular contraction that forces blood flow into a resistant peripheral vascular system produces pressure waves in the blood. These pressure waves reflect back toward the heart, unrestricted by the stiffened walls of the proximal aorta. The reflected pressure waves, aortic stiffness, and increased systemic vascular resistance collectively contribute to an increased afterload in the aging heart.[54,69] Increased afterload is thought to be a major factor in the age-associated decrease in maximum SV, hypertrophy of the left ventricle, and prolongation of myocardial relaxation (e.g., slowed relaxation in the presence of a persisting load on the heart).[12,13,15]

An unfortunate long-term consequence of increased afterload is weakening of the heart muscle itself, particularly of the left ventricle. Restricted blood flow out of the heart results in a large residual volume (RV) of blood in the heart at the end of systole, when ventricular contraction is complete. Large ESVs gradually increase the resting length of ventricular cardiac muscle, effectively weakening the force of contraction.[8,12,13,15,32,70]

Left Ventricular Ejection Fraction

Left ventricular ejection fraction (LVEF) is the proportion of blood pumped out of the heart with each contraction of the left ventricle, which is expressed by the following equation:

$$LVEF = (EDV - ESV) + EDV$$

At rest, the LVEF does not appear to be reduced in older adults. Under conditions of maximal exercise, however, the rise in LVEF is much less than that in younger adults.[30,71,72] This reduced rise in the LVEF with maximal exercise clearly illustrates the impact that functional cardiovascular age-related changes in preload and afterload have on performance.

A substantial reduction in EDV, an expansion of ESV, or a more modest change in both components may account for the decreased LVEF of the exercising older adult:

$$\downarrow EDV = \downarrow LVEF$$
$$\uparrow ESV = \downarrow LVEF$$

When going from resting to maximal exercise conditions, the amount of blood pumped with each beat for young healthy adults increases by 20% to 30% from a resting LVEF of 55% to an exercise LVEF of 80%. For a healthy older adult, in contrast, LVEF typically increases $<5\%$ from rest to maximal exercise.[72,73] The LVEF may actually decrease in adults who are 60 years of age and older.[72,74] As LVEF and CO decrease with aging, so does the ability to work over prolonged periods (functional cardiopulmonary reserve capacity) because the volume of blood delivered to active tissue decreases. Functional reserve capacity is further compromised by the long-term effects of inactivity and by cardiopulmonary pathology.[30,38,75–77] The contribution of habitual exercise to achieving effective maximum exercise LVEF is not well understood, but the decline may not be as substantial for highly fit older adults.[30]

Pulmonary Function in Later Life

Several important age-related structural changes of the lungs and the musculoskeletal system have a significant impact on pulmonary function.[78] These include changes in the tissues and structures making up the lungs and airways, alteration in lung volume, reduced efficiency of gas exchange, and a mechanically less efficient ventilatory pump related to changes in alignment and posture (Table 2.2).[79–82] Although a healthy adult at midlife uses only 10% of the respiratory system's capacity at rest, aging of the pulmonary system, especially when accompanied by chronic illness or acute disease, negatively affects the ability of the lungs to respond to increasing demands of physical activity (Fig. 2.3).[83] Age-related changes in the pulmonary and musculoskeletal systems also contribute to an increase in the physiologic work of breathing.

CHANGES WITHIN THE LUNG AND AIRWAY

The production of elastin, which is the major protein component of the structure of the lungs, decreases markedly in late life. The elastic fibers of the lung become fragmented, and, functionally, the passive elastic recoil or rebound important for expiration becomes much less efficient. The elastic fibers that maintain the structure of the walls of the alveoli also decrease in number. This loss of elastin means loss of alveoli and consequently less surface area for the exchange

Table 2.2 Summary of Age-Related Changes in the Cardiopulmonary System and Functional Consequences

Anatomic Changes	Physiologic Changes	Consequences	Change in Lung Function Tests
Rearrangement and fragmentation of elastin fibers Stiffened cartilage in compliant articulation of ribs and vertebrae Increasing stiffness and compression of annulus fibrosus in intervertebral disks Reduction of strength and endurance of respiratory musculature	Less elastic recoil for expiration Greater compliance of lung Decreased vital capacity, forced More rigid thoracic cage Decreased volume of maximum voluntary ventilation and maximum sustained ventilatory capacity Greater mismatch between ventilation and perfusion within lung	Greater airspace within alveoli, less surface area for O_2/CO_2 exchange thoracic cage Increased work of breathing Less force during inspiration Less efficient cough Diminished exercise tolerance Reduced resting PaO_2	Increased functional residual capacity and residual volume tissue Shorter, less vital capacity, and forced expiratory volume in 1 s (FEV_1) Decreased maximum inspiratory pressure, maximum expiratory pressure, and maximum voluntary ventilation

of oxygen as well as an increase in RV associated with more "dead space" within the lung, where air exchange cannot occur.[80–83] There may be as much as a 15% decrease in the total number of alveoli per unit of lung volume by the age of 70 years.[84]

With aging, there is also an increase in the diameter of major bronchi and large bronchioles as well as a decreased diameter of smaller bronchioles, often leading to a slight increase in resistance to airflow during respiration.[84] This contributes to greater physical work of breathing as age advances.

Starting at midlife and continuing into later life, there tends to be a growing mismatch between lung area ventilated with each breath and lung area perfused by pulmonary arterioles and capillaries, which is attributed to alteration in alveolar surface, vascular structures, and posture.[85] This mismatch compromises the efficiency of diffusion of oxygen across the alveoli into the capillary bed (i.e., decreasing arterial oxygen tension) within the lung and becomes less efficient from midlife into later life.[81,85] However, highly trained older adults can produce levels of maximum oxygen consumption that exceed those of untrained middle-aged males.[86] This suggests that pulmonary rehabilitation can play a large role in improving exercise tolerance in older adults.[82,87–89]

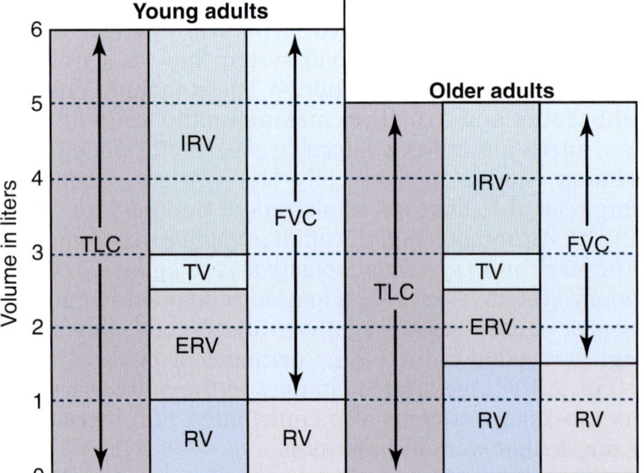

Fig. 2.3 Changes in the distribution of air within the lungs (volume) have an impact on an older adult's efficiency of physical work. Loss of alveoli and increasing stiffness of the rib cage result in a 30%–50% increase in residual volume (RV) and a 40%–50% decrease in forced vital capacity (FVC). FVC includes three components: inspiratory reserve volume (IRV) and expiratory reserve volume (ERV) tend to decrease with aging, whereas resting tidal volume (TV), the amount of air in a normal resting breath, tends to be stable over time. Total lung capacity (TLC) and inspiratory capacity (IRV + TV) also tend to decrease. Over time, the physiologic consequences of these changes make the older adult more vulnerable to dyspnea (shortness of breath) during exercise and physically demanding activity.

CHANGES IN THE MUSCULOSKELETAL SYSTEM

The decreasing elastic recoil and alveolar surface area for oxygen exchange may be further compounded by increased stiffness (loss of flexibility); "barreling" of the thoracic rib cage, which houses the lungs; and a decrease in height as intervertebral disks narrow and stiffen.[90] Much of this stiffness is attributed to changes in the articulation between ribs and vertebrae as well as decreased elasticity of the intercostal muscles and soft tissue.[91] Although the stiffened rib cage may be as much a consequence of a sedentary lifestyle as of advancing age, lack of flexibility compromises inspiration and also decreases the elastic recoil of expiration.[82,92] Furthermore, forward head and slight kyphosis alter the position of both ribs and diaphragm, thus decreasing the mechanical efficiency of inspiration.[83,90,92] The net effect of a stiffer thoracic cage is an increase in the work of taking a breath, since muscles of respiration must work harder during inspiration to counteract the stiffness.[83,90]

The striated muscles of respiration are composed of a combination of type I (slow twitch and fatigue resistant, for endurance) and type II (fast twitch, for power) muscle fibers and are susceptible to age-related changes in strength and endurance.[92] Normally type I muscle fibers are active during quiet breathing, whereas recruitment of type II muscle fibers is triggered by increasing physiologic demand as activity increases. Age-related decrements in the strength and efficiency of the diaphragm, intercostals, abdominal muscles, and other accessory respiratory muscles affect the effectiveness and work of breathing as well as functional capacity.[83,93,94] Altered posture and higher RV within the lung also contribute to an increased work of breathing; when the diaphragm rests in a less than optimal position and configuration for contraction, accessory respiratory muscles become active sooner as physiologic demand increases. Oxygen consumption in respiratory muscles, as in all striated muscles, decreases linearly with age, making older muscles more vulnerable to the effects of fatigue in situations of high physical demand, especially in the presence of lung disease or injury.[81]

CONTROL OF VENTILATION

The rate of breathing (breaths per minute) is matched to physiologic demand by input from peripheral mechanoreceptors in the chest wall, lungs, and thoracic joints, as well as centers in the brain stem of the central nervous system (CNS) and peripheral aortic and carotid bodies that are sensitive to concentration of CO_2, O_2, and hydrogen ions (pH) in the blood.[95] With aging, stiffness of the thorax tends to reduce the efficiency of mechanoreceptors, and the CNS and peripheral nervous system (PNS) centers that monitor CO_2, O_2, and pH to detect hypoxia during activity slowly begin to decline.[82]

Gradual loss of descending motor neurons within the CNS also occurs, with less efficient activation of neurons innervating muscles of respiration via the phrenic nerve to the diaphragm for inspiration and of spinal nerves to intercostals for expiration.[85] These three factors combine to compromise the individual's ability to quickly and accurately respond to increasing physiologic demand and increase the likelihood of dyspnea during activity.

FUNCTIONAL CONSEQUENCES OF PULMONARY AGING

With less recoil for expiration and reduced flexibility for inspiration, the ability to work is compromised in two ways (Fig. 2.3). First, vital capacity (VC), the maximum amount of air that can be voluntarily moved in and out of the lungs with a breath, is decreased by 25% to 40%. Second, RV, the air remaining in the lungs after a forced expiration, is increased by 25% to 40%.[81] This combination of reduced movement of air with each breath and increased air remaining in the lung between breaths leads to higher lung-air carbon dioxide (CO_2) content and, eventually, lower oxygen saturation of the blood after air exchange. The increase in RV also affects the muscles of inspiration: the dome of the diaphragm flattens, and the accessory respiratory muscles are elongated. As a result of these length changes, the respiratory muscles work in a mechanically disadvantageous range of the length-tension curve causing the energy cost of the muscular work of breathing to rise.[83]

Functionally the amount of air inhaled per minute (minute ventilation) is a product of the frequency of breathing and the TV (volume of air moving into and out of the lungs with each usual breath). In healthy individuals, the increased ventilatory needs of low-intensity activities are usually met by an increased depth of breathing (i.e., increased TV).[96] Frequency of breathing increases when increased depth alone cannot meet the demands of activity, typically when TV reaches 50% to 60% of the VC.[96] For the older adult with reduced VC who is involved in physical activity, TV can quickly exceed this level so that the frequency of breathing increases much earlier than would be demonstrated by a young adult at the same intensity of exercise.[97,98] Because the energy cost of breathing rises sharply with the greater respiratory muscle work associated with an increased respiratory rate, an important consequence of increased frequency of breathing is fatigue.[99] This early reliance on an increased frequency of breathing combined with a large RV and its higher CO_2 concentration in lung air results in a physiologic cycle that further drives the need to breathe more frequently. Overworked respiratory muscles are forced to rely on anaerobic metabolism to supply their energy need, resulting in a buildup of lactic acid. Lactic acid lowers the pH of the tissues (acidosis) and is a potent physiologic stimulus for increased frequency of breathing.[99–101] The deconditioned older person may be easily forced into a condition of rapid, shallow breathing (shortness of breath) to meet the ventilatory requirements of seemingly moderate-intensity exercise. Due to the combined effects of the age-related changes, the high incidence of cardiac and pulmonary pathologies in later life, and the deconditioning impact of bed rest and inactivity, older patients who require orthotic or prosthetic intervention may be vulnerable if physical activity is too physiologically demanding.

Implications for Intervention

Rehabilitation professionals must consider two questions about the implications of age-related changes in the cardiovascular and cardiopulmonary systems on an older person's ability to do physical work. First, what precautions should be observed to avoid cardiopulmonary and cardiovascular complications? Second, what can be done to optimize cardiopulmonary and cardiovascular function for maximal physical performance?

PRECAUTIONS

Rehabilitation professionals should consider whether the intervention is occurring after a recent major surgery, which may compound these age-related changes. High-complexity patients with a prolonged hospitalization who have undergone multiple procedures may demonstrate compromised airway protective responses and may be susceptible to diaphragmatic fatigue, which complicates mechanical ventilation weaning and overall recovery from surgery.[102,103] Although most older adults can tolerate and positively respond to exercise, there are a number of circumstances where exercise is not appropriate (Table 2.3).

Estimating Workload: Heart Rate and Rate Pressure Product

One of the readily measurable consequences of the reduced response of the heart to sympathetic stimulation in later life is a reduction in the maximal attainable HR.[54,95,104] This reduction in maximal HR also signals that an older person's HR reserve, the difference between the rate for any given level of activity and the maximal attainable HR, is limited as well. For older patients involved in rehabilitation programs, the difference between resting and maximal HR is narrowed. The commonly used method of estimating maximal (max) attainable HR is with the equation[11]:

$$HR_{max} = 220\text{–Age}$$

There are three primary concerns with this commonly used equation. First, this equation was derived from a sample consisting of males mostly under 55 years of age.[105] Second, the equation lacks clinical reliability.[106,107] Third, the equation may actually underestimate the HR_{max} in older

Table 2.3 Signs and Symptoms of Exercise Intolerance

Category	Cautionary Signs/Symptoms	Contraindications to Exercise
Heart rate	<40 bpm at rest	Prolonged at maximum activity
	>130 bpm at rest	
	Little HR increase with activity	
	Excessive HR increase with activity	
	Frequent arrhythmia	
ECG	Any recent ECG abnormalities	Prolonged arrhythmia or tachycardia
		Exercise-induced ECG abnormalities
		Second or third-degree heart block
BP	Resting SBP > 165 mm Hg	Resting SBP > 210 mm Hg
	Resting DBP > 110 mm Hg	Resting DBP > 110 mm Hg
	Lack of SBP response to activity	Drop in SBP > 10 mm Hg in low-level exercise
	Excessive BP response to activity	Drop in DBP during exercise
Angina	Low threshold for angina	Resting or unstable angina
		New jaw, shoulder, or left arm pain
Respiratory rate	Dyspnea > 35 breaths/min	Dyspnea > 45 breaths/min
Blood gas values	O_2 saturation < 90%	O_2 saturation < 86%
Other symptoms	Mild to moderate claudication	Severe, persistent claudication (8/10 pain scale)
	Onset of pallor	Cyanosis, severe pallor, or cold sweat
	Facial expression of distress	Facial expression of severe distress
	Lightheadedness or mild dizziness	Moderate to severe dizziness, syncope
	Postactivity fatigue > 1 h	Nausea, vomiting
	Slow recovery from activity	Increasing mental confusion, onset of ataxia, incoordination
Additional considerations	Fever > 100°F	Any acute illness
	Aortic stenosis	Digoxin toxicity
	Recent mental confusion	Overt congestive heart failure
	Abnormal electrolytes (potassium)	Untreated second- or third-degree heart block
	Known left main coronary artery disease	Acute pericarditis
	Idiopathic hypertrophic subaortic stenosis	<4–6 weeks after myocardial infarction
	Compensated heart failure	<2 days after pulmonary embolism
		Acute thrombophlebitis
		Acute hypoglycemia

BP, Blood pressure; *bpm*, beats per minute; *DBP*, diastolic blood pressure; *ECG*, electrocardiogram; *HR*, heart rate; *SBP*, systolic blood pressure.
Modified from Hillegass EA. *Essentials of Cardiopulmonary Physical Therapy*. 5th ed. Elsevier; 2022:664, 672–673.

adults. A revised equation derived from diverse age and gender populations has been recommended[83,107]:

$$HR_{max} = 208 - (0.7 \times Age)$$

For healthy individuals, the recommended target HR for aerobic conditioning exercise is between 60% and 80% of maximal attainable HR. For many older adults, especially those who are habitually inactive, resting HR may be close to the recommended lower range for exercise exertion.[108] Consider an 83-year-old individual with a resting HR of 76 beats per minute. The maximal attainable HR is approximately 150 beats per minute (208 – (0.7 × Age)). A target HR for an aerobic training level of exertion of 60% of maximal HR would be 90 beats per minute. The resting HR is within 14 beats of the HR for aerobic training. Functionally this means that an activity as routine as rising from a chair or walking a short distance on a level surface may represent physical work at the level of exertion equated with moderate to high-intensity aerobic exercise. Because of the reduction in maximal attainable HR with age, older adults may be working close to their VO_{2max} range even in usual activities of daily living (ADLs).[108,109]

Because HR essentially signals the work of the heart, with each beat representing ventricular contraction, increased HR relates closely to increased heart work and increased oxygen consumption by the myocardium.[104] Given that afterload on the heart increases with age, the overall work of the heart for each beat is likely greater as well.[30,53–55] A more representative way to estimate the work of the heart during activity for older adults is the rate pressure product (RPP),[110–113] using HR and SBP as follows:

$$RPP = HR \times SBP$$

The linear relationship between VO_{2max} and HR for younger adults actually levels off for older adults.[114] Because of this, HR alone cannot accurately reflect the physiologic work that the older patient experiences; the RPP provides a clearer impression of relative work.[111] For older individuals with HR reserve limited by age, adjusting activity to keep the rise in HR within the lower end of the HR reserve is wise, especially for those with known coronary artery compromise.

Blood Pressure as a Warning Sign

Blood pressure (BP) must also be considered prior to, during, and after intervention. Hypertension, particularly increased SBP, is common in older adults. SBP also provides a relative indication of the level of afterload on the heart.[55,115,116] Resting BP can be used to indicate whether an older person can safely tolerate increased physiologic work. Persons with resting BPs of more than 180/95 mm Hg may have difficulty with increased activity. A conservative estimate of the safe range of exercise suggests that exercise should be stopped if and when BP exceeds 220/110 mm Hg, although some consider 220 mm Hg too conservative a limit for older adults.[104] SBP should rise with increasing activity or exercise.[117]An older adult with limited HR reserve must increase SV to achieve the required CO.[30,54,72] SBP rises as SV increases and blood volume in the peripheral vasculature rises.[55] If SBP fails to rise or actually decreases during activity, this is a significant concern.[104] The drop or lack of change in SBP indicates that the heart is an ineffective pump, unable to contract and force a reasonable volume of blood out of the left ventricle. Continuing activity in the presence of a dropping SBP returns more blood to a heart that is incapable of pumping it back out to the body. Elevated diastolic BP (DBP) suggests that the left ventricle is maintaining a higher pressure during the filling period.[54,55,95] Early diastolic filling during preload will be compromised,[55,67] and the heart will be unable to capitalize on the Frank-Starling mechanism to enhance the force of ventricular contraction.[30,72]

Respiratory Warning Signs

Dyspnea, or shortness of breath, is another important warning sign that must also be considered during physical activity.[118] Age-related changes in the pulmonary system increase the work of breathing, and breathing becomes less efficient as work increases.[99] If an older person is prone to shortness of breath, recovering from shortness of breath during exercise may be difficult. Breathing more deeply requires a disproportionately greater amount of respiratory muscle work, which further increases the cost of ventilation.[100,101] The use of supplemental oxygen by nasal cannula for the postoperative or medically ill older adult who is beginning rehabilitation may be beneficial.

Oxygen supplementation may prevent or minimize shortness of breath, enabling an older person to tolerate increased activity better and to participate in rehabilitation more fully. During this oxygen-assisted time, any conditioning exercise to improve muscular performance (especially if combined with nutritional support) delivers blood to the working tissues and improves tissue oxygenation, ultimately aiding pulmonary function. Improved muscular conditioning and cardiovascular function may prevent or delay the onset of lactic acidemia and the resultant increased desire to breathe that would trigger shortness of breath.[99,119]

OPTIMIZING CARDIOPULMONARY PERFORMANCE

For most older adults, conditioning or training is an effective way to improve function, although some may need a longer training period than younger adults to accomplish their desired level of physical performance.[120–125] Physical conditioning in situations of acute and chronic illness enables the older person to do more work and better accomplish desired tasks or activities.

Older adults, including those who are very frail and deconditioned, experience improvement in physical performance as a result of conditioning exercises (Fig. 2.4).[121,122] For some, significant gains are made as aerobic capacity increases from an initial state below the threshold necessary for function, such that an older person appears to make greater gains than a younger individual in similar circumstances.[126,127] In many cases the cardiopulmonary system efficiency gained through conditioning means the difference between independence and dependence; functional recovery and minimal improvement; life without extraordinary means and life support; and, for some older individuals, life and death.

The physiologic mechanisms for achieving the conditioned responses of older adults may vary slightly from those of younger individuals. With increasing activity or exercise in the submaximal range, older adults demonstrate greater increases in SV and less rise in HR than do young adults.[30,55,67,72,104] This increase in SV is accomplished with an increased EDV, usually without change in the ESV.[30,55,67] Increasing the EDV enhances the force of ventricular contraction by the Frank-Starling mechanism, which, in turn, increases CO despite the age-related impairment of

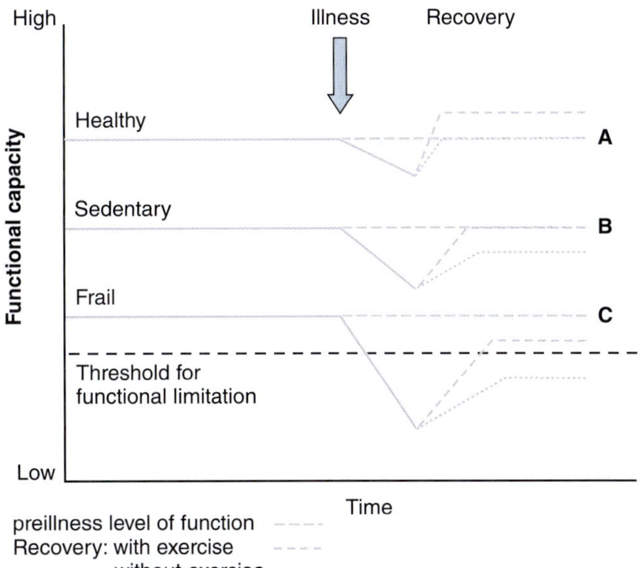

Fig. 2.4 Comparison of the impact of illness or prolonged inactivity or both on functional status and of exercise on recovery of premorbid functional levels of healthy, sedentary, and frail older adults. Each individual's functional reserve is represented by the distance between the threshold for functional limitation and the adult's functional capacity. *(A)* Healthy older adults have the most functional reserve and may recover preillness functional capacity without conditioning exercise; however, they often show improvement above baseline with exercise. *(B)* Sedentary older adults may not resume preillness functional capacity without the benefit of conditioning exercise. *(C)* Frail older adults have the least functional reserve, often falling below threshold for function when illness occurs and tending to remain below this threshold without conditioning exercise. However, even frail older adults can regain functional status with conditioning exercise.

the cardioacceleratory responses, which limits the rise in HR.[30,54,55,67,72] An increased preload, which improves CO, is the usual outcome of training at any age because improved conditioning of the peripheral musculature prevents distal pooling of blood and increased resting tension of the muscles assists blood return.[104]

Preparation for Activity and Exercise

Simple lower extremity exercise as a warmup before any functional activity or training session enhances the preload of the heart. Any gentle, repetitive, active lower extremity motions (e.g., ankle "pumps" in dorsiflexion/plantarflexion, knee flexion/extension, or cycling movements of the legs) before transfer or ambulation activities, before upper trunk and upper extremity activities, or as part of the warmup portion of an aerobic or strength training exercise, effectively improves the EDV. This increased EDV compensates in part for age-related preload problems, which might otherwise compromise aerobic capacity.

Additionally, the muscular work of preliminary lower extremity exercise initiates the electrolyte and hormonal changes that promote the metabolic changes and vasodilation in peripheral tissues necessary to support aerobic metabolism for meeting energy demands of the task.[104,122] Peripheral oxygen exchange improves as much as 16% with regular exercise training.[30] The peripheral vasodilation associated with exercise helps to regulate the rise in the heart's afterload and minimizes the development of lactic acidemia and the resulting drive to breathe more rapidly.[128]

As submaximal levels of exercise increase toward maximal exercise, SV continues to increase, maintaining CO.[30,67,72] When cardiopulmonary disease is present in addition to aging, however, this continued increase in SV is likely to be blunted.[54,104] Under these circumstances, the reduced sensitivity of the heart to sympathetic stimulation limits the force of contraction of the ventricle so that the ejection fraction decreases and the ESV rises slightly.[55]

MONITORING THE CARDIOPULMONARY RESPONSE TO EXERCISE

Consistent monitoring of the cardiopulmonary response is an essential component of rehabilitation interventions aimed at optimizing endurance and fitness of older frail or deconditioned individuals.[108,129] Positive effects of training occur when the older person is appropriately challenged by the exercise or physical activity. According to the principle of overload, functional improvements occur only when the body is asked to do more than the customary workload for that individual.[11] For an individual who is deconditioned due to prolonged bed rest, simple lower extremity exercises while sitting upright may be as challenging as training for a marathon in a healthy young adult. The level of physiologic exertion is relative to the individual's customary work. Providing the physiologic overload necessary to produce improvements in performance while avoiding a decline in performance because of exercise-induced fatigue or exhaustion requires that the therapist consistently monitor the individual's level of physical exertion.

Heart Rate and Blood Pressure

Maximum oxygen consumption (VO_{2max}) is the most accurate and sensitive measure of the individual workload.[104,108] Clinical availability of this measure is limited. A potential alternative is using consumer wearable devices (e.g., Fitbit, Garmin, Apple devices); additional psychometric evaluations are required prior to widespread clinical use.[130] Although the linear relationship between HR and VO_{2max} plateaus causes HR to become an inaccurate reflection of the workload for older adults, HR does partially indicate the work of the heart.[104,114] For a rapid clinical impression of the physiologic burden of an activity or exercise, HR is helpful as long as the clinician recognizes its limitations when the measure is being used with older adults. Preexercise or activity BP provides some indication of likely afterload against which the heart will be working.[55,104,117] Continuous BP monitoring during activity helps identify if the exercising cardiovascular system can meet the requirements of an increasing workload.[104] Calculation of the RPP (HR × SBP) may be a more accurate estimate of cardiac workload for older adults.[110,111,113]

Perceived Exertion

Ratings of perceived exertion (RPEs) are effective indicators of the level of physiologic exertion experienced by patients who are exercising or involved in a strenuous physical activity (Table 2.4).[104,131,132] These scales ask individuals to assess subjectively how much effort they are expending during an exercise session or activity, with higher ratings indicating greater effort. Many older adults using RPEs in the clinical setting tend to overestimate their true physiologic stress as indicated by their HR during exercise sessions.[104,131] Clinicians who appropriately recommend exercise for older adults relying on perceived exertion to limit the activity safely may find this phenomenon comforting.

Alternative scales have been developed to assess breathlessness, fatigue, discomfort or pain, or talking ability during exercise (Table 2.5). In the traditional version of the Talk Test, clients read a paragraph during various intensities of exercise and answer "yes," "not sure," or "no" to the following question, "Can you speak comfortably?"[133]

Table 2.4 Borg Scales: Ratings of Perceived Exertion

LINEAR SCALE		RATIO SCALE	
Value	**Description**	**Value**	**Description**
6	No exertion	0	No effort at all
7–8	Extremely light effort	1	Very little (very weak) effort
9–10	Very light effort	2	Light (weak) effort
11–12	Light effort	3	Moderate effort
13–14	Somewhat hard effort	4	Somewhat strong effort
15–16	Heavy or hard	5–6	Strong effort
17–18	Very hard effort	7–8	Very strong effort
19	Extremely hard effort	9	Extremely strong effort
20	Maximum exertion	10	Maximal exertion

Modified from Borg G, Ottoson D. *The Perception of Exertion in Physical Work.* London: Macmillan; 1986.

Table 2.5 Scales of Perceived Breathlessness, Fatigue, Discomfort or Pain, and Talking Ability During Exercise

				TALK TEST (VISUAL ANALOG SCALE)
Value	**Breathlessness/Dyspnea**	**Fatigue**	**Discomfort or Pain**	**Is It Easy or Hard to Talk?**
0	No breathlessness at all	No fatigue at all	No pain or discomfort	–
1	Very light breathlessness	Very light fatigue	Very little (weak) pain	Extremely easy
2	Light breathlessness	Light fatigue	Little (weak) discomfort	Very easy
3	Moderate breathlessness	Moderate fatigue	Moderate discomfort	Very easy
4	Somewhat hard to breathe	Somewhat hard	Somewhat strong discomfort	Slightly difficult
5	Heavy breathing	Heavy work/fatigue	Strong discomfort or pain	Slightly difficult
6	Heavy breathing	Heavy work/fatigue	Strong discomfort or pain	Hard
7	Very heavy breathing	Very heavy fatigue	Very heavy discomfort	Hard
8	Very heavy breathing	Very heavy fatigue	Very heavy discomfort	Very hard
9	Very, very breathless	Very, very fatigued	Very, very hard discomfort	Very hard
10	Maximum breathlessness	Maximally fatigued	Maximal discomfort or pain	Extremely hard

Modified from Dean E. Mobilization and exercise. In: Frownfelter D, Dean E, eds. *Principles and Practice of Cardiopulmonary Physical Therapy*. 3rd ed. Mosby; 1996:282; Orizola-Cáceres I, Cerda-Kohler H, Burgos-Jara C, Meneses-Valdes R, Gutierrez-Pino R, Sepúlveda C. Modified talk test: a randomized cross-over trial investigating the comparative utility of two "talk tests" for determining aerobic training zones in overweight and obese patients. *Sports Med Open*. 2021;7:1–8.

A "yes" or a "not sure" answer allows the client to advance to a more intense exercise; whereas, a "no" indicates the exercise intensity may be too difficult for the client. This test is a valid and reliable scale to assess and monitor intensity during exercise in a wide range of individuals.[117,134] In the visual analog scale version of the Talk Test, scores range from 1 to 10, with higher scores equating to more difficulty when reading a paragraph during exercise.[135] The Counting Talk Test works well with individuals who may have difficulty reading during exercise. For this test, a lower number means a higher exercise exertional level as participants take a deep breath in, and while exercising, state the following sequence with one breath: "1-one thousand, 2-one thousand, 3-one thousand, 4-one thousand..."[136] Among individuals on medication for cardiovascular disease, the Talk Test can indicate exertion levels when the HR response is blunted.[137] In summary, rehabilitation professionals can choose from a variety of scales to quantify various aspects of exertion while taking into account patient preferences to properly manage exercise intensity.

Exercise Testing Protocols

Standard exercise testing protocols are appropriate for the assessment of the status of conditioning of the cardiovascular system and exercise tolerance of older adults.[108,138] The "gold standard" treadmill test, a cycle ergometer, or a 2-Minute Step Test can be used to assess the cardiovascular performance of the older person unless the specific clinical setting or associated musculoskeletal dysfunction (e.g., balance problems, arthritic joints, or lower extremity muscle weakness) precludes this type of testing.[108] Alternatives for individuals who can walk distances include the 1-mile walk test and the 6-minute walk test.[139–141] For individuals unable to walk 1 mile or 6 minutes, an alternative is the 400-meter walk test or the 2-minute walk test.[142–144] The 2-minute walk test has been utilized in people with lower-limb amputation who are prosthetic ambulators.[145] For healthy individuals with low to average fitness levels, and individuals with unilateral TFA using a prosthesis, a VO_{2max} modified treadmill walking protocol with progressively increasing inclinations is suitable to measure exercise activity levels.[146] A brief step test performed while sitting in a chair has been developed for individuals who cannot otherwise be safely tested on a treadmill, with an ergometer, or by distance walked.[104,147]

Careful monitoring of HR, BP, and RPE before, immediately after, and a short while after completing the aerobic assessment provides a comprehensive picture of the cardiovascular function of the older patient. This information is paramount in clinical decision-making, exercise prescription, and program planning. Similarly, careful monitoring of HR, BP, and RPE before, during, and after a bout of exercise during rehabilitation allows the clinician to compare the pattern of responses with the expected pattern for conditioned adults.[148] Normal exercise-induced cardiovascular responses include a slow rate of rise of HR, a rise in SBP, and minimal (if any) rise in DBP during the exercise bout. For the conditioned older adult, HR and SBP should return toward preexercise values during the immediate postexercise recovery period on the order of 50% of the changes during exercise. The pattern of change in the RPP for the exercise bout and recovery period may be an even more descriptive measure of the cardiovascular response.

Expecting individuals to fully participate in gait and balance training activities seems unreasonable if they are significantly deconditioned, can barely tolerate sitting for 30 minutes, are short of breath after 10 repetitions of simple seated lower extremity exercises, or are fatigued after 5 minutes of a sitting step test. How can individuals who are working at 90% or more of their maximum target HR be truly concerned with much more than delivering oxygen to the working tissues? Deconditioned individuals who are working at a high intensity in simple, well-known tasks have seriously restricted energy reserves. They are likely to have difficulty with focus and attention, processing, and understanding the therapist's directions while supporting muscle activity—all necessary components for motor learning in performing a new skill such as gait training with a prosthetic device. Under these circumstances emphasis must first be placed on improving cardiovascular conditioning to improve energy reserves; then subsequent functional training with an orthosis or prosthesis will have a greater likelihood of a successful outcome.

PHYSICAL PERFORMANCE TRAINING

The same principles of training that are used with young adult athletes can be adapted and applied to frail or deconditioned older adults who are recovering from amputation in prosthetic rehabilitation or to a neuromuscular or musculoskeletal event that necessitates use of an orthosis. The primary goals of conditioning for frail individuals are (1) to develop enough aerobic capacity to do work and (2) to ensure efficient muscle function to produce work.[104,108,149] These concepts can guide any single rehabilitation session, as well as the progression of the rehabilitation program, over time. Understanding both exercise principles and cardiopulmonary age-related changes is necessary as a foundation for exercise prescription, which then is individualized on the basis of current exercise tolerance of a specific older patient. This strategy can likely optimize the performance and recovery of older adults in rehabilitation.

An effective strategy to improve cardiopulmonary response to activity for older patients who are deconditioned by bed rest, acute illness, or sedentary lifestyle begins with a warmup of continuous alternating movements using large muscle groups, particularly of the lower extremities. The goal of such activity is the facilitation of the preload and SV; any increase in SV realized through this training regimen helps an older patient maximize cardiovascular function despite age-associated limitations in HR, cardioacceleratory responses, and baroreceptor sensitivity.

For healthy adults, the aerobic physical activity recommendation is a minimum of 150 minutes of moderate-intensity activity or 75 minutes of vigorous activity per week in activities that use large muscles (i.e., running, cycling, swimming, brisk walking, dancing, or gardening) and keep HR in a target range between 60% and 80% of the individual's maximal attainable HR.[117,150,151] This amount of activity confers significant health benefits, including reduced risk of developing chronic diseases and reduced mortality. Strength training twice a week or more at a moderate to vigorous intensity is also recommended.[150] Additionally, older adults should do multicomponent physical activity that includes balance training.[150] For those who are deconditioned, evidence suggests that significant improvement in functional capacity can occur at exercise intensities as low as 40% of maximal HR.[125,152–154] Although high-frequency, high-intensity exercise can maximize an increase in aerobic capacity (VO_{2max}), high-intensity exercise performed less frequently and low-intensity exercise performed more frequently can also yield positive endurance training effects.[153,155]

Multicomponent rehabilitation programs are designed to address the impairments older adults may have prior to and develop during hospitalization. Rehabilitation for hospital-acquired deconditioning has been characterized as routinely low intensity in spite of evidence that older adults can tolerate and need more aggressive care during and after hospitalization.[156] Appropriately dosed intensities are required to increase muscle strength and mass to a level that allows activity and participation beyond basic ADLs.[129] For those who have lost muscle mass, the development of more lean body mass improves the basal metabolic rate, overall health, fitness, and functional status.[157,158] Flexibility exercises, another aspect of a multicomponent program, preserve or restore limited joint mobility that could compromise essential functions.[159] For example, hip, knee, or ankle contractures alter gait and have the potential to increase the energy cost of walking[160] A home-based multicomponent progressive high-intensity intervention including ADL training, walking endurance, strengthening at an eight-repetition maximum, and dual-task activities resulted in significantly better walking speed, modified Physical Performance Test, and Short Physical Performance Battery when compared to a usual care control group.[161] Similarly, in a skilled nursing facility pilot study, high-intensity strengthening, gait training, ADL, and balance interventions were found to be safe and resulted in significantly better patient satisfaction and improvement in gait speed during rehabilitation following acute hospitalization.[162]

Older adults who are inadequately active still benefit from physical performance training to reduce sedentary time or increase their physical activity, even if it does not reach the recommended guidelines.[163,164] Successfully completing any level of physical activity has multiple health benefits and can increase one's self-efficacy in performing additional physical activity.[5,150,165] In summary, an essential component of physical performance training is to aim for the recommended physical activity guidelines with the understanding that patient abilities may necessitate modifying the prescription.[166]

Energy Cost of Walking

The human body is designed to be energy efficient during upright bipedal gait. Muscles of the trunk and extremities are activated by the CNS in a precise rhythmic cycle to move the body forward while maintaining dynamic stability, adapting stride length and walking speed to the constraints and demands of the task, the force of gravity, and the characteristics of the environment in which walking is occurring.[167,168] The advancing foot is lifted just enough to clear the surface in swing, and muscle activity at the stance-side hip and lower torso keeps the pelvis fairly level and the trunk erect, thus minimizing vertical displacement of the body's center of mass.[169] Normal arthrokinematic and osteokinematic relationships between body segments ensure a narrow base of support in quiet stance and relaxed walking, and reciprocal arm swing counterbalances the dynamic pendular motion of the lower extremities, ensuring that the center of mass progresses forward with minimal mediolateral sway.[169-172] Much of the energy cost of walking is related to the muscular work performed to keep the center of mass moving forward with a minimum of vertical and mediolateral displacement.[173]

SELF-SELECTED WALKING SPEED

Since self-selected walking speed (SSWS) emerges from the interaction of the cardiovascular, pulmonary, musculoskeletal, and neurologic systems, it reflects the overall health and functional status of an individual.[174–177] Walking speed is recognized as a vital sign that not only captures current function but also can be used to predict the risk of functional decline, adverse health events and morbidity, length of stay and discharge location after hospitalization, and mortality.[176–195]

Energetic costs of walking predict the decline in SSWS in adults 65 years of age and older.[175] SSWS tends to decrease with aging, and therefore normative values considering age should be used for comparisons. Even with slower overall walking speeds, multiple studies have demonstrated that even into the ninth and tenth decades of life, healthy older adults are able to walk at speeds approaching 1 m/s (Table 2.6).[196–198] Values for typical walking speed are also becoming available for community-living older adults with impaired mobility and physical frailty.[175,190,199–202] There is also evidence that the ability to increase walking speed is an indicator of functional reserve.[90,200,203] In individuals with lower-limb amputation, those with better-expected walking potential (expressed as the Medicare Functional Classification Level or K levels) have demonstrated faster walking speeds at hospital rehabilitation discharge.[204]

Walking speed can be quickly and reliably measured using a stopwatch and either a 20- or 8-m walkway (Fig. 2.5).[205,206] The individual is instructed to walk over the entire distance of the walkway but is timed only while walking the middle distance (10 or 4 m, respectively) so that steady-state speed is more likely and the impacts of acceleration (at the start) and deceleration (at the end) are minimized. Reliability is strong at either distance for persons with amputation, stroke, and spinal cord injury (SCI) as well as for those with chronic disease, physical frailty, and other neurologic pathologies.[207–210] Minimal detectable differences/changes (MDD/MDCs) have been consistently reported between 0.04 and 0.1 m/s for community-living persons, those with cognitive impairment, and those with hip fractures.[211–214] MDC may be higher in those with neurologic pathology, sarcopenia, or during acute rehabilitation.[207,215,216] The minimal clinically important difference for walking speed following stroke is reported to be 0.16 to 0.175 m/s.[217,218] Walking speed has been successfully used to evaluate the outcome of interventions for persons with cognitive impairments as well as those with hip fractures and with patients in short-term rehabilitation.[211,213–215] It is important that the same distance and start/stop methods (acceleration/deceleration areas) are used each time as different testing protocols may yield results that exceed meaningful change values and could be statistically different.[205,206,219]

Table 2.6 Typical Self-Selected Walking Speed (SSWS; m/s) for Healthy Older Adult Populations Reported as Mean (Standard Deviation or 95% Confidence Interval)

RESEARCHER	BOHANNON AND ANDREWS[196]		KASOVIC ET AL.[198]		BOHANNON & WANG[197]	
METHODOLOGY[A]	METHODOLOGY VARIES, ALL INCLUDED ACCELERATION/DECELERATION[B]		1.5 M INSTRUMENTED WALKWAY, 4.5 M ACCELERATION/DECELERATION		4 M STOPWATCH TIMED, 1.5 M DECELERATION ONLY	
Gender	**Age Group**	**SSWS**	**Age Group**	**SSWS**	**Age Group**	**SSWS**
Females	60–69	1.24 (1.18–1.30)	60–65	1.36 (0.23)	60–69	1.05 (0.22)
			66–70	1.22 (0.30)		
	70–79	1.13 (1.07–1.19)	71–75	1.11 (0.25)	70–79	0.99 (0.22)
	80–99	0.94 (0.85–1.03)	≥76	0.98 (0.30)	80–85	0.95 (0.24)
Males	60–69	1.34 (1.27–1.41)	60–65	1.40 (0.18)	60–69	1.16 (0.22)
			66–70	1.31 (0.19)		
	70–79	1.26 (1.21–1.32)	71–75	1.19 (0.18)	70–79	1.07 (0.24)
	80–99	0.97 (0.83–1.10)	≥76	1.10 (0.23)	80–85	0.97 (0.20)

[a]Distance timed, timing method, acceleration/deceleration distances.
[b]Methodology varied across 41 studies including distances walked from 3.7 to 30 m, timing by stopwatch, photocells, instrumented walkways, distances used for acceleration and deceleration.

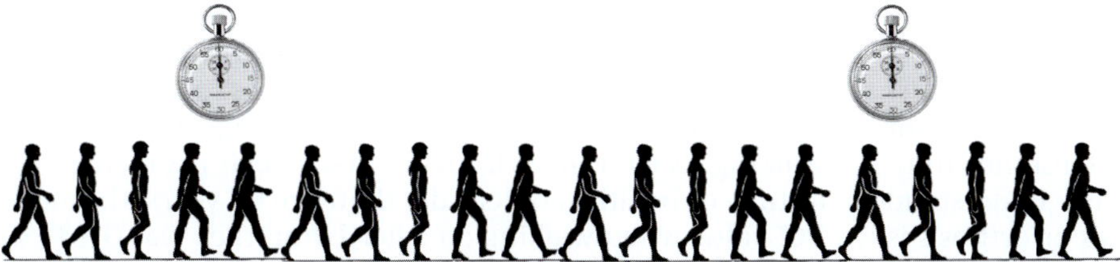

Acceleration Zone	Timed Walk	Deceleration Zone
1 m	2 m	1 m
5 m	10 m	5 m

Fig. 2.5 Strategy for assessing self-selected or fast walking speed timing either the central 10-m distance (10-m walk) or central 4-m distance (4-m walk) allowing for acceleration and deceleration at either end so that steady-state speed is better approximated.

Any pathologic condition that interferes with the alignment of body segments, the carefully controlled sequential activation of muscles, or the effectiveness of muscle contraction increases the energy cost of walking.[175] As vertical displacement and mediolateral sway increase and gait deviations occur, muscles must work harder to keep the center of mass moving forward despite extraneous displacing moments. As muscle work increases, the cardiopulmonary system responds to this physiologic demand with increased HR, SV, and respiratory rate. Any orthosis or prosthesis that adds mass to or alters movement of the lower extremity potentially increases the work of walking. However, in individuals with amputation or neuromuscular dysfunction, walking with an appropriate prosthesis or orthosis may actually require less energy than walking without it.[173,220,221]

MEASURING ENERGY COSTS OF WALKING

Measurement of physiologic energy expenditure by direct calorimetry is not realistic in all but the most sophisticated research laboratory settings. Instead, several indirect indicators have been found to be valid and reliable estimates of the energy cost and the efficiency of gait in research and clinical applications. These include calculation of oxygen consumption (VO_{2max}) and oxygen cost while walking, monitoring blood lactate levels, calculating the physiologic cost index (PCI) of walking, and monitoring heart and respiratory rates during activity.

Oxygen Rate and Oxygen Cost

The most precise indirect measurements of energy and gait efficiency use special equipment (e.g., a portable spirometer or a Douglas bag) to monitor ventilatory volumes and to measure how much oxygen is taken in and how much CO_2 is exhaled during physical activity. This type of testing is usually done while the subject or patient walks, runs on a treadmill or track, or cycles on a stationary bicycle. The rate of oxygen consumption (O_2 rate), measured as volume of oxygen consumed per unit of body weight in 1 minute (mL/kg/min), provides an index of intensity of physical work at any given time.[117,172] VO_{2max} is the highest rate of oxygen uptake possible and is determined by progressing the exercise test to the point of voluntary exhaustion, when the age-adjusted maximum attainable HR is approached or reached.[222,223]

If oxygen consumption during gait is low, an individual is likely to be able to walk long distances. If it is high, however, the distance of functional gait is likely to be limited. The oxygen cost of walking is determined by dividing the rate of oxygen consumption by the speed of walking. Oxygen cost is a precise indicator of efficiency of gait, or the amount of energy expended to walk over a standard distance (mL/kg/m).[172] Most of what researchers currently understand about energy expenditure when a prosthesis or orthosis is being used is based on studies that have measured oxygen rate and the oxygen cost of walking.

Serum Lactate

The energy efficiency of walking is also assessed by evaluating serum CO_2 and lactate levels as indicators of anaerobic energy production. The energy (adenosine triphosphate [ATP]) required for muscle contraction during gait can be derived from a combination of aerobic oxidative and anaerobic glycolytic pathways.[224] The aerobic oxidative pathway, which depends on oxygen delivery to active muscle cells, is the most efficient source of energy, producing almost 19 times as much ATP as the anaerobic pathway. In healthy, fit individuals, this aerobic pathway is more than able to meet energy requirements of relaxed walking. If energy demands of an exercise or activity are met by aerobic oxidation, the activity can be sustained for long periods with relatively low levels of fatigue. As activity becomes strenuous (i.e., as walking speed or surface incline increases) and the need for energy begins to exceed the availability of oxygen for aerobic oxidation, additional energy is accessed through anaerobic metabolism.[126] This transition to anaerobic metabolism is reported to begin at work levels of 55% of VO_{2max} in healthy, untrained individuals but may begin at 80% of VO_{2max} in highly trained athletes.[225]

When the ability to deliver oxygen is compromised by the physical deconditioning of a sedentary lifestyle or by cardiac, pulmonary, or musculoskeletal pathology, anaerobic glycolysis becomes a primary source of energy at lower levels of work.[226] Whenever the anaerobic pathway is the major source of energy, blood levels of lactate and CO_2 rise, lowering blood pH and increasing the respiratory exchange ratio (CO_2 production/O_2 consumption).[227] Under these conditions, the ability to sustain activity is limited, with an earlier onset of fatigue as workload increases.

Heart Rate and Physiologic Cost Index

High correlations between HR and oxygen consumption during gait have been reported for children and healthy young adults at a variety of walking speeds.[228–230] Although this suggests that HR monitoring may be a reliable substitute for oxygen consumption, it should be used with caution in older adults because of the age-related changes in cardiopulmonary function discussed earlier in this chapter. This is especially true for older adults with heart disease who are being managed with medications that further blunt HR response.[231,232] The RPP or the PCI may be a more appropriate indicator of the energy cost of walking in these circumstances. The PCI is calculated as follows[233]:

$$PCI = (HR\ walking - HR\ resting)/Walking\ speed$$

Measured in beats per meter, the PCI reflects the effort of walking; low values suggest energy-efficient gait. The PCI was originally used to assess gait restrictions in adults with rheumatoid arthritis or a similar inflammatory joint disease.[233] For children between 3 and 12 years of age, the mean PCI at self-selected or preferred walking speed has been reported to be between 0.38 and 0.40 beats per meter.[234] Typical PCI values for adolescents and young adults at usual walking speeds ranged from 0.3 to 0.4 beats per meter.[235] In a study of healthy adults older than age 65 years, the mean PCI value when walking on a flat 10-m track was 0.43 (SD = 0.13) beats per meter; when calculated while walking on a treadmill, mean PCI increased to 0.60 (SD = 0.26) beats per meter.[236] Additionally, PCI declines with increasing body weight–supported gait in both individuals with stroke and healthy age-matched controls.[237]

The PCI has been used to assess the effect of different assistive devices on the effort of walking,[236,238] evaluate the short- and long-term impact on neuromuscular stimulation on the ability to walk and run in older adults and in children with hemiplegia, assess outcomes of orthopedic surgery in children with cerebral palsy, and evaluate the efficacy of reciprocal gait orthosis (RGO)/functional electrical stimulation (FES) walking systems for individuals with SCI.[239–247] High correlation among the PCI, percent maximum HR, and oxygen rate ($r = 0.91$, $P > .005$) in nondisabled children and children with transtibial amputation (TTA) supports its validity as an indicator of energy cost for children.[248] A similar study of energy cost of walking in young adults using a microprocessor-controlled transfemoral prosthesis suggests that PCI is comparable with oxygen uptake as an indicator of the energy cost of walking.[249] The PCI has also been used to compare energy cost of walking in different types of transfemoral prosthetic sockets and to assess efficacy of a stance control knee orthosis.[250,251]

Studies of variability in PCI values on repeated measures have raised questions about its accuracy and sensitivity to change in energy cost of gait as compared with monitoring oxygen consumption and oxygen cost.[252–254] Although the relationship between PCI and the gold standards of oxygen consumption and oxygen cost may not be strong enough for researchers, it remains an important tool for clinicians who lack the resources necessary to directly monitor oxygen consumption and cost yet want to estimate the energy cost of walking and assess the impact of orthotic or prosthetic rehabilitation over time.

ENERGY EXPENDITURE AT SELF-SELECTED WALKING SPEEDS

The energy requirements of walking vary with age and walking speed.[253,255–261] Oxygen consumption is highest in childhood and decreases to approximately 12 mL/kg/min in healthy adults and elders.[258] When oxygen consumption during walking is expressed as a percent of VO_{2max}, a slightly different picture emerges. For a healthy, untrained young adult, oxygen consumption at a comfortable walking speed may be 32% of VO_{2max}, whereas for an older adult walking at a similar speed, oxygen consumption may be as much as 48% of VO_{2max}.[169,262] For functional gait, if walking is to cover long distances or is to be sustained over prolonged periods of time, oxygen consumption must be less than 50% of that individual's VO_{2max} so that aerobic oxidation will be used as the primary source of energy.[11] At comfortable walking speeds, older adults approach the threshold for transition to anaerobic metabolism faster than younger adults. If some form of gait dysfunction is superimposed, increasing the energy cost of gait, the work of walking will transition to anaerobic glycolysis unless a cardiovascular conditioning program is included in the rehabilitation program.[38,263–266]

For individuals without neuromuscular or musculoskeletal impairment, the relationship between the energy cost of walking and walking speed has been described as nearly linear (Fig. 2.6).[173,263] More recent data, in those both with and without amputation, suggest a U-shaped relationship, with higher energy requirements (O_2 rate/velocity) when walking both slower and faster than SSWS.[267] The lowest energy cost of walking is associated with SSWS; however, those with amputation often walk slower than their most economic or energy-efficient walking speed.[263,265,267–270]

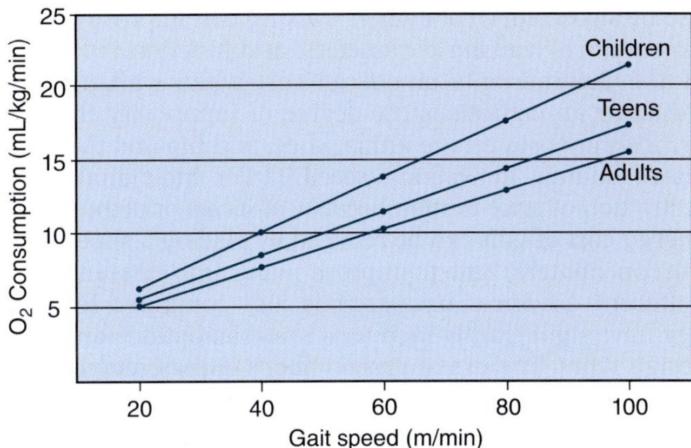

Fig. 2.6 Relationship between walking speed and oxygen consumption (O_2 rate). The differences in O_2 rate between children and adults (20 to 80 years) are attributed in part to differences in body composition. (From gait-velocity regression formulas reported by Waters RL. Energy expenditure. In: Perry J, Burnfield JM, eds. *Gait Analysis: Normal and Pathological Function*. Slack; 2010:483–518.)

This reduction in SSWS increases the energy cost of walking. In particular, those with vascular causes of amputation tend to walk slower, with higher energy costs, than those with nonvascular amputation, and those with TFA walk slower than people with TTA.[267,270,271] Individuals with limb loss are likely to have reduced aerobic capacity (secondary to complications from hospitalization and reduced activity), but individuals with vascular causes for amputation utilize a higher aerobic load at slower speeds than those with traumatic limb loss.[270] Slower chosen walking speeds are possibly a mechanism that prioritizes management of available aerobic load rather than energy costs of walking.[270] Unfortunately, improvement in aerobic capacity during rehabilitation has not been demonstrated and should be a priority intervention that could potentially reduce energy costs of walking in older adults with limb loss.[272]

The weight and design of the prosthesis or orthosis are also determinants of energy cost of gait. The impact of added mass on the energy cost of gait depends on where the load is placed. Extra weight loaded on the trunk (e.g., a heavy backpack) changes oxygen rate during walking less than would a smaller load placed around the ankle.[273] Adding weight to the prosthesis center of mass increases the energy cost of gait by 7%, whereas adding the same weight to the ankle increases the energy cost by 12%.[274] Despite theories that increasing prosthesis weight may improve gait symmetry, the increase in energy cost for the patient may not have been taken into account. This highlights the importance of minimizing weight of lower extremity orthoses and prostheses to keep the energy cost of walking within an individual's aerobic capacity.[274,275]

WORK OF WALKING WITH AN ORTHOSIS

When the energy cost of walking with an orthosis is being discussed, it is important to remember that, for those with significant neuromuscular or musculoskeletal impairments, the energy cost of walking without the orthosis is typically higher than that of walking with an appropriate orthosis.[276–282] For example, ankle/foot-orthosis (AFO) use by stroke survivors when walking can improve energy expenditure, walking parameters, and function.[283–285] One of the determinants of energy cost when walking with a cast or an orthosis is the degree of immobility that the orthosis imposes on the ankle, knee, and hip and the associated change in walking speed.[286] For individuals with restriction of knee motion because of a cast or orthosis, the energy cost of gait can be reduced by placing a shoe lift on the contralateral limb to improve swing limb clearance.[287]

Recent advances in materials and computer technology have significantly increased material options and AFO design types. The use of carbon fiber's energy return characteristics may improve walking speed and gait kinematics in patients after stroke, and the use of traditional thermoplastic material and an articulated joint may provide similar improvements when compared with a solid joint.[283,288–290] Newer technology including microprocessor-controlled knee-ankle-foot-orthosis (KAFO) may normalize gait kinematics and speed, and improve balance and function.[291–293] In one randomized controlled trial, participants using a microprocessor orthosis demonstrated significant improvements in self-selected gait speed, functional gait, distance walked, balance, stair assessment, quality of life, and physical health. After training, participants also reported significantly fewer falls during 1 month of use when compared to groups using a conventional KAFO or stance control orthosis.[291] Despite the differences in design, KAFOs consistently reduce energy expenditure with walking. The true key for the clinician is to determine which type of orthosis design is optimal based on the patient's individual deficits and resources.[294]

The movement dysfunction associated with neuromuscular impairments tends to reduce walking speed, with the degree of slowing determined by the severity of the impairment.[174,277,295] As abnormal movement patterns and impaired postural responses compromise the cyclic and dynamic flow of walking, the higher levels of muscle activity that are required to remain upright and to move forward increase the energy cost of gait.[296,297] Reduction of walking speed is a functional strategy to keep energy expenditure within physiologic limits in addition to maintain postural stability. Among stroke survivors walking at a reduced speed, oxygen rate (consumption) is close to that of older adults when walking at their SSWS, but oxygen cost is significantly higher.[173,278,298] When stroke survivors are able to improve their gait symmetry and walking speed, their overall oxygen consumption is reduced dramatically.[295] Orthosis use on the affected lower extremity may be one of the easiest methods to help facilitate improved gait quality and functional walking distance.

For individuals with SCI, regardless of age, the potential for functional ambulation appears to be determined by four conditions: the ability to use a reciprocal gait pattern, the adequacy of trunk stability, at least fair hip flexor strength bilaterally, and fair quadriceps strength of at least one limb.[297,299] This corresponds to an ambulatory motor index (AMI) score of 18 of 30 possible points, or 60% of "good" lower extremity strength.[261] In this instance, gait may be possible with bilateral AFOs or an AFO and a KAFO combination. Those with SCI at mid- to low-thoracic levels with AMI scores of less than 60% often require bilateral KAFOs with Lofstrand or axillary crutches in a swing-through gait pattern to ambulate. Waters[173] reports a near linear positive relationship between AMI scores and gait velocity as well as a somewhat curvilinear inverse relationship between AMI score and oxygen rate (percent above normal) and oxygen cost. For persons with SCI who have the potential for functional ambulation, continued cardiovascular conditioning after discharge from rehabilitation improves the efficiency of walking as reflected in lower oxygen cost and improvement in walking speed.[299–301]

The development of RGOs, at times augmented by FES, and robotic exoskeletons has demonstrated improved health, user satisfaction, comfort, and made modified ambulation safe and feasible for patients with neurological pathology such as SCI including tetraplegia, stroke, multiple sclerosis, and Parkinson disease.[302–308] A recent scoping review of exoskeleton training in persons with incomplete SCI lesions reported improvements in walking ability, spasticity, pain, and cardiovascular endurance. Consistent recommendations regarding the use of exoskeletons to minimize adverse events include selecting the type of robotic device, preparation/training, considering the diagnosis including the level of lesion, and possible comorbidities.[308] The clinician must consider the potential energy requirement of using a functional orthosis such as an RGO, FES, and exoskeleton with gait for a patient with an SCI (Table 2.7).[309–313] An individual ambulating at a normal walking speed of 1.3 m/s will use 3.4 times the average amount of oxygen at rest, or 3.4 metabolic equivalents (METs).[313] One MET is equal to 3.5 mL O_2/min/kg—essentially the amount of oxygen consumed while sitting at rest. When tasked with gait using a functional orthosis, patients with SCI demonstrate significantly higher energy requirements to complete the task. It is important to note that the energy expenditures listed in Table 2.7 were mostly performed at nonfunctional walking speeds.

WORK OF WALKING WITH A PROSTHESIS

The characteristics of gait and the energy cost of walking with a prosthesis are related to the etiology, level of amputation, and type of prosthesis.[314–316] The walking speed, stride length, and cadence of persons with lower extremity amputation who walk with a prosthesis are typically lower than those of individuals without impairment regardless of the cause of amputation,[317] although individuals with a traumatic etiology tend to walk faster than those with a dysvascular etiology.[314,318,319] Additionally, biomechanical and energy efficiency of prosthetic gait decreases as amputation level increases. Therefore preservation of the anatomic knee joint appears to be especially important.[314,317,320]

A classic study by Waters and colleagues[319] (Table 2.8) demonstrated that, for young adults with traumatic TTA, walking speed, oxygen rate, and oxygen cost were quite close to the normal values reported by Perry.[169] Studies by Esposito and colleagues[321] and Jarvis and colleagues[316] support the initial findings of Waters and colleagues[319] demonstrating similar metabolic demands for the same velocity of walking between young adults with traumatic TTA and controls. For those with traumatic transfemoral or dysvascular amputation, diminishing walking speeds kept oxygen consumption close to that of normal adult gait; however, oxygen cost increased well beyond the normal value of

Table 2.7 MET level for SCI Versus Able Body While Using Functional Orthosis

	Able Body, No Device[299]	Paraplegia w/FES[362]	Paraplegia w/RGO[363]	Paraplegia w/ Exoskeleton[364]	Able Body w/ Exoskeleton[365]
Walking speed (m/s)	1.3	0.5	0.27	0.27	1.2
MET level	3.4	8	4.4	3.3	6.5

FES, Functional electrical stimulation; *MET*, metabolic equivalent of the task; *RGO*, reciprocal gait orthosis; *SCI*, spinal cord injury.

Table 2.8 Walking Speed, Oxygen Consumption, and Oxygen Cost in Prosthetic Gait: Comparison of Etiology and Level of Unilateral Amputation

Etiology and Level	TRAUMATIC		DYSVASCULAR		Other Pathology
Parameter	Transtibial	Transfemoral	Transtibial	Transfemoral	Hip Disarticulation
Waters et al.[319]					
Walking speed (m/min)	71	52	45	36	
O_2 rate (mL/kg/min)	12.4	10.3	9.4	10.8	
O_2 cost (mL/kg/m)	0.16	0.20	0.20	0.28	
Torburn et al.[318]					
Walking speed (m/min)	82.3	—	61.7	—	
O_2 rate (mL/kg/min)	17.7	—	13.2	—	
O_2 cost (mL/kg/m)	0.22	—	0.21	—	
Jarvis et al.[316]					
Walking speed (m/min)	81.6	73.2			
O_2 rate (mL/kg/min)	12.3	13.3			
O_2 cost (mL/kg/m)	.15	.18			
Chin et al.[327]					
Walking speed (m/min)					30.5
O_2 rate (mL/kg/min)					18.3
O_2 cost (mL/kg/m)					.64

0.15 mg/kg/m.[286] In fact, Jarvis and colleagues reported a 20% (0.18 mL/kg/m) and 60% (0.24 mL/kg/m) increase in oxygen costs for those with unilateral and bilateral TFA, respectively.[316] Collectively, studies report oxygen costs of prosthetic gait at between 16% and 28% above normal for individuals with TTA and between 60% and 110% above normal for individuals with TFA.[316,322–326] For hip disarticulation due to pathology, the oxygen cost of prosthetic gait can be more than 60% above normal, even at a significantly lower walking speed.[327]Although the relationship between walking speed and oxygen rate (consumption) in prosthetic gait is linear, just as it is in unimpaired gait, the slope is significantly steeper.[328]

In a 2019 meta-analysis by van Schaik et al.,[271] level of amputation (transfemoral and transtibial) and walking speed were significant predictors of mean oxygen consumption and mean HR. Curvilinear relationships from the meta-analytic data were demonstrated between oxygen consumption and walking speed and between HR and walking speed. Both oxygen consumption and HR increased as walking speed increased and with more proximal amputation. In a 2021 meta-analysis by Ettema et al.,[267] significant differences were found in the energy cost of walking between persons without amputation and all four subgroups of people with lower limb amputation. In order of the highest to lowest between group differences, significant differences were found between persons without amputation and those with vascular TFA (102% higher), nonvascular TFA (41% higher), vascular TTA (36% higher), and nonvascular TTA (12% higher).[267]

The clinical implication of this relationship is that the rate of energy consumption and of cardiac work at any walking speed is higher for those with amputation and that the threshold for transition from aerobic to anaerobic metabolism is reached at lower walking speeds.[329]

Several explanations are possible for the differences in prosthetic gait performance after traumatic versus dysvascular amputation. Because those with dysvascular amputation are typically older than those with traumatic amputation, differences in performance may be the result of age-related changes and concurrent cardiovascular disease in the dysvascular group.[324,330,331] For many older patients with dysvascular amputation, the energy source for walking with a prosthesis may be anaerobic rather than the more efficient aerobic metabolic pathways.[318] A larger cardiac and respiratory functional reserve capacity in younger persons with traumatic TTA may permit them to meet the increased metabolic demands of prosthetic use because proximal muscle groups work for longer periods at higher intensities to compensate for the loss of those at the ankle.[318,328,332]

Importantly, for most individuals with unilateral TTA or TFA, regardless of age or etiology of amputation, the energy cost of walking with a prosthesis is less than that expended when walking without it, using crutches or a walker[319,333] For most persons with a new TTA, the ability to ambulate before amputation is the best predictor of tolerance of the increased energy cost of walking with a prosthesis after surgery.[331] For some older individuals with TFA and concurrent cardiovascular or respiratory disease, and for those with bilateral amputation at transfemoral/transtibial or bilateral TFA levels, wheelchair mobility may be preferred.[334–336]

Technological Advances Impacting Energy Demands

Significant efforts have been made to reduce the energy cost of prosthetic gait by developing dynamic-response (energy-storing) prosthetic feet and cadence-responsive and microprocessor-controlled prosthetic knee units.[337–342] The flexible keels of most energy storage and return prosthetic feet are designed to mimic those of normal ankle mobility, such that mechanical energy stored by compression during stance is released to enhance push-off in the terminal stance.[343] However, the impact of different prosthetic foot designs on the energy cost is limited and only under specific conditions.[315] The 1M10 Adjust demonstrated significant improvement in the energy cost of walking and perceived exertion for hypomobile adults with TTA.[344] Other studies on adults with TTA found that the FlexFoot functioned more like an anatomic ankle than did four other dynamic-response feet and the SACH foot, but little difference in stride, velocity, or energy cost was noted.[318,332] However, the materials and designs of most dynamic-response feet may enable transtibial prosthetic users to jump, run, and use a step-over-step pattern in stair climbing; these activities are difficult or impossible with a traditional SACH foot.[319,320,322–326,328] Additionally, many individuals with TTA wear their prosthesis for longer periods during the day and report less fatigue in prolonged walking when using a prosthesis with a dynamic-response foot.[331]

Recent research into dynamic ankle and foot system for TTA provides promise of improved performance of ADLs and even sports. Microprocessor ankle systems like the Proprio have demonstrated both objective and subjective improvements with slope ascent and descent.[345] However, with the varied designs of transtibial prostheses, the research has been mixed in determining whether active push-off reduces walking energy expenditure.[346–350] Some of the variables within the research has been the lack of subjects, weight of the prosthesis, gait analysis on a treadmill versus open ground, and the length of time of gait analysis, which may lead to fatigue becoming another factor. Much focus with these transtibial prostheses has been to replace 80% of the mechanical work to complete the gait cycle performed by the gastrocsoleus complex.[351,352] However, researchers are realizing that there are more factors besides energy return at toe-off to improve energy expenditure with gait.[353] New designs consider the entire gait cycle to reduce overall energy expenditure while improving gait kinematics. Updated analytical methods examine internal friction, the association between tendon work and apparent efficiency, the role of energy recovery and internal work in pathological gait, and analysis of human walking in simulated low gravity conditions.[354]

Promising research looking at microprocessor-controlled active joints has demonstrated a significant reduction in energy expenditure when climbing stairs, even allowing subjects with a TFA to perform a step-through gait.[355,356] Further research on the functional application of this latest generation of "smart" joints will definitely improve the overall functional capability of patients with transfemoral prostheses in the future.

Additional technological advances will likely change how orthotics and prosthetics are designed and manufactured. Breakthroughs in computer modeling and 3D printing are allowing devices to be designed exactly for the wearer and "built" via a 3D printer in precise detail.[357–360] A recent systematic review on the feasibility of 3D-printed AFOs concluded that its biomechanical effects and mechanical properties are comparable to traditionally manufactured AFOs.[360] In addition, 3D printing allows for the development of novel designs to optimize stiffness and weight to improve comfort and function.[360] This holds promise for patients with unique or less common amputations (such as a Syme or Pirogoff amputation) to have devices designed specifically for their needs, thereby maximizing walking efficiency and reducing energy expenditure.[361]

Summary

An understanding of normal cardiopulmonary and cardiovascular function and how they change due to the cumulative effects of aging, a sedentary lifestyle, and/or pathologic conditions provides a necessary foundation for rehabilitation professionals working with patients who require an orthosis or prosthesis to walk. This chapter reviews the anatomy and physiology of the cardiopulmonary and cardiovascular systems with attention to age-related changes, energy expenditure, and principles of aerobic conditioning for older adults.

Optimal performance of the cardiopulmonary and cardiovascular systems is influenced by three interrelated factors. First, the patient must have sufficient flexibility and mobility of the trunk for efficient and uncompromised ventilation. Second, adequate mobility of the extremities and excursion of the joints must be present for efficient performance of functional tasks. Third, the individual must have enough muscle mass, strength, and endurance to support the performance of the activity and function of the heart. Immediate and ongoing individualized interventions that functionally enhance preload by returning blood to the heart with age-related changes, and avoidance of potentially detrimental activities that unnecessarily increase afterload (e.g., isometric muscle contractions and Valsalva maneuvers) can result in marked improvement in activity tolerance and physical performance in older adults. With these conditions and compensation for the β-adrenergic receptor–reduced sensitivity with a prolonged period of warmup exercises, an older adult is capable of physical performance quite similar to younger adults and essential for functional recovery as the optimal outcome of rehabilitation.

The energy cost and efficiency of gait are negatively affected by the aging process, deconditioning from inactivity, chronic diseases, and neuromuscular and musculoskeletal impairments that alter motor control or the biomechanics of walking. Although an orthosis that restricts joint motion increases the energy cost in unimpaired individuals, the same orthosis leads to more efficient gait in those with neuromuscular impairment. Determinants of energy efficiency of prosthetic gait include the level, cause of the amputation, and walking speed. Reduction of walking speed when using an orthosis or prosthesis helps maintain oxygen consumption at close to normal levels; however, this tends to compromise overall efficiency of gait, as indicated by oxygen cost. Attention to the principles of cardiovascular conditioning-including monitoring the response to exercise so that patients are challenged appropriately-optimizes the outcomes of rehabilitation programs. Further research needs to be performed to assess the efficacy of newer materials and "smart" joints regarding gait kinematics and energy expenditure for both orthotics and prosthetics, especially in older adults.

References

The complete listing of the References are available in the accompanying enhanced eBook version included with the print purchase of this textbook. Visit Elsevier eBooks+ (eBooks.Health.Elsevier.com) to access this content.

3 Motor Control, Motor Learning, and Neural Plasticity in Orthotic and Prosthetic Rehabilitation

DANIELE PISCITELLI, KEVIN K. CHUI, AND DONNA M. BOWERS

LEARNING OBJECTIVES

On completion of this chapter, the reader will be able to do the following:

1. Discuss the strengths, limitations, and implementation for practice of current models of motor control.
2. Compare and contrast the tenets of current motor learning theories.
3. Discuss the role of physical therapy interventions based on knowledge of motor control and motor learning in augmenting neural plasticity after brain injury.
4. Apply principles of practice conditions in the design of therapeutic interventions for individuals using orthoses or prostheses.
5. Appropriately use augmented feedback in therapeutic situations with individuals using orthoses or prostheses.
6. Describe the role of mental practice and imagery on skill acquisition for individuals using orthoses or prostheses.

Why Think About Motor Control, Motor Learning, or Neuroplasticity?

Physical therapists and colleagues in rehabilitation assist individuals with movement dysfunction in enhancing or adapting their movement patterns. This ensures safety, efficiency, and satisfaction with their functional abilities in activities they consider significant for their quality of life.[1] Various body structure impairments, including physiologic structures and multiple systems, might lead to motor disorders, atypical patterns of movement, or lack of movement. These impairments interfere with an individual's performance of relevant activities and self-selected participation endeavors.[2,3]

Several underlying principles influence current thinking about how people move.[4] The first is that *movement is goal directed*. Individuals engage in movement to achieve specific tasks or activities, whether it is related to self-care, activities of daily living (ADLs), work responsibilities, leisure pursuits, or social participation.[5] The second is that there are *many different ways to accomplish any task*: the central nervous system (CNS) orchestrates elemental variables (i.e., individual joints and forces/moments or muscle) using available degrees of freedom in the context of the environment to accomplish any given task; there is no a unique solution (i.e., a single "best" way) of moving.[6–8] The third is that *each individual develops preferred movement patterns*. While there are many possible movement strategies available, people tend to adopt ways of moving that are most efficient for their own individual physical characteristics.[9] Preferential movement patterns, however, are not always optimal. For instance repetitive motion injuries may be the result of preferential movement patterns that are not biomechanically effective, stressing tissues until inflammation or permanent deformation occurs.[10] The fourth is that people move when they have self-efficacy regarding their movement. Self-efficacy stems from competence with movement (capability) plus confidence in performing such movement.[11] Finally, evidence suggests that rehabilitation interventions *promote neural plasticity* and enhance recovery following CNS lesions.[12]

When there are impairments of musculoskeletal, neuromuscular, or cardiopulmonary systems, the resources that an individual can bring to movement may be altered, limited, or constrained.[13] As movement is goal directed, individuals with impairments will find ways to accomplish movement goals that "work," often using compensatory movement strategies. These altered strategies are clinically referred to as movement dysfunction.[13] The use of ineffective or abnormal movement patterns can, over time, lead to inflammation, tissue remodeling, or even deformity.[14] For example, in an individual recovering from stroke who is walking, an "abnormal" extensor synergy of the lower extremity (i.e., extension, internal rotation, and adduction of the hip; knee extension; and ankle extension and inversion) may provide stance-phase stability, but it will impair swing limb advancement, leading to a compensatory circumduction or vaulting step.[15] Abnormal tone may contribute to habitual plantarflexion and eventually an equinus deformity.[16] Someone with a painful knee or back will modify the way they use those joints as well as the limbs or trunk when walking and transitions between sitting and standing.[17–21] Over time, this can lead to secondary musculoskeletal disorders at distal or proximal joints or physical deconditioning, exacerbating movement dysfunction.[22,23] Individuals experiencing pain, shortness of breath, or a sense of fatigue (whether from disease or deconditioning) may choose to reduce their activity to "conserve" energy and, as a result, become even more deconditioned, develop soft tissue tightness that impairs flexibility, and lose muscle mass, ultimately limiting functional strength and decreasing quality of life.[24–28] Individuals who are concerned about pain, falling, injury, or age-related comorbidities may also limit their physical activity and have a similar decline in physiologic capacity and resources.[29–31] Physical and occupational therapists use various types of therapeutic exercise (e.g., strengthening, endurance programs, flexibility, and balance activities) as well as functional training (often with assistive devices or ambulatory aids, orthoses, and prostheses) to minimize and improve movement dysfunction and recover or accommodate the underlying impairments.[32] To effectively implement these interventions, rehabilitation professionals must have a comprehensive understanding of exercise principles and the impact of exercise on the human body.[33–35] They must also be knowledgeable about the purpose of orthoses, prostheses, or assistive devices and how the design of these devices can enhance or constrain movement and function as well as how they can affect the patient psychologically.[36,37] If the goal of rehabilitation professionals is to help those with movement dysfunction learn more effective ways to accomplish what is important to them, they must also be aware of the process of learning, both on a cognitive and a motor level, and incorporate this understanding into their interventions.[38]

This chapter provides an overview of current perspectives on motor control using a dynamic systems perspective. It also examines the fundamental principles of motor learning and considers practice, augmented feedback, and mental imagery as tools to facilitate the development of new or adapted movement skills. This chapter also considers how physical therapy intervention, founded on knowledge of motor control and motor learning, can enhance neural plasticity and contribute to recovery after brain injury. The case examples at the end of the chapter are intended to assist readers in integrating a growing understanding of the principles of motor control and motor learning into the formulation of interventions for movement dysfunction.

Theories of Motor Control

Before reviewing the current theoretical frameworks of motor control, it is crucial to begin with a precise definition of the terminology. Motor control extends beyond the mere generation of muscle forces and encompasses the processes underlying voluntary control of movement, involving the coordinated actions of muscles and joints and the interaction with the environment.[6] Recently, motor control has been defined as *"an area of physics exploring laws of nature defining how the nervous system interacts with other body parts and the environment to produce purposeful, coordinated actions."*[7] While motor action takes place within a physical environment, it is important to recognize that various other disciplines contribute to the understanding of motor control, including anatomy, physiology, neuroscience, biomechanics, philosophy, psychology, and engineering. Notably motor control theories and principles are considered a foundational basis for rehabilitation.[39,40] Recently a crucial step in motor control science was made in a theoretical paper by Levin and Piscitelli[41] that discussed the two current contrasting theoretical frameworks of motor control, that is, the biomechanical and the physical framework. The biomechanical framework posits that the CNS directly activates muscles to generate muscle force. Conversely, the physical framework suggests that force production is indirect, with the CNS specifying parameters that determine the conditions and context in which muscles can act to accomplish a specific task within a given environment. Both frameworks consist of models and theories of motor control that share similar approaches but are referred to by different names.[41]

Under the biomechanical framework, several concepts can be grouped, including the computational approach,[42] the notion of internal model representation in the brain,[43] and the concepts of direct programming of electromyography (EMG) output. Within the physical framework, concepts align with neural control of movement proposed by Bernstein,[44] the equilibrium point, threshold control and referent body configuration theory,[45,45a] the dynamic action theory,[46] and the ecological theory.[47,48]

Notably, human movement has traditionally been examined from two distinct fields of study: a neurophysiological control approach and a motor behavioral approach.[4,41–45] The traditional neurophysiological approach explained movement within a hierarchic system of control on the basis of the development of neural mechanisms within the CNS and peripheral nervous systems and the interaction of sensory-motor systems. The motor behavioral approach examined movement performance from the perspectives largely from the field of psychology. In the past few decades, these two fields of study converged to develop new theories that more fully explain human movement and performance, taking into account environmental and task constraints.[4,41,45–48] Recently there has been an increasing emphasis on the use of therapeutic intervention as a means of driving neural plasticity as a mechanism of recovery following brain injury.[11,38,41]

The motor behavioral approach and neurophysiologic control approach are further integrated in the study of functional movement disorder (FMD). Recent literature highlights an emerging understanding of the neurobiology of FMD and the importance of developing behavioral models to address abnormal motor control patterns that are atypical of known organic disease processes.[49,50] It is thought that abnormalities in attention, personal agency, and beliefs and expectations about symptoms contribute to the manifestation of abnormal movement based on emotional triggers from prior traumatic events.[50] Evidence suggests that "fear" can be a cause of psychiatric disorders leading to FMD. Recently several case reports have been reported about FMD such as psychogenic tremor triggered by the "fear" of severe acute respiratory syndrome coronavirus 2 (SARS-CoV-2) responsible for the new coronavirus disease 2019 (COVID-19) pandemic.[51,52] Findings suggest that targeted motor reprogramming using a coordinated interdisciplinary approach is a promising intervention for the resolution of this disorder.[49,53] Interdisciplinary collaboration among neurology, rehabilitation services, and psychiatry is particularly important. Recent research in psychology emphasizes the likelihood of missing relevant stressors in the absence of a thorough psychiatric evaluation.[54] While not all patients may experience stressful life events, when they do occur, they become a significant focus of interdisciplinary treatment.[55] This growing body of research using integrated models from the fields of psychology and physiology advances our comprehension of motor control and motor learning. The importance of these findings is highlighted when considering complex presentations, including traumatic events frequently associated with traumatic brain injury, spinal cord injury, and limb amputations.

DYNAMIC SYSTEMS PERSPECTIVES

Rehabilitation professionals think about the human body as a complex biologic system with many interacting elements and subsystems (Fig. 3.1). These components have an infinite number of ways to work together in accomplishing a goal-directed motor act.[56,57] Due to the dynamic, adaptive, and inherently complex nature of the human body's subsystems, motor behaviors and movement patterns become more efficient with practice and experience. Motor systems can consistently generate simple and well-organized movement from a complex array of movement possibilities.[58,59] The dynamic systems perspective of motor control is founded on an understanding of the behaviors that physical systems of various types have in common: the ability to change over time, the ability to be adaptive yet have preference for habitual tendencies, and the context of interaction with the environment in which movement occurs.[44,60–62] In the human movement system, there is great "motor abundance." Each person has a wide variety of ways to accomplish an intended movement task (i.e., solve a functional movement problem) in whatever environmental conditions or circumstances that function occurs.[63,64]

According to Bernstein's model of motor control, individuals possess the ability "to make a choice within a multitude of accessible trajectories…of a most appropriate

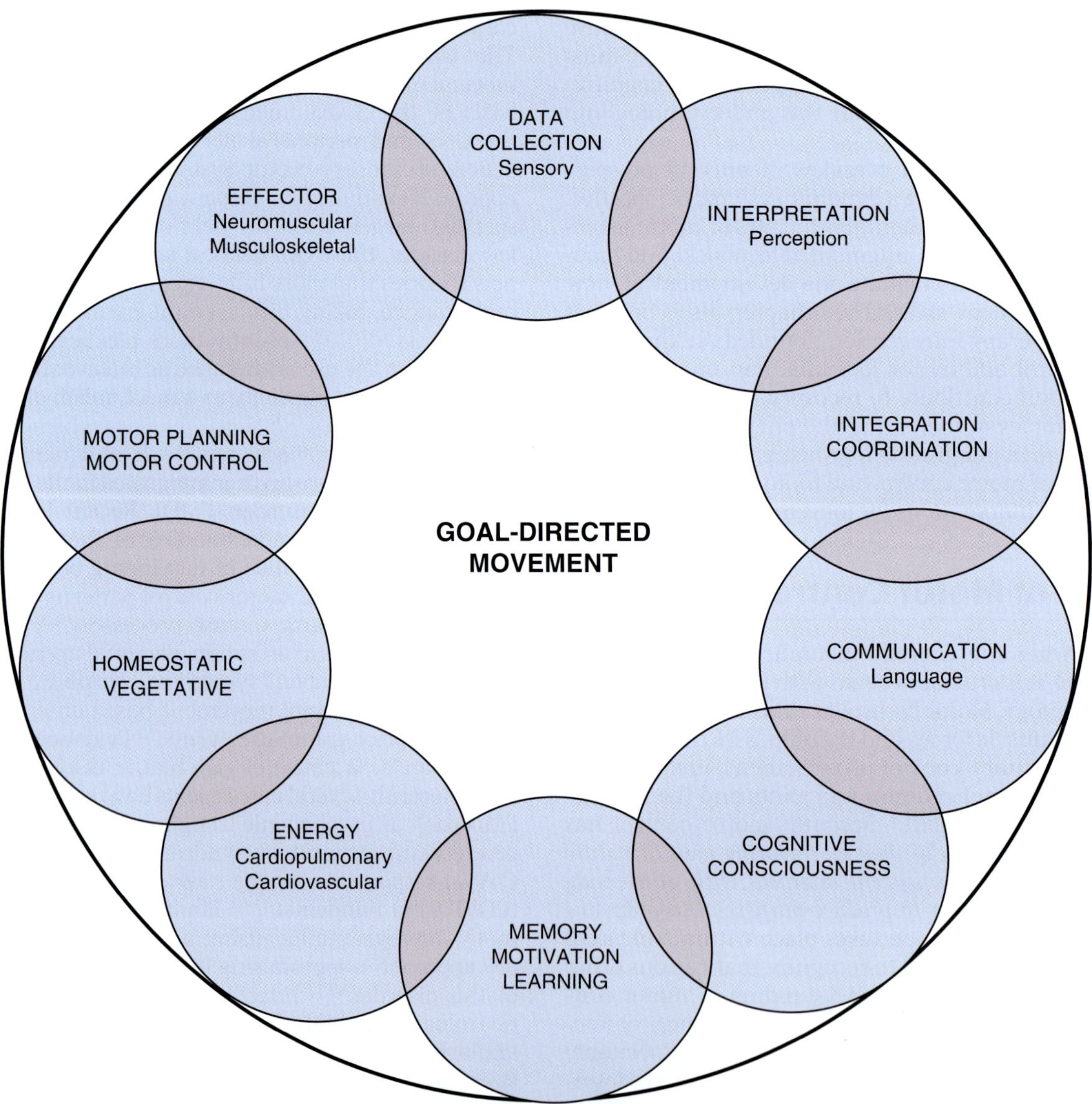

Fig. 3.1 The interactive physiologic systems of the body contribute to an individual's ability to carry out goal-directed (functional) movement. Sensory and perceptual systems contribute by monitoring the environment as well as the position and condition of the body during movement. Interpretive and integrative systems for perception work together with coordination, cognitive, memory, motivational, and planning systems to determine how a goal-directed task might be best implemented, corrected, or adapted for success (action). Homeostatic, vegetative, and energy systems anticipate physiologic demand and ensure that oxygen and glucose supplies are sufficient to meet task demands. The neuromuscular system fine-tunes postural control, tone, and recruitment so that the musculoskeletal system can be used effectively to accomplish the movement goal. Continuous communication and interaction among physiologic systems occur before, during, and in response to movement so that both feedforward and feedback can instantaneously influence task performance.

trajectory."[65] Notably, within the Uncontrolled Manifold (UCM) analysis,[6,7] it is possible to compute the inter-trial variability to measure the stability of a performance task during movement repetition.[65a,65b] Dynamic systems theory suggests that there are both opportunities and challenges presented by the interaction of the environment and the individual's will to move.[65] Unlike systems that are purely physical, the human biologic system is a smart, special-purpose machine able to instantaneously and efficiently work to meet many parallel and serial functional demands.[66–68] In addition, biologic systems such as the human body are self-organizing[67,69]; the mutually dependent and complex processes within the body's subsystems allow this wonderfully dynamic structure to enact efficient functional movement patterns. Even though it is an inherently multidimensional biologic system, the human body prefers to be in a state of relative equilibrium.[45,70] Recently, according to the theory of referent control of motor actions, it has been proposed that locomotion may arise from feedforward shifts of the referent body configuration (R) within the surrounding environment.[70,71] These shifts of the R position give rise to motor actions based on the degree to which the actual body configurations (Q) deviate from R. The speed of locomotion is determined by the rate at which shifts occur in the referent body configuration. The transition from walking to running occurs as a result of an increased rate of referent body configuration shifts in the environment.[72] This is likely to be the underlying reason why the gait cycle at self-selected (comfortable) walking speed tends to center around one cycle per second and why most individuals transition from walk to run at nearly the same velocity as gait speed increases.[73] The human body, as a smart and dynamic biological system, also exhibits intentional behavior characterized by purpose, goals, and a task-oriented nature in most motor behaviors.[6,7]

The dynamic systems model characterizes an intention as a purposeful or desired act that exerts influence (attracts) the human system to organize motor behavior toward the desired outcome within the contextual environment of the movement.[74] The organism and the environment are interdependent with each being defined in relation to the other.[66,73,74] While much research focuses on the physical characteristics of the environment in goal-directed movement studies, it is important to acknowledge that the social-emotional environment can also influence the emergence of goal-directed movement.[75] The combination of resources available to the organism-environment interaction, in conjunction with the individual's intention, shapes (constrains) how task-oriented motor behavior is organized.

Motor control was described by Shumway-Cook and Woollacott[4] as "the ability to regulate or direct the mechanisms essential to movement." However, this definition overlooks important elements. Specifically, motor control encompasses a domain of study in physics that explores the fundamental laws of nature governing how the nervous system interacts with other body parts and the environment to generate purposeful and coordinated actions.[6,7,41] Notably the interactive systems that provide resources that an individual uses to initiate and regulate goal-directed movement include the neurologic, musculoskeletal, sensory/perceptual, cardiorespiratory, and cardiopulmonary systems as well as the cognitive, learning, and memory

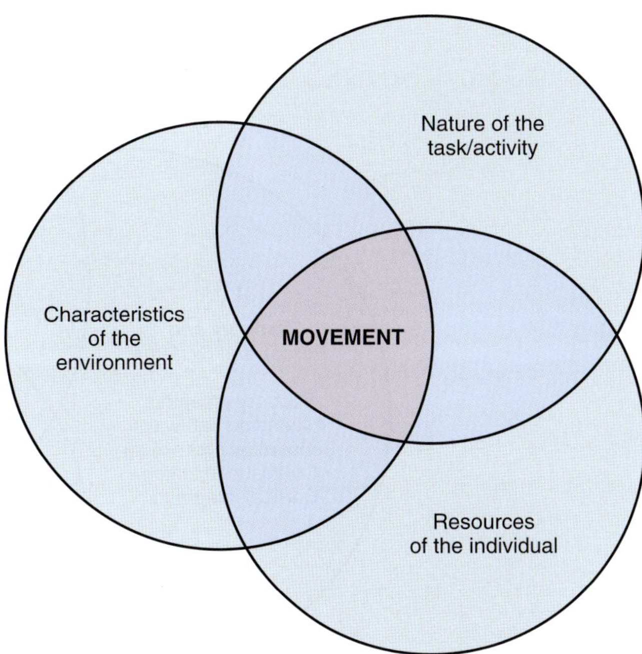

Fig. 3.2 A contemporary model of motor control: movement emerges from the interaction of the individual, the environment, and the task being attempted. Therapists must consider how the characteristics, resources, and constraints of each influence the ability to move and how each might be manipulated during intervention to enhance motor learning and effectiveness of movement.

systems. Human movement is a product of the interaction of the individual (with all of his or her subsystems), the characteristics of the environment, and the nature of the specific task or goal that the individual is involved in Fig. 3.2.[41] Movement, then, is goal directed and purposeful; it utilizes both inherent and acquired abilities of the individual and is influenced by the surrounding environment. By acknowledging each of these fundamental contributors to functional movement, healthcare and rehabilitation professionals can evaluate potential sources of movement dysfunction and/or impairments, investigate alternative movement strategies, and modify or adjust the task or environment to enhance movement outcomes.[76,77] To this end, motor control should drive rehabilitation interventions.[12,40] Below are presented the highlighted aspects by Shumway-Cook and Woollacott[4] of motor control related to resources of the individual, nature of the task, and the characteristics of the environment.

Resources of the Individual

The first component to consider when studying motor control is the individual, with their ability to think and reason, to sense and perceive, and to actively respond or initiate movement (Fig. 3.3). An individual's cognitive capabilities encompass critical thinking and conceptual integration, organization and delayed gratification, assigning emotional significance to activities or circumstances, problem solving, accessing and utilizing memory, managing attention and focus (especially when engaged in concurrent tasks), and learning.[78–80] Perceptual resources, on the other hand, stem from the ability to receive and process many different types of sensory information (i.e., data) and to integrate and interpret this data at both subcortical and cortical

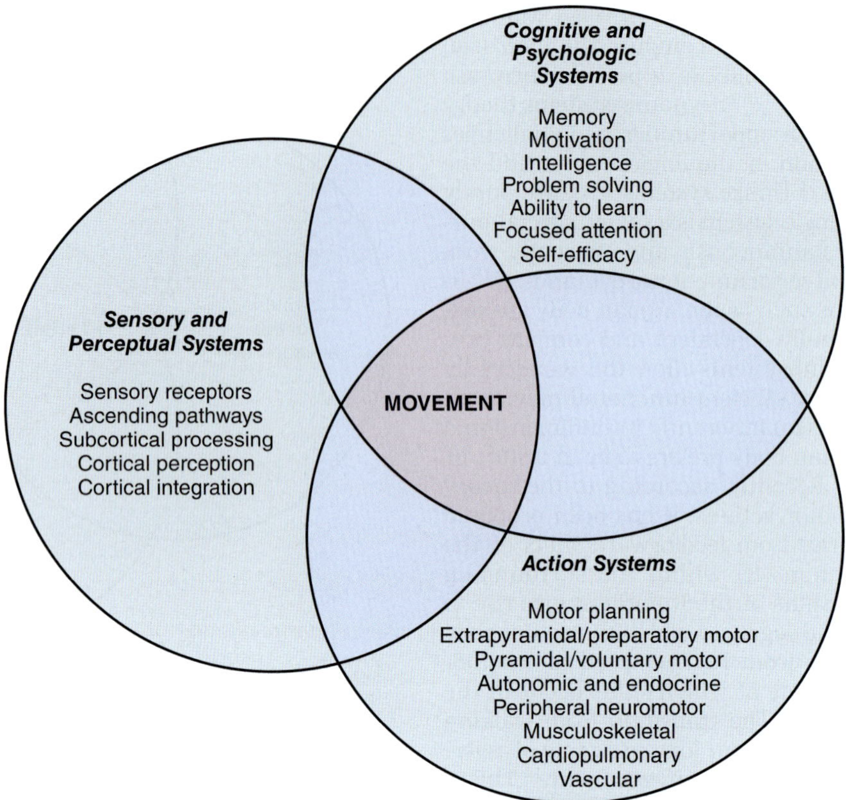

Fig. 3.3 The individual resources that contribute to movement include those in the sensory/perceptual systems, the cognitive systems, and the action systems. For persons recovering from central nervous system insult, the therapist must understand whether dysfunction in any of these systems has occurred and consider how intervention might enhance neural plasticity and recovery of function in each of these areas.

levels of information processing.[81–85] Action-related resources involve planning motor functions and refining motion at cortical and subcortical levels; controlling errors through the cerebellum, pyramidal, and extrapyramidal motor systems; and the contributions of the neuromuscular, musculoskeletal, and cardiopulmonary/cardiovascular systems to "effector" systems.[86–101] Perception influences motor action (feedforward movement), while action, in turn, leads to movement monitoring and refinement (feedback refinement).

To illustrate the impact of individual resources on movement, consider two individuals who are walking back to their cars after a Major League baseball game. Their pathway moves across a gravel-surfaced parking area with a slightly sloped and slightly unstable support surface. One person exhibits sensory and motor impairment known as "stocking-glove" neuropathy, commonly associated with diabetic polyneuropathy. The other person has consumed a few too many beers while enthusiastically supporting their team, making his thinking and motor behavior less efficient than normal. Both individuals are likely to exhibit less efficient postural responses and unsteady walking patterns as they make their way to their vehicles, but for very different reasons. The quality of the sensory data that the individual with diabetic neuropathy can collect may not be sufficient for accurate perception of environmental conditions, and, complicated by distal weakness, her patterns of movement may not meet the challenges presented by the sloped and slightly movable ground surface. On the other hand, the tipsy individual retains normal sensory data collection capabilities. However, the temporary impairment in cognitive function including judgment and perception, coupled with reduced efficiency in "error control" resulting from alcohol consumption, leads to motor behaviors that fail to align with environmental demands. Both baseball fans may stumble, walk with a wider base of support, or reach out for stable objects as they make their way toward their cars. Nevertheless, the underlying individual contributors to these motor outcomes are quite distinct.

Nature of the Task

The task is the second component to the overall outcome or motor action performed. A functional task may require an individual to organize goal-directed movement to address one or more of the following control processes (Fig. 3.4):

- Maintaining or adjusting antigravity body posture (static, anticipatory, or reactionary postural control)[102–104]
- Transitioning from one stable position to another (quasimobility; e.g., moving from sitting to standing)[105,106]
- Moving a limb or the whole body through space (e.g., reaching, lifting, carrying, walking, stair climbing, walking on inclines, avoiding obstacles, hopping, running)[107–109]
- Using or manipulating tools appropriate to the task (e.g., assistive devices, objects needed for ADLs)[110,111]

Any task can be described along a number of different dimensions or continua: it can have a *discrete* beginning and end point (e.g., transferring from bed to chair) or be

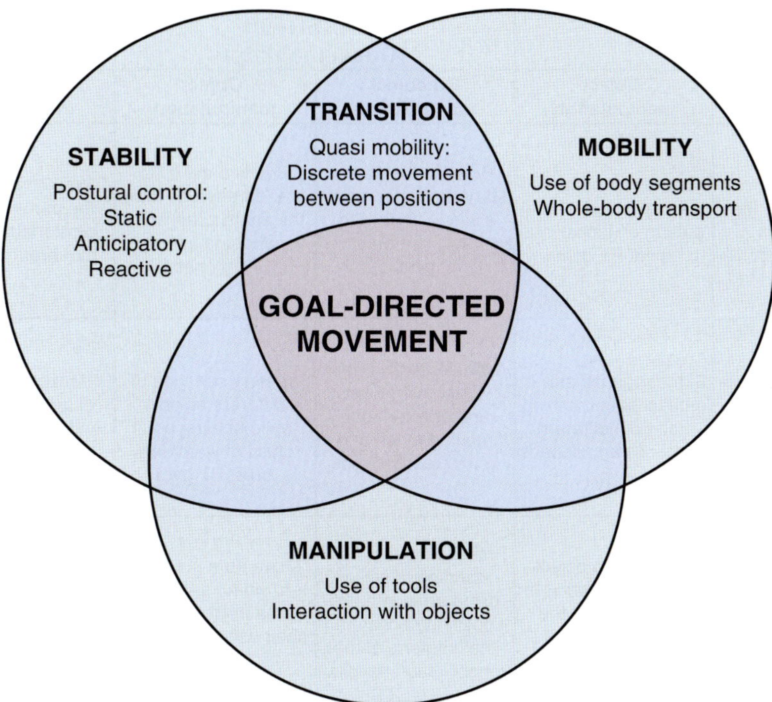

Fig. 3.4 The components or nature of the task being attempted also influences the movement that emerges. The task can include or combine goals of stability, transitions, mobility, and manipulation of tools or objects.

Box 3.1 Descriptors of Movements Based on the Attributes/Nature of a Task

- Discrete: The beginning or end point of movement, or both, as determined by the task itself (e.g., stepping onto a curb, donning a prosthesis, catching a ball).
- Serial: An ordered sequence of discrete movements, defined by the task itself (e.g., climbing a flight of stairs).
- Continuous: The beginning and end points of the task are determined and controlled by the individual (e.g., riding a bicycle, deciding when to start or stop).
- Stability: The primary task goal is to maintain position of body segments (often against gravity or in response to perturbation) or to keep the body's center of mass within the available base of support during functional activity (e.g., to provide a secure base in sitting or standing for subsequent skilled use of extremities).
- Transitional (quasimobility): The primary task goal is to move the body from a starting position of stability to a different ending position of stability (e.g., moving from sitting to standing, rolling from supine to prone, getting up from the floor).
- Mobility: The primary task goal is to move a body part, or the entire body, through physical space (e.g., rolling over in bed, walking or running, reaching for an object on a shelf or on the floor).
- Manipulation continuum: The degree to which a task requires the individual to use (manipulate) or interact with one or more external objects to complete the activity successfully (e.g., fastening buttons or handling clothes during dressing, donning/doffing a prosthesis or orthosis, opening doors during mobility, and locking the brakes on a wheelchair).
- Automaticity: The degree to which the task is well understood and can be carried out automatically or requires attention because of high task demand (level of preciseness, consequence of error) or the changing nature of the task or environmental conditions (e.g., threading a sewing needle, walking down an icy sloping walkway, catching a thrown object).
- Variability in performance: The degree to which an individual is able to adapt the performance of a learned task in response to differences in environmental conditions or changes in task constraints; the flexibility to apply what has been learned to similar or novel situations.

continuous (e.g., walking or running over large distances). Tasks can involve *stability and agility*[112] or require *mobility*, occur at *various speeds*, require different levels of *accuracy* or *precision*, and demand different levels of *attention* or *focus* (Box 3.1). Repetitive and overlearned tasks performed in predictable (closed or fixed) environments are often executed on a nearly automatic level, with minimal attention; this allows the individual to focus attentional resources on other priorities.[113]

On the other hand, tasks occurring in a changing (dynamic or open) environment necessitate flexibility and adaptability for successful completion and require a higher degree of attention during performance.[114,115] Finally, the complexity of the task and the attention it requires are crucial factors to be taken into account for effective task execution.[116]

An interesting way to understand the nature of a task (either broken into components or as a whole) is to examine or classify the task using Gentile's Taxonomy of Movement Tasks (Fig. 3.5).[114] The first component considered in the taxonomy is the movement task's outcome goals: does the task primarily focus on the stability of the body, transition between stable positions, or transport (movement) of the body through space? As an example of a body stability

		BODY STABILITY		TRANSITION (Quasi-mobility)		BODY TRANSPORT	
		No object manipulation	Object manipulation	No object manipulation	Object manipulation	No object manipulation	Object manipulation
CLOSED ENVIRONMENT	No variability	Stand in prosthesis unsupported in the parallel bars in a quiet PT gym	Stand in prosthesis unsupported while putting on jacket in a quiet PT gym	Practice the sit-to-stand transition from a single chair with armrests in a quiet PT gym	Practice the sit to stand transition from the same chair while managing axillary crutches	Walk the length of the parallel bars at comfortable speed, turn around, repeat	Walk forward with crutches using a 2-point gait pattern in an empty hallway
	Trial variability	Stand in prosthesis in parallel bars with diagonal weight shifts on command	Stand in prosthesis in parallel bars catching ball from different directions and speeds	Transfer to and from wheelchair, toilet, and shower seat, moving to left and right in random order	Transfer between seating surfaces of different heights while holding a full glass of water in a quiet PT gym	Practice stepping in different directions and distances in the parallel bars	Walk up to a closed door, opening it, and walking through while using a cane
OPEN ENVIRONMENT	No variability	Remain standing upright as people walk by at regular intervals from similar directions	Retrieve an object repeatedly from the same spot on the floor in a corner of a busy PT gym	Practice moving from standing to sitting using arms in a pre-positioned chair in the cafeteria of the rehabilitation hospital	Move from standing to sitting and vice versa from a rocking chair while managing crutches	Practice ascending and descending a set of training stairs in the corner of a busy PT gym	Approach and ascend a full flight of stairs in a quiet hallway, using bilateral canes
	Trial variability	Remain upright while standing in line in a busy public area	Retrieve various randomly dropped objects throughout an active PT gym	Rise repeatedly from a seat in the movie theater so that other people (of various height and weight) can move past into the row	Scoot sideways while sitting, managing the blankets on a soft mattress so that grandchildren can climb into bed to hear a story	Ascend and descend stairs using the railing in a busy public space	Walk from car to supermarket door, pushing the grocery cart across the busy parking lot

Fig. 3.5 Examples of therapeutic activities for an individual learning to use bilateral transtibial prosthesis based on a modified version of Gentile's Taxonomy of Movement Tasks. *PT,* Physical therapy.

task, consider the ability of an individual learning to use a transfemoral prosthesis to control hip and pelvic position while in a single-limb stance on the prosthetic side, while slowly lifting the "intact" limb to place it on a stool or step placed in front of him or her. A transitional (quasimobile) task for this person might be practicing moving between sitting and standing position from various seating surfaces or heights.[4] A body mobility task for the same individual might be to learn to use a cadence-responsive prosthetic knee unit by altering gait speed, changing direction, or navigating through a crowded public space.

The next consideration is whether the task involves use of, or interaction with, a tool or object (i.e., is object manipulation part of the task?). In working with persons with spinal cord injuries to develop postural control in sitting, for example, physical therapists often use catching and throwing activities with balloons and balls of various weights, thrown at different speeds and in varying directions, to provide an opportunity to master this body stability skill.[117–119] Managing assistive devices (e.g., cane, crutches) during transfers or operating orthotic knee locks or prosthetic knee units during transfers are examples of object manipulation during transitional motor tasks. Learning to use an ambulatory assistive device (e.g., crutch walking in a four-point reciprocal pattern; managing crutches when ascending or descending stairs) is a prime example of a body mobility task that requires object manipulation.[120,121]

Characteristics of the Environment

The final aspect of the Shumway-Cook and Woollacott model of motor control is the setting, environmental context, or conditions in which the goal-directed movement takes place. The physical therapist must examine (and, during intervention, purposefully manipulate) the environmental context in which functional movement occurs. Is the physical environment comfortable to be in while taking part in exercise and other rehabilitation interventions? Is it visually interesting and stimulating but not too distracting or challenging? Is the motor task occurring in an environment that is predictable (i.e., in a closed environment), or is there a degree of variability and possibility of change external to the individual (i.e., an open environment) that will require the individual to monitor and respond more carefully while performing the task?[122–124] Therapists should also consider the social-emotional context of the environment, which is established through interpersonal interactions. Will the individual feel nurtured and motivated as they venture into new territory and encounter challenges while developing skills in salient activities? Or does the emotional environment contribute to anxiety about receiving negative criticism (or negative feedback) or a fear of failure?[125,126]

For the therapeutic application of environmental variables, therapists can consider both macroenvironmental influences (e.g., actual physical conditions that influence task demand, the therapeutic setting, or the involvement of family members) and microenvironmental influences (e.g., the level of visual and auditory "noise" present in the therapy room or variations in surfaces over which a client may be sitting or walking). It is important to note that mastering a motor task within a single, simple environment does not directly translate into safe performance of the same task under more complex and demanding environmental conditions. For instance, being able to navigate up and down a set of training steps in the physical therapy gym does not ensure that the individual with stroke or paraplegic-level spinal cord injury will be functional and safe on a wet, leaf-covered, uneven brick staircase (with no railings) when entering or leaving his best friend's house or favorite neighborhood spot.[127,128]

When working with persons with acquired brain injury functioning at cognitive levels 4 (confused and agitated), 5 (confused inappropriate), or 6 (confused appropriate) on the Rancho Los Amigos cognitive continuum, therapists must provide a structured and predictable environment for functional and rehabilitative activities. This ensures that the demands of the environment do not exceed the individual's ability to monitor and respond to the challenges that the environment presents.[129,130] A complex environment can be overwhelming to the individual recovering from brain injury; the structured environment provides an opportunity to complete key tasks with minimal frustration and behavioral complications. As the individual progresses toward discharge, the complexity of the environment should be gradually increased. Being able to cross the street safely at a crosswalk with real traffic is a more complex task than managing curbs and walking over a distance within the rehabilitation gym.

Gentile's taxonomy offers an organizational framework for rehabilitation and healthcare professionals working with individuals with musculoskeletal or neuromuscular impairments and limitations in performing functional activities. For example, a key goal for a male who recently experienced a stroke may be to regain the ability to climb stairs to access his bedroom and bathroom located upstairs. In the early stages of rehabilitation, it may be necessary to first concentrate on static postural control and controlled weight shifting in sitting and standing on a firm support surface (body stability, no object manipulation, predictable environment). As the quality and performance of these motor tasks become more consistent, intervention expands to include ambulation in the parallel bars (body mobility, no object manipulation, unvarying environment), then with an assistive device in a quiet hallway (body mobility, object manipulation, and predictable environment), and finally in a busy rehabilitation gym in which the individual must anticipate and react to others in the environment (body mobility, object manipulation, and changing environment). As postural control becomes more efficient on level surfaces, task demand is increased by increasing speed or attempting more challenging surfaces such as stairs, inclines, and stepping over obstacles; this may initially occur in a relatively predictable environment but must eventually occur in an "open" situation in which the individual must dynamically react to or navigate around other persons and objects.

SKILL ACQUISITION MODELS

Movement has also been investigated from a behavioral perspective, with a focus on quality of motor performance and acquisition of relatively permanent skilled behavior. Researchers with this perspective are interested in the influence of cognitive information processing and cognitive psychology on motor behavior. They emphasize the acquisition of skills, the learning processes associated with skill development, the enduring changes in skills (retention), and the refinement of skills across different applications. Initially, studies of skill acquisition focused on orientation to the task; as the field developed and expanded, the focus shifted toward understanding the process of skill development. This led to the formulation of the concepts of motor memory and schema. Adams's theory of feedback-based learning was a catalyst for later research, which gave rise to Schmidt's schema theory for motor learning.

Currently motor learning theory has become a blend of the various bodies of study presented in this section, integrating neurophysiologic, dynamic systems/ecologic, and behavioral models.[38,40] This convergence of interests has fostered the study of motor learning, which explores the adaptation and application of movement strategies in altered or novel functional, behavioral, and environmental contexts. Notably in recent decades, significant attention has been devoted to understanding the process that enhances the relationship between perception and action, taking into account the specific demands of tasks and the environment. Essentially, within the dynamic approach has been conceptualized a model that considers the interplay of organismic, environmental, and task-related constraints, resulting in the emergence of novel patterns of movements. In this context, skill learning is manifested in the mastery of the abundant degrees of freedom, as initially proposed by Bernstein.[65] The acquisition of the abundant degrees of freedom is accomplished by employing problem solving. The dynamic approach places significant emphasis on actively exploring the perceptual and motor domains to develop optimal strategies for executing a task, resulting in adaptability that combines the requirements and restrictions of the given task and the environment.[38]

Theories of Motor Learning

While motor control frameworks focus on how the biologic system organizes and adapts movement as it occurs, theories of motor learning consider how the individual comes to understand and consistently performs a particular behavioral task.[131] The outcome of effective motor learning is mastery of skilled behaviors so that the individual can function appropriately in his or her physical and social environment. Most models of motor learning are founded on four distinct notions about learning:

1. Motor learning is a dynamic process that leads to acquisition of ability for skilled actions.
2. In order for motor learning to occur, there must be an opportunity to practice and build experience. Making errors is a necessary part of the learning process; as learning occurs, motor memories are established.

3. Motor learning itself cannot be observed directly; it is inferred by observing changes in motor behavior that become consistent over time.
4. Learning produces sustainable, relatively permanent changes in the capacity for skilled behavior by building motor memory; as a result, what has been learned can be applied or adapted when altered task or environmental constraints occur.

To effectively master a novel motor task or remaster a previously learned motor task with altered motor function from disease or injury, the individual must have the following[131,132]:

- Focused attention to develop sensory and perceptual strategies for collecting information relevant to the task and the environment in which it is occurring.
- Active problem solving to understand key features of the task, the performance environment, and any tools required to complete the task successfully.
- Motor ability to activate the components of the motor control system (anticipatory, guiding, corrective, and reactive) necessary for skillful performance of the task.
- Self-efficacy to apply (transfer) knowledge of the task, environment, and tools to perform skilled movement in conditions that are different from the one in which learning took place.

Rehabilitation professionals must be careful to distinguish between the concepts of motor learning and motor performance. *Motor performance* is the observable action or behavior that can be measured (rated) qualitatively or quantitatively by an observer.[38,40] It is a temporary execution of a motor task at a specific point in time when being measured. As healthcare professionals who focus on function, therapists are quite skilled at examining motor performance and determining whether an individual is moving effectively and efficiently or is coping with some form of movement dysfunction. Physical therapists use both subjective ratings (e.g., ratings of perceived exertion; using Likert-based anchors such as terms "poor, fair, good, normal/excellent" to describe static postural control, dynamic balance ability, or endurance) and objective performance-based assessments (e.g., trunk-based index of performance, self-selected and fast walking speeds, timed up and go times, trunk control measurement scale, dynamic gait index scores, 6-minute walk test distance, gross motor functional measure scores, among many others).[133–138]

On the other hand, *motor learning* pertains to the process that leads to relatively permanent changes in the quality, consistency, and efficiency of motor performance of a given individual.[131] Assessing this process is challenging, primarily relying on factors such as consistency or alterations in various aspects of task performance over a duration. Comparisons of baseline performance to postintervention performance indicate changes in the quality of performance. While motor performance may exhibit temporary enhancements after a single practice session, it is only when performance becomes consistently stable across multiple sessions over an extended period that we can confidently ascertain the occurrence of learning.[139,140] Improvement in motor performance to a level of consistency implies that effective motor learning has occurred; motor learning has occurred when the task is sustainable, long-lasting, and adaptable to situational demand and environmental changes.[141]

EVOLUTION OF MODELS OF MOTOR LEARNING

Initial models of motor learning were published in the early 1970s, the most prominent being Adams's closed-loop theory and Schmidt's schema theory.[142,143] Both models assume that, as a result of the motor learning process, the brain develops *generalized motor programs:* rules for timing and sequencing of muscle activity for key tasks.[139] The closed-loop theory proposes that sensory information generated from movements occurring during the performance of functional tasks provides *feedback* necessary to build the memory and perceptual traces that guide and refine subsequent performance of the task.[142] In contrast, schema theory suggests that an open-loop process occurs in which a general set of rules for a particular movement is developed (motor recall and sensory recognition schema) over time. Such schemas allow the individual to continuously compare actual outcomes of movement with anticipated (feedforward)/predicted outcomes via error detection and correction mechanisms.[143,144] According to schema models, variability of practice must occur to establish and strengthen the movement schema over time.[144,146]

In the 1990s, Newell proposed an alternative ecologic model of motor learning (resonant with Bernstein's dynamic systems model of motor control) that suggests that individuals use a problem-solving approach to discover the optimal strategy to produce the task (performance) given both environmental and task influences.[147,148] By exploring the *perceptual motor work space* during practice, individuals begin to recognize salient sensory/perceptual cues as they explore movement options that might lead to successful task completion.[149] In viewing a demonstration, perceptual information helps the learner better understand the nature of the task and task-related movements that need to be mastered. Perception during (knowledge of performance [KP]) and perception after (knowledge of results [KR]) task-related movement provides intrinsic feedback that assists the problem-solving process in the development of optimal strategies for the task at hand. Therapists can provide augmented information (explicit cues and extrinsic feedback) to facilitate an individual's search for optimal strategies. In this way, the perception (salient cues about the task and the environment) and action (adaptive motor performance of the task) are linked so that a task-relevant connection is established.[149]

Recent evidence highlights the importance of active participation and task relevancy in the learning process. Winstein and colleagues[141] described the necessity of both psychologic elements and motor capabilities for motor learning to occur. To acquire a motor skill, an individual requires a sufficient voluntary neuromotor capability and relevant motivation. These two elements drive active engagement in the acquisition of the skill (motor learning process). Motivation is a a multifaceted behavior that encompasses self-efficacy (competency plus confidence), social relatedness, and autonomy.[11] The level of motivation is influenced by the person's sense of involvement, which includes control, choice, and collaboration in the selection of the task activity. Additional insights regarding this subject will be presented in the section dedicated to feedback.

TEMPORAL CONSIDERATIONS

Motor learning has also been examined through a temporal perspective in which learning occurs in stages over time. Various three- and two-stage models have been proposed to describe the process of acquisition of skill and adaptability or generalization/transfer of the skill (Table 3.1).

Three-stage models generally describe the earliest stage as the discovery stage, in which an understanding of the nature of a task is developed through trial and error, sometimes with guidance.[145–153] During the initial stage of motor learning, the need for attention is high, and there is a significant a notable amount of trial and error in task performance early on with an eventual understanding or selection of the best plan for the task for that individual. The presence of performance variability during this stage is considered undesirable. Once a plan has been settled on, the second stage of motor learning focuses on refinement of the performance. Variability and errors during performance decrease while efficiency of performance increases. However, attention attention remains crucial and distraction is often problematic, interfering with performance.[150] In the third and final stage of motor learning, the individual attains the ability to generalize or adapt the learned skill to meet changing environmental demands. At this stage, performance variability becomes desirable, as it enables the task to be effectively executed in different ways to accommodate various environmental demands. [150]

Building on the work of Lereijken and colleagues, Shumway-Cook and Woollacott described a system-oriented three-stage model, integrating principles of dynamic systems motor control, human development, and the ecologic model of motor learning.[140,153] Early in motor learning, individuals constrain (freeze) the degrees of freedom among limb segments (joints) involved in the task as a means of reducing task difficulty; this freezing co-contraction around joints results in relatively accurate movement, although the movement typically has a high energy cost.[154] As learning occurs, there is a tendency to "unfreeze" joints sequentially such that movement becomes more fluid and

Table 3.1 Comparison of Concepts in the Major Models of Motor Learning

Models	Descriptive Stages/ Movement Characteristics
THREE-STAGE MODELS	
Fitts and Posner[150]	
Early skill acquisition through trial and error; high undesirable variability to find most effective strategy for task	Cognitive
Refinement of skill; performance less variable and more efficient	Associative
Low attention necessary for task; transfer or adapting skill to other environments; performance of skill during multiple task demands; desired variability	Autonomous
Vereijken, Whiting, and Beek[62]	
Discovery of task constraints; restriction of degrees of freedom to simplify task	Novice
Release of some degrees of freedom to coordinate movement; adaptation of tasks to environmental demands	Advanced
All degrees of freedom released; exploitation of mechanical forces to complement environmental forces	Expert
Larin[153] (refers to children)	
Verbal-cognitive stage; physical and verbal guidance necessary	Discovery
Motor stage; independent performance, greater consistency	Intermediate
Skilled performance; economy of effort; task adaptable to environment	Autonomous
Shumway-Cook, Woollacott Systems Model[139]	
Co-contraction to constrain degrees of freedom to reduce the number of body segments or joints to be controlled during movement, undesired variability	Stage 1
Gradual release of degrees of freedom of limb segments results in gradual increase in control and flexibility of the body during movement	Stage 2
Mastery of the skilled movement with automaticity and desired variability during performance, allowing adaptation and transfer of skill in response to changing conditions/demands	Stage 3
TWO-STAGE MODELS	
Gentile[114]	
Attainment of action-goal; conscious mapping of the movement's structure; rapid stabilization of performance	Explicit Learning
Dynamics of force generation; active and passive force components finely tuned unconsciously; gradual change in performance	Implicit Learning
Manoel and Connolly[155]	
Formulation of the action plan; understanding task and how to accomplish it; stabilization of action	Acquisition
Task and environment interaction; task is fluid with range of options to cope with new situations; breakdown of stable task and reorganization for new action plans	Adaptation

energy efficient. With mastery, the individual exploits the freedom of movement to fluidly perform the task and can adapt to changing characteristics of the environment.[155]

Two-stage models of motor learning focus on (1) acquisition of the skill and (2) adaptation or application of the skilled motor behavior.[156,157] The initial phase consolidates the first two components of the three-stage models: acquisition and refinement of performance occur within the same stage. Undesired variability of performance occurs through internal demands within the individual's attempts to find and select a preferred action/strategy before refinement. In the second stage, performance has desired variability due to external demands of the environment. The person must adapt the task accordingly; this is quite similar to the final component of each of the three-stage models.[158]

IMPLICIT AND EXPLICIT ASPECTS OF MOTOR LEARNING

To understand the process of motor learning, it is important to consider the fundamental principles underlying all learning processes. This entails understanding how new information is transformed into memory, ultimately becoming useful. Learning can be perceived as the process of acquiring new information and new skills; memory, then, is the product or outcome of the learning process.[131] Learning is one of the major drivers of plasticity within the CNS, stimulating the formation of new synapses as well as refinement of existing neural connections throughout the brain.[159,160] This plasticity is evident as information is moved from our short-term (working) memory into initial long-term memory stores, which become better established and more resistant to disruption with practice and experience (Fig. 3.6).[161]

Learning theorists describe two major categories of learning: implicit (nondeclarative) and explicit (declarative) learning (Fig. 3.7).[162] Both categories lead to functional and physiologic changes in synapses of involved areas of the spinal cord, brainstem, and forebrain.[163] One aspect of motor learning falls into the category of implicit procedural learning: it requires trial and error (discovery) in a relevant and functional context.[163] Focused attention is an important requirement during this discovery stage.[11,141] Consistently improved task performance over time and situation provides evidence of effective procedural learning. Neural structures thought to be necessary for implicit procedural learning include cortex of the frontal and parietal lobes, nuclei of the basal ganglia, and cerebellar cortex and nuclei.[163–166] Recent work has also identified that the hippocampus is involved in perceptual components of procedural learning.[167] Explicit (declarative) learning is founded on attention and conscious thought and can be described or demonstrated by the learner.[168] Neural structures involved with explicit learning include the prefrontal

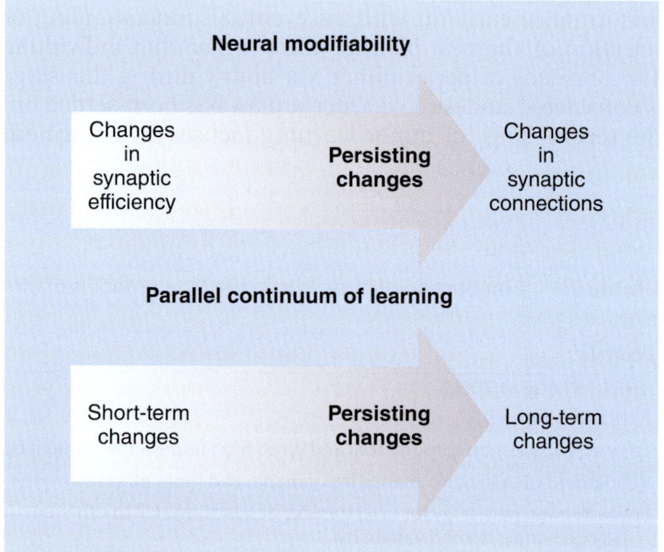

Fig. 3.6 The gradual shift from short-term (acquisition) to long-term (retention) learning and memory is reflected in a move along the continuum of neural modifiability. Short-term changes, associated with an increased synaptic efficiency, persist and gradually give way to structural changes, the underpinnings of long-term learning.

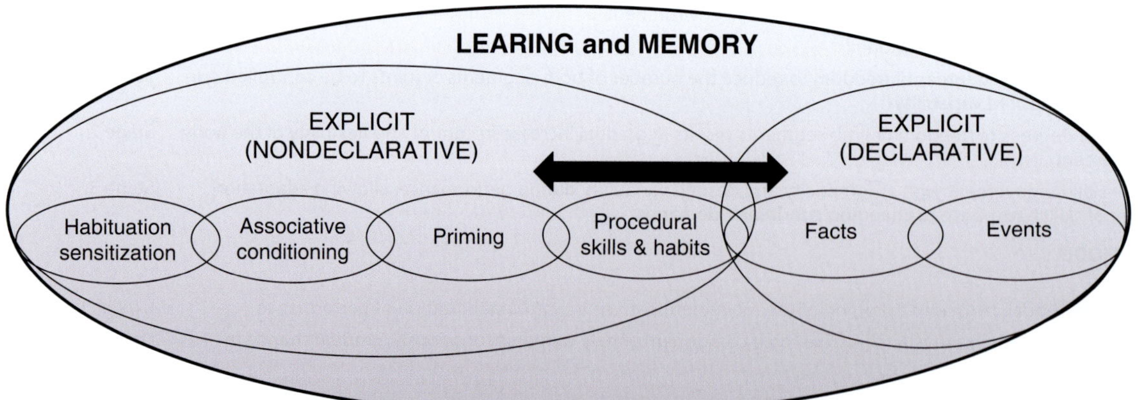

Fig. 3.7 Learning is the process of acquiring information or skill while memory is the product of the learning process. Traditionally, the learning process has been described as having two separate domains: explicit (or declarative) learning, which is primarily involved in acquisition of knowledge about facts and events, and implicit or nondeclarative learning. Much of motor learning falls into the category of procedural implicit learning, or the mastery of skills and habits. Recent research evidence using functional magnetic resonance imaging suggests that there are interactions between explicit and implicit processes (*arrow*) regardless of whether the focus is on fact or movement.

cortex, cingulate gyrus (limbic system), head of the caudate nucleus, medial temporal lobes, and hippocampus.[169] The hippocampus plays a key role in motor learning because it contains a cognitive-spatial map of the typical areas in which humans function.[170] Early motor learning is strengthened, as evidenced by changes in output of the primary motor cortex, when explicit learning of sequences is associated with implicit learning.[171–173]

Once sequential aspects of the task are well understood, the need to pay close attention during motor performance diminishes, and the skill becomes less effortful as it progresses toward automatization. [174] As automaticity increases, the ability to attend to simultaneous tasks also increases.[170,175] There is growing evidence that the transition from early motor learning of complex, sequentially organized tasks to automaticity requires more time and practice as a person ages.[176–179] Encouragement and feedback that focus on building perceptions of capability (self-efficacy) with respect to better performance than that of peers appear to enhance motor learning in both young and older adults.[180] Recently the critical addition of support for the psychologic needs of the learner has been shown to be an important element of the motor learning process. A person's sustained behavioral commitment to learning the skill leads to competence, which leads to self-efficacy and ultimately to retention.[11,141] Notably the level of self-efficacy has an impact on an individual's motivation to engage in the behaviors required to attain desired rehabilitation outcomes.[11]

Box 3.2 **Summary of the Dimensions or Characteristics of Practice**

- Contextual interference: The work of keeping many options available in working memory over time when involved in discovering solutions to movement problems during the acquisition of skill in motor learning.
- Blocked: A single motor behavior (task) is repeated multiple times in unchanging environmental conditions. Performance improves within the practice session, but less than optimal retention is demonstrated across sessions.
- Random (variable): Practice of the targeted motor task is interspersed or embedded within trials of different motor behaviors. Although performance in a single practice session is less consistent, there is better retention of skills across practice sessions and environmental conditions.
- Serial: A series of separate (related or unrelated) tasks is performed in the same sequence for multiple trials.
- Massed: Time for active practice exceeds rest time between trials.
- Distributed: Time for active practice is less than rest time between trials.
- Part task training: Each component of a motor behavior is practiced separately; this assists accuracy or efficiency of performance of the single-task component.
- Whole-task training: The entire motor behavior is practiced as a single task. Enhances the individual's ability to solve problems and adapt task performance across practice sessions and differing environmental conditions.

ROLE OF AEROBIC EXERCISE IN MOTOR LEARNING

Recent evidence suggests that aerobic exercise and possibly resistance training play key roles in the motor learning of individuals who have had a stroke. Aerobic exercise leads to upregulation of the protein called brain-derived neurotrophic factor (BDNF), which is involved in neuroprotection, neurogenesis, and neuroplasticity.[181] It has been suggested that BDNF influences the CNS by improving its capability for motor learning. Two different effects on the CNS and motor learning were described in relation to aerobic exercise: (1) exercise that happens immediately prior to motor task practice assists with improved detection and encoding of information relevant to the motor task and (2) exercise that happens immediately following motor task practice strengthens the motor memory process.[181]

Key motor learning concepts that are employed by physical therapists and healthcare professionals working with individuals new to prosthetic or orthotic use include *practice* conditions and schedule; appropriate level of *challenge*; the role of *motivation* and *self-efficacy*; the role of *variability*, *contextual interference*, and *feedback* on skill acquisition; development of *automaticity* of performance; as well as *retention* and *transfer* of the newly learned motor skill (Box 3.2).[136,140] Each is discussed in the following section.

The Importance of Practice

A fundamental aspect found in all motor learning models is the concept of practice. Motor learning cannot occur unless the individual has an opportunity to gain experience through repeated attempts (both successful and unsuccessful) at accomplishing the desired movement task.[182] A substantial portion of the research conducted in the field of motor learning focuses on investigating various aspects of practice and the optimal conditions or configurations in which it occurs. Different types of practice can impact the effectiveness of motor learning and its transferability or applicability to similar tasks or environmental conditions.

APPROPRIATE LEVEL OF CHALLENGE

Therapists have long recognized the importance of determining the optimal level of challenge for patients undergoing rehabilitation. This involves selecting the correct intensity of practice (labor) that will keep a patient engaged and motivated and the correct frequency of repetitions to drive neuroplastic changes in the CNS. Maintaining an appropriate level of challenge is crucial for patients during tasks, ensuring their physical and psychological well-being. A task that is too easy will not drive the physiologic conditioning that leads to neurocognitive changes for motor learning. Conversely, an excessively difficult task can pose a risk of potential harm or injury. A high frequency of repetitions in practice is necessary for neuroplasticity.[183] Research suggests that the neuroplasticity necessary for motor learning requires a range of several hundred to thousands of repetitions. However, therapeutic sessions often fall short of this target. To address this practice gap, telehealth modalities are currently being investigated for stroke rehabilitation.[184] Gaming, avatars, wearable sensors, and remote monitoring and feedback are being studied to increase intervention intensity and patient compliance, aiming for improved functional outcomes. This line of research is relatively new, however, and there is currently no strong evidence regarding the effectiveness and cost of telehealth for stroke rehabilitation in terms of improving functional outcomes.[184,185] When determining the suitable and optimal level of challenge for a patient, therapists need to take various factors into account including but not limited to the patient's physiologic conditioning, motor capabilities to meet the challenge, constraints on both patient and therapist time limitations imposed by the healthcare setting, and evidence-based findings regarding the recommended frequency and intensity of interventions.

MOTIVATION AND SELF-EFFICACY

Relevancy and meaningfulness of a task are critical for motor learning. The choice of a task for practice must include consideration of the person's desire to change.[41] A task that is not meaningful can lead to disengagement and lack of motivation on the part of the person performing the task. Effective practice occurs only when tasks are meaningful to the patient and the challenge of the task is optimal for learning.[11] Sustained practice leads to increased capability for performing the task; increased capability leads to confidence in performing the task; and the combination of capability (skill) and confidence leads to self-efficacy in acquisition of a new skill. Self-efficacy with a skill is necessary to sustain the use of that skill long enough for a person to get to the late stages of motor learning in which the skill can be adapted as needed for function.

VARIABILITY

In a complex and unpredictable environment, there are innumerable ways to respond to challenges that are encountered. Over the life span, typically developing individuals explore many movement options to accomplish salient task goals. This process leads to the formation of a collection of action strategies that showcase both automaticity in performance and adaptability to variations in task or environmental constraints (i.e., the mastery of bipedal locomotion, over different surfaces, at various speeds, in closed versus open environments).[186,187] Discovery learning and the feedback/feedforward provided by error during repeated practice across conditions with differing constraints allow the individual to develop an understanding (perception) of the common elements of the task wherever and whenever it is performed.[182,188,189] This perception provides the flexibility to select from a range of task-specific options and to adapt movement in response to variations encountered in daily life; variability in skilled movement is an adaptive resource responsive to variation in environmental demands.[190]

The movement patterns of individuals with neurologic or neuromuscular dysfunction, however, often demonstrate hyper- or hypovariability.[187,191] Excessive or insufficient variability can present challenges: it can limit or distort our perception of the task and the relationship between the task and the environment. Additionally, the acquisition of skills may be hindered by the limitations imposed by changes in muscle performance and motor control.[192,193] Functionally, this contributes to a reduced ability to adapt (vary) performance in response to changing environmental conditions.[39] The presence of rigidity and freezing episodes in individuals with Parkinson disease can be attributed to the inability of the CNS to modulate the "stability" during movements.[194] This interference with stability negatively impacts mobility (locomotion) and postural control when task conditions change (i.e., the need to increase speed, navigate through doorway, or to walk on inclines).[192,195] In persons with stroke, impaired ability to move the involved upper extremity has been found to be accompanied by difficulty recognizing action of the corresponding limb when observing others or a computer model.[196] Additionally, motor control studies in stroke survivors showed that stability and coordination during reaching are disrupted.[197] In persons with right hemispheric stroke, impairments of attention and perception challenge the ability to develop the set of task-specific movement options necessary for adaptive function in response to variations in environment and context.[198] Although implicit motor learning can be successful after a stroke, movement during acquisition stages is often slower and more variable in both blocked and random practice conditions.[199] Variability in movement is also altered in children with hypertonic and dyskinetic cerebral palsy and in those with developmental coordination disorder.[190,193,200]

In rehabilitation, therapists set up opportunities for the discovery of motor learning for their patients. These opportunities are specifically designed to enhance the likelihood of discovering, from among all possible movement options, the set of movements most likely to result in successful task performance.[186,187] This is accomplished by manipulating the environmental and task constraints in relevant and meaningful ways to actively engage the individual in iterations of the task with the goal of promoting both perceptual understanding and a usable set of action options to effectively accomplish the task.[186,201,202]

PRACTICE CONDITIONS: BLOCKED, RANDOM, OR SERIAL?

Practice can be categorized based on whether it follows a blocked or random sequence. *Blocked practice* (also known as constant practice) involves repeating the same task in separate but consecutive trials.[139,182] In blocked practice, the task is repeated in consistent environmental conditions. Modified blocked practice, on the other hand, entails repeating the motor task three or more times in one condition before altering conditions or context in which practice of the same task is repeated. During blocked practice, the individual focuses on performing a single task, which reduces the overall demand on working memory. As a result, the quality of performance tends to improve substantially over successive bouts of blocked practice. In healthy adults, acquisition of skill appears to be effective (performance becomes more accurate over a single practice session) with blocked practice; however, retention of the skill over time and transfer of the skill to differing conditions is not as strong.[203] For children under the age of 10, blocked practice seems to have a positive impact on skill retention. This is attributed to the development of information-processing abilities in late childhood and early adolescence.[204,205] In the case of an individual with transfemoral amputation focusing on stance control using a prosthetic limb, a blocked practice session could involve performing 10 trials (repetitions) of stepping up onto a stool with the intact limb while standing in the parallel bars. The level of difficulty of the activity could be advanced by setting up an additional practice session, asking the individual to perform a similar task while supporting himself or herself with a straight cane to a practice curb or to step outside the parallel bars. Theoretically, practice in the parallel bars would provide a model to use when performing a similar activity outside the parallel bars.

Random practice (also described as variable practice) is characterized as practicing a set of tasks in which order and perhaps difficulty of tasks vary across bouts of practice.[144,182] Because of the variation encountered during random practice, there is less improvement of performance in a given practice session (compared with blocked practice); however, there is greater retention of what has been learned over time. Theoretically, random practice creates *contextual interference* (the work of keeping many options available in working memory over time) that actually enhances learning and mastery over time despite poorer immediate performance.[182,203] Although this may be counterintuitive, the efficacy of contextual interference on mastery of complex movement tasks is well supported.[206–210] One of the proposed mechanisms for enhanced retention in random practice is increased attentional demand, which results in better use of perceptual understanding to prepare for movement.[208,210] The degree of similarity of tasks (distraction) undertaken during a practice session can also be a source of contextual interference; greater attention is required to discriminate between tasks with similar but distinct characteristics.[209] The improvement of retention occurs even when the context or characteristics of the task are somewhat altered; thus random variable practice may enhance the transfer of learning.[182]

To engage in random practice order for practicing the primary task of stance-phase stability, an individual with a transfemoral prosthesis would participate in an ongoing gait training session. As this person walked the length of the parallel bars (or across the gym), he or she might be asked to step up onto a stool or over an obstacle at a different point in the walk and to change direction or speed on randomly delivered commands. The entire walk might be repeated 10 times (practice trials), with a step up onto or over the stool and changing speed and direction at a different point in each of the 10 trials of walking. These trials of stepping up or over and altering speed and direction do not occur sequentially but instead are interspersed throughout the entire walking activity.

A third practice condition called *serial practice* can be seen as a combination of the blocked and random practice order. In serial practice, a series of different tasks are performed sequentially, starting from a specific point and progressing toward a predetermined end point.

These tasks are always executed in the same order and repeated as a complete set of movement tasks.[139,182]

In a serial practice session for an individual learning to use a transfemoral prosthesis, the therapist may instruct him or her to repeat a specific sequence of movements such as the following:

1. Rise from a seated position and take three steps toward an obstacle in your pathway.
2. Step over the stool (obstacle) with your intact (right) foot, bringing your prosthetic limb around the object in a small arc.
3. Complete three more gait cycles and turn around to the right.
4. Walk back toward the obstacle, stepping over it with the prosthesis first on the return.
5. Continue walking back to the chair, turn, and sit down.
6. Rise to stand once again and repeat the entire sequence until you have done it a total of × number of times.

The original task of stepping onto the stool with the right foot has been embedded into a series of different (but somewhat related) tasks performed in the same order over multiple trials.

Another way to classify practice is by the relative period of time spent in active practice versus rest time between practice sessions. In conditions of *massed practice*, there is more time spent over a practice trial than there is rest time between trials. Massed practice often increases intensity level. Fatigue may be a factor in decreases in performance over repeated practice sessions if rest periods are insufficient. In conditions of *distributed practice*, the amount of practice time is less than or equal to the amount of rest time between trials.[139,182] Given evidence of better retention and transfer of skills with longer rest periods between practice trials (i.e., distributed practice), rest and sleep appear to be more than a period of physical recovery; these periods may also enhance the consolidation of perceptual schemas and action rules associated with the skill that has been practiced into memory.[211] What is not yet understood is how much practice time and how much rest are optimal for tasks of different complexity or learners with various resources or impairments.

PART- VERSUS WHOLE-TASK TRAINING

Numerous functional tasks consist of identifiable subcomponents that occur in a specific sequence. The task of rising from a chair, for example, may require moving forward toward the edge of the seat, changing foot position, leaning forward to shift body weight from the ischial tuberosities toward the feet, lifting off the seat, rapidly accelerating upward into a standing position, and finally attaining postural control while upright.[212] The task of walking can be divided into stages, which include weight acceptance during the early stance, maintaining stability while in a single-limb stance, preparing for the swing phase at the end of stance, and initiating and completing limb advancement throughout the swing phase.[213] When therapists are working with individuals who have neurologic, neuromuscular, or musculoskeletal-related movement dysfunction, they often use task analysis to determine what subcomponents of the task are problematic. The therapist might opt to practice the problematic components of the task to build skill before attempting the entire task *(part-to-whole training)* or to practice the entire task repeatedly *(whole-task training)*. In partial-task training, the task is divided into separate parts, and each part is explained or modeled as a distinct component of the whole, whereas in whole-task training the entire task is explained verbally or modeled (demonstrated) in its entirety from beginning to end. The decision to structure training as part versus whole is influenced by the level of difficulty of the task, the degree to which the individual has already mastered some of the task's components, the individual's ability to attend to the task, his or her level of motivation and frustration, and safety considerations as the task is attempted. Tasks that are serial in nature lend themselves to part-to-whole training; spending time practicing complex or difficult task components (ending the session by putting all of the components together to perform the whole task) often leads to better retention and transfer than the same amount of time spent practicing the entire task.[182,213,214] Tasks that are continuous, such as carrying a tray while walking through a cafeteria, are not as easily separated into components because of the degree of coordination and interplay necessary among task components. When coordination, timing, and interaction must be learned, whole-task training appears to be more efficacious.[182,214,215]

RELATIONSHIPS: PRACTICE, RETENTION, AND TRANSFER

The impact of different practice conditions on motor learning has been extensively studied in psychology, movement science, and rehabilitation. When evaluating the evidence presented by these studies to assess their clinical relevance and potential application, it is crucial to consider the specific outcome of practice being investigated. Are the researchers focused on change in quality of performance during practice trials (i.e., skill acquisition within a session) or in carryover of understanding of the task from one practice session to another (i.e., postpractice performance or retention over time)? This distinction holds particularly significance for rehabilitation professionals, and it is important for them to be mindful of it. How do rehabilitation professionals assess the effectiveness of their interventions in promoting motor learning and skill development? Rather than focusing on improvement in a single session, we look instead at the development of *automaticity* and the ability to adapt performance across sessions and circumstances. Although performance over repeated trials within a practice session is often observed, this is not a reliable indicator that motor learning has occurred. Rather, consistency in motor behavior over multiple sessions and time suggests the presence of retention or a lasting change in motor behavior. The ability to *transfer* what has been learned and apply the set of movement options across situations appears to be related to the opportunity to practice under a variety of environmental conditions and constraints.

Scientists who study motor learning hypothesize that individuals who develop flexible learning strategies through random practice and whole-task training are better able to transfer learned skills to novel situations. This is particularly significant for individuals in rehabilitation, who will ultimately need to perform skills beyond the rehabilitation practice environment (rehabilitation settings) as they return to the real-world environment of their homes and community. This concept is connected to self-efficacy, as individuals need confidence in their ability to perform skills in their daily routines.[11] With these considerations in mind, rehabilitation professionals need to carefully consider and choose the practice conditions that will lead to the best possible functional outcomes for the individual under their care.

Intrinsic and Extrinsic Feedback

A second key concept in motor learning paradigms centers on the provision of feedback during practice trials (Box 3.3).[216] As movement occurs, it generates *intrinsic (inherent or unconscious) feedback* that the CNS (especially the

Box 3.3 Definitions for Feedback in Motor Learning

Basic Definitions

- Intrinsic (inherent): Sensations generated by movement of the body itself, monitored by sensory receptors (exteroception, proprioception, vestibular, visual, auditory), and transmitted to the brainstem and brain via sensory pathways.
- Extrinsic (augmented): Information provided about the movement task by sources external to the individual who is moving. Extrinsic feedback can be provided by another individual (e.g., the therapist or coach), or by an external device (e.g., biofeedback, other types of signals) that would not necessarily be present during the usual performance of the task. It can be provided before, during, or after movement.

Dimensions of Extrinsic Feedback

- Knowledge of performance (KP): Information about the quality of the movement, provided during or following performance.
- Knowledge of results (KR): Information about the outcome (success) of the movement or task, provided after it has been completed.

Variations of Extrinsic Feedback

- "Feedforward": Prompts or clues provided prior to movement to assist the learner's active engagement in problem solving or preparation for the motor task.
- Concurrent: KP information about the movement provided as it occurs.
- Terminal: KP or KR information provided after the movement task has been completed. This can be provided either as soon as the movement is finished (immediate) or after a period of time (delayed).
- Distinct: KP or KR information about one specific practice trial.
- Accumulated (summary): KP or KR information that reflects multiple attempts to perform the task or movement.

Channels Used for Extrinsic Feedback

- Verbal: Questions or statements made by the therapist or coach about the movement.
- Nonverbal: Gestures and facial expressions made by the therapist or coach; touch or guidance used to direct or redirect attention or movement; lights, whistles, or other sounds used to guide or influence the learning during or following the movement.

Timing for Extrinsic Feedback

- Consistent (100%): KR or KP distinct information provided after every practice trial.
- Reduced (50%, 33%, 25%): KR or KP distinct or summary information provided after every other, every third, or every fourth practice trial.
- For poor trials: Providing feedback for trials with large errors during practice.
- For good trials: Providing feedback for trials with relatively small or few errors during a practice trial.

cerebellum as a system interested in coordination and error control) compares with the sensation that it "anticipates" (feedforward) will or should result from the movement. Intrinsic feedback involves proprioceptive information associated with the movement and is connected to implicit learning. *Extrinsic (augmented or conscious) feedback* refers to information about the movement performance that is provided by an external source before, during, or after the movement. Extrinsic feedback may refer to sensory information such as auditory, visual, verbal, and environmental contextual information related to movement that is associated with explicit learning. If rehabilitation professionals understand the "what, when, why, and how" of extrinsic feedback (combined with well-structured practice), they will be much more effective in facilitating motor learning as well as the individual's ability to solve problems or adapt a motor skill. Rehabilitation professionals assess the most suitable type of information (KP or KR) for the person they are working with, as well as determine the optimal way and timing to provide feedback (feedback mode and schedule).

To begin a therapy session, the therapist can engage the individual by asking how they would approach a functional motor problem and what they anticipate during task performance: for example, "We're going to practice moving from the bed to the chair. How can you prepare to do this? What is the first thing you need to do? Are you ready to do it?" This provides extrinsic augmented *feedforward* information encouraging the person to explore potential solutions for the initial stages of the transfer task. If the therapist prompts the person to assess their sensations or experiences during performance, they are providing concurrent extrinsic feedback. If the therapist asks or comments on performance after the task is completed, it constitutes *terminal* extrinsic feedback. Therapists provide extrinsic feedback, sometimes spontaneously, in each intervention encounter when they say, "Good job!" or "Did that work out the way you expected?" or "What could you do differently next time?" In providing extrinsic information, the therapist drives the person's attention to and enhances the use of intrinsically generated feedback or sometimes the substitution of an alternative source of information when sensory impairment is present.

KNOWLEDGE OF PERFORMANCE AND KNOWLEDGE OF RESULTS

Extrinsic information can provide the individual who is learning a new motor strategy or skill with either KR, information about the outcome of the movement (i.e., whether it was successful), or KP, information about the quality or execution of the movement (accuracy of the performance).[216,217] Much of the research on feedback in motor learning has focused on KR (outcome); however, in rehabilitation, we often use KP (quality; e.g., "Do you think that you were leaning far enough forward as you began to stand up?") to help individuals recognize and respond to movement errors.

Evidence in the literature suggests that, although KR does not necessarily lead to better performance during practice conditions, this type of augmented feedback information contributes to better task performance during retention tests.[141,216,217] The individual learning a new skill may benefit most by considering whether he or she has accomplished a movement goal (KR), especially in the early and middle stages of motor learning, rather than how accurately or efficiently the goal was attained (KP). This correlates with supporting the psychologic needs of the patient through celebration of the patient's progress and attention to the patient's success (KR).[11] Early on, details about quality of performance may interfere with the individual's developing understanding of the nature of the task and ability to sort through possible strategies that might be used. In later stages of motor learning, when the focus shifts to refinement or improved precision of performance, KP is a more appropriate and powerful form of feedback information as long as the task is consistently accomplished.[218] It appears that augmented and intrinsic KP feedback leads to better quality and consistency of performance during practice but perhaps to less accurate performance in retention tests.[173,216] Although KP may not enhance retention as much as hoped, it has been found to be both effective and necessary in the acquisition of complex motor tasks as compared with mastery of simple motor tasks.[216–218] Use of KR to support a patient's self-efficacy may lead to more frequent use of the skill in multiple settings, enhancing activity and participation levels of functioning.

How and When Should Feedback Be Used?

An additional aspect explored in the study of motor learning investigates the effectiveness of various frequencies and timing when delivering augmented information. Offering excessive anticipatory cues prior to the task or excessive feedback during task execution and completion can actually be detrimental to the learning process. Frequent KR-focused feedback, provided on nearly every trial of the task, often contributes to dependence on external guidance and ultimately hampers performance on retention tests.[219] Summarized KR-focused feedback given at infrequent intervals (after multiple trials) appears to improve performance during practice as well as on retention testing.[219–221] Delaying the timing of KR appears to have a positive effect on performance during practice and on retention tests. Providing feedback after trials that are relatively successful appears to enhance motor learning more than when trials are full of error.[222–224] Researchers have noted that KR, like random practice and whole training methods, better prepares individuals for adapting motor performance to changing environmental demands, resulting in better performance on retention tests. These findings are consistent across individuals with no neurologic impairment; stroke survivors, those with a head injury or Parkinson disease; children with cerebral palsy and developmental delay; and persons with mild cognitive impairment and early dementia.[225–230] Increasing evidence suggests that allowing individuals to regulate or control feedback frequency also has a positive impact on the retention (effectiveness) of what has been learned.[231–233]

What Modality for Feedback Is Appropriate?

Extrinsic feedback (augmented information) can be provided in a number of ways, using the visual system (e.g., demonstration and modeling, targets and other visual cues); the auditory system (e.g., informational verbal prompts or questions, use of tone of voice); and the somatosensory-tactile systems (e.g., manual contacts, tapping/sweeping motions, compression of limb segments to cue stability response, traction/elongation of limb segments to cue mobility, appropriate resistance to guide movement).

Early in the motor learning process, therapists judiciously use all three modalities, keeping in mind that early stages of motor learning are periods of experimentation and trial/error as the individual becomes familiar with the nature of the task and develops strategies that lead to accomplishment of the task. Although it is tempting to explicitly direct and "tell" someone with movement dysfunction how to move more efficiently, prompting by using questions often can more effectively engage the individual in an active learning process. Active engagement in the problem-solving aspect of activity is a key motivator.[11] It appears that certain tasks are more responsive to particular modalities of feedback than others.[234,235] In persons with stroke, for example, visual feedback about weight distribution is useful for balance activities and auditory feedback about force production positively affects learning the sit-to-stand transition; the efficacy of verbal and kinesthetic feedback is not as well understood.[236]

Music and rhythm are frequently used in gait rehabilitation for persons with Parkinson disease.[237] Recent research suggests that the rhythmic variation fundamental to Argentine tango is an especially useful mode of extrinsic feedback for persons with Parkinson disease, requiring on-the-spot responses to variable stimuli. Outcomes have been positive for balance, functional mobility, and Parkinson-specific motor symptoms using Argentine tango as an intervention.[238,239] Recent research investigates rhythmic cueing further in the form of self-generated rhythm through singing aloud while walking. Results show decreased gait variability for people with Parkinson disease who sing aloud while walking.[240] Music has shown positive effects in the recovery of walking for post-stroke survivors.[241]

Simple tasks appear to be learned more easily following demonstration or physical practice with or without KP-focused feedback. The learning of more cognitively and motorically complex tasks, on the other hand, benefited from a combination of demonstration and practice with KP feedback.[237] Many previous studies suggest that an *external focus* of attention (success or quality of the movement) has a more beneficial effect on motor learning than an internal (kinesthetic) focus of attention during practice.[242–245] However, recent work suggests that focused attention is another key motivator and factor to increase motor learning.[141] Perhaps *prompting* a patient to pay close attention to internal kinesthetic cues is a good method to combine proven elements of previous and newer studies.

As individuals move into the later stages of motor learning, therapists must be aware of the need to wean the amount and frequency of augmented information as the individual moves toward becoming adept at the task. In the final stages of motor learning, augmented information becomes less and less essential or effective as mastery of the motor task is achieved.

Using Normative Feedback

There is increasing evidence that providing information that is normative (social comparative, social relatedness) has a positive impact on motor learning.[141,242] Providing feedback that suggests that the individual is doing as well or better than others in similar situations, when paired with KR information about outcomes of the individual's actual practice, appears to improve trial-to-trial performance as well as retention.[246,247] Making a statement at the start of a therapy session focused on a difficult motor task indicating that persons facing similar challenges typically do well and are able to master the task with practice enhances the individual's expectations of their own ability (self-efficacy) and reduces anxiety associated with risk of failure; this enhances motor learning as well.[248]

Mental Practice and Imagery

Another resource available to assist the process of motor learning is the incorporation of mental practice and imagery into therapeutic interventions. Mental practice is defined as the imagined execution of a task-related movement without actual movement or muscle activation.[249] Mental practice of a motor task is thought to activate the same areas and networks of the CNS that actual movement does, especially if the task has been previously practiced.[249,250] Growing evidence in both the human performance and rehabilitation literature indicates that mental practice and the use of imagery enhance learning effects of physical practice and improve motor performance and retention and decrease chronic pain.[251–253] Mental practice and motor imagery that focus on ease and quality of movement have been found to be particularly helpful in acquisition of motor skills in persons recovering from acute and chronic stroke.[253,254] Recently, mental practice was combined with a brain-computer interface in subacute stroke, providing promising results on the recovery of sensory-motor impairments in the most affected upper limb.[255]

Imagery and mental practice seem to have a more powerful influence on enhancing performance during skill acquisition; however, their influence on retention of skills is not thoroughly comprehended. This has implications for application to practice in therapeutic settings. Given high-volume patient caseloads and the realities of multiple patients per therapist during sessions, mental imagery can serve as an effective tool for maintaining the involvement of the client in activities, even when the therapist is attending to other patients.

Role of Sleep in Motor Learning

Newly acquired motor memory becomes more stable (more resistant to disruption or interference) during sleep.[256] The procedural memory consolidation process appears to reduce the need for neocortical (prefrontal lobe) input into the neuronal representation of the movement, making it easier to recall the movement and increasing the efficacy of retention.[257] Although early research suggested that consolidation during sleep actually improved learning (offline learning) and enhanced motor performance, more recent work proposes that it instead provides protection against forgetting by counteracting both physical and neuronal fatigue associated with practice.[258,259] Whichever perspective will prove to be accurate, it appears that sleep is a key component in the motor learning process.[260]

The positive effect of sleep on the retention of newly learned skills appears to be true for motor skills that have been physically practiced as well as those reinforced by mental imagery both in persons who are healthy and in those with a pathologic condition of the CNS.[260,261] The opportunity for uninterrupted overnight sleep, which allows for offline consolidation of motor memory, is a crucial aspect of the rehabilitation process for individuals with stroke.[262,263] This is particularly important since research has indicated that poor sleep quality is associated with lower functional levels in stroke survivors.[262,264] Individuals with prefrontal lobe damage (e.g., after traumatic brain injury), who typically are quite challenged by novel motor tasks presented during rehabilitation, appear to benefit significantly from the opportunity for offline learning and memory consolidation that occurs during a night of sound sleep.[263]

However, sleep disturbances are quite common for people with traumatic brain injury (TBI) and mild traumatic brain injury/concussion (mTBI). These sleep problems lead to symptom exacerbations and difficulties participating in rehabilitation.[265] Animal model research suggests that sleep deprivation affects neuroplastic processes negatively, which could further affect functional motor recovery for those with TBI who are experiencing sleep disorders.[265] A coordinated interdisciplinary approach is needed to effectively treat sleep disorders so that persons with TBI or mTBI can benefit optimally from rehabilitation treatments. Rehabilitation professionals should pay particular attention to the sleep habits of clients who have TBI or mTBI and coexistent post-traumatic stress disorder (PTSD). This is common in war veterans. Sleep problems are a diagnostic feature of PTSD, and veterans with PTSD commonly experience sleep problems at a rate much higher than that of veterans without PTSD.[265] For best outcomes, motor learning interventions for these individuals will likely need to occur along with an interdisciplinary strategy that addresses sleep disturbances.

Importance of Patient/Client-Centered Goals

Rehabilitation goals focus on improving an individual's ability to participate in meaningful activities. One aspect of the motor learning process that is often taken for granted is the salience of the task to the learner; therapists may assume that the goals they have developed for a given patient (e.g., to walk 150 ft safely and efficiently using an assistive device and a prosthesis or orthosis) are consistent with the goals of the individual with whom they are working, when in fact there may be a mismatch.[266,267] New findings suggest that focusing attention toward tasks that hold the greatest personal significance can enhance motivation and concentration. These factors are essential components of the motor learning process and can also promote neural plasticity and facilitate recovery following brain injuries.[11,268,269] A sense of empowerment and increasing self-efficacy contributes to efficacy of learning when an individual works toward a goal that is particularly meaningful to him or her.[11,270–273]

How does a rehabilitation professional help an individual identify salient personal goals and use these goals to inform the design of appropriate opportunities for motor learning (Fig. 3.8)? Framing goals at the level of activity and participation is the first step.[274] The next is to ensure that stated goals reflect consensus (as much as possible) of the patient and the health professional.[275] Such consensus is a key influence on the relationship between the patient and the health professional; being "on the same page" creates a level of trust that provides a solid foundation for risking failure in the rehabilitation learning environment.[275] Goals for motor learning are most effective if they reflect both expertise of the therapist and expectations of the individual beginning rehabilitation. Achieving a consensus sometimes necessitates educating patients and their families, as well as engaging in negotiations to establish priorities.[276–278] Effectively defined goals are (1) specifically related to the task to be accomplished or mastered; (2) measurable (i.e., use quantifiable metrics of distance, time, effort or difficulty, and frequency of performance); (3) ambitious yet achievable within the forecasted episode of care; (4) relevant, realistic, and congruent with the individual's potential and expectations; and (5) include a time line for achievement.[278] Establishing clearly stated and measurable goals provides a framework for assessment of outcomes of interventions as well as the revision or progression of activities that will further improve functional capacity and the individual's ability to participate in meaningful activity. Such attention to the early establishment of functional goals has been found to have a positive effect on outcomes of rehabilitation for children with cerebral palsy and persons with spinal cord injury, stroke, and traumatic brain injury.[279–284]

NEURAL PLASTICITY IN MOTOR CONTROL AND MOTOR LEARNING

Rehabilitation professionals are on the cusp of significant expansion in the understanding of the neurobiologic/physiologic basis of recovery after neurologic and neuromuscular injury.[285,286] The developing science suggests that we can use our understanding of motor control and motor learning to *drive neural plasticity* in both acute and chronic stages of many neurologic and neuromuscular diseases. Emerging scientific findings indicate that our understanding of motor control and motor learning can be utilized to *drive neural plasticity* in both early and long-term stages of various neurologic and neuromuscular disorders.[287–290] Learning-induced neuroplasticity involves three processes: (1) strengthening existing neural connections, (2) stimulating the formation of new neural connections, and (3) preferentially selecting neural connections and pathways, which is known as *pruning*.[291] This science also challenges us to reassess whether our interventions are satisfactory—in relation to therapeutic methods, intensity, and duration—to elicit the neuroplastic changes necessary for enhancing function and quality of life.[291–293]

The term *neural plasticity* refers to the dynamic ability of the brain to structurally and functionally reorganize neural circuits in response to activity and environmental demand: such plasticity occurs during development in children, during adulthood as one masters new motor skills and builds knowledge base, as well as after any type of brain injury or insult.[288,291] Plasticity is driven by (i.e., is dependent on) the process of learning, whether it be focused on new knowledge or skills or relearning of skills disrupted by illness or injury. Although the mechanisms underlying neuroplastic change are not fully understood, exposure to learning opportunities of sufficient intensity and duration contributes to the remapping of motor, perceptual,

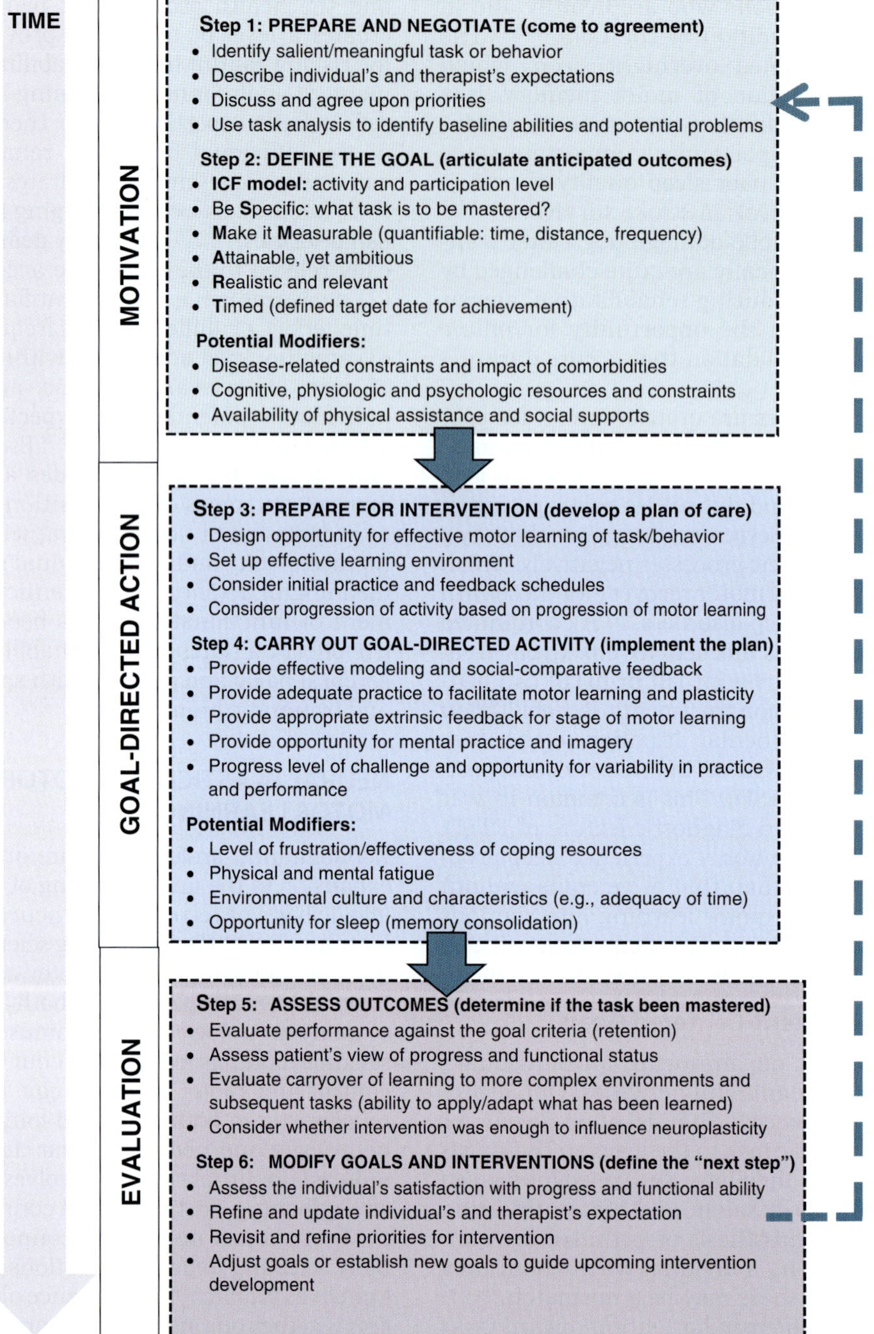

Fig. 3.8 A patient-centered model for setting goals for the effective motivation and facilitation of motor learning in rehabilitation. Initial efforts focus on building consensus between patient and therapist on the establishment of appropriate meaningful goals and on the articulation of such goals so that they can be later used to assess outcomes. Given understanding of motor learning, motor control, neuroplasticity, and recovery of function, the therapist then designs and implements task-specific, goal-directed rehabilitation interventions. Both the patient and therapist use agreed-upon goals as markers of efficacy of intervention; they modify or progress therapeutic activities and practice based on achievement of the goals. *ICF*, International Classification of Functioning, Disability and Health.

and communication areas within the brain.[288–291,294] Early in rehabilitation, as the effects of inflammation and edema associated with CNS infarct or injury diminish, activity-based interventions may help to revive and restore function in neural structures that were initially compromised; this is *neural recovery*.[295] In addition to brain plasticity new evidence suggests that activity-dependent plasticity is also observed in the spinal cord below the level of lesion in patients with spinal cord injury.[296] Even if there is potential for neural recovery, at times the effort required to activate recovering neural circuits is intensely difficult and frustrating. Without encouragement and opportunity to practice, function may continue to be compromised because of *learned nonuse* of a body part.[297] As rehabilitation progresses, continued activity-based interventions may facilitate the recruitment of intact neighboring neural structures to supplement the function of damaged brain structures. Even though this is actually a mechanism of *neural compensation*, it may be perceived by the individual, family, and rehabilitation professional as *functional recovery (i.e., restitution)* at the International Classification of Functioning, Disability and Health (ICF) levels of body function and activity.[288] If brain injury has been so extensive that alternative ways of performing key functional tasks are necessary, retraining leads to *functional compensation (i.e., adaptation or substitution)*.[288]

Historically, the medical approach to treating recently injured or compromised CNS has primarily aimed to prevent or minimize secondary complications arising from various insults such as trauma, ischemia, or infection.[163,298] However, as medical practices continue to advance, there is a growing emphasis on pharmacological and interventional strategies (e.g., noninvasive brain stimulation) that target functional recovery and activity in ADL.[299-301] Currently, the most potent facilitator of neural plasticity is rehabilitation based on motor learning principles. This approach effectively triggers neuroplastic processes in damaged CNS, similar to how they occur in developing brains, by addressing the behavioral, sensory/perceptual, and cognitive aspects of functional and skilled movement.[38,217,302]

Kleim and Jones[287] have described a set of 10 principles that translate current best evidence about experience-dependent neural plasticity from animal and human basic science studies to inform the development of motor learning-based interventions for clinical rehabilitation practice. New evidence from multiple authors adds weight to these principles.[296,302] A recent study by Mawase et al. demonstrates that task success reinforcement is an additional principle to consider (Table 3.2).[303] Discussion of each principle follows.

Table 3.2 Principles of Experience-Dependent, Use-Dependent, and Activity-Based Neural Plasticity

Principle	Description
Use it or lose it	Failure to drive specific brain functions can lead to functional degradation.
Use it and improve it	Training that drives a specific brain function can lead to the enhancement of that function.
Specificity	The nature of the training experience dictates the nature of the plasticity.
Repetition matters	Induction of plasticity requires high levels of repetition.
Intensity matters	Induction of plasticity requires high-intensity training.
Time matters	Different forms of plasticity occur at different times during training.
Exercise matters	Different forms of plasticity occur with exercise prior to and following training.
Salience matters	The training experience must be sufficiently salient to induce plasticity.
Age matters	Training-induced plasticity occurs more readily in younger brains.
Transference	Plasticity in response to one training experience can enhance the acquisition of similar behaviors.
Interference	Plasticity in response to one experience can interfere with acquisition of other behaviors.
Success reinforcement	Both internal reinforcement and external validation of success are necessary.

Modified from Mang CS, Campbell KL, Ross CJD, Boyd LA. Promoting neuroplasticity for motor rehabilitation after stroke: considering the effects on aerobic exercise and genetic variation on brain-derived neurotrophic factor. *Phys Ther.* 2013;93(12):1707–1716; Milton JG, Small SS, Solodkin A. On the way to automatic: dynamic aspects in the development of expertise. *J Clin Neurophysiol.* 2004;21(3):134–143; and Landers M. Treatment-induced neuroplasticity following focal injury to the motor cortex. *Int J Rehabil Res.* 2004;27(1):1–5.

Use It or Lose It

Basic science research has clearly shown that impaired performance and eventual loss of skill and ability are likely if neural circuits are not consistently activated by functional activity. This is the underlying assumption of the learned nonuse theory that forms the foundation for constraint-induced therapy targeting upper extremity use for adults and children with hemiplegia.[304,305] Furthermore, a similar concept has been proposed to explain the decline in muscle performance and endurance observed in individuals with a sedentary lifestyle or those confined to bed rest.[306] During the early stages of rehabilitation, individuals with CNS dysfunction or disease may develop compensatory or alternative movement strategies that are less difficult or frustrating, considering the alterations in brain function and the resulting paresis or altered muscle tone.[197,202] However, these different movement patterns also affect muscle performance and flexibility, increasing the likelihood of developing secondary impairments. Thus over time, not only is neural circuitry necessary for normal movement degrade but also the individual's physical resources for movement change. Both of these factors reinforce the altered or abnormal movement pattern and the loss of premorbid skill and activity.

Use It and Improve It

Animal models consistently show that, in both nonimpaired and impaired circumstances, consistent or extended training induces cortical plasticity as evidenced by reorganization of cortical motor and sensory mapping and synaptogenesis.[307] The expectation is that behavioral experience will optimize neural plasticity in humans as well.[290] Participating in extended training (i.e., practice, experience) of specific skills and functions enhances performance in areas of the brain associated with those functions; this is the outcome expectation for constraint-induced therapy and task-specific paradigms used in stroke, brain injury, and spinal cord injury rehabilitation programs.[304,308,309]

Specificity Is Significant

In humans, the acquisition of particular motor skills (e.g., finger tapping) through physical practice leads to changes in neural activity only in particular areas of the motor cortex and cerebellum (e.g., areas mapped to hand and fingers) as evidenced on functional magnetic imaging.[310] This demonstrates that the training experience that leads to the acquisition of a specific behavioral skill determines the resulting type and extent of plasticity. Task-specific training has been evaluated extensively as an intervention for recovery of upper extremity function and of locomotion after stroke.[311,312] It is important to note, however, that neuroplastic changes associated with training of one skill do not necessarily contribute to improvement in other skills or changes in other areas of the brain. Nonskilled movement appears to have little, if any, impact on neural plasticity.

Repetition, Repetition, and Repetition

One successful performance of a motor task does not mean that the task has been skillfully mastered. In motor learning, evidence of mastery is the transition to automaticity.[113,174] An individual moves toward automaticity only after many practice sessions. Sufficient repetition of new or relearned behaviors is necessary for neuroplastic changes to become well established.[186] The underlying assumption is that the outcome of such repetition is the establishment of neural circuitry that makes the effectively learned behavior less likely to decay over time when practice is infrequent.[287] The role of repetition for driving learning and neural plasticity is a critical one.

In the context of rehabilitation after stroke, spinal cord injury, and multiple sclerosis, body weight–supported treadmill (TM) training is specifically designed to enable repeated practice of locomotion, which may not be feasible during early stages of recovery when walking without assistance is challenging.[313,314] TM training has the added benefit of inducing cardiopulmonary/cardiovascular fitness, adding to overall resources for movement available to the individual whose CNS dysfunction may carry an associated secondary risk of deconditioning. [315]

Intensity Is Important

In persons without brain injury, training intensity (dose, number of repetitions, number of practice sessions) influences both degree and stability of the neuroplastic change induced by practice.[287] Both constraint-induced therapy for upper extremity rehabilitation and TM training for the recovery of locomotion are high-intensity interventions. Although the optimal "dosage" for rehabilitation intervention is not well defined and may differ across diagnoses, mounting evidence suggests that outcomes of intervention are influenced by dose, with high-intensity programs having the largest effect.[316] Rehabilitation interventions that span a duration of 4 to 5 weeks appear to yield greater improvements in upper limb impairments in stroke survivors. Interestingly, the duration of individual sessions, specifically those lasting less than 60 minutes, does not appear to have a significant impact on the upper limb recovery.[293] Intensity includes a high number of repetitions and high frequency of practice sessions.[183,293] Current rehabilitation practice models do not always provide the number of repetitions or dose intensity that might be necessary to induce neural plasticity and cortical reorganization.[317] Much of the research on intensity of intervention has involved persons who are medically stable and in the chronic period after their neurologic event. These individuals appear to tolerate intense interventions with little adverse consequence. What is not well understood, however, is whether there may be sensitivity to overuse in newly injured brains that is detrimental after a threshold level of repetitions is exceeded.[287,318] In the absence of guidelines about level intensity for persons with recent CNS insult, careful monitoring for signs of activity intolerance of the brain and body (e.g., fatigue, irritability, distractibility, change in attention or alertness, and a greater-than-anticipated decrement in performance, among others) may assist the therapist in keeping the intensity of intervention within safe ranges.

Time and Timing

There are many molecular, cellular, structural, and physiologic contributors to the process of neuroplasticity; the relationships and timing of changes at each of these levels continue to be explored.[287] Consolidation of motor memory, for example, requires "offline" time after practice for a newly learned skill to be effectively retained.[299] As in development, there may be windows of opportunity within the typical pattern of recovery when interventions targeting neuroplasticity are likely to be most effective.[317,318] Delaying intervention (or providing intervention at suboptimal levels of intensity) may allow abnormal compensatory movement patterns to become established, thus rendering rehabilitation less effective.[287] Interestingly, in individuals who have experienced an acute stroke, early mobilization should be considered within 24 hours following the onset of the attack.[319] Certainly, there is much more investigation needed regarding when neuroplasticity-focused rehabilitation intervention would be best implemented during the course of recovery following CNS insult.

Salience Is Substantial

Neural plasticity cannot be effectively induced in a well-practiced activity unless the individual perceives it as meaningful and important. The motivation, attention, and ability to learn are influenced by the relevance of and perception of potential reward associated with a specific movement task.[302] Participating in rehabilitation interventions that are based on motor learning and neural plasticity requires a significant investment of effort from the patient.[277] If the goal and level of effort needed to achieve it outweigh the perceived potential benefits or rewards of participation, is it any wonder that little will be accomplished in terms of skill development or facilitation of neural plasticity? It is essential that there be discussion and, optimally, consensus between the individual and the therapist about the likelihood of improved functional performance at a level that the individual perceives as valuable and important as a result of intervention. Increased motivation is noted in individuals who are allowed some choice and control over interventions and when collaboration with the therapist is embedded into treatment planning.[11] Attention to task and intrinsic motivation strengthen learning when individual goals are connected to tasks.[300] Furthermore, the salience or meaningfulness of a task appears to impact motor learning and recovery through the cholinergic system of the basal ganglia.[320]

Considering the Life Span

Although the brain is clearly most "plastic" in early life—during periods of rapid motor, perceptual, and cognitive development—the brains of older adults continue to be responsive to experience-driven catalysts of neural plasticity.[321–324] Rich physical, emotional, and cognitive experiences over the life span appear to protect the older individual against decrements in brain function typically thought to be the result of aging.[325,326] There are differences in the process of motor learning and neural plasticity, however, at both ends of the life span. Children may require longer periods of practice and a more gradual reduction in frequency of feedback for effective motor learning than adults to effect neuroplastic change and the consolidation of newly learned skills.[327] Older adults also require longer periods of practice and increased number of repetitions, especially when they are attempting to replace competing compensatory movement strategies after CNS insult.[328] When such individuals are compared with younger adults, the efficacy of the motor learning process (and by extension, neural plasticity) appears to be somewhat less for older adults in both acquisition and retention of skilled sequential movements and retention.[329] This may be associated with age-related declines in visuospatial working memory and attentional focus.[330] Nevertheless, older adults with stroke and other CNS diseases do respond to appropriately targeted complex motor skill training, demanding environmental contexts, and exercise interventions in both the acquisition and reinforcement of skilled movement.[313,331–333]

Transference

Kleim and Jones[287] refer to the ability of plastic changes in one set of neural circuits to enhance concurrent or future neuroplastic changes in other neuronal circuits. Incorporating repetitive transcranial magnetic stimulation or EMG-triggered/controlled neuromuscular electrical stimulation to physical practice of salient motor skills appears to enhance acquisition and retention of motor skills and promote more extensive restoration of function during both acute and chronic stages of stroke recovery.[294,334] Animal studies suggest that living and functioning in complex enriched environments may also potentiate neuroplastic changes in the cortex after brain injury.[335] In humans, both enriched environments and physical exercise appear to have a potentiating neuroplastic effect on the damaged brain, brainstem, cerebellum, and spinal cord, contributing to angiogenesis mediated by the release of brain-derived neurotrophic factors during activity.[336,337] Further studies are needed to evaluate the effects of environmental enrichment on motor function, activity, and participation following a stroke.[338] Repetitive physical activity and exercise during rehabilitation hold significant potential to enhance neural plasticity and improve muscle performance, as well as enhance cardiovascular and cardiopulmonary conditioning. The principle of transference has been the basis for recent works aimed at investigating if motor training could lead to improvements in other related behaviors. For example, Pournajaf et al.[339] reported improvements in gait and postural outcomes in individuals with total knee replacement who underwent a nonimmersive virtual reality–based serious games rehabilitation program. Moreover, promising evidence suggests that respiratory training with intermittent positive-pressure breathing ventilation in individuals with brain injury may lead to improvements in dysphonia and dysarthria.[340]

Interference

Just as some neuroplastic changes enable reorganization in the process of transference, they also may block, interfere with, or otherwise impede operation or reorganization of other circuits, with a negative impact on the ability to learn.[287] Kleim and Jones[287] define interference as the ability of plasticity in a particular neural circuit to impede the generation of novel circuits or enactment of established circuits. How does this translate into rehabilitation? The clearest example is the detrimental impact that self-discovered compensatory movement strategies (a neuroplastic change in which persons with stroke have learned to move functionally using alternate movement strategies) have on learning more effective strategies of movement during therapy.[197,202] This interference has also been demonstrated in persons with acute or chronic pain who have learned to move in ways that avoid discomfort but are not kinematically effective and are associated with likelihood of additional dysfunction.[341,342]

Neuroplastic interference as described by Kleim and Jones[287] is a different concept than the contextual interference that occurs during random practice discussed earlier in the chapter as a facilitator of motor learning. Contextual interference occurs as a result of the need to keep many options that might solve a motor problem available in working memory over time.[182,203] The increased attentional demand associated with contextual interference appears to augment, rather than interfere with, the learning (and hence the neuroplastic) process.[208–210] From a motor learning perspective, neuroplastic interference might occur if the type of practice or feedback provided during a rehabilitation session is not appropriate for a learner's specific needs or characteristics.[343,344] Another example of neuroplastic interference might be the impact of learning of an additional novel complex motor task soon after practice of a newly learned complex motor task; having little offline time may interfere with motor memory consolidation of the newly learned task.[345]

A history of trauma can add an obstacle to the restoration of normal motor control by causing interference in neuroplasticity. In persons with FMD, learning is negatively affected because of the influence of priors, or past trauma, on the active inference process. "Top-down" predictions about "bottom-up" sensory input become invalid; there is a failure of inference.[346] Consequently, the resulting movements appear purposeful but deviate from neuroanatomic and physiologic constraints. However, individuals with FMD report a lack of control or agency over these movements.[50] The rehabilitation professional is challenged with selecting the best task, environment, and feedback to promote the reestablishment of normal motor control. To address FMD, current literature suggests diverting attention away from the specific motor task during rehabilitation interventions.[50,53]

Task Success Reinforcement

One additional principle has been identified by Mowase et al. in a 2017 study.[303] It was found that when a person receives internal reinforcement through successful performance of a newly learned motor task during trials, plasticity changes occur in the motor cortex. This was termed use-dependent plasticity (UDP). UDP was observed significantly more often in participants who experienced success reinforcement than in those who did not.[303] This may suggest that successful performance during learning trials reinforces the learning, which in turn increases plasticity.[302]

AEROBIC EXERCISE, NEUROPLASTICITY, AND NEUROPROTECTION

Exercise may be a rehabilitation professional's most potent tool for facilitating neural plasticity.

Notably neural plasticity plays a key role not only in neurological disorders but also in musculoskeletal impairments.[347] Fitness (aerobic) exercise causes a cascade of events, at both molecular and cellular levels, that support the health and development of neural circuits.[348] This is thought to be due to the interplay of central and peripheral mechanisms supporting energy metabolism and homeostasis.[349,350] During and for a short time following a bout of aerobic exercise, the level of circulating neurotrophic factors increases and is more available for support of neuroplastic and neuroprotective changes in the brain.[46,348,351] Resistance (strengthening) exercise does not lead to the degree of increase in neurotrophic factors that aerobic exercise does.[352] While rehabilitation professionals commonly recommend aerobic exercise to enhance functional capacity and activity tolerance, we may overlook its potential impact on the brain's readiness to learn. As mentioned earlier in the chapter, engaging in exercise prior to motor task practice can aid in the enhanced detection and encoding of information relevant to the task. Similarly, participating in exercise immediately following motor task practice strengthens the motor memory process.[46] These are two powerful reasons that aerobic activity should be included in plans of care for all persons with CNS dysfunction as well as any individual who must develop new motor skills (e.g., learning to walk with a prosthesis).

Participation in TM training during rehabilitation after stroke or incomplete spinal cord injury enhances motor learning and neural plasticity in several ways: it is task specific, provides repetitive practice at high dosage, builds cardiovascular/cardiopulmonary fitness, and (as a result) readies the brain for functional modification of neural circuits.[313,348] Aerobic fitness is associated with greater neuroplasticity and better cognitive performance in persons with multiple sclerosis.[353,354] There is growing evidence that aerobic exercise can enhance motor performance, improve quality of life, decrease caregiver burden,[355] and possibly slow progression of mobility impairment in persons with Parkinson disease.[356–358] Current animal model research demonstrates upregulation of neurotrophic factors through aerobic exercise that may contribute to dopaminergic survival in those with Parkinson disease. It is not yet clear whether forced intensity of aerobic exercise provides more benefit than self-selected intensity in terms of sustained improvements in motor performance and function for persons with Parkinson disease.[359,360] Engaging in a single session of fitness exercise appears to transiently improve cognitive function in older adults. Furthermore, participation in habitual cardiovascular fitness training appears to have a neuroprotective effect on cognition and enhance learning abilities during the later stages of life.[361–363] The neuroplastic and neuroprotective effect of aerobic conditioning also appears to improve or stabilize cognitive function and learning in persons with mild cognitive impairment and dementia.[364–368]

Considering the current evidence regarding the potential of aerobic exercise to potentiate and protect brain well-being and function, it is crucial for rehabilitation programs to include a fitness or conditioning element. Neglecting this aspect might lead to a missed chance of improving motor learning and restoring functionality. This applies to persons with neurologic problems as well as those who may be learning to use an orthosis or prosthesis as a result of neuromuscular and musculoskeletal impairment from trauma, overuse, or disease.[369]

Application: Case Examples

The following case examples are presented as opportunities for readers to apply the information presented in this chapter. Readers are urged to take time to develop an appropriate plan of care/therapeutic intervention within the framework of the ICF model, using the interactive person-task-environment (systems model) framework of motor control and the context of the modified version of Gentile's Taxonomy of Movement Tasks presented in the chapter.

Furthermore, readers are encouraged to consider the principles of exercise/activity-based neuroplasticity, which include setting relevant goals to engage the patient, establishing practice conditions that provide an appropriate level of challenge, and providing feedback to facilitate effective motor learning and the acquisition of skills. These considerations also contribute to the development of self-efficacy, as discussed in earlier sections.

QUESTIONS TO CONSIDER

The authors suggest that readers consider the following strategies and questions to guide their planning.

Functional Considerations

- What tasks or activities are most appropriate or important to address in developing a physical therapy plan of care for the individual described in the case? (Prioritize three or four tasks to be targeted by physical therapy intervention.)
- How can the therapist incorporate the goals and priorities of the person into the development of goals and plan of care to make it salient?
- Motor control considerations.
- What resources/buffers and impairments/constraints does this individual bring to the situation? In what ways are these helpful or constraining, given the person's neuromotor and musculoskeletal condition, cognitive and emotional status, and level of fitness?
- What is the nature of the tasks that have been selected (stability, mobility, or quasimobility with or without object manipulation)? What are the foundational skills necessary to perform the task? What skills or abilities may be difficult, given the impairments/constraints described in the case? What skills are most feasible to improve to increase patient competence?
- Under what environmental conditions would this individual be best able to function at this time (closed/predictable versus open/variable)? In what type of

environment does this individual need to be able to eventually function? How might you manipulate activities and environmental conditions to achieve function in the real environment to set an appropriate level of challenge?

- What is the emotional context of the environment? Can you manipulate the emotional context to facilitate better learning conditions? Does your patient require more "emotional press" to problem solve with you on the task? Does your patient require a stressful environmental context to be reduced to have an appropriate ready-to-learn context? Does the patient require encouragement and validation of success to increase confidence?
- How might you organize/prioritize a sequence of activities, using the modified Gentile's Taxonomy of Movement Tasks (stability/transitional/mobility), to prepare or progress the individual toward safe independent function in the least restrictive environment?

Motor Learning Issues

Identify the purpose of the task trials that will be designed by the therapist.

- Is this a task that needs to be acquired (or reacquired postamputation or postincidence), or is this a task that needs to be refined?
- At what stage of motor learning is the individual in relation to the defined task?
- Does the individual have an understanding or familiarity with the task, or is it completely novel?
- Is current task performance sufficient for the task to be functional?
- Is performance efficient or optimal?
- Is performance automated, and does it demonstrate desired variability? Can the individual use a variety of motor strategies to accomplish or address this task under changing environmental demands?
- Can this task be broken into discrete parts? Would it be better to practice the task as a whole? Why or why not?
- Is performance of a particular part of the task problematic (mechanics of the task, fluidity between the components of the task)?
- Is performance of the task as a whole problematic (completion, speed, and endurance)?
- On the basis of your thoughts about the task trials, identify the best practice conditions for achieving the desired outcome.
- Is the primary goal of practice *retention (learning)* of motor behavior across practice sessions or *improving performance* within a practice session?
- Which practice condition or combination of practice conditions (blocked, random, or serial; massed or distributed; part- or whole-task training) would you use to assist retention of the skill? Why have you chosen these strategies?
- Which practice condition or combination of practice conditions (blocked, random, or serial; massed or distributed; part- or whole-task training) would assist improved performance *(competence)*? Why have you chosen these strategies?
- How might contextual interference influence the learning process?
- What type of augmented information should be included during practice of the tasks to achieve the desired outcome?
- What modes of information should be used for this individual (visual cues and demonstration, verbal prompting, physical prompt/facilitation)? Why has this augmented information strategy or combination of strategies been selected?
- What effect will the information have on the client's ability to recognize errors and self-correct motor behavior *(intrinsic feedback)*?
- What delivery scheme (KR or KP) should be used to provide augmented feedback?
- What is the anticipated effect of the selected delivery scheme (KR or KP) on retention versus performance of the motor skill being targeted?
- Can visual imagery or mental practice enhance the performance? What images would a rehabilitation professional want the client to visualize? What effect will imagery have on performance and on retention of the motor skill?
- What components can the client practice mentally? What effect will mental practice have on performance and on retention of the motor skill?
- How can the therapist incorporate understanding of neural plasticity into goal-directed activity and intervention? What strategies can be used to validate success and increase self-efficacy?
- Are the activities and tasks included in the plan of care sufficient in repetition and intensity to appropriately challenge the patient and influence neural plasticity?
- What evidence is available to guide decisions about potential windows of opportunity to time intervention for optimal neuroplastic effect in patients with similar diagnoses?
- How should the plan of care be influenced by the age of the patient in terms of facilitation of motor learning and neural plasticity?
- What additional medical interventions, environmental conditions, or principles of exercise can potentiate motor learning and neural plasticity for recovery of function?

Summary

This chapter explores the concepts that shape current understanding of human motor control, focusing on the dynamic and adaptive characteristics of the body as a biologic system. Rehabilitation professionals use their understanding of (1) an individual's resources and characteristics, (2) environmental conditions, and (3) the nature and constraints of functional tasks to design appropriate interventions aimed at enhancing or adapting an individual's ability to move effectively, safely, and efficiently, enabling them to accomplish what is personally meaningful.

This chapter also delves the process of motor learning, which encompasses how individuals acquire skills for novel tasks or adjust their approach to familiar tasks in different environmental conditions, or after experiencing injury or illness that affects their abilities. By understanding the stages of motor learning, the purpose of augmented information, types and timing of feedback/feedforward information, and types of practice conditions and other factors that optimize motor learning, physical therapists and other rehabilitation professionals can construct effective interventions. These interventions promote better retention of motor learning and refine performance for individuals with movement dysfunction.

This chapter concludes with a discussion of the emerging field of neuroplasticity, which connects the recovery of motor control and motor learning. It considers rehabilitation as a mechanism to trigger neural plasticity and recovery of function following insult or injury to the CNS. As our understanding of neuroplasticity evolves, rehabilitation professionals must reassess whether the interventions designed to enhance motor learning are also capable of driving neural plasticity and facilitating recovery of function for individuals facing events and diseases that impact the structure and function of the brain.

References

The complete listing of the References are available in the accompanying enhanced eBook version included with the print purchase of this textbook. Visit Elsevier eBooks+ (eBooks.Health.Elsevier.com) to access this content.

Case Example 3.1 **Adult With Right Hemiparesis Who Is Learning to Use an Ankle-Foot Orthosis and Ambulatory Assistive Device**

A.F. is a slightly obese 78-year-old African American female with a history of type 2 diabetes mellitus; she had an ischemic stroke of the left middle cerebral artery 3 weeks earlier. A computed tomography scan revealed a lacunar-shaped infarct from an embolic occlusion of a deep branch of the middle cerebral artery serving the internal capsule. A.F. was recently transferred to a skilled nursing facility for rehabilitation, particularly to address transfers and ambulation. She had received a prefabricated solid ankle-foot orthosis (AFO) just before her arrival. She says that the brace is intended to help control her "bad knee" and "lazy foot" position so she can walk better. She has not had much opportunity to use the orthosis and is concerned that it may actually make it more difficult for her to walk. She indicates that she prefers to use a rolling walker, although her therapist in the hospital insisted that she use a straight cane.

Chart review, interview, and physical therapy examination reveal the following:

- *Psychosocial*: A.F. lives alone in a two-story walk-up apartment. Her immediate family lives out of state. She retired 10 years ago from a position as a legal secretary and is heavily involved in the outreach ministry of her evangelical church.
- *Baseline vital signs*: heart rate: 82 beats/min; blood pressure: 132/94 mm Hg; respiratory rate: 16 breaths/min.
- *Cognitive status*: alert and oriented times 3.
- *Communication*: some slurring of words; has trouble finding the words she wants to say, but comprehension appears intact.
- *Vision*: intact; typically wears trifocals.
- *Sensory system*: cranial nerves intact; normal responses to light touch, pin prick, proprioception in all extremities.
- *Neuromotor status: See details below.*
- *Tone*: moderate spasticity of right (R) upper extremity (UE) and lower extremity (LE); 1+ on the Modified Ashworth Scale.
- *Range of motion (ROM)*: Passive ROM within normal limits for all extremities.
- *Strength:* L extremities 4+/5 throughout.
- *R UE:* shoulder elevation 2+/5; hand grip 2/5; elbow flexion 2/5; *R LE:* function strength grades include ankle plantarflexion 3/5; ankle dorsiflexion 1/5; knee extension 2+/5; knee flexion 3/5; hip flexion 3/5; hip extension 3/5; hip abduction 3/5; and hip adduction 3+/5.
- *Postural control*: able to sit upright against gravity, asymmetric weight distribution with more weight borne on left side. Anticipatory posture changes are adequate when reaching toward right, inadequate when reaching toward left. Stands with supervision; requires verbal and tactile cues to bear weight on R LE.
- *Functional activities*: rolls independently to both sides; supine to sit over edge of bed with supervision; transfers from bed to wheelchair with supervision; sit-to-stand transitions with supervision.
- *Ambulation:* uses straight cane with moderate assist, requiring both verbal cueing and physical prompt to improve loading response on right leg and to minimize genu recurvatum during forward advancement over right foot.

Goal: Design a physical therapy plan of care that will focus on the development of motor skills necessary for safe and efficient locomotion using the AFO and straight cane.

Case Example 3.2 **Child With Cerebral Palsy Who Has Just Received New (Bilateral) Articulating Ankle-Foot Orthoses**

T.D. is a delightful 2½-year-old boy with cerebral palsy and spastic diplegia of moderate severity. He was born prematurely at 27 weeks' gestation and remained in the neonatal intensive care unit for 10 weeks. By the time he was 18 months old, there were increasing indications of developmental delay and abnormal motor control. He currently attends an early intervention program (EIP), receives individual home visits from a physical therapist, and attends a therapeutic playgroup run by an educator and occupational therapist weekly.

EIP examination findings include the following:

- *Social:* T.D. lives with both parents and an older brother in a two-story, single-family home. He interacts well with his family members and is on target for social development. He plays side by side with peers and occasionally interacts with them appropriately.
- *Cognition:* T.D. scores age appropriately for cognitive tasks including cause and effect, object permanence, means to end, early numeration, and sorting by categories. His play with objects includes variety and imagination.

- *Language:* T.D.'s comprehension, expression, and pragmatic use of language are on target for his age. He has an extensive vocabulary and uses language appropriately in various situations.
- *Fine motor/activities of daily living (ADLs):* T.D.'s reach, grasp, and release skills are within the age-expected range. Bimanual skills and object manipulation are also on target. Feeding skills are appropriate; T.D. uses utensils and drinks from a cup as expected for his age. His dressing skills are slightly below age expectations largely because of balance concerns in standing for putting on pants.
- *Gross motor:* T.D.'s gross motor skills fall below age expectations. He has been walking independently with bilateral solid ankle-foot orthoses (AFOs) for 6 months. He can walk on multiple terrains including tile or wood floors, carpets, grass, asphalt, and wood chips. He has some difficulty with stairs, requiring a railing or one hand held. Tripping and falling are issues with increasing speeds during ambulation and with attempts at running. T.D.'s mother is most concerned about his safety in ambulation at this point.

T.D. was having increasing difficulty with squatting and transitioning into and out of standing from the floor. The rehabilitation team, discussing the problem, decided that articulating AFOs would increase the availability of ankle range of motion for these transition tasks. T.D. just received bilateral articulating AFOs with a plantarflexion stop set at 10 degrees. He is currently having trouble descending stairs in the new orthoses, refusing to go down stairs unless both hands are held. He also has increased frequency of tripping outside while ambulating on the grass and rock driveway at home.

Goal: Design a physical therapy plan of care to help T.D. master locomotion and transitional activities with the less constraining articulating AFOs in the environments of a typical 2½-year-old child.

Case Example 3.3 **Child With Congenital Upper Limb Deficiency Learning to Use a Myoelectric Prosthesis**

T.L. is a 3-year-old girl who has had a congenital right upper extremity limb deficiency since birth. She has an intact humerus and musculature of the upper limb with a functional elbow joint. Her forearm is incomplete, with a shortened ulna, missing radius, and no wrist or hand complex. T.L. has been wearing a prosthesis with a passive terminal device since she was 6 months old and uses her prosthesis well in mobility tasks and to stabilize objects against her body or a support surface during bimanual activities. T.L. began a preschool program 2 months ago and has adjusted well to socialization. She engages in play with her peers appropriately. She has good functional use of her left upper extremity (intact limb) and uses the residual limb to assist herself in tasks, particularly for stabilizing objects.

T.L. has been working with her prosthetist and therapists to learn to use a two-channel (voluntary closing/voluntary opening) myoelectrically controlled terminal device for the past 2 weeks. When she wears the myoelectric prosthesis throughout the day, she primarily uses it as she did her previous passive prosthesis. She has not attempted to use the "hand" for play or activities of daily living unless prompted by her parents or therapists. During her therapy sessions, she is intrigued with her new ability to open and close her "hand" but is inconsistent in controlling force of grasp and has difficulty initiating release. In today's session, she practiced picking up 1-inch blocks and placing them in a bowl, achieving the desired result in two of five trials. She was unsuccessful (and became frustrated) at picking up pegs that were much narrower than the blocks. The rehabilitation team's goals for T.L. include functional use of the prosthesis for grasp and release of household objects for feeding and self-care and school objects for play and participation in preschool activities. The team would like to increase the use of bimanual manipulation of various-sized objects.

Goal: Design a rehabilitation plan of care to help T.L. master grasp and release of objects of various sizes and levels of durability in activities meaningful for a 3-year-old child.

Case Example 3.4 **Adolescent With Transtibial Amputation Working on Returning to Competition in Track Events**

W.P. is a 16-year-old junior in high school who has been a star track athlete since he was a freshman. He currently holds his high school records in the 100- and 200-m events, which he achieved during his sophomore year. He also finished third in the state championships that same year.

Three months ago, during the summer, W.P. was seriously injured when the garden tractor/lawnmower he was operating rolled over and down an embankment as he was making a fast turn while mowing the lawn. He sustained deep lacerations to his right foot and lower leg from the mower's blade as well as third-degree burns from the muffler. His injured limb was pinned under the tractor in a pile of leaves and debris. In the emergency department, trauma surgeons concluded that he did not meet the criteria for limb salvage and performed a long open transtibial amputation. After an intensive course of antibiotics, W.P. returned to the operating room a week later for closure to the standard transtibial level with equal anterior/posterior flaps. When his residual limb healed without difficulty, W.P. was fitted with a patellar tendon-bearing prosthesis with a sleeve and pin suspension and a Seattle Systems dynamic response foot. He quickly mastered ambulation without an assistive device and returned to school in the winter of his junior year.

W.P. is eager to return to track for his senior year. His prosthetist has fabricated a special prosthesis for him to wear in competition, an Otto Bock Healthcare Sprinter prosthetic foot designed for track-and-field athletes. He has begun training for his events and is pleased that he can run again. He has two goals: to decrease his performance time (hoping to meet the records he set the previous year) and to become much more efficient at leaving the starting block. He wants to master the new prosthesis this year so that he can concentrate on conditioning for his senior year.

Goal: Develop a prosthetic training regimen focusing on improving W.P.'s performance as he prepares to return to track competition.

4 Evidence-Based Approach to Orthotic and Prosthetic Rehabilitation

RENÉE M. HUTH AND KEVIN K. CHUI

LEARNING OBJECTIVES

On completion of this chapter, the reader will be able to do the following:

1. Describe the basic principles of evidence-based practice and apply these principles to orthotic and prosthetic rehabilitation.
2. Ask well-formulated, clearly defined, and clinically important questions applicable to orthotic and prosthetic rehabilitation.
3. Efficiently locate meaningful research specific to orthotic and prosthetic rehabilitation.
4. Critically appraise the evidence for reliability, validity, and clinical importance.
5. Use the orthotic and prosthetic research evidence to make evidence-based clinical judgments that affect your practice.
6. Describe strategies to encourage practitioners to engage in greater use of evidence to inform holistic clinical decision-making and thus practice.

What Is Evidence-Based Practice?

This chapter provides the tools to support the evidence-based practitioner of contemporary practice. Providing effective health and rehabilitative care requires that practitioners be well-informed about advances in assessment, medical management, technology, theory, and effective rehabilitation interventions. Relying on experience is not enough. An evidenced-based health provider regularly updates their knowledge base by accessing the current practices generated by professionals in their field and beyond.[1] Challenges to remaining current include lack of time, resources, and dated skills to accurately locate, appraise, and apply scientific evidence.[1] Healthcare professionals who routinely access current and research their practice demonstrate improved quality of care with earlier access and referrals to improved outcome measures helping patients realize their full potential of function to engage in life.[2,3]

David Sackett, MD, the father of evidence-based medicine, described this approach as the "integration of best research evidence with clinical expertise and patient values."[4] Evidence-based practice (EBP) is a broader concept that applies Sackett's physician-oriented concepts to a wide range of health professions. Both models identify three major elements of evidence that are interactive and valuable, as well as a set of skills necessary to integrate each resource into an effective and informed clinical decision (Fig. 4.1). The three major elements are the following:

1. Best available information from up-to-date, clinically relevant research.
2. The skilled and experienced practitioner who can accurately perform diagnostic procedures and interventions, integrate findings to efficiently determine correct diagnosis, and engage in reflective clinical practice.
3. The integration of the patient or family issues and psychosocial concerns into the care plan.[5–8]

To make an informed clinical decision, the evidence-based rehabilitation professional must possess the skills to do the following:

1. Effectively search for and access relevant scientific evidence in the professional literature.[2,3,9]
2. Assess the strength and value of the scientific evidence that will support the decision to be made.[3]
3. Apply the results of an accurate clinical examination and the evidence from the literature in the process of diagnosis, evaluation, prognosis, and development of an appropriate plan of care.[10]
4. Assess and incorporate the patient's or client's values, knowledge, preferences, and motivation into the intervention and anticipated outcomes[8,11]

Process of Evidence-Based Practice

EBP is essentially an orientation to clinical decision-making that incorporates the best available sources of evidence into the process of assessment, intervention planning, and evaluation of outcomes. The skill set necessary for effective EBP develops over time, with practice and experience.

An EBP approach to the scientific literature is a systematic process with four primary steps.[1,3,4,12]

1. Posing a well-formulated, clinically important question.
2. Locating meaningful research that is well-targeted to the question (i.e., developing effective and efficient search strategies).
3. Critically appraising the available evidence for validity and clinical importance.
4. Using the findings to make an evidence-based clinical judgment about examination or intervention options based on the clinical relevance of the information applied to the needs of the individual patient.

Step 1: Formulating an Answerable Clinical Question

The questions posed by researchers and the questions posed by clinicians, although similar in many respects, are asked and answered at quite different levels. Research questions

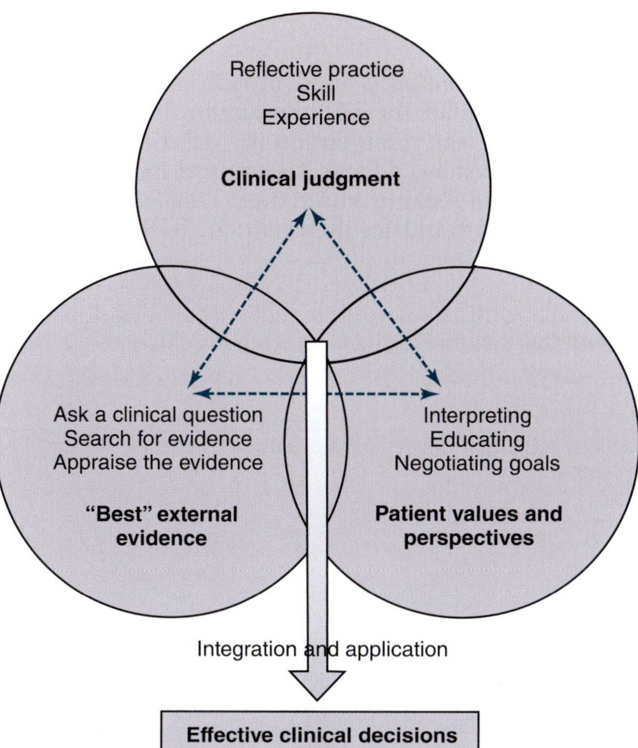

Fig. 4.1 Model of three essential and interactive components necessary for effective evidence-based healthcare approach to guide clinical decision-making, as well as the dimensions of each.

P	Patient	Patient diagnostic category or key characteristic
I	Intervention	Treatment group, diagnostic tool, or prognostic marker
C	Comparison	Applicable if comparison is wanted between or among interventions, diagnostic tools, or prognostic markers
O	Outcome	What is the outcome of interest: presence of disease? Impairment? Functional limitation? Disability?

Fig. 4.2 The PICO system for formulating clinical questions includes consideration of the patient (*P*) who is receiving care; the intervention (*I*) being considered; and, if available, the reference standard with which it is being compared (*C*) and the anticipated outcomes (*O*) (positive and negative) of the intervention being considered.

combine information from groups (samples) of individuals to develop evidence about relationships among characteristics, effectiveness of examination strategies, or effectiveness of intervention strategies for the group as a whole.[13] In contrast, clinical questions seek to apply this knowledge to a single person with individual characteristics.[2–4,9] For example, clinicians ask, "Which examination strategy will provide the information most important for the clinical decision-making process for this particular individual?" and "Which intervention is likely to have the optimal outcome for this particular individual?"

The first essential step in the EBP process is developing a well-formulated, clinically important question. Sackett identifies two categories of clinical questions: broad background questions and specifically focused foreground questions.[4] *Background questions* expand our knowledge or understanding of a disorder, impairment, or functional limitation; they are often concerned with etiology, diagnosis, prognosis, or typical clinical course. Patients and their family members often ask healthcare practitioners background questions. Answers to background questions expand the general knowledge base used in clinical decision-making. Students and novice clinicians ask many background questions as they develop expertise in their field. Even expert clinicians routinely need to seek answers to basic background questions when they encounter an unfamiliar pathologic condition or novel category of intervention. However, answers to background questions do not provide the specific evidence necessary to make individualized patient care decisions. Examples of broad background questions that might be asked by clinicians providing prosthetic and orthotic rehabilitation care include the following:

- What is the typical postsurgical rehabilitation program following a dysvascular transtibial amputation?
- What is peripheral arterial disease, and why can it lead to limb amputation?
- What neurologic functions are affected by a C7 spinal cord injury?
- What are the typical motor milestones of the first 2 years of life, and when is the achievement of these milestones considered delayed?

Foreground questions, in contrast, seek specific information to help guide management for an individual patient.[2–4,9,12] The most effective way to frame an answerable foreground clinical question follows the PICO model (Fig. 4.2). It identifies the patient population of interest (P), noting specific characteristics (e.g., age, sex diagnosis, acuity, and severity) that will link the evidence to the patient care situation prompting the question. It then identifies the predictive factor, examination, or intervention (I) that is being considered. If appropriate, it identifies what comparisons (C) are being made to inform the choice of examination or intervention. Finally, it clearly defines the outcomes (O) that might be expected for the given patient on the basis of the best available evidence. Using the PICO model,[14,15] foreground questions that rehabilitation professionals might ask as they care for a specific individual in need of a prosthesis or orthosis include the following:

- How much does advanced age (I) affect the ability to become a functional ambulator (O) in an individual who has a dysvascular transtibial amputation (P)?
- Does supported treadmill gait training (I) improve ambulation endurance with a prosthesis (O) in older patients with dysvascular transtibial amputation (P)?
- Does the addition of functional neuromuscular stimulation (I) to a typical early rehabilitation intervention (C) enhance active muscle control (O) in individuals with incomplete spinal cord injury (P)?
- What factors predict (I) ambulation ability (O) in a young child with spastic diplegic cerebral palsy (P)?

PATIENT CHARACTERISTICS

A well-focused clinical question narrows the scope of possible patient characteristics to ones most applicable to a specific clinical problem or situation.[4,12] It defines the key characteristics that will best differentially guide the search for evidence. Characteristics of categories that help to focus a clinical question related to orthotic or prosthetic management are summarized in Table 4.1.

INTERVENTION

The term *intervention* is used broadly in the evidence-based literature. In the EBP paradigm, the intervention (I) and comparison intervention (C), described according to the PICO system, refer to the central issue for which the clinician is seeking an answer. This issue can typically revolve around an intervention, a diagnosis, or a prognosis.

Table 4.1 Patient Characteristics That May Be Used to Help Focus Literature Searches for Prosthetic and Orthotic Rehabilitation

Domain	Characteristics	Search Terms
Underlying condition	Etiology	Acquired (traumatic injury, infectious process, autoimmune disease, ischemia, vascular disease, neoplasm, cancer)
		Congenital condition
		Developmental delay
		Hereditary disease
	Systems affected	Musculoskeletal
		Neuromuscular
		Cardiovascular
		Pulmonary, respiratory
		Integumentary
		Endocrine
		Systemic physiologic
	Nature of condition	Chronic
		Progressive
		Degenerative
		Developmental
		Requiring remediation
		Requiring accommodation
	Comorbid conditions	Peripheral vascular disease
		Diabetes mellitus
		Systemic infections
		Cancer care, chemotherapy, radiation
		Heart disease
		Pulmonary disease
		Obesity
		Depression, anxiety
		Cognitive dysfunction
		Smoking
	Confounding factors	Alcohol use
		Other substance abuse
		Nutritional status
Lifespan development	Age category	Infant
		Toddler
		School-age child
		Adolescent
		Young adult
		Midlife adult
		Older adult
Psychosocial Health	Individual health and well-being	Mental
		Emotional
		Physical
		Social well-being
		Sense of community

Table 4.1 Patient Characteristics That May Be Used to Help Focus Literature Searches for Prosthetic and Orthotic Rehabilitation—Cont'd

Domain	Characteristics	Search Terms
Interpersonal Health		Roles Responsibilities Caregiver Community Service
Physical Health	Level of activity Fitness/conditioning	Frail Sedentary Active Elite athlete
Mobility	Use of assistive device	None Ambulatory aid (cane, crutch, walker) Wheelchair Adaptive equipment Requiring human assistance
Environmental issues	Environment	School Home Work Leisure Accessible/inaccessible
	Living arrangements	Community dwelling (alone, independent, with caregivers or family) Assisted living setting Skilled nursing

1. Intervention: a procedure or technique (e.g., a physical modality, surgical procedure, medication) (I) that is compared with alternative procedures or techniques (C).[12,16]
2. Diagnostic test: a test or measure (e.g., a bone mineral density test for identification of osteoporosis; the Berg Balance Scale for identification of fall risk) (I) that correctly differentiates patients with and without a specific condition (C).[16–18] Prognostic marker: a specific set of characteristics or factors (I) that effectively predicts an outcome (O) for a given patient problem (P).[19]

DEFINING THE OUTCOME

A good clinical question focuses on the outcome that is most relevant to the patient care situation at hand. The Nagi model of disablement[20] or the World Health Organization International Classification of Function (ICF) model[21] provides a framework for clinicians to define the outcome they are most interested in pathology or disease at the cellular level, impairment of a physiologic system, functional limitation at the level of the individual, or disability or handicap that interferes with the normal social role (Fig. 1.6).[22,23]

Case Example 4.1 **Elderly Female With Recent Transtibial Amputation**

F.H. is an 89-year-old female who had an elective transtibial amputation 4 days prior due to peripheral artery disease (PAD) unrelated to diabetes. Her postoperative pain is being managed with a narcotic, and she has been mildly disoriented and distractible during rehabilitation visits. At present, she requires moderate assistance in rising to stand and minimal assistance and directive cues to ambulate in a "hop to" pattern with a rolling walker. Her medical history includes mild congestive heart failure managed effectively with diuretics, hypertension managed effectively with beta-blockers, and a compression fracture (2 years ago) of the midthoracic spine secondary to osteoporosis. She recently had lens implants for cataracts. Before her hospitalization, she lived somewhat independently in an assisted living complex, walking long functional distances within the sprawling facility using a straight cane and eating her noon and evening meals in the communal dining room. She served as vice-chair of the Resident Council and was the organizer of an active bridge club and book discussion group. Her nearest living relative is a granddaughter who is finishing her medical residency at the hospital. The amputation/prosthetic clinic team has been charged with developing a plan for prosthetic rehabilitation, including determining her potential for prosthetic use, the optimal setting for rehabilitation intervention, the likely duration of rehabilitative care, and preliminary prosthetic prescription.

QUESTIONS TO CONSIDER

Possible clinical questions that the team would ask to guide her plan of care include the following:

- Which strategies (pharmacologic and nonpharmacologic) for postamputation pain management (I, C) will minimize the risk of delirium and assist motor and cognitive learning (O) in elderly individuals with multiple comorbidities (P)?
- Which functional and cognitive characteristics (I) provide the best indication of potential for prosthetic use (O) in elderly individuals with multiple comorbidities?
- What intrinsic and extrinsic factors (I) influence the duration of preprosthetic and prosthetic care (O) for older adults with recent transtibial amputation (P)?
- Which prosthetic foot option (nonarticulating, articulating, or dynamic response) (C, I) and suspension system (silicone suspension sleeve with a pin, supracondylar cuff, waist belt, and forked-strap extension aid) (C, I) would maximize the potential for safe community ambulation (O) in older patients with transtibial amputation, impaired postural control, and limited cardiovascular endurance (P)?
- What support systems and community resources (I) are available to reinforce self-purpose, self-care, patient motivation, return to role fulfillment, activities, and participation in life (O)?

Case Example 4.2 **Young Adult With Incomplete Spinal Cord Injury**

S.K. is a 19-year-old with an incomplete C7 level spinal cord injury who has just been admitted to the rehabilitation facility, 2 weeks after injury. S.K. was a backseat passenger injured in a driving-under-the-influence motor vehicle accident following a Thanksgiving homecoming football game victory at his high school. He was unconscious at the scene and for several hours afterward. He was given methylprednisolone in the emergency department 2 hours after injury. Radiographs revealed an anterior wedge fracture of C6 vertebra. After intubation, he was admitted to the neurologic intensive care unit; 2 days later he a had surgical fusion of C4 through C7 with immobilization in a cervical halo. During the postoperative period, pneumonia developed and has since resolved. Sensation is intact in all sacral and lumbar 3 to 5 dermatomes, and he has 2/5 strength in dorsiflexion and plantar flexion bilaterally, with hyperactive deep tendon reflex at the knee. He can tolerate sitting in a bedside recliner or high-back reclining wheelchair for approximately 45 minutes. He is anxious to know whether he will be able to walk again and, although frightened by what has occurred, appears to be motivated to begin his rehabilitation. Before his injury, S.K. lived at home while attending a nearby state university as a biology major. His intention was to eventually apply to medical school to become an orthopedic surgeon. His parents and younger sister are involved in his care; a family member is with him for most of the day. He has a cousin, now in law school, who was born with spina bifida and uses a wheelchair for primary mobility.

QUESTIONS TO CONSIDER

Possible clinical questions that the team might ask to guide his plan of care might include the following:

- What are the most powerful indicators (I) of potential for return to functional ambulation (O) in patients with incomplete cervical spinal cord injury (P)?
- Which physical therapy interventions (I, C) will best improve functional lower extremity strength (O) in patients with incomplete cervical spinal cord injury who are immobilized in a cervical halo (P)?
- What strategies (pharmacologic and nonpharmacologic) (I, C) are effective in managing abnormal tone without compromising potential for strengthening (O) in patients with incomplete cervical spinal cord injury (P)?
- Will functional neuromuscular stimulation (I) reduce the orthotic need and improve the quality of gait (O) in patients with incomplete cervical spinal cord injury (P)?
- What psychosocial and environmental factors (I) may hinder, and support participation in life, goals, and outcomes (O)?

Case Example 4.3 **Toddler With Spastic Diplegic Cerebral Palsy**

E.C. is an 18-month-old with spastic diplegic cerebral palsy being cared for by an interdisciplinary early intervention team. E.C. was born prematurely at 34 weeks of gestation after her mom's high-risk first pregnancy. Her course in the neonatal intensive care unit was relatively uneventful: She did not require ventilatory assistance but did have periodic episodes of apnea and bradycardia until she reached a weight of 4 lb. She was discharged to home at 3 weeks of age and appeared to be developing fairly typically until approximately 8 or 9 months of age. Her parents noted increasing "stiffness" of her lower extremities when in supported standing, a tendency toward "bunny hop" rather than reciprocal creeping, and overreliance on her upper extremities to pull to stand (as compared with her cousins and babies in her playgroup). Her pediatrician referred the family to a pediatric neurologist, who found mild to moderate hyperreflexia and decorticate pattern hypertonicity in her lower extremities. She has been followed in the early intervention program for 7 months; the team is charged with determining whether this is an appropriate time for orthotic intervention because she is ready to begin gait training.

QUESTIONS TO CONSIDER

Questions that might be asked to guide her plan of care include the following:

- What are the minimal levels of muscle performance and range of motion at the hip and knee (I) necessary for effective ambulation with an articulating ankle-foot orthosis (O) in children with spastic diplegic cerebral palsy (P)?
- Which type of therapeutic activity or approach (e.g., neurodevelopmental, sensory integration, proprioceptive neuromuscular facilitation) (I) is most effective in assisting dynamic postural control of the lower trunk and lower extremities during transitional and locomotor tasks (O) in children with spastic diplegic cerebral palsy (P)?
- What accommodations or adaptations of the home environment (I) will best assist safety, as well as developmental progression (O), in children with spastic diplegic cerebral palsy (P)?
- What financial, psychological, and social support resources (I) are available to determine the most efficacious treatment options available (O)?

Step 2: Locating and Accessing the Best Evidence

Once the clinical question has been clearly identified and articulated, the next step is to search the rehabilitation research literature for relevant information. The second step is to access full-text articles, assess their quality, and read those that might inform decision-making.[24–27] Among the many ways to find citations and (hopefully) the full text of the article are the following:

- Regularly visit key journal websites to review what has been recently published or published ahead of print that might be relevant to the question. This strategy can be somewhat "hit or miss" in terms of effectiveness.
- Use the index in the back of up-to-date textbooks as a reliable secondary source of information; this can be especially useful to answer background questions.
- Use an internet search engine such as Google Scholar (http://scholar.google.com; free access), which provides both unjuried and juried resources and requires the ability to carefully assess the quality of the source and of the information that has been located.
- Use electronic databases of peer-reviewed journals such as PubMed/Medline/OVID (http://www.ncbi.nlm.nih.gov/

pubmed; free access) or the Physiotherapy Evidence Database (PEDro; http://www.pedro.org.au/; free access) using appropriate keywords. Many medical libraries maintain subscriptions to multiple medical databases through services such as EBSCO (https://www.ebsco.com/; subscription access), or ProQuest (http://www.proquest.com/products-services/pq_health_med_comp.html), among others.

- Access professional organizations such as the American Physical Therapy Association (APTA) provides organization members links to search engines (directly or through EBSCO Discovery Service for the American Physical Therapy Association [https://www.apta.org/patient-care]).
- Subscribe to electronic table of content alerts from research journals relevant to their practice areas. For example, *Physical Therapy* (http://academic.oup.com/ptj), the *Journal of Geriatric Physical Therapy* (http://www.jgpt.org), the *Journal of Neurologic Physical Therapy* (http://www.jnpt.org), *Clinical Biomechanics* (clinbiomech.com), and the *Archives of Physical Medicine and Rehabilitation* (archives-pmr.org), among many others will send table of contents for current issues to email, cellular phones, tablets, e-readers, and other devices.
- The Directory of Open Access Journals accessed at doaj.org is a valuable resource for primary and secondary journal articles. The website FreeBooks4Doctors! (http://www.freebooks4doctors.com) provides hyperlinks to many key medical textbooks free of charge online. Many other online textbooks are available for purchase.

Each strategy has pros and cons in terms of efficiency and availability. Health professionals who use an evidence-based approach to patient care develop, over time, an information-seeking strategy that works within their time constraints and accessible resources.[28–30]

SOURCES OF EVIDENCE

Research studies are the foundation of meaningful evidence. Clinicians can access information from a variety of sources and formats. Academic textbooks, journals, and Internet websites aimed at health professionals and biomedical researchers are common sources of research evidence.

Sources of information are either primary or secondary. Primary sources are the reports of original scientific works. Secondary sourced articles describe, interpret, or synthesize primary sources. Examples of secondary sources include textbooks, review articles, systematic reviews (such as meta-analyses, and critical reviews of individual articles), clinical practice guidelines (CPGs), commentary or opinion papers, and website summaries.

Textbooks

Secondary sources like academic textbooks can be a good starting point for locating background information, particularly for content areas that change slowly (e.g., gross anatomy or biomechanics). EBP textbooks are well-referenced, go through a review process, and are typically updated every 3 to 5 years. Textbooks summarize clinical studies and opinions of experts and analyze/synthesize the impact of the research and expert opinion on the topic. Some textbooks are currently available online, which provides the advantage of frequent updating of specific sections as new research evidence emerges and allows the reader to immediately hyperlink to primary research article sources. Box 4.1 lists key indicators of quality in academic textbooks.

Journal Articles

Journal articles may serve as either primary or secondary literature sources. They can be useful for both background and foreground clinical questions. Journals often contain clinical research focused on issues most relevant to the particular professional group. Journal articles may be primary like case reports,[31–33] or secondary sources like systematic reviews[34–36] and scoping reviews.[37–41] Table 4.2 includes

Box 4.1 Quality Indicators for Textbooks and Internet Sources of Evidence

- Credentials of the authors
- Quality of references
- Recent/regular updating
- Endorsement by respected groups
- Peer reviewed
- Disclosure of funding source

Table 4.2 Journals Relevant to Orthotic and Prosthetic Rehabilitation

Journal Title	Abbreviation
American Journal of Occupational Therapy	*Am J Occup Ther*
American Journal of Physical Medicine & Rehabilitation	*Am J Phys Med Rehabil*
American Journal of Podiatric Medicine	*Am J Podiatr Med*
American Journal of Surgery	*Am J Surg*
American Rehabilitation	*Am Rehabil*
Annals of Physical Medicine	*Ann Phys Med*
Archives of Neurology	*Arch Neurol*
Archives of Physical Medicine and Rehabilitation	*Arch Phys Med Rehabil*
Archives of Surgery	*Arch Surg*
Assistive Technology	*Assist Technol*
Journal of Athletic Training	*J Athl Train*
Australian Journal of Physiotherapy	*Aust J Physiother*
Biomechanics	*Biomechanics*
British Journal of Sports Medicine	*Br J Sports Med*

Continued

Table 4.2 Journals Relevant to Orthotic and Prosthetic Rehabilitation—Cont'd

Journal Title	Abbreviation
Bulletin of Prosthetic Research	*Bull Prosthet Res*
Canadian Journal of Occupational Therapy	*Can J Occup Ther*
Clinical Biomechanics	*Clin Biomech*
Clinics in Orthopedics and Related Research	*Clin Orthop Rel Res*
Clinics in Podiatric Medicine and Surgery	*Clin Podiatr Med Surg*
Clinics in Prosthetics and Orthotics	*Clin Prosthet Orthot*
Developmental Medicine & Child Neurology	*Dev Med Child Neurol*
Diabetes Care	*Diabetes Care*
Diabetic Foot	*Diabet Foot*
Diabetic Medicine	*Diabet Med*
Disability and Rehabilitation	*Disabil Rehabil*
Foot and Ankle Clinics	Foot Ankle Clin
Foot and Ankle International	Foot Ankle Int
Frontiers in Neurology	*Front Neurol*
Frontiers in Neuroscience	*Front Neurosci*
Frontiers in Rehabilitation Sciences	*Front Rehabil Sci*
Frontiers in Sports and Active Living	*Fron. Sports Act Living*
Frontiers in Robotics and AI	*Front Robot AI*
Gait and Posture	*Gait Posture*
Interdisciplinary Science Reviews	*Interdisc Sci Rev*
International Journal of Rehabilitation Research	*Int J Rehabil Res*
Journal of Allied Health	*J Allied Health*
Journal of Applied Biomechanics	*J Appl Biomech*
Journal of Biomechanical Engineering	*J Biomech Eng*
Journal of Biomechanics	*J Biomech*
Journal of Bone and Joint Surgery	*J Bone Joint Surg*
Journal of Geriatric Physical Therapy	*J Geriatr Phys Ther*
Journal of Head Trauma and Rehabilitation	*J Head Trauma Rehabil*
Journal of Medical Engineering and Technology	*J Med Eng Technol*
Journal of Musculoskeletal Medicine	*J Musculoskel Med*
Journal of Neurologic Physical Therapy	*J Neuro Phys Ther*
Journal of Orthopaedic and Sports Physical Therapy	*J Orthop Sports Phys Ther*
Journal of Pediatric Orthopedics	*J Pediatr Orthop*
Journal of Prosthetics and Orthotics	*J Prosthet Orthot*
Journal of Rehabilitation	*J Rehabil*
Journal of Rehabilitation Medicine	*J Rehabil Med*
Journal of Rehabilitation Research and Development	*J Rehabil Res Dev*
Journal of Spinal Disorders	*J Spinal Disord*
Journal of the American Geriatrics Society	*J Am Geriatr Soc*
Journal of the American Medical Association	*JAMA*
Journal of the American Podiatry Association	*J Am Podiatry Assoc*
Journal of Trauma	*J Trauma*
Journal of Medical and Biological Engineering	*J Med Biol Eng*
Open Journal of Orthopedics	*Open J Orthoped*
Orthopedic Clinics of North America	*Orthop Clin North Am*
Paraplegia	*Paraplegia*
Physiotherapy Canada	*Physiother Can*
Physical and Occupational Therapy in Geriatrics	*Phys Occup Ther Geriatr*
Physical and Occupational Therapy in Pediatrics	*Phys Occup Ther Pediatr*
Physical Medicine & Rehabilitation Clinics of North America	*Phys Med Rehabil Clin North Am*
Physical Medicine & Rehabilitation: State of the Art Reviews	*Phys Med Rehabil State Art Rev*
Physical Therapy	*Phys Ther*
Physiotherapy	*Physiotherapy*
Physiotherapy Research International	*Physiother Res Int*
Prosthetics and Orthotics International	*Prosthet Orthot Int*
Rehabilitation Nursing	*Rehabil Nurs*
Rehabilitation Psychology	*Rehabil Psychol*
Scandinavian Journal of Rehabilitation Medicine	*Scand J Rehabil Med*
Spinal Cord	*Spinal Cord*
Spine	*Spine*
Topics in Stroke Rehabilitation	*Top Stroke Rehabil*

a list of some relevant orthotic and prosthetic rehabilitation journals that include primary and secondary sourced articles.

Primary Sources

Primary journal research articles are those in which the author presents the findings of a specific original study.[25] It is best to use this category of evidence when dealing with rapidly evolving areas of healthcare (which many clinical practice questions fall into). Identifying two or three high-quality primary research articles allows for an integration of concepts of reflective practice inclusive of a variety of perspectives, and comprehensive generalizations of the evidence on which to base a clinical decision.[13,25,26,30] Searching, critiquing, and synthesizing primary research sources is a time-intensive task.

Secondary Sources: Integrative and Systematic Review Articles

The use of high-quality secondary source journal articles to guide evidence-based determinations can be a time-efficient strategy for clinicians.[13,42,43] Quality indicators for secondary source articles include a comprehensive search of the literature (using an explicit search strategy) to identify existing studies, an unbiased analysis of these studies, and objective conclusions and recommendations on the basis of the analysis and synthesis.[13,44,45] Secondary sources are available in a variety of formats: integrative narrative review, systematic review, meta-analysis, and CPG. Each of these summative resources can be an effective and time-efficient method to obtain a critical assessment of a specific body of knowledge. However, there are benefits and drawbacks associated with each type of summative resource.

In an *integrative review article*, the author reviews and summarizes, and sometimes analyzes or synthesizes, the work of several primary authors.[46] These narrative reviews are often broad in scope, may or may not describe how articles were chosen for inclusion in the review, and present a qualitative analysis of previous research findings. The quality (validity) of the narrative review varies with the expertise of the reviewer and requires careful assessment by the reader.

Systematic reviews are particularly powerful secondary sources of evidence that typically analyze and synthesize controlled clinical trials.[47–50] Well-done systematic reviews are valuable sources of evidence and should always be sought when initiating a search. Box 4.2 lists key indicators of a quality systematic review. Systematic reviews are typically focused on a fairly narrow clinical question, are based on a comprehensive search of relevant literature, and use well-defined inclusion and exclusion criteria to select high-quality studies (typically randomized controlled trials) for inclusion in the review. Each study included in the review is carefully appraised for quality and relevance to the specific clinical topic. The author attempts to identify commonalities among study methods and outcomes, as well as account for differences in approaches and findings. Systematic reviews are being published relevant to orthotics and prosthetics. For example, a PubMed search of the literature using the terms "limb amputation" AND "rehabilitation" with filters applied: Full text, Systematic Review, in the last 5 years (2018–23), Humans, and English yielded 12 applicable Systematic Reviews (Appendix 4.1).

A *meta-analysis* is a type of systematic review that quantitatively aggregates outcome data from multiple studies to analyze treatment effects (typically using the "odds ratio" statistic) as if the data represented one large sample (thus with greater statistical power) rather than multiple small samples of individuals.[19,51,52] The limitation to performing a meta-analysis is that to combine studies, the category of patients, the interventions, and the outcome measures across the studies must all be similar. Meta-analyses can provide more powerful statements of the strength of the evidence either supporting or refuting a given treatment effect than the separate assessment of each study. Because of the difficulty in identifying studies with enough similarity to combine data, only a small subset of systematic reviews has been carried to the level of a meta-analysis. Four meta-analyses were identified in PubMed using the terms "'limb amputation' AND 'rehabilitation' with filters applied: Full text, Meta-Analysis, in the last 5 years (2018–23), Humans, and English yielded four applicable Meta-analyses" (Appendix 4.1).

Secondary Sources: Clinical Practice Guidelines

Another secondary resource for clinicians may be CPGs that have been developed for application to clinical practice on the basis of the best available current evidence.[53] Most existing CPGs have been developed for screening, diagnosis, and intervention in medical practice. CPGs are intended to direct clinical decision-making about appropriate healthcare for specific diseases among specific populations of patients. The best available evidence upon which CPGs are typically based combines expert consensus and a review of clinical research literature.[54,55] Most are interpreted as prescriptive, using algorithms to assist decision-making for appropriate examination and intervention strategies for patients with given characteristics. The National Guidelines Clearinghouse was the most comprehensive database in the United States for CPGs but lost funding in 2018. CPGs may now be accessed at many online sources. Some of these sources are listed in Appendix 4.2.[10,43,54,56–63]

ELECTRONIC RESOURCES AND SEARCH STRATEGIES

A number of electronic databases can assist clinicians in quickly locating primary and secondary sources of evidence to guide clinical decision-making (Table 4.3). When seeking articles, it is often helpful to use several different databases.

Using an electronic database effectively is a two-step process. First, the searcher must locate applicable citations that provide the title of the article, author, and other

Box 4.2 Quality Indicators for Systematic Review Articles

- Exhaustive search for evidence
- Identified quality criteria for inclusion
- Multiple authors with independent judgments
- Impartial, unbiased summary
- Clearly stated conclusions: ready for clinical application
- If meta-analysis: statistical manipulation across studies

Table 4.3 Electronic Databases Used to Search for Relevant Evidence

Acronym	Database Information	Access
—	Academic Search Premier	By library access
CCTR	Cochrane Controlled Trials Register	By subscription or library access
CDSR	Cochrane Database of Systematic Reviews	By subscription or library access
CINAHL	Cumulative Index of Nursing and Allied Health Literature (citations and abstracts)	By subscription or library access (https://guides.library.uab.edu/CINAHL)
DARE	Cochrane Database of Abstracts of Reviews of Effectiveness	By subscription or library access
EBM Online	Evidence-based Medicine for Primary Care and Internal Medicine (critical reviews and systematic reviews)	By subscription (http://www.ebm.bmj.com)
Embase	Embase/Elsevier Science (citations and abstracts)	By subscription (https://www.elsevier.com/solutions/embase-biomedical-research)
Medline	National Library of Medicine (abstracts)	By library access
NIH	National Institutes of Health Library	https://www.nih.gov/research-training/library-resources
OVID	A collection of health and medical subject databases (abstracts and full text)	By subscription or library access (http://www.ovid.com)
PEDro	The Physiotherapy Evidence Database (systematic reviews)	http://www.pedro.org.au
PubMed	National Library of Medicine (abstracts)	http://www.ncbi.nlm.nih.gov/pubmed (no charge)

key identifying information (e.g., journal, issue, year, and pages). Most often, these citations also provide an abstract of the article. Sometimes the searcher can gather enough information about the applicability of the article for his or her needs purely on the basis of the information found in the title and abstract. However, most often the searcher must access the full-text article to adequately assess the findings of the study. Citations and abstracts are readily available free of charge from numerous databases. However, access to the full text of articles often requires a paid subscription to search databases.

Locating Citations

The National Library of Medicine, through the database PubMed, produces and maintains Medline, the largest publicly available database of English-language biomedical references in the world. PubMed references approximately 7000 journals, including many key non-English-language biomedical journals. This database is also a rich source of citations for quality systematic reviews. Journals indexed in PubMed must meet rigorous standards for their level of peer review and the quality of the articles published in the journal; this gives the searcher some confidence in the information that is located through PubMed. PubMed can be accessed through the National Library of Medicine's website (http://www.nlm.nih.gov). OVID is a second database produced by the National Library of Medicine resource typically accessed via library subscription and often links full-text articles for the professions of nursing, medicine, healthcare administrators, and allied health professionals (https://ovidsp.ovid.com/).

The Cumulative Index of Nursing and Allied Health Literature (CINAHL) includes journal citations from a larger pool of nursing and allied health fields than is found in Medline. This database includes 3800 active indexed and abstracted journals available only to paid subscribers via library or individual subscriptions. Many of these journals have a much smaller circulation than the typical medline-cited journals, and the quality of these smaller circulation journals may not meet PubMed requirements. The reader must remain cognizant of validity and methodologic citation quality. However, the greater inclusion of rehabilitation-focused journals in the CINAHL database makes this an important database for rehabilitation professionals.

PEDro is a database of the Centre for Evidence-Based Physiotherapy at the University of Sydney, Australia, and is available to the public free of charge (http://www.pedro.org.au). PEDro lists CPGs, systematic reviews, and clinical trials. An advanced search allows the searcher to select the type of therapy, problem, body part, and subdiscipline. The PEDro database focuses on high-quality studies related to physical therapy search. The research question should be fairly broad, using synonyms that represent words in the title. PEDro contains only a fraction of the citations found in PubMed; however, all of the citations are directly applicable to rehabilitation. A search of PEDro using "orthoses" AND "clinical practice guidelines" identified 54 records. By selecting each one of the references accessed through the original PEDro search, full text (free and purchasable) may be available using the source link(s) provided, for example, DOI, PubMed, PDF locator, or publisher. Appendix 4.3 includes references freely accessed using this two-step process further limited to articles published in 2018–23.

The Cochrane Database of Systematic Reviews (http://www.cochranelibrary.com) is widely accepted as the "gold standard" for systematic reviews. Groups of experts perform comprehensive and quantitative analysis and synthesis of the existing research on well-focused topics and distill the findings into scientifically supported recommendations. Cochrane reviews use a standardized format and carefully follow rules to decrease bias in the choice of articles to review and in the interpretation of the evidence. Although few address physical therapy exclusively, rehabilitation procedures and approaches are a component of many of these reviews. The findings are reported in structured abstracts that summarize the key aspects of the full review including the authors' conclusions about the strength of the evidence and their recommendations. These structured abstracts are available free online. Appendix 4.4 includes a list of five references resulting from a Cochrane Database of Systematic Reviews search using the keyword, "orthotics," filtered to publication dates 06/01/2018 to 06/01/2023. However, access to full-text review articles requires a paid subscription.

Finding valuable secondary references on the web is increasingly possible. However, searchers must carefully scrutinize these materials because there is wide variability in the accuracy and objectivity of the published information.[13]

This evidence represents such varied sources as reports of original research, research reviews from trusted experts, student summaries that are non–peer reviewed, marketing advertisements, opinion papers, commentaries, and lobbying groups' perspectives and persuasive arguments. There are many patient-focused sites and fewer practitioner-focused ones. The quality indicators identified in Box 4.1 apply to internet websites and textbooks.

Executing Search Strategies

Often, the first search for citations results in one of two extremes: hundreds or thousands of citations with only a few related to the clinical question being asked, or almost no citations focused on the topic of interest. Searchers should look carefully at the citations that result from a search. In a search that is too broad, the searcher must examine closely what he or she is looking for, comparing titles and keywords that have resulted from the search. Often, it may be productive to repeat a search by rewording or setting limiters to narrow results. A searcher who uses the search term *prosthesis* may find that the results include articles about such diverse topics as joint prostheses, dental prostheses, and skin prostheses, as well as limb prostheses. Search terms should be as applicable to the specific clinical question being posed as possible; using more precise search terms such as *limb prosthesis, leg prosthesis, arm prosthesis*, or *artificial limb* is typically more effective.

Searchers should recognize that the search engine is simply matching the search words that the searcher has entered with subject headings linked to the article by the database administrator or librarian using predefined medical subject heading names or words included in the title or abstract. Searchers may need to adjust search terms to find applicable references. For example, using the database, PubMed (http://www.ncbi.nlm.nih.gov/pubmed/) to search the terms *below-knee amputation* AND *prosthetic rehabilitation* with filters applied: Full text, Systematic Review, 5 years (between 2018 and 2023), Humans, English yielded one citation.[64] A follow-up search using the same filters and search terms, below-knee amputation AND rehabilitation AND prosthetics, yielded the same citation.[64] However, a third search with the same filters using the term *transtibial amputation*, rather than *below-knee amputation*, AND prosthetic rehabilitation yielded three citations,[65–67] with no citations overlapping between the two searches.

A search can be unforgiving to misspellings or, as described earlier, slight differences in search terms. If the searcher finds one citation that is on target for the topic of interest, repeating the search using terms from that article's title or abstract, as well as subject headings (keywords), may yield additional appropriate citations. Using a variety of synonyms or Medical Subject Headings from the MeSH database (http://www.ncbi.nlm.nih.gov/mesh) when repeating the search can help the searcher to be more confident that the correct concepts are being targeted. Searchers should note the search terms that result in successful searches so that future searches can be most efficient. Searchers using PubMed can set up a permanent search by establishing a "cubby." This service is free and fully available via an internet connection to PubMed. Online directions help users set up cubbies that save search terms.[68] Searchers can periodically check their cubbies and ask for literature updates on the topic.

In addition to the search topic, a good clinical question will often focus on one of three broad categories of clinical questions: treatment/intervention/therapy, diagnosis, or prognosis.[13] Searchers can use these terms to narrow their search as needed. Searchers must recognize that each database uses its own set of keywords and may (or may not) include the title words, abstract words, or common sense clinical terms in their electronic search process. Familiarity with key headings used by the database can minimize frustration during the search process; combining words from the title or abstract (e.g., by using Boolean operators such as "AND," "OR," or "NOT"), as well as using synonyms for the clinical terms or concepts of interest, can also assist the search process. In many databases, searchers can choose to limit the search to systematic reviews addressing their topic of interest.[69]

Searching for Interventions

Chosen words in your key search term may limit the search to studies that focus on the specifics of the research question intent.[70–72] For example, key search terms focused on therapeutic interventions may include the following:

- Physical therapy
- Rehabilitation
- Modality
- Technique
- Interventions
- Therapeutic
- Clinical trials
- Randomized controlled trial (to limit the search to articles of the highest quality, only if there are many relevant articles)

  More specific terms added to the search increase the likelihood of accessing meaningful therapeutic interventions commonly used in prosthetics and orthotics. Additional key terms search may include:
- Prosthetic rehabilitation
- Orthotic use
- Prosthetic fitting
- Prosthetic training
- Mobility
- Gait training
- Therapeutic exercise
- Edema management
- Balance training
- Skincare
- Strength training

Diagnosis as the Intervention

If the primary clinical question relates to making an accurate and efficacious diagnosis about some aspect of the patient's condition or to screening patients to determine the need for a more specific assessment, the health practitioner may search the "diagnosis" literature for relevant studies. General search terms that help limit the search to general studies focusing on diagnosis include the following[73]:

- Diagnosis (disease or disorder)
- Diagnostic tool
- Differential diagnosis
- Sensitivity

- Specificity
- Accuracy
- Predictive value
- Construct validity

Natural History or Prognosis

Studies of the prognosis of medical pathologic conditions and impairments are becoming increasingly available. Such studies attempt to predict who is most likely to benefit from specific treatment interventions or determine whether specific characteristics of patients or their environment predict outcomes. Search terms that are likely to limit the citations to those focused on the general category of prognosis include the following[55,58,74]:

- Experimental cohort studies
- Prognosis
- Prognostic factors
- Disease progression
- Recurrence
- Morbidity
- Mortality
- Incidence
- Prevalence
- Clinical course
- Outcomes

Systematic Review

Currently PubMed allows the researcher to limit the search by article types by checking one or up to all of the following:

- Books and documents
- Clinical trial
- Meta-analysis
- Randomized controlled trial
- Review
- Systematic review

Articles commonly identified as review-academic, CPGs, review-tutorial, meta-analysis, guideline, and consensus development conference are all categorized in PubMed under the term systematic review. The researcher who is seeking to limit the citations to ones focused on true systematic reviews would check the boxes next to clinical trial, meta-analysis, randomized controlled trial, review, and systematic review, then include the following key search terms:

- Systematic review
- Systematic
- Meta-analysis
- Development
- Validation

LOCATING FULL-TEXT ARTICLES

Once appropriate citations have been found via a search of the literature, the next step is to locate the full text of articles that appear to be most closely related to the clinical question of concern. Individual journals are published and owned by publishing companies that support themselves with paid journal subscriptions. Each journal has its mechanism for providing access to the articles it contains. If the journal is published by a specific professional organization, members of that organization typically have access to a delivered hard copy of the journal or access via the organization's website (by entering an assigned user name and password).

Libraries purchase hard copy and online access to specific journals, either bundled together as part of an intermediary company service (e.g., EBSCO or ProQuest), as stand-alone subscriptions, or as a publisher aggregated offering of several or all of its journals at a specified price. Libraries make online copies of these journals available to their library patrons, either free of charge or for a specified library fee. Some journals provide full text free to the public via the internet, either for all issues or for articles published after a certain period (e.g., 1 to 2 years after publication). Most journals provide full text of individual articles for a fee; this fee may be as much as $20 to $25 per article. One benefit of searching the literature on PubMed is that this database provides a link to any online access to a specific citation, both those with free access sources and those with a fee attached. The website http://www.freemedicaljournals.com lists the various biomedical journals that provide full text free, provides the hyperlink to the journal website, and identifies any limitations to free access (often time since publication). Healthcare practitioners should search out the availability of full-text biomedical journal articles (either hard copy or online) from the libraries to which they have regular access. Access will vary widely based on the work setting and the mission of the library at the health facility or in the community.

Step 3: Critically Appraising the Evidence

Once the clinician has located and screened the article to ensure that it is reasonably focused on the clinical research question of interest and applicable to the patients in his or her clinical practice, the clinician must critically appraise the methodologic and analytic quality of the research process used in the study.[13,36,53,72,75–78] This is a skill that clinicians can develop with consistent practice, over time, and is well worth the effort involved.[13,29,53] Participation in study groups or journal clubs often helps development of this useful EBP skill.[77,79]

OVERALL METHODOLOGIC QUALITY

The best-quality research evidence comes from studies with a carefully articulated research question, an appropriate design and methodology, and a sample representative of the population of interest. No clinical research study or article is perfect, and the critical appraiser of the research literature must develop skills to *weigh the evidence* that an article provides to determine whether the information is accurate, relevant, and clinically important for his or her patients.[80–86] Just because something is published and in print does not ensure that it provides valuable or accurate information. Whether the clinical study focuses on treatment/intervention, prognosis, or diagnosis, the overall purpose of critical appraisal is to determine the extent to which threats to the internal and external validity of the study bias, and potentially invalidate, the findings of the study.[81,87] The clinician is interested in determining whether, and to what degree, the findings of the study truly represent the answer to the research question asked in the study. Box 4.3 lists a series of questions about the overall quality and applicability of primary research studies. Some questions are applicable across all categories of primary research; others are specific to certain categories. Box 4.4 identifies quality assessment questions applicable to the secondary source category of systematic review.

Box 4.3 Questions to Consider in the Critical Appraisal of a Research or Review Article

For All Studies

- What criteria were in place in the database used to find the study (e.g., journals referenced in PubMed have met stringent quality criteria)?
- How up-to-date (recent) is the study?
- Is the purpose of the study clearly stated? How closely does the purpose of the study address the clinical question of concern?
- How comprehensive is the review of the literature? How up-to-date and relevant are the references cited in the article? Does the review of the literature support the need for the study that is being reported?
- Are the outcome measurement tools used in the study described sufficiently? Are they appropriate to the clinical question of concern?
- Is evidence of the reliability and validity of each outcome measurement tool presented? Is the evidence adequate for the clinical question of concern?

For Studies of Interventions/Treatments/Therapy

- Have subjects been randomly assigned to groups?
- Is there a control group (or placebo or standard care group) used to compare with the experimental group?
- Are the researchers collecting outcome data blind to subject group assignment?
- As feasible, are subjects blinded to their group assignment?
- How similar are the experiment and control groups? Optimally, the only difference should be the intervention.
- Do confounding variables make the groups different before intervention?

For Studies Concerned With Prognosis

- Are the researchers collecting outcome data blind to each subject's score on prognostic factors?
- Is the period of follow-up sufficiently long to ensure that the outcome of interest is captured?
- Is there evidence from repeated analysis with a second group of subjects with similar results to confirm the prognostic factors being investigated?

For Studies Concerned With Diagnosis

- Has the new diagnostic test been compared with an accepted reference standard?
- Is the researcher performing the new diagnostic test blind to each subject's score on the reference standard?
- Is there evidence from repeated analysis with a second group of subjects with similar results to confirm the accuracy of the new diagnostic test?

Box 4.4 Questions Used to Assess the Quality of a Systematic Review

Formulation of Objectives

- Is the topic (purpose of the review) well defined?
- Intervention
- Patients
- Outcomes of interest

Literature Search for Studies

- Was the search for papers thorough?
- Use of search terms that fully capture key concepts
- Identification of databases or citation sources used
- Search methods exhaustive, international in scope
- Search methods described in enough detail to replicate
- International in scope
- Search terms that fully capture search concepts

Study Selection

- Were study inclusion criteria clearly described and fairly applied?
- Explicit inclusion and exclusion criteria
- Criteria should apply to the topic
- Selection criteria are applied in a manner that limits bias
- Account for studies that are rejected

Assessing Quality of Design and Methods

- Was study quality assessed by blinded or independent reviewers?
- Was missing information sought from the original study investigators?
- Do the included studies seem to indicate similar effects?
- Were the overall findings assessed for their robustness?
- Was the play of chance adequately assessed?

Data Gathering

- Was information from each article extracted using a standardized format?
- Does the information gathered from each article include the following?
- Type of study (e.g., randomized, controlled trial)
- Characteristics of the intervention for experimental and control groups
- Key demographics of all subjects
- Primary outcome of importance
- An accounting for missing data

Pooling Method

- Are selected studies similar enough to be pooled for analysis?
- In design
- In interventions
- In the operational definition of the outcome variable

Discussion, Conclusions, and Recommendations

- Are recommendations based firmly on the quality of the evidence presented?
- Are conclusions and recommendations justified based on the analysis performed?

Sample: Adequacy and Appropriateness

Sample size plays a major role in the study design, methodologic quality, and interpretation.[13,88] In studies with small sample sizes, a few nonrepresentative subjects can skew data substantially and lead to statistical findings that are nonrepresentative of the parent group.[88,89] In addition, the natural variability between subjects may end up masking real differences when the sample size is low. There is no absolute minimum number of subjects identified quantitatively as the minimum needed for a legitimate study. However, research textbooks often recommend 8 to 15 subjects per group as a minimum number to ensure that the statistical analysis has at least a reasonable opportunity to demonstrate real differences or real relationships if they are present.[13] The larger the sample size, the more likely that the sample will represent the population from which it has been drawn.

Researchers, as well as readers of research articles, can use a power analysis to evaluate the adequacy of the sample size. A power analysis provides an objective estimate of the minimum sample size necessary to demonstrate real differences or relationships between and among groups.[88,90,91] The inclusion of power analysis as a standard part of the research design is a fairly new concept. Thus although the presence of a power analysis is helpful in assessing the adequacy of the sample size, the lack of a specifically identified power analysis—particularly in older studies—does not necessarily indicate a weak study.

A power level (β) of 0.8 (80%) is generally considered acceptable in ensuring that, if real group differences (or relationships) are present, the study design is sensitive enough to pick them up. A power analysis considers five factors in the determination of power. Knowing any four of these five factors allows the reader to calculate the final factor.[88,90]The five factors include the following:

1. The significance level (α coefficient) set for the statistical analysis of the outcome variable.
2. Anticipated variance (e.g., standard deviation) within each group of subjects related to the outcome variable.
3. Sample and group size.
4. The anticipated effect size for the intervention or relationship; how large a difference or a correlation does there need to be to ensure that the outcome under review is important or clinically meaningful?
5. The desired level of power (β coefficient), an estimate of the likelihood that a real difference between groups will be demonstrated if it exists (avoiding a type II error).

Power analysis performed in preparation for a study (i.e., before subject recruitment, data collection, or analysis) identifies the ideal number of subjects that should be in each group.[13,88–90] When a power analysis is performed after the data analysis has been completed, it is used to determine the likelihood that a small sample size affected the statistical analysis when insignificant findings occurred.[13,89,91]

When a power analysis is performed before implementation of a study, most use a significance level of $\alpha = 0.05$ or lower and the power level of $b = 0.8$ or higher. The score for effect size and anticipated group variance will be study specific. Typically researchers provide references from prior research or their pilot data to justify their choices of effect size and variance. This use of power analysis provides evidence of a rigorous research design and helps the clinician to trust the findings of the study.

The next important appraisal of the sample concerns its representativeness: to what extent are the subjects in the sample similar to (and therefore representative of) the "population" of interest and to the individual for whom the clinician is caring? The goal of all research studies is to make decisions about a general population of people based on the findings of a representative sample from that population. How well a sample represents the larger group to which results will be generalized is a function of subject recruitment, selection, and retention.[13,92–94] When appraising articles applicable to clinical decision-making, the health professional must consider how subjects were recruited and assigned to groups (random assignment is best), exclusion and inclusion criteria, and the reasons that subjects who started the study dropped out before data collection was completed. Study results will be biased if the sample used for the study is not representative of the underlying population. Small variations randomly occurring across all subject groups may be acceptable; however, larger variations, particularly ones that systematically affect one group more than others, may introduce unacceptable levels of bias.

The evidence-based practitioner must be on the alert for sampling bias.[13,81,95,96] Ideally, any subject in the patient population of interest is equally likely to be chosen to be a subject in the study. Realistically, this is rarely the case. Instead, participant recruitment results from matters of convenience with subjects recruited from previously formed groups, for example, by migratory and settlement patterns, geography, occupations or work environments, systems accessed, social interactions, activities, or hobbies, and individual characteristics such as diagnosis, or personal interests, beliefs, or values. This recruitment strategy introduces bias, and outcomes are less generalizable. No one researcher has access to each older adult who has had a transtibial amputation, each child with cerebral palsy, or each young adult with an incomplete spinal cord lesion. The researcher should provide enough evidence in his or her discussion of the study's methodology that the reader can be reasonably comfortable that the methods implemented for choosing subjects provided access to subjects reasonably representative of the breadth of subjects with the target characteristics under investigation.

Descriptive evidence from previous studies of the common characteristics of patients with the pathologic condition of interest may be compared to the descriptive characteristics of subjects in their particular study. Any differences should be identified and presented. The critical appraiser must use professional judgment to determine the extent to which potential biasing factors influence the methodologic rigor of the study. If inequalities are detected, it is possible to add steps to the statistical analysis to account for the inequality and report.

Attrition (subject dropout rate) also influences the researcher's ability to generalize the findings of the study to the larger population of individuals with the diagnosis or impairment.[13,97,98] A useful rule of thumb for readers who are critically appraising an article is that, if more than a 20% dropout rate has occurred, then the findings of the study are likely suspect. The researcher should always explain the rationale and when subjects were lost. Evidence-based practitioners want to know whether subjects chose to leave the study because the intervention made them worse, were too difficult or painful to complete, or too burdensome to follow-through compared with its potential benefits. Subjects in the sample who completed the study may be the most persistent. Researchers attempt to account for dropouts either by performing an "intention-to-treat" analysis or presenting descriptive statistics that compare key characteristics of subjects who completed the study with those who did not complete the study.[99] If the researcher can confirm that both groups of subjects are not significantly different, particularly in terms of any characteristic that might bias outcomes, then a study may still be identified as having adequate methodologic quality.

In an intention-to-treat analysis, all subjects who started a study but did not finish it are assigned the most negative outcome likely to occur with the measurement tool for the purposes of statistical analysis.[99–101] If a statistically significant finding still occurs in the presence of an intention-to-treat analysis, then even assuming that all dropouts had a bad outcome, the study still demonstrated significant effects.

Outcome Measures

In assessing the quality of a study's outcome measurement tools, three questions must be addressed:

- Are the outcome tools described well enough for the evidence-based practitioner to make an informed and realistic judgment about their appropriateness for assessing the variables of interest for this study?
- Are the outcome tools reasonably valid and reliable?
- Are the outcome tools reasonably responsive and sensitive to change?

A high-quality study describes the outcome measures in enough detail for the reader to understand exactly what was measured and to determine whether the tools are appropriate to answer the research questions addressed in the study.

The article should also provide sufficient detail to confirm the reliability and validity of each outcome measurement tool. Reliability represents the consistency with which scores are reproduced given repetition of the test with the same tester or across numerous testers.[13,53,102] Validity represents the accuracy with which the measurement tool taps into the construct or characteristics that the test is purported to measure.[13,53,102] Table 4.4 lists the various aspects of reliability and validity.

If a test is reliable, it should perform consistently under similar testing situations regardless of who performs the test. Studies of reliability usually report either correlation coefficients or intraclass correlation coefficients as the statistical measure of the accuracy with which scores are reproduced.[103–105] There is no absolute standard of minimally acceptable reliability.[106,107]. A score of 1 indicates complete reliability (and is rarely achieved); a score of 0 represents a complete lack of reliability. A general benchmark is that a score of $r = 0.9$ or better is strong evidence of the reliability of that measure[13,53,108]. Coefficients between 0.75 and 0.89 suggest that the measure has a moderate risk of error but may be acceptable. Correlations of less than $r = 0.75$ are not typically perceived as having acceptable reliability.

The researchers who are reporting their study should provide an adequate description of the methodology of the study for the critical appraiser to determine which aspects of reliability are most important in this study (and therefore to determine whether the authors provided evidence of the appropriate reliability). Intertester reliability should be reported when more than one tester measures the same outcome, and intratester reliability should be reported when the same tester measures outcomes on more than one occasion. Test-retest reliability provides evidence that the test performs consistently when repeated under similar conditions.

In addition, readers are interested in whether the validity of the measure has been assessed. To be considered valid, there must be sufficient evidence to demonstrate that the test or tool measures what it is purported to measure.[13,53,109] The researchers who have written the article must provide this evidence about the measure so that the critical appraiser can be comfortable that concerns about validity have been adequately addressed. Just because a tool is reliable (consistent in its measurement properties) does not mean that it is also valid (measures what it intends to measure). However, a tool cannot be valid if it is not reliable in its measurement.[13,53,110] Ideally, the tests or measures used in the study demonstrate great consistency with high reproducibility (i.e., reliability) and accurately assess the targeted characteristic (validity).

Evidence of validity is especially important when the test or tool measures an abstract concept (e.g., quality of life or functional independence) rather than a physiologic phenomenon (e.g., heart rate, range of motion). A valid test or measure contains enough items or questions related to the concept or characteristic being evaluated that the clinician can be confident that the results of testing will represent the subject's status in relation to the construct being assessed.

A test or measure found to be reliable in one patient population is not automatically reliable in other populations.[13,77,102,111,112]

Step 4: Applicability to Patients and Clinical Practice

The final component of an EBP approach to rehabilitative care is just as essential to the provision of quality care as the ability to access and use available evidence and clinical expertise. Without consideration of the unique goals, expectations, values, and concerns that an individual in our care brings to the healthcare encounter, even the "perfect" plan of action will not be as efficacious as it might otherwise be. An individual's perspective and values are influenced by a number of factors, including their beliefs, values, motivation and drive, coping styles and strategies, psychosocial factors, developmental issues, social determinants of health, settlement patterns, family and work roles, support structures, culture, knowledge and access to resources, and social and community participation and engagement.[113,114] To be as effective as possible in providing care, evidence-based practitioners consider what the pathologic condition, impairment, functional limitation, or disability means to the individual with respect to self-concept and sociocultural roles, their lived experiences, and future goals.

Table 4.4 Validity and Reliability

DETERMINATION OF A TEST OR MEASURES RELIABILITY

Type of Reliability	Question Being Addressed
Intrarater	Will the same examiner make consistent ratings of the same individual?
Test-retest	Is the measure stable/accurate over time?
Interrater	Will different examiners make consistent ratings of the same individual?
Internal consistency	How well does each of the items contribute or reflect what the test intends to measure (how well do the items hang together)?
Parallel forms	Are different versions of the test or measure equivalent?

RELIABILITY COEFFICIENTS

Parametric Analyses		Nonparametric Analyses		
Strategies for Continuous Measures	Types of Reliability Evaluated	Strategies for Nominal Measures	Strategies for Ordinal Measures	Types of Reliability Evaluated
Pearson product moment (Pearson *r*) (0.0–1.0)	Intrarater Test-retest Interrater Parallel forms	Percent agreement (includes chance agreement)	Percent agreement (includes chance agreement)	Test-retest Interrater Parallel forms
Coefficient of variation (standard deviation/mean) (<10% suggests reliability)	Intrarater Interrater	Kappa coefficient (agreement beyond chance)	Weighted percent agreement (magnitude of disparity) (includes chance agreement)	Intrarater Test-retest Interrater Parallel forms
Intraclass correlation coefficient (ICC) (association and agreement)	Intrarater Test-retest Interrater Parallel forms		Weighted kappa (agreement beyond chance)	Intrarater Test-retest Interrater Parallel forms
Cronbach alpha	Internal consistency			

DETERMINATION OF A TEST OR MEASURE'S VALIDITY

Type of Validity	Question Being Addressed	Continuous Measures
Content	How well are items on the test sample from the domain being evaluated?	Content expert review of items
Concurrent or Criterion	How well does the measure reflect a particular event, characteristic, or outcome?	Correlation (with reference to a standard measure of characteristic or construct)
Predictive	How well does the measure predict a future event or outcome?	Correlation (with the outcome variable, measured after some time)
Construct	Does the test measure a single underlying theoretical concept or construct?	Correlation (with variables theoretically related to the construct of interest)
	How many underlying constructs are included in the measure?	Confirmatory factor analysis
Discriminant or Divergent	How well does the test or measure differentiate between/among groups?	*t*-Test or analysis of variance

CLINICAL RELEVANCE

Assessing the clinical importance of a study has both objective and subjective considerations. The clinician must look beyond the statistical significance of the findings and engage the patient as the center of the healthcare team.[115–117] Often this assessment is based on professional judgment about the impact of the extent of change.

- Does a statistically significant change in a functional test score or pain level translate into a change that the patient will perceive as important in daily life?
- Does long-term follow-up occur? That is, does the author examine the effectiveness of a given intervention 3 months, 6 months, or 1 year following the intervention?
- If the article only provides evidence of the short-term benefits of the intervention, are these short-term benefits worth the time and effort in the long run? Would other interventions have had a better long-term outcome?

Making the decision to implement new approaches to care supported by the research literature requires the evidence-based practitioner to answer several questions related to his or her specific clinical environment.[53,79,80]

- How similar are the subjects used in the study to those in his or her clinical practice?
- How do the patient's values and expectations interact with or relate to effort, risks, and likely outcomes of the intervention being considered?

For studies of interventions/therapy/treatment, consider the following:

- How likely is it that the patient will be willing and able to comply with intervention activities suggested in the study?

For studies of diagnosis, consider the following:

- Is the diagnostic test adequately available, affordable, accurate, and precise for use in the clinician's setting?
- Is it likely that the patient will be willing and able to comply with the testing procedures?

For studies of prognosis, consider the following:

- Will knowing the predictor factors make a clinically important difference in the way the clinician will care for his or her patients?

Integrating Clinical Expertise and Skill

Although research literature is a valuable and important resource for evidence-based decision-making, using evidence from the literature is not sufficient for effective EBP. Practitioners must also have strong examination, evaluation, and diagnostic skills and should be able to incorporate these skills into reflective experience and current research findings.[13,53,77]

What is clinical expertise? In physical therapy, it is the core competencies that combine and integrate (1) a multidimensional knowledge base that is grounded in basic science, medical science, psychologic/sociocultural sciences, and movement sciences; (2) effective clinical reasoning skills and an orientation toward function; (3) well-developed and efficient psychomotor skills for examination and intervention; and (4) the desire or commitment to provide patient-centered care (Fig. 4.3).[118,119]

The first chapter of this text explores the educational preparation, roles, and responsibilities of individual health professionals involved in orthotic and prosthetic rehabilitation. Each has a particular body of knowledge to bring to the care of individuals needing a prosthesis or orthosis, as well as shared understanding (albeit at various depths) of anatomy, kinesiology, biomechanics, gait analysis, mobility training, motor control and motor learning, and principles of exercise. The authors have established that effective interdisciplinary teaming, in which each profession's perspective interacts so that the team becomes "more than the sum of its parts," is an essential component in the provision of successful orthotic or prosthetic rehabilitative care.

The background knowledge important in orthotic and prosthetic rehabilitation that enables clinicians to ask sound clinical questions and apply evidence to patient care includes a strong foundation in the following areas:

- Anatomy and physiology of the musculoskeletal, neuromuscular, cardiovascular, and cardiopulmonary systems
- Kinesiology and biomechanics of the human body
- Properties of orthotic and prosthetic materials
- Principles of motor control and motor learning
- Lifespan development
- Exercise prescription and assessment of exercise tolerance
- Determinants of normal gait and methods of gait assessment

How does the clinician gain the knowledge necessary for expert practice? Entry-level professional education and core competencies are the baseline, and on-the-job experience via trial-and-error practice and discussion/debate/collaboration with colleagues moves clinicians from students toward novices.[13,53,118–120] They become more competent in their roles and responsibilities as their experience grows; they support and enhance their developing mastery and expertise with continuing education, participation in journal clubs perusal of the clinical research literature, and

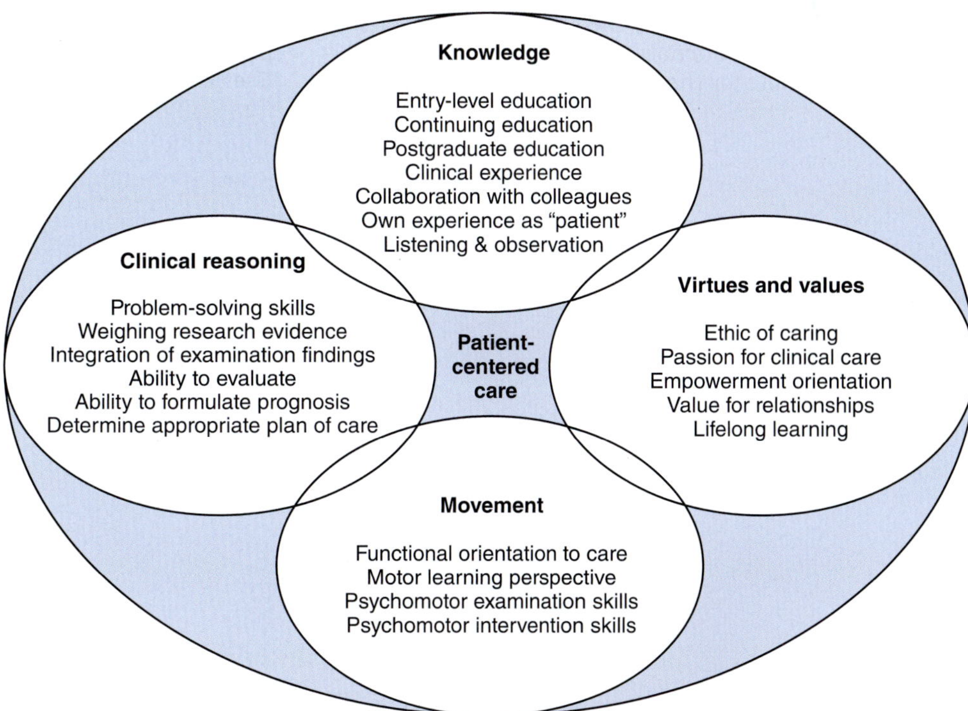

Fig. 4.3 Expert patient-centered physical therapy practice requires integration and interaction of a provider's underlying knowledge, values, examination, and intervention skills as well as clinical reasoning.

postgraduate education. Another important component of increasing competence and developing expertise is the ability to actively listen to the hopes and concerns of those they work with and incorporate these into decision-making and plans of care.

Clinical expertise, then, allows healthcare providers to quickly and efficiently identify an individual's rehabilitation diagnosis and, based on their constellation of impairments and functional limitations, select the strategies for remediation or accommodation that will assist the individual's return to a preferred lifestyle.

STAYING CURRENT WITH THE LITERATURE

One proactive way that a clinician can keep informed about new studies focused on his or her area of practice is to sign up for an online service that automatically sends weekly or monthly electronic updates of new articles from journals that the clinician feels are important to read or content areas that he or she wants to stay informed about. Professional organizations often offer this service as a membership benefit. Many journals allow readers to sign up for a service that electronically sends the table of contents via email whenever a new issue of the journal is released. Another valuable service (without charge) for evidence-based practitioners is available from an information management company, Amedeo (http://www.amedeo.com). When an evidence-based practitioner subscribes to Amedeo, he or she chooses from a list of topics for notification of newly published articles linked to those selected topics. Amedeo topics include rehabilitation, pain management, vascular surgery, and stroke, among many others. Amedeo routinely searches a large variety of high-quality journals for new publications on the topics selected by subscribers and sends weekly updates via email. This is a valuable resource for busy clinicians who may not have ready access to a medical library.

Two strategies, if routinely used, help health professionals to update and expand their expertise. The first is to select two or three journals (see Table 4.2) that are particularly appropriate for the clinician's area of professional interest and practice and arrange (via the journal's website) to receive an electronic copy of the table of contents of each issue. When the update arrives, it will be well worth the clinician's time and effort to scroll through the listing of articles and authors to determine which would be worth tracking down to read. The second strategy is to use whatever electronic literature update service is available through professional organizations, PubMed, or Amedeo to arrange to be notified regularly of research reports published in the clinician's area of interest. The final step is to actually (and consistently) make time to read the resources that have been identified and discuss and debate them with colleagues to effectively integrate the new information into clinical practice.

Summary

This chapter explores the concepts underlying evidence-based healthcare practice and illustrates strategies to develop clear clinical questions that are relevant to an individual patient who is receiving care. This chapter also identifies various sources of evidence available to clinicians and illustrates how electronic databases can assist the search process. The authors suggest strategies that clinicians can use to develop critical appraisal skills and to update and expand their clinical expertise. Although much of the chapter focuses on evidence available in the research literature, it is the integration of the best available scientific evidence; clinical expertise, and judgment; and engaging the patient where possible in care decisions by incorporating their concerns, values, and expectations that determines the effectiveness of clinical decision-making.

References

The complete listing of the References are available in the accompanying enhanced eBook version included with the print purchase of this textbook. Visit Elsevier eBooks+ (eBooks.Health.Elsevier.com) to access this content.

Appendix 4.1

Side-by-Side Comparison of Database Searches Using the Same Filters Except for Systematic Reviews and Meta-analysis. On the left, the search included PubMed Electronic Research Database Published from 2018 to 2023, Identified by Using Search Terms "Limb Amputation" AND "Rehabilitation" with the following filters applied: Full text, Systematic Review, in the last 5 years, Humans, English yields 12 Systematic Review articles. On the right, are the results of a separate search maintaining all previous filters and replacing systematic review with meta-analysis (a specific type of systematic review), yielded four meta-analysis articles.

Systematic Reviews

1. Manz S, Valette R, Damonte F, et al. A review of user needs to drive the development of lower limb prostheses. *J Neuroeng Rehabil*. 2022;19(1):119. https://doi.org/10.1186/s12984-022-01097-1
2. Young M, McKay C, Williams S, Rouse P, Bilzon JLJ. Time-related changes in quality of life in persons with lower limb amputation or spinal cord injury: protocol for a systematic review. *Syst Rev*. 2019;8(1):191. https://doi.org/10.1186/s13643-019-1108-3
3. Crane H, Boam G, Carradice D, Vanicek N, Twiddy M, Smith GE. Through-knee versus above-knee amputation for vascular and non-vascular major lower limb amputations. *Cochrane Database Syst Rev*. 2021;12(12):CD013839. https://doi.org/10.1002/14651858.CD013839.pub2
4. Escamilla-Nunez R, Michelini A, Andrysek J. Biofeedback systems for gait rehabilitation of individuals with lower-limb amputation:a systematic review. *Sensors (Basel)*. 2020;20(6):1628. https://doi.org/10.3390/s20061628
5. Guémann M, Olié E, Raquin L, Courtet P, Risch N. Effect of mirror therapy in the treatment of phantom limb pain in amputees: a systematic review of randomized placebo-controlled trials does not find any evidence of efficacy. *Eur J Pain*. 2023;27(1):3–13. https://doi.org/10.1002/ejp.2035
6. Arora M, Harvey LA, Glinsky JV, et al. Electrical stimulation for treating pressure ulcers. *Cochrane Database Syst Rev*. 2020;1(1):CD012196. https://doi.org/10.1002/14651858.CD012196.pub2
7. Miller MJ, Jones J, Anderson CB, Christiansen CL. Factors influencing participation in physical activity after dysvascular amputation: a qualitative meta-synthesis. *Disabil Rehabil*. 2019;41(26):3141–3150. https://doi.org/10.1080/09638288.2018.1492031
8. Thibaut A, Beaudart C, Maertens DE Noordhout B, Geers S, Kaux JF, Pelzer D. Impact of microprocessor prosthetic knee on mobility and quality of life in patients with lower limb amputation: a systematic review of the literature. *Eur J Phys Rehabil Med*. 2022;58(3):452–461. https://doi.org/10.23736/S1973-9087.22.07238-0
9. van Schaik L, Geertzen JHB, Dijkstra PU, Dekker R. Metabolic costs of activities of daily living in persons with a lower limb amputation: a systematic review and meta-analysis. *PLoS One*. 2019;14(3):e0213256. https://doi.org/10.1371/journal.pone.0213256
10. Schober TL, Abrahamsen C. Patient perspectives on major lower limb amputation – a qualitative systematic review. *Int J Orthop Trauma Nurs*. 2022;46:100958. https://doi.org/10.1016/j.ijotn.2022.100958
11. Limakatso K, Bedwell GJ, Madden VJ, Parker R. The prevalence and risk factors for phantom limb pain in people with amputations: a systematic review and meta-analysis. *PLoS One*. 2020;15(10):e0240431. https://doi.org/10.1371/journal.pone.0240431
12. Lathouwers E, Díaz MA, Maricot A, et al. Therapeutic benefits of lower limb prostheses: a systematic review. *J Neuroeng Rehabil*. 2023;20(1):4. https://doi.org/10.1186/s12984-023-01128-5

Meta-analysis

1. Arora M, Harvey LA, Glinsky JV, et al. Electrical stimulation for treating pressure ulcers. *Cochrane Database Syst Rev*. 2020;1(1):CD012196. https://doi.org/10.1002/14651858.CD012196.pub2
2. Miller MJ, Jones J, Anderson CB, Christiansen CL. Factors influencing participation in physical activity after dysvascular amputation: a qualitative meta-synthesis. *Disabil Rehabil*. 2019;41(26):3141–3150. https://doi.org/10.1080/09638288.2018.1492031
3. van Schaik L, Geertzen JHB, Dijkstra PU, Dekker R. Metabolic costs of activities of daily living in persons with a lower limb amputation: a systematic review and meta-analysis. PLoS One. 2019;14(3):e0213256. https://doi.org/10.1371/journal.pone.0213256
4. Limakatso K, Bedwell GJ, Madden VJ, Parker R. The prevalence and risk factors for phantom limb pain in people with amputations: a systematic review and meta-analysis. PLoS One. 2020;15(10):e0240431. https://doi.org/10.1371/journal.pone.0240431

Appendix 4.2

Select Sources and Examples of Current Clinical Practice Guidelines. Note that this is not an exhaustive list.

Author, Year	Title	Access
American Physical Therapy Association, 2023	*Clinical Practice Guidelines*	https://www.apta.org/patient-care/evidence-based-practice-resources
APTA Academy of Orthopaedic Physical Therapy, 2023	*Published CPGs*	https://www.orthopt.org/content/practice/clinical-practice-guidelines/published-cpgs
Brosseau L, Toupin-April K, Wells G, et al., 2016	*Ottawa Panel Evidence-Based Clinical Practice Guidelines for Foot Care in the Management of Juvenile Idiopathic Arthritis*	https://www.archives-pmr.org/article/S0003-9993(15)01480-X/fulltext
Martin, 2014	*Heel Pain—Plantar Fasciitis: Revision 2014*	https://www.jospt.org/doi.org/10.2519/jospt.2014.0303
Chou et al., 2014	*Nonpharmacologic Therapies for Low Back Pain: A Systematic Review for an American College of Physicians Clinical Practice Guideline*	https://doi.org/10.7326/M16-2459
Moore et al., 2018	*A Core Set of Outcome Measures for Adults With Neurologic Conditions Undergoing Rehabilitation*	https://doi.org/10.1097/NPT.0000000000000229
Johnston et al., 2021	*A Clinical Practice Guideline for the Use of Ankle-Foot Orthoses and Functional Electrical Stimulation Post-Stroke*	https://doi.org/10.1097/NPT.0000000000000347
Daley et al., 2021	*Clinical Guidance to Optimize Work Participation After Injury or Illness: The Role of Physical Therapists*	https://www.jospt.org/doi.org/10.2519/jospt.2021.0303
Hanger Clinic, 2023	*Clinical Practice Guidelines*	https://hangerclinic.com/for-professionals/hanger-institute/clinical-affairs/clinical-practice-guidelines/
Osborne et al., 2022	*Physical Therapist Management of Parkinson Disease: A Clinical Practice Guideline From the American Physical Therapy Association*	https://doi.org/10.1093/ptj/pzab302
van Doormaal et al., 2020	*A Clinical Practice Guideline for Physical Therapy in Patients With Hip or Knee Osteoarthritis*	https://onlinelibrary.wiley.com/doi/abs/10.1002/msc.1492
Veterans Affairs, 2023	*VA/DoD Clinical Practice Guidelines*	https://www.healthquality.va.gov/index.asp

Appendix 4.3

Results of Search Using Pedro Database a Keyword: Orthoses AND Limited to Articles/abstracts Published 2018–23.

- Santos EJF, Duarte C, Ferreira RJO, et al. Portuguese multidisciplinary recommendations for non-pharmacological and non-surgical interventions in patients with rheumatoid arthritis. *Acta Reumatol Port.* 2021;46(1):40–54.
- Jung C, Tepohl L, Tholen R, et al. Rehabilitation following rotator cuff repair. *Obere Extrem.* 2018;13(1):45-61. https://doi.org/10.1007/s11678-018-0448-2
- Logerstedt DS, Scalzitti DA, Bennell KL, et al. Knee Pain and mobility impairments: meniscal and articular cartilage lesions revision 2018. *J Orthop Sports Phys Ther.* 2018;48(2):A1–A50. https://doi.org/10.2519/jospt.2018.0301
- Gignoux P, Lanhers C, Dutheil F, Boutevillain L, Pereira B, Coudeyre E. Non-rigid lumbar supports for the management of non-specific low back pain: a literature review and meta-analysis. *Ann Phys Rehabil Med.* 2022;65(1):101406. https://doi.org/10.1016/j.rehab.2020.05.010
- Kitamura K, Iwase S, Komoike Y, et al. Evidence-based practice guideline for the management of lymphedema proposed by the Japanese Lymphedema Society. *Lymphat Res Biol.* 2022;20(5):539-547. https://doi.org/10.1089/lrb.2021.0032
- Erickson M, Lawrence M, Jansen CWS, Coker D, Amadio P, Cleary C. Hand pain and sensory deficits: carpal tunnel syndrome. *J Orthop Sports Phys Ther.* 2019;49(5):CPG1-CPG85. https://doi.org/10.2519/jospt.2019.0301
- Caserta AJ, Pacey V, Fahey MC, Gray K, Engelbert RH, Williams CM. Interventions for idiopathic toe walking. *Cochrane Database Syst Rev.* 2019; (10): CD012363. doi:10.1002/14651858.CD012363.pub2
- Simonds AH, Abraham K, Spitznagle T. Clinical Practice Guidelines for Pelvic Girdle Pain in the Postpartum Population. *JWomen's Pelvic Health Phys Ther.* 2022;46(1):E1. https://doi.org/10.1097/JWH.0000000000000236
- Valdes K, Boyd JD, Povlak SB, Szelwach MA. Efficacy of orthotic devices for increased active proximal interphalangeal extension joint range of motion: a systematic review. *J Hand Ther.* 2019;32(2):184–193. https://doi.org/10.1016/j.jht.2018.05.003
- Wallis JA, Roddy L, Bottrell J, Parslow S, Taylor NF. A systematic review of clinical practice guidelines for physical therapist management of patellofemoral pain. *Phys Ther.* 2021;101(3):pzab021. https://doi.org/10.1093/ptj/pzab021
- Martin RL, Chimenti R, Cuddeford T, et al. Achilles Pain, Stiffness, and Muscle Power Deficits: Midportion Achilles Tendinopathy Revision 2018. *J Orthop Sports Phys Ther.* 2018;48(5):A1–A38. https://doi.org/10.2519/jospt.2018.0302
- Williams G, Singer BJ, Ashford S, et al. A synthesis and appraisal of clinical practice guidelines, consensus statement,s and Cochrane systematic reviews for the management of focal spasticity in adults and children. *Disabil Rehabil.* 2022;44(4):509–519. https://doi.org/10.1080/09638288.2020.1769207
- Ringold S, Angeles-Han ST, Beukelman T, et al. 2019 American College of Rheumatology/Arthritis Foundation Guideline for the Treatment of Juvenile Idiopathic Arthritis: therapeutic approaches for non-systemic polyarthritis, sacroiliitis, and enthesitis. *Arthritis Care Res.* 2019;71(6):717–734. https://doi.org/10.1002/acr.23870

Appendix 4.4

Results of Search Using Cochrane Database of Systematic Reviews

- French HP, Abbott JH, Galvin R. Adjunctive therapies in addition to land-based exercise therapy for osteoarthritis of the hip or knee. *Cochrane Database Syst Rev*. 2022;(10). https://doi.org/10.1002/14651858.CD011915.pub2
- Chiu HC, Ada L, Bania TA. Mechanically assisted walking training for walking, participation, and quality of life in children with cerebral palsy. *Cochrane Database Syst Rev*. 2020;(11). https://doi.org/10.1002/14651858.CD013114.pub2
- Blumetti FC, Belloti JC, Tamaoki MJ, Pinto JA. Botulinum toxin type A in the treatment of lower limb spasticity in children with cerebral palsy. *Cochrane Database Syst Rev*. 2019;(10). https://doi.org/10.1002/14651858.CD001408.pub2
- Mehrholz J, Thomas S, Kugler J, Pohl M, Elsner B. Electromechanical-assisted training for walking after stroke. *Cochrane Database Syst Rev*. 2020;(10). https://doi.org/10.1002/14651858.CD006185.pub5
- Hoe VC, Urquhart DM, Kelsall HL, Zamri EN, Sim MR. Ergonomic interventions for preventing work-related musculoskeletal disorders of the upper limb and neck among office workers. *Cochrane Database Syst Rev*. 2018;(10). https://doi.org/10.1002/14651858.CD008570.pub3

5 Clinical Assessment of Gait

MARIE B. CORKERY, JESSICA M. MARENGO, SHENG-CHE YEN, AND KEVIN K. CHUI

LEARNING OBJECTIVES

On completion of this chapter, the reader will be able to do the following:

1. Describe the major functional tasks of the gait cycle and their corresponding subphases.
2. Identify the muscle activity, ground reaction forces, and joint angles during each of the subphases of the gait cycle.
3. Define the time and distance parameters used to describe and assess normal gait.
4. Describe common pathological gait patterns, including contributing factors, compensatory deviations, and when these are likely to occur in the gait cycle.
5. Compare and contrast the type and quality of information gathered with various quantitative, qualitative, instrumented, and function-based gait assessment tools.
6. Differentiate between pathological and compensatory gait characteristics typically observed in individuals with lower motor neuron disease, hemiplegia, spastic diplegic cerebral palsy, and spina bifida.
7. Discuss how prosthetic components and alignment influence the efficacy and quality of gait for individuals with amputation at the transtibial and transfemoral levels.

Normal Gait

Walking requires numerous physiological systems (neurologic, musculoskeletal, cardiopulmonary, and cognition) to work congruently. Understanding normal gait is a prerequisite to understanding pathological gait, as it will provide the standard against which the gait pattern (GP) of an individual could be compared. Normal walking requires stability to provide body weight support against gravity during stance, mobility of body segments, and motor control to sequence multiple segments while transferring body weight from one limb to the other. The primary goal in gait is forward progression by using a stable kinetic chain of joints and limb segments working congruently to transport its passenger unit, consisting of the head, arms, and trunk in a continuously changing environment and varied task demands.

Clinical gait assessment identifies primary or pathological gait problems and helps differentiate them from compensatory strategies. It is necessary for selection of appropriate orthotic or prosthetic components, alignment parameters, and identification of other variants that might enhance an individual's ability to walk. Clinical gait assessment also contributes to the development of a comprehensive treatment plan with the ultimate goal of optimal energy efficiency and appropriate pathomechanical control, balancing cosmesis, and overall function.

A comprehensive system to describe normal and abnormal gait has been developed by the Pathokinesiology and Physical Therapy Departments at Rancho Los Amigos Medical Center over the past several decades.[1,2] Based on this system, a comprehensive manual for normal and pathological observational gait analysis has been published to offer a practical guide for clinical gait assessment.[3]

Kinetic and Kinematic Descriptors of Human Walking

The mechanics of human movement and related biomechanical behavior is studied by individuals desiring to know more about the loading experienced by the body, the body's response to loading, overall motion of the body, as well as the motions of its unique body segments, and ultimately the forces required to produce motion. *Kinematics* is the study of motion, whereas *kinetics* is the study of the forces that produce motion. Studying kinematics and kinetics in unison provides knowledge and understanding of human movement that is far-reaching and comprehensive.

Step length, stride length, cadence, and velocity are important quantitative, interrelated kinematic measures of gait.[1] Step length and stride length are not synonymous. *Step length* is the distance from the floor-contact point of one (ipsilateral, originating) foot in early stance to the floor-contact point of the opposite (contralateral) foot—in normal individuals, the distance from right heel contact to left heel contact. *Stride length* is the distance from floor contact on one side to the next floor contact on that same side—the distance from right heel contact to the next right heel contact. A reduction in functional joint motion or the presence of pain or muscle weakness can result in decreased stride or step length, or both. Pathological gait commonly produces asymmetries in step length between the two lower limbs.

Cadence is the number of steps taken in a given unit of time, most often expressed in steps per minute. *Velocity* is the distance traveled in a given unit of time (the rate of forward progression) and is usually expressed in centimeters per second or meters per minute. Velocity is a valid index to measure walking ability.[4] Decreased joint motion, pain, and/or muscle weakness can reduce cadence and/or velocity.

Velocity can also be qualitatively categorized as free, slow, or fast. Free walking (self-selected) speed is an individual's normal self-selected (comfortable) walking velocity. Fast walking speed (WS) describes the maximum velocity possible for a given individual while being safe. Slow WS describes a velocity below the normal self-selected WS. In people with musculoskeletal and neuromuscular impairments that affect gait, often much less difference is found between free and fast gait velocity. *Double limb support* is the period of time when both feet are in contact with the ground. It occurs twice during the gait cycle, at the beginning and the end of each stance phase. As velocity increases, double limb support time decreases. When running, the individual has rapid forward movement with little or no period of double limb support. Individuals with slow WS spend more of the gait cycle in double limb support. *Step width*, or width of the walking base, typically measures between 5 and 10 cm from the heel center of one foot to the heel center of the other foot. A wide walking base may increase stability but also reduces energy efficiency of gait.

Ground reaction force (GRF) in gait is established between the contact of the limb and the supporting surface; the point of application of the GRF and the supporting surface is called the *center of pressure*. The GRF is a vector quantity comprised of both magnitude and direction and can be resolved into perpendicular force vectors, normal force, and tangential force components, respectively. The magnitude is a result of the combination of the gravitational and inertial effects on all the body segments while the foot is in contact with the ground, and the direction is the result of the angle of application of the combination of gravitational and inertial forces when the foot is in contact with the ground.[5] Kinetic and kinematic measurements can be assessed through the combination of force plates, electromyography (EMG), and motion capture analysis. *Force plates* are platforms set on or into the ground that a person is traversing. The force plates measure the amount of force exerted on them during the respective steps taken across the platforms.[5] *EMG* captures the electrical signals produced by muscle activation. EMG data is implied from muscle activation patterns and can be compiled with correlating force plate data to directly produce kinetic data in real time.

The spatial relationship between the GRF and a given joint center influences the direction of its rotation and measurements. The rotational potential of the forces that act on a joint is called a *torque* or *moment*. *Torque (or moment)* is the tendency to produce rotational motion as a result of a force being applied across a distance from the pivot point. Torque produces displacement of the lever or limb segment with a particular angular velocity. The measure that assesses the quantity of work occurring over a particular time or the rate of change of energy in a particular system is known as *power*. Power is useful in both kinetic and kinematic assessments of joint motion. Joint power is found by multiplying the magnitude of torque and the angular velocity for the respective joint.

Kinetic and kinematic descriptors of human motion are not only helpful in describing motion but also in the quantification and qualification of both static and dynamic assessment, providing feedback to the client and clinician, and informing modification to both technique and equipment, respectively. This allows for adequate evaluation and adaptation to ultimately improve performance and reduce the risk of injury.

Gait Cycle

The *gait cycle* is the time interval between two successive occurrences of one of the repetitive events of walking. Conventionally the time from initial contact to initial contact of the same foot is selected as the starting and completing event of a single cycle of gait. Each cycle is divided into two periods: stance phase and swing phase. *Stance* is the time when the foot is in contact with floor during one gait cycle (0%–60%).[1] For adults, it constitutes approximately 60% of the gait of the gait cycle. *Swing* denotes the time when the foot is in the air during one gait cycle and constitutes the remaining 40% of the gait cycle. There are five subphases within the stance period: initial contact (IC), loading response (LR), midstance (MSt), terminal stance (TSt), and preswing (PSw). Swing phase is divided into three subphases: initial swing (ISw), midswing (MSw), and terminal swing (TSw). Single limb support (SLS) is the time when only one foot is in contact with the ground during one gait cycle. Double limb support (DLS) is the time when both feet are in contact with the ground during one gait cycle. A variety of conceptual approaches describe the walking process. Saunders and colleagues define the functional task of walking as translation of the center of gravity through space in a manner that requires the least energy expenditure.[6] They identify six determinants, or variables, that affect energy expenditure in sustained walking: pelvic rotation, pelvic tilt, knee flexion in stance phase, foot interaction with the knee, ankle interaction with the knee, and lateral pelvic displacement. Individually and collectively, these determinants have an impact on energy expenditure and the mechanics of walking. Although they help us understand the process of walking, the determinants do not themselves offer a practical clinical solution to address the problems of gait assessment. Three functional tasks are achieved during these eight gait phases: weight acceptance in early stance, SLS in MSt to TSt, and limb advancement during swing (Fig. 5.1).

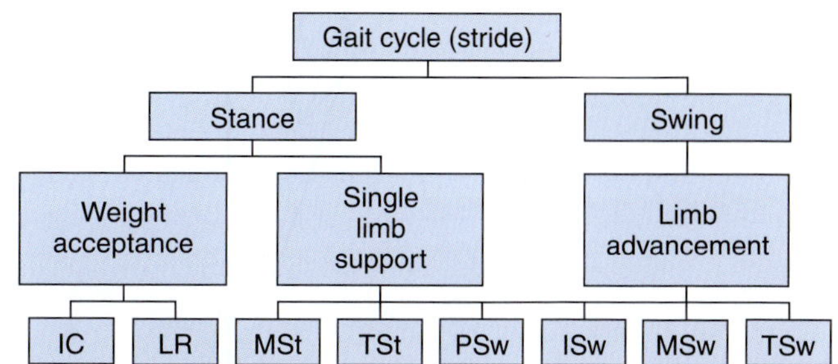

Fig. 5.1 A complete gait cycle divided into three functional tasks of weight acceptance, single limb support, and limb advancement. The gait cycle can also be described in phasic terms of initial contact *(IC)*, loading response *(LR)*, midstance *(MSt)*, terminal stance *(TSt)*, preswing *(PSw)*, initial swing *(ISw)*, midswing *(MSw)*, and terminal swing *(TSw)*. The PSw phase is a transitional phase between single limb support and limb advancement.

FUNCTIONAL TASK 1: WEIGHT ACCEPTANCE

IC and LR are the subphases of stance where weight acceptance is accomplished. Effective transfer of body weight onto the limb as soon as it makes contact with the ground requires initial limb stability, shock absorption, and the preservation of forward momentum.

Initial Contact

IC is the instant the foot of the leading lower limb touches the ground. Most motor function during IC is preparation for LR. At IC, the ankle is in a neutral position, the knee is close to full extension, and the hip is flexed 30 degrees. The sagittal plane GRF vector lies posterior to the ankle joint, creating a plantarflexion moment (Fig. 5.2A). Eccentric contraction of the pretibial muscles (tibialis anterior and long toe extensors) holds the ankle and subtalar joint in neutral position. At the knee, the GRF vector is anterior to the joint axis, which creates a passive extensor torque. Muscle contraction activity of the three vasti of the quadriceps and hamstring muscle groups continues from the previous TSw to preserve the neutral position of the knee joint. A flexion moment is present around the hip joint because the GRF vector falls anterior to the joint axis. Gluteus maximus and hamstring muscles are activated to restrain the resultant flexion torque.

Loading Response

LR occupies approximately 10% of the gait cycle and constitutes the period of initial double limb support (see Fig. 5.2B). Two functional tasks occur during LR: controlled descent of the foot toward the ground and shock absorption as weight is transferred onto the stance limb.

The momentum generated by the fall of body weight onto the stance limb is preserved by the *heel rocker* (first rocker) of stance phase.[1] Normal IC at the calcaneal tuberosity creates a fulcrum about which the foot and tibia move. The bony segment between this fulcrum and the center of

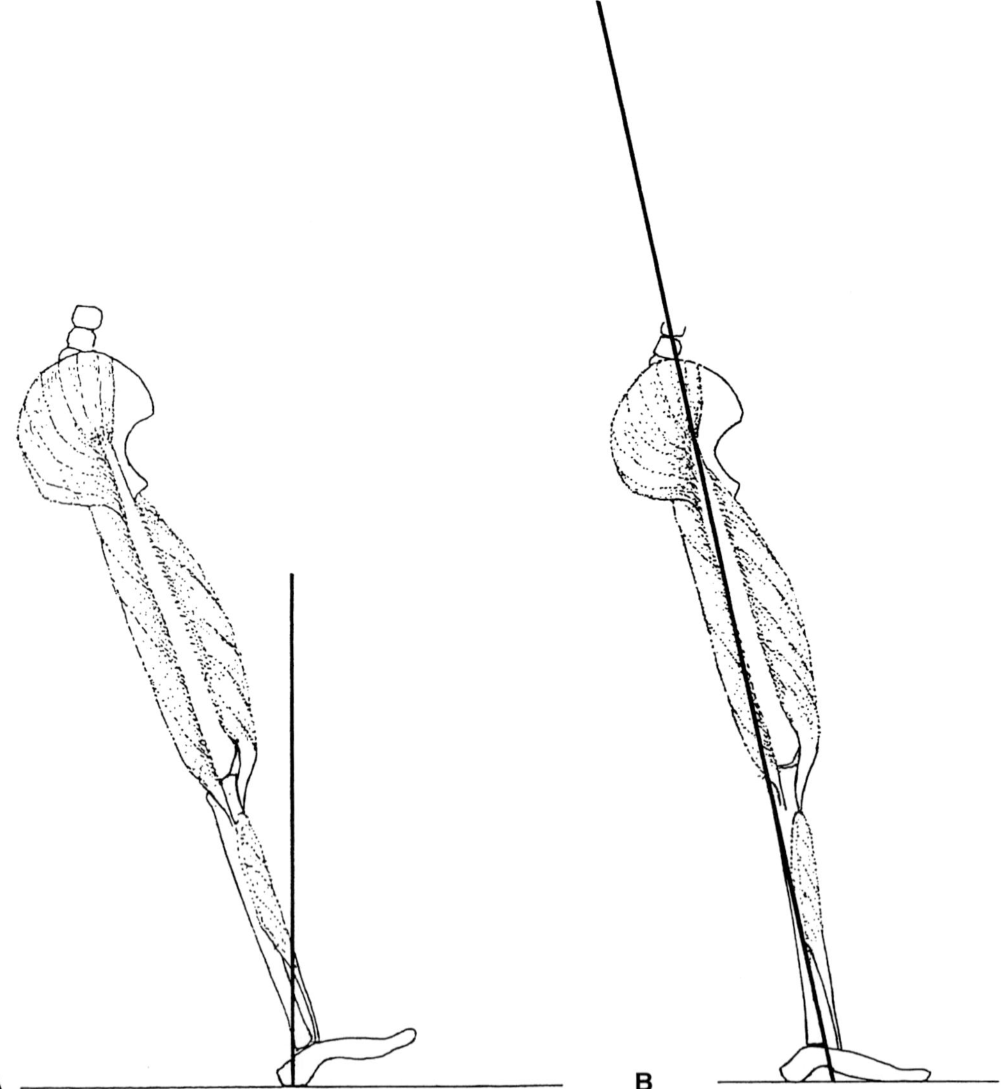

Fig. 5.2 The two subphases of gait involved with the functional task of weight acceptance are initial contact (IC) and loading response (LR). (A) At IC, the ground reaction force (GRF) line is posterior to the ankle and anterior to the knee and hip with activation of pretibial, quadriceps, hamstring, and gluteal muscles. Note that the length of the GRF line represents its magnitude. (B) The LR phase results in an increased magnitude of the vertical force, which ultimately exceeds body weight. Activity of the same muscle groups elicited at IC increases steadily with the vertical force.

the ankle rolls toward the ground as body weight is loaded onto the stance foot, preserving the momentum necessary for forward progression. Eccentric action of the pretibial muscles regulates the rate of ankle plantarflexion, and the quadriceps vasti contract to limit knee flexion. The action of these two muscle groups provides controlled forward advancement of the lower extremity unit (foot, tibia, and femur). During the peak of LR, the magnitude of the vertical GRF exceeds body weight. To absorb the impact force of body weight and preserve forward momentum, the knee flexes 15 to 18 degrees and the ankle plantar flexes to 10 degrees. The hip maintains its position of 30 degrees of flexion. Contraction of the gluteus maximus, hamstrings, and adductor magnus prevents further flexion of the hip joint.

FUNCTIONAL TASK 2: SINGLE LIMB SUPPORT

Two phases of stance are associated with SLS: MSt and TSt. During this period, the contralateral foot is in swing phase, and body weight is entirely supported on the stance limb. Forward progression of body weight over the stationary foot while maintaining stability must be accomplished during these two subphases of stance.

Midstance

MSt begins when the contralateral foot leaves the ground and continues as body weight travels along the length of the stance foot until it is aligned over the forefoot at approximately 20% of the gait cycle (Fig. 5.3A). This pivotal action of the *ankle rocker* (second rocker) advances the tibia over the stationary foot.[1] Forward movement of the tibia over the foot is controlled by the eccentric contraction of the soleus assisted by the gastrocnemius.

During this phase, the ankle moves from its LR position of 10 degrees of plantarflexion to approximately 5 degrees of dorsiflexion. The knee extends from 15 degrees of flexion to a neutral position. The hip joint moves toward extension, from 30 to 10 degrees of flexion. With continued forward progression, the body weight vector moves anterior to the ankle, creating a dorsiflexion moment. Eccentric action of the plantar flexors is crucial in providing limb stability as contralateral toe-off occurs, transferring body weight onto the stance foot. By the end of MSt, the body weight vector moves anterior to the knee (creating passive extensor stability at the knee) and posterior to the hip (reducing the demand on the hip extensors). The gluteus maximus, active in early MSt, ceases its activity and now stability relies on passive structures as the hip nears vertical alignment over the femur. Vertical GRF is reduced in magnitude at MSt because of the upward momentum of the contralateral swing limb. In the coronal plane, activity of hip abductors during MSt is essential to provide lateral hip stability and an almost level pelvis.

Terminal Stance

TSt, the second half of SLS, begins with heel rise of the stance limb and ends when the contralateral foot makes contact with the ground. As the body vector approaches the metatarsophalangeal joint, the heel rises, and the phalanx dorsiflexes (extends). The metatarsal heads serve as an axis of rotation for body weight advancement (see Fig. 5.3B). This is referred to as the *forefoot rocker* (third rocker).[1] The forefoot rocker serves as an axis around which progression of the body vector advances beyond the area of foot support, creating the highest demand on calf muscles (gastrocnemius and soleus). During TSt, the ankle continues to dorsiflex to 10 degrees. The knee is fully extended, and the hip moves into slight hyperextension. Forward fall of the body moves the vector further anterior to the ankle, creating a large dorsiflexion moment. Stability of the tibia on the ankle is provided by the eccentric action of the gastrocnemius and soleus muscles.

The trailing posture of the limb and the presence of the vector anterior to the knee and posterior to the hip provide passive stability at hip and knee joints. The tensor fascia latae serves to restrain the posterior vector at the hip. At the end of TSt, the vertical GRF reaches a second peak greater than body weight, similar to that which occurred at the end of LR.

FUNCTIONAL TASK 3: LIMB ADVANCEMENT

Four phases contribute to limb advancement: PSw, ISw, MSw, and TSw. During these phases, the stance limb leaves the ground, advances forward, and prepares for the successive IC.

Preswing

PSw, the second period of double limb support in gait, comprises the last 10% of the stance phase. It begins when the contralateral foot makes contact with the ground and ends with ipsilateral toe-off. During this period, the stance limb is unloaded, and body weight is transferred onto the contralateral limb (Fig. 5.4A). This is referred to as the *toe rocker* (fourth rocker). The toe rocker, the most anterior aspect of the medial margin of the forefoot and the great toe, serves as the base for accelerated limb advancement.[1] The ankle moves rapidly from its TSt dorsiflexion into 20 degrees of plantarflexion. During this subphase, plantar flexor muscle activity decreases as the limb is unloaded. Toward the end of PSw, the vertical force is diminished such that plantar flexors rapidly decrease their activity to complete quiescence. There is minimal muscle contraction for "push off" in normal reciprocal, free walk, bipedal gait.[7] The knee also flexes rapidly to achieve 35 to 40 degrees of flexion by the end of PSw.[8] The GRF vector is at the metatarsophalangeal joints and posterior to the knee, creating passive knee flexion with toe clearance. Knee flexion during this phase prepares the limb for toe clearance in the swing phase. PSw hip flexion is initiated by the rectus femoris and the adductor longus, which also decelerates the passive abduction created by contralateral body weight transfer. The sagittal vector extends through the hip as the hip returns to a neutral position.

Initial Swing

Approximately one-third of the swing period is spent in ISw. It begins the moment the foot leaves the ground and continues until maximal knee flexion (60 degrees) occurs, when the swinging extremity is directly under the body (see Fig. 5.4B). Concentric contraction of pretibial muscles initiates foot dorsiflexion from its initial 20 to 5 degrees of plantarflexion. This is necessary for toe and foot clearance as swing phase begins. Knee flexion, resulting from action of

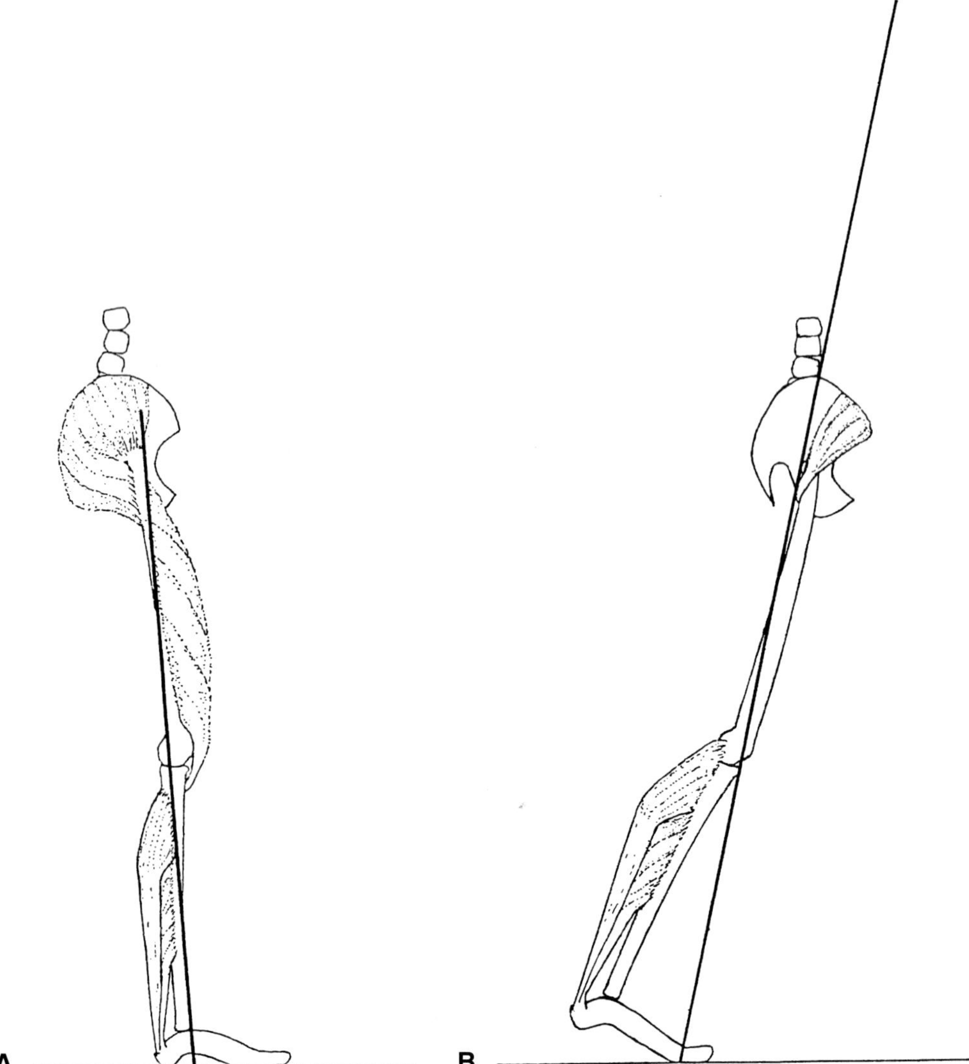

Fig. 5.3 The subphases of gait involved in the functional task of single limb support are midstance (MSt) and terminal stance (TSt). (A) In early MSt, the vertical force begins to decrease and the triceps surae, quadriceps, and gluteus medius and maximus are active. (B) During TSt, there is a second peak in vertical force, exceeding body weight, with high activity of the triceps surae, which maintain the third rocker. The tensor fascia lata restrains the increasing posterior hip vector.

the short head of the biceps femoris, also assists in toe clearance. The knee continues to flex until it reaches a position of 60 degrees of flexion. Contraction of the iliacus advances the hip to 20 degrees of flexion. Contraction of the gracilis and sartorius muscles during this phase assists hip and knee flexion.

Midswing

During MSw, limb advancement and foot clearance continue. MSw begins at maximum knee flexion and ends when the tibia is vertical. Knee extension, coupled with ankle dorsiflexion, contributes to foot clearance while advancing the tibia (see Fig. 5.4C). Continued concentric activity of pretibial muscles ensures foot clearance and moves the foot toward the neutral position. Momentum creates an extension moment, advancing the lower leg toward extension from 60 to 30 degrees of flexion, with the quadriceps quiescent. Mild contraction of hip flexors continues to preserve the hip flexion position.

Terminal Swing

In the final phase, TSw, the knee extends fully in preparation for heel contact (see Fig. 5.4D). Eccentric contraction of the hamstrings and gluteus maximus decelerates the thigh and restrains further hip flexion. Activity of the pretibial muscles maintains the ankle at neutral to prepare for heel contact. In the second half of TSw, the rectus femoris is quiescent but the rest of the quadriceps vasti become active to facilitate full knee extension. Hip flexion remains at 30 degrees.

A comprehensive system to describe normal and abnormal gait has been developed by the Pathokinesiology and Physical Therapy Departments at Rancho Los Amigos Medical Center over the past several decades.[1,2,9] Because velocity affects many parameters of walking, the description of normal gait assumes a comfortable self-selected velocity. At free walking velocity, the individual naturally recruits strategies and assumes the speed that provides maximum energy efficiency for their physiological system throughout the gait cycle.

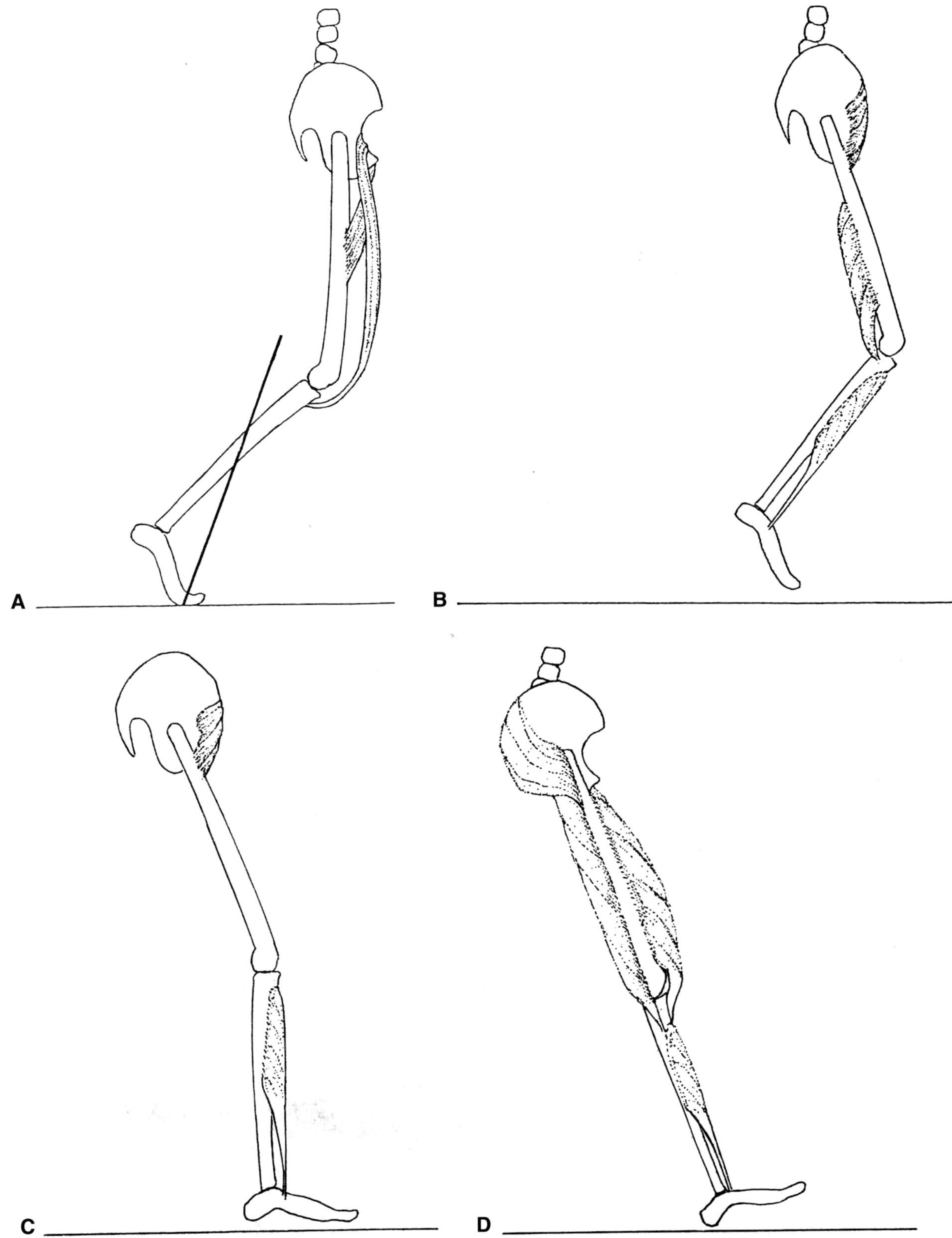

Fig. 5.4 The subphases of gait involved in the functional task of swing limb advancement include preswing (PSw), initial swing (ISw), midswing (MSw), and terminal swing (TSw). (A) During PSw, contralateral loading results in limited muscle activity in the limb transitioning from stance to swing. The rectus femoris and adductor longus initiate hip flexion. Knee flexion is passive, resulting from the planted forefoot and mobile proximal segments. (B) During ISw, the pretibial muscles, short head of the biceps femoris, and iliacus are active in initiating limb advancement and providing swing clearance. (C) A vertical tibia signals the end of the period of MSw. Here contraction of the iliacus preserves hip flexion while pretibial muscle activity maintains foot clearance. (D) At TSw, the gluteus maximus, hamstrings, quadriceps, and pretibial muscles are active to prepare for limb placement and the ensuing loading response.

Describing Pathological Gait

Qualitative descriptors are often used to characterize gait deviations and compensations. Some of these terms help identify specific primary impairments; others describe compensatory strategies adopted by individuals to address gait difficulties created by various primary impairments. Pathological gait mechanisms can be rooted in one of five primary areas: deformity, muscle weakness, sensory loss, pain, and impaired motor control.[1]

COMMON GAIT DEVIATIONS OBSERVED DURING STANCE

One common gait deviation observed in the stance phase is *increased contralateral pelvic drop or Trendelenburg gait pattern*.[10] This deviation can result from musculoskeletal complications or impaired motor control and is observed when the hip abductors are unable to generate sufficient torque to prevent excessive femoral adduction during LR. Increased contralateral pelvic drop is observed when the trunk leans to the same side as the hip pathology (ipsilateral lean), coupled with pelvic rotation. This is a compensatory strategy used when the gluteus medius muscle and its synergists (gluteus minimus and tensor fascia latae) cannot adequately stabilize the pelvis during stance.[11] Normally the drop of the contralateral pelvis is limited to 5 degrees by the eccentric control of the strong hip abductor muscles. To support the pelvis, the hip abductor muscles must generate a force that is about two times the body weight.[12] Weak or absent gluteus medius musculature leads to a postural substitution observed as an ipsilateral trunk lean over the weight-bearing hip joint. This reduces the external adductor moment created by a GRF line that falls medial to the joint center. Without this postural compensation, clearance of the distal portion of the contralateral limb becomes difficult in swing. Rarely, a positive Trendelenburg sign is caused by overactive hip adductors (adductors longus, magnus, brevis, and gracilis).

Vaulting may be a result of deformity or impaired motor control. Vaulting is observed through excessive plantarflexion of the stance foot, occasionally occurring with simultaneous stance limb hip and knee extension, with the goal of raising the pelvis to clear the contralateral swing limb.[13] It occurs when the functional length of the swing limb is relatively longer than that of the stance limb. It also occurs when swing limb advancement is impaired or delayed by inadequate motor control of hip or knee flexion, or both, or in the presence of a plantarflexion contracture of the swing leg. It may compensate for pelvic obliquity or leg length discrepancy.

Antalgic gait is a strategy used to avoid pain during walking. It is frequently observed in LR when the individual reduces SLS time on the affected limb. If the pain occurs during a particular interval in stance phase, that time interval is avoided. Antalgic gait caused by pain that originates around the hip might translate into a lateral lean to permit the individual to position the center of gravity over the support point, the head of the femur. If pain occurs during the extreme end range of a particular joint motion, that motion is diminished. For example, if full extension produces pain, the knee would be maintained in slight flexion throughout the gait cycle. It is important to note that while gait deviations are intended to lessen or avoid pain altogether, the compensatory movement patterns and altered mechanics can subsequently cause pain, dysfunction, and damage to the surrounding anatomy.[1]

COMMON GAIT DEVIATIONS OBSERVED DURING SWING

One common gait deviation observed in the swing phase is *circumducted gait*. Circumduction is described as hip abduction combined with a wide arc of external pelvic rotation. Circumduction can be observed as a lateral arc of the foot in the transverse plane that begins at the end of PSw and ends at IC on the same limb; the arc typically reaches the apex of its lateral movement at MSw. Most often, circumduction occurs as a compensatory pattern when there is a relatively longer swing limb compared with the stance limb. A plantarflexion contracture at the foot or a stiff knee or hip joint can necessitate a circumduction pattern during swing in an effort to achieve toe and foot clearance. The combination of abduction and pelvic rotation is a compensatory strategy to advance the limb through swing phase.

The typical pattern is a mixture of a wide base of support with the foot abnormally outset and may include an ipsilateral pelvic drop. In addition, it is possible for a contracture of the contralateral adductors to create this deviation by pulling the pelvis toward the contralateral femur and demanding a compensatory ipsilateral abducted position relative to the pelvis. A severe leg length discrepancy can result in an exaggerated pelvic tilt from the contralateral stance leg, which obligates the swing limb to an increased abduction position. Circumduction and abduction create a significant energy cost penalty, increasing lateral displacement of the center of gravity.

GAIT DEVIATIONS ASSOCIATED WITH ABNORMAL MUSCLE TONE

Gait deviations associated with abnormal muscle tone or weakness can be seen in both stance and swing phases and are also abnormalities produced by primary pathologies that present in the form of abnormal mechanics of one or more of the five functional areas (deformity, muscle weakness, sensory loss, pain, and impaired motor control).[1] A variety of abnormal GPs are associated with abnormal muscle tone—most commonly spasticity, rigidity, hypotonicity, or abnormal motor control or muscle weakness.

Ataxic gait is a complication in gait that is seen as a failure of coordination or irregularity of muscular action of the limb segments, commonly caused by cerebellar dysfunction. Ataxia often becomes accentuated when the eyes are closed, or vision is impaired or distracted.

Crouch gait is seen as excessive ankle dorsiflexion and exaggerated knee and hip flexion occurring throughout the stance phase of the gait cycle. Crouch gait is often seen in combination with toe-walking in children and adults with spastic diplegic cerebral palsy.[14] It has been attributed to a combination of overactivity of the hamstrings and weakness of calf muscles.

Scissor gait describes a pattern of poor control in limb advancement or tracking of the swing leg often characterized by the crossing, or scissoring (hip adduction, flexion, and medial rotation), of the lower limbs. It is most often observed in individuals with spastic or paretic pathological conditions such as hemiplegia, spastic diplegia, and cerebral palsy.[15]

Steppage gait occurs when there is weakness or paralysis of the dorsiflexor musculature, such as in persons with peroneal palsy or peripheral neuropathy, demanding exaggerated hip and knee flexion of the proximal joints to accomplish swing clearance; this gait deviation is most easily observed in late MSw.

Although orthosis use can successfully control abnormal motion in the sagittal plane as in steppage gait, orthoses are less effective in controlling the abnormal transverse, rotational, or coronal plane limb placement problems observed in ataxic, scissoring, or crouched GPs.

Qualitative Gait Assessment

Qualitative methods for identification and recording of gait deviations have played a role in patient care for decades. In 1925 Robinson described pathological GPs and attempted to correlate them with specific disease processes.[16] In 1937 Boorstein identified 14 disease processes that could be diagnosed with gait assessment.[17] He described seven major gait deficit groups, attributing the term *steppage gait* to the French physician Charcot and the identification of *waddling gait* in hip dysplasia to Hippocrates. In the late 1950s Blair Hangar, the founder of Northwestern University's School of Prosthetics and Orthotics, and Hildegard Myers, a physical therapist at Rehabilitation Institute of Chicago, collaborated to develop the first comprehensive system of clinical gait analysis for persons with transfemoral amputation.[18]

Brunnstrom's comprehensive gait analysis form for hemiplegic gait, published in 1970, is a checklist of 28 deviations seen at the ankle, knee, and hip that are common after stroke.[19] Many other assessment tools have evolved; many are used but only a few have been assessed for validity and reliability. The Gait Assessment and Intervention Tool (GAIT) is a 31-item objective measure of the movements of persons following stroke that provides a comprehensive assessment of the coordinated components of gait pre- and postintervention.[20] This tool has been shown to be reliable and valid in the assessment of gait and the assessment of the success of intervention following neural injury.[21,22]

Early work in observational gait analysis received a significant impetus from Perry as an outgrowth of basic research data published in 1967.[23] In the late 1960s Perry and a group of physical therapists from the Rancho Los Amigos Medical Center Physical Therapy Department developed an organized format for systematically applied observational gait analysis. Their work initially focused on the development of an in-house training program for students and personnel who were new to the rehabilitation hospital. Subsequent revisions have included additional gait data and gait interpretation and uses parameters of normal gait as a comparative standard for abnormal or pathological gait.[2] Subsequently Adams and Cerny have designed a similar but more simplified observational gait analysis form (KAKC's Observational Gait Analysis) that includes only major, most commonly occurring gait deviations.[3] It focuses on identifying gait deviations that affect the three functional tasks of walking: weight acceptance, SLS, and swing limb advancement. Problems in each of the major body segments are noted with a check in one of the bubbles, beginning with the ankle, calcaneus, toes, knee, thigh, pelvis, and trunk. This format allows the clinician to systematically consider critical questions to illuminate the deviations and complications present in each unique client presentation.[3]

Qualitative gait assessment is an important component of preorthotic assessment because it assists the clinician in identifying the functional task and the subphase of gait that are problematic and can be addressed with orthotic intervention. Similarly, qualitative assessment can inform preprosthetic choices, as well as identify deviations observed during gait analysis, illuminating the need for adjustment of prosthetic design and alignment.

Instrumented Gait Analysis

Instrumented gait analysis records the process of walking with measurable parameters collected through the use of computerized equipment with the goal of enhancing the interpretive quality of clinical gait analysis. Gait parameters can be recorded with instruments as common as a stopwatch or as complex as the simultaneous integration of three-dimensional kinematics, kinetics, and EMG methods. The primary emphasis of clinical assessment has been on accessible techniques and inexpensive technologies. A simple, inexpensive footprint mat has been used for decades to record barefoot plantar pressures. Clinics use individual or multiple mats to record step and stride length, as well as walking base width. Early on, video technology with slow-motion capabilities made more precise qualitative description of the gait cycle possible. The continued development of inexpensive video gait assessment software has made clinical quantitative applications more practical as well. Most quantitative and qualitative video systems, however, measure joint angles in two dimensions, which does not offer a complete analysis of the three-dimensional walking activity.

TECHNOLOGY IN GAIT ASSESSMENT

The high-tech side of quantitative gait analysis has traversed a surprisingly long road. The birth of instrumented kinematic, EMG, and temporal performance analysis began in the 1870s with E.J. Marey, who first performed movement analysis of pathological gait with photography.[24] He also developed the first myograph for measuring muscle activity and the first foot-switch collection system for measuring gait events related to the temporal parameters. The foot-switch system was an experimental shoe that measured the length and rapidity of the step and the pressure of the foot on the ground. Modern gait technology began in 1945, when Inman and colleagues initiated the systematic collection of gait data for individuals without impairment and with amputation in the outdoor gait laboratory at the University of California at Berkeley.[6] Since then, researchers and clinicians have increasingly used the wide array of gait technologies to measure the parameters of human performance in normal and pathological gait. A full-service gait laboratory gathers information on six performance parameters in walking: temporal, metabolic, kinematic, kinetic, EMG, and pressure.[5]

MEASURING TEMPORAL AND DISTANCE PARAMETERS

Temporal parameters (time and distance) enable the clinician to summarize the overall quality of an individual's gait. Temporal data collection systems might be one of the most effective components available for assessment in the clinical setting. In the gait laboratory, microswitch-embedded pads taped to the bottom of an individual's shoes or feet can record the amount of time the individual spends on various anatomical landmarks over a measured distance. Portable pressure-sensitive gait mats, connected to a laptop computer with gait analysis software for time and distance parameters, are also commercially available to use in clinical settings.[25,26] For example, the GAITRite system, which consists of an electronic walkway connected to a computer, records the temporal and spatial characteristics of individuals while walking, as well as while performing other functional or occupational tasks.[27] The GAITRite mat is flexible and can be rolled and transported in a hard case, which enables data collection at different clinics or sites. Rao and colleagues used the GAITRite system to collect temporal and spatial data to compare the effects of two unique and different ankle-foot orthosis (AFO) designs on the GP of individuals following acute hemiparetic cerebrovascular accidents (CVAs). In this study, they compared stride length, velocity, cadence, and step length, while also surveying the clients' perceptions between walking with no device, an off-the-shelf carbon AFO, and a custom plastic AFO. The GAITRite system data collection was consistent with the client perceptions; velocity, cadence, stride length, and step length increase with either the carbon AFO or the custom plastic AFO compared to no AFO.[26]

Gait deviations related to excessive inversion, eversion, or prolonged heel-only time can be recognized and should be considered when modifying the alignment or components of prostheses or orthoses. A temporal data collection system is particularly cost effective and clinically meaningful. Temporal data are usually a product of another measuring system such as EMG or motion analysis. Temporal data systems are commercially available, covering a wide range of costs, technical sophistication, and time required to analyze the summarized data. Some of the temporal parameters, however, can be recorded to a lesser degree of accuracy using a stopwatch and basic video camera.[28]

ASSESSING THE ENERGY COST OF WALKING

Metabolic data reflect the physiological "energy cost" of walking. The traditional measures of energy cost are oxygen consumption, total carbon dioxide generated, and heart rate. Other relevant factors include volume of air breathed and respiratory rate. All these parameters are viewed in relation to velocity and distance walked over the collection period. Historically, metabolic data were collected while the individual walked on a treadmill, wearing umbilical devices. In recent years, because of the known influence of treadmill collection in altering normal gait velocity, energy cost data are more likely to be obtained on an open track of a measured distance with the individual ambulating in a free walk or natural cadence. With the cardiopulmonary monitor device market continually growing and advancing, there is a wide array of versatile testing equipment to choose from. This equipment allows the individual to negotiate their normal environments with little or no interruption due to the testing and collection setups. Some of the newest products on the market couple the traditional oxygen and carbon dioxide (VO_2 and VCO_2) measurement with the capability of collecting telemetry data, indirect calorimetry, and integrated electrocardiogram, among other addons to standard systems. The primary limitation of energy cost as an assessment tool is that although it can inform the investigator about body metabolism relative to the individual's gait, it cannot explain why or how an advantage or disadvantage was obtained. Dr. Weinert-Aplin found that through the analysis of the center of mass in all three plans for participants with amputations there could potentially be a correlation between metabolic cost and the center of mass positioning during gait. The study revealed the base of support, and the medial-lateral positioning of the center of mass had the most significant correlation with the subject's metabolic requirements, suggesting that increases in base of support and medial-lateral center of mass displacement reduce walking efficiency.[29] Energy cost measures alone cannot easily differentiate between the impact of varieties of components, muscle activation, or a combination of both with regard to metabolic energy, whereas a combination of kinematic, kinetic, and EMG data typically can.[30] The COSMED K4b2 system has been used in many studies; in particular, one study utilized the wearable metabolic analysis system to assess the impact of new technologies in prosthetics and the associated energy requirements. The comparison was made between the standard energy storing prosthetic feet and the relatively new concept of crossover prosthetic feet.[31] The MetaMax 3B system was utilized to demonstrate that the movement of the center of mass, as well as the base of support, were significant indicators of the metabolic cost of walking in persons with amputations.[29]

Perhaps the best kept secret in the energy cost arsenal is the *physiological cost index* (PCI). It is easily calculated as follows:

$$\text{PCI} = (\text{walking pulse} - \text{resting pulse})/\text{gait speed}$$

The PCI is one of the most sensitive indicators of energy cost of gait. Tanabe and colleagues compared two different orthotic designs by measuring a wide variety of metabolic parameters as well as the PCI.[32] Their results demonstrated statistically significant differences in PCI between the two devices when all other measured parameters failed to produce such differences.

KINEMATIC AND KINETIC SYSTEMS

Most *kinematic* systems provide joint and body segment motion in graphic form. This information includes sagittal, coronal, and transverse motions that occur at the ankle, knee, hip, and pelvis. The individual is instrumented with reflective markers that are placed on well-recognized anatomical landmarks (Fig. 5.5). Typically, an infrared light source is positioned around or integrated into each of several cameras. This light is directed to the reflective spheres, which in turn are reflected into the cameras. Each field of video data is digitized, the markers are manually identified, and the coordinates of the geometric center of each marker are calculated with computer software. Resultant data are displayed as animated figures that represent the actual motions produced by the individual. The operator can freeze any frame and enlarge the image at any joint to examine GPs in greater depth. The operator can extract raw numbers that represent joint placement and motion in space or produce a printout showing joint motion in all planes plotted against the percentage of the gait cycle (Fig. 5.6). Angular velocities, accelerations, and joint and segment linear displacements can be calculated. Data from other systems (force platforms and EMG) collected during the same time sequence as the motion data are often integrated with the kinematics. Advanced systems like these can be a very expensive component of the gait lab, but the information collected provides some of the most in-depth and valid data. In the gait lab or a clinical lab, the motion system setup serves as the technological core. A variety of optical motion systems have been used to evaluate the joint motion in individuals with spastic diplegic cerebral palsy and various other client populations.[33] More recently, a marker-less motion capture system has been developed to avoid marker placement during motion tracking in clinical use.[34] An inertial-based motion capture system has been developed to track motion in the field, rather than a confined lab space.[35] In addition, the EvaRT motion analysis system has been used to collect data comparing mechanical and microprocessor knees in individuals with gait and balance deficits associated with transfemoral amputations.[36]

The Dartfish system is another motion analysis tool that is used in gait laboratories and clinical settings.[37] The Dartfish system allows for two- and three-dimensional joint motion analysis. It is portable, less expensive, and requires less time to set up when compared with other motion analysis systems. In one study, the Dartfish system demonstrated excellent validity and reliability as well as agreement between 2D and 3D motion analysis in participants demonstrating postural control of varying capabilities, as well as balance deficits.[38]

When an individual takes a step, they are exerting force against the surface they are walking on. This kinetic information is obtained from one or more force platforms, which collect data on the three components of the GRF: vertical, fore-aft (anterior-posterior), and medial-lateral (Fig. 5.7). The contribution of kinetic data can be significant. Fore-aft shear is quite useful in establishing appropriate transtibial prosthetic alignment in the sagittal plane. For this purpose, the clinician would anticipate a balanced magnitude and timing of the braking and propulsive patterns. Data collection from two consecutive steps, one gait cycle, requires dual force plates. Some kinetic software packages also offer specialized programs for specific purposes such as stability analysis, which provides information about center of gravity shift relative to time.

Although the typical force platform system provides data about forces and moments occurring at the ground, or center of pressure progression, it can be combined with kinematic data to provide additional information. By combining these two data sets, the moments and powers acting at the joints can be calculated. This information is useful

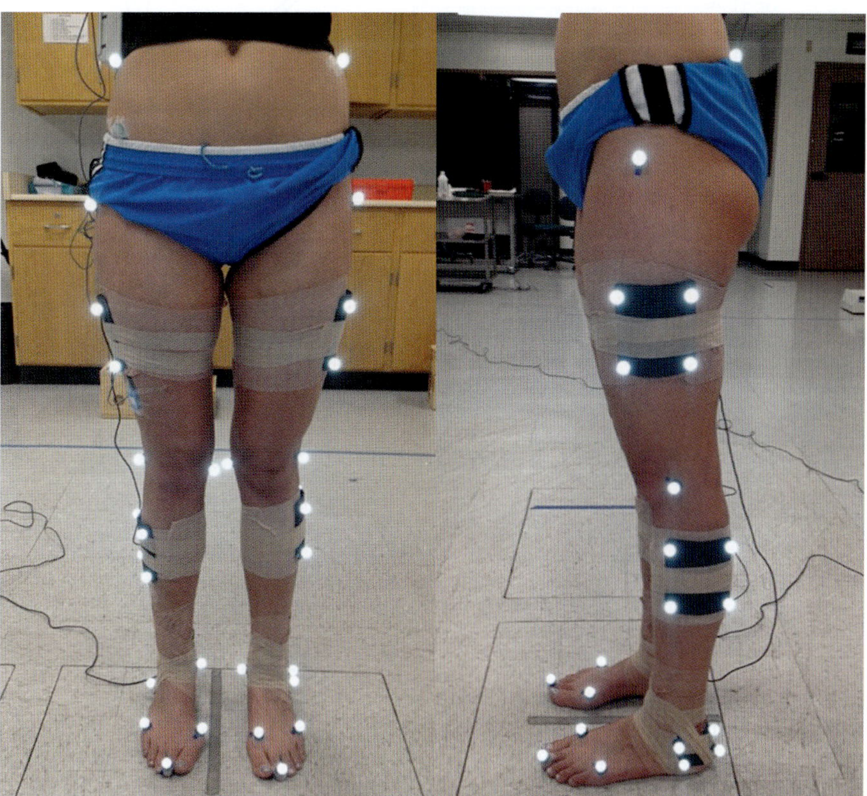

Fig. 5.5 This individual is wearing reflective spheres. An infrared camera system can track limb segment motion as the patient walks across the field of view.

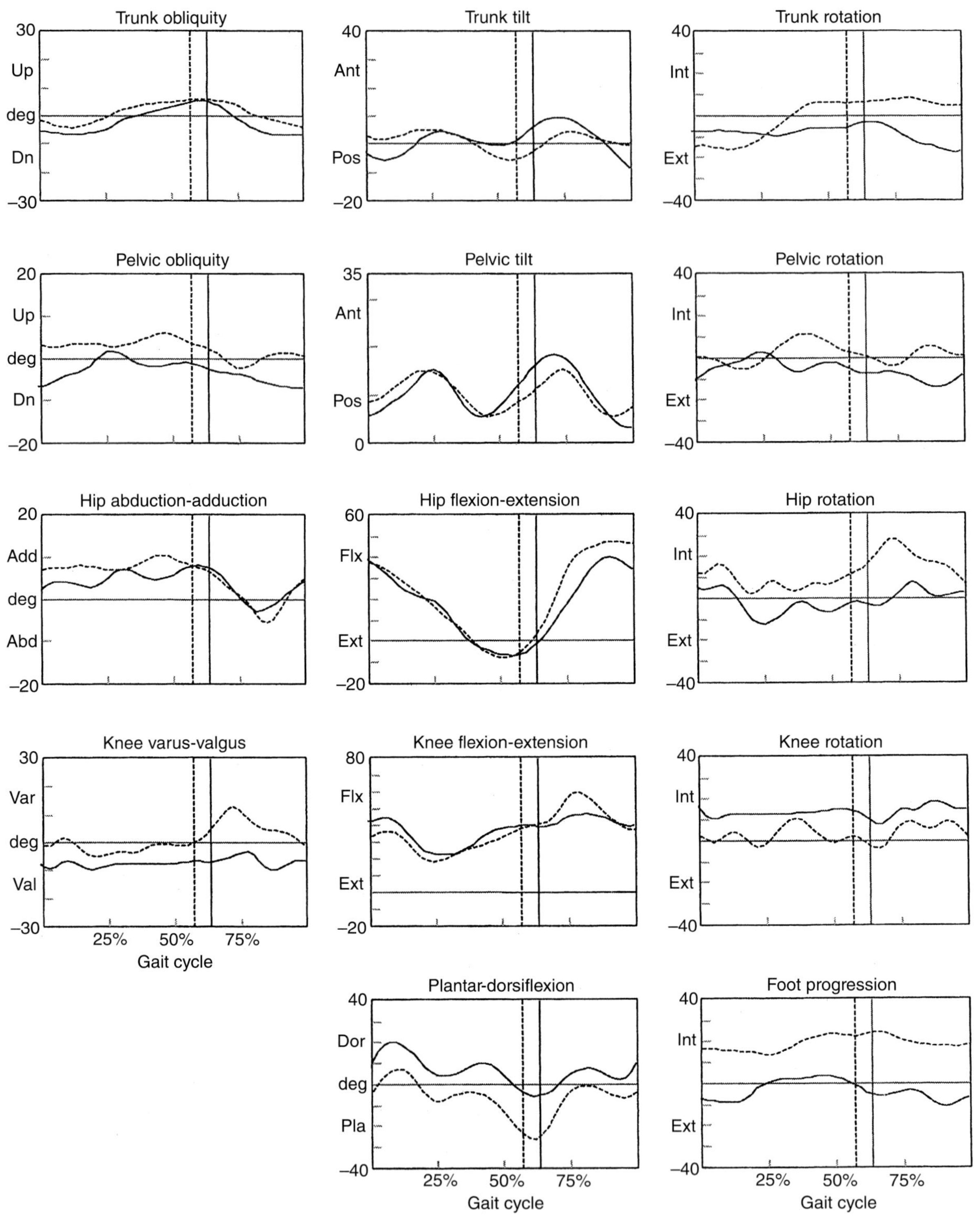

Fig. 5.6 The output generated by a computer-based motion analysis system includes graphs of the mean range of motion at each body segment or joint (trunk, pelvis, hip, knee, and ankle) in coronal *(left column)*, sagittal *(middle column)*, and transverse *(right column)* planes as the individual being evaluated progresses through multiple gait cycles. This is the output of an 8-year-old child with spastic diplegic cerebral palsy. (Courtesy the Center for Motion Analysis, Connecticut Children's Medical Center, Hartford, Connecticut.)

in measuring the dynamic joint control of an individual throughout stance, particularly when used in conjunction with EMG. Similarly, information about joint moments, sometimes referred to as *torque*, is also often reported as an outcome measure in research studies. Although this information can be potentially important in the evaluation of pathological gait, it is also necessary to have a basic understanding of how these values are derived. As mentioned,

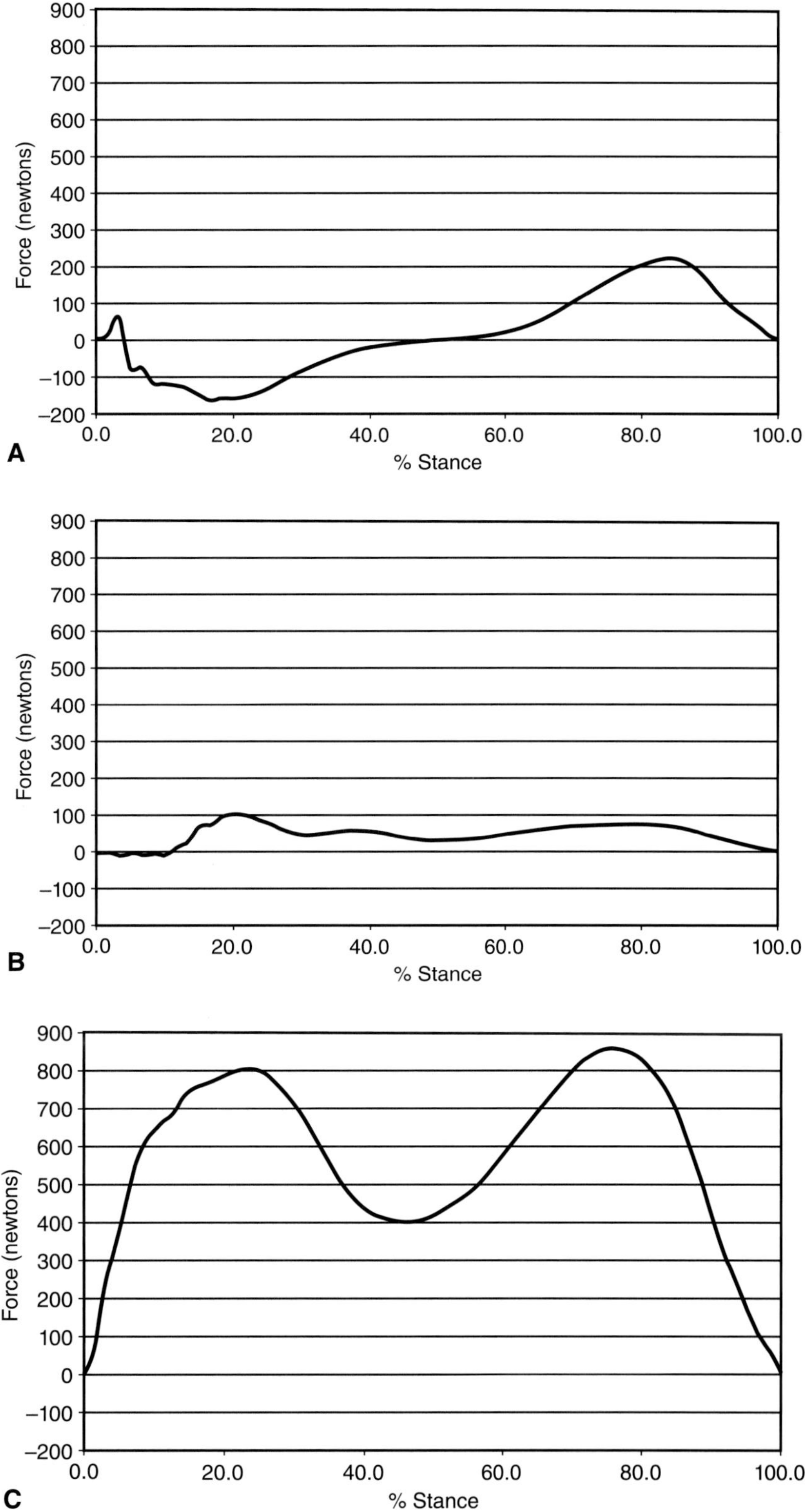

Fig. 5.7 Example of output generated by a forceplate as the individual being tested progresses through stance phase. (A) The anteroposterior component of the ground reaction force (GRF). (B) The medial-lateral component of the GRF. (C) The vertical component of the GRF. (Output courtesy the Motion Analysis Laboratory, Department of Physical Therapy and Human Movement Science, Sacred Heart University, Fairfield, Connecticut.)

when a person ambulates, the individual exerts force on the walking surface; differing degrees of this force are similarly exerted on each of the joints in the lower extremity. With the exertion of these forces comes an associated moment that is also acting at the joint, along with a power value. In its most basic form, a moment is the result of a force multiplied by the moment (lever) arm.[5] The moment arm is calculated as the perpendicular distance from the rotation center of the joint to the line of action of the force acting on the associated segment. Joint power is then calculated by multiplying the moment acting at a joint by the joint's angular velocity. In order to calculate these values, the lower extremity must be broken down into segments—often the ankle, shank or calf, and thigh. By doing this, a link-segment model is being applied and the parameters of interest can be calculated. One study utilized a multilink segment model to evaluate the kinetics, kinematics, and energetics associated with energy storage and return (ESAR) prosthetic feet used in high impact sports. The study revealed there were some flaws in merging unaffected limb and affected limb parameters; this should be taken into consideration when studying the kinematics and kinetics of persons with unilateral amputations.[39]

To further illustrate the interrelated nature of these measures, the calculation path for forces, moments, and power is also presented in a flowchart (Fig. 5.8). It is important to note within the diagram where the different data sources originate. There are very few directly measured values that are then combined with biomechanical models to calculate these variables.

The calculation process begins with the determination of the GRFs, which are obtained through the direct measurement of an individual stepping on a force platform. Once that information is available, it is combined with kinematic data and derived from a two- or three-dimensional motion capture system for each lower extremity body segment so that the joint reaction forces can be calculated. As the forces at each of the joints are determined, then the associated moments acting on each segment can also be calculated. Ultimately, the power can be calculated as well (Fig. 5.9).

In many cases, instrumented kinetic and kinematic systems have included an inverse dynamics model that is applied to determine the forces acting at each of the lower extremity joints. Like virtually all biomechanics models, certain assumptions must be made in order for the calculation to be carried out in a practical manner. With assumptions come the opportunity for the introduction of additional error throughout the process. Because of the high potential for induced error, it is important to understand the limitations associated with them. A fundamental point is that these calculations frequently rely upon data that are calculated using general body proportions and anthropometric models for whole-bodied individuals. Because of this, certain assumptions are made about the mechanical properties of the segments and joints being evaluated. For example, many of the commonly used models assume that the subject has no limb deficiencies and essentially normal musculature. While this may be acceptable for evaluations of individuals without pathology, these assumptions can become a source of error

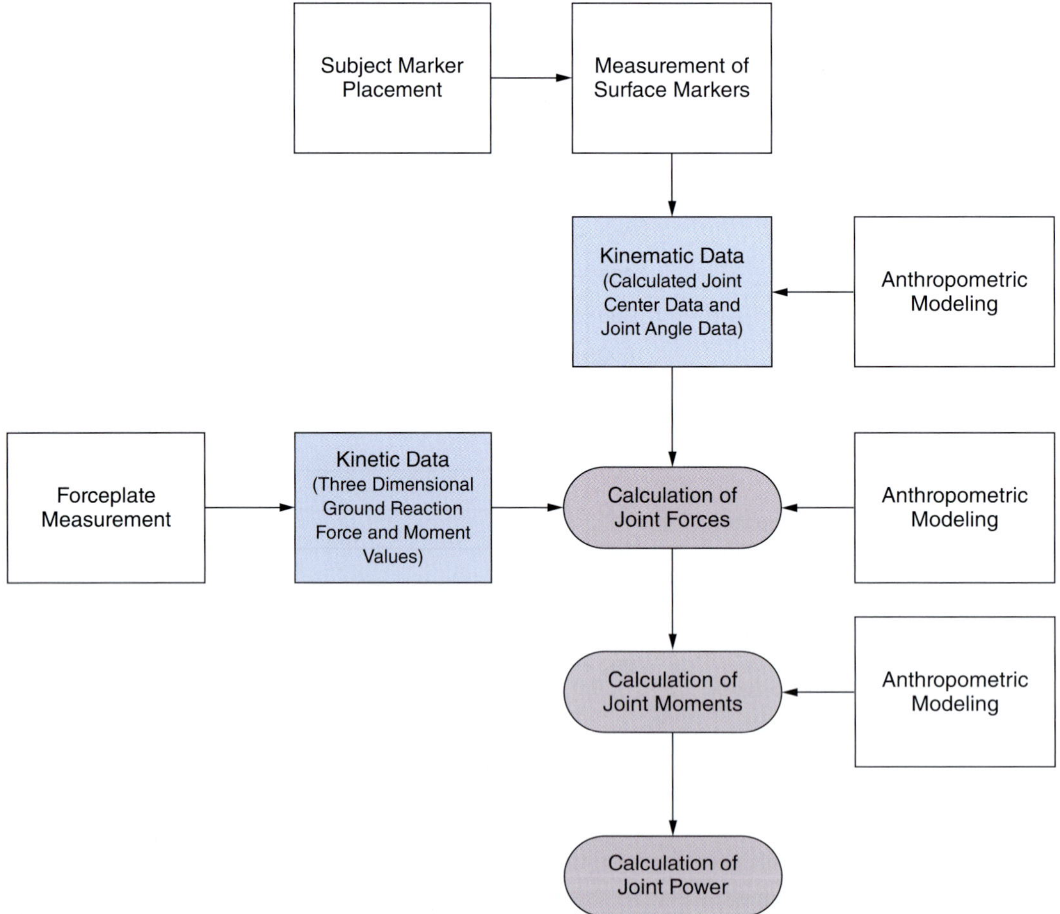

Fig. 5.8 Calculation flowchart: the kinematic data collected from the motion analysis system is entered into a series of calculations based on the person's anthropometric data to produce the instantaneous position of every joint and segment. These data are then combined with force plate data collected at the same time to calculate joint forces, moments, and powers.

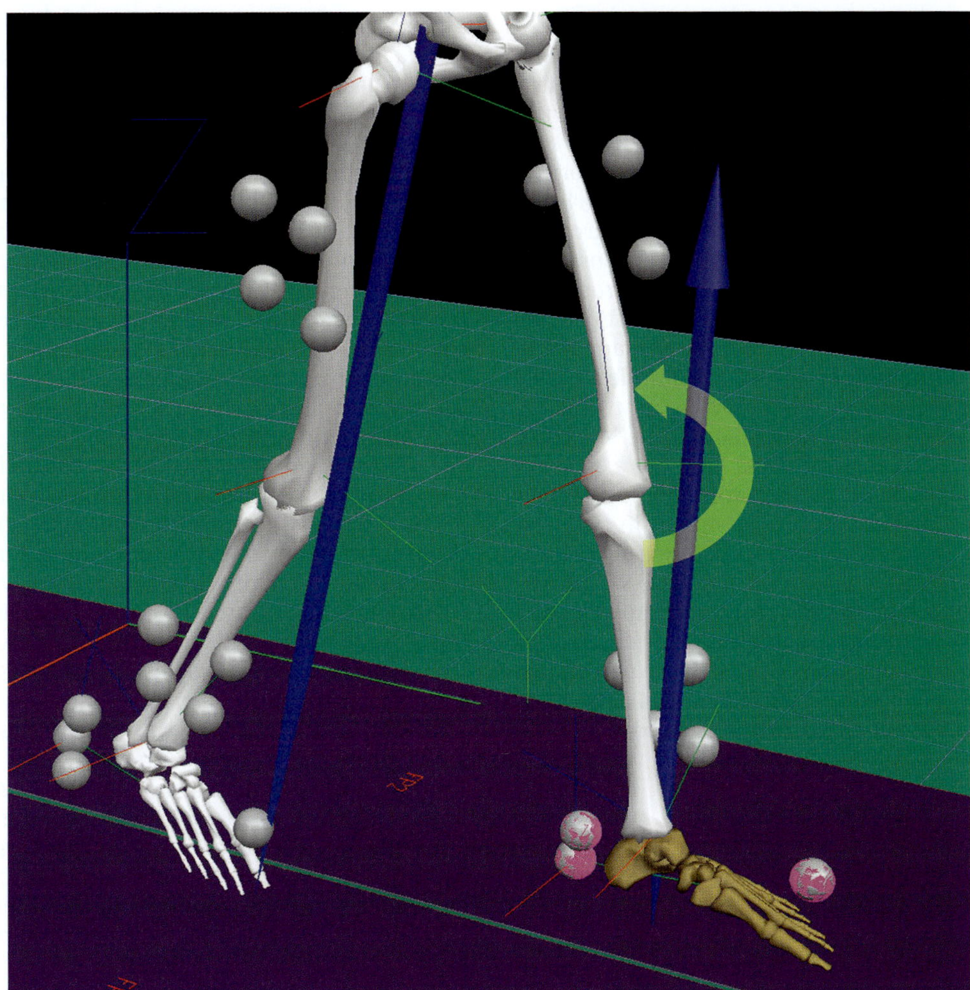

Fig. 5.9 Example of knee joint moment (yellow arrow) calculation based on the ground reaction force (blue arrow) and kinematic data.

when evaluating an individual with an amputation or other limb dysfunction. There is also the issue that the knee and ankle joints are frequently modeled as simple hinge joints. Doing this makes the calculations more practical to perform but does not completely represent the anatomical reality. Particularly in the case of the knee, the joint center does not stay in a fixed position during stance, but many of the models for calculating joint moments assume that it does. As a result, there can be variation in the distance used to calculate the moment at the knee. Considering the physical location, even a small variation in the estimated joint center could result in a significant change in the value calculated. Because many of the calculations rely upon model assumptions, the inherent errors can be easily compounded. This is not to say that these variables should be ignored, but that their value should be tempered with an understanding of the process for obtaining them.

ELECTROMYOGRAPHY

Muscle action beneath skin and subcutaneous tissue cannot be directly measured but through the use of EMG, the activity can be approximated and studied in relation to the action, size of muscle, and signals obtained. EMG records the muscle activity by the electrical signal detected from the contraction and chemical stimulation of the respective musculature.[40]

EMG instrumentation can vary, as is seen with surface EMG (sEMG) or fine-wire EMG. With sEMG, the electrode pad is adhered to the skin above the muscle being studied, while fine-wire EMG uses wire electrodes directly inserted into the belly of the respective muscle. Intrasocket EMG is a relatively new technique, employing traditional sEMG techniques as well as the use of transcutaneous electrical nerve stimulation (TENS) techniques to allow for EMG to be worn by amputees underneath their prosthesis. This technique allows for EMG information to be gathered on amputees during walking and other dynamic activities, including the use of human intent and control of powered prosthetic devices.[41,42]

EMG records the motor unit activation of muscle fibers in the specific muscle being studied. This is very useful, but can be problematic with surface electrode applications in that they can pick up the signal from surrounding musculature during testing. EMG characterization allows for timing and relative intensity of muscular effort, as well as resultant muscle force, all of which are necessary to understand normal and pathological gait. EMG data are normalized against maximum contraction data for each respective muscle. Without normalization, the data collected may be invalid and can lead to erroneous interpretation. Maximum contraction is dependent on joint angle as well as the duration of the contraction, both of which are influential to the overall information extracted from analysis.

Patterns of muscle activity in individuals with abnormal gait are compared with well-established norms. Knowledge of the timing and intensity of the muscle activity throughout the gait cycle may guide gait training, orthotic or prosthetic prescription, and dynamic orthotic or prosthetic alignment aimed at reduction of excessive, ill-timed, or prolonged muscle activity. EMG is exceedingly adaptable with the most basic function of superficial muscle activity data to intramuscular fine-wire sensor technology, which is all cohesive to the implementation of many other complex clinical or gait lab technologies.[28] EMG data are also helpful in guiding decisions about surgical intervention (dorsal rhizotomy, tendon lengthening, or osteotomy) in children with cerebral palsy. Some myoelectric prosthesis users have benefitted from increased device control as a result of targeted muscle reinnervation (TMR). TMR procedures intend to create additional EMG sites in higher level candidates with upper extremity amputations (transhumeral or shoulder disarticulations), where the user would benefit from intuitive, physiological, and overall improved control of the myoelectric device.[43]

PRESSURE-SENSING TECHNOLOGY

Pressure-sensing technologies offer the clinician tremendous insights into the treatment of individuals at risk for amputation because of vascular disease and diabetic neuropathy. They can also assist vascular surgeons and orthopedic foot specialists in limb salvage through more appropriate custom-designed prophylactic orthoses. In some systems, a thin plastic array can slip nearly unnoticed between the plantar surface of the foot and an orthosis or insole of the shoe (Fig. 5.10). This array, connected to a computer by a lead wire or Bluetooth technology, can measure dynamic pressure patterns and record critical events throughout the walking cycle. A prosthetic version can provide various measurements at 60 individual sites within a socket and record those measurements during multiple events of the gait cycle. Pressure is expressed in terms of a force distributed over the area on which the force is acting.

$$\text{Pressure} = \text{Force}/\text{Area}$$

Plantar pressure and temperature measurements in the foot contribute to the identification of abnormal values and the risk for potential ulcers.[44] These measurements transition critical feedback from subjective to objective clinical measurements offering a way to break out of the cycle of trial and error that is often necessary to find the correct solution to an individual's problem.[45] Currently, surface pressure measurement systems exist in various forms ranging from in-shoe, barefoot, seating and positioning, joint, and prosthetic and orthotic floor-based models. Over the years, Perry and colleagues have collected data on the most common types of pressure testing systems that consist of a "force plate" that uses ink and paper to record the areas of peak pressures during ambulation. This type of system is inexpensive and provides reliable, easily interpreted data. Instrumented insoles, however, are positioned inside the individual's shoes and worn during ambulation and activity performance. The insoles record pressures and various forces on the plantar surface of the foot through an integrated array of sensors.[40,44] The diversity of treatment applications has promoted these systems to be some of the most valuable in the laboratory setting.[28] An example of the application of pressure sensing technology is in the area of detecting plantar ulcers in the diabetic population.[44] The compilation of data gathered from a six-camera motion capture system for kinematic data, kinetic data collected from two-force plates, data from a two-dimensional plantar pressure finite element model, and EMG data corresponding to the respective lower extremity musculature is used to predict the internal stresses experienced prematurely that ultimately present as plantar surface ulcers.[46] This area is one of the more recent and clinically promising technologies for future use in the clinical assessment setting.

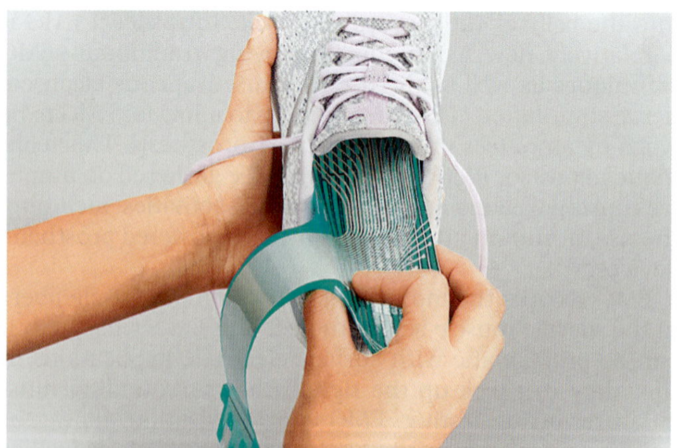

Fig. 5.10 An in-shoe pressure-sensing array can help identify areas of high pressure concentration. This information assists in the design of an orthosis to modify pressure dynamics during the stance phase of gait. (Courtesy of Tekscan™, Inc., Norwood, MA USA.)

Choosing the Appropriate Assessment Tool

Over the past several decades, technologies have advanced and aided in providing a significantly improved understanding of pathological gait. They have also assisted clinicians in providing strong evidence for the efficacy of various treatment approaches and ultimately helped enhance patient care. Advocates of a more universal application of the high-end technologies in the clinical setting have made a compelling case for implementation in gait laboratories and clinical settings alike across the field of rehabilitative care. Determining the extent and necessity for various high-end devices, such as full featured motion analysis systems, in the clinical setting can be a very extensive process requiring the evaluation of the advantages and disadvantages to both the individual and the clinic, particularly in the current climate of cost containment. Perhaps the strongest argument for gait technology in our present era lies in its use for outcome measurement to justify legitimate therapeutic treatment approaches, as well as orthotic and prosthetic applications.

Recognizing the need, benefits, and drawbacks of technology in the clinical setting is very important. Appropriate instrumented evaluations will need to be made by the rehabilitation team to help optimize client outcomes.

Function-Based Assessment

Functional measures are performance-based tools directly related to specific activities and linked to "real-world" domains of function. For example, walking in the community requires meeting the demand of varied distance, terrain, illumination, obstacles, stair-climbing, and multitasking. The results of these functional measures are usually compared with established "norms," which characterize the full spectrum of a specific population. Results of functional measures help specify level of function, evaluate progress after intervention, and establish goals and benchmarks.

Holden and colleagues suggest that gait performance goals for individuals with neurological impairments are best measured against values from impaired rather than healthy participants.[47] Treatment goals are adjusted for the individual's diagnosis, etiologic factor, ambulation aid, and functional category. In separate studies, Brandstater and colleagues and Holden and colleagues found that individuals with the greatest number of gait deviations did not have the lowest temporal values.[47,48] A great deal of energy is often expended by physical therapists, prosthetists, and orthotists in an attempt to help individuals achieve optimal GPs. Holden and colleagues suggest that hard-won qualitative gait improvements may cause secondary losses in time-distance parameters, such as slower velocity and reduced step length.[47] The fundamental issue is whether temporal gait efficiency or cosmesis should be the preferred goal. Certainly, in cases in which individuals are nominal walkers and in which therapy, surgery, and orthotics or prosthetics have been optimized, gait efficiency is far more important than reducing compensatory gait deficits.

In the past, symmetry and reciprocal movement patterns have been significant treatment goals. Wall and Ashburn maintain that "an ideal objective in the functional rehabilitation of hemiplegia is the reduction of the asymmetrical nature of movement patterns."[49] Measuring pathological gait against normal gait values is a useful means of providing an overall clinical picture. In setting treatment goals, however, measuring an individual's performance against their own best possible outcome is more reasonable. This requires collection of accurate data to establish pretreatment and posttreatment profiles for a wide variety of involvement levels within each pathological condition. Olney and Richards suggest that large groups of instrumented studies be undertaken to identify clusters of biomechanical features associated with functional performance during walking.[50]

Time-distance parameters have enormous potential for setting outcome goals. Variations in time-distance values are often specific to pathological condition. Asymmetries in hemiplegia, for example, are obviously greater than in most other types of pathological conditions. Variables that are reported to affect temporal measurements in normal healthy participants include age, sex, height, orthotic use, or type of assistive device. In separate studies of individuals with pathological conditions, Brandstater and colleagues and Holden and colleagues found no significant difference in temporal performance based on sex or age.[47,48]

Corcoran and colleagues measured temporal parameters of participants with hemiplegia under two gait conditions: with and without their AFO. Individuals with hemiplegia had significantly faster gait velocity when wearing their orthoses than when walking without them.[51] Another similar study of healthy unimpaired participants wearing AFOs found reduced step length. Apparently participants without central nervous system involvement altered their movement strategy to decrease movements at the knee in an effort to minimize shearing forces in the AFO.[52] Reduced step length can minimize force exerted by the brace along the posterior aspect of the calf band.[53]

FUNCTION-BASED ASSESSMENT

Understanding pathophysiological mechanisms associated with gait and posture as well as underlying reasons for impairment including diagnosis, changes in sensory-motor integration, impaired postural control, alterations in motor control, and psychological conditions can influence strategies for treatment and rehabilitation.[54] Physical therapists, prosthetists, and orthotists strive to help individuals achieve optimal gait patterns. Historically, emphasis has been placed on achieving symmetrical and reciprocal movement patterns in treatment.[49] Time-distance parameters established through gait analysis have potential for setting outcome goals. Variations in time-distance values are often specific to pathological conditions. Asymmetries in hemiplegia, for example, are typically greater than in most other conditions. Variables that are reported to affect temporal measurements in normal healthy subjects include age, sex, height, orthotic use, or type of assistive device.

There remains debate in the literature regarding a causal relationship between energy expenditure and spatiotemporal parameters of gait.[55,56] However, some evidence suggests that improvements in performance on functional assessment measures may not arise from betterments in spatiotemporal gait asymmetry, nor may these changes translate to increased community mobility.[57] Therefore, a central debate ensues; should temporal gait efficiency or cosmesis be the preferred goal? Following therapeutic and/or surgical intervention, as well as the optimization of orthotics or prosthetics, gait efficiency should be prioritized, rather than establishing a reduction in compensatory gait deviations.

While observational gait analysis is valuable in identifying gait deviations throughout the phases of the gait cycle, functional measures provide information about how these gait deviations impact engagement in necessary life tasks. Innumerable gait-specific functional measures have been developed to evaluate performance-based metrics that may impact community participation. These functional measures provide information about the ambulatory abilities of individuals with varying neuromuscular, musculoskeletal, cardiopulmonary, or metabolic diseases and conditions. Functional measures can be performed in most settings, as they do not require specialized equipment or instrumentation.

Commonly used gait-specific outcome measures include (1) Walking Speed (WS), (2) Timed Up and Go Test (TUG), (3)

Dynamic Gait Index (DGI), (4) Tinetti Performance Oriented Mobility Assessment (POMA), (5) Functional Ambulation Classification System (FAC), and (6) The Modified Gait Abnormality Rating Scale (GARS-M). To ensure accuracy in tool utilization and application of psychometric implications, testers often benefit from training in outcome measure administration. Oftentimes clinicians combine several of these measures to collect sufficient information to render a clinical decision regarding functional level, safety, and/or need for a specific intervention.

WALKING SPEED

Walking speed (WS), also known as gait speed, has been termed both the "sixth vital sign" and the "functional vital sign."[58,59] WS is the time required for a person to traverse a specific distance. To follow the International Standards of Measurement, gait speed should be expressed in meters/second (m/s). Reported norms for WS of older adults are typically around 1.3 m/s.[60,61] WS is most commonly tested during the middle 10 m of a 20-m course, allowing for 5 m of acceleration and deceleration. This allows for the capture of an individual's self-selected or comfortable WS. A self-selected walking speed is often one that optimizes mechanical efficiency and stability during gait.[62] In the gait laboratory, this preferred speed is referred to as "free walking velocity" to be distinguished from "fast walking velocity." In gait laboratory investigations, researchers have used a variety of state-of-the-art equipment including portable computerized walkways, motion analysis systems, and foot switch technology to measure WS. Clinicians, however, can reliably measure WS in almost any clinical setting using a stopwatch and a walkway.

Numerous factors contribute to WS, including joint mobility, muscle strength, sensory function, neural control, cognitive status, and energy level, so it can be utilized to reflect overall health. WS is largely viewed as a valid and reliable outcome measure, but it is important to note that variations in starting, distance, timing, surface, walkway, and finishing procedures can have a clinically significant impact on calculated speed.[63] Gait speed differs between groups defined by sex, age, race, ethnicity, and health status.[60,64] Additionally, slow gait status is predictive of 4-year mortality.[64] In patients requiring hemodialysis, gait speed is correlated with poor quality of life and risk for all-cause mortality and cardiovascular events.[65] Decline in gait speed has also been shown to precede cognitive decline and correlate to Alzheimer's diagnosis.[66] Perhaps most importantly, there is robust literature connecting WS with risk of falling. Among community-dwelling adults, decline in WS over 12 months is associated with increased likelihood of falls, regardless of cognitive status.[67] Faster gait speed is associated with decreased risk of falling in community-dwelling older adults with and without mild cognitive impairment.[68]

TIMED UP AND GO

The Timed Up and Go (TUG) is a useful and valid measure for determining the risk of falls in older adults.[69,70] A 2021 systematic review concluded that the TUG is reliable across multiple patient populations.[71] To perform the test, individuals are asked to rise from a seated position in a standard height chair, walk 3 m on a level surface, turn, walk back to the chair, and return to a seated position, moving as quickly as they are safely able. Performance is based on the total time necessary to complete the task. It is important to note that the TUG is a measure of overall functional mobility, assessing the ability to transfer, walk, and change direction.

Several studies have assessed the utility of the TUG in anticipating risk of morbidity and mortality in a variety of populations. In older adults, the TUG is a relevant predictor of all-cause mortality.[72] Individuals who require more time to complete the TUG are at greater risk of developing myocardial infarction and congestive heart failure, and are at increased risk of mortality.[73] Additionally, individuals with a history of falls are likely to require more time to complete the TUG than counterparts without a history of falls.[74] In community-dwelling older adults with preserved functionality, TUG scores were correlated with age and sex with slightly lower times in males.[75] A systematic review and meta-analysis sought to evaluate reference values for the TUG in healthy people over the age of 60. They identified that age affects the results of the TUG; the mean TUG results for adults in their 60s, 70s, and 80s were 7.91s, 8.67s, and 11.68s, respectively.[76] Clinical utility has been demonstrated in the utilization of the TUG for patients with normal pressure hydrocephalus, arthritis, and Parkinson's disease, among other conditions.[77–79]

The TUG dual-task tests have the same basic instructions as the TUG, but the participant simultaneously performs another task. Most commonly this involves a secondary cognitive test such as counting down from 100 by threes or some similar task. TUG dual-task tests are promising for diagnostic and predictive purposes.[80] There is also evidence to demonstrate that neurodegeneration, as in the case of Alzheimer's disease, negatively impacts TUG dual-task performance.[81]

DYNAMIC GAIT INDEX

The Dynamic Gait Index (DGI) tests the ability of the participant to maintain walking balance while responding to dynamic balance challenges. It includes eight items: walking on level surfaces, changing gait speeds, ambulation while performing both horizontal and vertical head turns, walking followed by a pivot 180 degrees to stop, stepping over and around obstacles, and stair negotiation. Each item is scored on a scale of 0 to 3, with 3 indicating normal performance and 0 representing severe impairment. The best possible score on the DGI is a 24. The DGI has been utilized in multiple patient populations; it has been demonstrated to be a reliable and valid outcome measure for the assessment of patients with cerebellar ataxia.[82] In a small sample of patients with chronic stroke, the DGI was more responsive than the TUG or the Berg Balance Scale.[83] Additionally, the DGI has been utilized in pediatric populations and was demonstrated to be valid and reliable for the assessment of children with hemiplegic cerebral palsy.[84]

A short form of the DGI includes only four items: walking on level surfaces, changing gait speeds, and ambulation while performing both horizontal and vertical head turns. A 2006 study demonstrated that the clinical psychometric properties of the 4-item DGI were equivalent or superior to those of the 8-item test, suggesting its potential for clinical use.[85] However, there is notably scarce recent research that utilizes the short-form DGI. There is some evidence that the 4-item DGI can assist in prediction of a fall in individuals with a history of a stroke with a cut-off score of 9.5/12 indicating increased risk.[86]

The Modified Dynamic Gait Index (mDGI) expands on the original 8-item DGI, accounting for the level of assistance, gait pattern, and time required for each of the eight items. The mDGI also accounts for four environmental dimensions: temporal, postural, terrain, and density. The total possible score of the mDGI is 64 points.[87] People with mDGI scores greater than 49 points have low or minimal fall risk.[88] The minimal clinically important difference of the mDGI is 6 points.[89] The mDGI has been demonstrated to be a reliable and valid clinical gait measurement for patients with vestibular disorders.[90]

TINETTI PERFORMANCE ORIENTED MOBILITY ASSESSMENT

The Tinetti Performance Oriented Mobility Assessment (POMA) is a screening modality that has balance and gait subcomponents that can be utilized in a variety of patient populations including older adults, patients with Parkinson's disease, multiple sclerosis, traumatic brain injury, or following stroke.[91,92] If a patient scores less than or equal to 18, the patient is deemed to be at high risk for falls. There are age-related norms documented in the literature.[92] In a study of older adults the POMA had satisfactory reliability and validity; however, the authors note that a high ceiling effect may limit applicability in all community settings.[93] The balance subcomponent of the POMA is associated with mortality in adults with late-onset Parkinson's disease.[94]

FUNCTIONAL AMBULATION CLASSIFICATION

The Functional Ambulation Classification (FAC) was first utilized at Massachusetts General Hospital for the purpose of categorizing patients by their ability to ambulate. The FAC classifies patients ranging from "nonfunctional ambulator" to "independent ambulator." There are six total categories.[47,95] Although the FAC is a general ambulation test, its scores showed a positive linear relationship with such variables as gait velocity, step length, and the 6-minute walk test.[95,96] The FAC has been used most extensively in the assessment of functional locomotion and as a rehabilitation outcome measure for individuals who have experienced a stroke.[97–101] Contemporary evidence regarding the FAC is limited. One 2022 study found that in individuals post-stroke, increased physiological cost index values related to ambulation may imply lower functional mobility scores on FAC.[102]

MODIFIED GAIT ABNORMALITY RATING SCALE

The original Gait Abnormality Rating Scale was developed to quantify abnormal gait performance of frail institutionalized older adults in an effort to identify those most as risk of falling.[103] The scale has since been modified (GARS-M) for use in community settings.[104] The GARS-M is a 7-item version of the original 16-item GARS; 11 items were removed for reasons including redundancy, inconsistent visual rating among raters, and ineffective discrimination between fallers and nonfallers.[104] While performing the GARS-M, the participant is videotaped ambulating at a self-selected pace on a level surface of 8 m, pivoting, and returning to the starting point. The evaluator then examines the videotape and scores the individual on seven dimensions: variability, guardedness, staggering, foot contact, hip range of motion, shoulder extension, and synchrony of arm movement and heel strike. Total GARS-M scores range from 0 to 21. Gait variability is one of the unique measures of the GARS-M, which has been linked to increased fall risk in older adults and in individuals with varying neurological disorders.[104–106] The GARS-M has been determined to be valid and reliable.[104,107,108] Current literature regarding the utility of the GARS-M is limited.

CHOOSING AN ASSESSMENT STRATEGY

Gait can be assessed in a myriad of ways; selection of an appropriate assessment depends on the underlying objectives. Observational gait analysis assists in the systematic identification of phase-specific gait deviations. Instrumented gait analysis provides quantitative kinematic and kinetic information about joint movement and forces. Performance-based measures attempt to characterize how variations in gait impact an individual's ability to meet the mobility demands of their environment. Functional measures capture current functional status and assist in documenting change over time or demonstrating response to interventions. Appropriately selecting an assessment strategy requires attention to clinical aims, available technology, and assessment feasibility.

CLINICAL EXAMPLES OF GAIT DEFICIENCIES: IMPACT OF FUNCTIONAL TASKS DURING GAIT

Upcoming case examples illustrate variations in gait associated with conditions that commonly alter gait performance: pretibial flaccid paralysis, hemiplegia, cerebral palsy, and spina bifida. Each case example demonstrates common gait characteristics specific to the particular condition while presenting variants from that profile. The discussion is based on information gathered by foot-switch stride, kinematic, and observational gait analysis.

CLINICAL CHARACTERISTICS OF GAIT IN HEMIPLEGIA

Following stroke, improvement in the quality of the gait is often central for gait retraining in rehabilitation. In the weeks immediately following a stroke, only 53% of individuals are able to ambulate independently after intensive rehabilitation training.[109] After weeks of rehabilitation, approximately 75% of individuals are able to walk without assistance, especially if using an assistive device, including AFOs and canes.[110] Six months following stroke, more than 80% of individuals ambulate independently.[111]

There is significant variation in the gait of individuals who have experienced a stroke, which can be due to differences in limb control including: primitive locomotor patterns, impaired postural responses, abnormal postural

Case Example 5.1 A Patient With Flaccid Paralysis of Pretibial Muscles

J.J. is a 37-year-old male with inherited sensorimotor neuropathy due to Charcot-Marie-Tooth disease who has been referred to the gait assessment clinic for evaluation of his orthotic intervention. Examination of muscle function and strength reveals relatively symmetrical distal impairment. Manual muscle test scores include trace activity of dorsiflexion muscles bilaterally, poor plantarflexion on the left, and fair + plantarflexion on the right. Knee and hip strength are normal.

CONSIDER

- Given J.J.'s muscle weakness, what deviations might you predict during the functional tasks of weight acceptance (IC and LR), SLS (MSt and TSt), and swing limb advancement (PSw, ISw, MSw, and TSw)?
- Given J.J.'s muscle weakness, what compensatory strategies might he use to accomplish these functional tasks of gait?
- What quantitative measures, indicators of energy cost, qualitative measures, or function-based assessments would you use to determine whether a change in orthoses would be warranted? Why would you select those measures?

EXAMINATION AND EVALUATION

During a foot-switch stride analysis, J.J. walks without his usual orthoses. In the trailing left limb, the posterior compartment fails to support the forefoot lever arm so that the tibia progresses forward with limited heel-off in late stance. This creates excessive knee flexion and limits the step length of the contralateral limb. The net effect of this inadequate forefoot rocker is a reduction in velocity. Lack of support of the trailing forefoot allows depression of the center of gravity. At the same time, dorsiflexion weakness on the right creates early abrupt plantarflexion (foot slap) with premature contact of the first metatarsal. The variance between plantar flexor strength of the left and right limbs is demonstrated by difference in SLS times. The stronger right calf participates in 39.8% (0.416 s) of the gait cycle, whereas the weaker left calf commits itself to only 31.4% (0.328 s). This subtle timing discrepancy in gait was not readily identifiable in observational analysis.

In right MSw, while the left foot is in a supporting posture, the classical steppage gait characteristics of a flail forefoot are observed. Compensatory swing clearance is accomplished through excessive hip and knee flexion.

When J.J. wears his orthoses (a dorsiflexion assist thermoplastic AFO on the right and a dorsiflexion stop-plantarflexion resist thermoplastic AFO on the left), results of foot-switch temporal analysis are quite different. Velocity, cadence, and stride length increase slightly. The asymmetry between right and left SLS times decreases because the AFO provides external support of the trailing left limb. The energy-inefficient steppage gait and right foot flat at initial contact are improved as well.

QUESTIONS TO CONSIDER

- What specific problems do the examination and evaluation identify in each of the functional tasks of gait: weight acceptance (IC and LR), SLS (MSt and TSt), and swing limb advancement (PSw, ISw, MSw, and TSw)?
- In what ways do J.J.'s orthoses address the functional problems observed when he walks without his orthoses in each of the functional tasks of the gait cycle: weight acceptance (IC and LR), SLS (MSt and TSt), and swing limb advancement (PSw, ISw, MSw, and TSw)? In what ways do his orthoses potentially limit each of the functional tasks of gait? Do the benefits outweigh the limitations?

tone in the presence of spasticity or rigidity, inappropriately timed muscle contractions, or diminished muscle strength. A key determinant of gait pattern in individuals with hemiplegia following stroke is whether the individual has some degree of selective control of specific muscles or experiences the activation of abnormal flexor or extensor synergistic patterns. Individuals with hemiplegia often have difficulty grading the magnitude of a particular muscle contraction with respect to other muscle contractions. The ability to move toward dorsiflexion with forward progression of the tibia during stance may be counteracted by contraction of plantar flexors into a position of equinus due to hyperactivity of the muscle spindle/stretch reflex in the presence of spasticity. Clinically, spasticity is often described via the Modified Ashworth Spasticity Scale, ranging from 0 (no measurable tone) to 4 (marked rigidity).[112]

In the presence of hypertonicity of the lower extremity following stroke, orthotics can be utilized to control ankle motion and preposition for tibial advancement. Two orthotic strategies are commonly used: (1) provision of an AFO with a locked ankle component set in slight dorsiflexion or (2) use of an articulated AFO that allows slight ankle motion around a neutral position. When ankle joint motion is limited or restricted by an orthosis, stability in stance improves; however, forward progression of the tibia is compromised and step length is reduced. Modifications to the shoe such as application of a rocker bottom sole or elevation of the heel can compensate by mimicking the forefoot and toe rockers of gait.[1] There is evidence to support that change of tibia to vertical angle at initial contact, foot flat, and terminal contact may correlate with increased walking speed in individuals following stroke, suggesting the importance of orthotic strategy and alignment.[113]

Over the course of rehabilitation, the individual with hemiplegia often experiences changes in tone, joint flexibility, pain or discomfort, fear or confidence, motor strength or weakness, and quality of proprioception. In 1970, Brunnstrom characterized six stages of motor recovery in hemiplegia progressing from absence of volitional movement in the first stage to coordinated controlled movement in the sixth stage.[19] Clinically, the International Classification of Functioning assists in the provision of a framework to maximize functional recovery of patients following stroke in several domains. A combination of interventions and approaches can yield better clinical outcomes throughout the course of care, facilitating optimal motor recovery.[114] There is a growing interest in nontraining approaches to the restoration of motor function following stroke, including epidural or deep brain stimulation, but these potential interventions are still in early propositional stages.[115] Because of the dynamic nature of the recovery process, the ability to adjust orthotic alignment or characteristics is very desirable. It is not unusual that an orthosis prescribed early in rehabilitation becomes inappropriate at a later stage. Once rehabilitation is complete and the individual has achieved stability in walking patterns, definitive biomechanical needs are identified deemphasizing the need for adjustability of the orthosis.

The extensor synergy pattern is characterized by excessive extension at the hip and knee with the foot in equinovarus. This reduces the amount of knee flexion and dorsiflexion achieved during swing phase, necessitating a compensatory strategy such as circumduction to provide foot clearance.[116] Rigidity of the ankle results in inadequate dorsiflexion mobility and reduced plantarflexion excursion during PSw and early swing. Stance time is considerably reduced on the affected side, and the quadriceps, gastrocnemius, gluteus maximus, and semitendinosus muscles are excessively active throughout stance.[117] Activity of lower limb muscle groups on the affected side is increased as compared with typical patterns of muscle activation. Excessive hip flexion at MSt on the affected side shifts the GRF line anteriorly, producing a knee extension moment that interferes with forward progression. The affected side also achieves less hip adduction in SLS, which compromises lateral shift.[118] SLS time on the affected side is shortened following stroke.[119]

The use of an appropriate AFO improves the quality of gait, increasing step length and stance time, as well as reducing swing time of the affected side by correcting foot drop.[120] Velocity of gait improves when the AFO is placed in slight dorsiflexion to assist with ground clearance. When spasticity is not limiting, an AFO that permits some plantarflexion normalizes IC to LR timing and prevents an unstable knee flexion moment in early stance. Knee extensor strength often equals or exceeds hip extensor strength after stroke; therefore, most individuals with hemiplegia can be adequately managed with an AFO alone, rather than a knee-ankle-foot orthosis.[118] Retraining of normal movement patterns in gait should be prioritized over muscle strengthening for achieving improved walking characteristics in the presence of hemiplegia.[121] There is emerging evidence to support using virtual reality-based interventions to improve walking speed and for the negotiation of environmental challenges, which may facilitate carryover to independent community ambulation.[122,123] Other novel technological approaches to gait rehabilitation in patients following stroke include the use of robot-assisted gait training, body weight support training, and high-intensity interval training.[120,124,125]

Case Example 5.2 **A Patient With Hemiplegia**

M.G. is a 67-year-old male referred to the gait laboratory for evaluation 13 months after a stroke with resultant damage to the sensorimotor cortex of the left hemisphere. Currently, he is a community ambulator (MGH Functional Ambulation Classification level 6) who walks with the use of an AFO and quad cane (FIM Locomotion score 6). In the clinical examination, his spasticity becomes apparent when his ankle moves toward a neutral position (Ashworth Spasticity Scale level 3). The orthosis he received early in rehabilitation and continues to use is a traditional double upright, which locks his ankle in slight plantarflexion. Although this ankle angle delays tibial advancement and forward progression in stance, M.G. has come to rely on its contribution to stability at proximal joints.

CONSIDER

- Given M.G.'s pattern of spasticity and weakness, what deviations might you predict when he is not wearing his orthosis during the functional tasks of weight acceptance (IC and LR), SLS (MSt and TSt), and swing limb advancement (PSw, ISw, MSw, and TSw)?
- Given M.G.'s pattern of spasticity and weakness, what compensatory strategies might he use to accomplish these functional tasks of gait?
- What additional quantitative measures, indicators of energy cost, qualitative measures, or function-based assessments would you use to determine if a change in orthosis would be warranted? Why would you select those measures?

EXAMINATION AND EVALUATION

M.G.'s gait with the AFO is evaluated by foot-switch testing. Extensor synergy patterns contribute to function by providing a degree of stability in stance but also reduce efficiency of gait by limiting normal stance progression beginning with the first rocker period. The duration of heel-only time of the first rocker (IC to the foot-flat position at the end of LR) is approximately one-sixth of a second on the hemiplegic side, which is significantly less than normal heel-only time. Heel-only time on the intact side is roughly three times greater than that on the hemiplegic side. Forward progression during MSt is halted at the second rocker when spasticity prevents the necessary dorsiflexion of the ankle.

As M.G. moves into TSt, when metatarsophalangeal break (concurrent with heel-off) should allow progression onto the forefoot, the third rocker is also relatively blocked. This lack of mobility of the metatarsophalangeal joints and inadequate third rocker result in a loss of knee flexion necessary for an effective PSw, for which M.G. is unable to compensate. Of the 60 degrees of knee flexion necessary for swing phase clearance, 35 degrees should be achieved passively during PSw. For individuals with hemiplegia, the loss of this positional flexion is an additional challenge to clearance beyond that produced by the equinus position of the ankle. Any attempts to compensate by "hip hiking" are likely to be inefficient and unsuccessful. These rocker limitations reduce step length of the sound side, leading to premature double limb support. The corresponding MSw knee flexion on the hemiplegic side is also reduced.

MG demonstrates a much-reduced stance time on the affected side (62% gait cycle) versus the sound side (71% gait cycle) and a reduced SLS time on the affected side (28% gait cycle) versus the sound side (38% gait cycle).

QUESTIONS TO CONSIDER

- What specific problems has the examination and evaluation identified in each of the functional tasks of gait: weight acceptance (IC and LR), SLS (MSt and TSt), and swing limb advancement (PSw, ISw, MSw, and TSw)? How do these problems relate to M.G.'s abnormal tone and motor control?
- In what ways does M.G.'s orthosis address or constrain each of the functional tasks of the gait cycle: weight acceptance (IC and LR), SLS (MSt and TSt), and swing limb advancement (PSw, ISw, MSw, and TSw)?

CLINICAL CHARACTERISTICS OF GAIT IN SPASTIC DIPLEGIC CEREBRAL PALSY

Children with spastic diplegic cerebral palsy often have significant spasticity and marked weakness of the antigravity muscles in both lower extremities. This combination is a precursor for joint contracture. The clinical term often used to describe the typical gait pattern of an individual with diplegia is *crouched gait*, which is characterized by marked internal rotation of the femur and tibia, excessive knee flexion throughout stance phase, and ankle plantarflexion during both stance (toe walking) and swing phases. Energy cost does increase with this excessive knee flexion, which may decrease efficiency, but kinematics alone may not be the single most important indicator of energy consumption in these individuals.[126] The combination of an equinus ankle, positive Trendelenburg hip, and stiff knee gait often produces various combinations of compensatory hiking of the pelvis, external rotation of the foot, and circumduction of the swing limb. This pattern has been attributed to overactivity of the distal hamstrings alone or in combination with the hip flexors.[127–129]

Some individuals with diplegia ambulate with a *jump gait* pattern, using somewhat less hip and knee flexion than individuals with crouch gait, but with excessive ankle dorsiflexion rather than plantarflexion.[130] Jump gait often manifests following surgical lengthening of bilateral Achilles tendons without concurrent release of hip and knee contractures. Common compensatory strategies in jump gait include vaulting and circumduction. In both crouch and jump gait patterns the GRF line falls progressively behind the knee joint during SLS, creating an excessive demand on the quadriceps for stance phase stability. One surgical strategy utilized in the presence of jump gait includes hip flexion releases, lengthening of the distal hamstrings, and correction of external rotation. Postoperatively, the individual is fitted for floor reaction AFOs.[131] Ideally, the Achilles tendon is lengthened to neutral dorsiflexion and the individual is protected in AFOs for one year postoperatively.

The *scissoring* pattern, which is also common in children with diplegia, is aggravated by spastic hip flexors and adductors because the smaller base of support reduces the efficiency of their line of pull. Orthotic solutions provide limited assistance in limb tracking and rotational control. Those that attempt to control rotation must cross the hip joint, adding significant weight and bulk, increasing difficulty in donning and doffing. Notably, there is emerging, though not conclusive, evidence that robotic-assisted interventions can assist in gait training of children with spastic diplegic cerebral palsy.[132,133]

Case Example 5.3 A Patient With Spastic Diplegic Cerebral Palsy

K.E. is a 10-year-old boy with spastic diplegic cerebral palsy who has been referred to the gait laboratory for evaluation to assist his orthopedist in deciding whether corrective surgery is indicated. K.E. currently ambulates independently, without assistive devices, wearing bilateral solid ankle AFOs (WeeFIM Locomotion score of 6).

CONSIDER

- Given K.E.'s pattern of spasticity and weakness, what deviations might you predict when he is not wearing his orthoses during the functional tasks of weight acceptance (IC and LR), SLS (MSt and TSt), and swing limb advancement (PSw, ISw, MSw, and TSw)?
- Given K.E.'s pattern of spasticity and weakness, what compensatory strategies might he use to accomplish these functional tasks of gait?
- What additional quantitative measures, indicators of energy cost, qualitative measures, or function-based assessments might help determine whether further surgical or orthopedic intervention is warranted? Why would you select those measures?

EXAMINATION AND EVALUATION

K.E. is fitted with reflective markers for three-dimensional motion analysis of his gait. A typical crouch gait pattern is observed during observational gait analysis. His gait is also being recorded for more detailed kinematic and kinetic analysis by computer software. Foot-switch analysis confirms diminished heel contact with no heel-only time on the left and no heel contact at all on the right.

Clinical examination of K.E.'s lower extremity function reveals a combination of overactive hamstrings and weak gastrocnemius and soleus muscles. Flexion of hips and knees increases the need for proximal stabilization, resulting in compensatory hyperextension of the trunk and posterior arm placement. Because the ankles are held in equinus, the final rocker propels tibial advancement, despite limitation in ankle mobility. K.E. spends most of the stance phase in TSt and PSw; consequently, double limb support time is vastly increased.

K.E. has not had previous surgical release of his gastrocnemius muscles. Even with surgery, impairment of motor control may continue to be problematic so that dorsiflexion may not work in concert with knee flexion to provide a heel-toe gait pattern. Gastrocnemius release without concurrent release of the hip and knee contractures usually leads to short step length with a compensatory increase in cadence. Spastic hip flexors, also serving as adductors, create a mild scissoring effect during each swing limb advancement. Ambulation with bilateral AFOs, which the client prefers, increases step length and reduces knee flexion compared with ambulation without orthosis.

QUESTIONS TO CONSIDER

- What specific problems does the examination and evaluation identify in each of the functional tasks of gait: weight acceptance (IC and LR), SLS (MSt and TSt), and swing limb advancement (PSw, ISw, MSw, and TSw)? How do these problems relate to K.E.'s abnormal tone and motor control?
- In what ways do K.E.'s orthoses address or constrain each of the functional tasks of the gait cycle: weight acceptance (IC and LR), SLS (MSt and TSt), and swing limb advancement (PSw, ISw, MSw, and TSw)? What is the interaction of his abnormal tone and impaired motor control with his orthoses on the efficacy and energy cost of his walking?

CLINICAL CHARACTERISTICS OF GAIT IN CHILDREN WITH SPINA BIFIDA

Myelomeningocele is the most significant form of spina bifida, which occurs when the vertebral arches fail to unite very early in gestation. Clinically, this leads to partial or complete paralysis at or below the level involved. The most common impairment is flaccid paralysis with loss of proprioception and exteroception including impaired pain, temperature, light touch, and pressure sensation. Many children with spina bifida have resultant gait deviations and benefit from individualized orthotic management.[134] Assessment for orthotic support begins early in childhood.

Severity of gait dysfunction depends on the level of involvement of the spinal cord. When the L5 and S1 nerve roots are impacted, the gluteus maximus, hip abductors, and triceps surae are unable to function, the hamstring strength is diminished, and sensory loss affects the plantar surface of the feet. Given the lack of plantar flexor activation, impacted individuals benefit from orthotic joint control that limits dorsiflexion range of motion, which allows the individual to establish hip stability though hip extension that is accomplished via exaggerated truncal lordosis. Without it, the individual would fall forward, unopposed. Lateral stability is often achieved through the use of crutches and a wide base of support.

When the L3 and L4 nerve roots are affected, there will be absent hamstring, hip extensor, knee flexor, plantar flexor, and dorsiflexor function. The resultant foot drop cannot be sufficiently compensated in swing phase by hip and knee flexion. Hip flexion, adduction, and knee extension are intact, but may be weak. At the L3 level, the gracilis may contribute to a limited amount of knee flexion. These children benefit from the early utilization of standing frames; later in life, they are often able to ambulate with orthotic assistance. Orthotic application can be utilized to facilitate adequate stabilization of the foot and ankle via a locked ankle joint mechanism in neutral or slight dorsiflexion. The hip is often stabilized in stance via excessive trunk lordosis. The individual is at risk of hip flexion contracture due to muscular imbalance at the hip; this may perpetuate the need for even more compensatory lordosis. Extreme hip flexion contracture may ultimately preclude ambulation. If contractures at the hip, knee, and ankle are minimal and the child gains trunk control, they will be able to stand erect but will rely on trunk alignment for static balance and forearm crutches for further stability.

When the L1 and L2 levels are impacted, the individual will have little lower limb function. They may have some preservation of weak hip flexors. These children often begin upright function with a parapodium or swivel walker and can later progress to reciprocal gait orthoses. The swing-through gait with bilateral hip-knee-ankle-foot orthosis has been shown to be less efficient than a reciprocal gait orthosis for thoracic level spinal bifida.[135] Dias et al. have proposed a new functional classification system for individuals with myelomeningocele that may serve as a gait prognosis guide and assist in the anticipation of orthotic needs.[136]

Gait Patterns in Individuals With Amputation

Qualitative observational gait analysis is a broadly accepted approach to achieving a clinically optimal gait in individuals with amputation. Instrumented gait analysis provides a more repeatable accurate assessment of prosthetic function. In its broadest scope, the data derived increasingly serve as foundational guidelines for both prosthetic design and clinical application. The daily practice of assessment and management of prosthetic gait, however, depends on the subjective skills of the prosthetist and the targeted treatment protocol of the therapist.

The University of California at Berkeley prosthetic project, which began in the mid-1950s, represented the most concentrated period of prosthetic advancement. The comprehensive basic gait studies and their application to the biomechanics of amputee gait for transtibial and transfemoral amputations established fundamental design criteria.[137] Contributions of subsequent investigators continued to be largely based on the Berkeley criteria. Extensive calculations and interpretations were required to relate normal and prosthetic gait data to the problems of prosthetic design. Data reduction was a slow process before relatively recent technological advancements because all motion measurements had to be performed by hand. There were no automated film analyzers to identify the motion patterns and no computers to perform rapid data processing. Therefore, the number of subjects studied was limited. The project also had the additional depth of considering all three planes of motion, in contrast to prior studies that analyzed only the sagittal plane of gait progression.[40]

TRANSTIBIAL PROSTHETIC GAIT

In 1957 the Berkeley project was specifically commissioned to reconsider transtibial prosthetic gait and biomechanics. Basic transtibial prostheses at that time were attached to the limb with a thigh lacer that included articulated knee joints and a foot with an articulated ankle. Detailed review of the normal and transtibial amputee-gait data resulted in a totally new approach that led to two developments: the patellar tendon-bearing (PTB) prosthesis and the solid-ankle, cushion heel foot.[28] The improved transtibial socket was a PTB design that closely followed the contours of the proximal tibia. The PTB prosthesis replaced the thigh lacer with supracondylar fixation, again with the advantage of anatomical contour and total contact.

Studies of Transtibial Prosthetic Gait

Most studies of individuals with transtibial amputation, instrumented and noninstrumented, have focused on foot design, with the general exclusion of alignment. In more recent years, an increase in studies focusing one prosthetic alignment, specifically the impact of the alignment of the socket to the foot and the associated energy cost, have evolved in number and depth of meaning and implication for the overall well-being of the client.

Prosthetic foot designers attempt to passively reproduce, by material quality and design, the normal dynamic

Case Example 5.4 A Child With Spina Bifida

N.P. is an active 9-year-old boy with myelomeningocele at L5 who returns to the gait laboratory as part of an ongoing research study to document changes in gait characteristics over time. He currently ambulates wearing bilateral AFOs set in a neutral ankle position using forearm crutches in a four-point reciprocal gait pattern.

CONSIDER

- Given N.P.'s pattern of weakness and sensory loss, what deviations might you predict when he is not wearing his orthoses, during the functional tasks of weight acceptance (IC and LR), SLS (MSt and TSt), and swing limb advancement (PSw, ISw, MSw, and TSw)?
- Given N.P.'s pattern of weakness and sensory loss, what compensatory strategies might he use to accomplish these functional tasks of gait?
- What additional quantitative measures, indicators of energy cost, qualitative measures, or function-based assessments might help determine if further surgical or orthopedic intervention is warranted? Why would you select those measures?

EXAMINATION AND EVALUATION

Comparative foot-switch testing reveals that without crutches, stride length and velocity are reduced. External rotation of both limbs is present throughout the gait cycle (Fig. 5.11). With or without crutches, N.P. has no measurable fifth metatarsal or toe contact on either limb in his typical stance phase weight-bearing patterns. Passive external rotation is present at the hip as well as abducted limb placement as he advances over the forefoot. His abducted limb placement and wide-based gait provide increased stability at a cost of excessive loading on the posteromedial aspect of the feet (see Fig. 5.11). Like many children with spina bifida, he spends excessive time in heel contact, largely to the exclusion of lateral forefoot weight bearing. This loading and shear pattern often leads to callusing and eventual neuropathic breakdown in adult life. His fastest gait velocity (0.92 m/s) is approximately 60% of normal free-gait velocity. During swing phase, external rotation of the limb is marked. The flail foot is held in slight dorsiflexion during TSw through the support of the AFO.

QUESTIONS TO CONSIDER

- What specific problems does the examination and evaluation identify in each of the functional tasks of gait: weight acceptance (IC and LR), SLS (MSt and TSt), and swing limb advancement (PSw, ISw, MSw, and TSw)? How do these problems relate to N.P.'s flaccid paralysis and sensory impairment?
- In what ways do N.P.'s orthoses address or constrain each of the functional tasks of the gait cycle: weight acceptance (IC and LR), SLS (MSt and TSt), and swing limb advancement (PSw, ISw, MSw, and TSw)? What is the interaction of his flaccidity and sensory changes with his orthoses on the efficacy and energy cost of his walking?

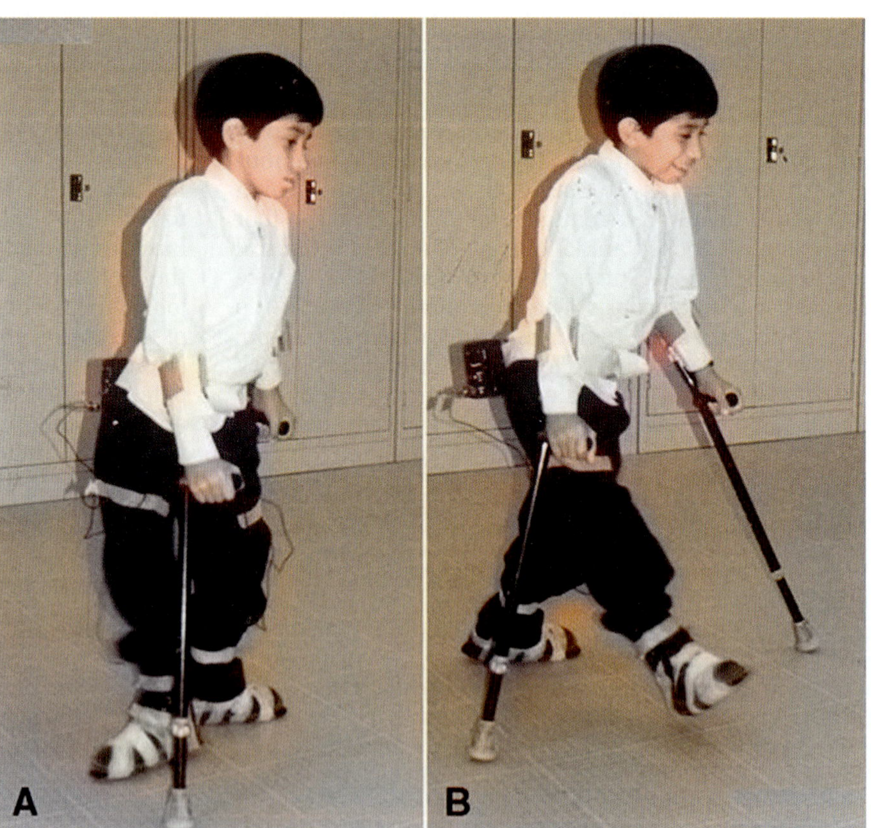

Fig. 5.11 In this child with myelomeningocele, weakness at the hip results in external rotation of the limbs in both stance and swing phase (A), which contributes to altered forward progression from the heel to the medial forefoot, with minimal weight bearing on the lateral foot (B).

functional balance between mobility and stability provided by the anatomical foot. The greatest difference is between the relatively rigid compressible heel-type feet and the mobile hinge of the single-axis foot.[137] Optimization of prosthetic foot stiffness has been studied in relation to the associated metabolic costs in unilateral transtibial amputee walking. For people navigating the challenges of a unilateral amputation, the development of gait abnormalities and compensations, as well as elevated metabolic cost, is unavoidable. Therefore, studies modeling the variable impact of foot stiffness on metabolic cost is an integral part of optimizing the prosthetic device. Modeling analyses showed optimization in foot stiffness through stiffening the toe and forefoot while making the heel and ankle less stiff. The optimization improved prosthetic foot performance by offloading the sound side knee during early to MSt decreasing the metabolic cost.[138] Motion analysis has shown that the articulated ankle improves weight acceptance stability by providing significant plantarflexion, allowing an earlier foot flat posture; however, the arc of knee flexion and the timing and intensity of the quadriceps do not differ from that of the compressible heel-type foot.[139,140]

Kendell and colleagues identified six factors that that can be related to dynamic stability in lower limb prosthesis users: shifts in anterior-posterior center of pressure, shifts in mediolateral center of pressure, cell triggering, maximum lateral force placement, stride time, and double limb support time. These parameters influenced the adoption of GPs, which facilitated forward progression without compromising the location of the center of pressure in either direction.[141] Stance phase limb progression is enhanced by an articulating ankle in two ways. In footswitch analysis, the mobile ankle had a longer period of single limb stance time, whereas total stance time was shorter compared with solid-ankle designs.[140] In addition, there was more prolonged hamstring action with the compressible heel foot; this implies that a forward lean was used to improve progression over the less yielding foot. These functional advantages of a mobile prosthetic foot would be significant in a marginal walker, but the heaviness of a single-axis foot creates an energy-cost penalty that must also be considered. The relationship between the body, specifically the musculature of the limb involved with controlling a prosthetic device, and the device and its respective components work in synergy to provide body support, forward propulsion, and limb-swing initiation, and mediolateral balance impacts the metabolic costs required.

Since the 1980s, the use of elastic materials and designs has been increasingly applied to prosthetic feet. The initial objective was to facilitate running because the presence of normal knee control gives the individual with transtibial amputation considerable functional potential.[142] Foot designs all emphasize controlled dorsiflexion mobility for greater push-off. It has been assumed that these dynamic, elastic prosthetic feet would be advantageous for the average walker by reducing the greater-than-normal energy cost currently experienced by individuals with amputation.[31] The most mobile designs, in terms of dorsiflexion range, are those with a long-bladed shaft such as the Flexfoot and Springlite. These bladed shaft designs have not lessened the muscular demands of weight acceptance. Their simulated "ankle plantarflexion" during limb loading is no better than the solid-ankle, cushion heel foot. Both result in a plantarflexion that is markedly less than the normal controlled, yet rapid, ankle plantarflexion of 12 degrees used to reduce the propulsive effect of the heel rocker by allowing early forefoot contact. Both prosthetic feet cause a significant delay in attaining the stability of foot flat.[143] One modeling study demonstrated that the prosthesis as a whole provided body support in the absence of ankle muscles, braking from early to late MSt, decreasing the body's need to provide compensation for missing anatomy, and propulsion in late stance, decreasing the energy recruitment needed. GRF and the associated muscle recruitment and activation identified the ability of the prosthesis to transfer energy from the residual limb to the trunk implying greater overall propulsion of the trunk, furthering the perception of improved efficacy of ESAR feet over solid ankle cushion heel feet. Relieving the body in part by decreasing the musculoskeletal deficit as well as lessening the metabolic burdens influences the perceived quality and the functional quality in the design of the prosthesis.[144] Finite element analysis (FEA) has been used more recently to investigate the implications of ESAR feet without the cofounding factors of gait deviations. FEA modeling standardized the mechanical characteristics of ESAR feet through simulation. The FEA demonstrations showed impressive consistencies with older data surrounding the relationship between stiffness and energy stored and returned to the user.[145]

The intact limb uses a modest arc (15–20 degrees) of knee flexion to absorb the shock of contact with the floor, whereas prosthetic feet rely on a cushion heel.[1] The time needed for adequate cushion compression delays the drop of the forefoot to the floor. This perpetuates an unsteady, heel-only source of support that requires increased active muscular control of the knee and hip to ensure weight-bearing stability. This subtle source of instability is obscured by two findings. The stiffness of the foot, particularly the heel, can contribute to increased prosthesis range of motion and increased energy storage in early stance and energy return in late-stance; however, the decrease in propulsion and swing initiation as a result increases the net metabolic requirements for additional muscle activation and body support maintenance. In addition, the mechanical efficiency of the device is influenced by the adjustment of the stiffness of the device.[146] Heel cushion compression delays the rate of initial tibial advancement, resulting in reduced weight acceptance knee flexion for the transtibial amputee compared to normal. This difference is reflected in calculations of subnormal moments and powers.[147,148] These findings have been interpreted as a sign of reduced muscle demand, and a corresponding conservation of energy has been attributed to the development and implementation of dynamic ESAR feet. Direct EMG recordings, however, showed significantly higher than normal muscle demand for the five different feet tested.[149,150]

Transtibial Alignment

The positional relationship between the socket and prosthetic foot is critical to achieve optimal progression in stance, yet is also highly subjective. The goal is to promote tibial progression in stance and place the knee in a stable (minimally flexed) weight-bearing posture without causing hyperextension in late stance and to encourage the lower limb to follow a normal path of motion in swing.

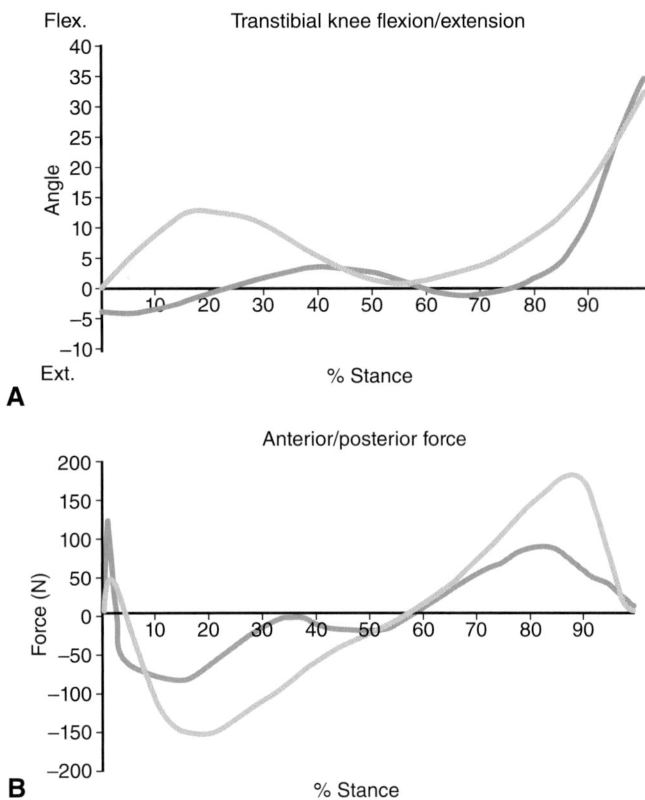

Fig. 5.12 (A) Patients with dysvascular transtibial amputation typically shift the weight line anterior to the knee early in stance, which results in reduced knee flexion throughout stance phase and delayed flexion in swing. (B) Patients with dysvascular transtibial amputation typically shift the weight line anterior to the knee early in stance, which results in typical midstance hesitation in the progression of rollover, reflected in the shear pattern. (Courtesy VA Long Beach Gait Laboratory.)

Static or "bench" alignment uses the subcutaneous crest of tibia (tibial blade) to establish alignment of the residual limb within the prosthesis. In the sagittal plane, this landmark, at its origin at the tibial tubercle, is typically angled approximately 5 degrees forward of the perpendicular to the tibial plateau that serves as the supporting surface for the knee joint. Hence, if the socket is aligned by the tibial blade, the socket is set so that the tibia is tilted slightly forward to avoid a backward thrust during stance. This angular posture of the prosthetic socket, in conjunction with a deliberate anterior displacement (translation) of the socket relative to the foot, generally succeeds in encouraging tibial progression.

Even with this alignment, the individual with dysvascular transtibial amputation who typically exhibits some degree of weakness will likely shift the weight line anterior to the knee by simply leaning forward during LR in a postural movement akin to a quad avoidance gait. This results in reduced knee flexion throughout stance phase and delayed flexion in swing (Fig. 5.12). A hesitation of stance progression (the MSt dead spot) is a common phenomenon. A delay in the rollover pattern, common to the dysvascular transtibial amputee, is reflected in the shear pattern (see Fig. 5.12B).

Final positioning of the socket-foot relation is determined by observational analysis of the subject's gait and feedback from the prosthesis user. This process, referred to as *dynamic alignment*, examines smoothness of the rollover pattern and medial-lateral verticality of the foot, avoiding both extremes of inversion and eversion during progression. The absence of abnormal motions in swing such as a whip, compensatory motions to avoid scuffing the foot in swing (e.g., degree of pelvic elevation or vaulting), and an erect trunk posture are additional observational criteria used for assessment. Comfort and ease of walking are criteria of the individual with amputation. A study on individuals with transtibial amputation evaluated whether or not the client could perceive and effectively communicate feedback regarding induced perturbations to the prosthesis alignment. The data reported that subjects were able to communicate extreme malalignments and demonstrated the ability to unknowingly shift loading and balance to compensate for smaller perturbations. Data analysis revealed that coronal adjustments were more noticeable to the subjects than sagittal or transverse adjustments; the data did not indicate whether or not the perception had anything to do with residual limb tissue volume or not. Overall, coronal translation and angulation alignment changes were perceived more often than sagittal alignment changes; however, the subjects were not able to detect small changes in alignment that could be clinically significant.[151] Socket alignment changes and disruptions can be compensated for through balance and center of mass adjustments, as well as compensatory gait motions; however, the effects of malalignments on the kinetics and kinematics should not be ignored. Malalignments of the socket have been shown to propagate statistically significant changes in the socket reaction moments experienced in persons with transtibial amputations. Coronal perturbations caused significant changes in socket reaction moments at 30% and 75% of stance while sagittal perturbations triggered significant changes at 45% of stance phase.[152]

In optimizing the alignment in the coronal plane, there is an attempt to mimic the slight varus moment seen at the knee during MSt of normal human locomotion. This moment is usually achieved by a slight medial inset of the prosthetic foot relative to the socket, taking advantage of the tolerant weight-bearing areas in the proximal-medial and lateral-distal regions of the residual limb where pressure is well tolerated. Inadequate inset of the foot, or worse, outset of the foot, will generally result in excessive pressure on the very superficial cut end of the tibia (medial-distal) and the fibular nerve and bony prominence of the head of the fibula (lateral-proximal). Alignment affects the transmission of forces and moments from the limb through the prosthesis, as well as from the ground up through prosthesis, and ultimately to the limb; however, the relationship between alignment and the generation of reaction moments is not well established or implemented into the alignment process. The kinematic assessment is predominantly completed through observational gait analysis and client feedback. One study looked at the implications of a methodical alignment of the coronal plane first followed by the sagittal plane to study the associated socket reaction moments and observed gait deviations. The data revealed sagittal plane alignment (and malalignment) significantly affected coronal reaction moments in early stance while coronal plane alignments (and malalignments) did not produce significant sagittal reaction moments. This study concluded that implementing a systematic alignment approach would positively influence the reproducibility and consistency of the alignment process, with the recommendation to complete sagittal plane alignment first without concern that subsequent coronal plane alignment might alter or negate the prior adjustments.[153] Although observational analysis is appropriate for general clinical care, the alignment of individuals with amputation with complex fitting problems is best resolved through objective confirmation with force plate and motion data.

Initial Contact and Loading Response

Prosthetic control and success are achieved through several individual attributes, as well as the interaction between them, including the fit of the prosthetic socket, the alignment of the prosthesis, the prosthetic component choices utilized, and the contributions of the prosthetic user in the patterns of gait. Gait assessment for individuals with transtibial amputations must be critically assessed with these areas in mind, as well as the interdependent symbiotic relationships thereof.

Prior to early stance, the prosthetic foot swings through in anticipation of heel-first contact. As the prosthetic foot approaches contact with the floor the ball of the prosthetic foot is intended to be no more than an inch and a half above the ground's surface. Complications can arise if the prosthetic heel is not the primary aspect to come in contact with the ground; if the client's stride lengths are too long as a result of poor gait habit, if the suspension of the prosthesis is too tight not allowing full extension of the knee, or if the socket exhibits excess flexion restraining the knee from full extension, an inappropriately positioned foot at IC may result. One case study found significant improvement in observed gait, mobility potential, and overall range of motion of the knee following a multidisciplinary therapeutic approach. The Amputee Mobility Predictor increased from a score of 5 to 29, center of pressure data improved, passive range of motion steadily increased, activity level assessment revealed progression from K0 initially to K3 at the end of the study, and overall ambulation function improved.[11]

During IC, normal gait knee flexion ranges from 0 to 5 degrees after which the knee begins to flex.[1] Transtibial gait assessment strives to evaluate the achievement of similar metrics. Knee flexion in stance may be absent at times when full extension or excess flexion of the knee are observed. Full extension of the knee at IC can be a result of suspension issues, poor flexion alignment of the socket, or if the relative alignment of the foot in relation to the socket is inappropriate. Excess knee flexion at IC is measured as flexion greater than 10 degrees and can be produced by deficient suspension or a flexion contracture at the knee.[154] Kim and colleagues found that excess knee flexion negatively impacts gait ability, quality of life, and the potential eligibility for newer prosthetic technology.[11]

The spatial measurement of stride length in nondisabled gait reveals nearly equal lengths. In transtibial gait kinematics equal stride lengths are desired; however, unequal stride lengths can result from prosthesis-related factors such as socket fit and suspension efficiency, or patient-related compensatory mechanisms adopted by individuals with amputation.[155,156] One study by Sinitski and colleagues looked at the spatial characteristics of subjects with transtibial amputations in varied walking environments. The subjects adjusted their stride length and stride time to maintain stability in unfamiliar conditions; when walking on a self-paced treadmill, participants consequently adjusted their WS and walking strategy in climbing a moderate slope compared with level walking. Stride length and stride time subsequently affect WS and ultimately metabolic cost; therefore, the spatial parameters of gait are important to monitor and control throughout the gait cycle.[157] Viewed in the sagittal plane, the desired characteristics of LR include smooth controlled knee flexion and minimal vertical movement or piston action of the limb-socket relationship. Erratic, abrupt, uncontrolled, or delayed knee flexion can be detected when gait is viewed laterally. Erratic flexion of the knee may result from weak hip or knee musculature.[162] Abrupt and uncontrolled knee flexion may arise from malalignment of anteroposterior positioning of the foot in relation to the socket or deficient alignment of the dorsiflexion-plantarflexion positioning of the foot relative to the socket, if the heel of the prosthetic foot is excessively stiff or firm, or if the shoe does not house the prosthetic foot in a way that allows the needed movement and support.[158]

Occasionally, clients can display an extended knee with delayed progression through LR, sometimes described as "riding the heel" or continual pressure felt on the anterior distal aspect of the tibia. This presentation can be a product of malalignment of anteroposterior positioning of the prosthetic foot relative to the socket, inappropriate prosthetic foot selection, unsatisfactory socket flexion, or due to a client who markedly utilizes the knee extensors.[158]

Knee control during gait is critical in the prevention of falls. Schafer and colleagues conducted a study of the impact of personalized training regimens on the rate of falls, as well as associated gait biomechanics.[159] This study concluded that subjects who received the personalized training plans had a significant reduction of falls over the 1-year study period compared with average annual fall rates. In addition, gait speeds increased from baseline, indicating potential impact of exercise interventions on gait kinematics.

Pistoning is described as the vertical motion between the limb and the socket, which mimics the motion of a piston in the cylinder of an internal combustion engine. Piston action is produced in LR due to insufficient suspension, which allows the limb to slip vertically in relation to the socket as when weight is borne down through the limb. In addition, if the fit of the prosthesis does not maintain appropriate suspension, pistoning may also result.[158]

Midstance

At MSt, relative component alignment, alignment of the prosthesis relative to the body, and alignment of the body in space are observed to qualify gait parameters as well as the function of the device. Coronal plane observation yields superior views of MSt gait.

At MSt, the verticality of the pylon or shank of the prosthesis is evaluated. A pylon that leans medially can be produced by excess adduction in the alignment of the socket or a prosthetic foot that is excessively outset. Alternatively, a pylon that leans laterally is produced by either a socket aligned in insufficient adduction or a prosthetic foot that is unduly inset. Consequently, with a vertical pylon, the sole of the shoe (and the prosthetic foot) should be completely in contact with the ground at MSt. Commonly, a nonvertical pylon will be accompanied by a shoe that is not completely seated on the ground surface.[158] A device that is not optimally aligned, particularly at MSt when the maximum weight is born on the residual limb, implies the magnitude and means of weight transfer to the residual limb is directly impacted. One study looked at how the alignment of transtibial prosthetic devices influences the socket reaction moment impulse. Data showed alignment changes indicate significant alterations in the magnitude of the moment, as well as the stance duration time, both of which may impact gait speed, metabolic cost, and long-term health of the residual and contralateral limbs.[160]

Width of the walking base is viewed in the coronal plane. The walking base is anticipated to be a minimum of 2 in. and a maximum of 4 in. when measured between the medial aspect of the heels as the foot passes the stance foot. A walking base that is less than the target minimum is said to have a narrow walking base and is typically a result of the prosthetic foot being excessively inset relative to the socket alignment.[154] If the walking base exceeds the target maximum, it is described as a wide walking base and is commonly a result of the foot being too outset in relation to the socket. Additional causes may include poor gait habit, improper length of prosthesis, or an undetected hip pathology.[154,158] Aside from the biomechanical implications a wide walking base can have, there are additional interconnected costs that can be derived from the width of a client's walking base. In a study conducted by Weinert-Aplin and colleagues, the relationship between center of mass motion in all three directions of motion, base of support and WS, and the metabolic cost of walking in both in nondisabled individuals and different levels of lower limb amputee was considered. This investigation revealed that base of support and mediolateral center of mass displacement were the strongest correlates to metabolic cost and the positive correlations suggest increased mediolateral center of mass displacement or base of support will reduce walking efficiency.[29] Metabolic efficiency is a key consideration during all phases of gait, but is of particular interest during the stance phase of gait as the kinematics and kinetics directly contribute to the efficacy and acceptance of the device through associated quality-of-life implications.[161]

In normal human locomotion a varus moment at the knee is present at MSt as a result of the orientation of the GRF in relation to the knee. The GRF is present in disabled gait as well; however, the addition of the prothesis presents additional challenges and variables. At MSt, lateral displacement of the socket up to half an inch is an indication that the GRF is appropriately interacting with and influencing the body producing the desired varus moment at the knee. Lateral displacement exceeding half an inch indicates an excess varus moment at the knee. Excess lateral displacement can be produced by the prosthetic foot being disproportionately inset or the mediolateral dimension of the socket being too large.[154,158] Kobayashi and colleagues concluded that the varus moment impulse is a potential indicator of gait instability at MSt.[160] In contrast, if no displacement or medial displacement of the socket is observed at MSt, the desired varus moment at the knee is lacking and reveals the inappropriate or insufficient interaction between the GRF and the body. Medial displacement of the socket at MSt may result from a prosthetic foot that is extremely outset relative to the socket, pain on the residuum, a very short residuum, or an undetected knee pathology.[154] In addition, varus moment impulse is related the presence and magnitude of lateral trunk bending during stance on the prosthetic side.[160]

Lateral bending of the trunk toward the prosthetic side at MSt, displacing the head more than 1 in., is an indication of the presence of complications with the alignment and fit of the prosthesis. A prosthesis that is of inappropriate length, a prosthetic foot that is disproportionately outset, or socket-induced pain can result in compensatory trunk and head motion.[154,158]

Terminal Stance

TSt prepares the limb for initiation of swing phase. TSt is characterized by the completed progression over the prothesis accompanied by smooth flexion of the limb, with a flexion magnitude equal to the contralateral limb. As the heel of the prosthesis leaves the ground, the motion should be smooth and without any additional exertion; timing of this sequence is accomplished prior to IC of the contralateral limb.[154,158] Early or abrupt heel-off can be produced when the sagittal plane alignment of the foot in relation to the socket is incongruous; this compensation is commonly assessed by the perceived "drop-off" of the client at the end of stance. If heel-off is delayed, and the client experiences the feeling of "walking up a hill" or "being unable to get over the toe," the sagittal plane alignment of the foot in relation to the socket is most likely inappropriate. [154,158]

For new and seasoned clinicians alike, understanding the influence of prosthetic socket fit, prosthetic alignment, prosthetic component selection, and the contributions of the prosthetic user in the success of the prosthesis and ambulatory function cannot be understated. Alignment and alignment changes affect socket moment impulse, impulse time intervals, and overall efficacy. When socket impulse exceeds the acceptable range, either defined by the wearer or physiological limits, compensations in GP or reduction of daily activity level result to decrease residual limb discomfort ultimately affecting overall function and quality of life.[160]

Preswing

As the limb continues to prepare for swing phase, body weight transfers smoothly to the contralateral limb without any perceptible rise or fall of the head and torso and the magnitude of flexion of the prosthetic knee is equal to that of the contralateral knee. Suspension of the socket retains the limb securely within the socket in preparation for the prosthesis to leave the ground. Sagittal plane assessment will reveal the rise or fall of the head and torso during PSw.

Inappropriate movement of the head and torso during PSw indicates that the alignment of the foot in relation to the socket may be misaligned or the provided socket flexion may be unwarranted; clients may describe this motion as falling too quickly to the contralateral side or "drop-off." Ineffective suspension or poor socket fit can result in the socket dropping away from the limb as body weight if offloaded from the residual limb, described as pistoning, as swing phase is initiated.[154,158]

Swing Phase

Once the limb leaves the ground swing phase commences with the goals of heel rise equal to the contralateral limb and swinging the limb through on the line of progression free of any motion of the limb in the transverse plane (circumduction, medial, or lateral whips), with ample ground clearance of the prosthetic foot and adequate socket suspension. Swing phase assessment is best viewed in the sagittal plane and the coronal plane viewed posteriorly. Sagittal plane viewing provides feedback regarding heel rise and toe clearance as the prosthetic foot passes over the ground surface and for assessing device suspension. ISw is characterized by heel rise of the prosthetic limb equal to that of the sound limb. Insufficient suspension or socket flexion can inhibit the appropriate heel rise during ISw.[154] At MSw, the limb passes over the ground without contact or additional force or energy to accomplish the task. Improper prosthesis length or device suspension can lead to the prosthetic foot not clearing the ground. In addition, limited knee flexion resulting from socket interference or physiological complications can also produce the same complication.[154,158] Socket suspension is imperative at all phases of the gait cycle; however, during the swing phase, should suspension be ineffective, the client will lose confidence in the device's safety and effectiveness, which may potentially lead to significant harm. If pistoning is observed during swing phase, common causes may be socket fit or inadequate primary suspension.[154,158] Prosthetic toe clearance is imperative for protection from increased fall risk. Individuals with a lower limb amputation have an increased risk of falling at all stages of their clinical course.[162] One study found that transtibial prosthesis users with low minimum toe clearance may be at increased risk of experiencing a trip-related stumble in the community[163] Tripping is a cause of falls and the rate of tripping increases with prosthetic use and even more so when adequate toe clearance or socket suspension is deficient.[164,165] Toe clearance is a function of proximity of the prosthetic foot to the ground, swing limb velocity, and forward progression of the center of mass relative to the base of support. Research has deduced that the WS-related toe-ground clearance changes on the prosthetic side compared with the contralateral side may potentially increase the risk of tripping, further highlighting the need to adequately assess prosthetic fit and function as it relates to GPs.[166]

Coronal observations allow for assessment of the path of the limb relative to the line of progression, as well as detection of motion in the transverse plane as the limb travels through swing phase. Smooth acceleration and progression of the limb along the line of progression can be influenced negatively by a prosthesis that is too long, a prosthesis that is donned improperly and is internally or externally rotated, or if the suspension is not adequate or appropriate for the client. [154,158]

COMMON GAIT DEVIATIONS IN TRANSTIBIAL PROSTHETIC GAIT

Our understanding of prosthetic gait deviations and the dynamic alignment process has evolved over many decades. The important early work of Inman, described previously, served as a basis for subsequent development.[40] As the field of prosthetics has progressed, the refinement of the various prosthetic gait deviations has continued to evolve. A brief description of the most common transtibial gait deviations is given in Table 5.1

TRANSFEMORAL PROSTHETIC GAIT

Initial research of transfemoral amputation by the Berkeley group focused on unilateral amputation because the problems of this group appeared more critical at that time.[167]

Motion analysis showed a fully extended knee starting in TSw and continuing through stance. The inadequate ankle plantarflexion that followed heel strike and threatened knee stability was attributed to dependence on an ankle bumper in place of the lost pretibial muscle control. Active ipsilateral thigh control and postural adaptation by the sound limb and trunk were identified as the variable mechanisms used by the individual with transfemoral amputation to ensure knee extension stability. Rotation of the fully extended limb rolling over the ankle before heel rise caused a maximum rise of the hip (and thus center of gravity), which was interpreted as vaulting. Compensatory actions by the sound limb were identified.

In swing, the inability of the prosthetic foot to generate a propelling force to initiate limb advancement was interpreted as a need to restrict the weight of the prosthesis so that the work of hip flexors would not be excessive. The individual with transfemoral amputation also demonstrated rapid hip extension in TSw to use tibial inertia as a means of completing knee extension in preparation for stance. These findings of excessive knee extension in stance and excessive hip action in swing formed the basis for others to design more sophisticated knee joints to replace the then-dominant, single-axis constant friction joint.

The biomechanical response to the problem of residual limb discomfort was twofold. Torque absorbers were designed, but the solution was the combination of improved socket design, in addition to more normal joint mechanics. The loss of knee control creates compensatory kinematic and kinetic changes that result in asymmetries reflected in a variety of gait parameters. As the individual wearing a transfemoral prosthesis with a compressible heel-type foot levers over the heel rocker during LR, the knee may be at an increased risk of destabilization. When challenged by the potential for knee instability, the prosthetic wearer will attempt to preposition the hip before LR, with a change in body mechanics to shift the GRF to a more anterior position. These typical compensatory patterns can be measured directly through EMG, kinematics, or kinetics, or inferred by measuring heel-only load-bearing time through a temporal analysis.

Temporal Values

Individuals with unilateral transfemoral amputation (TFA) have a slower walking speed and wider step width and a shorter step length on the nonprosthetic side, compared to individuals without an amputation.[158,168] Gait speed in individuals with a transfemoral amputation varies depending on patient and prosthetic factors. Gait characteristics such as cadence and step length vary based on prosthetic knee components and body size.[168] Individuals with more advanced

Table 5.1 Common Gait Deviations in Transtibial Prosthetic Gait

Gait Cycle Phase	Gait Deviation	Description	Patient Cause(s)	Prosthetic Cause(s)
Initial contact	Abnormal narrow base (stance and swing)	Stance between heels is less than 2 in.	Hip adductor contracture or spasticity Genu varum	Prosthetic foot too far inset
	Abnormal wide base (stance and swing)	Stance between heels is greater than 4 in.	Hip abductor contracture or spasticity or weakness Instability (patient has neuropathy and uses the wide base of support to avoid falling) Genu valgum	Leg length discrepancy—prosthesis too long Prosthetic foot too outset
	Excessive medial or lateral weight on the foot (stance phase)	Excessive weight or time spent on medial or lateral side of foot	Genu valgum (medial) Genu varum (lateral)	Foot too inverted/everted Uneven wear of shoe heel Insufficient accommodation for toe-out
	Excessive knee flexion (stance phase)	Knee flexed greater than 10°	Knee flexion contracture Hip flexion contracture	Keel too soft allowing excessive knee flexion to occur late in stance Stiff or long heel lever Foot too dorsiflexed Socket in flexion/anterior tilt
	Hyperextended knee (IC and TSt)	Excessive extension of knee in stance	Quadriceps weakness or spasticity Genu recurvatum Ligamentous laxity Gastrocnemius weakness Compensation of contralateral hip or knee contracture or skeletal shortening	Heel height of shoe too low (this usually occurs when the patient changes shoes after the prosthetic fitting) Insufficient socket flexion Socket in extension/posterior tilt Foot plantarflexed Plantarflexion bumper too soft
Initial contact	Anterior trunk bending (IC, LR, MSt, TSw)	Patient flexes trunk Possible hands on thighs	Quadriceps weakness or paralysis Flexor spasticity Tight iliotibial band Knee and/or hip flexion contracture	Heel height too low Excessive socket flexion
	Foot rotation on initial contact	External rotation of prosthetic foot at initial contact	Extension of residual limb is too vigorously at initial contact Amputee has poor muscle control of residual limbAmputee does not put enough weight on the heel during initial contact to compress the heel	Plantarflexion bumper too stiff Heel wedge too hard Socket fit is loose allowing for rotation Too much toe-out in prosthetic alignment
Midstance			Amputee has poor muscle control of residual limb	Socket fit is loose allowing for rotation Too much toe-out in prosthetic alignment Adducted (varus) or abducted (valgus) socket
	Lateral trunk bending (MSt, occasionally swing)	Stance lean toward involved side with weight Swing lean toward unaffected side	Hip abductor weakness Hip dislocation/coxa vara Hip pain Scoliosis	Mediolateral dimension of socket too wide Prosthesis too short Pain from the prosthetic socket
Preswing	Insufficient push-off (early heel off)	Weight on heel and entire foot leaves ground for swing	Fear of placing full weight on prosthesis	Foot is too far posterior, causing shortened anterior lever arm Foot is too dorsiflexed
	Delayed heel off	Patient feels he or she is walking uphill		Long toe lever Foot too plantarflexed
Swing phase	Vaulting	Exaggerated plantarflexion of contralateral side	Poor gait habit—desire to keep knee locked during ambulation	Dorsiflexion bumper too soft Prosthesis too long
	Circumduction	Foot follows laterally curved path	Poor gait habit—desire to keep knee locked during ambulation	Inadequate prosthetic suspension Prosthesis too long Foot plantarflexed

IC, Initial contact; *LR*, loading response; *MSt*, midstance; *TSt*, terminal stance; *TSw*, terminal swing.

From Spires MC, Kelly BM, Davis AJ. *Prosthetic Restoration and Rehabilitation of the Upper and Lower Extremity*. Springer Publishing Company; 2013; Adapted from Kapp S. Visual analysis of prosthetic gait. In: *Atlas of Amputations and Limb Deficiencies*. American Academy of Orthopedic Surgeons; 2004:388–394; Gitter A, Bosker G. Upper and lower extremity prosthetics. In: DeLisa JA, ed. *Rehabilitation Medicine: Principles and Practice*. 4th ed. Lippincott Williams & Wilkins; 2005.

Case Example 5.5 A Patient With a Unilateral Transtibial Amputation

W.T. is a 59-year-old with a transtibial amputation secondary to peripheral vascular disease. After he underwent the amputation, he subsequently experienced a fall, causing secondary injuries to the residual limb. Previously, he underwent bilateral total knee arthroplasty, most recently on the right side two years prior to the amputation. W.T. started physical therapy for gait training 6 months postoperatively and completed 4 months of physical therapy. He has been referred for a gait evaluation due to complaints of right knee pain, as he has continued to become ambulatory with the prosthesis.

CONSIDER

- Given W.T.'s history of a total knee arthroplasty and common gait deviations associated with transtibial amputation, how might his residual limb be impacted during gait?
- What options could be considered to minimize the impact on his intact joints? With this, consider the role of client education and adherence to the treatment plan.
- What type of qualitative and quantitative information would you use to support your decision(s)?

EXAMINATION AND EVALUATION

On the day of evaluation, W.T. presented using a single-point cane and, after discussion with the staff, complained of intermittent pain at the distal end of his residual limb. A further chart review revealed that since the time that he completed physical therapy, multiple prosthetic feet have been trialed, along with additional modifications to the prosthetic socket to help increase comfort. There were also documented limitations in client adherence to the prosthesis wear schedule. The individual had periodically developed areas of redness on his residual limb and was advised to pay particular attention to this area and to document it when it occurred.

An initial assessment with video-based data collection was determined to be an appropriate first step. During the evaluation, the client was asked to walk multiple times over level ground at his self-selected WS while being videotaped. The principal findings were as follows: (1) Periodic knee hyperextension during MSt on the involved side, (2) the involved side knee is often not fully extended at IC, and (3) for the times that the knee is flexed going into stance, there is a rapid extension during MSt.

Taking into consideration the individual's history and current complaints about exacerbated knee pain with ambulation, it was determined that a trial of a custom knee brace modified to fit in conjunction with his prosthesis would be the next alternative. He was subsequently casted over the prosthesis to help ensure the device would contour appropriately and not interfere with its function. By doing this, the brace would provide additional support when combined with the single-point cane.

QUESTIONS TO CONSIDER

- Given the situation with this client, would further, instrumented, kinetic, and kinematic testing be warranted?
- If so, how would you conduct the testing session, and in which specific variables would you look for changes?

swing control such as microprocessor-controlled knees tend to have faster walking speeds and more efficient gait.[169]

Chang et al. analyzed changes in spatiotemporal gait parameters after 12 weeks of prosthetic gait training in 10 individuals with a unilateral TFA compared to 10 healthy individuals as controls. Individuals with a TFA had an average age of 44.8 ± 7.9 years. They demonstrated a baseline average walking speed of 54.2 ± 18.7 cm/s and average step width of 19.8 ± 2.9 cm. Step length ratio (SLR), which is the value on the prosthetic side divided by the value on the intact side, was 1.19 ± 0.22. In comparison, walking speed of healthy controls was 126.0 ± 8.7 cm/s, step width 11.6 ± 3.3 cm, and step width ratio 0.99 ± 0.05. After 12 weeks of training, walking speed of individuals with TFA improved to 88.2 ± 16.6 cm/s but was still slower at 70% of that of the control group. Step width decreased to 17.3 ± 2.3 cm at week 12, which was 12.6% less than that at the beginning. However, the step width was still 149.1% wider than that in the control group. As training progressed, the SLR in the TFA group gradually declined and approached 1, indicating improved symmetry, and was not significantly different from the control group at the end of training. However, patients with a TFA still had a longer stance time and single limb support time on the intact limb than on the prosthetic limb.

A study by Batten at al. examined gait speed at discharge from inpatient rehabilitation among individuals prescribed a prosthetic leg after unilateral lower limb amputation. They also examined the relationship between gait speed and prosthetic potential (K-level classifications)[170] Gait speed was considerably faster among each higher K-level classification at the point of discharge from hospital rehabilitation. The study included 30 individuals with a transfemoral amputation. The average walking speed for those individuals was 0.35 (0.23–0.51)m/s. This speed is slower than 0.8 m/s, which is the minimum gait speed associated with successful community ambulation.

Transfemoral Alignment

As previously mentioned, prosthetic control and success is achieved through several individual attributes as well as the interaction between them including the fit of the prosthetic socket, the alignment of the prosthesis, the prosthetic component choices utilized, and the contributions of the prosthetic user in the patterns of gait. For persons with transfemoral amputations not only must the clinician take into consideration the socket-foot relationship, but also the socket-knee relationship and the knee-foot relationship. Gait assessment for persons with transfemoral amputations must be critically assessed with the areas mentioned, as well as the interdependent symbiotic relationships thereof.

Initial Contact and Loading Response

Prosthetic alignment assessed during IC of the gait cycle yields optimum achievement of smooth controlled plantarflexion and knee extension as well as equal stride length to the contralateral limb. Knee instability may be observed as a result of inadequate positioning or mechanical adjustment of the prosthetic knee, deficient socket alignment decreasing the efficiency of the hip extensors, or prosthetic user error. Prosthetic user error or interference is common throughout the life of the prostheses affecting comfort, efficacy, and safety. User interference resulting in knee instability can include inappropriate shoe wear producing alignment changes or an undetected hip pathology or weakness. In addition to knee instability, plantarflexion that is uncontrolled or erratic may be detected. Erratic and uncontrolled plantarflexion can be produced by use of inappropriate distal components or component adjustment, as well as the client lacking trust in the safety and stability of the prosthetic device. At times unequal step length may be assessed; step length is a function of alignment and trust. Inappropriate socket flexion alignment or prosthetic knee adjustment can lead to a shorter prosthetic step, while residual limb pain and lack of trust can also produce asymmetric stride lengths.[154,158]

As the limb continues to progress from IC to LR, a stable foot that remains on the line of progression during plantarflexion, an upright trunk with minimal lateral displacement of the head, and the presence of sufficient pelvic stabilization are anticipated. Commonly, the prosthetic foot may externally rotate and deviate from advancement along the line of progression. External rotation of the foot may be produced by ineffective socket contouring and fit and inappropriate prosthetic foot choice or alignment, or weak musculature may be present, preventing necessary control of the prosthesis. Similar to lateral trunk bending observed in transtibial gait, excessive lateral deviation of the trunk or forward bending of the trunk is undesired and should be addressed.

The initiation of heel contact at the beginning of stance phase in transfemoral gait has been reported to be characteristically delayed on the prosthetic side, which typically demonstrates a longer swing phase.[171] Contemporary hydraulic knee units, particularly those that provide a programmable chip that can establish optimal swing phase timing characteristics, have the potential to overcome this limitation. However, probably because of cost, they do not represent a typical prosthesis. Early gait studies of single-axis prosthetic feet showed that as the prosthetic limb made contact with the ground and began to load, an exaggerated knee extension was seen in the prosthetic limb that continued throughout early stance.[171] This phenomenon depends somewhat on knee design. There is little evidence that polycentric knees such as four- and six-bar linkage knee units and others that have been designed to be stable with a few degrees of built-in flexion compliance during stance provide normal kinematics of the knee in stance. Most individuals with transfemoral amputation who use the polycentric designs walk with a nearly extended knee.

The total vertical forces occurring on the prosthetic side are less during the initial double limb support period than on the contralateral side during the terminal double limb support period. It has been theorized that this loading restraint requires costly compensations of the sound limb.[172] Knee instability, which produces these costly compensations, generally results from inappropriate positioning of the knee joint relative to the socket and prosthetic foot. The individual with transfemoral amputation relies on hip extensor strength and the reduced lever arm of the transected femur to stabilize the prosthetic knee by restraining the limb during LR. Profound hip extensor weakness can be catastrophic and preclude functional ambulation. Anterior translation of the prosthetic socket relative to the knee and foot has the effect of shifting the GRF anterior to the knee joint axis, thereby increasing stability. Socket flexion affects knee stability as well. Because efficient use of the gluteus maximus as a hip extensor requires the muscle group to be on stretch, the prosthetist deliberately places the socket in a position of flexion. Five degrees of socket flexion are generally considered clinically optimal in an individual with no contracture at the hip. In cases of hip contracture, the amount of flexion is limited by the length of the femoral remnant.[167]

Stability of the knee joint is unquestionably the most important factor in considering a knee unit. Uncontrolled knee flexion renders an otherwise perfect prosthesis useless. A slight degree of socket flexion is also a factor affecting stability because socket flexion slightly elongates hip extensors, rendering them more effective. The relative positions of the prosthetic foot, knee, and socket to this line significantly affect stability of the knee when the individual walks. When the ground reaction line passes posterior to the knee center, the knee will collapse unless resisted by another force, usually the hip extensors forcing the femur against the socket wall.

Another potential destabilizing factor is limitation of free plantarflexion at heel contact, which may produce a knee flexion moment in early stance. This is why an articulated prosthetic foot (as opposed to a prosthetic foot, which attains a plantar grade position by means of heel compression) provides increased stability for those with transfemoral amputation. A general clinical guideline on an individual who demonstrates minimal knee stability is that the prosthetic foot should reach foot-flat position (mimicking plantarflexion during LR) as quickly as possible, short of demonstrating a foot slap characteristic. As soon as the foot plantarflexes fully during stance phase, the ground reaction line moves anteriorly from the point of foot-floor contact at the heel to approximately midfoot, enhancing stability at the knee. Because of this, a single- or multiaxis foot with a soft plantarflexion bumper is preferred for those with a short transfemoral residual limb, who have limited muscular control for knee stability. At times, the single-axis function can be combined with that of dynamic ESAR foot.

Midstance

As the individual moves into MSt, sound-side hip elevation and trunk lean toward the affected side provide balance, limit the force on the lateral aspect of the residual limb, and reduce the demands of the residual limb abductors. The transition from braking to propulsive shear on the ipsilateral limb is characteristically delayed and unsteady (Fig. 5.13A). It is necessary to maintain optimal alignment to reduce any further potential to negatively influence the MSt transitions. Prosthetic device causes of excess lateral trunk bending during LR and MSt include inadequate socket or prosthetic foot alignment and incorrect prosthesis length. Additional client causes can include weak hip musculature, short residual limb length decreasing available strength necessary for hip stabilization, or a painful residuum with pain being located distally and laterally.[158] Individuals with transfemoral amputation exhibit muscle weakness, which is partly due to residual limb disuse and altered forces within the socket.[173] Heitzman et al. found moderate correlations between gait deviations and strength deficits in individuals with a unilateral transfemoral amputation. Individuals with the transfemoral amputation demonstrated a lean of the trunk to the involved side with a linked pelvic drop and increased hip abduction on the involved side.[173]

MSt gait is most effectively observed in two planes, the sagittal plane and coronal planes respectively; these two vantage points allow the clinician to observe the degree of presence of pylon verticality and prosthetic foot contact with the ground, appropriate width of walking base, and reasonable lateral trunk flexion. Pylon verticality is affected when socket discomfort exists, poor socket fit and alignment are not corrected, or when the individual has weak musculature and does not feel safe using the device. Typically, in addition to a nonvertical pylon, the prosthetic foot will not be flat on the floor. Inversion and eversion of the prosthetic foot can be produced by inappropriate socket alignment or socket fit. Transfemoral walking base is best viewed in the coronal plane. A width of 2 to 4 in. when measured between the medial aspect of the heels as the foot passes the stance foot is desired. Excess or insufficient walking base is both unesthetic, inefficient, and unsafe; undesired widths are caused by inappropriate device alignment.[158]

When both limbs are intact, the momentum of the contralateral swing limb results in a reduced vertical force at MSt of the stance limb. This is not so, however, for individuals with dysvascular transfemoral amputation, in which the reduced upward velocity and momentum of the contralateral swing limb does not have the vigor necessary to decrease vertical force of the prosthetic limb during MSt (see Fig. 5.13B). Maximum knee flexion and swing velocities of the sound side during swing phase, as well as the involved side during swing phase, can be positively improved through the use of microprocessor-controlled knee units for some individuals.[174]

Stance phase knee flexion of the affected side is significantly reduced throughout stance (see Fig. 5.13C). During PSw, delayed and reduced knee flexion and consequent reduced heel rise on the ipsilateral limb are characteristic of the transfemoral amputee. Except in the case of those fitted with microprocessor stance control knees, it can be anticipated that many individuals with transfemoral amputation will progress through MSt with a nearly extended knee. Microprocessor-controlled knees have shown improvements in stance knee flexion as well as increased velocity in stair descent.[175,176] This is an important development because it may provide increased energy efficiency in gait and avoid compensatory mechanisms, such as prepositioning of the femur before LR and MSt.

Terminal Stance

TSt is characterized by the smooth advancement of the center or mass without any observable rise or fall of the torso and head. In addition, step length of the uninvolved limb should be normal length and without excess lumbar lordosis. Pelvic rise or "hill climbing" and "drop off" are undesirable consequences observed in the sagittal plane. Pelvic rise is detected by noticeable elevation of the head and torso and is sometimes described by the individual as "difficult to ride over the foot." Pelvic rise is produced by inappropriate prosthetic foot alignment. Drop-off is evidenced when the torso and head drop markedly and is accompanied by a shorter rapid step on the uninvolved side. Drop-off is commonly a result of inadequate prosthetic foot alignment or compensatory gait habit. Increased lumbar lordosis is common in individuals with transfemoral amputation as a compensatory strategy to overcome the constraints induced by traditional socket models.[177] During TSt the individual may exhibit additional lumbar lordosis in an effort to overcome insufficient socket alignment, improper socket fit, inherent hip musculature weakness or pathology, or a short residual limb which inadvertently decreases the function of the available lever arm.[158]

TSt on the prosthetic side is noted for its premature cessation. The prosthetic side generally shows a decrease in SLS time, whereas the sound side shows a concurrent increase in SLS time.[174] There is a persistence of knee extension on the prosthetic limb during contralateral sound side deceleration.[178,179] Delayed and reduced knee flexion, and consequent reduced heel rise on the ipsilateral limb, are characteristic of transfemoral prosthetic gait (see Fig. 5.13C). A failure to limit dorsiflexion in a single-axis foot at this juncture will have a destabilizing effect on the prosthetic knee joint during TSt. Without an appropriately placed dorsiflexion stop, nothing will dampen the forward progression of the tibia, and the tibial section may continue its anterior progression to the point of knee collapse.

Preswing

Characteristics of transfemoral gait in PSw include the hip, knee, and foot swinging through on the line of progression, heel rise of the prosthetic foot equal to the contralateral limb, and necessary suspension to maintain the socket securely on the limb. Typical causes for prosthesis progression that deviates from the line of progression are malalignment of the prosthetic knee or socket alignment and fit issues. A medial whip is observed when the prosthetic heel rises medially from the floor accompanied by lateral movement of the prosthetic knee. In contrast, a lateral whip is observed when the prosthetic heel rises laterally from the floor, accompanied by medial movement of the prosthetic knee. Excessive external and excessive internal rotations of the knee axis are to blame respectively. Socket rotations resulting in medial and lateral whips can result from inappropriate donning of the prosthesis or inadequate socket contouring and fit. Deviation from the line of progression can also be a result of weak musculature and inability to provide the necessary muscle control. Inadequate, delayed, or uneven heel rise is best observed in the sagittal plane. Heel rise deficiencies result from inappropriate prosthetic knee adjustment, a prosthesis that is aligned with too much inherent stability, or the individual may lack confidence to adequately operate the device. Lack of suspension can be detected in both the sagittal and coronal planes. As the body weight transfers to the contralateral limb and the prosthetic limb prepares to leave the ground the prosthesis must remain secure. Lack of adequate suspension may result in lack of toe clearance later in swing.[158]

During PSw in transfemoral gait, the vertical force of the sound side is abnormally high and greater than that of the prosthetic side.[172] Abrupt reversal from hip extension to hip

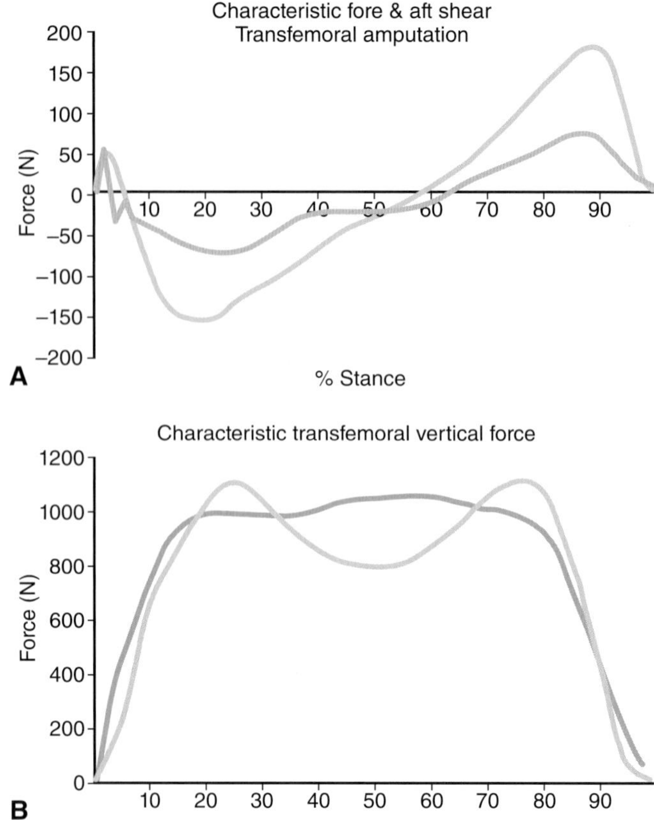

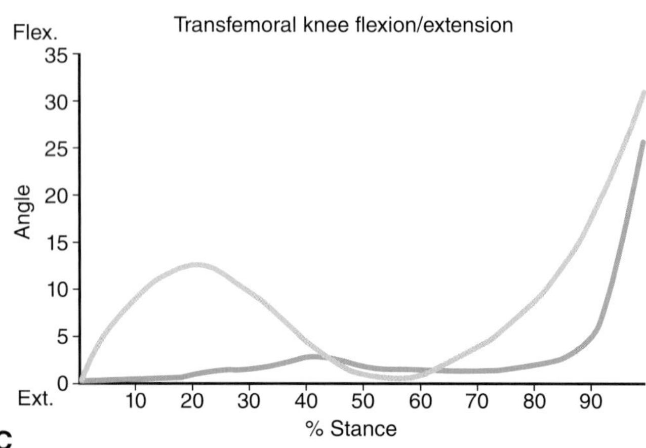

Fig. 5.13 (A) The transition from braking to propulsive shear on the ipsilateral limb during transfemoral prosthetic gait is characteristically delayed and unsteady. (B) Although there is a reduction in vertical force at midstance (Mst) of the sound limb as the prosthetic limb advances in swing, the prosthetic transfemoral limb demonstrates reduced upward velocity because the momentum of the contralateral swing limb lacks the vigor to lessen the vertical force of the affected stance limb during MSt. (C) Knee flexion of transfemoral prosthetic limb is reduced throughout stance. During preswing, delayed and reduced knee flexion, and consequent reduced heel rise on the ipsilateral limb is characteristic. (Courtesy VA Long Beach Gait Laboratory.)

flexion occurs because some hip extension is required for knee stability until the moment when the prosthetic knee has to flex to initiate swing. In normal gait, half the knee flexion required for swing phase is obtained passively during PSw.

During prosthetic PSw, inadequate forefoot support can lead to costly compensations in the double limb support period.[172] PSw is characterized by a rapid transfer of body weight to the contralateral limb. In normal gait, this transfer begins at 50% of the gait cycle and continues until the end of stance phase (approximately 62% of the gait cycle).

Individuals with transfemoral amputation often have a shortened sound side step length. This may be aggravated by insufficient socket flexion because the individual with transfemoral amputation uses any and all available lumbar lordosis to advance the sound limb. Failure to place the socket in flexion limits the availability of lumbar lordosis and prohibits a sound side step length that is at least somewhat close to normal. Even in an optimal prosthetic gait, typical sound side step length is reduced compared with the prosthetic side or that of normal gait.

Swing Phase

Similar to transtibial gait assessment, swing phase is observed through the lens of three smaller periods of time in the overall phase. ISw, MSw, and TSw compose the swing phase, and each subphase is categorized by unique attributes and expectations. Desired criteria of ISw include smooth hip and knee flexion, while MSw criteria boasts a rhythmic progression over the prosthetic foot produced by the smooth peaking of the center of mass, as well as symmetric GPs for both limbs. Circumduction can be observed during swing phase resulting from inadequate knee unit adjustment, inappropriate prosthesis length or fit, insufficient suspension effectively lengthening the prosthesis, or lack of trust in the function of the device. Excessive elevation on the sound side limb during swing phase of the involved limb, also known as *vaulting*, may result from inadequate knee unit adjustment, inappropriate prosthesis length, insufficient suspension effectively lengthening the prosthesis, or poor gait habit. In conjunction with circumduction and vaulting, occasionally, asymmetric gait is observed; the prosthetic foot may rise too high and as a result, additional time is spent on the sound side limb. Asymmetric gait during swing phase results from an adequate adjustment to the prosthetic knee.

Deceleration of the prosthetic limb is paramount in preparation of IC of the subsequent gait cycle. Deceleration should occur smoothly and without perceptible noise of knee extension or terminal impact, and equal step length is desired. Terminal impact is produced when the distal portion of the prosthetic limb travels with excess velocity as the knee reaches full extension. Terminal impact is a result of insufficient prosthetic knee adjustment, a knee unit that is in need of repair, or poor gait habit to ensure the knee is fully extended to prevent buckling. During TSt, unequal step length can result for many reasons. Component adjustment issues can produce knee hyperextension, elongating deceleration: a knee that does not reach full extension shortening deceleration and prematurely instigating IC or a knee that bounces back after full extension allowing premature flexion prior to IC. Inappropriate socket alignment can produce a long sound side step or a short prosthetic step, or lack of accommodation for a hip pathology, whereas an individual who lacks confidence and trust may exhibit slow stride velocity, delayed contact with the floor to ensure full knee extension, or a short sound side step.[158]

Gait characteristics during swing phase when wearing a transfemoral prosthesis can be profoundly influenced by prosthetic alignment and design variations. The most challenging factor in achieving a functional swing phase is the lack of active dorsiflexion in most prosthetic designs. The Stewart-Vicars knee developed in 1947 and the more recent Hydracadence knee, couple knee flexion with ankle dorsiflexion. However, this design concept has been largely ignored in recent years. With the prosthetic incorporation of active dorsiflexion in early swing many costly postural substitutions, including vaulting and abducted or circumducted gait, could be minimized.

The swing phase of the prosthetic limb is often longer than that of the sound limb.[180] The presence or lack of fluid control mechanisms variations in alignment stability, extension assist, and joint friction alignment mechanisms can all influence swing phase timing. During MSw, the individual with transfemoral amputation demonstrates exaggerated hip elevation of the prosthetic side to enable swing clearance. In TSw, prosthetic swing time is much greater than sound limb swing time or normal gait swing time. Excessive prosthetic swing flexion is one of the commonly reported transfemoral prosthetic gait deviations. Contradiction in results of maximum knee flexion can easily be attributed to the wide variety of prosthetic dampening and extension assist designs, as well as other variations in prosthetic adjustment.[174]

COMMON GAIT DEVIATIONS IN TRANSFEMORAL PROSTHETIC GAIT

A brief description of the most common transfemoral gait deviations is given in Table 5.2.

Table 5.2 Common Gait Deviations in Transfemoral Prosthetic Gait

Gait Cycle Phase	Gait Deviation	Description	Patient Cause(s)	Prosthetic Cause(s)
Initial contact	Abnormal narrow base (stance and swing)	Stance between heels is less than normal	Hip adductor contracture or spasticity Genu varum	Proximal-lateral device discomfort Hip joint excessively adducted
	Abnormal wide base (abducted gait) (stance and swing)	Stance between heels is abnormally far apart	Hip abductor contracture or spasticity Instability (patient has neuropathy and uses the wide base of support to avoid falling) Genu valgum	Proximal-medial device discomfort Improperly shaped lateral wall fails to support femur Leg length discrepancy—prosthesis too high
	Foot rotation on initial contact	External rotation of prosthetic foot at initial contact	Extension of residual limb is too vigorous at initial contact Amputee has poor muscle control of residual limb Amputee does not place enough weight on the prosthetic foot to compress heel	Plantarflexion bumper too stiff Heel wedge too hard Socket fit is loose allowing for rotation Too much toe-out in prosthetic alignment
	Excessive medial or lateral weight on the foot (stance phase)	Excessive weight or time spent on medial or lateral side of foot	Genu valgum (medial) Genu varum (lateral)	Foot too everted Uneven wear of shoe heel Insufficient accommodation for toe-out
	Excessive knee flexion (knee buckling) (stance phase)	Knee flexed greater than 20 degrees	Knee flexion contracture Involved limb relatively longer Hip flexion contracture	Stiff or long heel lever Foot too dorsiflexed Foot keel too soft—allows knee flexion late in stance Knee joint can be aligned anterior to weight line or TKA line Socket too posterior Heel height too high
Initial contact	Hyperextended knee (IC and TSt)	Excessive extension of knee in stance	Quadriceps weakness or spasticity Genu recurvatum Ligamentous laxity Gastrocnemius weakness Compensation of contralateral hip or knee contracture or skeletal shortening	Excessive socket flexion Socket too anterior Foot plantarflexed Plantarflexion bumper too soft Heel height too low
	Anterior trunk bending (IC, LR, MSt, TSw)	Patient flexes upper trunk Possible hands on thighs to lock knee for stability	Quadriceps weakness or paralysis Flexor spasticity Tight iliotibial band Knee and/or hip flexion contracture	Knee axis too far anterior Inadequate socket flexion
	Unequal step length	Short prosthetic side step	Painful socket causing a quick transfer of weight to intact limb Patient insecurity, lack of balance, or insecurity	Insufficient knee friction or extension aid Unstable knee

Table 5.2 Common Gait Deviations in Transfemoral Prosthetic Gait—cont'd

Gait Cycle Phase	Gait Deviation	Description	Patient Cause(s)	Prosthetic Cause(s)
Midstance	Varus/valgus thrust	Knee pops into a varus or valgus position during midstance	N/A	Foot too inset (varus) or too outset (valgus) Abducted (varus) or adducted (valgus) socket Mediolateral dimension of socket too wide
	Lateral trunk bending (MSt, occasionally swing)	Stance lean toward involved side with weight Swing lean toward unaffected side	Hip abductor weakness Abduction contracture Hip dislocation/coxa vara Hip pain Scoliosis	Hip joint excessively abducted Prosthesis too short Device discomfort Mediolateral dimension of socket too wide Prosthesis is aligned in too much abduction leading to a wide base of support
Preswing	Insufficient push-off (excessive pelvic drop with forward progression)	Weight on heel and entire foot leaves ground for swing	Fear of placing full weight on prosthesis	Foot is too far posterior, causing shortened anterior lever arm Dorsiflexion bumper too soft
Swing phase	Vaulting	Exaggerated plantar- flexion of contralateral side	Habit—desire to keep knee locked during ambulation Forceful hip flexion to put knee into extension	Prosthesis too long Knee locked in extension Excessive friction or stability at the knee Inadequate suspension
Swing phase	Uneven heel rise	Prosthetic heel rising quite markedly and rapidly when the knee is flexed at the beginning of swing phase	Patient uses more power to force knee into extension	Knee joint with inadequate friction
	Terminal swing impact	Knee extends rapid forward movement of the shank to reach maximum extension with too much force before initial contact of the heel	Patient wants to ensure the prosthesis will be there for full weight acceptance so they will not fall Poor gait habit	Inadequate knee friction Knee extension aid too strong
	Circumduction	Foot follows laterally curved path. Mainly in swing phase as foot returns to the normal base of support foot position in stance	Habit—desire to keep knee locked during ambulation Poor gait habit Abduction contracture	Extension aid too strong Prosthesis too long Foot plantarflexed Inadequate suspension Excessive knee flexion resistance or too much stability in alignment
	Whips	Rapid motion of heel into internal or external rotation A medial whip: the heel travels medially on initial flexion at the beginning of swing phase Lateral whip: the heel travels laterally on initial flexion at the beginning of swing phase		Medial Whip—knee too externally rotated with respect to socket Lateral Whip—knee too internally rotated with respect to socket Improperly contoured socket
	Uneven timing	Characterized by a short stance phase on the prosthetic side	Muscle weakness Poor balance with prosthesis Fear and insecurity	Weak extension aid or insufficient knee friction can cause excessive heel rise and result in a longer time spent on the sound side Knee instability Poor fitting socket

IC, Initial contact; *LR*, loading response; *MSt*, midstance; *TSt*, terminal stance; *TSw*, terminal swing.
From Spires MC, Kelly BM, Davis AJ. *Prosthetic Restoration and Rehabilitation of the Upper and Lower Extremity*. Springer Publishing Company; 2013; Adapted from Kapp S. Visual analysis of prosthetic gait. In: *Atlas of Amputations and Limb Deficiencies*. American Academy of Orthopedic Surgeons; 2004:388–394; Gitter A, Bosker G. Upper and lower extremity prosthetics. In: DeLisa JA, ed. *Rehabilitation Medicine: Principles and Practice*. 4th ed. Lippincott Williams & Wilkins; 2005.

Case Example 5.6 **A Patient With a Hemipelvectomy Amputation**

L. is a 38-year-old female with a right hemipelvectomy amputation secondary to osteosarcoma. She has been referred to the gait laboratory for evaluation as a possible candidate for a microprocessor-controlled knee unit. For the past several years, she has been ambulatory without the use of assistive devices.

CONSIDER

- Considering L.'s level of amputation, what types of difficulties or deviations might you expect during the course of level overground ambulation?
- What quantitative measures would serve as indicators of the likely gait deviations?

EXAMINATION AND EVALUATION

L. was fitted with reflective markers and underwent three-dimensional kinetic and kinematic testing. This testing was performed at her self-selected WS, and she was given a suitable amount of time to become acclimated to the testing environment before data collection. Observational assessment indicates a significant amount of vaulting and excessive pelvic movement, but no indication of circumduction.

The temporal data show that she walks at a rate of 92 steps per minute and a velocity of 0.96 m/s. Along with this, her step length on the left side is 0.58 m, and the right side is 0.70 m, even though the total stride length for both sides is 1.24 m. Similarly, the total stride time for both sides was 1.3 s; however, the single limb support time was 0.55 s on the left side and 0.41 s on the right. The step time for the left was 0.59 s, and the right was 0.71 s. Similarly, toe-off occurred at 68.8% of the gait cycle on the left side, and it occurred at 57.9% on the right.

Kinematic data at the ankle showed a consistent pattern of abnormal plantarflexion on the left side occurring from approximately 14% of the gait cycle through 60% of the gait cycle. Overall knee flexion on the left side was within the overall expected range, as was hip flexion in swing. The right side knee flexion showed approximately 5 degrees of knee flexion during LR and a peak average knee flexion of 53 degrees. Exaggerated anterior-posterior pelvic tilt was also documented (Fig. 5.14).

Kinetically, the left side consistently showed greater anterior/posterior shear forces compared to the contralateral side, usually twice as much force exerted on the left compared to the right. Along with this, there was no clear twin peak maximum in the vertical component of the ground reaction force. Instead, there were multiple maxima over the course of a single stance phase (Fig. 5.15).

QUESTIONS TO CONSIDER

- Based on what is presented here, what possible advantages could a microprocessor-controlled knee unit have over a conventional mechanical unit? When considering this, bear in mind that the specific microprocessor knee unit she is being evaluated for is designed to allow for adjustments in both flexion and extension resistance based on the individual's walking velocity.
- What kinematic, kinetic, and temporal changes could you expect to see with a change in knee unit?
- Considering that the potential improvements are not absolute, do the potential benefits warrant the issuance of the device?

Summary

The examples of gait deficiencies typical of neuromuscular conditions and in prosthetic gait that we have considered demonstrate the complexity and variety that challenge orthotists, prosthetists, and physical therapists working with individuals with gait deviations. Each individual presents unique combinations of pathological and compensatory deficits that require a combination of the essential tools of simple quantitative measure (cadence and velocity, step length, stride length and width, and double support time), systematic qualitative gait analysis (Rancho Los Amigos observational gait assessment protocol), measures of energy cost (PCI), LOA (FAC), and functional measures (the TUG or GARS-M). These tools help the clinician differentiate primary pathological conditions from secondary compensations, guide orthotic recommendation and therapeutic intervention, and assess efficacy of treatment. Instrumented gait assessment is an important part of preoperative assessment and research in orthotic and prosthetic design. In addition, the data collected in gait laboratories are accumulating into a database that can provide information necessary to build accurate outcome estimations for many groups of clients. The current challenge is for the clinic team to gain the broadest possible knowledge base in analytical gait assessment and to serve each client as a team, considering them as an individual.

References

The complete listing of the References are available in the accompanying enhanced eBook version included with the print purchase of this textbook. Visit Elsevier eBooks+ (eBooks.Health.Elsevier.com) to access this content.

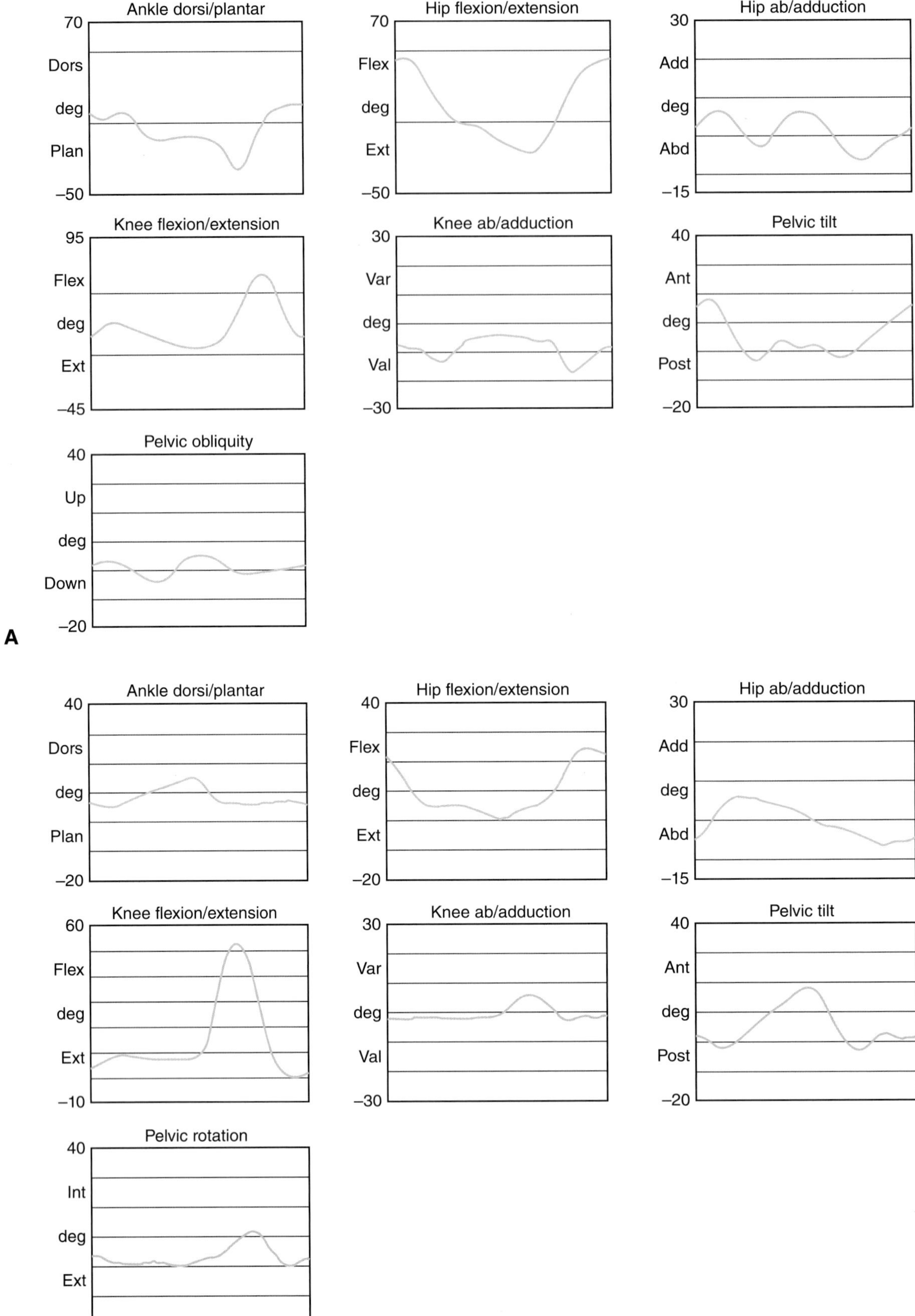

Fig. 5.14 A patient with right hemipelvectomy amputation: average motion data results for the left (A) and right side (B). Particularly note the ankle motion on the left side indicating the vaulting pattern.

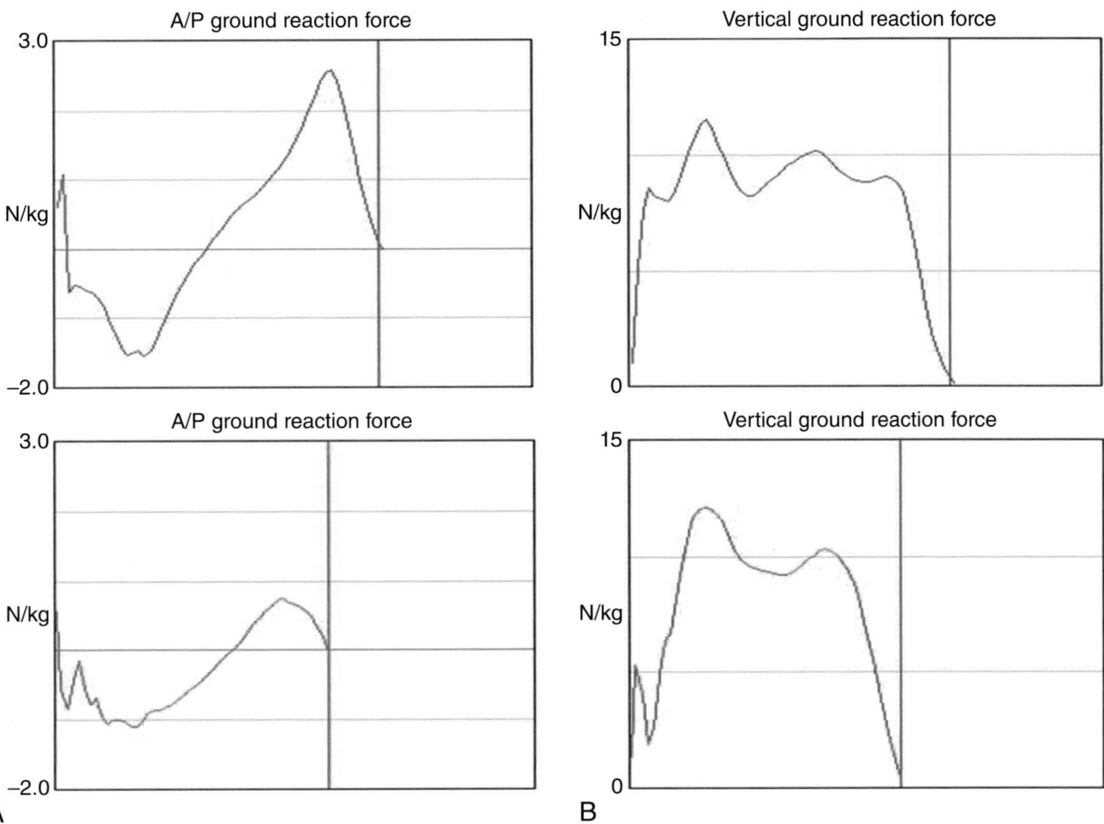

Fig. 5.15 A patient with right hemipelvectomy amputation: vertical and anterior-posterior (A/P) ground reaction force data for the left side (A) and right side (B). Note the difference in the vertical force patterns, especially the lack of two well-defined force peaks on the left side and the difference in magnitudes between the two peak force values on the left.

6 Materials and Technology

DUFFY FELMLEE AND KEVIN K. CHUI

LEARNING OBJECTIVES

On completion of this chapter, the reader will be able to do the following:

1. Compare and contrast the materials most often used in current orthoses and prostheses.
2. Describe how the basic mechanical properties of commonly used materials determine how they will be used in orthotic and prosthetic devices.
3. Describe the process of, and measures used in, the formulation of a biomechanically appropriate orthotic or prosthetic prescription that will address a patient's functional deficits.
4. Describe how a prosthetist or orthotist determines the appropriate prosthetic or orthotic controls needed for the management of a patient's impairments or functional limitations.
5. Delineate the steps in the fabrication or production of a custom orthosis or prosthesis.
6. Discuss the use of computer-aided design/computer-aided manufacture in the measurement for and fabrication of orthoses and prostheses.
7. Describe the factors influencing the development of central fabrication centers and the manufacture of prefabricated components, orthoses, and prostheses.

A fundamental concept and common goal within the professions of orthotics, prosthetics, and rehabilitation is the restoration of optimal form and function after injury or disease. In many cases, movement and mobility are compromised and the use of orthoses and prostheses can enable improved function. To accept this challenge, the fields of orthotics and prosthetics have evolved into uniquely specialized professions. In addition to training in the basic biologic and medical sciences, orthotists and prosthetists have an understanding of biomechanics, kinesiology, and the material sciences complemented by highly developed technical skills. Knowledge of the physical properties of materials and the techniques to manipulate and use them is essential to the design and fabrication of orthoses and prostheses. The topic is presented here as a general overview so the rehabilitation clinician can develop a basic understanding of current design and fabrication processes used by orthotists and prosthetists.

Orthotics and Prosthetics in the 20th Century

Orthotics and prosthetics have a rich history of research and development. Many innovative devices have been designed to restore function and provide relief from various medical ailments. Although progress can be documented throughout human history, the most significant contributions to orthotics and prosthetics were made in the 20th century, stimulated by the aftermath of the world wars. Injured veterans who returned home from battle with musculoskeletal and neuromuscular impairments or traumatic amputation dramatically increased the demand for orthotic and prosthetic services. Although World War I stimulated some clinical progress in the two disciplines, notable scientific advancements did not occur until World War II. To improve the quality and performance of assistive devices at the end of World War II, particularly for veterans with amputation, the US government sponsored a series of research and development projects under the auspices of the National Academy of Sciences (NAS) that would forever change the manner in which orthotics and prosthetics would be practiced.[1]

An extensive research effort was initiated by the NAS in late 1945, when a consensus conference revealed that few modern scientific principles or developments had been introduced in prosthetics.[2] Research and educational committees were formed between 1945 and 1976 to advise and work with the research groups. Universities, the Veterans Administration, private industry, and other military research units were subcontracted to conduct various prosthetic research projects. In summarizing the most notable achievements in prosthetics during this period, Wilson[3] cites the development of the total contact transfemoral socket; the quadrilateral socket design and hydraulic swing-phase knee-control units for the transfemoral prosthesis; the patellar tendon–bearing (PTB) transtibial prosthesis; the solid-ankle, cushioned-heel prosthetic foot; several new designs for the Syme prosthesis; and the Canadian hip-disarticulation prosthesis. He also notes the implementation of immediate postsurgical and early fitting as having a significant impact on the rehabilitation process for persons with lower extremity amputation. The most notable improvements in upper extremity prosthetics were the lyre-shaped three-jaw chuck terminal device and more efficient harnessing systems. In addition, modular components and advances in bioengineering have permitted increased use and availability of the myoelectric prosthesis since it was first proposed in 1950.[4]

Of the wealth of scientific advances made during this intensive research period, the most important is the greater attention paid to the biomechanics of prosthetic alignment and socket design.[5] According to Wilson,[2] "The introduction of socket designs based on sound biomechanical analyses to take full advantage of the functions and properties of the stump in conjunction with the rationale for alignment undoubtedly represents the greatest achievement in prosthetics since World War II."

Although the focus of the NAS Artificial Limb Program was in prosthetics, it was anticipated that these efforts would also benefit orthotics. A formal research directive in orthotics did not begin until 1960. Biomechanical principles developed for the PTB prosthesis were immediately introduced in orthotics at the Veterans Administration Prosthetic Center, with the PTB orthosis to unload the foot-ankle complex axially.[6] The concept of fracture bracing or cast bracing began at approximately the same time and is now common practice for orthopedic management of fractures.[7,8] Clinical aspects of orthotic practice were also considered; a systematic approach to prescription formulation was established with the development of the technical analysis forms. Nomenclature to describe orthoses and their functions was standardized to identify the body segments they encompassed with the desired biomechanical control mechanisms.[9]

The introduction of new materials led to further advances in the field shortly after World War II. The use of thermosetting plastics in prosthetics permitted the development of the suction socket suspension system.[10] Transparent plastics offered a new approach to diagnostic and fitting evaluation techniques, such as the transparent prosthetic socket (test socket) and the transparent face mask for patients with thermal injuries. In orthotics, the addition of thermoplastics led to numerous innovative designs of ankle-foot orthoses (AFOs) in the 1960s and 1970s. The custom plastic AFO was an important technologic advance in lower extremity orthotics. The physical characteristics of thermoformable plastics allowed biomechanical controls to match the prescription for improved function. The mechanical properties of an orthosis could be controlled by the layout of the trimlines of a device or structural reinforcements through specially placed corrugations that could be incorporated into its surface geometry. Advances have been steady in the area of material engineering and continue to have an impact on orthotics and prosthetics.

Numerous prosthetic feet have been introduced as elite athletes demand increased performance capabilities from their prosthetic components. Innovative designs for some prosthetic feet have been possible in part because of the diversity of carbon composite technology complemented by sound engineering design.

The development of computer-aided design/computer-aided manufacture (CAD/CAM) systems for orthotics and prosthetics, which began in the 1970s, was another major technologic advance, considering the long tradition of custom hand-crafted devices in the profession. In the late 1980s and early 1990s, as computers became more economical, facilities began to integrate CAD/CAM systems into their practices. CAD/CAM systems have now been designed for most orthotic and prosthetic applications, often with specialized digitizers, scanners, and milling equipment to accommodate the unique needs of a particular device. The one trend within the profession is that orthotists and prosthetists use the CAD portion to digitize and manipulate the data, then subcontract the production of a device from a central fabrication company for the CAM or traditional fabrication portion. The art and workmanship that have distinguished the orthotists and prosthetists from other health professionals for most of the 20th century continue to evolve as CAD/CAM technologies improve the design, manufacture, and diagnostic aspects of the field.

Orthotics and prosthetics have played an important historical role in the development of medical and surgical orthopedics and rehabilitation. Fundamental concepts that evolved from orthotic and prosthetic advancements are now basic principles in rehabilitation. Orthotics and prosthetics have evolved as sister professions because the technical skills and knowledge base to prescribe, fabricate, and fit the respective mechanical devices are similar. Because of this, material and technologic advancements have been shared between these two rehabilitation specialties.

Materials

In the first part of the 20th century, orthoses were constructed primarily of metal, leather, and fabric, and prostheses were manufactured from wood and leather (Fig. 6.1). In the last 60 years, however, tremendous technologic advancements have been made in the material sciences. The demand for strong and lightweight components in the aerospace and marine industries has produced a variety of new materials that possess mechanical properties suitable for use in the construction of orthoses and prostheses. New plastics have led to revolutionary advancements in the profession, permitting increased durability and strength and significant cosmetic improvements. Although a multitude of materials are currently available, traditional ones are still in wide use; material selection depends in part on the individual needs of each patient. In a rehabilitation team setting, the orthotist and prosthetist are responsible for choosing the appropriate materials and components for fabrication because their experience and training are specialized in this area.

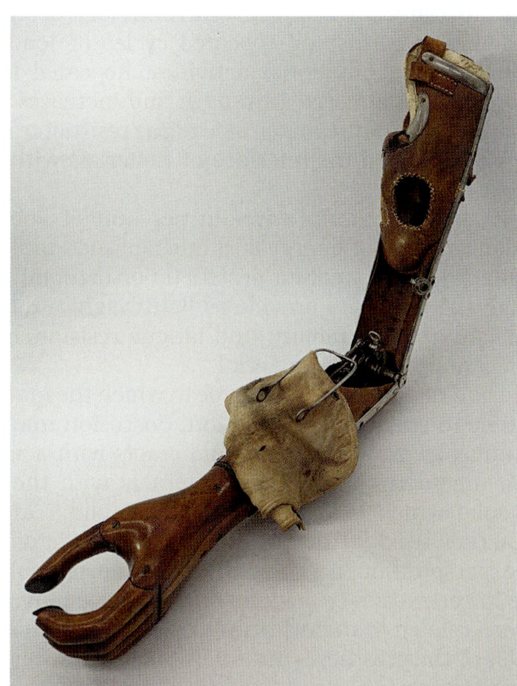

Fig. 6.1 Transhumeral prosthesis. Leather, metal, wood construction c.1940. (Courtesy Matthew Parente.)

This chapter presents an overview of the general types of materials used in orthotics and prosthetics for rehabilitation professionals. Publications by the American Society for Testing and Materials contain specific technical information.[11] Industry standards established by the International Organization for Standardization for consumer and patient protection give the strength requirements for orthotic and prosthetic components.[12]

The types of materials used most commonly in current orthotic and prosthetic practice include leather, cork, wood, metal, thermoplastic and thermosetting materials, foamed plastics, and viscoelastic polymers. In deciding which materials are most appropriate for a patient, the orthotist or prosthetist considers the five important characteristics of materials: strength, stiffness, durability, density, and corrosion resistance.

A material's strength is determined by the maximum external load that the material can support or sustain. Strength is especially important in lower limb devices, in which loading forces associated with gait can be very high, or when heavy use of the orthotic or prosthetic device is anticipated. Materials may have higher strength in different loading scenarios. Some materials may be more effective under tensile load while others may be better under compressive loads.

Stiffness is a measure of the resistance of the material to relative atomic separation. This measurement, named the Young modulus, is larger when materials are stiffer and is related to the amount of force that is required to displace the atomic structure of the material.[13] The stiffer a material, the less flexible it is and the less likely that deformation will occur during wear. When significant external stability is desirable (e.g., in a fracture brace or a rigid prosthetic frame), a stiff material is often chosen. When co nformation to body segments is necessary (e.g., in a posterior leaf-spring AFO or a flexible transfemoral prosthetic socket), a more flexible material is used.

Durability (fatigue resistance) of a material is determined by its ability to withstand repeated cycles of loading or unloading during functional activities. Repeated loading compromises the material's strength and increases risk of failure or fracture of the material. Fatigue resistance is especially problematic in the interface of materials with different characteristics.

Density is the material's weight per unit of volume, a prime determinant of energy cost during functional activities while a patient wears a prosthetic or orthotic device. Although the goal is to provide as lightweight a device as possible, strength, durability, and fatigue resistance needs may necessitate a denser material.

Corrosion resistance is the degree to which the material is susceptible to chemical degradation. Corrosion may occur in a number of ways when a liquid reacts with a solid. In general, the surrounding liquid interacts with the bonds of the solid which in turn weakens the solid.[13] Many of the materials used for orthoses or prostheses retain heat, making perspiration a problem. For some patients who require lower extremity devices, incontinence may also be a concern related to the urine interacting with the various materials of the prosthesis. Materials that are impervious to moisture are easier to clean than porous materials.

The ease of fabrication in another important consideration for materials. Certain materials can be easily molded or adjusted for a custom fit; others require special equipment or techniques to shape the material.

NATURAL MATERIALS

Leather

Leather is manufactured from the skin and hides of various animals. Tanning methods and the type of hide determine the final characteristics of the leather. As an interface material for an orthosis or a prosthesis, vegetable-tanned leather is used to protect the skin from irritation.

Chrome-tanned leather is used for supportive purposes when strength and resiliency are needed. Additional chemical processes can be incorporated during manufacturing to produce leathers that are waterproof, porous, flexible, or stiff. Useful qualities of leather include its dimensional stability, porosity, and water vapor permeability.[14] These features have made leather a frequently used material within orthopedics, and it continues to be a material of choice in many current devices. Currently, leather is used for supportive components such as suspension straps, belts, and limb cuffs. Leather is also used to cover metallic structures such as pelvic, thigh, and calf bands (Fig. 6.2). For foot orthoses and shoe modifications, leather is often preferred over synthetic substitutes because of its superior "breathability" characteristics.

Another important attribute of leather is its moldability. Although numerous techniques are available to mold leather, the most common one in orthotics and prosthetics is to stretch it over a plaster cast after it has been mulled (dampened or soaked) in water. When the water evaporates from the molded leather, its dried shape is maintained, and the leather can be trimmed to the desired dimensions. To increase strength and durability, leather can be reinforced

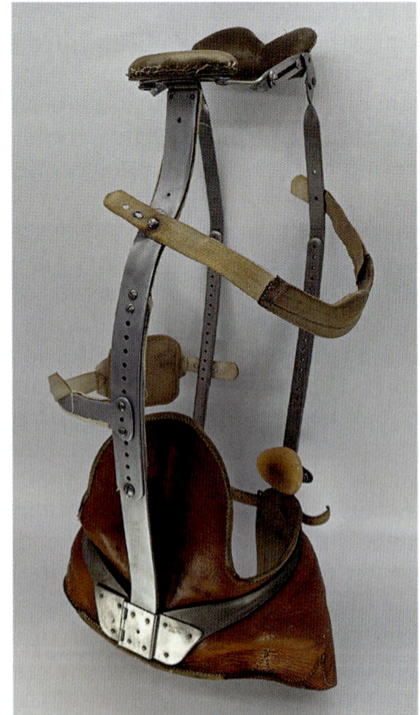

Fig. 6.2 Custom fabrication CLTSO (Milwaukee) c.1960. (Courtesy Matthew Parente.)

by lamination with plastics or other leathers. Similarly, if padding is desired over bony regions of the body, foamed plastics or felt can be sandwiched between layers of leather for comfort or to distribute applied forces over a larger surface area. Three basic skills are required for crafting orthotic or prosthetic components of leather: cutting, sewing, and molding. A technique specific to leather work is that of skiving, or thinning the edge on the flesh side of the hide. Finishing methods such as these contribute to the final appearance of the leather work and the device.

Wood

Wood possesses many desirable characteristics for use in prosthetics. Its wide availability, strength, light weight, and ability to be shaped easily have continued to be of benefit in prosthetic socket and component construction, even with the introduction of thermoplastics. The wood used in prosthetics must be properly cured, free of knots, and relatively strong. Yellow poplar, willow, basswood (linden), and balsa are most commonly used. Hardwoods have been reserved for prosthetic applications in which structural strength is essential, most often in certain types of prosthetic feet or as reinforcement for knee units. The keel prosthetic foot is fabricated of maple and hickory. The solid-ankle, cushioned-heel prosthetic foot has a hardwood keel that is bolted to the prosthetic shank, creating a solid structural unit for standing and ambulation.

Cork

Cork is a renewable, natural material that is primarily used within foot orthotics. Related to the porosity of the materials cork performs on par with synthetic materials when evaluated for comfort and antifungal characteristics.[15,16] To optimize functional characteristics, such as thermoformability, self-adhesion, and variable density, cork has increasingly become a blended final product. Examples include Mutlicork (Acor Orthopaedic, Inc.), Birkocork, and Thermocork (Apex Foot Products).

METALS

The types of metal used in the fabrication of orthoses and prostheses can be categorized into three groups: steel and its alloys, aluminum, and titanium or magnesium alloys. These metals may or may not share similar characteristics. If metals are incorporated into an orthosis or prosthesis, the choice of metal is determined by the needs and preferences of the particular patient.

Steel

The general term *steel* refers to any iron-based alloy material. Carbon alloys have carbon added to the iron ore. The term *alloy steel* is used when other materials are included in the material manufacture. Alloy steels are further defined as low-alloy or high-alloy steels. Steels are strong, rigid, ductile, and durable, but their high density (weight) and susceptibility to corrosion are major disadvantages. Many different types of steel are available to meet various engineering needs. To assist in identifying the composition and type of material, the American Iron Steel Institute-Society of Automotive Engineers has established a four-digit numbering system. The first two digits in the number indicate the type of steel, and the last two digits identify the carbon content. For alloy steels, the first digit identifies the major alloy and the second digit indicates the percentage of the major alloying element.

The carbon content of steel is the major determinant of its ductility and yield strength characteristics. Yield strength is the point where the amount of stress applied to a material corresponds with that material's elastic limit, the point where any extra load plastically changes the material and it will not return to its original shape.[13] Ductility is the property of a material to deform in the inelastic or plastic range under load before failing. Low carbon content (0.05%–0.10%) produces high ductility and a low yield strength.[15] As the carbon concentration increases, yield strength increases and ductility is reduced. Heat treatments can alter the properties of carbon steel by increasing yield strength and reducing ductility. The mechanical properties of low-alloy steels fall between those of carbon steels and high-alloy steels. High strength/weight ratios are possible with the high-alloy steels, an important characteristic for repetitive loading situations. These types of steels are used for some orthotic and prosthetic joint components.

High-alloy steels are not very resistant to corrosion and are often more difficult to fabricate. Stainless steel is a steel alloy that contains 12% or more of chromium, a material that increases resistance to corrosion and oxidation. Chromium produces a light oxide film on the surface that deters deterioration of the base metal. Because durability and protection from corrosion are highly desirable, stainless steels are used extensively within orthotics and prosthetics to enhance longevity of devices. Two types of stainless steel, martensitic steel and ferritic steel, have chromium as the predominant alloying element, but martensitic steel is the only one used in orthotics and prosthetics because it can be hardened by heat treatment. Stainless steel is used for orthotic and prosthetic joints, support uprights, and band material.

Aluminum

Aluminum alloys are well suited for orthotics and prosthetics because of their high strength/weight ratio and resistance to corrosion. As with steels, the properties of aluminum depend on alloying compositions, heat treatments, and cold working. *Wrought* and *cast* are terms used to describe the two ways to produce aluminum devices. Wrought metals are hot or cold worked, meaning they are formed using tools like a large roller, a stamp, or even a hammer around a mold.[13] The shape of the piece is mechanically formed from the outside force of the forming device. Casting is a process where liquid metal is poured into a mold, oftentimes made out of sand, and the final device takes the shape of the mold. Alloys are further subdivided into those that are heat treatable and those that are not. The low ductility and low strength of cast aluminum are ideal for prefabricated prosthetic components and in some assemblies for moving parts.

Wrought aluminum alloys are used in orthotics and prosthetics for structural purposes such as prosthetic pylons, orthotic uprights, and upper extremity devices. The high-compression bending stresses of lower extremity prosthetics are well suited to the use of wrought aluminum alloys.

Although aluminum alloys are very resistant to atmospheric and some chemical corrosion, the acids and alkalis in urine, perspiration, and other bodily fluids deteriorate the natural protective oxides on the material's surface, making the aluminum susceptible to corrosion. To deter corrosion in aluminum and to resist abrasive wear, various hard coatings, such as anodic or oxide finishes, can be applied. Mechanical finishes, such as polishing, buffing, and sandblasting, offer attractive cosmetic appearances for devices.[15,17]

Titanium and Magnesium

Components made of titanium alloys have become more prevalent in prosthetics but are rarely used in orthotics. Although titanium alloys are stronger than those of aluminum and have comparable strength to some steels, their density is 60% that of steel.[18] Because prosthetic components made of titanium are lighter in weight than steel counterparts, they require less energy expenditure by the patient during use. Titanium alloys are also more resistant to corrosion than are aluminum and steel. However, it is important to note that titanium alloys are often more difficult to machine and fabricate. Consequently, titanium is most often used in prefabricated prosthetic components, when strength and light weight are of concern. Titanium is also more expensive than aluminum and steel, which has been a limiting factor for its use.

Magnesium alloys are lighter than those of aluminum and titanium, are corrosion resistant, and have a lower modulus of elasticity than does aluminum. The modulus of elasticity (Young modulus) is defined as the ratio of unit stress to unit strain in a stress-strain curve's elastic range; materials with low modulus values are associated with lower rates of fatigue under conditions of repeated stress. Although some of these features are promising, magnesium alloys have not yet been widely used in orthoses and prostheses.

PLASTICS AND COMPOSITES

One of the most important production-related characteristics of an orthotic or prosthetic material is its ability to be molded over a positive model. Because plastics can be readily formed, they are a very popular, widely used material for orthoses and prostheses. Plastics are grouped into two categories: thermoplastics and thermosetting materials.[17,19–21]

Thermoplastics

Thermoplastic materials are formable when they are heated but become rigid after they have cooled. Thermoplastics are classified as either low-temperature or high-temperature materials, depending on the temperature range at which they become malleable. Low-temperature thermoplastics become moldable at temperatures less than 149°C and can often be molded directly on the patient's limb, whereas high-temperature materials require heating to much higher temperatures and must be molded over a positive model of the patient's limb.[20] One advantage of thermoplastic materials is that they can be reheated and shaped multiple times, making possible minor adjustments of an orthosis or prosthesis during fittings. Thermoplastics are the material of choice for "shell" designs in which structural strength is required. Some of the more popular materials used are acrylic, copolymer, polyethylene, polypropylene, polystyrene, and a variety of vinyls.

Certain low-temperature thermoplastics, those moldable at temperatures less than 80°C can be applied and shaped directly to the body. Some of the most commonly available materials include Kydex (Kleerdex, Aiken, SCCurbell Plastics, Bloomsburg, Pennsylvania); Orthoplast (Johnson & Johnson, Raynham, Massachusetts); and Polysar (Bayer, Pittsburgh), X-LITE (New Jersey). These materials are most often reserved for orthotic devices that are designed to provide temporary support and protection. Their susceptibility to repetitive stress, high loads, and temperature changes usually limits their use to spinal and upper extremity orthoses. Because these devices are molded directly on the patient, no casting is necessary, and the time required from measurement to finished product is greatly reduced. Another important convenience of low-temperature thermoplastic materials is that no special equipment is required; hot water heated in an external heat source, a heat gun, and sharp scissors are all that are necessary to produce a functional splint or orthosis.[21,22]

High-temperature plastics are frequently used in the production of orthotics and prosthetics. The most commonly used materials include polyethylene, polypropylene, polycarbonate, acrylic, acrylonitrile butadiene styrene (ABS), acrylics, polyethylene vinyl acetate, polyvinyl chloride, and polyvinyl alcohol.

Polypropylene is a rigid plastic material that is relatively inexpensive, lightweight, and easy to thermoform. Polypropylenes, which can be further characterized as homopolymers or copolymers, are one of the most widely used plastics in orthotics. The raw material form has a white, opaque color, though this can vary with additional pigments and designs, and is available in sheets of various thicknesses, from 1 mm to 1 cm.

Polypropylene is impact resistant and can endure several million cycles of repetitive flexes. This attribute has been extremely useful in orthotics as the primary material within lower extremity interventions.

However, the material is susceptible to ultraviolet light and extreme cold and is sensitive to scratches and nicks. In prosthetics, the light weight of polypropylene makes it ideal for components such as sockets, and pelvic bands. Polypropylene is commonly used for orthoses which require structural rigidity and the ability to make minor adjustments to shape without affecting the integrity of the material such a majority of custom lower extremity orthoses. Copolymers address the cold-temperature notch sensitivity though lack the rigidity seen in polypropylene. Copolymers are utilized in prefabricated AFOs and preformed modular orthotic systems. The long fatigue life of polyethylene during repeated loading situations makes this material suitable for a number of orthotic and prosthetic applications. Prosthetic sockets, orthotic hinge joint components, and compression shells for clamshell design orthoses are common uses of polyethylene plastics. Several densities of polyethylene are available from various manufacturers. Low-density polyethylene is used for upper extremity and spinal orthoses under the trade names Vitrathene (Stanley Smith & Co, Ltd, Isleworth, United Kingdom) and Streifen (FG Streifeneder KG, Munich, Germany). High-density polyethylene, Subortholen (Wilhelm Julius Teufel GmbH, Stuttgart, Germany), is used for spinal and lower extremity orthoses. The ultra-high-density polyethylenes such as

Ortholen (Wilhelm Julius Teufel) are used principally for lower extremity orthoses.

A thermoplastic material that is commonly used in conjunction with thermoset plastics is EVA (polyethylene vinyl acetate). Adjustable volume prosthetic sockets combine a rigid external frame of thermosets, discussed in a subsequent section of this chapter, and a flexible inner socket allowing for volumetric adjustments to be made (Figs. 6.3 and 6.4).[23]

Foamed Plastics

Foamed plastics can be used as a protective interface between the orthotic or prosthetic and the skin, especially over areas that are vulnerable to pressure, such as bony prominences. Foamed plastics are commonly referred to as "Foams" and are grouped into two classes: open and closed cell. Cells are created in rubber or polymers in a high-pressure gassing process.[20] The microcell structure allows the foamed plastic material to be displaced in several planes, which is an ideal physical property for the reduction of shear forces. In an open-cell foam, the cells are interrelated (as in a kitchen sponge); in a closed-cell foam, the cells are separate from each other. Because closed-cell foams are impervious to liquids, they are less likely to absorb body fluids such as perspiration or urine; however, they do act as insulators and can be hot when worn for extended periods.

An orthopedic grade of polyethylene foam was introduced in the 1960s by a British subsidiary of the Union Carbide Company.[24] These closed-cell foams are available in a wide array of durometer hardness. (Durometer refers to a spring indenture post instrument that is used to measure the resistance to the compression/hardness of a material.) Polyethylene foams are commercially available under trade names such as Plastazote (Hackettstown, New Jersey); Pe-Lite Evazote (Bakelite Xylonite Ltd., Croydon, United Kingdom); and Aliplast (Alimed Inc., Dedham, Massachusetts). Various polyethylene foams are used in the manufacture of soft and rigid orthoses, depending on the

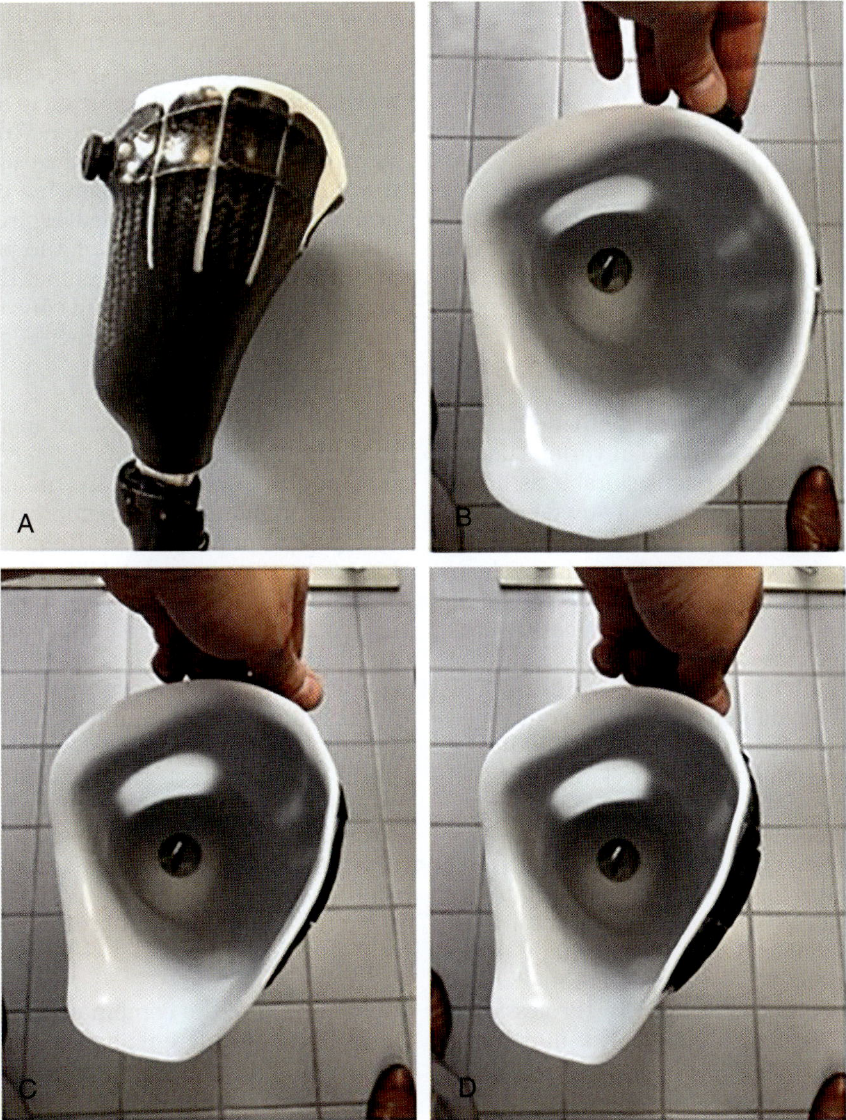

Fig. 6.3 Example of volume adjustability in a transfemoral socket with a rigid external frame and flexible inner socket. Socket views both in the sagittal (A) and transverse planes (B, C, D). Image B shows the socket fully opened; image C shows the socket halfway tightened; and image D shows the socket fully tightened. (Courtesy Katie Johnson, R.J. Rosenberg Orthopedic Lab, Inc.)

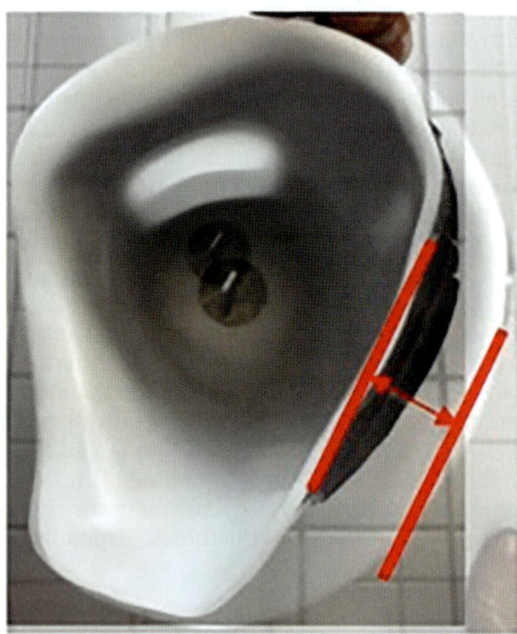

Fig. 6.4 An overlay of images B and D in Fig. 6.3A, in the transverse view of the socket fully opened and fully tightened. (Courtesy Katie Johnson, R.J. Rosenberg Orthopedic Lab, Inc.)

density of the material. Plastazote is a low-temperature, heat-formable foam that has been used successfully in the treatment and prevention of neuropathic foot lesions.[25–28] Its light weight and forgiving quality to bony prominences make it a desirable interface for the insensate foot.

See Hertzman[25] for a complete review of the use of Plastazote in lower limb orthotics and prosthetics.

Closed-cell foams are also made with synthetic rubber or polychloroprene. Neoprene is available in various densities, making the low-durometer versions suitable as liners for orthoses, whereas the firmer materials are used for posts or soling for shoes. Spenco (Spenco Medical Corp., Waco, Texas) is a microcellular neoprene foam that reduces shear forces to the foot's plantar surface and the occurrence of foot blisters in athletes.[29] The nylon (polyamide)-covered neoprene acts as a shock absorber while also reducing friction on the foot's plantar surface.[24] Although few of these materials are heat moldable, most can be conformed without difficulty to the shallow contours of foot orthoses. Lynco (Apex Foot Health Industries, Teaneck, New Jersey) is an open-cell neoprene foam that dissipates heat more efficiently than its closed-cell cousin; however, it does not attenuate shock as well as Spenco.[24]

Polyurethane open-cell foams are alternatives for top covers for foot orthoses. They provide good shock absorption and dissipate heat well. Some of the commercially available open-cell polyurethane foams include Poron (Rogers Corporation, Rogers, Connecticut); PPT (Professional Protective Technology, Deer Park, New York); and Vylite (Steins Foot Specialties, Newark, New Jersey).

Several studies that compare materials used to fabricate orthoses have been conducted.[30–36] In 1982, Campbell and colleagues[30] conducted compression tests on 31 materials to determine their suitability for insoles in shoes. Materials were classified according to stiffness into the categories "very stiff," "moderately deformable," and "highly deformable." The moderately deformable group of plastics, which included 19 of the tested foamed plastics, was deemed the most beneficial as an insole material. Campbell and colleagues[30] concluded that these materials could relieve stress from bony prominences and transfer the loads to the adjacent soft tissues more effectively than could the very stiff or highly deformable materials. Studies evaluating shoe insole materials also report them to be effective at attenuating shock during walking in various ways.[36]

Thermoforming

Thermoforming is one of the most common techniques used in orthotic and prosthetic laboratories to fabricate the "user" interface components of a device (e.g., prosthetic socket, AFO). The process of thermoforming entails heating a sheet of thermoplastic material in an oven until it has reached its "plastic" state (i.e., ability to distort) and then forcing the material over a prescribed shape (i.e., positive mold) under pressure until it has cooled. Negative air pressure or vacuum is the typical method used to apply pressure and form the plastic over the mold, hence the terms "vacuum-form" are also used to describe the process. Once the plastic has cooled and returned to its solid state, the perimeter of the formed components (negative mold) is determined. Using a cutting tool the excess material is removed from the negative mold following the previously identified perimeter; the remaining edges are commonly referred to as "trimlines." The edges of the plastic are then finished on specialized grinding machines that have a diverse set of abrasive sanding and buffing cone options that are used to achieve a high-polish smoothed edge.

Thermosetting Materials

Thermosets are plastics that are applied over a positive model in liquid form and then chemically "cured" to solidify and maintain a desired shape. To enhance their structural properties, thermosets are often impregnated into various fabrics by a process of lamination. Although this group of plastics has inherent structural stability, their rigidity precludes modification by heat molding; their shape can only be changed by grinding. Thermosetting plastics cannot be reheated without destroying their physical properties. Some of the most common thermoset resins used to produce rigid orthoses are acrylic, polyester, and epoxy. Because acrylic resins are strong, lightweight, and somewhat pliable, they offer a different set of characteristics than those of polyester resins. With lamination, acrylic resin can create a thin but strong structural wall for a prosthetic socket or component of an orthosis. However, if frequent adjustments are anticipated, thermoforming plastics would be indicated; as thermosets structural integrity is compromised with repeated heating.

Composites

Composites are the combination of two or more materials with distinctly different physical or chemical properties that together produce a material with enhanced performance characteristics relative to their material properties as a single substance. Numerous types of composites exist under this broad descriptive term, ranging from natural materials such as wood to manmade materials such as concrete. This chapter focuses on the combination of fibers and matrices associated with thermosetting plastics.

Fiber-reinforced plastics (FRPs), also referred to as *composites*, have revolutionized orthotics and prosthetics, primarily because they can be engineered to have mechanical properties with strength characteristics optimized for specific types of loading situations, thereby greatly improving the functionality of many types of orthoses and prostheses. The mechanical properties of reinforcement fibers, for the most part, dictate the mechanical properties of a composite through the orientation and position of the fibers. In general, FRPs offer high strength and stiffness qualities yet are also capable of incurring compressive or flexural stresses. Plastics can also be reinforced with other fillers, particulates, and short or chopped fibers, but FRPs are most widely used. This section focuses on fiber reinforcement for thermosets.

Polymer composites are made of a binder material (i.e., resin), referred to as the *matrix*, which is reinforced with fibers to improve strength and stiffness. The matrix of a composite encapsulates the fibers to maintain their desired orientation and position and ensure that load sharing of fibers is well distributed through the material. The volume fraction of resin to fiber is an important determinant of the mechanical properties of a composite and its performance. In general, the volume of fiber should be higher than the volume of resin matrix. A fiber volume fraction that approaches 90.7% with a matrix volume fraction of 9.3% is considered an ideal ratio.[37]

By comparison, the fibers in composite materials are stronger than the matrix material and can handle stresses applied to them better than the weaker matrix material. Typical fiber reinforcements used in polymer composites are fiberglass, carbon/graphite, and Kevlar aramid fibers (DuPont, Wilmington, Delaware). Grades of different fiberglass include E, C, and S glass, which stand for electrical (E), chemical (C), and strength (S), respectively. S glass has a higher tensile strength than E and C glass. Carbon fiber is widely used in orthoses and prostheses having strength properties greater than steel while also being lightweight and very stiff. Carbon fiber has superior stiffness properties in both compression and tension but, because it has relatively low impact strength, it is often combined with other reinforcement fibers like fiberglass or Kevlar to improve its performance. Aramid fibers (e.g., Kevlar) have tensile strength properties that are five times greater than steel for the same weight.

Laminar composites or laminates are fabricated out of "continuous fibers" that may extend the length of a given part and are one of the most common FRPs used in orthotics and prosthetics. Continuous fiber reinforcements can be woven into the form of a fabric in many different weave patterns. By combining different types of fiber fabrics (e.g., carbon graphite; Kevlar) and stacking these plies into layers, the resultant laminate can possess properties for particular modes of loading. When engineering laminates for orthoses and prostheses, the practitioner or technician must understand the manner in which loads will be transmitted through a device so that appropriate layering and orientation of plies will be incorporated into the composite to meet its functional performance duties. A laminate code system is used to describe the direction and ply layer with the longer dimension of the laminate serving as the *x*-axis and the width serving as the *y*-axis. A fiber orientation angle is used to describe the orientation of plies with respect to the *x*-axis, which is designated as 0 degree. A laminate code describes the sequencing of each layer from top to bottom. An example of a laminate code where the top ply is 0 degree followed by subsequent plies oriented, respectively, at 45, 90, 45 degrees, with the bottom ply at 0 degree would be written as follows: $[0/45/90]_2$. Brackets define the code's beginning and end, and the subscript indicates the adjacent plies are oriented the same, which is essentially one half of the ply description. The purpose of having a variety of different fiber orientation angles in a composite is to optimize the strength and dynamic functionality of the definitive intervention.

Preimpregnated composites

Preimpregnated composites have emerged as a valuable material in the field of orthoses and prostheses, offering numerous benefits and advancements in patient care and mobility. These composites, commonly referred to as prepregs, are composite materials that consist of reinforcing fibers impregnated with a precisely controlled amount of matrix resin. The controlled impregnation process ensures uniform distribution of the resin within the fibers, resulting in a highly homogeneous and consistent material with enhanced mechanical properties.

One significant advantage of preimpregnated composites in orthoses and prostheses is their exceptional strength-to-weight ratio. These materials exhibit superior stiffness and strength characteristics, allowing for the fabrication of lightweight yet robust devices.[38] The ability to customize the ratio of resin within certain elements of the componentry optimizes the mechanical properties, which may be difficult to achieve in a traditional lamination process. In the case of an AFO, the forefoot could have a dynamic characteristic as not to impede third or fourth rocker, but the uprights and calf portion could have increased rigidity to resist excessive sagittal plane movement across the talocrural joint. This variation in stiffness be completed within a single lamination, differing from the traditional fabrication techniques which results in a uniform resin-to-matrix ratio. This consideration is particularly advantageous in orthotic and prosthetic applications, where the reduction of weight and bulkiness is beneficial for patient comfort and overall mobility.

Processing Technologies and Composite Fabrication

Orthotic and prosthetic devices often are a compilation of custom-molded interface shell components combined with additional premanufactured parts (e.g., prosthetic foot, pylon). Practitioners and their technical staff have the capability to fabricate the human interface portions of a device within their laboratories, although the processes and equipment in their labs are limited to only a few techniques. Manufacturers, on the other hand, have the capacity to consider a much wider variety of processing techniques for mass producing composite parts and thus take advantage of processing technologies that can maximize the performance potential of the material.

The most common method for processing FRP composites in orthotic prosthetic laboratories is a contact molding technique called a "vacuum bag" lamination. The technique is relatively simple and does not require any specialized equipment aside from ventilation and vacuum system. A flexible membrane bag of plastic is tightly stretched over the positive mold part and sealed; then negative air pressure (i.e., vacuum) is applied between the bag and the mold, drawing the bag tightly to the surface of the mold. A hand layup of fiber cloth is placed on the mold in a predetermined manner with regard to the orientation and position of the fibers with an understanding of how loads will be transmitted through the structure when it is incorporated into a device. After the desired layup of fiber and cloth is achieved, a second flexible membrane bag is pulled over the mold, creating an enclosure that can accommodate the wet liquid resin (matrix) part of the composite. After the resin is poured into an opening of the second bag and sealed, vacuum inside the enclosure draws the outer bag toward the mold, pressing the resin through the fiber in a uniform manner to create a thin-walled structure of composite that has a high fiber-to-resin ratio. If the atmospheric pressure that presses on the outside bag is not adequate to achieve the desired fiber-to-resin ratio, then the vacuum bag mold construct can be placed into an autoclave to create higher pressures on the external bag. Because most orthotic prosthetic laboratories do not have autoclaves for such procedures, central fabrication laboratories equipped with such equipment are being used to a greater extent to maximize the benefits of pressure processing in composites. Upon curing or cross-linking of the resin within the overlayed model, the mold and "layup" are removed from the vacuum. The trimlines are determined for the intervention, and various cutting tools are used to remove the negative model (composite layup) from the positive model (mold of patient anatomy), completing the process by grinding and smoothing the edges. In Fig. 6.5, it can be observed that the outermost layer can include an esthetic element of textile, which is laminated into the definitive socket.

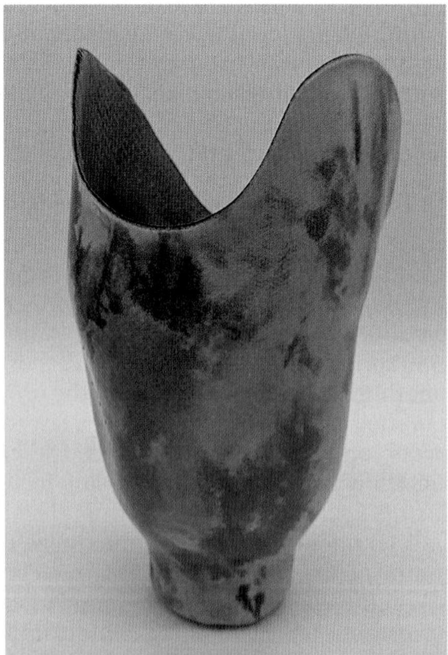

Fig. 6.5 A transtibial definitive socket with an esthetic multicolor outer laminated layer. (Courtesy Duffy Felmlee.)

Viscoelastic Polymers

A viscoelastic solid is a material that possesses the characteristics of stress relaxation and creep. Stress relaxation occurs when a material that is subjected to a constant deformation requires a decreasing load with time to maintain a steady state.[39] Creep refers to the increase in deformation with time to a steady state as a constant load is applied.[39] Sorbothane (Sorbothane, Inc., Kent, Ohio), widely used as an insole material, is made of a noncellular polyurethane derivative that possesses good shock-attenuating characteristics.[39] Viscolas (Viscolas Corp., Soddy Daisy, Tennessee), another type of viscoelastic solid, has been found to attenuate skeletal shock at heel strike in the tibia to half the normal load.[15,40] Two other viscoelastic polymers used to fabricate orthotic prosthetic components are Viscolite (Polymer Dynamics, Inc., Allentown, Pennsylvania) and PQ (Riecken's Orthotic Laboratories, Evansville, Indiana).

Prescription Guidelines

The formulation of a prescription for an orthosis or prosthesis greatly influences the potential functional outcome for the patient. It is critical that rehabilitation objectives and design criteria be carefully considered. Physicians, physical and occupational therapists, orthotists, and prosthetists who are involved in developing a prescription for an orthotic or prosthetic device must have a sound understanding of orthotics and prosthetics to be successful in effectively treating patients with these devices, although there is currently a degree of variability regarding best practice guidelines in the literature.[41] The American Academy of Orthotists and Prosthetists publication the *Journal of Prosthetics and Orthotics* has adopted the AGREE II assessment instrument for identifying the rigor of proposed clinical guidelines for the publication consideration. These types of developments demonstrate the value of standardization and accountability within the specialty of orthotic and prosthetic patient care.[42]

Assessment of functional deficit includes a thorough evaluation of the patient's present physical status, including muscle strength testing, range of motion measures, and documentation of other physical impairments that would affect the fit or performance of the device. Equally important to the physical examination is the consideration of any individual needs of the patient and an understanding of how the treatment will affect daily activities and the patient's ability to navigate the home environment. Included in these considerations must be an individual's ability to don and doff an orthosis or prosthesis and any related components.[43,44] To increase the success of treatment, the patient and other rehabilitation team members must reach a consensus on the type of device and the associated training and education required for optimal functional outcome.

More recently, Clinical Practice Guidelines have been established for specific areas of clinical focus within the subsets of patient population, componentry, outcome measures, etc., through expert consensus and literature review. Organizations such as the American Academy of Orthotists and Prosthetists,[45] Department of Veteran Affairs/Department of Defense,[46] and Hanger Clinic[47–49] have provided open-source guidelines to practioners for methodological strategies for optimizing various aspects of the rehabilitation process with respect to the orthotist/prosthetist. The multidisciplinary approach to patient- centered care includes various members of the rehabilitation team, with the independent assessment of each care expert supported by evidence-based practice on a case-by-case consensus to determine improved outcomes for the patient.[50–53]

ORTHOTIC PRESCRIPTION

The Committee on Prosthetics and Orthotics of the American Academy of Orthopaedic Surgeons developed a technical analysis form to standardize the process of patient evaluation. This evaluation protocol documents the biomechanical deficits of the patient and provides the basic information needed for orthotic prescription formulation. This systematic approach has two major objectives: to define the anatomic segments the orthosis will encompass and to accurately describe the biomechanical controls needed for treatment. The underlying principle of this assessment is that orthoses should be designed to control only those movements considered abnormal while permitting free motion in anatomic segments that are not impaired.

Technical analysis forms were developed for three general regions of the body: the upper limb, lower limb, and spine. The forms are four pages long with the same basic approach for formulating an orthotic prescription. The first page has sections for recording general patient information and noting major physical impairments (Fig. 6.6). The major impairment section characterizes any functional limitations, such as skeletal structure, sensation, or joint contracture. This information provides an overview of the patient's clinical presentation.

The second and third pages of the technical analysis form (Fig. 6.7) contain diagrams of the respective anatomic (limb or trunk) segments for which an orthotic prescription is being considered. Each skeletal region is represented in three planes of motion: coronal, sagittal, and transverse. On either side of the figures, square boxes at the level of the joints are used to note volitional force, hypertonicity, proprioception, and range of motion. The fourth page consists of a summary of the functional disability, treatment objectives, orthotic recommendation, and a key for the biomechanical controls of function.

Voluntary movements of muscles are assessed by conventional muscle testing techniques. Muscle strength can be recorded with either the standard descriptive or numeric muscle grading systems, depending on regional preferences.

Two types of joint (limb) motion are recorded on the forms: rotary and translatory. According to McCollough,[54] all points of the distal segment move in the same direction, following the same path shape and distance during translatory motion. During rotary motion, one point of the distal segment (or its imaginary extension) remains fixed while other points move in an arc around it. Translatory motion is recorded with linear arrows in the direction of the distal segment's movement relative to its proximal counterpart. The linear arrows are placed below the circle (representing the joint axis) for translatory motion. If translatory force acts in the vertical axis, the linear arrow is placed to the side of the circle. Rotary motion and the related degree of range of motion are documented by an arrow within a protractor-type arrangement for each joint. The established normal range of motion for each joint is shaded on the form for comparative reference. If a fixed contracture or fusion of the joint is present, a double linear arrow is used.

Hypertonicity of muscle groups in each of the body segments is described by a functionality based letter scale.[54] A designation of mild tonicity is given when any hypertonus that is present is thought to be functionally insignificant. Moderate tonicity indicates that tone might have some functional value, such as assisting the patient in holding an item during minor tasks. A designation of severe tonicity indicates that normal function is not possible. The patient's proprioceptive ability is described in a similar way, as absent, impaired, or normal for each of the body segments of interest.

The final page of the technical analysis form (Fig. 6.8) contains space for an overview of functional impairments, a checklist of the orthotic treatment objectives, and a chart that details the orthotic recommendation. The desired orthotic control for each body segment is indicated by a specific letter; as many as seven types of orthotic controls can be incorporated into the design of an orthosis. The terms and descriptions of these controls are indicated in the key. If the orthotic recommendation section is completed correctly, the chart will indicate the body segments the device will encompass and the desired biomechanical control of function needed. Any comments on the specific design requirements or materials, or both, can be detailed in the remarks section of the form. Although an in-depth biomechanical assessment may not always be necessary, a system based on these principles is a logical and objective method for formulating an orthotic prescription.

For the orthotic care provider, the prescription is the initiation of the clinical assessment and required component for the provision of an intervention to the individual patient.

PROSTHETIC PRESCRIPTION

The formulation of a prosthetic prescription requires a different evaluative process. Prosthetic prescription depends on an in-depth understanding of components and materials as well as their indications and contraindications for use. Ideally, prosthetic prescription begins before amputation surgery, so the residual limb is of appropriate length and healing is adequate for optimal prosthetic use. Factors such as vascular supply, anticipated activity level, intelligence, vocation, social support, and age are also important to consider.[55] Range of motion, flexible and fixed contracture, functional strength, skin condition, girth measurements, pain, and sensation of the residual limb and the intact limb are evaluated.

An important part of prosthetic prescription is component selection.[56] The diversity of prosthetic foot-ankle units and knee mechanisms for lower extremity prosthetics, and the variety of terminal devices for the upper extremity, can present difficult decisions for those who are unfamiliar with their intended application. Various socket designs, suspension methods, and activity-specific componentry considerations require synthesis of both qualitative and quantitative evidence for which the prosthetist is trained. Therefore, prosthetists are often relied on for recommendations on components because they are usually most familiar with the specifications

Technical Analysis Form **Lower Limb** **Revised March 1973**

Name ______ No. ______ Age ______ Sex ______

Date of onset ______ Cause ______

Occupation ______ Present lower-limb equipment ______

Diagnosis ______

Ambulatory ☐ Nonambulatory ☐

Major impairments:

A. Skeletal
1. Bone and joints: Normal ☐ Abnormal ______
2. Ligaments: Normal ☐ Abnormal ☐ Knee: AC ☐ PC ☐ MC ☐ LC ☐
   Ankle: MC ☐ LC ☐
3. Extremity shortening: None ☐ Left ☐ Right ☐
   Amount of discrepancy: ASIS-Heel ______ ASIS-MTP ______ MTP-Heel ______

B. Sensation: Normal ☐ Abnormal ☐
1. Anesthesia ☐ Hypesthesia ☐ Location: ______
   Protective sensation: Retained ☐ Lost ☐
2. Pain ☐ Location: ______

C. Skin: Normal ☐ Abnormal: ______

D. Vascular: Normal ☐ Abnormal ☐ Right ☐ Left ☐

E. Balance: Normal ☐ Impaired ☐ Support: ______

F. Gait deviations: ______

G. Other impairments: ______

Legend

= Direction of translatory motion

= Abnormal degree of rotary motion (60°)

= Fixed position (30°, 1 cm.)

= Fracture

Volitional force (V)
N = Normal
G = Good
F = Fair
P = Poor
T = Trace
Z = Zero

Hypertonic muscle (H)
N = Normal
M = Mild
Mo = Moderate
S = Severe

Proprioception (P)
N = Normal
I = Impaired
A = Absent

D = Local distension or enlargement

= Pseudarthrosis

= Absence of segment

Fig. 6.6 The technical analysis form provides a systematic method of data collection for the development of prescriptions for lower extremity orthoses. The first page of the form is used to record the patient's history and current impairments. *AC,* Anterior cruciate ligament; *ASIS,* anterior superior iliac spine; *LC,* lateral collateral ligament; *MC,* medial collateral ligament; *MTP,* medial tibial plateau; *PC,* posterior cruciate ligament. (From Committee on Prosthetics Research and Development. *Report of the Seventh Workshop Panel on Lower Extremity Orthoses of the Subcommittee on Design and Development.* National Research Council–National Academy of Sciences; 1970; McCollough NC III. Biomechanical analysis systems for orthotic prescription. In: American Academy of Orthopaedic Surgeons, ed. *Atlas of Orthotics: Biomechanical Principles and Application.* Second ed. Mosby; 1985:35–75.)

and limitations. Many prosthetic teams have developed data collection forms to standardize the prosthetic prescription process. Redhead[57] suggests that the prescription for a prosthesis consider each of the major "prescription options." Examples of the specifications delineated by Redhead for a transfemoral prosthesis are type of limb, socket material and design, suspension, knee joints, knee controls, ankle joints, feet, and cosmesis. Additionally, Clinical Practice Guidelines

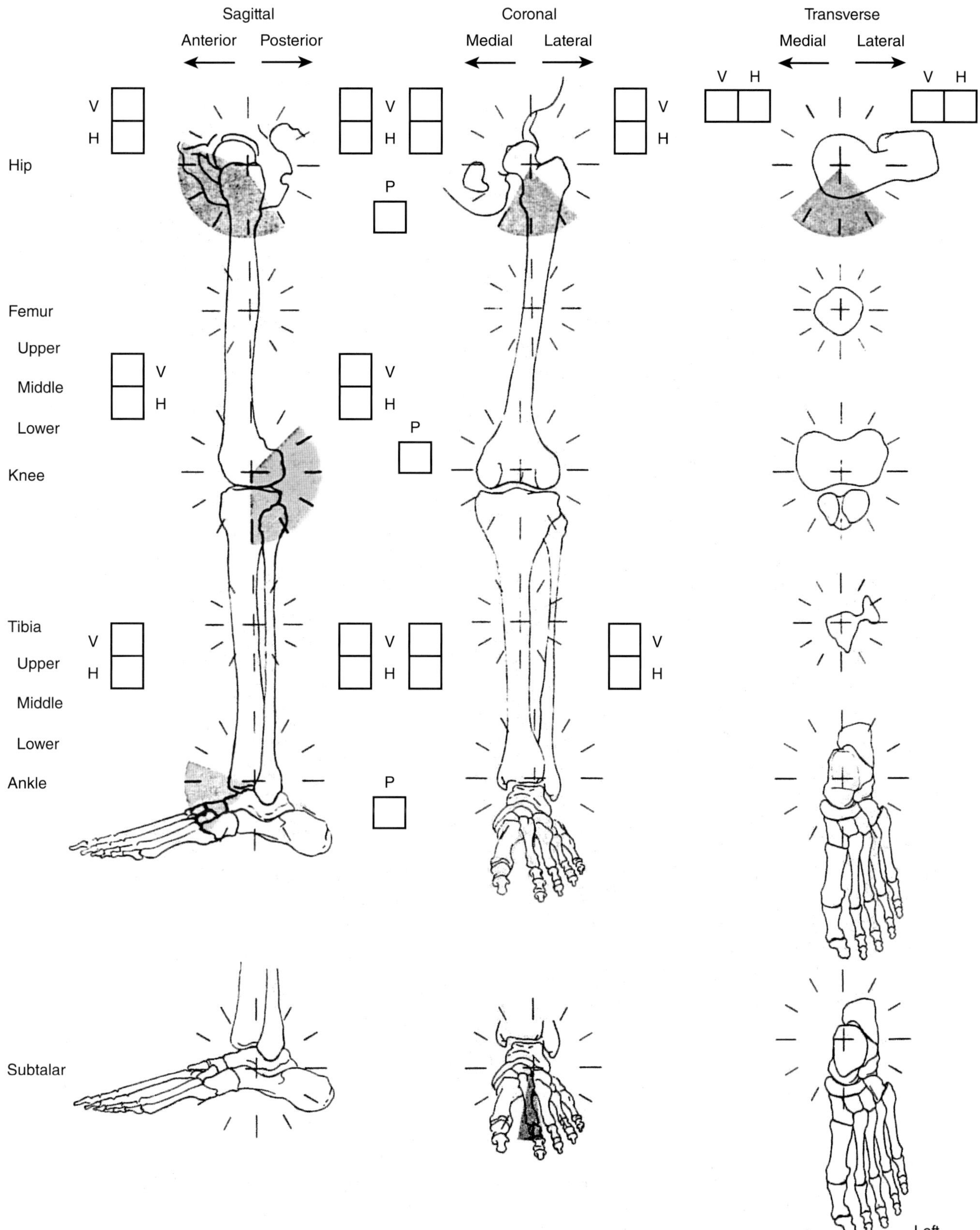

Fig. 6.7 Subsequent pages of the technical analysis form are used to detail characteristics of each limb or body segment for which the orthosis or prosthesis will be made. Information recorded on these pages includes existing deformity, proprioceptive capacity (P), restriction or hypermobility of joint rotary, and translatory range of motion in all three planes of movement, volitional strength (V), and the level of hypertonicity (H). (From Committee on Prosthetics Research and Development. *Report of the Seventh Workshop Panel on Lower Extremity Orthoses of the Subcommittee on Design and Development.* National Research Council–National Academy of Sciences; 1970; McCollough NC III. Biomechanical analysis systems for orthotic prescription. In: American Academy of Orthopaedic Surgeons, ed. *Atlas of Orthotics: Biomechanical Principles and Application.* Second ed. Mosby; 1985:35–75.)

Summary of functional disability ______________________

Treatment objectives:

Prevent/correct deformity ☐ Improve ambulation ☐
Reduce axial load ☐ Fracture treatment ☐
Protect joint ☐ Other ______________________

Orthotic Recommendation

Lower limb		Flex	Ext	Abd	Add	Rotation Int	Rotation Ext	Axial load
HKAO	Hip							
KAO	Thigh							
	Knee							
AFO	Leg							
	Ankle	(Dorsi)	(Plantar)					
FO Foot	Subtalar					(Inver)	(Ever)	
	Midtarsal							
	Met-phal							

Remarks:

Signature ______________________ Date ______________________

Key: Use the following symbols to indicate desired control of designated function:

F = Free Free motion
A = Assist Application of an external force for the purpose of increasing the range, velocity, or force of a motion
R = Resist Application of an external force for the purpose of decreasing the velocity or force of a motion
S = Stop Inclusion of a static unit to deter an undesired motion in one direction
v = Variable A unit that can be adjusted without making a structural change
H = Hold Elimination of all motion in prescribed plane (verify position)
L = Lock Device includes an optional lock

Fig. 6.8 The final page of the technical analysis form details the goals for the orthosis and the specific prescription for the desired device. Once the prescription is developed, the form serves as a guideline for fabricating and fitting the orthosis. *AFOs*, Ankle-foot orthoses; *FO*, foot orthosis; *HKAO*, hip-knee-ankle orthosis; *KAO*, knee-ankle orthosis; *V*, volitional force. (From Committee on Prosthetics Research and Development. *Report of the Seventh Workshop Panel on Lower Extremity Orthoses of the Subcommittee on Design and Development*. National Research Council–National Academy of Sciences; 1970; McCollough NC III. Biomechanical analysis systems for orthotic prescription. In: American Academy of Orthopaedic Surgeons, ed. *Atlas of Orthotics: Biomechanical Principles and Application*. Second ed. Mosby; 1985:35–75.)

for both lower and upper limb amputation specifications have been developed though literature review, expert consensus, and patient reported outcomes.[45–49]

The prescription serves as the starting point for prosthetic care providers when conducting a clinical assessment and delivering interventions to patients. It is an essential document that outlines the specific requirements and recommendations for prosthetic intervention, to be optimized with the input of each member of the rehabilitation team and the patient.[50–53]

Fabrication Process

Once a prescription for a custom orthosis or prosthesis has been created, the fabrication process begins. The traditional fabrication process is composed of six steps:

Step 1: Taking accurate measurements of the limb
Step 2: Making a negative impression (cast)
Step 3: Creating a three-dimensional (3D) positive model of the limb or body segment
Step 4: Modifying the positive model to incorporate the desired controls
Step 5: Fabricating the orthosis or prosthetic socket around the positive model
Step 6: Fitting of the device to the patient

In some instances, further modification or adjustment is necessary to achieve optimal fit and function of the device.

MEASUREMENT

Measurements are most often referenced from readily palpable bony landmarks. Important anthropometric measurements include the residual limb length, successive circumferences, and mediolateral and anteroposterior dimensions of the body segment for which the orthotic or prosthetic device is being created. Using this method, bony landmarks are identified as reference points and measurements are obtained at fixed distances from this reference. For instance, Boonhong performed this in subjects with transtibial amputation by identifying the tibial tubercle and obtaining circumferential measurements in 4-cm increments down to the distal end of the residual limb;[58] others have elected to measure in 4-cm increments beginning at the distal end of the residual limb.[59] Measurements are recorded on forms that are specific to the body segment being treated, such as the technical analysis form previously described. These measurements are used in two ways: as a reference when modifications to the positive cast are needed and as a way to determine the placement of the perimeter or "trimlines" of the device.

Although clinically practical and easily performed with simple tools such as a tape measure, caution needs to be exercised when using anthropometric measurement methods, because they have been shown to have poor intrarater and interrater reliability.[60] Water immersion has also been described to determine residual limb volume. To perform this in patients with a transtibial amputation, de Boer-Wilzing et al. used a 15-cm glass cylinder filled with water that was placed on a hand-operated elevator. The distal part of the residual limb was inserted into the water-filled cylinder and the elevator raised until specified reference points touched the water's surface, thus displacing an amount of water equal to the volume of the residual limb.[59] However, although results are less variable, this method cannot be used when open wounds are present or if a patient has bilateral leg amputations.[61] In addition, a recent systematic review indicated that there are inadequate data for drawing conclusions in patients with other types of limb amputations.[62]

New technologies, such as laser scanning methods (including CAD/CAM scanning), have helped to decrease fitting errors, manufacture time, and overall cost of prosthetic sockets.[63] One group of authors reported a mean percentage error of 1.4% using a 3D scanner and very low intrarater and interrater reliability coefficients (05.% and 0.7%, respectively).[63]

NEGATIVE MOLD

A negative impression is a mold taken of an actual body part that is used to create the 3D-positive cast or model necessary for fabrication of the orthosis or prosthesis. This negative impression is most often taken with a plaster-of-Paris bandage or fiber resin tape, although in some instances direct impressions are used as an alternative. Creation of a negative impression has four steps. First, a layer of tubular stockinet or a stocking is placed over the skin to create a protective interface and control the position of soft tissue structures within the cast (Fig. 6.9). Tubular stockinettes are available in sizes that range from small diameter for the pediatric limb to large diameter for the adult torso. When a direct impression technique is being performed, a topical separator such as petroleum jelly can be used as an interface to minimize the risk of capturing cuticle hair in the impression. Second, bony prominences or other important guiding landmarks are marked on the body segment with indelible ink. These marks transfer to the inside of the negative mold and from there to the surface of the positive model.

Once the limb or body segment has been prepared, a thin layer of plaster of Paris or fiber resin tape is applied (see Fig. 6.9B). This procedure differs from that of fracture casts in one important way: the goal is to achieve an "intimate" fit that captures the actual contours of the limb or body segment so that no protective padding is required. Failure to achieve a successful interface between the wearer and the device may result in discomfort, excessive tissue stress, skin irritation and destruction, and potential amputation revision.[64] Rolls of elasticized plaster can be wrapped circumferentially in no more than two or three layers. Alternatively, strips of the material can be laid along the length of the limb or body segment. Most impression casting materials are readily available in roll form, although special versions have been produced for specific types of impression procedures, such as the fiber resin sock for an AFO. As the molding material is applied, the clinician smooths the surface, following the normal shape of the limb.

While the mold hardens, the clinician supports the limb or segment in the desired position, sometimes applying a light corrective force. As an example, the desired limb position of an orthosis incorporating the ankle joint might be in subtalar and talocrural neutral. If a PTB socket design is desired for a transtibial prosthesis, an extra force applied just distal to the patella marks its desired location on the resulting positive mold.

Once the cast is hardened sufficiently, it is carefully removed from the limb segment, preserving its shape and contours, and checked for alignment (see Fig. 6.9C and D). It is essential that the clinician who takes the negative impression has a thorough understanding of the forces that will be applied to the anatomic segments involved to ensure optimal fit and function of the orthosis or prosthesis. Estimates of soft tissue compression and skeletal alignment changes need to be carefully considered during the negative

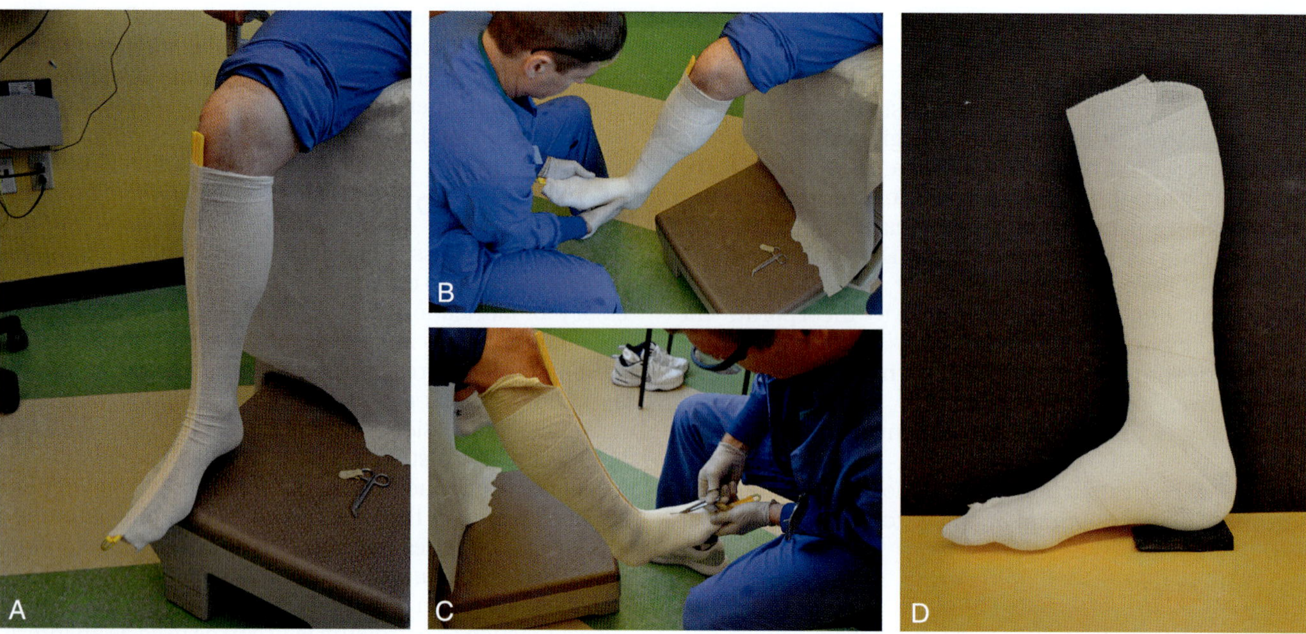

Fig. 6.9 Casting for ankle-foot orthosis using fiberglass. (A) Tubular stockinette places over the foot and calf with placement of cutoff strip. (B) Application of 3″ fiberglass circumferentially around the involved limb. (C) Removal of the fiberglass cast (negative model) from patient with bandage scissors. (D) Negative model set in neutral alignment. Photo Mr. Kei Takamura, MSOP. (Courtesy Shriners Hospital for Children Portland, Oregon.)

impression procedure. A skilled and experienced professional uses clinical judgment to create a negative impression, not only to capture the shape of the anatomic segment but also to apply an efficient force system to improve or maximize function. Basic design decisions must be made before the impression procedures so that any special accommodations required for the desired functional outcome can be incorporated.

Special negative impression techniques have been developed for specific purposes. Polystyrene foam impression blocks are one of the common methods of acquiring an impression of the plantar surface of the foot.[65] For patients who are recovering from facial burns, fabrication of a facial orthotic designed to deliver even, steady pressure during the period of scar maturation requires a highly detailed mold of the face. Alginate impressions, also referred to as *moulage techniques*, similar to those used in dentistry, are often used.

FABRICATING AND MODIFYING THE POSITIVE MODEL

Conventional methods for creating a positive cast are well established. The negative impression is prepared by sealing the mold so that it can accept liquid plaster of Paris. A separator material (e.g., silicone, soap) is added to the inner walls of the mold before the plaster of Paris is poured so that it can be removed more easily once the positive model has set. Once the cast has solidified, the negative impression is stripped away and discarded. The anatomic landmarks and reference points marked on the limb or body segment with indelible pencil and transferred from the patient to the negative impression are again transferred to the positive model. A mandrel (post) is embedded into the setting plaster of the positive model. This mandrel is used to hold the model for cast rectification and the rest of the production processes.

Model rectifications remove artifacts produced during the molding or impression process and bring the cast to specification of the measured values taken from the patient. Once the positive model has been rectified, further modifications can be made on the basis of the design of the orthosis or prosthesis being fabricated. During the negative impression procedure, soft tissue may have been manipulated for specific applications of force or pressure to be incorporated into the final orthosis or prosthesis. Although the positive model represents a 3D shape of a respective body segment, it cannot relay information about the density of the tissue that it will interface. In general, additional plaster is added where relief of pressure is desired (e.g., over bony prominences) (Fig. 6.10) or is removed where additional forces are to be applied. When the orthosis or prosthesis is formed over the model, an area of relief for a more intimate fit is achieved. Although some guidelines have been established regarding the amount of material to be removed or added to the positive model, the clinical experience of the prosthetist or orthotist is essential in this stage of the process. The positive model can also be modified to reconfigure surface geometry to improve the strength of the finished product.

Once design changes have been incorporated into the model, its surface is prepared for component production. This involves removing any surface imperfections with abrasive tools and abrasive sanding screen to ensure the surface in contact with skin will be smooth. The positive cast is then ready to be used as a form from which different materials can be shaped to produce an interface component.

FABRICATING THE ORTHOSIS OR PROSTHETIC SOCKET—THERMOFORMING

The fabrication process used with the positive model depends on the material selected for the device. Thermoforming is a common production method used in orthotics and

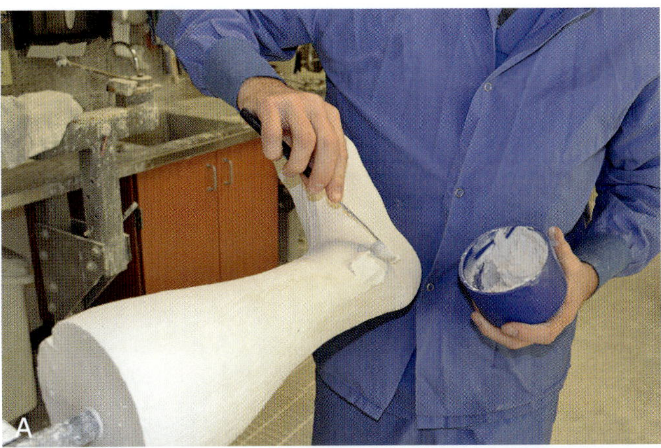

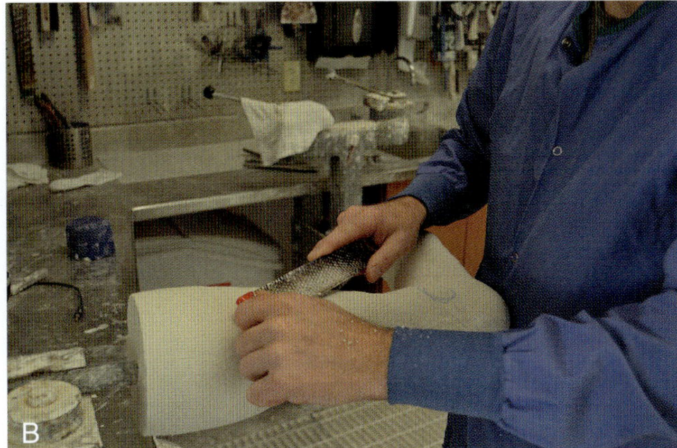

Fig. 6.10 Modification of a positive model for a solid ankle-foot orthosis. (A) Plaster additions to the positive model over area (lateral malleolus) requiring pressure relief. (B) Final plaster removal prior to definitive smoothing of positive model. Photo Mr. Kei Takamura, MSOP. (Courtesy Shriners Hospital for Children Portland, Oregon.)

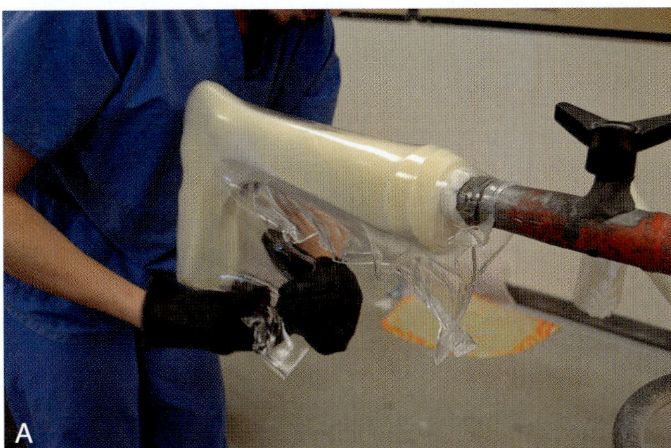

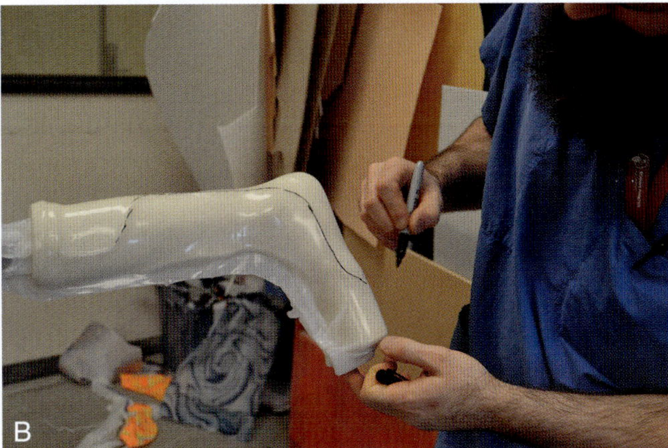

Fig. 6.11 Drape thermoforming of a PLS AFO (posterior leaf spring ankle-foot orthosis). (A) Creation of the anterior seam of the PLS AFO from a sheet of 3/16" polypropylene. (B) Transfer of the trimlines from the positive mold through the translucent polypropylene plastic. Photo Mr. Kei Takamura, MSOP. (Courtesy Shriners Hospital for Children Portland, Oregon.)

prosthetics. Thermoplastic sheet material is heated in an oven until it has reached its "plastic" state, then shaped over a positive model by changing the air pressure difference across its surface (vacuum forming). The method of thermoforming pictured in Fig. 6.11 is that of drape forming. The drape-forming approach is common in orthotics as it yields a more uniform wall thickness, though a seam is created. This seam is usually outside of the trimlines and will not be present in the definitive orthosis. Thermoforming prosthetic componentry is most common in the area of diagnostic fitting or "check sockets." This step within the fabrication process allows for the patient to provide feedback to the clinician regarding the fit and function of the prosthesis prior to definitive fabrication of the socket. Blister or bubble forming frequently used in check socket fabrication requires a vacuum-forming station of different orientation than that of drape forming, but operates on the same atmospheric pressure principles. An implication for the use of blister forming is that there is no seam in the finished component allowing for a uniform interior surface. Prosthetic sockets which are blister formed with the use of copolymer did demonstrate a decrease in ISO strength testing as compared to drape forming.[66] Fig. 6.12 is a demonstration of the final stages of a blister forming methodology for a transfemoral socket. With both thermoforming methods once the plastic has cooled and returned to its solid state, trimlines are delineated on the formed plastic before the edges are finished and smoothed. An overview of the fabrication process for thermosetting materials can be found earlier in this chapter (page 8) within the section titled "Processing Technologies and Composite Fabrication."

Computer-Aided Design/ Computer-Aided Manufacture

In the 1960s an alternative method of prosthetic fabrication that used computers was first introduced. Early CAD/CAM methods used stereophotography and digitization to create a numeric model, which guided a milling machine in the creation of a positive model of the residual limb.[2] A more complete concept of fabrication and manufacture of a prosthesis was developed at the University College London

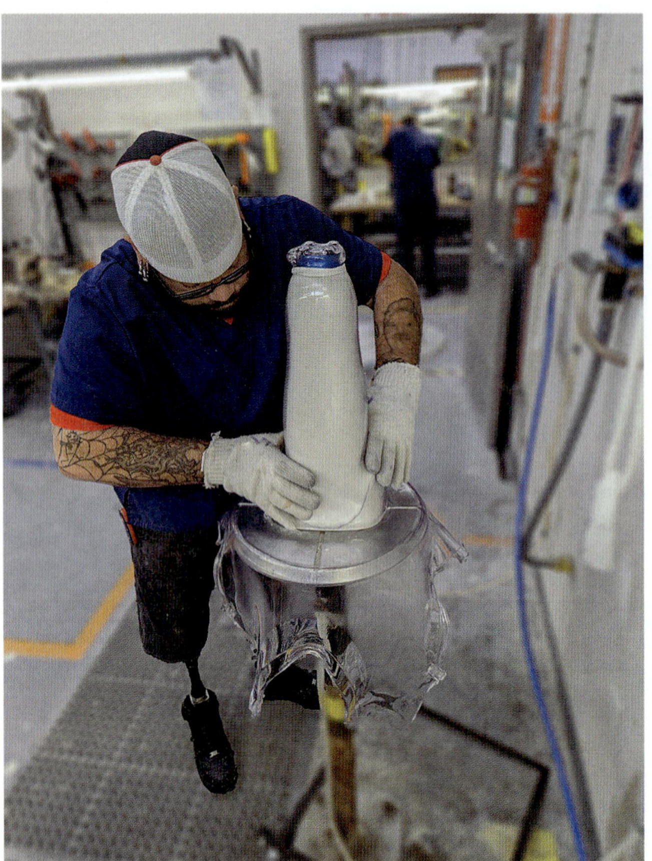

Fig. 6.12 Blister forming of a transfemoral diagnostic socket. (Courtesy of Hanger Fabrication Network.)

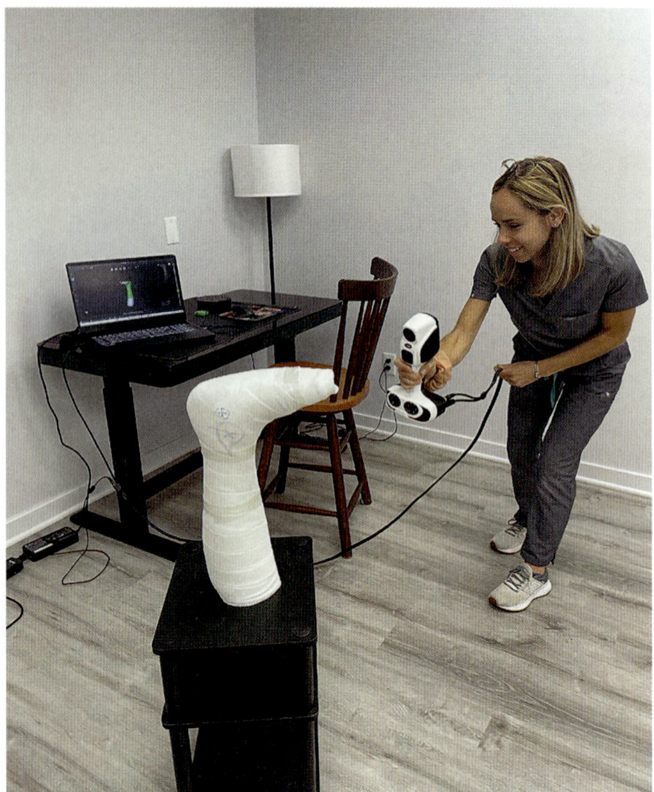

Fig. 6.13 Clinician scanning a negative mold of an ankle-foot orthosis into CAD (Computer-Aided Design) software using a handheld scanner. (Courtesy Macy O&P LLC, East Lyme, Connecticut.)

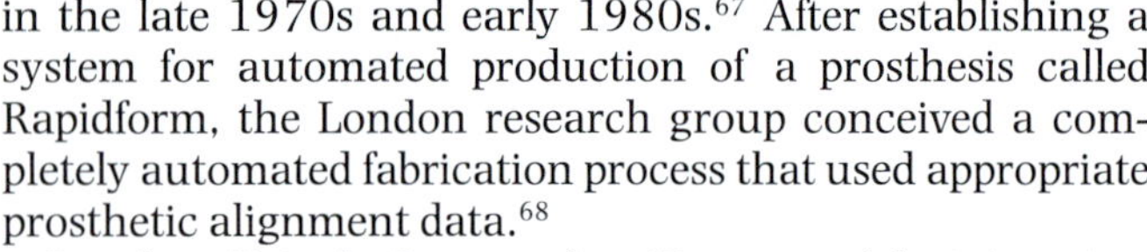

in the late 1970s and early 1980s.[67] After establishing a system for automated production of a prosthesis called Rapidform, the London research group conceived a completely automated fabrication process that used appropriate prosthetic alignment data.[68]

In the United States, the Veterans Administration began funding research projects in the 1980s to investigate the potential of CAD/CAM in orthotics and prosthetics. Advances were also made in private industry as the availability of personal computers became widespread. Beginning in the late 1980s, manufacturers designed a multitude of CAD/CAM systems for various applications in orthotics and prosthetics. Advances in computer hardware, processors, and software have made CAD/CAM systems fast and efficient, and are economical alternatives for fabrication of devices for many orthotic and prosthetic practices.

Currently, most CAD systems use a scanning device to record digital information of a body segment for CAM. The primary components of a CAD/CAM system consist of a digitizing device, computer, and milling machine. Surface contours of the anatomic segment are recorded with various digitization devices: optical-laser scanners, surface-contacting stylus, and pneumatically operated mechanical posts. Digital information acquired from a scan of a body segment is processed by the computer and translated into a tricoordinate data point file. This file is used by the computer to create a graphic image in the form of a surface contour plot.[69] The data are then relayed to a milling unit to carve an orthosis or prosthesis for a positive model.

DATA ACQUISITION

Each of the many digitizers used for data acquisition is designed for a specific task or to handle certain anatomic regions. Noncontact laser digitizers capable of circumferential scanning are well suited for measurement of cylindrical shapes such as those found in limb prosthetics or spinal orthotics. An optical-laser camera mechanism images the surface topography of the body segment and records the measured data points in a computer. Special holding fixtures and bars to aid in patient comfort and safety are part of each system. An apparatus designed to scan the torso for a spinal orthosis usually requires a different setup than that of a limb prosthesis. Some scanners are capable of digitizing directly from the patient's body segment, whereas other systems take measurements from a negative impression or mold of the segment (Fig. 6.13).

Compact, handheld contact digitizers have been introduced by several CAD/CAM manufacturers. These units allow the clinician to digitize a body segment by direct contact with the skin. Handheld contact digitizers are described as a wand, pen, stylus, or pointer. Contact digitizers often have special attachments to scan certain shapes or measurement tools, such as calipers, for acquiring anteroposterior or mediolateral dimensions. Their versatility permits data acquisition of complex shapes. In some systems, handheld digitizers can be used in conjunction with a laser scan.

The use of digitizers in the production of foot orthoses is also becoming more common. Several systems based on differences in technique and philosophy in foot orthosis design have been developed for data acquisition of the foot. For full weight–bearing or partial weight–bearing techniques, pneumatically operated mechanical posts are used to digitize the foot's plantar surface (Amfit Corp., Vancouver, Washington). Orthotic contoured shapes such as metatarsal domes can be evaluated during the digitization procedure to determine optimal position and comfort before fabrication. An optical-laser scanner situated under an acrylic platform has also been used for scanning the foot when a weight-bearing technique is desired (Bergmann Orthotics Lab, Northfield, Illinois). Because this system is also capable of scanning the foot with non–weight-bearing methods without the platform, it is quite versatile in clinical practice.

In many instances, orthotists and prosthetists are restricted to surface geometry and palpation of underlying anatomic structures to interpret the position of skeletal and soft tissue structures of the body segment. Magnetic resonance imaging and computed tomography have been used to create a 3D computer model and assist in making design decisions for a mechanical device. Data from these scans are converted to a working format for specific graphic and modeling programs. Although this capability may not be practical for all applications, it may offer insight into areas of further research and development in the field.

3D Scanners and Shape Manipulation Software

Inherently, the portion of the orthosis and prosthesis that interfaces with the body is often custom-molded to achieve an exacting fit. Traditionally, a facsimile of a limb segment or body part is created by taking a mold or capturing the shape by tracing the contour combined with a series of relevant measurements to duplicate the geometry. Developments in laser-based scanners, structured light technology, and photogrammetry have offered more options for digital imaging of surfaces for prosthetics and orthotics.[70–72] Handheld portable scanners with both technologies allow more diverse applications to which 3D scanning can offer clinical advantages for custom-molded devices. 3D scanners are becoming more accessible for the clinical practice setting since the cost of scanners has significantly decreased for a number of applications. Some versions of structured light scanners can be attached to tablets or mobile phones (Fig. 6.14). Both scanner technologies are portable, have fast scan times, and take highly accurate measurements. Although these new scanner technologies can help to streamline capturing the shape of body part, computer software to modify the topography of the interface is crucial to perfecting fit and function.

Numerous industry-specific CAD/CAM software programs are available for the design and manufacture of prostheses and orthoses. Because orthotic and prosthetic applications are diverse, ranging from cranial helmets to spine and extremity orthoses and limb prosthetics, the software programs for each region of the body are often different. As such, a clinical practice has to have several distinct software programs to accommodate the full range of clinical services it may offer. Hence, the costs associated with having multiple systems has contributed to a slow adoption of CAD/CAM in clinical practices and is why traditional processes and methods are still in wide use.

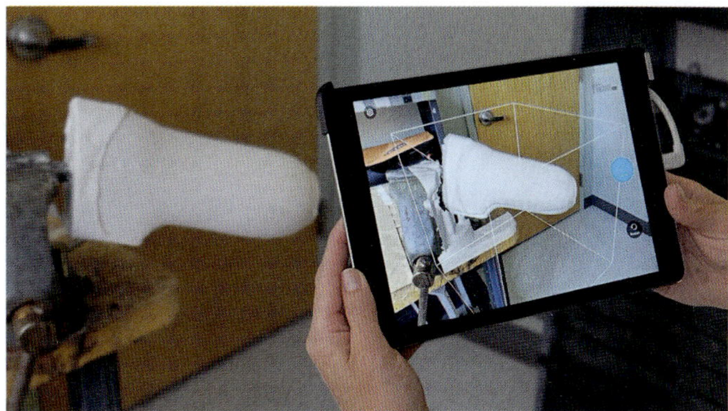

Fig. 6.14 Clinician scanning a negative model of a transtibial model into CAD (Computer-Aided Design) software using a tablet-mounted scanner. (Courtesy Orthotics and Prosthetic Labs, Springfield, Massachusetts.)

Multiple software programs, scanners, and printers may be needed for a prosthetic and orthotic service to have a fully integrated CAD/CAM operation in prosthetics and orthotics. Each region of the body presents with a unique set of conditions in which a practitioner may need to capture the shape of an anatomic surface. For individuals with limb loss, a handheld scanner can be ideally suited to capture the shape of the residuum. For orthotic management of the foot, clinicians may prefer scanning the foot in partial weight bearing (e.g., seated) because the plantar soft tissues compress during loading and the shape of the foot changes dramatically compared with its shape in non–weight bearing. Practitioners may scan a negative impression (i.e., mold) or a positive model of a body part rather than the actual patient to acquire a digital image file. Thus, traditional prosthetic and orthotic techniques are blended with CAD/CAM technologies as practitioners try to maximize the advantages of both approaches.

MILLING AND PRODUCTION

Once the digital model is in place, the milling apparatus creates the actual orthotic or prosthetic device. Because each type of orthosis or prosthesis usually has specific milling parameters, a different setup may be required for each. For instance, the long, rounded shape of a transtibial or transfemoral socket is often manufactured with a lathe-type milling machine (Fig. 6.15). In contrast, foot orthoses are manufactured by an end mill setup because their plate-like structure and production processes create different finishing needs. The volume or scale of the production laboratory may find benefit in having separate milling stations for certain type of orthosis or prosthesis. This manufacturing limitation has led to the establishment of laboratory production companies that mill the positive models and manufacture the orthoses or prostheses from computer data. Computer production networks can often reduce fabrication time and decrease production times, making the use of CAD/CAM economically feasible even for small orthotic/prosthetic facilities. Special production equipment is available that partially automates the thermoforming processes of some components. In the thermoforming machine for prosthetic sockets, a preformed polypropylene shell travels upward on a mechanical platform to an oven that heats the plastic to its

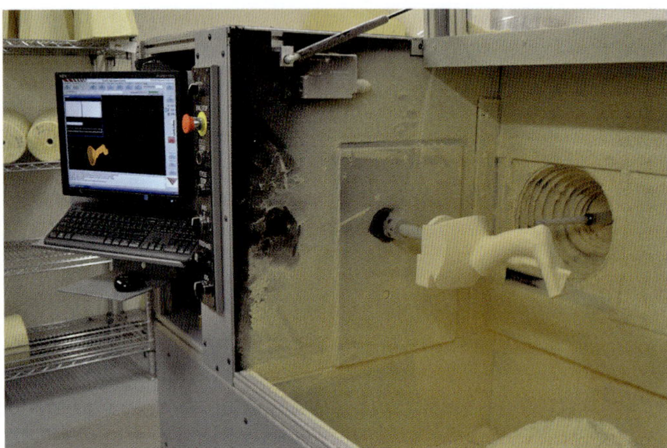

Fig. 6.15 CAM milling machine carving the positive model for an ankle-foot orthosis from CAD (Computer-Aided Design) software. Photo Mr. Kei Takamura, MSOP. (Courtesy Shriners Hospital for Children Portland.)

formable temperature. The heated shell is then lowered over the positive model of the residual limb and vacuum formed for an intimate fit.

CAD/CAM in orthotics and prosthetics will play an important role in clinical and research settings. Although the development of CAD/CAM in orthotics and prosthetics has a history that spans more than two decades, only since the 1990s has it become an integral part of some clinical practices. Systems that have been designed for virtually all prosthetic and orthotic applications can be integrated with computed tomography, magnetic resonance imaging, and other medical imaging technologies. The technological advancements of CAD/CAM offer orthotists and prosthetists an additional clinical fabrication and research tool. Although this sophisticated equipment can contribute greatly to certain clinical and manufacturing tasks, successful fitting of a device depends on proper data input and prescription formulation.

Central Fabrication and Mass Production

The techniques and processes associated with the fabrication of orthoses and prostheses described in this chapter can be relatively labor intensive and expensive. As managed care and insurance companies strive to reduce medical costs, the profession is under greater pressure to remain competitive by finding alternative production methods that are cost effective. One option is to maximize the clinical productivity of orthotists and prosthetists and limit their technical responsibilities. Central fabrication operations allow practitioners to develop clinical practices that do not require large technical facilities and space. Depending on the size of the practice, outsourcing the production portion of the business can be a more economical way to run an orthotic/prosthetic clinic. Some practitioners do not want to manage in-house technical operations that include additional technical staff, specialized equipment, and increased space requirements. Another advantage is that central fabrication may offer improvements in consistency and quality of devices.

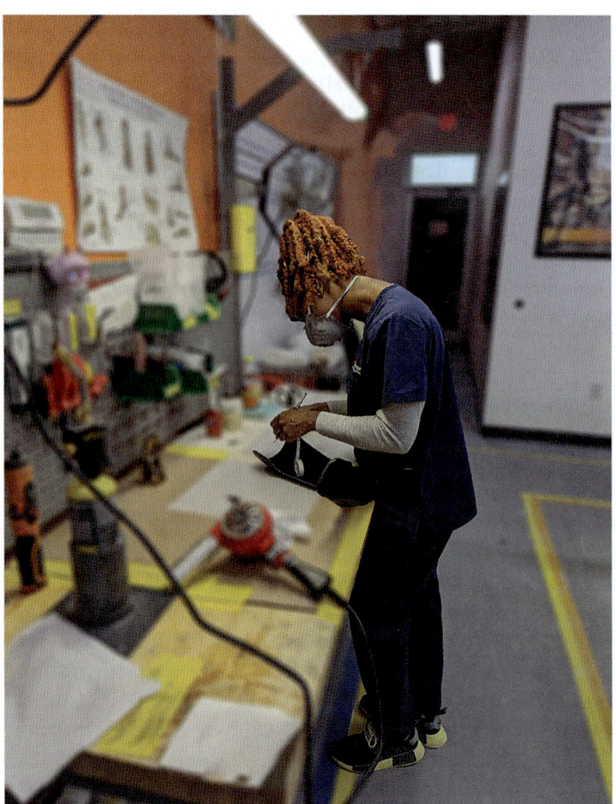

Fig. 6.16 Technician finishing a polypropylene solid ankle-foot orthosis. (Courtesy of Hanger Fabrication Network.)

CENTRAL FABRICATION FACILITIES FOR CUSTOM DEVICES

Central fabrication facilities typically specialize in the manufacture of custom orthoses and prostheses, often serving a large number of orthotic and prosthetic practices. These manufacturing services are available to produce almost every kind of orthosis and prosthesis, with many companies specializing in a specific area (e.g., spinal orthoses, knee orthoses, transtibial prosthetics). Central fabrication facilities have the capability to optimize the skillsets of technicians to improve the good manufacturing processes which may be more challenging to implement at the individual clinic level (Fig. 6.16). The 2022 ABCOP National Practice Analysis shows a trend toward increased utilization of central fabrication facilities. The two most recent analyses (2015 and 2022) differentiated between the percentages of orthoses and prostheses fabrication completed at a central fabrication center: Orthotics—43% (2015) to 61% (2022) Prosthetics—31% (2015) to 39% (2022).[73] Some central fabrication operations offer the advantage of producing a device without the need for a negative impression, an additional cost savings in time and materials. A series of conventional measurements of patients combined with height and weight data is entered into a computer to generate a milled positive model for production. Orthotic systems in particular have been refined to produce excellent fitting devices that are comparable in function to custom-molded orthoses produced from a patient model. Although there will always be a need for custom-molded devices, technologic advancements in human factors, ergonomics, and computer modeling will improve generic sizing and contoured interface systems, permitting a larger portion of the population to be fit with prefabricated devices and components. Modular components of varying material properties are already a part of general practice in prosthetics.

MASS PRODUCTION

Mass-produced, prefabricated orthoses are still a smaller proportion than custom-molded lower extremity orthoses fitted to patients as reported by ABCOP-certified individuals, though there is an increasing trend.[73] Orthopedic companies continue to develop orthotic and prosthetic products whose fit and performance approach that of custom-molded devices through diverse sizing systems and modular components. In the future, prefabricated modular component systems may bridge the gap between prefabricated and custom-molded devices by improving performance outcomes with custom-fitted systems and expanding their use in clinical practice. Although these advances in fit and function are possible for some problems, certain deformities and pathologic conditions will almost always require custom-molded or measured orthoses and prostheses made by traditional or CAD/CAM methods of production.

Maintenance of Orthoses and Prostheses

Routine care and maintenance of orthoses and prostheses are important for proper function and long-term use of a device. An orthotic or prosthetic maintenance program usually includes servicing by the orthotist or prosthetist and the patient. The service schedule depends on the specific orthosis or prosthesis, the materials from which it is made, the durability of the components, and the knowledge and ability of the patient and caregivers. Patient instructions for the daily care of an orthosis or prosthesis should include cleaning and inspection. Proper patient education of basic fitting criteria and instructions on donning and doffing a device allow the patient to evaluate the fit of a device during routine use. Professionals in orthotic and prosthetic work environments also need to adopt strategies to decrease the risk of cross-contamination from devices such as hand washing (frequency and time spent), cleaning devices and tools, and implementation of an infection control coordinator.[74]

Orthoses and prostheses should be inspected weekly for any defects, stress risers (nicks, scratches), loose screws, or weakened rivets. Any device that has mechanical components and moving parts and is subjected to repetitive loading requires periodic servicing; it is less expensive to recognize and fix early signs of a problem than it is to replace a device that has failed because of a lack of proper maintenance. Informing patients of potential problems associated with the use of their orthoses or prostheses and how to resolve these problems can prevent serious situations from arising.

Most plastic components should be cleaned with a mild antibacterial soap and rinsed thoroughly with cold water. Extra moisture should be absorbed with a towel and the orthosis or prosthesis air dried. Heat can distort some plastics; patients should be warned not to use electric hairdryers to dry their devices. Similarly, devices should not be left near direct heat sources, such as radiators, wood/pellet stoves, or any appliance that generates heat when running. They must also be protected from intense direct sunlight.

Leather liners and covers are cleaned weekly with a leather "saddle" soap. Leather softeners should not be used unless directed by the orthotist, because they can compromise function of some straps and cuffs. Water-repellent treatments and protectants for leather often contain skin irritants and should not be used on leather components that have direct contact with the body. Most orthoses and prostheses are designed to apply a corrective or stabilizing force to a body segment during wear. For some patients, especially those with fragile skin or scarring, this pressure may increase the risk of skin irritation or damage. The risk of skin problems differs from device to device and depends on the general health and skin condition of the individual who is wearing the orthosis or prosthesis. To minimize problems with skin intolerance of these extra forces, most new orthotic or prosthetic users begin with an intermittent wearing schedule. A treatment plan that incorporates a gradual buildup of orthotic or prosthetic use can avert complications such as excessive redness, chafing, and blisters. For a patient with a high risk for or a history of skin problems, a variety of preventive measures (e.g., foam or silicone interface liners) can be incorporated into the orthotic or prosthetic system.

Most custom orthoses or prostheses are designed to achieve a very intimate fit with the body segments that they encompass. Changes in the physical condition of a patient can significantly alter the fit and function of a device. Compromised fit occurs most often when the patient has had significant growth, weight gain or loss, muscle atrophy, edema, structural degeneration, or trauma. Periodic evaluations are necessary to ensure that fit and function are maintained in the months and years after the initial fitting. Semiannual or annual checkups should be part of the treatment plans for definitive orthotic and prosthetic devices.

To maintain proper function of a lower extremity prosthesis, special attention is needed in several areas. The alignment of a prosthesis is usually based on a specific heel height; variation from the prescribed heel height (when footwear is changed) often leads to functional problems during gait. In the same way, moderate to excessive wear of the shoe at the heel also compromises performance. The condition of footwear must be carefully and frequently monitored. The prosthesis should be free of dirt, sand, and other debris to ensure that joint mechanisms and their movements are not inhibited. Socket attachment and suspension systems need daily attention because they are usually prone to accumulation of lint, dirt, and other debris. If the prosthesis or any of its components are subjected to water, the device should be thoroughly dried to prevent permanent damage. Rubber bumpers in prosthetic feet deteriorate over time and with use and must be replaced regularly. The prosthetist can advise patients on specific parts that require regular maintenance.

The socket portion of a prosthesis should be faithfully cared for to avoid potential skin problems, especially infection, on the residual limb. When a special liner is used with a prosthesis, specific instructions for cleaning are necessary because materials used vary greatly. For patients who are fitted with suction sockets or special socket attachment mechanisms, the joining components or threads should be cleaned with a soft brush or rag to remove debris.

TECHNOLOGIES POISED TO TRANSFORM PROSTHETICS AND ORTHOTICS AND REHABILITATION

Healthcare economics and reimbursement issues have impeded the pace of technologic advancements and patient access to new technologies in prosthetics and orthotics. The transfer of science and technology from other medical and engineering disciplines to prosthetics and orthotics will be important for continued innovation. Biosensor technologies, power actuation, and CAD/CAM are three areas primed to advance prosthetics, orthotics, and rehabilitation in the next decade. Orthotic and prosthetic practices are slowly transitioning from experiential practice-driven decision-making to one founded on biomedical sensor data from the user and their respective devices. Clinically relevant measures offer improved reliability to assess user performance and to determine treatment prognoses. Actuators can provide power assistance to augment movement and offer advantages that conventional passive prosthetic and orthotic systems cannot offer. Advances in 3D scanners and printers offer an alternative means for capturing the shape of a body segment for custom-fitted interfaces, and 3D printers and computer numerically controlled milling machines and lathes could replace some of the traditional methods and processes (e.g., plaster-of-Paris molds) of fabrication. Although the application of newer technologies may be feasible, their adoption within the field will ultimately rest on treatment outcome results and monetary benefits to our healthcare delivery systems.

Biosensors

In comparison with other areas of medicine, prosthetics and orthotics have lagged behind in the use of biomedical instrumentation to assist in clinical decision-making, diagnostics, and monitoring user performance and outcomes. Considerable advances have been made in sensor technology, microprocessors, and data analyses that are applicable to orthotics and prosthetics. The reduction of sensor size and cost has permitted them to be embedded into orthoses and prostheses without compromising functionality for the user. Wireless systems (e.g., Bluetooth) that communicate through user-friendly interfaces (e.g., tablets) allow sensing systems to be used in the clinical setting, remotely in the home and community. Data on the actual use of an orthosis or prosthesis are important to monitor because compliance and dosage parameters (i.e., time of use) can help with treatment prognoses. In the orthotic management of scoliosis, temperature and force sensors embedded in thoracic lumbosacral orthoses provide clinicians with a relatively accurate account of patient use but can also reveal if the orthosis postural support is being optimized when in use.[75,76] The combined data of several sensors characterize the duration of use (i.e., time) and the manner in which the desired orthotic control is being achieved. As more sensor data are collected and studied in all domains of orthotics and prosthetics, the efficacy and efficiency of treatment interventions can be refined and improved on a foundation of clinically relevant measures.

Prostheses and orthoses interact with a respective body segment (e.g., leg, residuum) via a socket or shell-like interface, respectively. The specified geometry of the interface controls the manner in which loads are transmitted from the device to the human user. Therefore transducers that can quantify pressure and force data coupled with sensors that detect movement provide vital information for practitioners to optimize fit and function for the user.[77–79] In addition to gathering information from the human subject user, instrumented orthoses and prosthesis can collect data from the device itself for feedback and control systems to optimize function, user intent, and safety. Electromyography (EMG) sensors measure muscle activity, and if embedded into the interface, practitioners can consider a user's neuromotor response mechanism to the use of an orthosis or prosthesis. EMG data can also be used to determine control parameters for power actuation systems in devices.[80] Some of the current challenges with surface EMG sensors are physical dimensionality and cost. A team at the MIT Media Lab has begun development on a low-profile Sub-Liner Interface for Prosthetics electrode to address these concerns.[81]

Pattern Recognition

Pattern recognition for prosthetic control is a sophisticated approach that has gained significant attention in the field of prosthetics. It involves the utilization of advanced algorithms and machine learning techniques to decipher the intentions and movements of the user, enabling intuitive control over the prosthetic device. By analyzing patterns of muscle activity, neural signals, or other relevant input data, pattern recognition systems can accurately decode the user's desired actions and translate them into appropriate prosthetic movements.

In 2019 a review of existing methods by Parajuli et al. outlined the following: the underlying principle of pattern recognition lies in the extraction of meaningful features from the input signals (EMG), followed by the classification and prediction of the user's intended movements. Various signal processing techniques, such as time-domain analysis, frequency-domain analysis, or time-frequency analysis, can be employed to extract relevant features from the acquired signals. These features are then fed into machine learning algorithms, such as artificial neural networks or support vector machines, which learn to recognize patterns and make predictions based on the training data. The system continuously adapts and updates its knowledge through iterative training processes, enhancing its ability to accurately interpret the user's commands and provide responsive control of the prosthetic device.[82] There are limited pattern recognition components currently available and are primarily upper extremity prosthesis componentry.[83] Through the integration of pattern recognition, prosthetic control can be significantly improved, offering individuals with limb loss greater autonomy, natural movement, and enhanced quality of life.[84]

Power Assistance and Actuation

Traditionally, most orthoses and prostheses have designs that feature "passive" motion control mechanisms.[85] For instance, most ankle-foot orthoses assist, resist, and/or limit ankle joint motion range mechanically with springs or elastic bands or through the controlled deflection of a strut element (e.g., posterior leaf-spring AFO). Furthermore, passive resistance can be also be achieved via friction, pneumatics, hydraulics, and magnetorheologic damping systems.[85] These types of damping methods can be controlled by microprocessors within the knee mechanism. Microprocessor-controlled prosthetic knees (MPKs) represent one of the most significant technologic advances made in prosthetics. In particular the Ottobock C-Leg (Ottobock, Duderstadt, Germany), introduced in 1997, was the first MPK that had microprocessor control stance and swing phases. Compared with non–microcontrolled prosthetic knees, users of MPKs report an improved perception of balance confidence, and scientific studies are currently showing the incidence of falls can be reduced between 64% and 80%.[86] There are now various manufactures and types of MPKs available addressing individual patient presentations regarding functional level,[87] activities of daily living,[88] and energy efficiency.[89] Similar control systems for knee control in knee-ankle-foot orthoses have also been developed.[86]

Although passive resistance and controlled motion has provided improvements in joint motion control in both orthotics and prosthetics, powered actuation is the next phase which can generate active joint movement. The use of different types of actuators to augment motion in orthoses and prosthesis is expanding at a rapid pace particularly with wearable exoskeletal robotic systems. Although technologic barriers still exist in creating systems for everyday use, there is promising applicability for powered assistance in the rehabilitation clinic/hospital setting for more controlled therapeutic interventions compared with traditional physical therapy techniques (e.g., caregiver-assisted resistance training).[90,91]

Exoskeletal Robotics

Computer-controlled robotic systems have some distinct advantages over traditional rehabilitation therapies. Exoskeletal robots are often ideally suited for repetitive strength and/or stretching routines or when prescribed target dosages are needed. Although hands-on therapist-administered treatments have proven to be effective, robots have the potential to be more efficient due to their precision-controlled movement, and if instrumented with sensors, they can provide valuable performance feedback data.

The biomechanical principles used to maximize fit, function, and comfort with orthoses are also applicable for exoskeletal robots. Actuators transmit power to mechanical armatures and levers linked to orthotic interface shells. Exoskeletal systems are unique as compared to most orthoses as they provide an external force on the users soft tissue. These forces are necessary to generate the required motion; though the clinician should be aware of the adverse events which could occur. Considerations for protective sensation, pressure distribution, and material selection are necessary for optimal performance.

3D Printers and Additive Manufacturing

Additive manufacturing and 3D printing are quickly gaining traction within the profession as the technologies and materials improve and can better meet the demands for clinical use. This is evidenced by the inclusion of an additive manufacturing specific item in the 2022 Practice Analysis (Table 6.1). The early plastics used in 3D printing lacked the strength and reliability of the conventional composites and thermoplastics used in the industry and slowed the application of 3D printing into clinical practice. However, advances such as carbon fiber–infused plastics and the ability to structurally engineer (e.g., vary thickness) a component have allowed some 3D-printed parts to be applicable for definitive use rather than for prototyping purposes. A diversity of materials is available with a wide variety of mechanical properties. Some of the most common filament materials used are polycarbonate, nylon, ABS, polylactic acid, polypropylene, thermoplastic elastomers (TPEs), thermoplastic polyurethane, polyethylene terephthalate with glycol (PETG), polyvinyl alcohol, and acrylic styrene acrylonitrile. The addition of carbon and wood fibers or metal powders infused into the base materials can further enhance properties of materials.[71] Fig. 6.17 demonstrates the integration of traditional and advanced materials and methods within the check and definitive stages of the same partial hand prosthesis. In this image, it is observed that significant changes have occurred between the two designs. This is the purpose of the diagnostic fitting procedure—to provide the patient the ability to interact with the intervention prior to finalizing the design. Fig. 6.16A is an initial diagnostic fit including milled (custom machined) silicone interface with blister formed PETG rigid frame; the patient and clinician identify markings on the frame and silicone interface to optimize functionality once multiarticular digits are added. Fig. 6.16B shows the definitive design, using milled silicone with integrated threaded anchor points and SLS printed Nylon 11 rigid frame. Notice that the method of suspension has significantly changed from the diagnostic as the wrist band has been removed due to the optimizing of the multidurometer silicone interface.

Rapid prototyping is a developing advancement for additive manufacturing. The ability to design and print across various materials[92] and within a small work environment allows the clinician and researcher the opportunity to test new designs without the requirement of having an onsite lab. Piloting an innovative design consideration on lower cost materials such as ABS prior to moving into a more advanced definitive materials allows for a more cost-effective method for the clinician and researcher. Furthermore, it offers the ability to outsource exotic material prints to third-party manufacturers without upfront cost of independently purchasing a printer. Fig. 6.18 shows a screenshot of

Table 6.1 Device Types Utilizing Additive Manufacturing

Percentage of Orthoses/Prostheses in Each Area	
Incorporating Additive Manufacturing (3D Printing)	
Upper Extremity	2%
Lower Extremity	6%
Foot (including diabetic inserts)	11%
Spinal	6%
Cranial	10%
	Prostheses
Lower Extremity	19%
Upper Extremity	5%

3D, Three dimensional.
Modified from ABCOP 2022 Practice Analysis

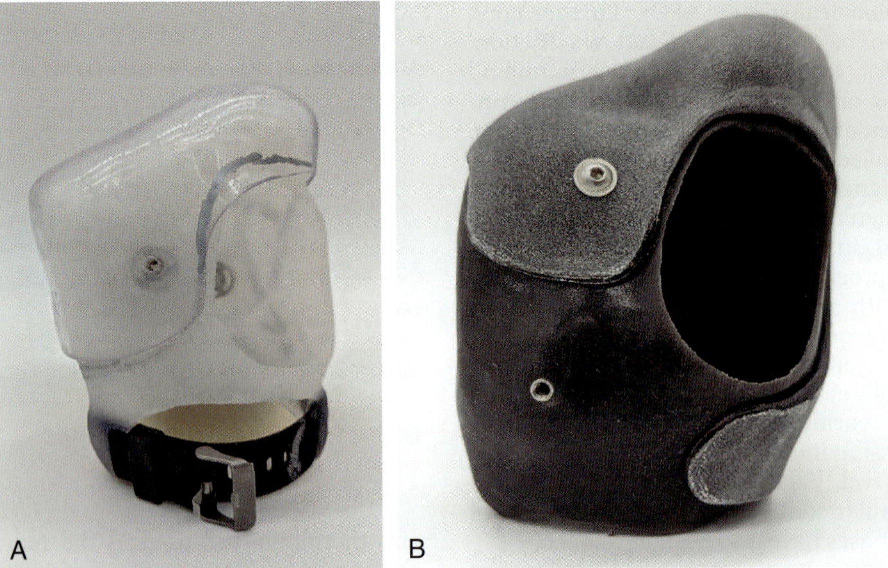

Fig. 6.17 Series of a partial hand prosthesis (frame and interface). (A) Diagnostic fit partial hand frame and silicone interface. (B) Definitive prosthesis (frame and interface) frame: Nylon 11 additive manufactured Interfaced: Milled silicone. (Courtesy of Hanger Fabrication Network.)

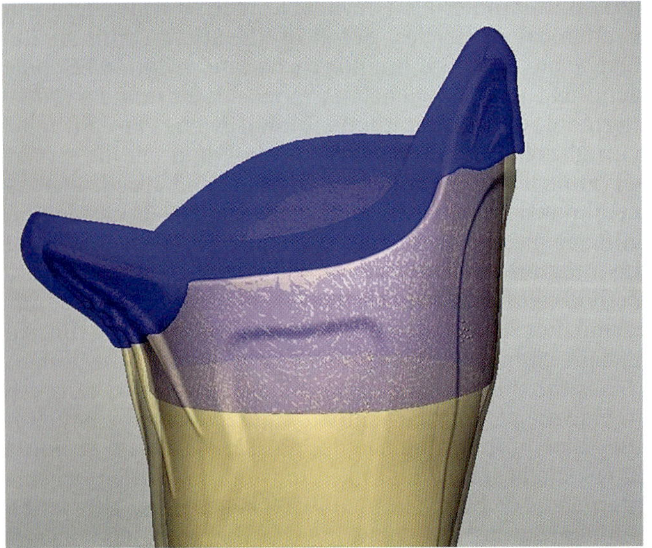

Fig. 6.18 Screenshot of custom CAD (Computer-Aided Design)–designed proximal brim for a transfemoral socket. (Courtesy Macy O&P LLC, East Lyme, Connecticut.)

a CAD design. This addition is a flexible proximal brim to a transfemoral socket to improve comfort of the patient, the initial design will be confirmed for fit and shape with a desktop printer. Once the shape is confirmed, a final print will be sent through an advanced standalone printer which will print a softer durometer shape that will provide control of the patient's anatomy yet be tolerated well during a variety of physical activities.

Summary

This chapter explored the materials and methods most commonly used in the prescription, measurement, and production of orthoses and prostheses. The type of design, materials, and components are selected to best facilitate the functional goals of the patient. The foundation for effectiveness of the orthosis or prosthesis is careful measurement of the body segment (by casting or by CAD/CAM) and careful modification of the resulting model for optimal fit. For an individual who is being fit for his or her initial orthosis or prosthesis, shared decision-making of the rehabilitation team, including the patient and caregivers, is essential. An orthosis or prosthesis that is difficult to don or is uncomfortable to wear is more likely to be found standing in a closet or pushed under a bed than on the patient for daily use.

References

The complete listing of the References are available in the accompanying enhanced eBook version included with the print purchase of this textbook. Visit Elsevier eBooks+ (eBooks.Health.Elsevier.com) to access this content.

7 Footwear: Foundation for Lower Extremity Orthoses

STANISLAW SOLNIK AND MILAGROS JORGE

LEARNING OBJECTIVES

On completion of this chapter, the reader will be able to do the following:

1. Determine the proper fit of standard footwear for a patient's foot based on the necessary function of the foot during gait and the contour and alignment of the foot.
2. Recommend appropriate footwear styles and characteristics for patients with foot deformities and those who wear orthoses or prostheses.
3. Describe the shoe modifications and accommodative orthoses that can be used to address musculoskeletal problems affecting the foot and lower limb.
4. Describe the effect of selected problems and deformity of the forefoot, midfoot, or rearfoot on weight bearing and efficiency of the gait cycle and suggest appropriate footwear or orthotic interventions to reduce pain and improve function.
5. Identify special footwear needs for individuals with arthritis, gout, diabetes, peripheral vascular disease, hemiplegia, and amputation or congenital deformity of the foot and leg.

It can be said that the most essential element of clothing in any person's wardrobe is the shoe. Unlike any other clothing item, it is specifically designed to provide a precise fit; additionally, continuous pressure from tight shoes can produce ulceration and deformities. Ill-fitting shoes can generate shear forces that lead to skin breakdown, toe and foot deformities, and even falls.[1] Shoes serve essential functions by transferring body weight to the ground during walking and safeguarding the wearer from environmental hazards. A well-designed shoe is a necessary foundation for many lower extremity orthotics, prosthetic alignment, and an energy-efficient gait. This chapter explores the components and characteristics of shoes, emphasizes the importance of proper fit, and guides the selection of suitable footwear for individuals with foot dysfunction and deformity.

Components of a Good Shoe

Properly designed shoes are crucial in reducing stress on various parts of the feet, offering support, and absorbing the impact of ground reaction forces.[2]

The basic parts of a shoe are the sole, upper, heel, and last. Each of these parts is further divided into components or areas that are required for ensuring the correct design of shoes (Fig. 7.1). Each component is crucial to the prescription of appropriate shoes for an individual's needs.

SOLE

The sole protects the plantar surface of the foot. The traditional method of constructing the sole involves sewing two pieces of leather together with a layer of compressible cork in between. An additional layer, the insole, is situated next to the foot in most shoes. A heavy thick sole protects the foot against irregularities in the walking surface. The rigidity or stiffness of the sole is also essential. Although durable, the sole must not be overly rigid as it can interfere with the toe rocker of the metatarsophalangeal (MTP) hyperextension during the terminal stance and preswing phases of gait.

Various areas of the sole are identified by location. The *welt* is the inside piece of the external sole; the *outsole* is the most superficial portion. The area that lies between the heel and the ball of the shoe, the *shank*, is commonly fabricated to provide reinforcement and shape using materials such as spring steel, steel and leatherboard, or wood strips between the welt and the outsole. The purpose of the shank is to prevent collapse of the material between the heel and the ball of the foot and to provide additional support. In most athletic shoes, rubber is commonly used for the sole to maximize traction. Rubber soles effectively absorb shock, thereby minimizing heel impact forces.

UPPER

The upper of the shoe, which includes the *vamp, tongue*, and *rear quarters*, covers the dorsum (top surface) of the foot. The vamp extends from the insole forward. The tongue is an extension of the vamp in a blucher-style closure. In contrast, in the Balmoral or Bal-type Oxford shoe design, the tongue is separate (Fig. 7.2). The blucher-style closure allows for slightly more opening than the Bal Oxford closure, facilitating the easy entry of the foot into the shoe. The front part of the vamp, known as the toe, is often covered with a separate piece of leather called the *tip*. The rearward line of the tip may be straight or winged. The vamp is connected to the quarters, which form the sides and back of the upper. The two quarters are joined together at a seam located at the back. The design of the shoe dictates the shape and size of the quarters. For the Oxford shoe, the outside quarter is cut lower than the inner quarter to avoid contact with the malleoli. In the Bal-type Oxford, the back edges of the vamp cover the front edges of the quarter. In the blucher style of shoe, the front edges of the quarters are located on top of the vamp.

For individuals wearing orthoses and those with foot deformity, the blucher closure is preferable over the Bal-style closure because of its construction. The blucher closure separates the distal margins of the lace stays, resulting in a wide inlet. This makes the shoes easier to put on and take off and allows for adjustable circumference. High shoes encase the malleoli and provide additional stability in the medial-lateral direction.

HEEL

The heel is located beneath the outer sole under the anatomic heel. Typically, the heel base is made of rigid rubber, plastic, or wood, featuring a resilient plantar surface. As heel height increases, the ankle range of motion necessary to lower the forefoot to the floor increases. Additionally, weight-bearing pressures on the forefoot and hallux (big toe) escalate from midstance to late stance.[3] The individual with limited ankle motion may benefit from a compressible heel base to absorb shock and achieve plantarflexion during the early stance phase. Opting for a wide and low heel enhances stability and minimizes stress on the metatarsal heads. Most lower extremity orthoses and prosthetic feet are designed for a specific heel height. The effectiveness of an orthosis or the quality of prosthetic gait can be significantly compromised if used with shoes with higher or lower heels.

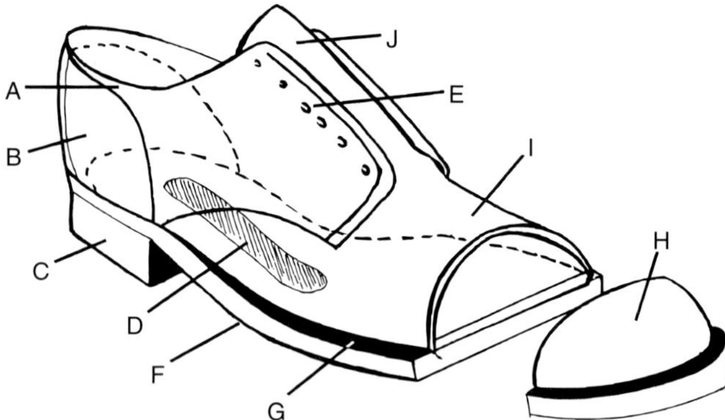

Fig. 7.1 Basic parts of a shoe. The upper is made up of the quarter *(A)* and its reinforcing counter *(B)*, which stabilize the rearfoot within the shoe; the closure *(E)* and the tongue *(J)* across the midfoot; and the shaft (vamp; *I*) and toe box *(H)*, which enclose the forefoot. The exterior outsole *(F)* is often reinforced with a steel shank *(D)* and is attached to the upper at the welt *(G)*. The standard heel *(C)* is ¾-inch high.

REINFORCEMENTS

Strategic shoe reinforcements contribute to foot protection. Toe boxing at the distal vamp shields the toes and prevents the vamp's anterior portion from losing shape. The toe box can also be increased in depth to protect and accommodate any toe deformities. The heel counter reinforces the quarters to help secure the shoe to the anatomic heel. The medial counter helps support the shoe's medial arch, and the heel counter aids in controlling the rearfoot. The convex shank piece stiffens the sole between the distal border of the shoe heel and the MTP joints and aids in supporting the longitudinal arch.

LASTS

Shoes are constructed over a model of the foot, called a *last*, which is styled from wood, plaster, or plastic. Manufacturers are now converting to computer-aided last designs. Regardless of the origin of the last, it determines the fit, walking ease, and appearance of the shoe. Commercial shoes are made over many different lasts in thousands of size combinations. Most shoes are made with a medial last, meaning the toe box is directed inward from the heel (Fig. 7.3). Shoes can also be made from conventional lasts, straight lasts, inflared or medial lasts, or outflared or lateral lasts.

ENHANCING FUNCTION

Shoes are essential to daily professional,[4] leisure, and recreational[5] life. Regardless of the reason for using a particular shoe, ensuring foot stability is critical to minimizing ankle injury, excessive pronation, and heel slippage during the gait cycle. A well-designed shoe incorporates a broad heel base, ankle collar, and close-fitting heel counter. An important feature of a good shoe is its ability to absorb shock. The construction of and materials used for the insole, midsole, and outer sole determine the level of shock absorption provided by the shoe.[6]

A good shoe should be flexible and provide stability with each step. Flexibility, particularly in the sole, enhances the toe rocker during the late stance phase. The sole should also provide adequate traction as it contacts the ground, especially in the early stance, as body weight is transferred onto the foot. A coefficient of friction that is sufficient to minimize slips and near slips is vital. The height of the heel can exert stress on the forefoot during walking. Heels of more than 1½ inches exponentially increase weight-bearing forces on the metatarsal heads.[7]

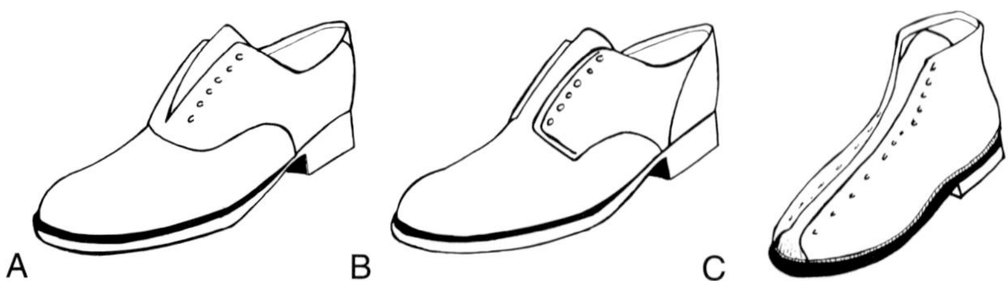

Fig. 7.2 Three types of shoe closures. (A) In the Bal Oxford, the tongue is a separate piece sewn to the vamp and anterior edges of the quarters. (B) In the blucher style, the tongue is an extension of the vamp and can be opened slightly wider. (C) For patients with rigid ankle orthoses, fixed deformity, or fragile neuropathic feet, the lace-to-toe (surgical) style may be necessary.

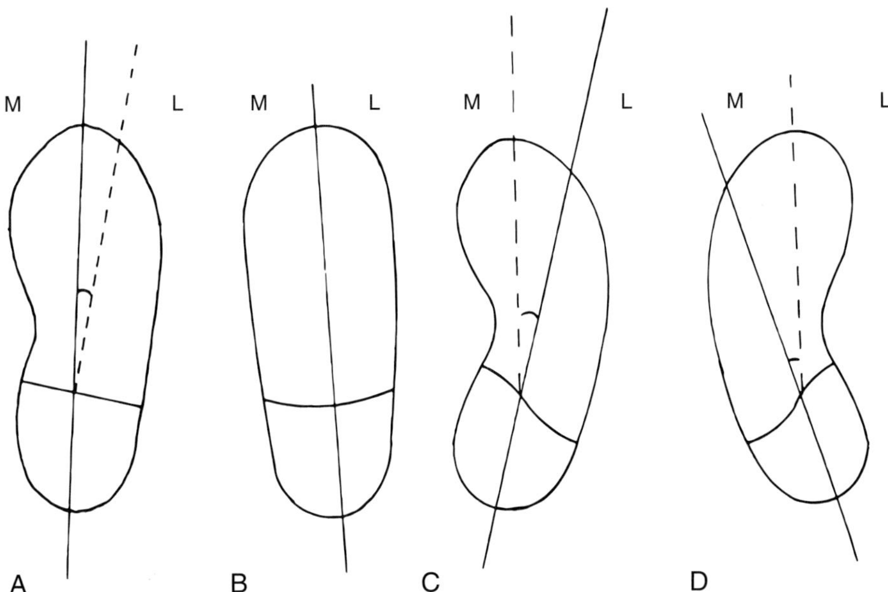

Fig. 7.3 The last determines the shape of the shoe. (A) In a conventional last, the forefoot is directly slightly lateral *(L)* to the midline. (B) A straight last is symmetric around the midline. (C) An inflared last directs the forefoot medially. (D) An outflared last directs the foot more laterally than a conventional last. *M*, Medial.

Moisture management is another important factor in shoe selection. For optimal foot health and comfort, perspiration must be wicked away while preventing external moisture from entering.

The upper should be soft and pliable. Modern tanning techniques enable the creation of strong yet pliable uppers that surround the feet supportively and protectively without rubbing and chafing while allowing the foot to breathe.

ORTHOTIC-RELATED FUNCTION

A molded insole contributes to foot stability, shock absorption, and a transfer of shear forces away from problem areas. Orthoses can enhance the function of the shoes. Chapter 8 presents the principles and practices of orthotic prescription in commonly occurring foot conditions.

Proper Fitting of a Shoe: "If the Shoe Fits"

The critical factors in ensuring a proper fit for shoes are their shape and size. *Shoe shape* refers to the shape of the sole and the upper. Proper fit is achieved when the shoe shape is matched to the foot shape. *Shoe size* is determined by arch length, not by overall foot length. The proper shoe size is the one that allows for comfortable accommodation of the first metatarsal joint at the widest part of the shoe. It is crucial to wear shoes that fit properly to avoid foot discomfort and deformities. This is particularly important for people with arthritis, diabetes, and other foot disorders.[8]

There is significant variation in the size and shape of human feet. Mass-produced shoes, however, are formed over fairly standard lasts that give a shoe its special size and shape. In the well-fitting shoe, the shape determined by the last approximates the human foot. The design and construction of the shoe should allow for a roomy toe box; it should be wide enough for normal toe alignment and be ½ inch longer than the longest toe. Ensuring a proper fit of the forefoot within the shoe is crucial for reducing the occurrence of bunions, hammertoes, and other deformities in the front part of the foot. The shoe should generally be wide enough to accommodate the widest part of the forefoot. When standing, a tracing of the foot should fit within the outline of the shoe bottom.

A proper fit relies on appropriate design, shape, and construction, and it is equally important to have a range of available widths and lengths. The clinician must cultivate a consumer mindset that realizes the medical importance of modifying the old cliché "if the shoe fits, wear it" to "if the shoe fits, wear it, and if it does not, order it in the correct size."

DETERMINING MEASUREMENTS

The average shoe salesperson does not offer to measure the foot, instead relying on the consumer to know their foot size. However, periodic measurement of both feet for length and width is essential because foot size changes over time. Many shoe styles available in retail shoe stores do not appropriately match the shape of an individual's foot. As a result, comfort and protection are compromised in the name of "style." This is especially problematic in the presence of foot deformity. Hallux valgus is a foot deformity aggravated by wearing shoes that are too narrow across the metatarsal heads and triangularly shaped in the toe box. Shoes should be wide enough to allow the material of the upper surrounding the widest region of the forefoot (i.e., the metatarsal heads) to be compressed at least 1/16 inch before bony contact is made. Likewise, it is important to have an ½ inch space between the longest toe and the front of the shoe's toe box when standing, which is usually the width of a thumb.

In the United States, 12 different standard shoe widths are manufactured.[1] They range from the very narrow AAAAA to the very wide EEEE—that is, AAAAA, AAAA, AAA, AA, A, B, C, D, E, EE, EEE, EEEE. Because most retail stores stock midrange width (A–E) shoes, patients with narrow or wide feet often have difficulty finding shoes of the optimal width.

Standard US shoes are available in half-size increments, from an infant's size 0 to a man's size 16. The difference in length between half sizes is 1/16 inch. Standard shoe-sizing classifications are made by groups and lasts: infants' sizes 0 to 2; boys' sizes 2½ to 6; girls' sizes 2½ to 9; women's sizes 3 to 10; and men's' sizes 6 to 12. Sizes larger than 'women's size 10 and men's size 12 must often be specially ordered. A US women's shoe size is usually three half sizes smaller than the corresponding men's size (e.g., a women's size 9 is the same as a men's size 7½).

European and UK manufacturers use a different numbering system. The comparison of European and UK women's to men's sizes is based on centimeters (e.g., women's size 38 EUR/5 UK is the same as men's size 40 EUR/5 UK). Table 7.1 compares the standard sizes for US, European, and UK shoe manufacturers and lists the measures for each size.

Table 7.1 Comparison of Standardized Shoe Sizes

United States	Europe	United Kingdom	Centimeters
WOMEN'S SIZES			
3	34	1	20
3½	34.5	1.5	20.5
4	35	2	21
4½	35.5	2.5	21.5
5	36	3	22
5½	36.5	3.5	22.5
6	37	4	23
6½	37.5	4.5	23.5
7	38	5	24
7½	38.5	5.5	24.5
8	39	6	25
8½	39.5	6.5	25.5
9	40	7	26
9½	40.5	7.5	26.5
10	41	8	27
MEN'S SIZES			
6	40	5	24
6½	40.5	5.5	24.5
7	41	6	25
7½	41.5	6.5	25.5
8	42	7	26
8½	42.5	7.5	26.5
9	43	8	27
9½	43.5	8.5	27.5
10	44	9	28
10½	44.5	9.5	28.5
11	45	10	29
11½	45.5	10.5	29.5
12	46	11	30

FOOT CONTOUR

Throughout our lives, the shape of our feet undergoes various changes. Aging, pregnancy, obesity, and everyday stresses can widen the foot. Deformities such as bunions increase the width and shape of the foot, and splaying of the metatarsal heads creates a collapse of the transverse arch, further expanding the width of the forefoot.[9] In the presence of toe deformities, the height of the forefoot may also increase. Deformities such as pes planus[10] (foot flattening) or pes cavus[11] (high arches) change the contour of the midfoot. The foot's shape must be considered and accommodated when an individual is measured for shoes. Often a "combined last" (where the last in the toe box is different from the rearfoot counter) is required to accommodate the foot's contour. The relationship between the forefoot and the rearfoot is crucial in determining whether the shoe shape, provided by the last, aligns with the shape of the foot.

To best meet the specific needs of patients, shoes with medial, straight, or lateral lasts can be ordered.

OBESITY AND EDEMA

Obesity can affect the foot's medial and lateral longitudinal and transverse arches, resulting in an increased length and width of the foot in both children[12] and adults.[13] The additional weight strains the plantar fascia and ligaments of the foot's plantar surface. Those structures begin to buckle under stress when engaged in weight-bearing activities such as standing and walking. Therefore overweight individuals often exhibit overpronation and collapsing arches. The additional mechanical stress of carrying excess weight takes its toll on the feet, often resulting in problems such as plantar fasciitis, arthritis and bursitis, heel pain, neuroma, and gait changes.[14]

Ensuring proper shoe fit is crucial in preventing secondary foot problems from wearing ill-fitting shoes. Overweight individuals should be encouraged to have their feet measured regularly, particularly if they have had a significant weight gain. It is often helpful to shop for shoes at the end of the day, when the feet are largest, and the shoe fitting should be done with the person standing to ensure that there is ½ inch between the end of the longest toe and the edge of the toe box. The shoes should feel comfortable from the moment they are worn.

Fluctuation in foot size in individuals with edema (e.g., those with kidney dysfunction or congestive heart failure or anyone taking diuretic medication) creates a challenge when shoes are being fitted. The contour of the foot constantly changes in these cases. For individuals with severe edema, a shoe/sandal with a Thermold Velcro closure (Fig. 7.4) is recommended to accommodate and support the foot and prevent the undue pressures imposed by a shoe that becomes too small throughout the day. The consequences of ill-fitting shoes—especially shoes with a narrow tow box—are foot problems such as bunions, valgus deformity, and neuromas. The regular use of properly fitting shoes can help prevent many of these issues.[1]

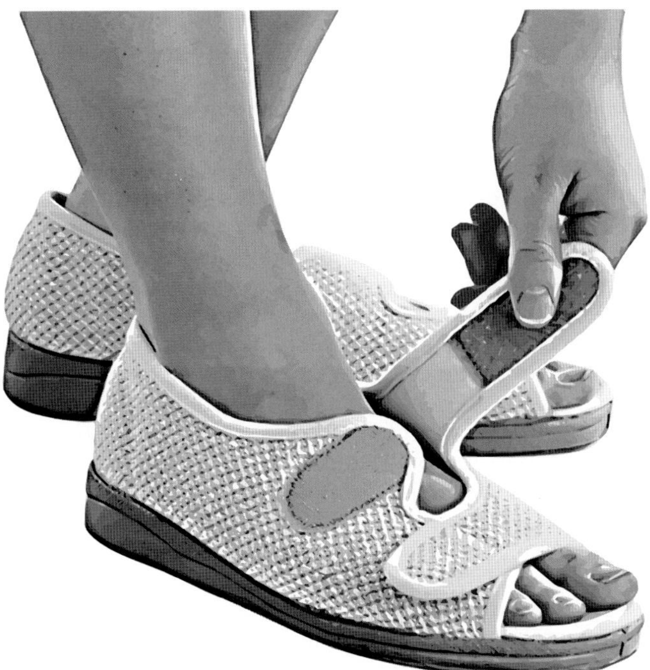

Fig. 7.4 Velcro closure shoe/sandal. Adjustable Velcro closures are recommended to accommodate edematous feet and prevent tissue damage due to high pressure. Courtesy Silvert's Stores, Concord, Ontario, Canada.

Special Considerations

The diversity of foot shapes, sizes, and health conditions necessitates considering these factors when selecting appropriate footwear. The biomechanical and functional characteristics of feet change over an individual's lifetime and must also be reflected in shoe choice. The foot gradually adapts to weight bearing in infancy, especially as walking becomes functional. During childhood, the foot continues to adapt as normal growth changes the alignment of the pelvis, femur, and tibia. Pregnancy introduces hormonal changes that affect the structure and function of the foot. Finally, the combined influence of the aging process, obesity, and diseases common in later life can create special footwear needs for older adults. Considering these various factors is essential to address the footwear requirements at different life stages.

PEDIATRIC FOOT

Many foot disorders in pediatric and lower extremity conditions may exhibit minimal symptoms and not require treatment, while others may require more aggressive management. Understanding the natural history of many of these disorders is essential in establishing the appropriate footwear for toddlers and children as they begin to walk and run.[15,16]

In-toeing is a problem caused by positional factors in utero and during sleep, muscle imbalances due to motor disorders, and decreased range of motion in the lower kinetic chain. It may also be due to metatarsus adductus, internal tibia torsion, or internal femoral torsion.

Metatarsus adductus is characterized by a foot with a bean-like shape due to forefoot adduction. In approximately 90% of cases, this condition resolves spontaneously.[15] If it does not improve over the first 6 to 12 weeks of life, the treatment of choice is manual stretching and an outflared shoe. The foot bones are soft and can be corrected with the positioning in the outflared shoe (reverse last) or Bebax shoe (Camp Healthcare, Jackson, Michigan).

Internal tibial torsion refers to a twist between the knee and the ankle, which typically resolves by the age of 5. Torsion can be exacerbated by abnormal sitting and sleep postures with the foot turned inward. In conjunction with a reverse last shoe, the Dennis Browne bar or the counter-rotation splint can help remodel the bones during growth. Persistent severe toeing created by internal tibial torsion requires a derotational osteotomy of the tibia/fibula in the supramalleolar region.

Internal femoral torsion can also cause in-toeing with a twist between the knee and hip. Neither splints nor shoes are effective in the treatment of torsion. Habitual sitting in the "W" position (e.g., when a child is watching television or playing games on the floor) can worsen the condition. Children with internal femoral torsion should be encouraged to sit cross-legged as an alternative.

Out-toeing occurs in children who sleep in the frog position and have soft tissue contractures around the hip. This condition is usually attributed to hip or long bone torsion and is not influenced by footwear.

Toe walking can be the result of an in utero shortening or a congenital shortening of the Achilles tendon but can also be an early sign of cerebral palsy, muscular dystrophy, or Charcot-Marie-Tooth disease.[17] Toe walking has been observed in children and adolescents with autism spectrum disorder.[18] Until 4 years of age, the ability to stretch the tendon is well preserved, and conservative treatment includes stretching, casting, ankle-foot orthoses, and a night splint. If conservative interventions fail, Z-plasty lengthening may be performed.[17] Shoe prescription objectives follow the same principles as those in older adults with Achilles tendinitis.

Flexible and Rigid Flatfoot

Flatfoot or pes planus is characterized by the loss of the medial longitudinal arch. Flatfoot is classified as either flexible or rigid. A flexible flatfoot exhibits an arch when the foot is not bearing weight (open kinetic chain). However, the arch disappears when weight is placed on it (closed kinetic chain). A rigid flatfoot has a loss of longitudinal arch height in open and closed kinetic chains.[19] Treatment of flatfoot disorders in children is approached through properly fitting shoes with good arch support and, if necessary, orthotic inserts in the shoes. Fitting children with standardized shoes that have good arches, be they dress shoes or athletic shoes, can support fallen arches and pronated feet. In cases where additional support is needed, insole orthotics can be added.[17,20] The shoe used to treat flatfoot is designed to correct heel valgus and support the arch. Forefoot pronation is achieved by using a lateral shoe wedge combined with a medial heel wedge. A scaphoid pad supports the arch, and a strong medial counter prevents medial rollover. A Thomas heel is often used to provide additional support for the arch.

In-shoe orthotics are prescribed to improve arch alignment, increase the duration of the stance phase of level walking, and reduce both the maximum foot pronation angle and tibial internal rotation.[18,19] Orthotics have demonstrated the ability to reduce foot pain in children with flatfoot.[19]

The *calcaneovalgus* deformity is a congenital condition that is usually secondary to the individual's initial position in utero. It is characterized by severe valgus (outward) angulation of the heel and excessive dorsiflexion, with the foot resting against the anterolateral aspect of the tibia. While most cases correct spontaneously, treating severe cases includes stretching and serial casting. In rare instances, if left untreated, severe cases can persist into adolescence and manifest as pes planus (flatfoot).

An *accessory navicular bone* is a small ossicle at the medial tuberosity of the navicular. Individuals with an accessory navicular bone often complain of pressure and discomfort while wearing shoes. Placing prefabricated arch support in the shoe can elevate the arch sufficiently to minimize friction and rubbing against the shoe.

Hallux valgus (bunions) is most often the consequence of rearfoot valgus, leading to varus of the first metatarsal. The conservative approaches to treating this condition in children are orthoses and comfortable shoes, with a good heel counter to maintain the heel in subtalar neutral.

Curly toes involve the congenital shortening of the flexor tendons. Treated conservatively, flexors are stretched, and a rocker-like insole is used in the shoe to support the toes in extension. Additionally, it is important that shoes have extra depth with plenty of room in the toe box.

Shoe prescription for these biomechanical problems of the foot and lower extremities in childhood is as valuable as a conservative corrective intervention. Overall, a soft-soled shoe is appropriate if a child's foot is developing normally and does not exhibit any signs of an abnormality. If some degree of abnormality exists, a more supportive, rigid shoe is indicated for toddlers. Generally, the stiffer the heel counter, the more effective the intervention.

The most common prescription shoe for young children is a straight-last shoe. This type of shoe is roomy enough to accommodate pads or wedges. In addition, a straight-last shoe does not generate any abnormal forces against the child's foot.

FOOT DURING PREGNANCY

Females may experience problems in their lower extremities during pregnancy, including edema, leg cramps, restless legs syndrome, joint laxity, and low back pain. As a result, foot pain is a common problem in pregnant females.[21,22] An important consideration is the provision of shoes with maximum shock absorption. Gel-cushioned running shoes are recommended, especially if females continue to jog or walk for exercise. Expectant mothers are also advised to exercise on soft surfaces to prevent problems caused by repetitive pounding on unforgiving surfaces.

High-heeled shoes exaggerate the lordotic curve and are inadvisable during pregnancy. As weight distribution shifts with advancing pregnancy, especially if edema occurs, many females choose to wear shoes with laces or a Velcro closure. Athletic and walking shoes provide good support, excellent cushioning, and a solid heel counter. If a heel is desired for special occasions, a 1-inch or lower-heeled shoe should be recommended. Even low but tiny tapered heels cause females to wobble as they walk.

Many females find that their feet have "grown" during pregnancy; after having returned to prepregnancy weight and clothing, their shoes no longer fit. Measurements often reflect an increase in shoe length of a half to a full size. The stress of extra body weight coupled with ligamentous laxity can reduce arch height, adding length to the feet. This process is a typical age-related change in foot structure, associated with wear and tear of the body over time, which is hastened during pregnancy. The hormonally induced tissue laxity of pregnancy leads to a broader forefoot as the metatarsal heads separate and the distal transverse arch flattens and to a longer foot as soft tissue structures less efficiently support the longitudinal arch. For this reason, pregnant females are advised to wear a larger shoe size, with a square or deeper toe box or both, especially if edema is also a problem.

Gabriel et al., in a research study titled *Anthropometric Foot Changes During Pregnancy*, concluded that "the foot of the pregnant woman tends to flatten during gestational weeks 12 to 34, taking a more pronated posture, and the anthropometric changes in late pregnancy result in increases in foot length and forefoot width, changes that seem to be moderate."[23] The hormonal changes during pregnancy—which cause ligamentous laxity, flattening of the medial longitudinal arch, excessive pronation of the foot, and pregnancy-induced forward displacement of the center of gravity—cause foot pain, increased strain on the axial skeleton, and reduced efficiency of gait. Foot orthotics to support the metatarsal heads and medial longitudinal arch, placed in shoes with good shock-absorbing ability, can help decrease foot discomfort and prevent injury to the low back during pregnancy.[24]

FOOT IN LATER LIFE

Foot problems are among the most common complaints of older adults. Nearly one-third of community-dwelling adults 65 years of age or older experience a fall.[25] Falls are the primary reason behind both fatal and nonfatal injuries in the aged population, leading to functional decline, institutionalization, and reduced quality of life. Researchers explain that the reasons for falls among older adults are multifaceted and often the result of a combination of intrinsic (e.g., preexisting disease or chronic conditions, polypharmacy, muscle weakness, functional limitations, and vision impairment) and extrinsic risk factors such as hazards in the home and poor footwear. Several outcome measures are used to assess the risk of falling.[25,26] The increased risk of falls among older adults has led to investigating factors that contribute to falls.[25] One of the factors associated with loss of balance and falls is the type of footwear worn.[27,28] To address the problem of frequent falls in the geriatric population, researchers studied the footwear worn by older patients.[27] Senior persons often wear poorly fitted shoes, slippers, and sandals, contributing to poor balance and increasing the risk of falls. Persons in hospital settings wearing hospital slippers are at greater risk for falls.

Gait and foot problems in older adults are associated with diseases that are common in later life and the natural aging process. Various conditions that can compromise gait and foot function include the residuals of congenital deformities, ventricular enlargement, spinal cord diseases, joint deformities, muscle contractures, peripheral nerve injuries, peripheral vascular disease, cerebrovascular accidents, trauma, ulcers, arthritis, diabetes, inactivity, and degenerative and chronic diseases. The anatomic and biomechanical considerations of podogeriatrics focus on the rearfoot, midfoot, and forefoot relationships established by osseous, muscle, and connective tissue structures. One joint's movement influences other joints in the foot and ankle. Soft tissue structures establish an interdependency of the foot and ankle to the entire lower limb. As tissues age, they tend to become stiffer, less flexible, weaker, and more susceptible to damage and breakdown.

Foot contour alters with aging; the foot gets wider, and bunions and splaying occur from the collapse of the transverse arch. Forefoot height increases in the presence of toe deformities. Fat pads under the metatarsal joints atrophy and shift position distally, whereas the calcaneal fat pad atrophies and shifts laterally. These changes leave bony prominences that are vulnerable to breakdown.

In persons with type 2 diabetes, the development of Charcot joints (neuropathic arthropathy) is a relatively painless, degenerative, progressive neuropathic destruction of the bony architecture. The ankle mortis and the tarsal and metatarsal joints are most frequently affected.[29]

With the sensory losses that are common in type 2 diabetes, these joints are subjected to extreme stresses without the benefits of normal protective mechanisms. Capsular and ligamentous stretching, joint laxity, distention, subluxation, dislocation, cartilage fibrillation, osteochondral fragmentation, and fracture can occur. Motor impairment contributes to the wasting of muscles in the feet and permits digital contractures as a compensatory mechanism for dynamic muscular imbalances. Thus Charcot collapse may lead to the development of a rocker-bottom foot and increases the likelihood of developing hammertoe deformities.[29]

Many older adults with type 2 diabetes attribute their problem with walking to pain or a sense of unsteadiness, stiffness, dizziness, numbness, or impaired proprioception. Preventing foot ulcers due to poor circulation, poor sensation, and ill-fitted footwear is critical for persons with diabetes. Persons with type 2 diabetes and dysvascular foot disease have a greater need for specialized footwear such as custom-molded shoes.[30,31]

Physical therapists work with older individuals to reduce pain, improve circulation through exercise, increase muscle strength, improve balance and flexibility, and modify the reaction times of movements to maximize the individual's functional abilities and upright mobility. Assessing old adults for appropriate footwear is a fundamental requirement for enabling them to become functional in ambulation.

Proper shoe fitting and minimal modifications to shoes are often sufficient to manage the majority of foot problems in the geriatric population. The most inexpensive footwear for this patient population comprises running or walking shoes. These are less expensive and fit within a fixed-income budget. They provide good foot support and can be purchased with Velcro straps for closure if hand function or foot edema is a problem. The Thermold shoe is also appropriate for many pathologic and structural deformities the older patient must deal with that do not involve unhealed foot ulcers. When foot ulcers are present, and prevention of limb becomes a critical concern, more extensive therapeutic interventions are required, such as removable or nonremovable foot casts.[32]

Choosing Appropriate Footwear and Socks

A vast and somewhat bewildering variety of "off-the-shelf" footwear is available to consumers. Many shoes are designed with certain types of activities in mind. Understanding their design and construction and ensuring proper fit can enhance foot health and minimize the risk of foot dysfunction, injury, and pain.

ATHLETIC SHOE GEAR

Many people jump into fitness activities "feet first" and develop blisters, calluses, and other foot injuries because of inappropriate footwear. A well-fitting, activity-appropriate athletic shoe enhances the enjoyment of the activity by protecting and supporting the foot and minimizing injury. Athletic shoes are designed for specific activities. A running shoe is designed with a high-force heel impact and forward foot movement in mind; the various shoe models have specific features for different surface conditions and distances in running. Basketball shoes do not provide as much cushioning as running shoes, but instead, focus on foot support during quick lateral movement. Aerobic shoes are also designed for lateral movement but offer more cushioning for the impact anticipated on the ball of the foot. Shoe soles are also designed for the surface on which the activity is performed. Some shoes are manufactured as cross-training shoes so they can go from the workout in the gym to jogging, but they are not designed for high-mileage runners.

Determining the foot type is essential in prescribing the best shoe. For individuals with a flat, low-arched foot, a shoe that provides maximum stability to prevent the foot from rolling in with each step is required. High-arched feet demand a more flexible shoe. "Normal" feet do best in a shoe that combines the last to accommodate the heel and the forefoot and has forefoot flexibility. The size and shape of the toe box must also be considered. Enough room should be available in the toe box to prevent blisters, ulcers, and chafing of the toes. Shoes made from "breathable" materials to promote airflow and prevent excessive sweating are desirable. Athletic shoes are best used only for their intended activity and should be replaced regularly to maximize their effectiveness.

Most athletic footwear is available in medium widths, although a few manufacturers provide shoes in several widths. Children's athletic footwear is available in narrow, medium, and wide widths. Women's athletic footwear may be available in AA, B, and D widths. Men's athletic footwear may be available in B, D, EE, and EEE widths. The key element in the proper fit of athletic shoes is comfort from the moment the shoe is put on, with no break-in period needed. The shoe should also provide adequate support and shock absorption for the sport or activity that is being pursued.

WALKING SHOES

A well-designed walking shoe provides stable rearfoot control, ample forefoot room, and a shock absorption heel and sole. This type of footwear may be specifically designed by an athletic footwear manufacturer or even by an orthopedic footwear manufacturer. Walking shoes are available in various widths and several different lasts. Long medial counters, Thomas heels, and crepe soles can be used to modify this type of shoe gear to meet specific needs.

DRESS SHOES

Despite the current trend favoring shoes with narrow or pointed toes and slim high heels, the most foot-friendly dress shoe for females is a rounded-toe Mary Jane style with boxy heels. An ideal dress shoe should mimic the shape of the individual's foot, offering flexibility and effective shock absorption. When selecting a good dress shoe, looking for a few key characteristics is essential. These include a roomy toe box, low and stable heel, proper width in the ball of the foot area, flexible outsole with skidproof bottoms, and adequate arch support.

It is advisable to steer clear of dress shoes with triangular toe boxes and high heels, regardless of their delicate appearance, as they can lead to foot deformities. A high-heeled shoe requires a snug fit around the toes to remain on the foot, resulting in no room for anything but the foot. The foot is virtually unsupported at the distal end of the shank, exerting excessive pressure on the metatarsal heads. Heels higher than 2 inches render any orthosis ineffective. Because the angle of the foot causes the heel of the orthosis to lift up, high heels can transform an orthosis into a catapulting device. Although orthoses can alleviate metatarsal and heel pain and provide arch support, they cannot correct the issues caused by shoes designed so unnaturally for the human foot.

SOCKS

Socks are frequently overlooked when shoes of any kind are prescribed. However, socks play a vital role in various aspects of foot care. They contribute to shock absorption, safeguard the skin against abrasion caused by shoe stitching and lining, and prevent irritation from dyes and synthetic leather materials. Additionally, clean, freshly laundered socks are crucial to a sanitary foot environment. Unbleached white cotton socks are ideal because they lack dyes, are hypoallergenic, and absorb perspiration readily. Unlike stretchable fabric socks that can crowd the toes, cotton socks provide sufficient room for the toes.

The size and style of socks also influence foot health. Socks that are too short crowd the toes; those that are too long wrinkle within the shoe, creating potential shear pressure points. When wearing knee-high socks, it is crucial to ensure that the proximal band is not overly restrictive. Likewise, circumferential garters to hold socks can impede circulation to the foot. Any holes worn into a sock also potentially create shear pressures, and such a sock should be discarded. Because of the difference in thickness and materials, mended holes in socks can irritate delicate or insensate soft tissue. An open hole at the toes pinches and constricts the digits, with excessive friction at the hole's edges.

Specially designed socks that support and cushion the insensitive foot or athletic/military foot that is exposed to repetitive frictional forces are commercially available.[33] These specialized socks reduce friction and shearing forces and significantly decrease vertical ground reaction pressure, thus preventing blisters and ulcers.[30] Extra high-density padding functions as a natural fat pad, reducing the destructive effects of shearing forces, pressure, and friction in the toe area. Supportive socks have proven beneficial for individuals with insensitive feet and are widely used in aerobic exercise, baseball, basketball, cycling, golf, hiking, trekking and climbing, skiing, tennis, walking, and running.

Prescription Footwear, Custom-Molded Shoes, Accommodative Molded Orthoses, and Shoe Modifications

Alteration of foot function and alignment can be accomplished with one or more of the following strategies: use of foot orthoses[34] or prescription shoes[35] and modifications of shoes themselves.[36] These strategies relieve pain and improve balance and function during standing and locomotion. Such alternatives are particularly recommended when a transfer of forces from sensitive to pressure-tolerant areas is needed to reduce friction, shock, and shear forces; to modify weight transfer patterns; to correct flexible foot deformities; to accommodate for fixed foot deformities; and to restrict motion in joints that are painful, inflamed, or unstable.

When considering special protective or prescription footwear, the functional objectives must be clearly stated to develop appropriate specific prescription. A careful, comprehensive examination of the foot allows the clinician to identify any pathologic conditions or mechanical factors that need to be addressed. Based on these findings, the clinician can choose the appropriate materials and footwear styles to meet the patient's specific needs.

MOLDABLE LEATHERS

Thermold is a type of prescription footwear designed to protect feet vulnerable due to vascular insufficiency, neuropathy, or deformity. It is a cross-linked, closed-cell polyethylene foam laminated to the leather upper of the footwear that can be heat-molded directly to the foot. This method is more cost-effective compared to custom molding options. Thermold shoes are also available in extra-depth styles with a removable ¼-inch insole. Extra-depth shoes enable adequate room for custom-made insoles or orthoses to become an intricate adjunct to the footwear. The Thermold, in some cases, can be used as an alternative to custom-molded footwear.

CUSTOM-MOLDED SHOES

Custom-molded shoes may be the most effective solution when certain foot problems cannot be addressed with conventional footwear.

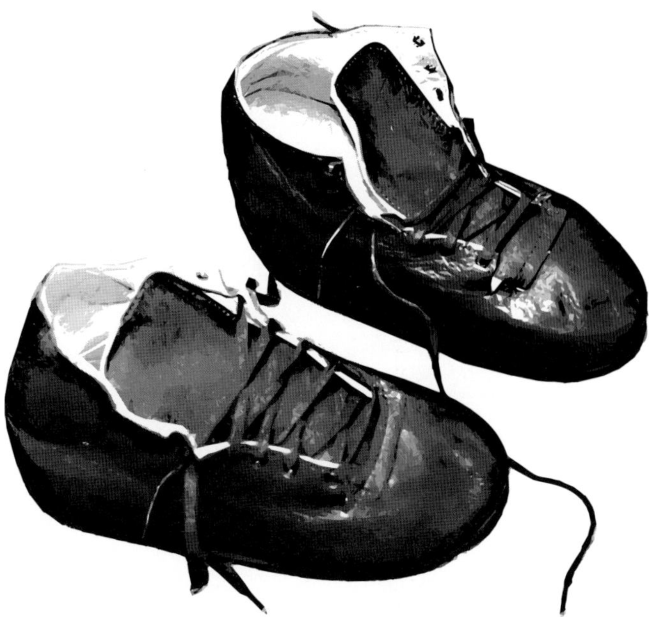

Fig. 7.5 **Examples of custom-molded shoes. These shoes are prescribed when foot deformities are too severe for accommodation in a conventional shoe.** Courtesy Ottawa Foot Balance, Ottawa, Ontario, Canada.

This footwear is molded directly over a plaster reproduction of the foot rather than a standard last. Special modifications—such as toe fillers, Plastazote, rocker bars, and elevations—can be added during manufacturing to meet the specific requirements of each foot. Because of this process, custom-molded shoes are made to conform to the foot shape in all respects (Fig. 7.5). Custom orthopedic shoes represent the ultimate combination of function and esthetics. By combining biomechanics and skilled craftsmanship, custom-molded shoes can redistribute weight, restrict joint motion, facilitate ambulation, and lower the risk of neuropathic ulceration.[34,37,38]

PLASTAZOTE SHOE OR SANDAL

A "healing sandal" or Plastazote shoe is often prescribed for patients with insensitive or ulcerated feet. This custom shoe is fabricated using a plaster cast of the individual's foot construction.[39] Temporary protective footwear, such as a Plastazote boot or shoe or a healing sandal, is often used, while a neuropathic ulcer heals to allow for ambulation without pressure on the healing area, especially for patients who are unable to walk or noncompliant with non–weight-bearing ambulation.

SHOE MODIFICATIONS

Various shoe modifications can be used to address functional and anatomic deformities of the foot and leg. Clearly stated objectives, based on careful evaluation, ensure that the appropriate shoe modifications are chosen.

Lifts for Leg-Length Discrepancy

For individuals with a leg-length discrepancy of ⅜ inch or more, a full-length external lift can be mounted to the shoe's sole on the shorter limb to equalize leg length and reduce proximal stresses at the hips and spine. If the length difference is less than ⅜ inch, the discrepancy can usually be accommodated with an orthotic heel wedge worn inside the shoe. If the discrepancy results from a unilateral equinus deformity, a heel wedge can be attached to the external surface of the shoe. The leg-length discrepancy is a common result of a hip fracture, congenital anomaly, or biomechanical imbalance such as pelvic rotation, hip anteversion or retroversion, or unilateral foot pronation. The level of the pelvis and absolute and relative measures of leg length should be part of a comprehensive gait evaluation.[40]

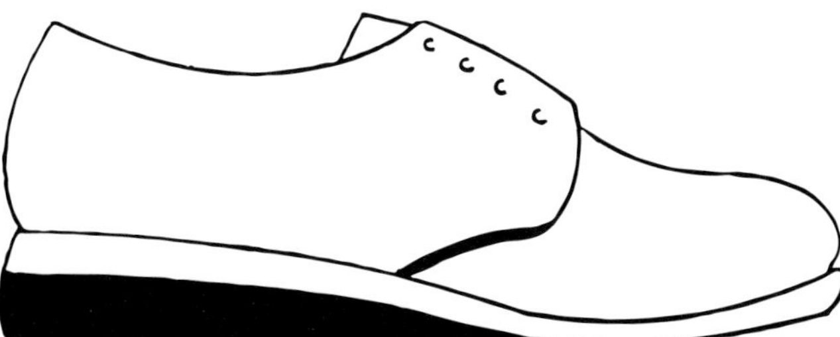

Fig. 7.6 **A heel wedge provides elevation of the heel for equinus deformity.** Courtesy Dr. Richard Blake of San Francisco.

Heel Wedging

Wedging is used to alter lines of stress to facilitate a more normal gait pattern. The most effective wedges range from ⅛ to ¼ inches in thickness at their apex. Larger wedges tend to cause the foot to slide away from the wedge toward the opposite side of the shoe, drastically reducing the effectiveness of the modification. Wedging is helpful for children with rotational problems, such as tibial torsion. In adults, wedges are used for accommodation in conditions such as a fixed valgus deformity of the calcaneus (Fig. 7.6).

A medial heel wedge is used when a flexible valgus of the calcaneus is present (Fig. 7.7A). As the wedge elevates the medial heel, a resultant varus tilt acts on the calcaneus, preventing excessive foot pronation. A lateral heel wedge is used when a flexible varus of the calcaneus is present (see Fig. 7.7B). Elevating the lateral heel decreases the medial drive on floor contact at heel strike, tipping the calcaneus into valgus. A full heel wedge is sometimes used in the presence of fixed or functional equinus deformity. The goal of wedging is to obtain a subtalar neutral position during the stance phase of gait.[41]

Sole Wedging

Wedging can also be used to modify midfoot and forefoot positions. A medial sole wedge produces an inversion effect on the forefoot. This wedge is positioned along the medial aspect of the footwear, from a point just proximal of the first metatarsal head to the midline of the footwear (see Fig. 7.7C). Conversely, a lateral sole wedge creates an eversion effect at the forefoot. This wedge is placed proximal to the fifth metatarsal head to the midline of the footwear. The apex of this wedge is the fifth metatarsal head (see Fig. 7.7D).

A Barton wedge (see Fig. 7.7E) is used in severe flexible pronation deformities, such as those seen in pes planus, when midfoot control is the goal. The Barton wedge, usually

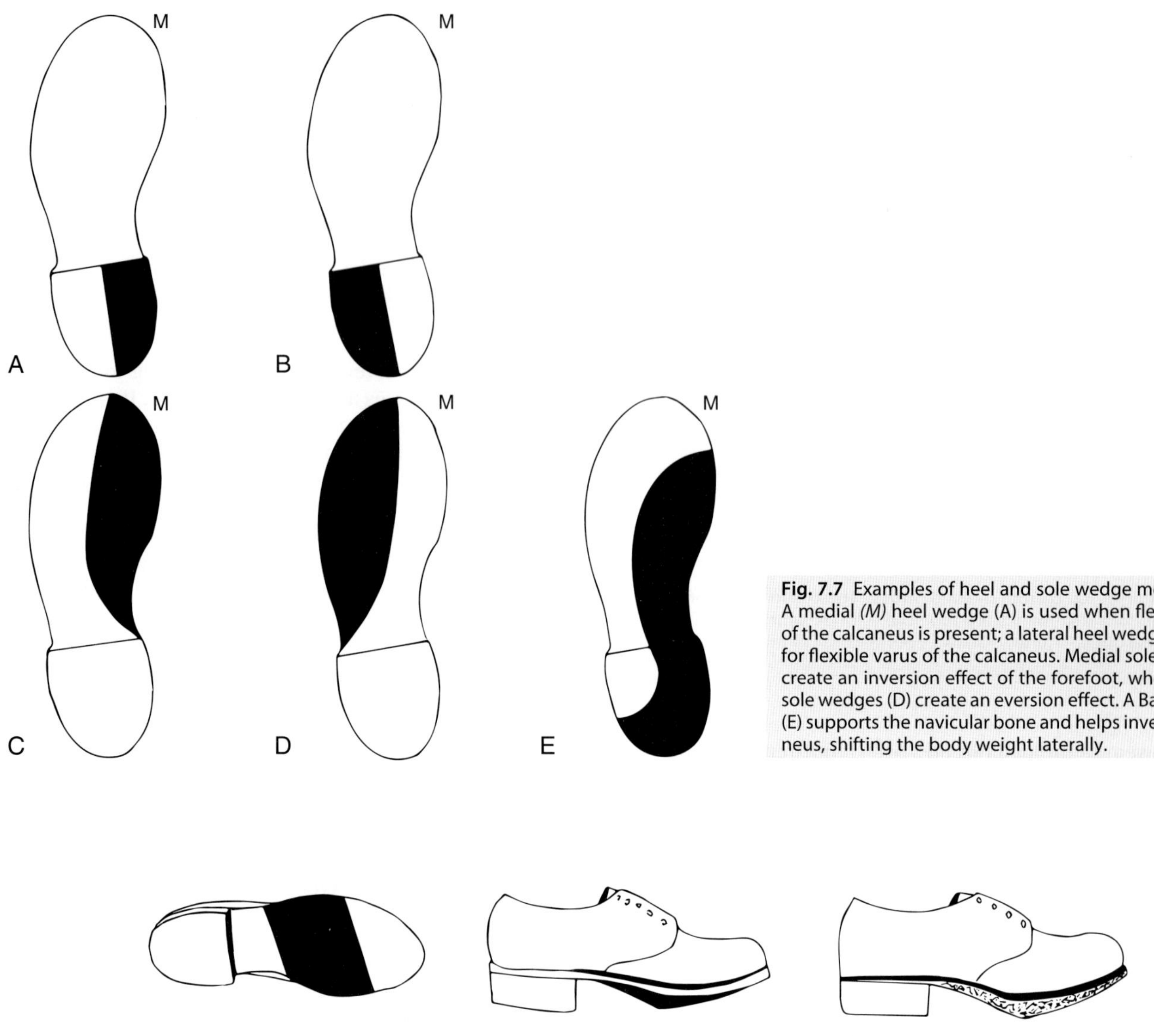

Fig. 7.7 Examples of heel and sole wedge modifications. A medial *(M)* heel wedge (A) is used when flexible valgus of the calcaneus is present; a lateral heel wedge (B) is used for flexible varus of the calcaneus. Medial sole wedges (C) create an inversion effect of the forefoot, whereas lateral sole wedges (D) create an eversion effect. A Barton wedge (E) supports the navicular bone and helps invert the calcaneus, shifting the body weight laterally.

Fig. 7.8 Examples of rocker-bottom soles. A metatarsal bar (A) prevents undue pressure at the metatarsal heads during push-off in late stance. A rigid leather rocker sole (B) or an extended crepe rocker bar (C) redistributes body weight over the entire plantar surface, facilitating a smoother and more normal gait pattern while reducing stress and trauma in the forefoot.

made with (1/16)-inch leather, extends along the medial side of the foot to the midtarsal joint and tapers laterally just anterior to the cuboid bone. It provides support to the navicular and helps invert the calcaneus. It is used when it is necessary to shift body weight laterally. The shoe must have a firm medial counter when a Barton wedge is used. The Barton wedge can be incorporated in an internally placed lateral heel wedge for patients with fixed calcaneal varus or clubfoot deformity. Because an internal wedge is closer to the target deformity, it creates a greater positive force than possible with the external Barton wedge. Instead of tilting the footgear, the wedge tilts the calcaneus into the desired position.[42]

Metatarsal Bars and Rocker Bottoms

A metatarsal bar is a solid piece of material, typically composed of stacked leather or rubber, affixed to a shoe's sole. Positioning proximal to the metatarsal heads is crucial in reducing the pressure exerted on these specific areas during the push-off phase of the walking cycle.[43,44] The curved distal edge of the metatarsal bar is designed to follow the curve of the metatarsal heads. It is commonly used to adapt shoes worn by patients with transmetatarsal amputations, fixed arthritic deformities, diabetes, and forefoot deformities such as hallux rigidus, and neuromas. The placement of a metatarsal bar or rocker facilitates push-off by simulating forward propulsion in the absence of metatarsal flexibility.

Rocker bottoms are made of either lightweight crepe or leather (Fig. 7.8). These modifications are flush with the heel and toe in an arch with an apex of ½ to ⅝ inch. The rocker bar redistributes body forces over the entire plantar surface of the foot while it bears weight. It facilitates a smooth roll during the stance phase of gait, reducing sheer stress and trauma to the midfoot and forefoot. It is often used to modify shoes worn by patients with partial foot amputations, arthritis, and diabetes. It is also used for patients with any lower extremity orthosis that limits the forward progression of the tibia over the foot and toes during the middle and late stance phases. For patients with diabetes, a rigid rocker sole (a steel-spring heel-to-toe with the toes extended and a rocking axis near the center of the foot) can be used to help distribute body weight and compel knee flexion at toe-off, thus reducing the length of stride and shear stress on the metatarsal heads.

Thomas Heels

The Thomas heel is a type of corrective shoe design that involves the heel being around 12 mm longer and 4 to 6 mm higher on the medial edge. This design induces varus positioning of the foot, effectively preventing depression of the head of the talus.[45] The Thomas heel is designed to improve foot balance and relieve excessive pressure on the shank portion of the footwear. Applied as either a lateral or a medial flare of the heel, its goal is to increase stability during gait by assimilating subtalar neutral. A laterally flared heel is used with a rearfoot varus to decrease the incidence of inversion injuries. A medially flared heel is used with a rearfoot valgus to decrease the incidence of eversion injuries (Fig. 7.9).

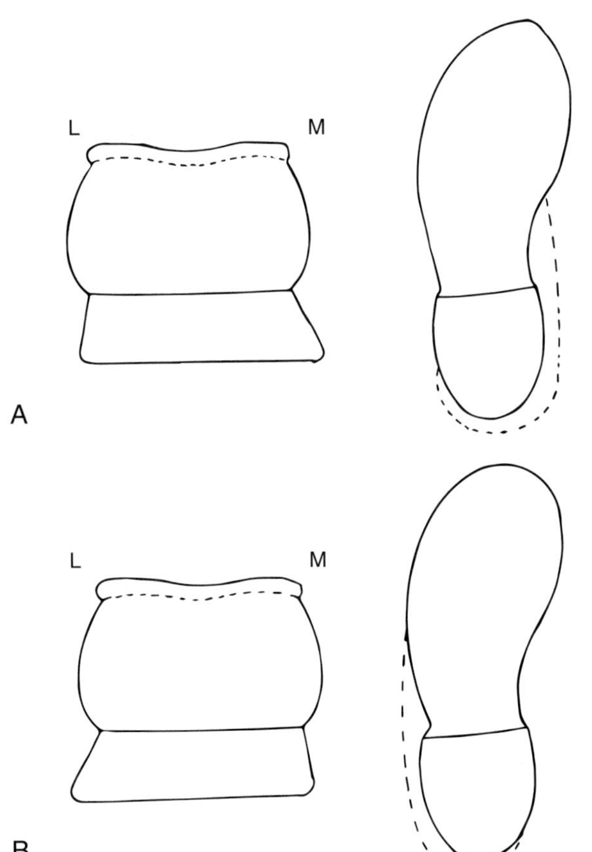

Fig. 7.9 Examples of Thomas heels. (A) A medial *(M)* flared heel provides a broader base of support and prevents eversion of the ankle. (B) A lateral *(L)* flared heel prevents inversion of the ankle.

For instance, a medial flare from the heel to the sustentaculum tali prevents excessive pronation of the foot during gait.

Offset Heels and Shoe Counters

The offset heel is a modification employed to address valgus or varus deformities. It provides a broad support base, especially at the superior surface of the heel, where the broad buildup against the shoe's counter provides reinforcement either medially or laterally. A heel counter is an extension along the medial or lateral borders of the shoe from the heel to the proximal border of the fifth or first metatarsal head. This shoe modification strengthens the shank portion of the footwear for better control of the hindfoot. The heel counter is often used in combination with the appropriate Thomas heel. A counter can also be placed medially or laterally in the midfoot region. In cases where the patient exhibits excessive pronation in their gait, as is common in rheumatoid arthritis (RA), a firm medial counter may be necessary to prevent the medial collapse of the shoe and aid in realigning the foot to a neutral position.

Attachments for Orthoses

For some patients with neuromuscular dysfunction (e.g., hemiplegia, paraplegia, multiple sclerosis), a traditional metal double-upright lower extremity orthosis can be prescribed. If so, the shoe must be modified: a U-shaped orthotic bracket (stirrup) is attached using three copper rivets, one on the heel and two on the shank. The metal is riveted through the outsole to the insole. To accomplish this, the heel is removed, and the stirrup plate is attached. The groove is then cut through the heel, and the heel is reattached. The appropriate orthotic ankle joint is then attached to the uprights of the stirrup.

Shoe Stretching

Shoes crafted with leather uppers can be stretched almost one full width. While it is not possible to physically lengthen a shoe, it can be made to feel longer with a toe box stretcher device that looks like the shape of the foot and is inserted into the shoe to expand it (Fig. 7.10). After the leather is moistened or softened, this device effectively raises and slightly rounds the toe box. The pressure exerted by a flat toe box on the toes often poses more issues than the shoe's actual length. To address this, specific points within the shoe can be softened and expanded by utilizing an "expansion knob" on the toe-box stretcher or a ball-and-socket device. Site-specific stretching particularly benefits patients with toe deformities such as hallux valgus, hammertoe, mallet toe, claw toe, overlapping toes, and Taylor bunion deformity.[1]

Blowout Patches and Gussets

Patients with foot deformities who prefer conventional shoes to Thermold shoes may find temporary pain relief if a blowout patch or gusset is applied to their shoe. The shoe leather around the area of deformity is cut away and replaced with a softer blowout patch or gusset of moleskin, soft leather, or suede.

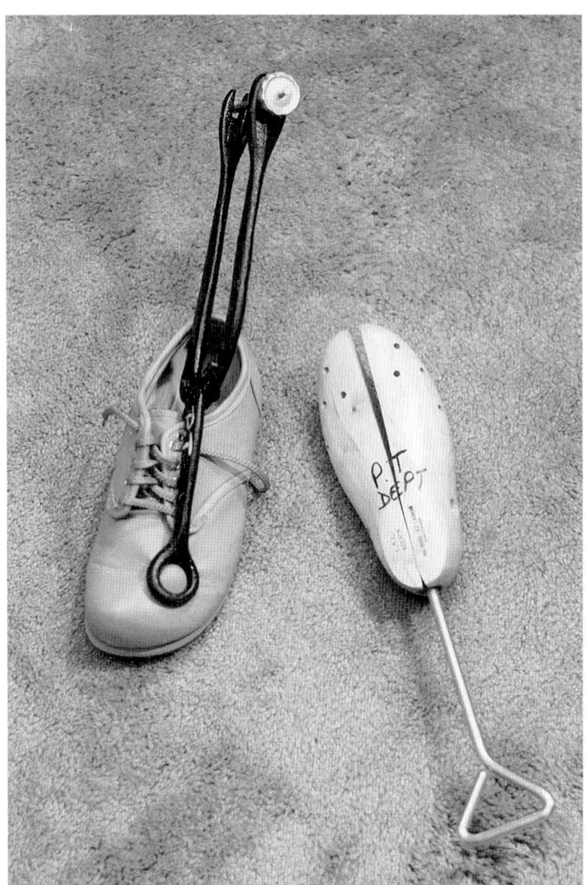

Fig. 7.10 Tools used to stretch leather shoes. Stretching often provides adequate accommodation for deformities in conventional shoes. Courtesy Colonial Medical Assisted Devices, Nashua, New Hampshire.

Footwear for Common Foot Deformities and Problems

Conservative management of common forefoot, midfoot, and rearfoot deformities often involves modification of shoes, prescription footwear, or both. Specific footwear strategies for several common foot problems are described in the following section.

PROBLEMS IN THE FOREFOOT

The most common footwear variation used for abnormalities in the forefoot is a high toe box. High toe boxes are available in various types of footwear, including athletic sneakers, comfort shoes, Thermolds, and prescription footwear. To best address any deformities in the forefoot, it is important to measure the maximum height of abnormal toes while weight-bearing. Tables of manufactured shoes by toe box space are available to guide the clinician in recommending shoes that most closely match a patient's needs.[46]

Metatarsalgia

Metatarsalgia is pain around the metatarsal heads that results from compression of the plantar digital nerve as it courses between the metatarsal heads. Excessive weight bearing with atrophy of the metatarsal fat pad can irritate the nerves and potentially lead to the development of a neuroma. The three major objectives in shoe prescription for patients with metatarsalgia are to (1) transfer pressure from painful, sensitive areas to more pressure-tolerant areas; (2) reduce friction by stabilizing the MTP joint; and (3) stabilize the rearfoot and midfoot to reduce pressure on the metatarsal heads.[47] Characteristics of the shoe that will accomplish these goals include wide width to reduce pressure on the transverse metatarsal arch, long fitting to eliminate plantarflexed MTP joints, cushion soles to enhance shock absorption, and a high toe box to allow forefoot flexion and extension. In addition, the shoe should feature a lengthy medial counter to provide stability to the rearfoot. A lower heel is recommended to reduce pressure on the metatarsal heads, and thermoldable leather is preferable for accommodating deformities. Shoe modifications often include a transverse metatarsal bar to redistribute pressure from metatarsal heads to metatarsal shafts and shorten stride and a rocker sole to reduce the motion of painful joints.[48]

Sesamoiditis

Sesamoiditis refers to inflammation around the sesamoid bones located beneath the first metatarsal head. It often results from a loss of soft tissue padding under the first metatarsal head and from toe deformities such as hallux valgus and hallux rigidus. The goal of prescribing shoes for patients with sesamoiditis is to redistribute weight-bearing forces from the first MTP joint and its sesamoids to the long medial arch and shafts of the lesser metatarsals. A transverse metatarsal bar is employed to redirect pressure from the metatarsal heads to the metatarsal shafts and shorten the stride. A rocker sole can be used to reduce the motion of the painful hallux joint.

Morton Syndrome

The Morton toe/Morton foot syndrome was first described by Dudley J. Morton, an orthopedic surgeon, researcher, physician, and author.[49] Morton syndrome is the configuration of the foot in which the second toe is either the same size as the great toe or slightly longer than the great toe. The increased length of the second ray causes lateral instability. The three major objectives in shoe prescription for patients with Morton syndrome are to (1) redistribute weight from the lesser metatarsals (especially the second and third) to the proximal phalanx of the hallux; (2) stabilize the rearfoot by maintaining subtalar joint neutral; and (3) accommodate forefoot varus as well as a possibly dorsiflexed first metatarsal. Shoe prescription includes a long medial counter for rearfoot support and stability, a straight or flared last to accommodate foot shape, a high wide toe box to reduce compression across the transverse metatarsal arch, a large enough shoe size to accommodate the long second toe, and a Thomas heel or wedge sole to support the medial longitudinal arch. In cases of severe symptoms, it may be necessary to incorporate a medial heel and medial sole wedge to provide additional support and relief.

Morton (Interdigital) Neuroma

Morton neuroma is a painful condition of the foot characterized by neural degeneration and perineural fibrosis, most commonly seen between the third and fourth or the second and third metatarsals.[50] Overstretching of the digital nerves during extreme extension of the toes at the proximal phalanx can also lead to the formation of a neuroma. Two objectives should be considered for patients with Morton neuroma. First, the patient must obtain relief from the pain and burning, especially in the third interspace of the MTP joint. Second, compression of the digital nerve as it passes between the heads of the third and fourth metatarsals must be reduced. To achieve these goals, the shoe should have a wide width to eliminate transverse compression and sufficient length to reduce plantarflexion of the MTP joints. A long medial counter can assist in reducing the pronation, a cushioned sole increases shock absorption, and a low heel unloads pressure on the metatarsals. Elastic laces may be beneficial in allowing expansion of the forefoot. Shoe modifications for Morton neuroma might include a metatarsal bar to elevate the metatarsals and redistribute weight, a metatarsal rocker bar to immobilize the metatarsals, or a combination of both approaches.[51,52]

Metatarsalgia of the Fifth Metatarsophalangeal Joint

Similar to the previously described condition of metatarsalgia described, metatarsalgia of the fifth MTP joint results in plantar digital nerve irritation at the interdigital space of the fourth and fifth metatarsal heads. When metatarsalgia of the fifth MTP joint is present, treatment objectives are to redistribute the weight forces onto the fifth metatarsal shaft and provide a wide base of support along the lateral border of the foot. The optimal shoe should have a last with enough lateral flare to accommodate the lateral aspect of the foot and fifth metatarsal shaft, along with a sturdy lateral counter and a firm sole made of leather or rubber. Possible shoe modifications include a lateral heel and sole flare ending proximal to the fifth metatarsal head to provide a broader base of support. Lateral heel and sole wedges may be useful for patients with flexible feet.

Hallux Rigidus (Limitus)

The degenerative joint disease of the first MTP joint causes pain, loss of mobility, and, eventually, joint fusion. Osteophyte formation on the dorsal aspects of the metatarsal head and base of the proximal phalanx can be quite painful and result in a loss of extension. For patients with hallux rigidus or limitus, the goals are to limit motion of the hallux and first MTP joint and to reduce pressure on the dorsal and plantar aspects of the hallux and first MTP joint.[53] To achieve this, the shoe should feature a high, wide toe box and uppers made of Thermold or soft leather. In cases where there is significant deformity, adding a steel shank extending from the heel to the phalanx of the big toe, along with a rigid rocker sole, and compensating heel elevation may be necessary.

Hallux Valgus (Bunions)

Hallux valgus is characterized by a lateral deviation (abduction) of the hallux with a corresponding medial deviation (adduction) of the first metatarsal.[54] The deformity tends to persist and worsen due to walking with a foot angle rotated outward and excessive foot pronation, which are common compensations during gait.[46] Hallux valgus deformity is often associated with long-term wearing of shoes with a triangular toe box. When prescribing shoes for patients with hallux valgus, five objectives should be considered in the prescription of shoes for patients with hallux valgus: (1) to reduce friction and pressure to the first MTP joint; (2) to eliminate abnormal pressure from narrow-fitting shoes; (3) to reduce pronation of the foot from heel strike to midstance; (4) to correct eversion; and (5) to relieve strain on the posterior tibial tendon ligament. Patients with hallux valgus benefit from shoes with high wide toe boxes and Thermold or soft leather uppers. A combined last with increased last width in the toe box and a smaller heel for better control of the subtalar joint may also be indicated. Additionally, choosing longer and wider shoes helps accommodate the deformity. A lower heel reduces pressure on the forefoot, and a reinforced medial counter helps prevent excessive pronation.[46]

Hammertoes, Claw Toes, and Mallet Toes

Hammertoe deformity is characterized by hyperextension of the MTP joint, flexion of the proximal interphalangeal (PIP) joint, and extension of the distal interphalangeal (DIP) joint. This leads to high load during weight bearing at the plantar metatarsal heads and at the plantar surface of the distal phalanx. Claw toe deformity involves hyperflexion of the PIP and DIP joints, with the MTP joint potentially being hyperextended or hyperflexed.[55] Mallet toe deformity results from hyperextension of the MTP joint, flexion of the PIP, and a neutral position of the DIP so that weight bearing is on the tip of the distal phalanx. Deformities of the lesser toes can be problematic, especially for patients with compromised circulation and neuropathy. For these individuals, there are two major footwear goals: (1) to transfer pressure away from the metatarsal heads, the PIP joints, and the distal phalanx joints and (2) to encourage flexion of the MTP joints and extension of the PIP joints.[46] Patients with lesser toe deformities should wear shoes with a high, wide toe box made of soft leather or Thermold material to minimize the risk of microtrauma over bony prominences. The shoe should also be long enough to allow flexion of MTP joints and extension of PIP joints rather than cramping the toes. Finally, a soft cushion outsole and low heel further reduce pressure on the metatarsal heads. Commonly used shoe modifications for lesser toe deformities include metatarsal bars to reduce pressure to metatarsal heads, shift weight bearing to metatarsal shafts, and a rocker bar or rocker sole to accommodate rollover on fixed deformity.

PROBLEMS IN THE MIDFOOT

Shoe prescriptions, modifications, or both are also helpful in managing midfoot dysfunction and deformity. The most commonly encountered problems include pes planus, pes equinus, pes cavus, and plantar fasciitis.

Pes Planus

Pes planus refers to the inward rolling of the midfoot that results in a failure of the foot to supinate during midstance. This causes the longitudinal arch to flatten, leading to splaying of the forefoot and the metatarsals deviating laterally. The deformity can be flexible or fixed (rigid). In cases of flexible pes planus, the intervention aims to reduce pronation from heel strike to midstance, correct eversion, alleviate tension on the posterior tibial tendon, and relieve strain on the ligaments.[10] To achieve these objectives, the shoe should offer a long medial heel counter, a Thomas heel (medial extension) or a firm wedge sole, and a straight last. Severe cases may require custom-made shoes. In extreme cases, shoe modifications may include a medial heel wedge to correct eversion and reduce pronation or a medial heel and sole flare.[46]

Because of the fixed nature of a rigid pes planus, the goals are somewhat different. The focus is on relieving ligamentous strain and arch pain and correcting foot eversion. The optimal shoe should offer a broad shank (extra wide midfoot), a straight last, and a long medial counter. Additionally, a wedge sole minimizes the load on the metatarsal heads, stabilizes the intertarsal joint, and assists with dorsiflexion.

Pes Equinus

In *pes equinus*, the plantarflexor muscles and Achilles tendon are tightened, which limits dorsiflexion of the ankle and results in a plantarflexion deformity.[56] In cases of flexible pes equinus, the footwear choice aims to minimize ankle plantarflexion, reduce pressure on the metatarsal heads, and stabilize the subtalar joint. This can be achieved in a shoe with a low heel. Adding a rocker bottom to the sole can assist with dorsiflexion and further alleviate pressure on the metatarsal heads.

When dealing with a rigid or fixed pes equinus deformity, the objectives of footwear intervention shift. Instead of reducing plantarflexion, a posterior platform supports the rearfoot from heel strike to midstance and mimics the dorsiflexion needed at toe-off. It is crucial to contain the entire foot in the shoe, thus reducing the load on the metatarsal heads. For patients with unilateral deformity, equalizing the relative leg-length discrepancy between the normal foot and the foot with equinus throughout the entire gait cycle is essential. The shoe prescription for patients with a fixed equinus deformity includes a Cuban (elevated) heel to provide a platform and deep quarter or high-top shoes. Modifications may consist of posterior heel elevation on the equinus side and the contralateral limb to facilitate swing of the involved limb and reduce pelvic obliquity.

Pes Cavus

Pes cavus refers to an exaggerated longitudinal arch that can cause the forefoot to be plantarflexed with retraction of the toes and severe weight-bearing stresses on the metatarsal heads and heel. Individuals with pes cavus benefit from shoes that provide a broad platform for stability; reduce loading at the heels, lateral borders, and metatarsal heads; and accommodate the deformed foot within the shoe. The shoe should also have a firm heel counter to maintain rearfoot stability and a modified curved last to accommodate foot shape. Custom-molded shoes are recommended in severe cases. Potential shoe modifications for individuals with pes cavus include a lateral flare to provide a platform for greater stability, a cushioned sole to absorb shock on the heel and metatarsal heads, and a metatarsal bar to redistribute weight from the metatarsal heads.[57]

Plantar Fasciitis

Plantar fasciitis is inflammation of the plantar fascia at its insertion to the medial aspect of the calcaneus.[58] This inflammatory process can result in calcification formation at the insertion point, commonly known as a *heel spur*. Plantar fasciitis often occurs due to a loss of the longitudinal arch in conditions such as pes planus or undue stresses created in the forefoot with the tightness of the gastrocnemius and soleus muscles or an elevated longitudinal arch. When dealing with plantar fasciitis, the goals of intervention are to reduce the painful signs and symptoms by transferring weight-bearing pressure from painful areas to more tolerant ones, reducing tension on the plantar fascia and Achilles tendon, controlling pronation from heel strike to midstance, and maintaining the subtalar joint in a neutral position. The shoe prescribed for plantar fasciitis has a long medial heel counter to limit heel valgus, a high heel to reduce tension on the plantar fascia and Achilles tendon, and adequate length to minimize compression and promote supination from midstance to toe-off. Beneficial shoe modifications may involve adding a raised heel at the back to alleviate the tension on the plantar fascia and Achilles tendon.[59]

PROBLEMS IN THE REARFOOT

The most common dysfunctions and deformities of the rearfoot that can be addressed by footwear prescription or modification include arthrodesis, Achilles tendinitis or bursitis, and Haglund deformity (pump bump).

Arthrodesis

Arthrodesis refers to the loss of mobility at the ankle mortise, which is the junction of the talus with the tibia and fibula. This deformity restricts ankle motion in all planes and alters progression through the stance phase of gait. It can also hinder the clearance of the limb during the swing phase. When arthrodesis of the ankle is present, the primary objectives are to provide effective shock absorption and controlled lowering of the forefoot at loading response, improve comfort and efficiency of push-off, and accommodate any shortening or residual equinus. Shoes designed for individuals with arthrodesis should feature a reinforced counter for stability. They may include a flared heel on the medial or lateral side (or a combination of both) to provide greater stability. Some patients benefit from a high-top shoe as well. Modifications that protect the foot and facilitate a more normal gait pattern include the application of a cushioned heel to absorb shock and simulate plantarflexion after heel strike, as well as a rocker sole to replicate the dorsiflexion required during the late stance phase.

Achilles Tendinitis, Bursitis, and the Haglund Deformity

Excessive strain on the Achilles tendon, inadequate shoe length causing direct pressure, and tightness in the gastrocnemius and soleus muscles can lead to tendinitis or bursitis. The *Haglund deformity* is an osseous formation at the insertion of the Achilles tendon at the calcaneus. The goals of shoe prescription for patients with Achilles tendinitis, bursitis, and/or Haglund deformity (pump bump) are similar: (1) to alleviate tension on the Achilles tendon, (2) to provide dorsiflexion assist at heel strike and at toe-off, (3) to reduce abnormal pronation, and (4) to reduce pressure and friction (shear) at the insertion of the calcaneus. Patients with these problems require a slightly higher heel to reduce dorsiflexion, a long medial counter to limit subtalar motion, a longer shoe size to reduce compression pressure, and a backless shoe to prevent irritation of the pump bump. Some beneficial shoe modifications may include adding a posterior heel elevation to reduce tension on the Achilles tendon or a foam-filled posterior heel counter.

Diagnosis-Related Considerations in Shoe Prescription

Prescription footwear and shoe modifications are also extremely useful tools to protect joints, prevent skin problems, and enhance the normal function of patients coping with arthritis, gout, diabetes, or peripheral vascular disease. Adaptations to footwear may also be helpful for patients with hemiplegia, partial foot amputations, or congenital deformities.

ARTHRITIS

Arthritis, whether degenerative, rheumatoid, or caused by trauma, causes joint damage. When working with patients with foot arthritis, intervention objectives are to prevent or limit abnormal motion, accommodate for deformities caused by arthritis, cushion impact loading, and reduce microtrauma within the joint.[60] A reinforced counter can help limit subtalar motion; a high-top shoe can also help limit ankle motion. Extra-depth shoes may be needed to accommodate deformities of the midfoot and forefoot. If deformities need further accommodation, it is preferable to use thermoldable leather. Applying a rocker bottom helps improve push-off by shortening the distance between the heel and the MTP joint. It also reduces the total ankle motion required for push-off. Shock-absorbing accommodative orthoses can be placed inside the shoe, and a cushioned heel can be added to absorb even more force at heel strike and limit ankle and subtalar motion. A flared heel can reduce medial and lateral movement at the subtalar joint. In 2008 a Cochrane review, "Custom-made foot orthoses for the treatment of foot pain,"[34] found that custom foot orthoses compared with supportive shoes in persons with juvenile idiopathic arthritis reduced foot pain after 3 months. Still, similar results were not achieved using prefabricated neoprene shoe inserts. Additionally, the review concluded that custom foot orthoses reduced rearfoot pain in adults with RA after 3 months compared to no treatment.

GOUT

In patients with gout, the treatment goals align with those for patients with arthritis. These objectives involve preventing or limiting the motion of painful or inflamed joints, accommodating foot deformities, and cushioning the impact of loading on the affected joints. It is worth considering using a reinforced counter to limit subtalar motion or a high-top design to restrict overall ankle movement. An extra-depth shoe of thermoldable leather can best accommodate deformities without creating pain and discomfort over sensitive joints. Applying a rocker bottom can facilitate push-off, prevent pedal joint movement, and reduce ankle motion. Additionally, shock-absorbing accommodative orthoses and cushion heels provide even more comfort and protection for inflamed joints during gait.

DIABETES

The loss of protective sensation in patients with diabetic neuropathy creates significant vulnerability to injury from repetitive microtrauma. Protection of the plantar surface of the diabetic foot from microtrauma is of paramount importance.[61] Patients with diabetic neuropathy often have significant weakness of intrinsic muscles. Forefoot deformities develop, including claw toes, which are susceptible to breakdown in areas of excessive shoe pressure. The risk of nonhealing, infection, and subsequent amputation is quite high; prevention is the most effective treatment strategy. Total-contact full-foot orthoses using soft, shock-absorbing materials help distribute weight-bearing pressures over the entire plantar surface of the foot away from the vulnerable bony prominences. A Thermold leather shoe is recommended for the insensitive diabetic foot.[62]

PERIPHERAL VASCULAR DISEASE

Due to compromised healing ability in individuals with peripheral vascular disease, the presence of any irritation or ulceration significantly raises the chances of infection and subsequent amputation.[34] Here, too, the primary goals are preventing skin breakdown and protecting the vulnerable foot.[63] The ability to fit and protect the foot effectively is further challenged by fluctuating edema. For patients with peripheral vascular disease–related edema, it is often recommended to use a Thermold sandal with Velcro closure as a safe and effective alternative to standard shoes. If edema is not a problem, a soft Thermold shoe can protext the plantar surface of the foot from repetitive pressures and accommodate deformities that are at risk for shoe pressure-related injuries. As hypersensitivity is frequently encountered in circulatory pathologic conditions in the lower extremities, a shoe that cushions the foot may be helpful. Elastic shoelaces allow for show expansion in patients with minimal edema-related fluctuations in foot size.

HEMIPLEGIA

The patient with hemiplegia after a cerebrovascular accident (e.g., stroke) may have an inadequate or excessive tone of the lower extremity. Many of these patients need orthotic intervention to control the foot and ankle in some or all phases of gait to accommodate for any fixed deformities and to cushion impact loading at initial contact.[64,65] Footwear is selected to enhance orthotic function or, in some instances, to control mild dysfunction directly. A reinforced heel counter can help to limit subtalar motion and stabilize the foot on heel strike. A flared heel or high-top shoe may be recommended to enhance foot placement and stance stability. A rigid shoe shank may be required for some lower extremity orthoses. In an equinus deformity, a heel lift on the shoe provides total contact during weight bearing and facilitates stability. A custom-molded shoe might be the only viable option in cases of severe ankle deformities. In hemiplegia, the most commonly utilized ankle-foot orthoses often increase shoe length, width, and depth by half to a whole size. The insole can be frequently substituted with an insert foundation to create additional space within the shoe for accommodating the orthosis. Extra-depth shoes are particularly beneficial for patients with difficulty donning their orthoses and shoes because of upper extremity dysfunction in hemiplegia.

AMPUTATION AND CONGENITAL DEFORMITY

The foot that is shortened surgically or is congenitally deformed is a management challenge because the weight-bearing surface is reduced or altered, increasing the likelihood of tissue breakdown with repeated loading in gait. The type of protective footwear used can range from an over-the-counter extra-depth shoe for a mild deformity to a custom-molded shoe for a severe deformity. When the feet are of unequal size, it is more difficult to fit them without buying two pairs of shoes or making custom footwear. If the difference between the feet is no more than one size in length, the larger size can be used with toe padding for the shorter deformed or amputated foot or with an orthosis to accommodate the deformity (Fig. 7.11). The shorter foot is frequently wider and must be accommodated by the appropriate orthosis custom-molded to the shoe. A toe filler will prevent the shortened foot from sliding within the shoe during gait but also increase the risk of skin breakdown. It is crucial that the first MTP joint be aligned with the "toe break" point in the shoe. If the foot falls posterior to the toe break, stress is concentrated at the distal end of the foot, increasing the chance of pressure imposition by the "filler."

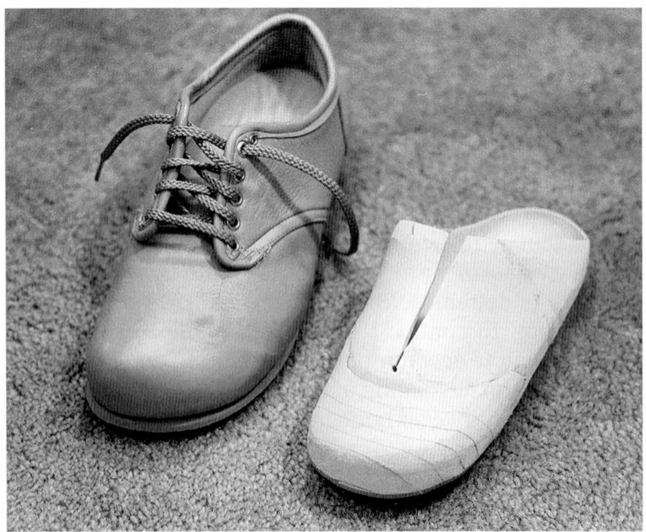

Fig. 7.11 A toe filler can be used on a foot that has been shortened by amputation or congenital deformity. Courtesy Marathon Orthotics, Inc.

Reading the Wear on Shoes

For the clinician who is faced with decisions about modifying, repairing, or replacing footwear, examination of patterns of wear and erosion provides essential information. The deterioration of the shoe itself not only hampers tactile sensibility but also impairs the judgment of position and sense of balance. Shoes that have outlasted their purpose often create abnormal forces and shearing that increase the risk of repetitive microtrauma to the skin and joints of the foot and ankle. Analyzing the wear and erosion of the shoe serves as a helpful tool in providing recommendations, prescriptions, and modifications to ensure a proper fit that meets the unique needs of each individual.

Accommodating shoe gear should be used by patients with diabetes, and walking barefoot should not be permitted. The shoe's upper should be soft so as not to irritate any prominence or developing deformity. The accommodative insole used should be adaptable to changes as well. A combination of an expanded polyethylene, such as Plastazote, which can be heat molded to provide total contact and then mounted on a shock-absorbing material such as poron performance technology or covered with a neoprene, such as Spenco, which is soft and retains its shape, makes an excellent accommodative insole. This type of accommodative orthosis protects the foot from trauma to prominent areas and redistributes the forces to provide even weight bearing through total contact on the plantar surface. When accommodative orthoses are used, the shoe must have adequate depth to accommodate it. Extra-depth shoes such as Thermold shoes or extra-depth sneakers allow not only the room needed for the accommodative insole but also modification of the upper through heat molding to accommodate lesser toe deformities. A rigid-sole rocker-bottom shoe might also be recommended to reduce pressures under the metatarsal heads during push-off. The apex of the rocker is positioned just proximal to the metatarsal heads, allowing for the shoe itself to provide forward propulsion of the foot.

Summary

The shoe serves as an essential interface between the foot and the ground, providing protection against trauma and offering support to the foot's structures during activities such as walking, running, and changing direction. Fashionable footwear, especially for females, often compromises foot function rather than enhancing it. Foot function and footwear must have a developmental aspect as well—an understanding of how the foot changes over the life span and of the special needs of children, pregnant females, and older adults is essential. Gaining knowledge about the various components of shoes, their diverse variations, the criteria for proper fitting, and the correlation between shoe design and the demands of different activities is an invaluable tool for clinicians in their practice. Therapists are often called on to recommend footwear for patients with special needs. Having a foundational understanding of shoe characteristics and modifications tailored to specific deformities or diagnoses greatly enhances their ability to fulfill this role effectively.

Case Example 7.1 A Patient With Diabetes Who Is Homeless and Has a Neuropathic Foot Ulcer

J.H. is a 71-year-old homeless living in a shelter with a 22-year history of type 2 diabetes mellitus treated with metformin. He presents with a large ulcer (6.552 cm^2) of the plantar surface of the midfoot with significant arch deformity of the right foot subsequent to an episode of Charcot arthropathy several years earlier. J.H. reports that the ulcer has been present for more than a year. He has complications resulting from diabetes, including retinopathy, peripheral neuropathy, and a history of numerous neuropathic ulcerations involving both feet. He also has a 24-year history of arterial hypertension and a documented myocardial infarction. He is currently managed with angiotensin-converting enzyme inhibitors and calcium antagonists. It is unclear how regularly he has taken his medications, although they are available at no cost through the shelter's clinic. J.H. has been homeless for 7 years.

J.H. is referred to the health clinic at the homeless shelter for diabetic and hypertensive assessment and conservative treatment of the foot ulceration.

QUESTIONS TO CONSIDER

- What tests and measures might the foot clinic team use to assess the current status and changes in J.H.'s neuropathic wound, the deformity of his feet, the circulation and sensory status of his limbs, and his functional status and gait? What is the evidence of reliability and validity of these measures?
- What does the team need to understand about his current health status and diabetes control? How will they gather this information?
- What are J.H.'s immediate needs in terms of footwear? How might his needs change over time as his wound heals?
- Given his current health status and lifestyle, what factors will likely affect (both positively and negatively) clinical decision-making about J.H.'s footwear, wound care, diabetes management, and follow-up care? How might the team prioritize goals and possible interventions?
- How would the team assess the efficacy of their interventions?

INITIAL RESULTS

Satisfactory metabolic control and blood pressure values were achieved during the initial week of medical management at the shelter clinic. J.H. was referred to Boston City Hospital (BCH) for a series of tests and measures on an outpatient basis. Although he was found to have bilateral diabetic retinopathy *(fundus oculi)*, there was no evidence of diabetic nephropathy. An echocardiogram pointed to left ventricular hypertrophy with a normal regional kinesis and an ejection fraction of 50%.

Electromyography showed normal conduction velocity and slight abnormalities of sensory action potentials in the nerves of both lower extremities. An elevated threshold of 40 V to the biothesiometer and a partial loss of sensitivity (nine of nine areas tested were insensitive bilaterally) to a Semmes-Weinstein 5.07 monofilament are recorded. The transcutaneous oxygen tension was 30 mm Hg at the dorsum of the involved foot (right) and 15 mm Hg at the perilesional site. In the ulcerated limb, the ankle-brachial index measured with the Doppler technique was 0.8. Duplex scanning showed widespread atheromasic lesions in the carotids and lower limb arteries without hemodynamically significant stenoses and no significant alterations in the venous distribution of the lower limbs.

J.H.'s ulcer on his right foot appeared superficial and was graded as a Wagner grade II ulcer. The ulcer was covered by a fibrinous exudate with keratotic margins. The microbiologic cultures were negative. A surgical debridement was performed at BCH, and then J.H. was sent back to the shelter with instructions for local treatment before and after daily sharps debridement, consisting of the daily application of sterile paraffin gauze, as well as for "evaluation and conservative treatment" by a physical therapist.

QUESTIONS TO CONSIDER

- How might the team interpret the results of the tests performed at BCH? How will this information influence or inform wound care and recommendations for footwear for this patient?
- What additional information will the physical therapist and foot care clinic team have to gather?
- What are the primary goals of physical therapy/foot care intervention? What is the prognosis and anticipated outcome? What is the anticipated duration of this episode of care? How frequently might J.H. receive care?
- What interventions would be most appropriate to address the goals of wound healing and prevention of future recurrence of neuropathic ulcers?

PHYSICAL THERAPY EXAMINATION, EVALUATION, AND INTERVENTION

J.H. was examined at the shelter by a physical therapist on the Foot Clinic Team. He arrived at the clinic ambulating independently, without any assistive devices. The ulcer on the plantar surface of his midfoot measured 6.552 cm^2 in the Charcot joint deformity region of the right foot. The ulcer was determined to be secondary to repetitive trauma to this region due to shoes that had large holes in the midsections of the soles.

A total contact cast was applied. Selective padding of the cast included foam padding over the toes and an ulcerated area of the foot; felt pads over the malleoli and navicular prominence; and cotton cast padding around the proximal and anterior lower leg, heel, sides, and dorsum of the foot. A rubber heel mount was applied to the cast for ambulation. Fiberglass casting material was used to decrease the effects of the elements (weather) on a plaster cast for this homeless individual who spends much time outdoors. The cast was also bifurcated to allow high galvanic electrical stimulation to be used as a local treatment modality to the wound and to provide access for daily debridement, the application of dressings, and monitoring for secondary lesions. The cast was secured with Velcro straps. The patient was allowed to walk freely and was highly compliant, wearing the cast continuously.

The ulcer responded favorably to a combination of periodic surgical debridement, local wound care, and daily sharps debridement, a modified total contact casting protocol, and high galvanic electrical stimulation. After 6 weeks the ulcer had completely closed and J.H.'s condition remained stable. He was subsequently fitted with a total contact foot orthosis bilaterally and provided with a pair of Reebok walking sneakers with an extra width to accommodate the Charcot foot deformity bilaterally.

With proper intervention and attention to J.H.'s social situation, it was determined that the prognosis for preventing recurrence of his neuropathic foot ulcer wound is good and that he can be integrated into appropriate home, community, and work environments within the context of his disability. J.H. was placed in a permanent shelter/housing residence and obtained part-time employment as a guide at the Boston Museum of Science.

Continued

Case Example 7.1 A Patient With Diabetes Who Is Homeless and Has a Neuropathic Foot Ulcer—cont'd

DISCUSSION

For individuals with neuropathic wounds, total-contact casting allows ambulation with protection from external stress and trauma. In addition, when such a cast is well molded and minimal padding is applied, the pressure is distributed evenly and maintained as long as the cast is worn. A total-contact cast also counteracts lymphatic congestion, which compromises the healing process. For J.H., the cast was bifurcated to allow for daily wound care while also providing consistent pressure relief and foot protection.

The primary objectives of treatment after J.H.'s diabetic neuropathic wound healed were to protect the plantar surface from repetitive microtrauma and accommodate deformities that could be traumatized by excessive shoe pressures, which could result in ulceration and subsequent injury. A total-contact full-foot orthosis using soft shock-absorbing materials helped to distribute weight-bearing pressures over the entire plantar surface of the foot and away from the vulnerable bony prominences. A Thermold leather shoe or good walking sneaker is recommended for the insensitive diabetic foot.

Accommodative devices are insoles placed in shoes to balance the feet, allowing pressure to be evenly distributed and permitting support and shock absorption of the foot. An orthosis, in contrast, supports and also controls the foot by neutralizing pronatory forces. Following wound healing, a total-contact orthosis (Plastazote with a layer of ⅜-inch Poron Performance Technology) was fabricated for J.H. and placed in a pair of extra-depth Reebok walking shoes.

References

The complete listing of the References are available in the accompanying enhanced eBook version included with the print purchase of this textbook. Visit Elsevier eBooks+ (eBooks.Health.Elsevier.com) to access this content.

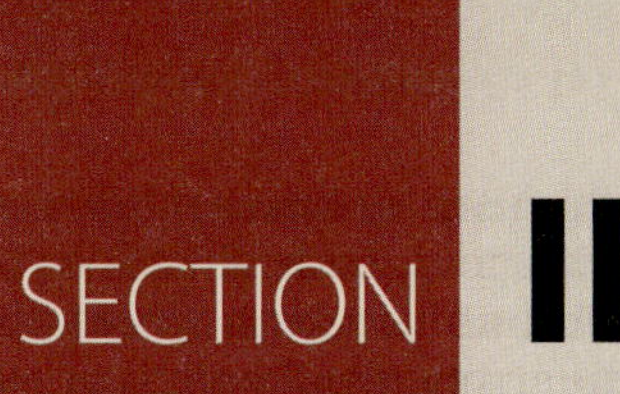

Orthoses in Rehabilitation

8 Foot Orthoses

ELICIA POLLARD AND DONNA SYLVESTER

LEARNING OBJECTIVES

On completion of this chapter, the reader will be able to do the following:

1. Describe the major anatomical structures of the foot as well as the basic biomechanical principles associated with these structures.
2. Describe the effects of extrinsic and intrinsic deformities and of abnormal pronation on the function of the foot during the various phases of gait.
3. Explain the strategies used to examine and evaluate intrinsic foot deformities.
4. Describe abnormal pronation and the pathological conditions that contribute to abnormal pronation in gait.
5. Describe components of a foot orthosis, goals of orthotic intervention, and specific purposes of the most common orthotic interventions.
6. Discuss the biopsychosocial considerations associated with foot pain and orthoses.
7. Discuss the controversy related to traditional orthotic theory.
8. Review literature related to the efficacy of foot orthoses for the management of common disorders.

History of the Functional Foot Orthosis

The use of foot orthoses as an effective treatment tool for biomechanical dysfunction of the feet evolved during the 20th century and continues to be the subject of research and technological advancements. A growing body of literature has found foot orthoses to be an effective component of treatment for lower extremity pain, lower limb dysfunction, and overuse injuries.[1–4] Early on, foot orthoses were used to redistribute plantar surface foot forces to alleviate discomfort in pressure-sensitive areas of the foot. Little consideration was given to the specific foot abnormality that led to the pathological condition.[5] In the early 1900s metal foot braces began to be used to control motion at specific joints of the foot and to prevent pathological conditions.[6] These devices, although functional, were often not well tolerated because of the rigidity of the materials and the mismatch between brace design and foot pathokinesiology. In 1948 Schreber and Weineman first identified forefoot invertus (varus) and evertus (valgus) as primary foot deformities that required correction by an orthosis.[7] In the 1960s Merton Root developed neutral impression casting techniques, positive cast modifications, and posting (mechanical correction) techniques.[8] The standards that Root established have enhanced orthotic comfort and function. Since then, the use of functional foot orthoses has evolved to include the consideration of the person-centered approach to care when addressing pathologies of the mechanics of the foot and ankle in musculoskeletal and neurological disorders.[9–14]

Triplanar Structure of the Foot

The foot is a complex of bones interconnected by a series of multiplanar articulations supported by soft tissue structures. It is subdivided into three functional components: the rearfoot, the midfoot, and the forefoot.

Several important articulations of the foot (talocrural, subtalar, midtarsal, first and fifth rays) are triplanar; the axis of rotation in these joints is not perpendicular to any of the cardinal planes (sagittal, horizontal, frontal) of the human body. As a result, motion about triplanar joints leads to simultaneous movement in all three of these cardinal planes.[8] The amount of motion evident in any single plane is related to the pitch (inclination) of the triplanar axis from the respective cardinal plane. Triplanar motion occurs in three-dimensional (3D) space; the breakdown of triplanar motion into its three constituent cardinal plane movements is artificial.

Because motion about a triplanar axis is 3D, motion occurs simultaneously in the three cardinal planes. Blocking any one component of triplanar motion in a single cardinal plane prevents movement in the other two planes as well. This "all-or-nothing" rule is the premise for orthotic posting or wedging.[8] Theoretically, the addition of a post or wedge to an orthosis blocks the frontal plane component of triplanar motion, which, in turn, blocks or limits the triplanar motion of pronation. The design principles of foot orthoses are founded on knowledge of the functional anatomy of the foot.

TALOCRURAL JOINT

The talocrural joint (TCJ) (articulation between tibia, fibula, and talus, connecting the foot to the lower leg) has a triplanar axis of rotation. In neutral position, the TCJ axis passes through the tips of the medial and lateral malleoli, pitched 10 degrees from the transverse plane and 20 to 30 degrees from the frontal plane (Fig. 8.1).[15–17] Although sagittal plane plantarflexion and dorsiflexion are primary motions at this joint, the slight inclination of the TCJ axis of rotation leads to concomitant transverse and frontal plane motion. During plantarflexion, the foot adducts and inverts; with

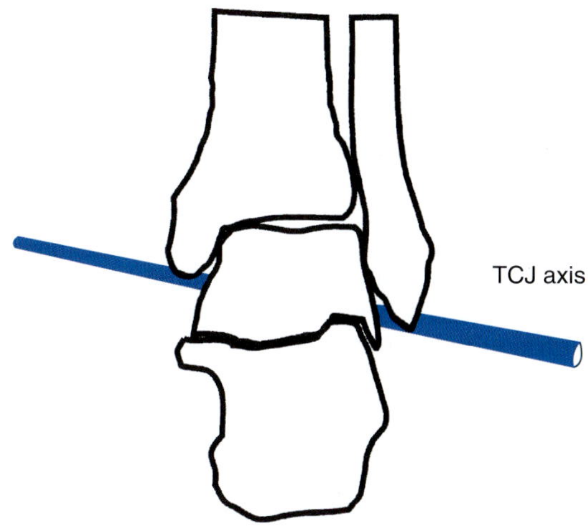

Fig. 8.1 Posterior view of the osseous components and axis of the talocrural joint *(TCJ)*. The osseous components of the TCJ are the tibia medially and superiorly, the fibula laterally, and the talus inferiorly. The axis of the joint passes in a posterolateral to anteromedial direction through the tips of the lateral and medial malleoli. (Courtesy Juan C. Garbalosa, University of Hartford, West Hartford, Connecticut.)

dorsiflexion it abducts and everts. Normal range of motion (ROM) of the TCJ is between 12 and 20 degrees of dorsiflexion and 50 and 56 degrees of plantarflexion.[18] The medial (deltoid) and lateral collateral ligaments stabilize and limit motion that occurs at the TCJ.[19]

REARFOOT

The osseous structures of the rearfoot are the calcaneus (inferior) and the talus (superior) (Fig. 8.2). The articulation between the calcaneus and talus is the subtalar joint (STJ). Three joint surfaces are present in this articulation: posterior, anterior, and middle. The posterior joint surface has a concave talar and convex calcaneal portion, whereas the anterior and middle joint surfaces have convex talar and concave calcaneal arrangements.[20] This structurally based articular geometry, along with the interosseous talocalcaneal ligament, limits the amount and type of motion occurring at the STJ.[21,22] The medial and lateral collateral ligaments and the posterior and lateral talocalcaneal ligaments also offer support to the STJ.[22,23]

At the STJ, the triplanar axis of rotation is oriented in an anterosuperior to posteroinferior direction, pitched approximately 42 degrees from the transverse plane, 48 degrees from the frontal plane, and 16 degrees from the sagittal plane (see Fig. 8.2). The location of the STJ axis in the human foot varies greatly. Manter[24] reported that the inclination from the transverse and sagittal planes varies from 29 to 47 degrees and from 8 to 24 degrees, respectively.

The triplanar motions at the STJ are supination and pronation. Supination of the weight-bearing foot leads to dorsiflexion and abduction of the talus with simultaneous inversion of the calcaneus. Pronation of the weight-bearing foot results in plantarflexion and adduction of the talus and eversion of the calcaneus.[8] Because of the variability in location of the axis of rotation of the STJ, the component motions of supination and pronation vary as well. As the axis becomes more perpendicular to a particular cardinal plane, the motion occurring in that plane becomes more pronounced,

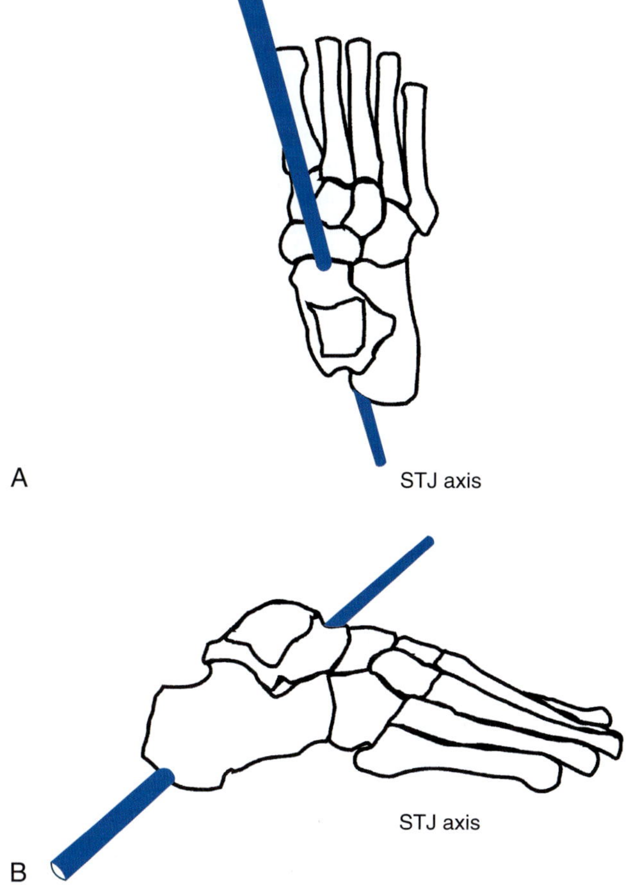

Fig. 8.2 Superior (A) and lateral (B) views of the osseous structures in the rearfoot: the superior talus and inferior calcaneus. Also pictured is the triplanar axis of the subtalar joint *(STJ)*. Note the inclination of the axis from all three cardinal planes of the body. (Courtesy Juan C. Garbalosa, University of Hartford, West Hartford, Connecticut.)

whereas the other motions become less prominent.[25,26] This variability affects coupled motion between the joints of the foot and the lower leg. During pronation and supination of the rearfoot, the tibia and fibula rotate internally and externally in the transverse plane.[8,27,28] An increase in the frontal plane motion of the rearfoot could cause a simultaneous increase in the transverse plane motion of the lower leg.

MIDFOOT

The midfoot is composed of two bones: the cuboid and the navicular. The talonavicular and calcaneocuboid articulations between the midfoot and rearfoot form an important composite joint: the midtarsal joint (MTJ) or transverse tarsal joint. The articular surfaces of the talonavicular joint are convex-concave, whereas the surfaces of the calcaneocuboid joint are sellar shaped.[16,24] MTJ movement is supported and restricted by the bifurcate, short and long plantar, and plantar calcaneonavicular (spring) ligaments. The short and long plantar ligaments and the plantar calcaneonavicular ligaments also support the longitudinal and transverse plantar arches of the foot.[29]

Because the MTJ is a composite joint, motion occurs about two separate triplanar joint axes: a longitudinal and an oblique axis (Fig. 8.3). Movement of the forefoot about each joint axis can occur independently of the other. Manter[24] reported that the longitudinal axis is inclined superiorly 15 degrees from the transverse plane and medially 9 degrees from the sagittal plane, whereas the oblique axis is pitched superiorly 52 degrees from the transverse plane and medially 57 degrees from the sagittal plane. The predominant motion about the longitudinal axis is frontal plane inversion and eversion. Because of the slight deviation of the longitudinal axis from the three cardinal planes, small amounts of forefoot plantarflexion and dorsiflexion and adduction and abduction occur during inversion and eversion. Plantarflexion and dorsiflexion and abduction and adduction are the predominant movements around the oblique MTJ axis, with little concomitant inversion and eversion.[8]

These two joint axes produce the combined motion of supination and pronation of the MTJ. During supination and pronation, the forefoot inverts and everts about the longitudinal axis. The motion around the oblique axis is plantarflexion with adduction and dorsiflexion with abduction. The amount of motion possible at these MTJ axes is determined by the position of the STJ. In STJ supination, the two joint axes are nearly perpendicular so that MTJ mobility is restricted. This mechanism helps convert the forefoot into a rigid structure for propulsion during the push-off phase of gait (from heel rise through toe-off).[24,30] When the STJ is pronated, the joint axes are more parallel, allowing a greater degree of MTJ mobility.

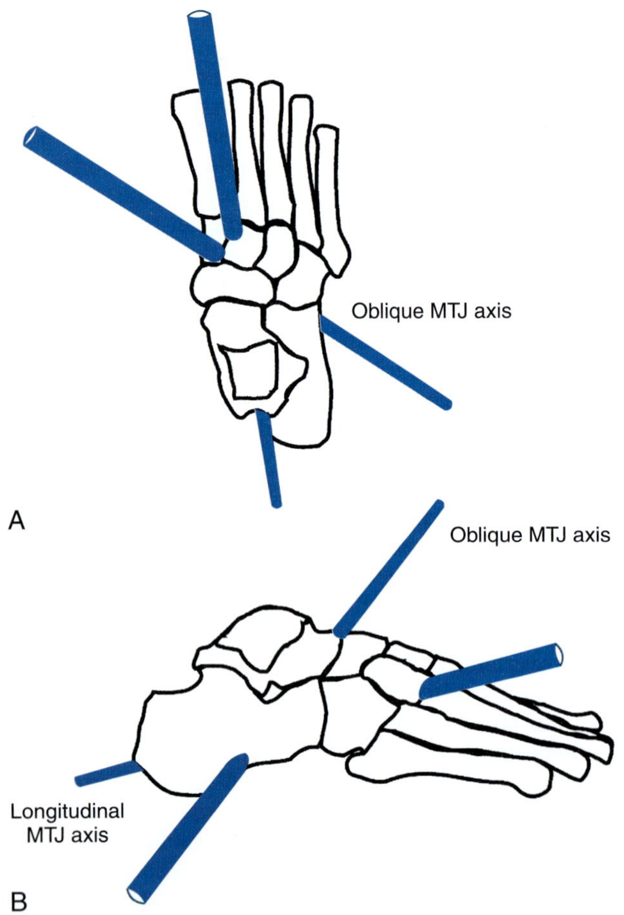

Fig. 8.3 Superior (A) and lateral (B) views of the osseous components of the midtarsal joint *(MTJ)*. The anterior portion of the MTJ is composed of the navicular and cuboid bones, whereas the posterior portion is composed of the calcaneus and talus. The two axes of the MTJ, the oblique and longitudinal axes, are also depicted. As in the subtalar joint, both axes of the MTJ are triplanar. (Courtesy Juan C. Garbalosa, University of Hartford, West Hartford, Connecticut.)

FOREFOOT

The forefoot includes all structures distal to the navicular and cuboid bones; it is subdivided into five rays and toes. The first through third rays consist of a cuneiform and its associated metatarsal bone; the fourth and fifth rays consist only of a metatarsal. The tarsometatarsal joints—the primary joints of the ray complexes—have two opposing planar surfaces.[8,29] The hallux, or first toe, has two bones (a proximal and distal phalanx) and two corresponding joints (metatarsophalangeal [MTP] and interphalangeal [IP]). The lesser toes have three bones (proximal, middle, and distal phalanges) and three associated joints. The proximal articular surfaces of the MTP and IP joints are convex, and the distal articular surface is concave.[8] Numerous soft tissue structures support these joints.[29,31]

Although each ray has its own axis of motion, the first and fifth rays are of particular interest. The triplanar axes of rotation of these two joints are nearly perpendicular. The axis of the first ray is pitched at a 45-degree angle from the sagittal and frontal planes; the primary motions possible are plantarflexion with eversion and dorsiflexion with inversion. Because the axis of the first ray is minimally pitched from the transverse plane, insignificant transverse motion occurs.[8] In contrast, the axis of rotation of the fifth ray is oriented at a 20-degree angle from the transverse plane and a 35-degree angle from the sagittal plane. The resulting motions combine inversion with plantarflexion and eversion with dorsiflexion. Less motion is present about the axis of rotation of the fifth ray than of the first ray.[8] MTP joints have two separate axes of rotation: the vertical axis (abduction and adduction) and the transverse axis (plantarflexion and dorsiflexion).[8,16,29] Typically, there is minimal motion in the frontal plane at the MTP joints, as excessive; frontal plane motion can result in subluxation.[8]

PLANTAR FASCIA AND ARCHES OF THE FOOT

The plantar aponeurosis, one of the most functionally important soft tissue structures of the foot, is a sheath of fascia spanning most of the foot's plantar surface. Arising from the medial process of the calcanean tuberosity, it passes distally along the plantar aspect of the foot, then divides into five slips for its distal attachment at the base of the proximal phalanges by the plantar pads.[32] This fascial sheath plays an extremely important role in providing the stability needed by the foot during the toe-off phase of stance during gait and in supporting the longitudinal arch of the foot.

The medial longitudinal and transverse arches are formed by the ligamentous and osseous structures of a "normal" foot.[33] The medial longitudinal arch (MLA) extends from the calcaneus (posterior) to the first metatarsal head (anterior) and is supported by the plantar aponeurosis, the short and long plantar ligaments, and the spring ligament. During weight bearing, the height of the arch is reduced as the supporting ligamentous structures are elongated. The transverse arch reaches across the foot from medial to lateral borders. The height of the arch varies along the length of the foot: its maximum height occurs at the cuboid-cuneiform bones of the midfoot, and its lowest point is at the metatarsal heads.

Function of the Foot in Gait

The foot and ankle complex has three major functions in the gait cycle: attenuating impact forces, maintaining equilibrium, and transmitting propulsive forces. For optimal biomechanical and energy-efficient performance, the joints of the foot and ankle must work in harmony. In early stance, the foot-ankle complex absorbs energy generated at initial contact (IC) and decreases forces transmitted to proximal structures during loading. The foot and ankle must also adapt to surface conditions encountered by the foot as stance begins. In late stance, the foot and lower leg transmit propulsive forces generated by muscles of the lower extremity onto the ground. The ability of the foot and lower leg to accomplish these functions depends on the integrity of the various structures of the foot. Gait abnormalities occur when the foot and ankle complex is unable to compensate for deficits in motion or structure.

The kinematic, kinetic, and neuromuscular events of the normal human gait cycle have been described in many ways.[8,34,35] Most focus on five distinct events: IC or heel strike, loading response (LR) or foot flat, midstance (MSt), terminal stance (TSt) or heel-off, and preswing (PSw) or toe-off. See Chapter 5 for a more detailed description of the gait cycle.

SHOCK ABSORPTION

Musculoskeletal structures of the lower limb act from IC to MSt to attenuate impact forces.[8,34,36] Force plate recording of ground reaction forces (GRFs) estimates the foot's ability to absorb energy and decelerate the lower leg. The push of the foot against the floor creates a GRF with three components: vertical, medial, and lateral; and fore and aft forces. The vertical component of a typical GRF record has a bimodal shape (Fig. 8.4). The brief first peak results from the impact of the heel with the ground. Some of the vertical GRF is attributed to the acceleration of the centers of mass of the foot and shank of the leg.

In early stance, from IC to LR, the STJ moves into pronation as the TCJ is plantarflexing.[8,34,37,38] The fibula and tibia internally rotate with respect to the foot.[26,27] Pronation of the STJ is controlled by eccentric contraction of the tibialis anterior, posterior tibialis, flexor hallucis longus, and flexor digitorum longus muscles.[8,34,39] Plantarflexion of the foot is controlled primarily by eccentric action of the tibialis anterior.[8,38] The combined muscle activity decelerates plantarflexion and pronation motion of the TCJ, STJ, and MTJ, slowing vertical and anterior movement of the center of mass of the foot and shank and decreasing impact forces encountered at IC.

The viscoelastic plantar fat pad absorbs some of the energy generated between IC and LR.[40] Pronation of the STJ flattens the arches of the foot, elongating plantar connective tissue structures. Because these tissues are viscoelastic, they also absorb some of the energy generated from IC to LR.

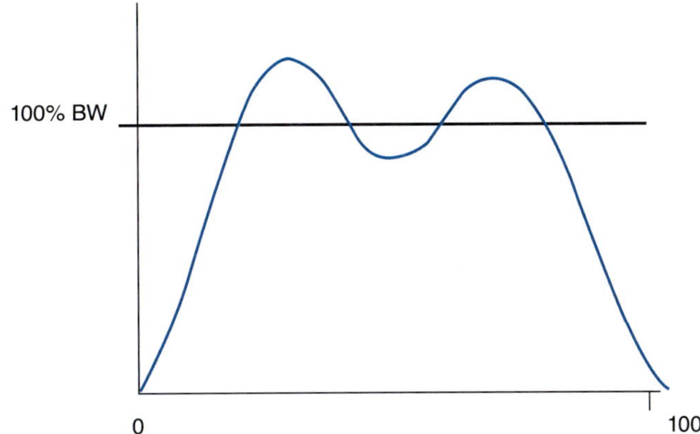

Fig. 8.4 Typical vertical ground reaction pattern during walking. Note the bimodal shape of the ground reaction force. The first peak occurs at initial contact, and the second peak occurs during the toe-off phase of gait. The recorded ground reaction force represents the whole-body center of mass acceleration. *BW*, Body weight. (From Valiant GA. Transmission and attenuation of heelstrike accelerations. In: Cavanagh PR, ed. *Biomechanics of Distance Running*. Human Kinetics; 1990:225–249.)

ADAPTATION TO SURFACES

In everyday walking, the foot must be able to adapt quickly to many types of terrains and uneven surfaces. The key contributor to surface adaptation is STJ pronation, which unlocks the MTJ, permitting the joints of the foot to function in loose-packed positions and enabling the osseous elements to shift their relative positions.

At IC, the forefoot is in a supinatory twist (inverted) about the longitudinal MTJ axis. Eccentric action of the anterior tibialis decelerates plantarflexion of the forefoot, lowering it to the ground. The MTJ becomes fully supinated at LR as a result of eversion of the STJ and GRFs acting upward on the foot's medial border. Contraction of the extensor digitorum longus and fibularis (peroneus) tertius abducts and dorsiflexes (pronates) the forefoot, locking it about the oblique MTJ axis and preparing the forefoot to receive the loading forces encountered at MSt.[8]

PROPULSION

During MSt (LR to PSw), the STJ is maximally pronated and begins to resupinate. At this time, the GRF maintains the MTJ in a pronated position about its oblique axis. At the same time, a pronatory twist is initiated at the longitudinal axis by concentric action of the fibularis muscles. The MTJ locks in a fully pronated position around the longitudinal axis just before heel rise as the STJ reaches its neutral position. The MTJ must remain locked in this position throughout propulsion as the fibularis muscles contract to lift the lateral side of the foot from the ground and transfer weight medially to the other foot. As the heel is raised from the ground, the rearfoot continues to supinate (talus abducts and dorsiflexes) as the lower limb rotates externally. This coupled motion necessitates supination of the MTJ about the oblique axis to maximize joint stability and to convert the foot into a rigid lever for propulsion.

Supination of the STJ occurs with concentric action of the tibialis posterior, flexor hallucis longus, and flexor digitorum longus and soleus, as well as the antagonistic functioning of the fibularis brevis.[8,34] The concentric activity of the gastrocnemius and soleus muscles causes vertical acceleration of the foot and lower leg. Propulsive forces generated by the foot and lower leg are transmitted to the floor.[8,34,38] The second peak of a GRF curve corresponds to propulsion in the late stance phase (see Fig. 8.4).

Supination of the STJ and locking of the MTJ about the longitudinal axis place the foot in a closed-packed position, transforming the foot into a rigid lever.[8,17,27,34,41] This transformation is aided by the action of the plantar aponeurosis as it wraps around the metatarsal heads. During TSt, the MTP joints extend (dorsiflex), creating a "windlass effect." This action compresses joints of the midfoot and forefoot, facilitating the transition from flexibility to rigidity required for effective push-off.

Biomechanical Examination

The biomechanical examination of the foot and ankle has three components: a non–weight-bearing assessment, a static weight-bearing assessment, and a dynamic gait analysis (Fig. 8.5). Five common intrinsic foot deformities

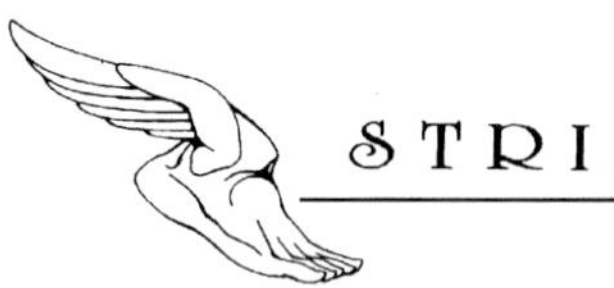

STRIDE, Inc.

Physical Therapy and Pedorthic Services
530 Middlebury Road • Suite 102 • Middlebury, CT 06762
TEL.: (203) 598-0070 • FAX: (203) 598-0075

BIOMECHANICAL FOOT EVALUATION

Patient: ______ Phone: ______
Address: ______
Age: ______ Height: ______ Weight: ______ Shoe size: ______ Shoe Style: ______
Occupation: ______ Activity level: ______ Sports: ______
Referring Practitioner: ______ Date of Evaluation: ______
Diagnosis: ______

I. NON-WEIGHTBEARING EVALUATION

	Left	Right
Rearfoot:		
STN position	______ varus	______ varus
calcaneal inversion	______ degrees	______ degrees
calcaneal eversion	______ degrees	______ degrees
rearfoot dorsiflexion	______ degrees	______ degrees
Forefoot:		
STN position	______ varus/valgus	______ varus/valgus
locking mechanism	poor fair normal rigid	poor fair normal rigid
MTJ dorsiflexion	______ degrees	______ degrees
First Ray:		
STN position and mobility		
hallux dorsiflexion	______ degrees	______ degrees
Arch Position:	low med high	low med high
Toe Position/Deformities:	______	______

Lesions/Shoe Wear:

R L

L R

Calluses:

L R

Fig. 8.5 Biomechanical examination form outlining components of the non–weight-bearing and weight-bearing assessment. *Ante*, Femoral anteversion; *ASIS*, anterior superior iliac spine; *DLS*, double-limb stance; *Gastroc*, gastrocnemius; *G.T.*, greater trochanter; *ITB*, iliotibial band; *M.M.*, medial malleolus; *MTJ*, midtarsal joint; *PSIS*, posterior inferior iliac spine; *RCS*, relaxed calcaneal stance; *Retro*, femoral retroversion; *SLS*, single-limb stance; *STN*, subtalar neutral; *T.T.*, tibial tubercle; *VAL*, valgus; *VAR*, varus. (Courtesy Stride, Inc., Middlebury, Connecticut.)

II. Weightbearing Evaluation

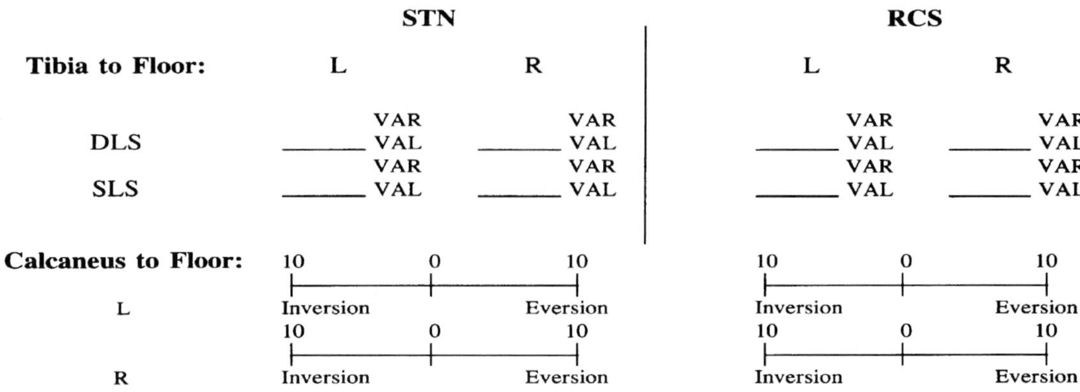

	STN L	STN R	RCS L	RCS R
Tibia to Floor:				
DLS	_____ VAR / VAL	_____ VAR / VAL	_____ VAR / VAL	_____ VAR / VAL
SLS	_____ VAR / VAL	_____ VAR / VAL	_____ VAR / VAL	_____ VAR / VAL

Calcaneus to Floor:

	STN	RCS
L	10 — 0 — 10 (Inversion — Eversion)	10 — 0 — 10 (Inversion — Eversion)
R	10 — 0 — 10 (Inversion — Eversion)	10 — 0 — 10 (Inversion — Eversion)

III. Soft Tissue Restrictions

	L	R
Iliopsoas	_____	_____
Rectus Femoris	_____	_____
ITB	_____	_____
Hamstring	_____	_____
Gastroc	_____	_____
Soleus	_____	_____

	L	R
Hip Rotation (Hips 90º, Knees 90º)		
Internal	_____	_____
External	_____	_____
Hip Rotation (Hips 0º, Knees 90º)		
Internal	_____	_____
External	_____	_____

IV. Postural Observations

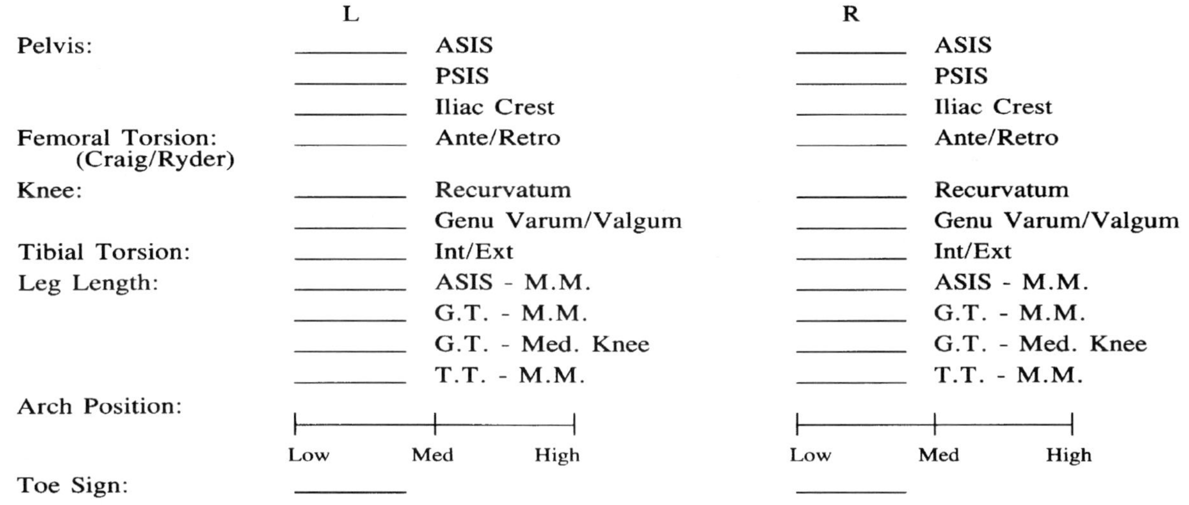

	L		R	
Pelvis:	_____	ASIS	_____	ASIS
	_____	PSIS	_____	PSIS
	_____	Iliac Crest	_____	Iliac Crest
Femoral Torsion: (Craig/Ryder)	_____	Ante/Retro	_____	Ante/Retro
Knee:	_____	Recurvatum	_____	Recurvatum
	_____	Genu Varum/Valgum	_____	Genu Varum/Valgum
Tibial Torsion:	_____	Int/Ext	_____	Int/Ext
Leg Length:	_____	ASIS - M.M.	_____	ASIS - M.M.
	_____	G.T. - M.M.	_____	G.T. - M.M.
	_____	G.T. - Med. Knee	_____	G.T. - Med. Knee
	_____	T.T. - M.M.	_____	T.T. - M.M.
Arch Position:	Low — Med — High		Low — Med — High	
Toe Sign:	_____		_____	

Fig. 8.5, Cont'd

are identified in the biomechanical examination: rearfoot varus, forefoot varus, forefoot valgus, equinus deformity, and plantarflexed first ray.

The theoretical model of biomechanical foot and ankle examination is based on the work of Root and colleagues.[8] Debate continues about the validity of Root's criteria for normalcy and the assumption that the STJ is in neutral position from MSt to TSt of the gait cycle. Reliability of the measurement techniques used to determine STJ neutral position has also been questioned.[42–45] Although controversial, Root's theory and his biomechanical evaluation and treatment techniques are used by many clinicians.

Root describes deviations from normal foot alignment as "intrinsic" foot deformities, which can lead to aberrant lower extremity function and musculoskeletal pathological conditions.[8,46] To prescribe an appropriate biomechanical foot orthosis, the source of the pathological condition or deformity must be determined by a detailed patient history and a comprehensive biomechanical examination.[47] This helps the clinician identify resultant pathomechanical abnormalities and determine the benefits of orthotic intervention.

Non–Weight-Bearing Open Chain Examination

During the non–weight-bearing open chain examination, the basic architecture of the foot and ankle is assessed. Any bony deformities or prominence of the joints or rays (toes) and any callosities are noted. The examiner uses a goniometer to locate the subtalar neutral (STN) position and identify any intrinsic foot deformities.

The non–weight-bearing goniometric examination is performed with the patient in the prone position, with the targeted lower extremity positioned with extended knee and the foot 6 to 8 inches off the treatment table. Placing the contralateral lower extremity in a figure-four position orients the ipsilateral lower extremity in the frontal plane, reducing the influence of proximal rotational limb disorders on measurement.[48]

EXAMINATION OF THE REARFOOT

Goniometric measurements of the non–weight-bearing examination assess the rearfoot with respect to STN position, as well as STJ mobility, based on calcaneal positioning in the frontal plane. Calcaneal frontal plane motion is the most readily examined component of triplanar STJ motion. To perform the examination, the stationary arm of a goniometer is aligned with an imagined bisection of the lower third of the limb (tibiofibular complex), the mobile arm is aligned with an imaginary bisection of the posterior surface of the calcaneus, and the axis of the goniometer is aligned at the STJ axis, just above the superior border of the calcaneus but beneath the level of the medial and lateral malleoli (Fig. 8.6).[48,49]

Subtalar Neutral Position

STN position can be manually estimated by palpation or by using a mathematical model developed by Root. If using palpation, the examiner identifies the anteromedial and anterolateral aspects of the talar head with the thumb and index fingers of the hand closest to the patient's midline, placing the thumb just proximal to the navicular tuberosity approximately 1 inch below and 1 inch distal to the medial malleolus (Fig. 8.7). In STJ pronation, the anteromedial talar head is most prominent beneath the thumb, and an anterolateral sulcus (the sinus tarsi) is apparent. The index finger is placed in this sulcus, where the talar head is found to protrude when the foot is fully supinated. The thumb and index finger of the other hand grasp the fourth and fifth metatarsal heads, moving the foot in an arc of adduction and inversion (supination) and abduction and eversion (pronation). STN is the point where the talar head is equally prominent anteromedially and anterolaterally.[46,48,49] The examiner then "loads" the foot by applying a dorsally directed pressure against the fourth and fifth metatarsal heads until slight resistance is felt. The loading procedure locks the MTJ against the rearfoot, mimicking GRFs of MSt.[8,50] The angular relation between the bisection of the calcaneus and the bisection of the lower third of the leg is measured with a goniometer (see Fig. 8.6), recorded on the evaluation form as rearfoot STN position.

Root's mathematical model for determining STN position uses a quantitative goniometric formula.[8,46] First, end ROM calcaneal inversion and eversion are determined by goniometric measurement. Total calcaneal ROM is the sum of the inversion and eversion values. The STN position is determined as the calcaneus is moved into inversion at one-third of the total calcaneal ROM. If end-range calcaneal

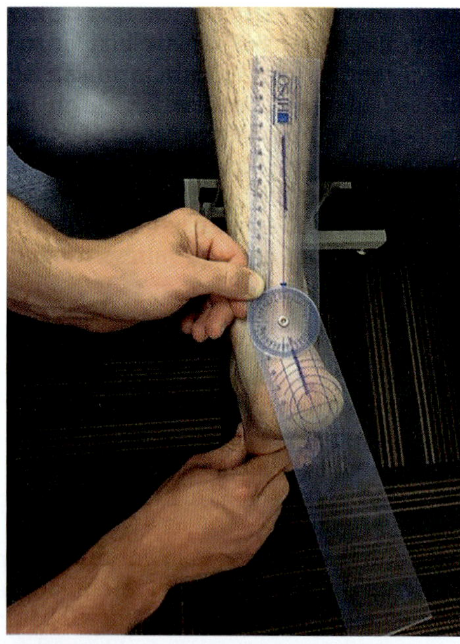

Fig. 8.6 Non–weight-bearing goniometric technique. A loading force applied by the examiner over the fourth and fifth metatarsal heads locks the forefoot on the rearfoot while the examiner's opposite hand operates the goniometer to measure subtalar neutral position and calcaneal range of motion. The examiner is seated at the distal end of the treatment table, with the chair height adjusted to position the patient's foot at chest level.

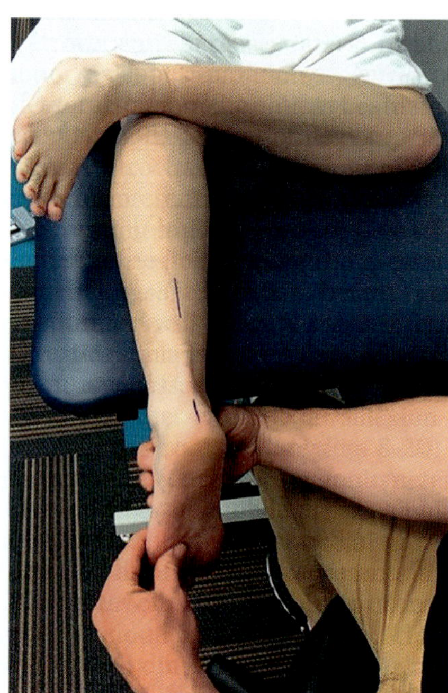

Fig. 8.7 To determine subtalar neutral position, the examiner moves the forefoot slowly between supination and pronation until the anteromedial and anterolateral surfaces of the head of the talus are equally prominent.

inversion is 25 degrees and end-range calcaneal eversion is +5 degrees, total calcaneal ROM would be 30 degrees. STN position is calculated to be at 5 degrees calcaneal inversion, one-third of the distance from its fully everted position.

Reliability and clinical validity of both models have been debated.[44,46,48,51–53] Although acceptable reliability is possible, it is influenced by examiner experience. Palpation to determine STN position is efficient in terms of time but requires more advanced manual skills and experience than the mathematical model. The mathematical model may be more reliable for the entry-level practitioner.

Calcaneal Range of Motion

Calcaneal inversion and eversion occur primarily at the STJ, with lesser contributions from the TCJ. Calcaneal ROM is assessed with the patient in the prone position with the same anatomical landmarks and lines of bisection as for STN assessment. The examiner grasps the calcaneus in one hand, fully inverts it in the frontal plane until end ROM is achieved, and then takes a goniometric measurement.[53] The procedure is repeated for calcaneal eversion. The TCJ must be maintained in a neutral to slightly dorsiflexed position while measuring to lock it in a closed-packed position and better isolate STJ motion.[54] Normative values of 20 degrees for calcaneal inversion and 10 degrees beyond vertical for eversion have been reported.[8]

Because values of calcaneal eversion are larger when assessed in a full weight-bearing position, some clinicians suggest that this position is more clinically valid.[42,53] Assessment of calcaneal eversion in the weight-bearing position represents a total “functional” pronation and eversion that is the summation of motion occurring at the STJ and compensatory motion occurring extrinsic to the STJ (e.g., TCJ, MTJ). Passive assessment of calcaneal eversion in a non–weight-bearing examination remains the most accurate method to determine the degree of composite pronation acquired from the STJ itself.

Talocrural Joint Range of Motion

In normal walking, the TCJ is maximally dorsiflexed just before heel rise when the knee is fully extended and the STJ is in a nearly neutral position.[8,55] When and whether an actual STN position ever occurs during gait is disputed.[42] However, the use of a standard position of knee extension and STN offers a consistent point of reference when assessing TCJ dorsiflexion. According to most sources, a minimum of 10 degrees TCJ dorsiflexion is required for normal gait; anything less is classified as an equinus deformity.[8,55–58] A minimum of 20 degrees of plantarflexion is also required for normal gait.[8]

Ankle dorsiflexion is measured in a non–weight-bearing position with the STJ held in the neutral position and the knee extended. The examiner forcefully dorsiflexes the ankle with active assistance from the patient. Active assistance encourages reciprocal inhibition of the calf muscle group and is essential for accurate measurement.[55] The proximal arm of the goniometer is positioned along the lateral aspect of the fibula, the distal arm along the lateral border of the fifth metatarsal, and the axis distal to the lateral malleolus.[59] An alternative placement of the distal arm of the goniometer along the inferolateral border of the calcaneus may more effectively isolate true TCJ dorsiflexion (Fig. 8.8).

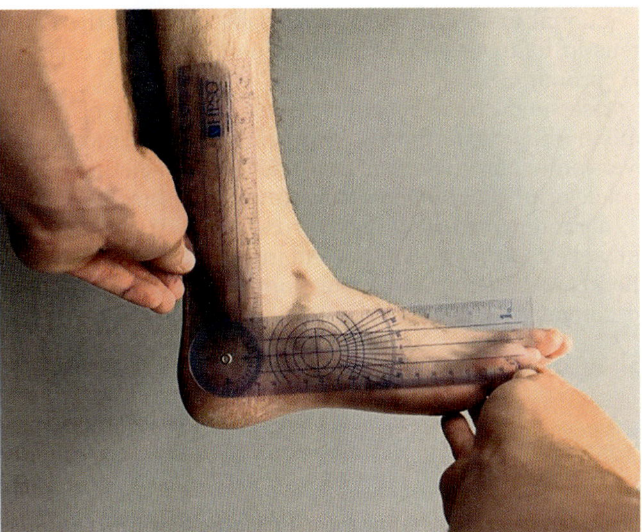

Fig. 8.8 Alignment of the distal arm of the goniometer along the inferior-lateral border of the calcaneus may provide a more accurate measure of talocrural joint dorsiflexion than the traditional alignment along the shaft of the fifth metatarsal used to measure overall ankle dorsiflexion.

This value is recorded as rearfoot dorsiflexion. Forefoot dorsiflexion is measured by repositioning the distal arm along the lateral aspect of the fifth metatarsal. This method allows the examiner to identify contributions or restrictions in sagittal plane motion from the oblique axis of the MTJ.

If ankle dorsiflexion is less than 10 degrees when measured with the knee extended, remeasurement with the knee flexed may rule out soft tissue restriction of the gastrocnemius-soleus complex.[8,55] If dorsiflexion values are consistent in both positions, the limitation is likely a result of osseous equinus formation of the ankle.

During gait, ankle dorsiflexion occurs in a closed kinetic chain as the tibia and fibula rotate forward over a fixed foot. On the basis of this, some have suggested that assessing ankle dorsiflexion may be more accurate with the patient in a weight-bearing position.[42,57] The weight-bearing technique measures the angle between the tibia and the floor as the patient leans forward with the foot flat on the floor. Unwanted compensations are often difficult to control during weight bearing and may mask true TCJ limitations. The non–weight-bearing technique allows the examiner to assess end-feel and joint play, as well as mechanical blocks or joint laxity, providing additional information not accessible in the weight-bearing examination.

Rearfoot Deformities

Normal rearfoot position is one in which STN is 1 to 4 degrees of varus.[43,44,52,53] Values of more than 4 degrees are described as a rearfoot varus deformity. This deformity may be the result of ontogenetic failure of the calcaneus to derotate sufficiently during early childhood development.[8,50,60] Because this deformity is a torsional structural malalignment of the calcaneus, not a joint-related problem, the TCJ and STJ lines remain congruent when observed in the non–weight-bearing STN position. As a structural deformity, it cannot be corrected or reduced by joint mobilization or a strengthening program. Instead, it is managed with a functional foot orthosis that partially supports the calcaneus in its inverted alignment while preventing excessive STJ pronation.

Assessment of calcaneal ROM predicts quality of motion and the integrity of the STJ. Measuring calcaneal motion into eversion allows the examiner to determine whether a rearfoot deformity is compensated or uncompensated (Fig. 8.9).

In a compensated rearfoot varus deformity, the calcaneus fully everts to vertical or beyond in weight bearing because the STJ possesses an adequate amount of pronatory motion to compensate for the deformity. A compensated rearfoot varus deformity of 10 degrees (STN position) requires that the STJ pronate or evert at least 10 degrees to enable the medial condyle of the calcaneus to achieve ground contact in weight bearing. Such excessive pronatory motion causes medial gapping and lateral constriction at the STJ line and a medial bulge of the talus as it moves into adduction and plantarflexion.

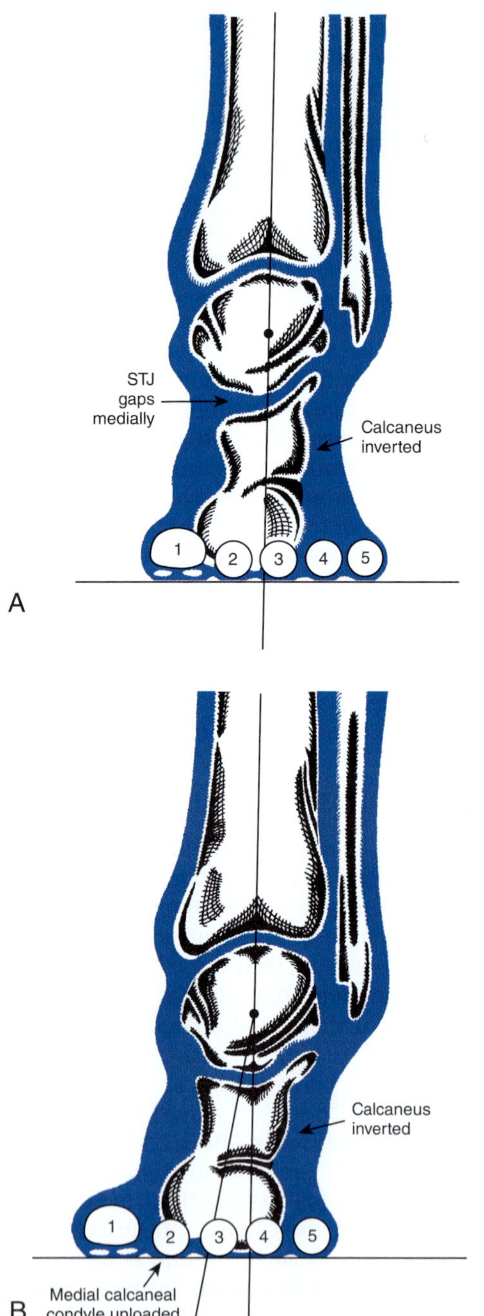

Fig. 8.9 (A) In relaxed calcaneal stance, compensation for a rearfoot varus is normally subtalar joint (STJ) pronation. (B) In an uncompensated rearfoot varus, the STJ cannot pronate and instead may develop compensatory midtarsal joint pronation about the longitudinal joint axis. (Courtesy Stride, Inc., Middlebury, Connecticut.)

In an uncompensated rearfoot varus deformity, the calcaneus remains fixed in its inverted STN position with no eversion motion at the STJ. A partially compensated rearfoot varus deformity allows for partial STJ eversion so that the medial condyle of the calcaneus does not make complete contact with the ground on weight bearing. Alternative compensatory motion, extrinsic to the STJ, is necessary to achieve weight bearing on the medial aspect of the foot. One common compensation is an acquired soft tissue (valgus) deformity of the forefoot caused by a plantarflexed first ray. Other sources of compensatory motion can occur at the MTJ or proximally at the knee, hip, or sacroiliac joints.

An equinus deformity occurs when fewer than 10 degrees of ankle dorsiflexion are available as a result of osseous or muscular problems.[56,58,61,62] Clubfoot (talipes equinovarus) is a congenital osseous deformity that includes varus deformity of both rearfoot and forefoot, rearfoot equinus, and an inverted and adducted forefoot.[63,64] The angular relation between the body and the head and neck of the talus is decreased, and the navicular is shifted medially. Muscular forms of equinus include congenital or acquired soft tissue shortening or muscle spasm.[58] Tissue contracture or shortening occurs in both contractile tissues (gastrocnemius, soleus, and plantaris) and noncontractile tissues (teno-Achilles and plantar fascia).[56,58]

Compensation for an equinus deformity occurs at the foot through pronation, perpetuating soft tissue contractures. The STJ is forced to pronate maximally to gain as much sagittal plane dorsiflexion as possible. Although foot pronation allows some dorsiflexion from the STJ, the amount is often inadequate. Pronation of the STJ unlocks the MTJ, creating an unstable midfoot while allowing further dorsiflexion and forefoot abduction from the oblique axis of the MTJ.[58] Other compensatory strategies for equinus deformity include knee flexion (especially in individuals with cerebral palsy), early heel rise, toe walking, shortened stride length of the contralateral lower limb, and toe-out walking.[34,46,58] Clinical consequences of long-term ankle equinus include many conditions normally associated with the excessively pronated foot: plantar fasciopathy, heel spurs, bunions, and capsulitis.[58]

EXAMINATION OF THE FOREFOOT

Forefoot position is assessed with the STJ in neutral position. Because the first and fifth rays have independent axes of motion, forefoot orientation is defined by the planar relation of the second, third, and fourth rays to the bisection line of the calcaneus.

NEUTRAL FOREFOOT POSITION

If the forefoot is properly balanced, the plane of the three central metatarsals is perpendicular to the bisection of the calcaneus when in STN (Fig. 8.10). In a forefoot varus

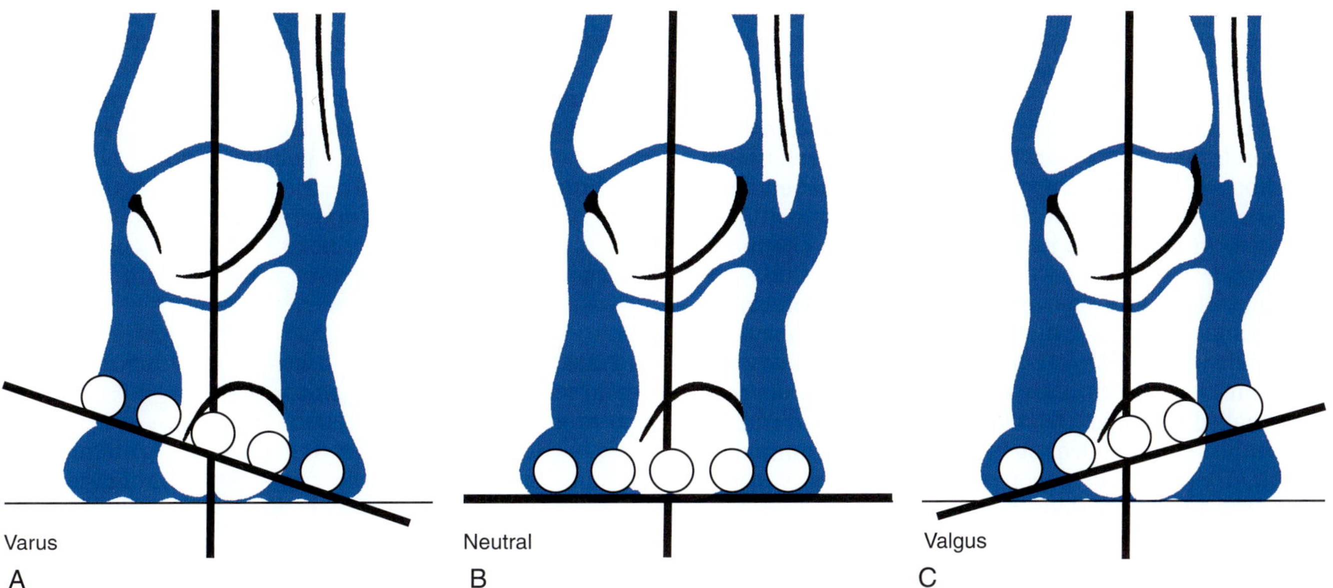

Fig. 8.10 In subtalar neutral position, the normal orientation of the forefoot to the calcaneus (B) is perpendicular. Excessive supination and inversion of the forefoot in subtalar neutral position indicates a forefoot varus (A), whereas excessive pronation and eversion of the forefoot indicates a forefoot valgus (C). (Courtesy Stride, Inc., Middlebury, Connecticut.)

deformity, the forefoot is excessively supinated or inverted, whereas in a forefoot valgus the forefoot is excessively pronated or everted.

Mobility Testing: Locking Mechanism

To isolate the STN position in the non–weight-bearing examination, the examiner attempts to lock the MTJ by applying a dorsally directed loading pressure with the thumb and index fingers over the fourth and fifth metatarsal heads of the patient's foot (see Figs. 8.6 and 8.7). Loading force must be gently applied over the fourth and fifth metatarsal heads until tissue slack is taken up from the normally plantarflexed resting position of the ankle.[8,60] Overload of the forefoot leads to dorsiflexion and abduction of the foot, placing the forefoot in an excessively pronated position and giving a false valgus orientation.

Although many forefoot measurement devices are available, forefoot orientation can be accurately assessed with a standard goniometer.[65] To assess the forefoot to rearfoot relation, the proximal arm of the goniometer is aligned along the bisection of the calcaneus, with the axis just below its distal border. The distal arm is positioned in the plane of the three central metatarsal heads (Fig. 8.11). The angular displacement is recorded on the evaluation form under STN position for the forefoot assessment (see Fig. 8.5).

In normal walking, the MTJ locks as heel rise begins so that the foot is converted into a rigid lever for propulsion. This lock requires that the STJ be in the neutral position. Clinical assessment of MTJ mobility and the locking mechanism is an advanced manual skill. Observations made during weight-bearing assessment (e.g., toe sign, navicular drop test, talar bulge) provide an elementary method to identify an MTJ unable to lock.

An ineffective locking mechanism at the MTJ is often more clinically significant than the absolute degree of forefoot deformity. For example, a forefoot varus deformity of 3 degrees with a poor MTJ locking mechanism may be symptomatic, whereas an 8-degree forefoot varus deformity with a normal MTJ locking mechanism may not be.

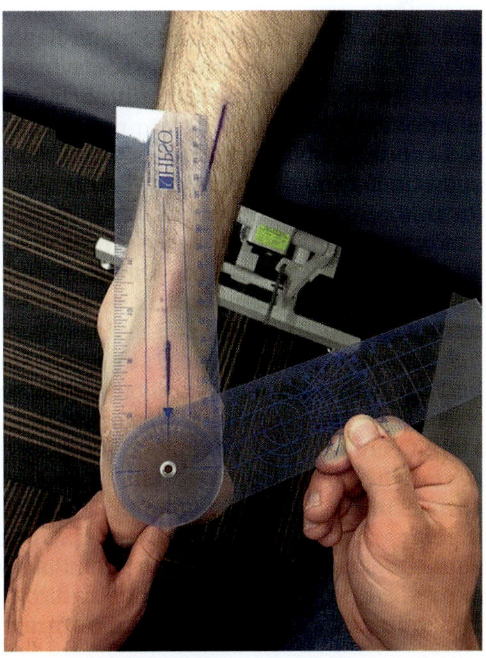

Fig. 8.11 Measurement of forefoot orientation in subtalar neutral position with a standard goniometer. The proximal arm of the goniometer is aligned with the bisection of the posterior surface of the calcaneus, and the distal arm parallels the plane of the metatarsal heads. The axis lies beneath the distal aspect of the calcaneus.

Identifying Forefoot Deformities

Although the prevalence of forefoot deformity, with or without symptoms, is well documented, less agreement exists regarding which types of deformity are most common.[52,66] If an individual has bilateral forefoot deformity, the deformities may not be of the same severity or type. MTJ deformities change the location of the lock of the forefoot against the rearfoot.[8] Although these osseous frontal plane deformities alter the direction of motion, they do not limit the total ROM of the MTJ.[8] In forefoot varus, locking of the forefoot occurs in an inverted position relative to the rearfoot.[8] Forefoot varus results from ontogenetic failure of the normal valgus rotation of the head and neck of the talus in relation to its body during early childhood development.[8,50,60]

Compensations for foot deformities are viewed in a relaxed weight-bearing position, which is referred to as relaxed calcaneal stance (RCS). When excessive pronation of the STJ compensates for the deformity on weight bearing, the condition is called a compensated forefoot varus (Fig. 8.12A). When the STJ cannot adequately pronate to accommodate an inverted forefoot, an uncompensated forefoot varus is present. The medial forefoot does not make contact with the ground, and the lateral forefoot is subjected to excessive pressure. A thick callus develops beneath the head of the fifth metatarsal, and the risk of stress fracture is increased. Plantarflexion of the first ray and pronation at the MTJ are common compensations that allow the medial forefoot to make contact with the ground (see Fig. 8.12B). Persistent MTJ stress may lead to joint damage and excessive forefoot abduction and eversion.

Forefoot valgus occurs in the frontal plane deformity, locking the forefoot in eversion relative to the rearfoot.[8] Root suggests that this deformity results from ontogenetic overrotation of the talar head and neck in relation to its body during early childhood development.[8,50,60] Forefoot valgus can be a rigid or flexible deformity. In rigid forefoot valgus, the compensatory weight-bearing mechanism occurs at the STJ as excessive supination or calcaneal inversion. It is a result of excessive premature GRFs at the first metatarsal head, causing rapid STJ inversion and increasing loading forces beneath the fifth metatarsal head. Thick callosities are often present beneath the first and fifth metatarsal heads. In contrast, flexible forefoot valgus is usually an acquired soft tissue condition. It most often occurs as a consequence of uncompensated rearfoot varus as an attempt to increase weight bearing along the medial foot. Because this deformity is flexible, no compensatory mechanism is necessary. Contact force beneath the first metatarsal head simply pushes it up out of the way, and the foot functions as if this condition were not present.

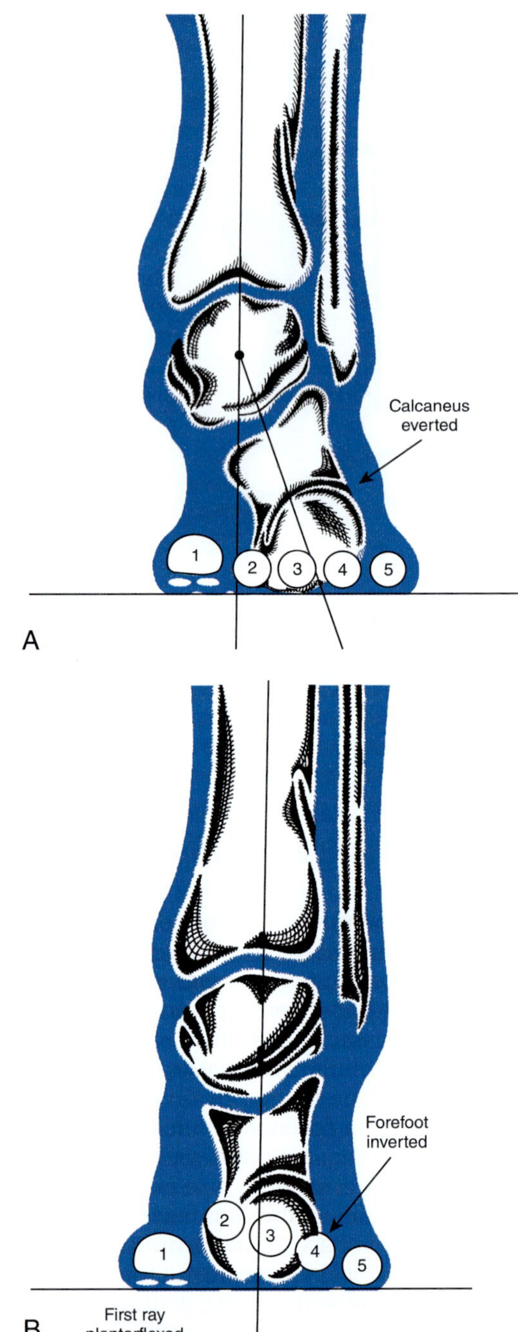

Fig. 8.12 (A) In relaxed calcaneal stance, compensation for a forefoot varus deformity is normally subtalar joint pronation, resulting in an everted calcaneus. (B) In an uncompensated forefoot varus, the subtalar joint is unable to compensate. Instead, the first ray plantarflexes to achieve weight bearing medially on the foot. (Courtesy Stride, Inc., Middlebury, Connecticut.)

The First Ray

Assessment of first ray position is also carried out in the STN position. Ideally, the first ray lies within the common transverse plane of the lesser metatarsal heads. To examine the mobility of the first ray, the examiner holds the first metatarsal head between the thumb and index finger and performs a dorsal and plantar glide while stabilizing the lesser metatarsal heads with the other hand. Normally, first ray movement is at least one thumb width above and below the plane of the other metatarsal heads.[8]

As the stance phase is completed, activity of the fibularis longus creates a pronatory twist of the forefoot, stabilizing the medial column of the foot on the ground, locking the MTJ about its longitudinal axis, and converting the foot to a rigid lever for propulsion. Adequate plantarflexion of the first ray must be present for conversion from flexible forefoot to a rigid lever. Three factors determine how much first ray plantarflexion must occur: the amount of inversion of the foot at propulsion, the width of the foot, and the length of the second metatarsal.[8] The more the foot inverts during propulsion, the further the first ray must plantarflex to make ground contact. Elevation of the medial forefoot is related to foot width; wide feet require more first ray plantarflexion. An excessively long second metatarsal also increases the distance the first ray must plantarflex to make ground contact.

In some instances, the first ray is inappropriately dorsiflexed above the plane of the other metatarsals, resulting in restriction of plantarflexion and impeding normal propulsion. The first ray may also be plantarflexed below the plane of the other metatarsals. In uncompensated rearfoot varus, for example, the eversion motion of the calcaneus is insufficient, the medial condyle fails to make contact with the ground, and excessive weight bearing is present on the lateral border of the foot. The fibularis longus contracts to pull the first metatarsal head toward the ground in an attempt to load the medial side of the foot. This action is possible because of the cuboid pulley system (Fig. 8.13).[8] When the STJ remains abnormally pronated in late stance phase, orientation of the cuboid tunnel is altered and the mechanical advantage of the fibularis longus is lost. The MTJ cannot lock, and the foot is unstable throughout propulsion.

The presence of a rigid plantarflexed first ray sometimes results in a functional forefoot valgus (Fig. 8.14). The compensatory mechanism for this condition is similar to that for rigid forefoot valgus: STJ supination or calcaneal inversion on weight bearing to lower the lateral aspect of the foot to the ground.

The Hallux

In normal gait, dorsiflexion of the hallux occurs during the late propulsive phase as the body moves forward over the foot. Sagittal plane motion of the hallux is assessed as passive ROM. The stationary arm of the goniometer is positioned along the medial first metatarsal and the mobile arm along the medial proximal phalanx of the hallux. The axis is medial to the first MTP joint.[54] Sufficient force is applied to bring the hallux to its end ROM. Normal range of hallux dorsiflexion is between 70 and 90 degrees.[8,59]

In hallux limitus deformity, pathomechanical functioning of the first MTP joint prevents the hallux from moving through its full range of dorsiflexion during propulsion. Repetitive trauma to the first MTP joint can lead to ankylosis, or hallux rigidus. Functional hallux limitus is a condition in which full first MTP ROM is present when non–weight bearing, but a functional restriction of hallux dorsiflexion occurs during gait. Functional hallux limitus disrupts the normal windlass mechanism previously described.[67,68]

Limitation of hallux dorsiflexion prohibits the normal progression of the foot and interferes with propulsion of the body over the hallux. Several gait compensations can overcome this limitation.[67,68] An abducted or toe-out gait pattern shifts propulsion to the medial border of the hallux. A pinched callus then develops from friction between the hallux and shoe during propulsion. Alternatively, the IP joint of the hallux may hyperextend, causing a callus in the sulcus of the IP joint and the forefoot may increase supination to compensate for the decreased dorsiflexion of the hallux.[67–69]

Hallux abductovalgus (HAV) is a progressive, acquired deformity of the first MTP joint that eventually results in a valgus subluxation of the hallux.[8,50] This deformity is caused by abnormal first ray pronation and hypermobility.[4] A common misconception is that HAV is caused by restrictive footwear. Although inappropriate or restrictive footwear can accentuate or speed the progression of HAV deformity when present, the deformity is frequently observed in populations that do not typically wear shoes.[8,50]

ADDITIONAL OBSERVATIONS

Several other important observations are made as the non–weight-bearing examination is completed. Non–weight-bearing arch height is observed for later comparison to weight-bearing arch height as a composite estimate of foot

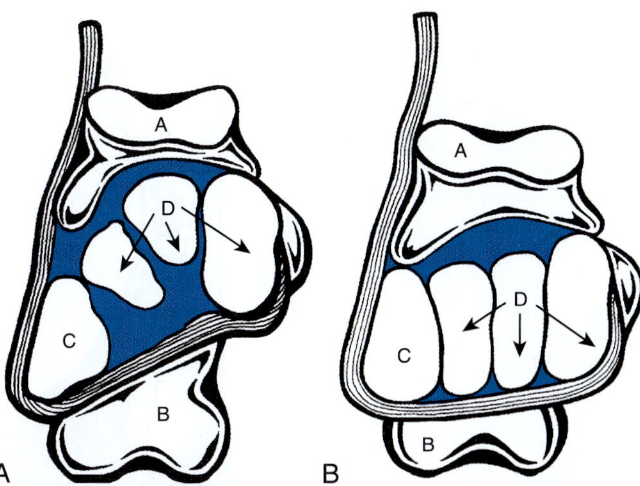

Fig. 8.13 (A) Cuboid pulley mechanism in a normal foot. (B) In an abnormally pronated foot, the mechanical advantage of the fibularis muscles is impaired. *A*, Talus; *B*, calcaneus; *C*, cuboid; *D*, the cuneiforms. (Courtesy Stride, Inc., Middlebury, Connecticut.)

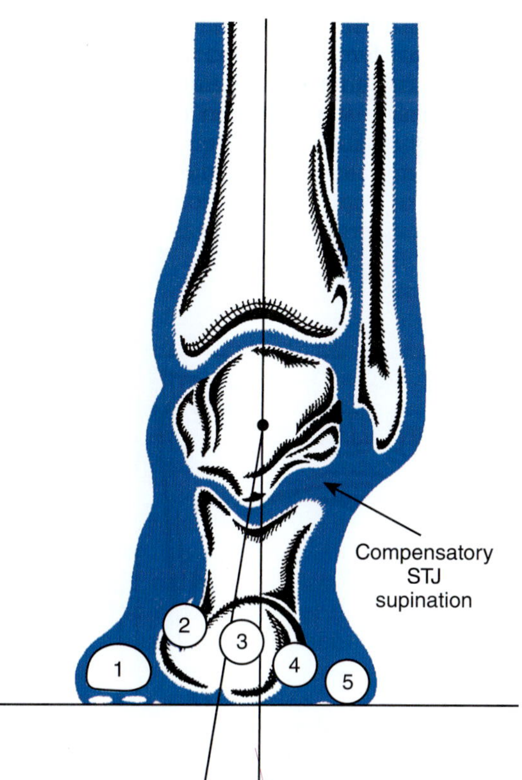

Fig. 8.14 Plantarflexed first ray deformity in relaxed calcaneal stance. Compensation occurs at the subtalar joint (STJ), with lateral gapping and medial compression. (Courtesy Stride, Inc., Middlebury, Connecticut.)

pronation. Toes are inspected for positional deformities such as hammertoe, claw toe, crossover deformity, and the presence of bunions or bunionettes. The foot is checked for calluses, plantar warts, retrocalcaneal bursitis, or other signs of excessive pressure. The shoes are inspected for excessive or uneven wear patterns.

Static Weight-Bearing Closed Kinetic Chain Examination

The open chain kinetic motion evaluated in the non–weight-bearing examination is dramatically different from the functional sequence of events in the closed kinetic chain of standing and walking. Open kinetic chain pronation (calcaneal dorsiflexion, eversion, and abduction) and supination (calcaneal plantarflex, inversion, and adduction) are triplanar motions around the STJ.[8,16,32] During closed kinetic chain pronation, internal rotation of the leg is coupled with talar adduction and calcaneal plantarflexion and eversion. Closed kinetic chain supination couples external rotation of the leg with talar abduction and calcaneal dorsiflexion and inversion. In the open kinetic chain, movement is initiated in the distal segment (the foot). In the closed kinetic chain, motion is initiated proximally (at the tibia and talus). A thorough closed kinetic chain examination includes static postural observations, dynamic motion testing, and gait assessment.

Compensatory mechanisms that result from intrinsic deformities are assessed as the foot is subjected to GRFs during the static weight-bearing examination. This provides valuable insight regarding how the body compensates for the intrinsic foot deformities or impairments of normal foot joint function identified in the non–weight-bearing examination. Improper foot functioning can lead to a complex series of compensations that influence the mobility patterns of the foot and lower leg, as well as the knee, hip, pelvis, and spine.

The patient stands in a relaxed, weight-bearing posture (RCS). The examiner observes the patient's preferred stance, noting postural alignment and foot placement angle. The patient then adjusts the stance position, if necessary, to assume equal weight-bearing double-limb support, with feet 5 to 10 cm apart and oriented in neutral toe-in and toe-out foot placement angle. This adjusted posture, with neutral foot placement angle, offers a better frame of reference for assessing planar alignment and enhances the reliability and consistency of the measurement.[46] Postural alignment or body symmetry of the patient is evaluated in the frontal, sagittal, and transverse planes. Recent research has suggested the use of additional biomechanical examination tools such as the Foot Posture Index (FPI) to reliably classify foot type.[70] Utilizing multiple methods may be beneficial. The FPI and RCS methods demonstrate moderate correlations and may be used in the biomechanical examination of the foot.[71]

FRONTAL PLANE

Static weight-bearing examination in the frontal plane focuses on the angular relation of the calcaneus and the tibia and fibula with respect to the floor and the relation between the pelvis and the lower leg.

Calcaneal Alignment to the Floor

With the patient in double-limb stance posture, a line bisecting the posterior surface of the calcaneus is visualized and the angular relation between the line and the floor is taken. Because the infracalcaneal fat pad often migrates (related to prolonged weight bearing), care must be taken to avoid errors in visual assessment (Fig. 8.15). Palpation of the osseous medial, lateral, and inferior borders of the calcaneus helps to factor out fat pad migration and to improve measurement accuracy. Calcaneal alignment also can be quantified with a protractor to measure the degree of calcaneal tilt relative to vertical.[72]

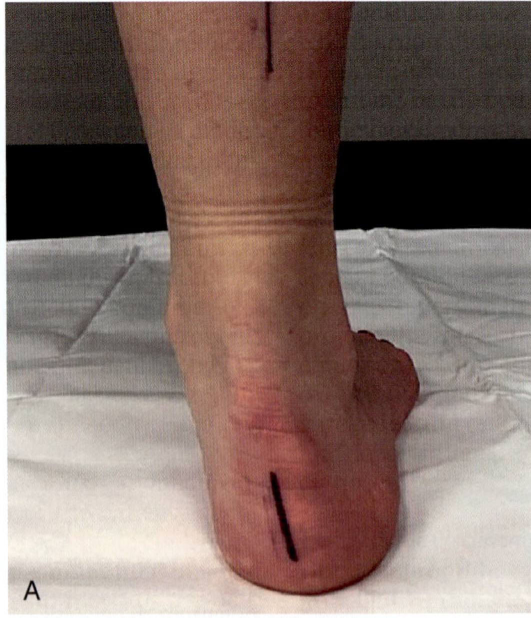

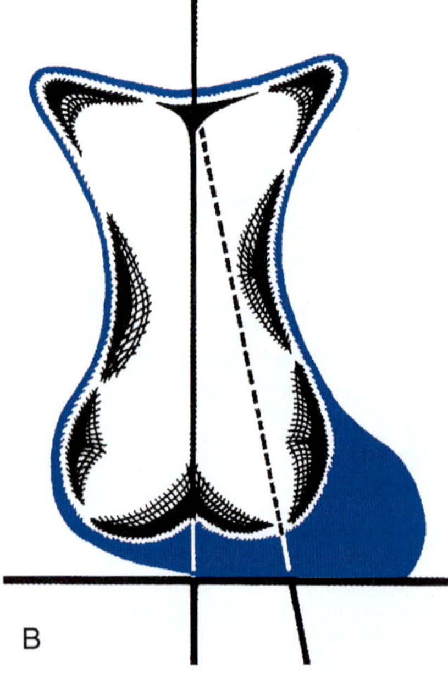

Fig. 8.15 (A) Calcaneal alignment to floor. (B) Lateral migration of the infracalcaneal fat pad can give the illusion of an everted calcaneal to floor alignment. (Courtesy Stride, Inc., Middlebury, Connecticut.)

The key question to answer is whether the calcaneus is inverted, vertical, or everted relative to the floor during stance; the actual angular degree is not as important as the relative orientation of the calcaneus. This component of the examination assesses the ability of the STJ to provide enough pronation to compensate for its neutral position. In the normal closed-chain STN position, the calcaneus is in 1 to 4 degrees of varus (inversion). The STJ must have an equal amount of compensatory pronation to lower the medial condyle to the ground for a vertical calcaneus. If a patient has uncompensated rearfoot varus of 10 degrees in STN as well as restricted calcaneal motion (−4 degrees) eversion, the STJ would not be able to achieve sufficient pronation or eversion in stance for normal calcaneal alignment. Instead, the calcaneus would be in an inverted alignment relative to the floor. Inverted calcaneal position also occurs when a rigid forefoot valgus or rigid plantarflexed first ray deformity is present. STJ supination is a compensatory mechanism for both deformities.

In contrast, forefoot varus deformity requires excessive compensatory STJ pronation; calcaneal eversion occurs in weight bearing. The position of the calcaneus with respect to the floor provides insight into the type of STJ compensation present and can be correlated with the biomechanical findings of the non–weight-bearing examination. If the STJ is unable to pronate enough to completely compensate for a deformity, additional pronatory motion occurs at the MTJ or by eversion tilting of the talus within the ankle mortise.[8,46,53] The functional rearfoot unit (calcaneus and talus) may assume a valgus (everted) position relative to the floor, even if calcaneal eversion is restricted.

Tibiofibular Alignment

Proximal structural malalignments, such as tibial varum or valgum, contribute to abnormal foot pronation and overuse injuries. In osseous congenital tibial varum, the distal third of the tibia is angled medially in the frontal plane, whereas in tibialvalgum, the distal tibia inclines away from the midline.[46]

Tibial alignment can be measured with either a standard goniometer (Fig. 8.16) or a bubble inclinometer; both assess the angular relation between the bisection of the distal third of the lower leg relative to the supporting surface.[46,73] Radiographic measurement of lower leg position is better correlated with clinically assessed tibiofibular position values than with isolated tibial position. Radiographic measurement may be the most accurate method to isolate true tibial varum.[73]

The test position is critical because variation in STJ alignment greatly influences tibiofibular varum measurement values. Tibiofibular varum values are larger in RCS than in the STN position because of the combined effects of osseous malalignment and varus leg alignment associated with compensatory STJ pronation in stance.[73–75] The incidence of tibiofibular varum appears to be high, although no clear normative values have been established.

The alignment of the distal third of the leg relative to the floor more accurately represents tibiofibular position than tibial position. Values assessed in STN reflect neutral tibiofibular alignment, whereas values assessed in RCS represent compensatory tibiofibular repositioning in response to STJ and MTJ pronation. High tibiofibular varum values measured in STN elevate the medial foot from the supporting surface, requiring excessive compensatory foot pronation during gait. High tibiofibular varum values in RCS suggest excessive foot pronation, although the source of that pronation cannot be isolated.

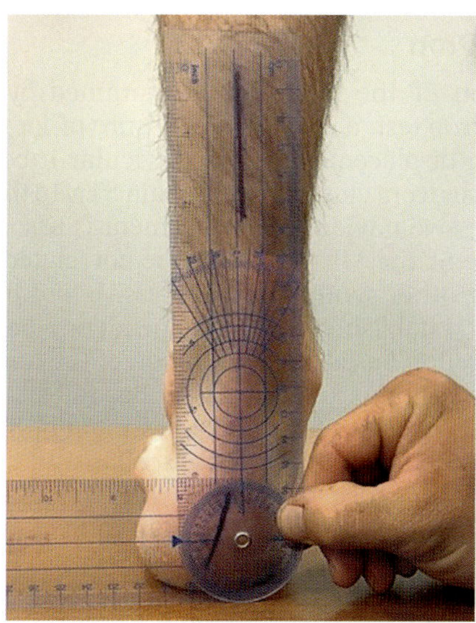

Fig. 8.16 Goniometric assessment of tibiofibular varum. The proximal arm of the goniometer is aligned with the bisection of the distal third of the tibiofibular complex, and the distal arm is level with the floor. The axis of measurement shifts with the degree of varum or valgum deformity and may not always fall directly behind the calcaneus.

Alignment of the Pelvis and Lower Leg

The final component of the frontal plane assessment evaluates symmetry of the anterosuperior iliac spines, iliac crests, greater trochanters, gluteal folds, popliteal creases, genu varum or valgum deformities, fibular heads, patellae, and malleolar levels. Asymmetry often indicates sacroiliac joint dysfunction or leg-length discrepancy, influencing foot position and function in the closed kinetic chain.

SAGITTAL PLANE

The second component of the weight-bearing examination considers function in the sagittal plane. The examiner looks for evidence of genu recurvatum or excessive knee flexion, navicular drop, talar bulge, and inadequate or excessive height of the longitudinal arch.

Knee Position

Viewing the patient's stance from the side, the examiner observes the verticality of the tibia. In genu recurvatum, the proximal tibia is aligned behind the axis of the TCJ, resulting in hyperextension of the knee and plantarflexion of the TCJ with relative shortening of the limb. Genu recurvatum also occurs as a compensation for equinus deformity at the ankle. When true leg-length discrepancy is present, two types of compensation are possible. If limb length difference is small, genu recurvatum may adequately shorten the longer limb. For larger limb length differences, knee flexion of the longer limb is often used to minimize asymmetry.

Navicular Drop

The position of the navicular is examined by using the navicular drop test, a composite measure of foot pronation focusing on displacement of the navicular tuberosity as a patient moves from closed kinetic chain STN to the RCS position.[76] Excessive navicular displacement is associated with the collapse of the MLA and may be correlated with midfoot pain or other symptoms of excessive foot pronation.[46] Subotnick[77] established an interdependency between MTJ and STJ function based on articulation of the navicular and cuboid with the talus and calcaneus. Brody[76] suggested that the navicular drop test is a valid assessment of STJ function in the closed kinetic chain. Zuil-Escobar and colleagues[78] further recommended the use of the navicular drop test as the first-choice examination tool in individuals with pes planus. Although navicular drop occurs with STJ pronation that stems from intrinsic foot deformity, it can also be the result of muscle insufficiency or ligamentous laxity.[46]

To measure navicular drop, an index card is held perpendicular to the medial foot, the level of the navicular tuberosity is marked in STN position and in RCS, and the distance between the marks is calculated.[42,46,78] Normative studies report a mean navicular drop of between 7.3 and 9 mm.[43,79] A navicular drop of more than 10 mm is considered abnormal.[79]

Talar Bulge and Arch Height

When excessive STJ pronation is present in stance, the talus moves into adduction and plantarflexion. Displacement of the talar head causes an observable medial bulge in the region of the talonavicular joint.[56] The height of the MLA normally decreases moderately in weight bearing as a result of normal STJ pronation. Pes planus deformity (flatfootedness) is characterized by excessive collapse of the MLA. In hereditary rigid flatfoot, the MLA is low or absent in non–weight-bearing and weight-bearing positions. In flexible flatfoot, the height of the MLA is normal in non–weight bearing but drops excessively in weight bearing because of abnormal STJ pronation. In normal foot alignment, the medial malleolus, navicular tuberosity, and first metatarsal head fall along the Feiss line.[56] In a severely pronated foot, the navicular tuberosity lies below the Feiss line. In extreme cases the tuberosity may even rest on the floor.[56,80]

TRANSVERSE PLANE

The final component of the static weight-bearing examination considers foot function in the transverse plane. The examiner looks for signs of excessive pronation or forefoot adduction and torsional deformities of the lower extremities.

Toe Sign

A positive toe sign indicates excessive pronation or abduction of the foot in the transverse plane (Fig. 8.17). The sign is determined by the number of toes that can be seen in a posterior view when the patient is standing in RCS with a neutral foot placement angle.[68] Normally no more than 1.5 toes are visible beyond the lateral border of the foot. If more toes can be seen, abnormal pronation may be present, causing excessive transverse plane motion or abduction of the foot. A false-positive toe sign can occur in the presence of a relative toe-out foot placement angle associated with lateral rotational deformities (e.g., femoral retroversion) or muscle imbalances that limit internal rotation of the hip (e.g., tight piriformis). Ensuring that the patient's patellae are oriented in the frontal plane before assessing toe sign reduces the risk of false-positive findings.

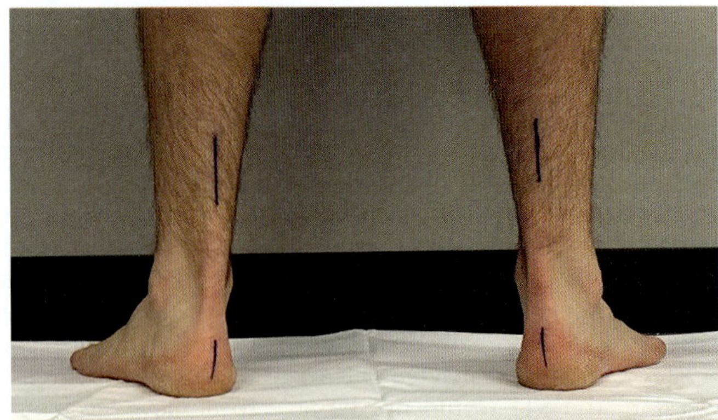

Fig. 8.17 Toe sign, demonstrating excessive transverse plane motion as evidenced by the abducted position of the forefoot.

Torsional Deformities

Transverse plane abnormalities of the femur and tibia also adversely affect normal foot functioning. The femoral shaft normally has approximately 15 degrees of medial rotation relative to the femoral head and neck (Fig. 8.18). In femoral anteversion more than 15 to 20 degrees of rotation are present, whereas in retroversion, fewer than the expected 15 to 20 degrees of medial rotation are present.[81] In normal transverse plane tibial alignment, the fibular malleolus is situated posterior to the tibial malleolus, for 20 to 30 degrees of lateral rotation.[21] Internal tibial torsion or femoral anteversion increase medial rotational forces, leading to abnormal foot pronation. Excessive external tibial rotation or femoral retroversion increases lateral rotational forces, leading to abnormal foot supination.

To assess femoral torsion, the patient lies in the prone position with the knee in 90 degrees of flexion.[46] The examiner palpates the greater trochanter as the lower limb is passively moved laterally (representing hip internal rotation) and medially (representing hip external rotation). Femoral torsion is measured at the point where the greater trochanter is most prominent (Fig. 8.19). When there is "normal" anteversion, tibial position will indicate slight internal rotation of the hip. A vertical tibia indicates femoral retroversion.

Tibial torsion is assessed with the patient in the supine position, with 90 degrees of ankle dorsiflexion and the leg placed neutrally in the frontal plane (Fig. 8.20). The examiner holds the stationary arm of the goniometer parallel to the table surface while the mobile arm is aligned with the TCJ axis as it passes through the medial and lateral malleoli. This angular displacement represents tibial torsion. Normally, 20 degrees of external tibial torsion are present.

Dynamic Gait Assessment

The final component of the clinical evaluation is the observation of foot function during walking. During the dynamic

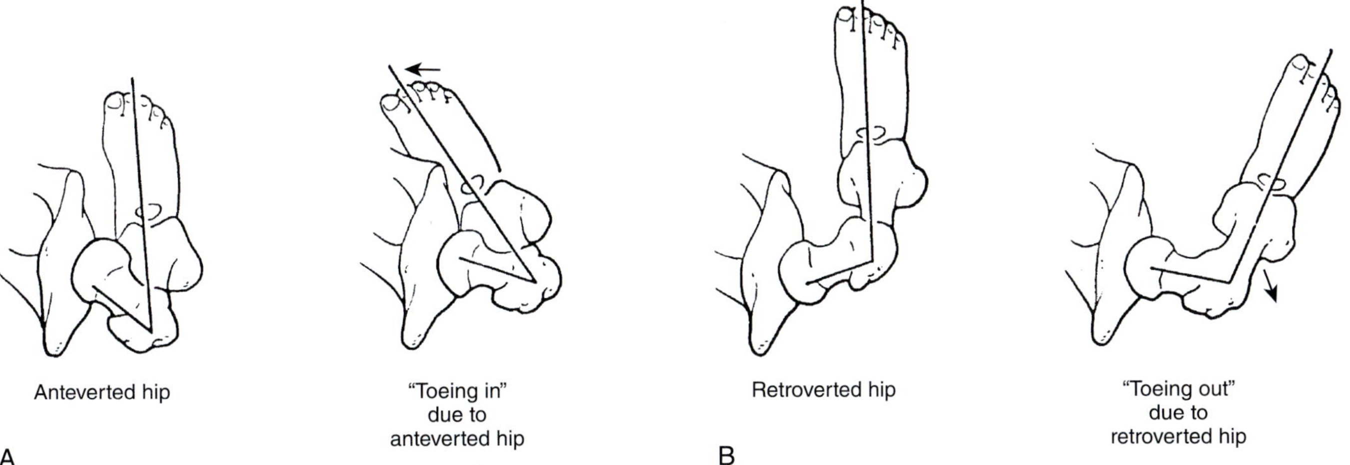

Fig. 8.18 (A) With excessive femoral anteversion, the limb appears to be internally rotated when the head of the femur is well seated in the acetabulum. (B) With femoral retroversion, the limb appears to be externally rotated when the femur is well seated in the acetabulum. (From Magee DJ. *Orthopedic Physical Assessment*. Third ed. Saunders; 1997:475.)

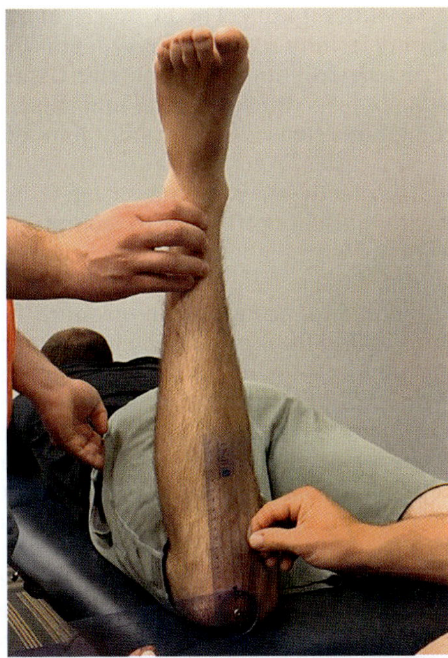

Fig. 8.19 Assessment of femoral torsion in prone position with a standard goniometer. The examiner palpates the greater trochanter and rotates the lower leg. Femoral torsion is measured at the point of greatest prominence of the greater trochanter.

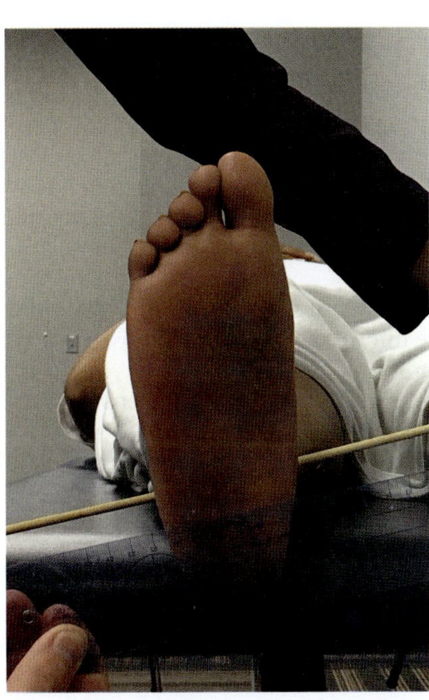

Fig. 8.20 Tibial torsion is measured as the angle between horizontal and the plane of the axis of the talocrural joint.

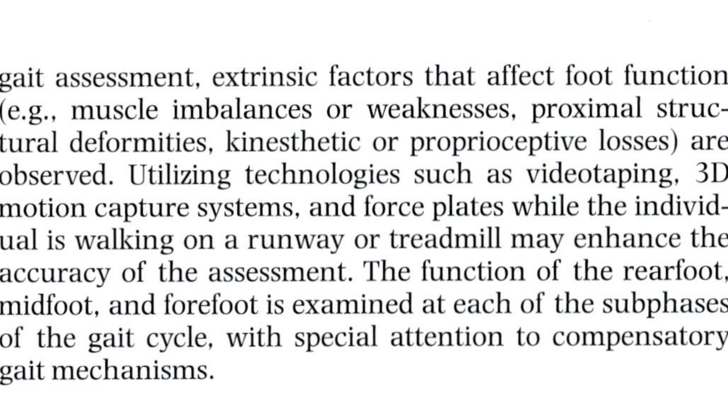

gait assessment, extrinsic factors that affect foot function (e.g., muscle imbalances or weaknesses, proximal structural deformities, kinesthetic or proprioceptive losses) are observed. Utilizing technologies such as videotaping, 3D motion capture systems, and force plates while the individual is walking on a runway or treadmill may enhance the accuracy of the assessment. The function of the rearfoot, midfoot, and forefoot is examined at each of the subphases of the gait cycle, with special attention to compensatory gait mechanisms.

Functional Foot Orthoses

Although 4 to 6 degrees of triplanar STJ pronation are necessary to provide adequate shock absorption and accommodation to uneven ground terrain, persistent or recurrent abnormal pronation disrupts normal temporal sequencing of the gait cycle. This disruption creates an unstable osseous and arthrokinematic situation that contributes to pathological musculoskeletal conditions.[8,49]

Compensatory motion occurs in the primary plane of a given deformity. In frontal plane deformities (e.g., rearfoot varus or forefoot varus), the typical compensatory motion is eversion at the STJ. In transverse plane deformities (e.g., torsional deformities of the hip, femur, or tibia), the typical compensatory motion is adduction at the STJ. In sagittal plane deformities (e.g., ankle equinus), the typical compensatory motion is dorsiflexion at the STJ. Root's model suggests that single-plane compensatory motion is beneficial, allowing adequate accommodation for a deformity.[8] However, because the STJ is a triplanar structure, movement in one plane leads to movement in the others as well. The associated motion of the other planes has the potential to become dysfunctional and destructive.[8]

A functional foot orthosis is an orthopedic device designed to promote structural integrity of the joints of the foot and lower limb by resisting the GRFs that cause abnormal skeletal motion during the stance phase of gait.[49] A functional foot orthosis attempts to control abnormal foot functioning during stance by controlling excessive STJ and MTJ motion, decelerating pronation, and allowing the STJ to function closer to its neutral position at MSt.[79–82] In contrast, an accommodative foot orthosis is used to distribute pressures over the plantar surface for individuals with fixed deformity or vulnerable neuropathic feet.

CRITERIA FOR ABNORMAL PRONATION

Five criteria are used to determine whether pronation is abnormal. Pronation is considered an abnormal mechanical condition when the following conditions are present:

1. STJ pronation is more than the normal 4 to 6 degrees.[8,39]
2. The foot pronates at the wrong time, disrupting the normal sequencing of events during closed kinetic chain motion.
3. Pronation is recurrent, with each step contributing to repetitive microtrauma to musculoskeletal structures.
4. Pronation happens at a location other than the STJ (e.g., when MTJ pronation compensates for limited STJ motion).
5. Unnecessary destructive compensatory motion occurs in the other planes of motion of the STJ.[8]

CAUSES OF ABNORMAL FOOT MECHANICS

Three pathological situations contribute to abnormal foot mechanics: structural malalignment, muscle weakness or imbalance, and loss of structural integrity.

Structural Malalignment

Structural malalignment can be intrinsic or extrinsic to the foot or caused by abnormal mechanical forces.[8] Rearfoot and forefoot varus and valgus, ankle equinus, and deformities of the rays are examples of intrinsic deformities. Congenital and developmental conditions, such as tibial varum or valgum, torsional deformities of the tibia or femur, and other conditions that occur above the foot and ankle are extrinsic deformities. The types of abnormal mechanical forces that might contribute to pathomechanical foot function include obesity, leg-length discrepancies, and genu valgum or varum. Orthotic management for structural malalignment is preventive; control of aberrant or excessive STJ and MTJ motion forestalls the sequence of mechanical events associated with abnormal pronation or supination, minimizing the consequences of painful foot conditions.

Muscle Weakness or Imbalance

A variety of upper and lower motor neuron diseases result in muscular weakness, abnormal muscle tone, or paralysis of the foot, with resultant instability of foot structure and reduced mechanical efficiency during gait.[47] In Charcot-Marie-Tooth disease (hereditary sensory motor neuropathy), for example, weakness of intrinsic, fibularis, and anterior tibial muscles contributes to development of a "cavus" foot, with claw toes, metatarsus adductus, or other deformities of the rays.[47] When muscle weakness or imbalance is present, the examiner must identify its origin and extent, the specific soft tissue structures involved, the resultant mechanical foot deformities, and the potential to reduce them. An effective foot orthosis for a patient with muscular weakness deters the pathomechanical sequelae that result from such induced structural foot deformities.

Compromised Joint Integrity

Compromised joint integrity and mechanical instability also can be caused by pathological musculoskeletal conditions of the foot or ankle, including arthritis, acute trauma, or chronic repetitive injury. For example, in rheumatoid arthritis, joint deformity results from synovitis and pannus formation. Autodestruction of connective tissue weakens tendons, contributes to muscle spasm and shortening, and erodes cartilaginous surfaces. Eventually, joint dislocations occur.[83]

The loss of protective sensation associated with peripheral neuropathy also contributes to compromised joint integrity. Patients with diabetes mellitus, chronic alcoholism, or Hansen disease (leprosy) are particularly vulnerable. The inability to perceive microtrauma because of sensory compromise, weakness of intrinsic muscles of the foot, compromised autonomic control of the distal blood flow, and the poor nutritional and metabolic state of soft tissues combine to increase the risk of plantar foot ulceration. If neuropathic osteoarthropathy (Charcot-Marie-Tooth disease) occurs, significant bone and joint destruction, collapse of the midfoot, and a fixed rocker bottom deformity can result.[84] Plantar ulceration at the apex of the collapsed cuneiforms or cuboid is common.[85] Whenever mechanical instability is present, normal joint orientation is altered, and gait compensation shifts weight-bearing forces. A foot orthosis can be used to reduce pain, reduce weight-bearing stresses, control abnormal or excessive joint motion, or compensate for restricted motion.

Goals of Orthotic Intervention

A functional foot orthosis attempts to improve foot mechanics during walking, regardless of the cause of foot dysfunction, by the following actions:

- Controlling velocity of pronation
- Redistributing plantar pressures
- Supporting abnormal structural forefoot positions that lead to abnormal rearfoot function in stance
- Supporting abnormal rearfoot deformities that lead to excessive STJ pronation
- Resisting extrinsic forces of the leg that lead to aberrant pronation and supination of the foot

- Improving calcaneal positioning at IC
- Repositioning the STJ in the neutral position just before heel rise
- Fully pronating the MTJ, when the STJ is in the neutral position, to lock and stabilize the foot, converting it into a rigid lever for propulsion
- Allowing normal plantarflexion of the first ray and stabilizing the forefoot in response to the retrograde GRFs sustained during propulsion
- Providing a normal degree of shock absorption during LR

A functional foot orthosis does not support the MLA of the foot; STJ pronation is controlled by the pressure of the rearfoot post on the calcaneus at the sustentaculum tali. The ultimate goal is to stop, reduce, or slow abnormal compensatory motion of the joints of the foot as the foot and leg interact with the GRFs.

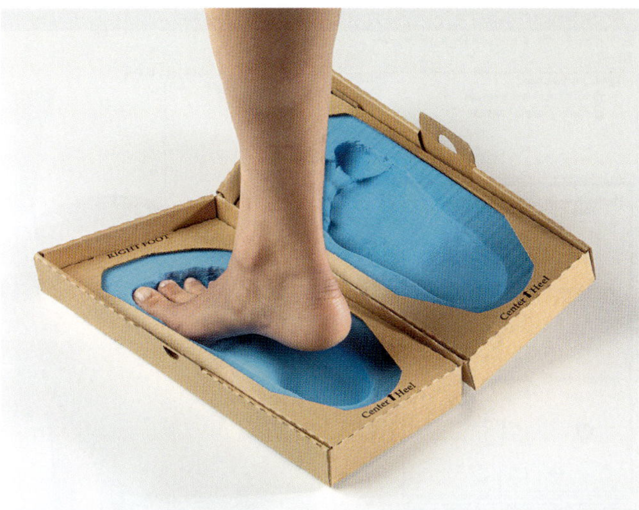

Fig. 8.21 Negative cast impression using the foam box technique. (Courtesy Amfit, Inc., Vancouver, Washington.)

Measurement and Fabrication

The information gathered in the non–weight-bearing and static weight-bearing examinations and in gait analysis provides direction for orthotic prescription. Traditionally, a simple plaster cast is used to make an accurate negative impression of the patient's foot in the STN position. A positive model based on this impression is then prepared. Thermoplastic materials are heat molded over the model to form an orthotic shell. Accommodative padding, soft tissue supplements, and covering materials are added to address the patient's functional foot problem. The orthosis is fitted to the patient, and its effect on foot function during gait is evaluated. An early wearing schedule is devised, and an appointment for a recheck visit is scheduled.

NEGATIVE IMPRESSION

If a foot orthosis is to control abnormal pronation and supination effectively and to minimize painful symptoms in gait, the negative foot impression must precisely duplicate the existing foot structure, including any intrinsic deformities. The goal of the foot impression is to capture the patient's STN position during the MSt phase of the gait cycle.

Comparison of Negative Casting Techniques Used for Fabrication of Foot Orthotics

Multiple strategies can be used to take negative impressions, including suspension techniques, modified suspension techniques, direct pressure techniques, foam impression systems, digital casting, and in-shoe vacuum casts. The negative impression techniques may be applied with the patient in semi–weight-bearing, weight-bearing, or non–weight-bearing positions. Foot measurements are greatly influenced by the technique used to obtain the impression.[86]

The foam box technique (Fig. 8.21) captures a negative impression of the foot with the patient in semi–weight-bearing positions. Typically, the patient is seated on a firm surface and the practitioner directs the foot to the foam box. After the foot makes contact with the foam and the desired position is established, the practitioner applies a downward pressure along the tibial axis moving the heel into the foam followed by the forefoot. The foot is then removed from the box leaving a negative impression in the foam. The foam box technique requires less technical skills and is more time efficient than plaster negative casting. It might be used when the goal is to fabricate an accommodative (soft) foot orthosis.[87]

The digital casting technique produces a digital foot impression and allows for a variety of positions depending on the scanning device, which might include a laser scanner, digitizer, pressure mat system, digital photography, or adapted video game systems.[88] Computerized images of the foot can be viewed by the practitioner from multiple angles, and some software allows the practitioner to modify the images (Fig. 8.22). The Computer-Aided Design and Computer-Aided Manufacturing (CAD/CAM) system uses a milling apparatus to create the actual orthosis.

Plaster casting has traditionally been the gold standard for obtaining negative cast impressions. However, newer techniques involving 3D scanning and printing of foot orthoses have produced similar outcomes.[89] Foot alignment during plaster casting is a critical factor for the effectiveness and quality of the foot orthoses. It is common practice to align the STJ in a "neutral" position.[90] Because maintenance of the STN position and correct loading of the forefoot are difficult to control in weight-bearing impression techniques, suspension and direct pressure non–weight-bearing techniques appear to be the most reliable methods for making accurate negative impressions. The direct pressure technique, one of the easiest procedures to learn, captures the STN position by loading the fourth and fifth metatarsal heads to mimic GRFs during MSt (Fig. 8.23). Alternative casting procedures are also available.[91]

Direct Pressure Impression Technique

The patient is placed in the prone position, in the figure-of-four position used for goniometric measurement. Two double-layer thickness wraps of 5-inch plaster bandage are used to make the negative cast. The first wrap is cut to surround the foot from just distal to the fifth metatarsal head, around the posterior heel, to just beyond the first metatarsal

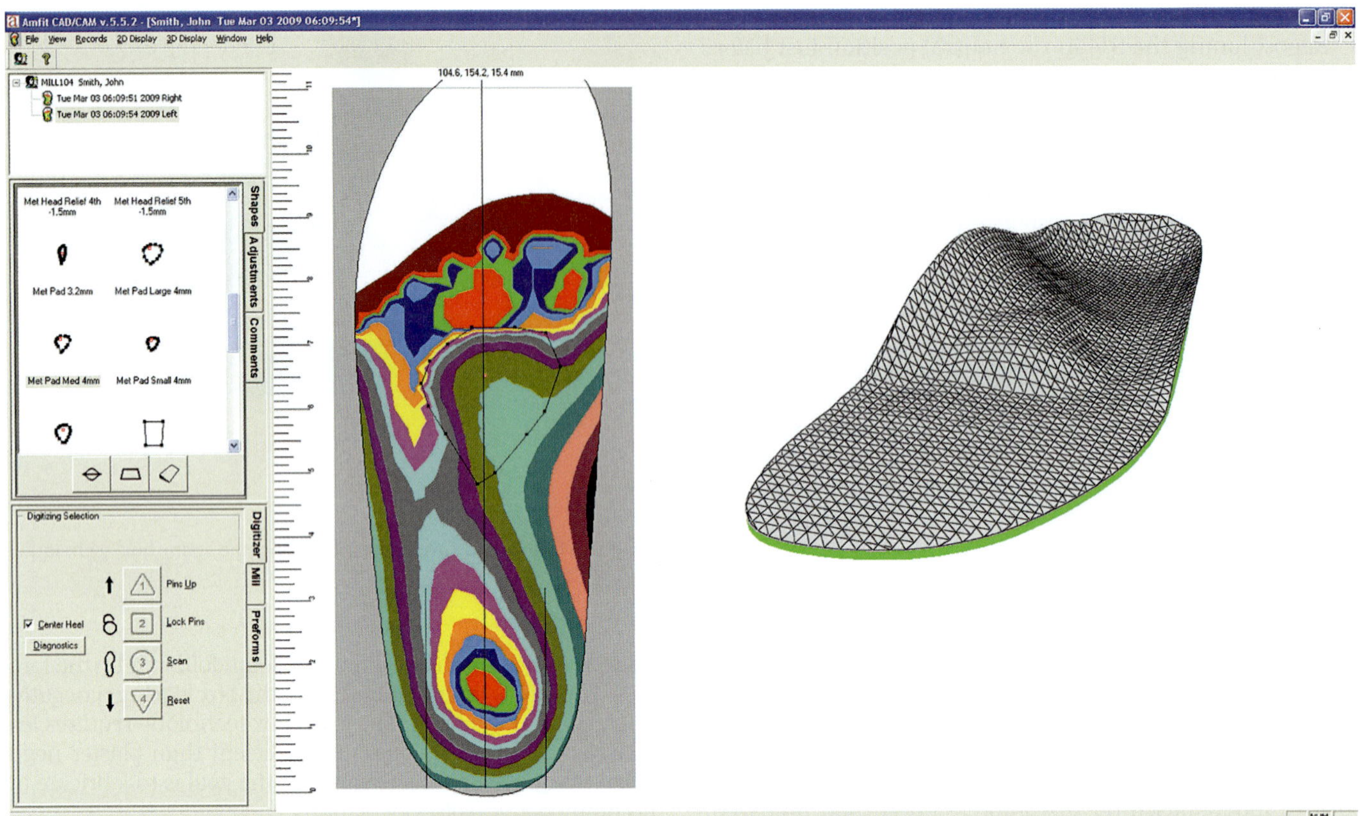

Fig. 8.22 Example of a negative cast impression using the digital casting technique. (Courtesy Amfit, Inc., Vancouver, Washington.)

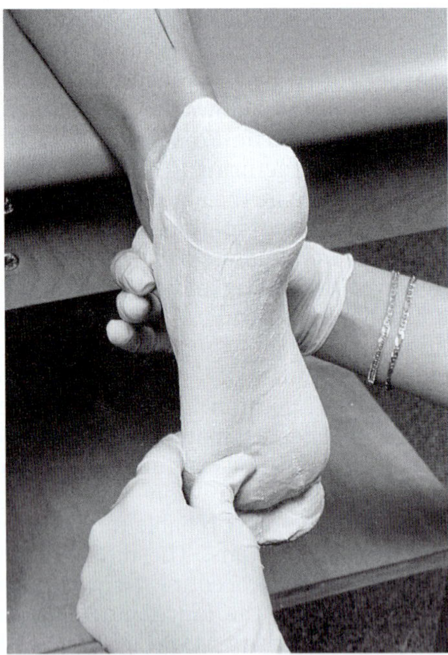

Fig. 8.23 Negative cast impression by the direct pressure technique. The foot is maintained in subtalar neutral position while the plaster hardens.

head. The second wrap is cut so that, when draped over the plantar surface of the forefoot, it overlaps the first wrap at the metatarsals.

The first wrap is thoroughly moistened with tepid water and any wrinkles in the mesh are smoothed. The top edge of the plaster splint is folded 0.5 inch, providing reinforcement to prevent distortion when the cast is later removed. The first wrap is draped over the heel, just below the malleoli, and along the borders of the foot to just beyond the first and fifth metatarsal heads. Because total contact with the sole of the foot is essential, the plaster is carefully smoothed along the sides of the foot, across its plantar surface, and around the curves of the malleoli. The second wrap is moistened and draped around the forefoot, overlapping the distal edges of the first layer. Any excess bandage is folded into the sulcus of the toes. This layer should also have wrinkle-free total contact with the foot and toes.

Once both wraps are in place, the foot is positioned in the STN position by maintaining appropriate forefoot loading pressure at the fourth and fifth metatarsal heads. The plaster splint is sufficiently hardened when an audible click is produced when it is tapped. The negative cast is then carefully removed. The skin is gently pulled around the reinforced top edge to loosen contact from the cast. A downward force over the superior border of the heel cup is exerted to free the heel from the cast. A gentle forward force is then provided to free the forefoot and remove the cast from the foot.

Errors in Negative Casting

Accuracy in the negative impression is the key to an effective orthotic. Although the casting procedure is simple, three types of errors during the process can compromise the efficacy of orthotic design.

First, the foot may be inadvertently supinated at the longitudinal MTJ axis as a result of contraction of the anterior tibialis while the patient "helps" hold the foot still. Alternatively, the loading force may be applied too far medially at the forefoot, creating a false forefoot varus. An orthosis manufactured from such a cast can cause excessive pressure plantar to the distal aspect of the first metatarsal shaft. It can also lead to lateral ankle instability or the development of a functional hallux limitus or HAV deformities.[92]

The second common casting error occurs when the foot is excessively supinated at the oblique MTJ axis. Improper loading at the fourth and fifth metatarsal heads results in insufficient dorsiflexion of the forefoot. When this happens, transverse skin folds can be seen inside the negative cast at the MTJ. An orthosis manufactured from this cast creates an excessive sagittal plane angulation plantar to the calcaneocuboid joint (lateral longitudinal arch), with pain and irritation on weight bearing.[92]

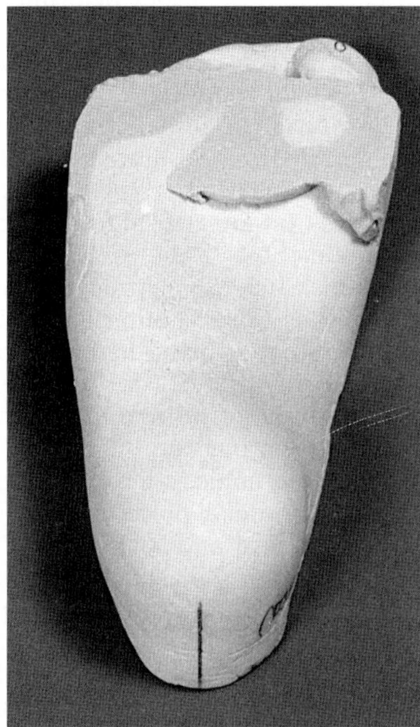

Fig. 8.24 The modification process of forefront position on a positive cast.

The third error occurs when the STJ is excessively pronated during casting, placing the foot in a false forefoot valgus position. An orthosis manufactured from this cast does not capture the STN position and is ineffective in controlling the symptoms of abnormal pronation.[92]

POSITIVE CAST MODIFICATIONS

Once a satisfactory negative impression of the patient's foot has been obtained, a positive cast is made and then modified. The hardened negative impression is filled with liquid plaster and allowed to dry. The negative cast is peeled away, leaving a positive mold of the foot (Fig. 8.24). Modifications to the positive cast ensure an effective correction in foot alignment and function by redirecting forces through the foot. Those made to enhance comfort include plaster additions to relieve pressure-sensitive regions of the forefoot and MLA. Because the negative cast is taken in a non–weight-bearing position, it is also modified to allow for the elongation of the foot and expansion of the soft tissues in weight bearing. The cast is also modified to allow for normal plantarflexion of the first metatarsal during propulsion.[50,93] Intrinsic or extrinsic posts can be added for further correction of forefoot or rearfoot deformities.

Forefoot Posting

Two techniques can be used to provide orthotic correction for forefoot deformity. Both are based on modification of the positive cast impression. The first, a traditional root functional orthosis, uses an intrinsic correction. A plaster platform is applied to the positive cast at the level of the MTP joints to balance the abnormal forefoot to rearfoot relation (Fig. 8.25). A lateral platform corrects forefoot valgus, and a medial platform corrects forefoot varus.[50] When the shell is pressed over the modified positive mold, it creates convexity at the distal anterior border of the orthosis. This posting technique achieves correction by effectively realigning the skeletal structure of the foot.[93] The intrinsic posting technique is often selected when shoe volume is limited, as in some women's footwear.

A second forefoot posting technique involves a variation of Root's original design, referred to as a standard

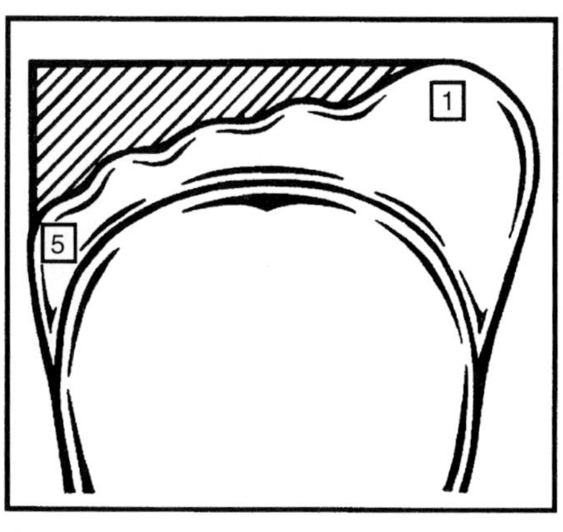

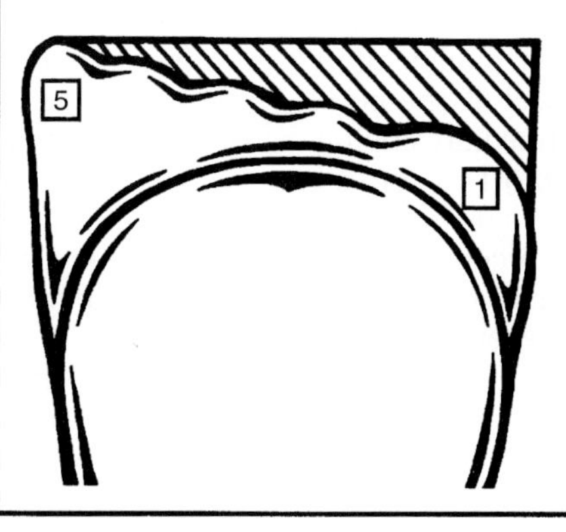

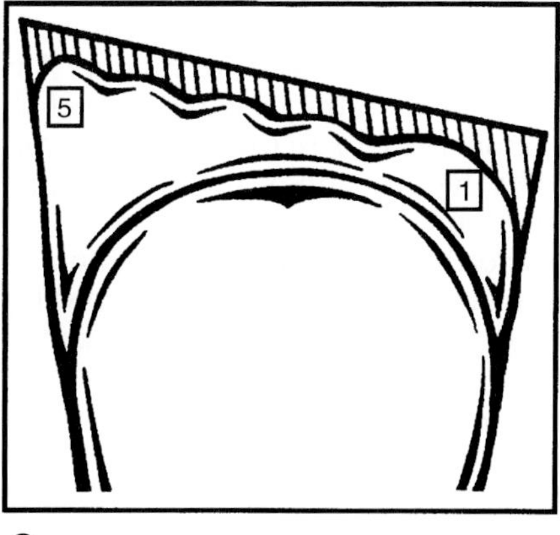

Fig. 8.25 Cross section at the level of the metatarsophalangeal joints, with first and fifth metatarsals labeled, demonstrating intrinsic modifications to the positive mold. (A) A lateral platform corrects forefoot valgus. (B) A medial platform corrects forefoot varus. (C) A neutral balancing platform maintains forefoot alignment and serves as a base for extrinsic posts. (Courtesy Stride, Inc., Middlebury, Connecticut.)

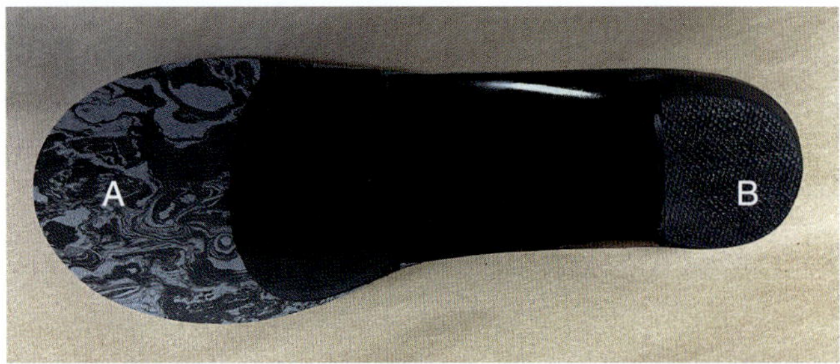

Fig. 8.26 Standard biomechanical orthosis with an extrinsic forefoot post (A) and an extrinsic rearfoot post (B).

biomechanical orthosis. In this technique, a neutral platform is formed on the positive mold, but the existing valgus or varus position of the forefoot is maintained. An extrinsic forefoot post or wedge is attached to the bottom of the orthotic shell to support the forefoot in its position of deformity. Unwanted compensatory motion is prevented by stabilizing the distal border of the orthosis (Fig. 8.26). Although an orthosis with an extrinsic correction takes up more space inside the shoe than an intrinsically corrected orthosis, it can be modified more easily if the individual has difficulty tolerating the original posting prescription.

Rearfoot Posting

As the foot makes contact with the ground and moves through stance during gait, GRFs act on the joints of the foot. An orthosis acts as an interface between the ground and the foot, creating its own orthosis reactive force. In a foot that pronates excessively, the foot orthosis is designed to decrease STJ pronation during weight bearing by creating a supination moment acting medial to the STJ axis.[6] This can be accomplished by adding an extrinsic rearfoot post or wedge to the inferior surface of the heel cup or by modifying the plaster mold to incorporate an intrinsic rearfoot post to the heel cup of the orthosis. A rearfoot post effectively reduces rearfoot pronation (eversion) during the contact phase of gait as well as the angular velocity of eversion.[6,94,95]

Extrinsic rearfoot posts are attached to the bottom of the orthosis shell beneath the heel (see Fig. 8.26*B*). A medial wedge or rearfoot post increases orthosis reactive forces at the sustentaculum tali (medial to the STJ axis) to reduce abnormal STJ pronation. It also promotes stability of the heel by increasing the contact surface of the orthosis beneath the heel.[92–94] An intrinsic rearfoot post can be made with a medial heel skive technique. A plaster modification is performed on the medial aspect of the heel of the positive mold to increase the amount of varus (medial) sloping within the heel cup of the orthosis in an effort to control pronation.[6] An intrinsic rearfoot post reduces overall bulk of the orthosis for optimal fit within a shoe. A combination of intrinsic and extrinsic rearfoot posting permits more correction than possible with either method independently.

THE ORTHOTIC SHELL

To be effective, a functional orthosis must be made on the basis of a neutral position model of the patient's foot. Prefabricated foot supports do not offer adequate control of foot motion or resistance to GRFs and cannot fulfill all criteria of functional foot orthoses. A custom orthosis, made of rigid or semirigid materials, can offer maximal resistance to weight-bearing forces and optimal realignment of foot structure. Accommodative orthoses, made of softer materials, support the arches of the foot and provide relief to pressure-sensitive areas while offering minimal control of STJ motion.[96,97] A semifunctional orthosis is a hybrid of functional and accommodative orthoses that combines the motion effectiveness of a semirigid shell with soft posting and accommodative material to cushion the foot.

Many studies have evaluated the effectiveness of the different types of orthotic materials in controlling rearfoot mechanics and clinical symptoms.[96–100] Some suggest that orthotic materials be classified by degree of rigidity (soft, semirigid, rigid), but standards for the classification of materials are not well established.[5]

A rigid orthosis achieves maximal motion control and biomechanical correction of a foot deformity; it is lightweight and takes up the least space within the shoe. Some clinicians are concerned that orthoses made of rigid materials are uncomfortable for the wearer. However, Anthony[50] suggested that those "who propose rigid devices to be patient intolerant are generally less acquainted with the theory of podiatric biomechanics and the correct diagnostics and prescription formularies that are critical for the provision of a truly functional foot orthosis."

Semirigid materials, such as polypropylene and TL-2100 (Performance Materials Corp., Camarillo, California), are attractive alternatives to rigid orthotic shells. Polypropylene is a flexible olefin polymer that resists breakage. TL-2100 is a thermoplastic composite of resin and fiber that is harder and more rigid than polypropylene.[5]

Soft orthoses are often made of closed-cell foams manufactured from heat-expanded polyethylene. Examples of such foams include Aliplast and Nickleplast (Alimed, Inc., Dedham, Massachusetts) and Plastazote (Bakelite Xylonite Ltd, Croydon, United Kingdom), cross-linked polyethylene expanded foams available in many densities. Pelite (Fillauer, Inc., Chattanooga, Tennessee) is a cross-linked, closed-cell foam that can be heat molded in the fabrication of semiflexible foot orthoses. Various rubberized or thermoplastic cork materials are also used. Lightweight and available in different densities, these materials are effective in orthotics for which accommodation and shock absorption are desirable. However, these same features limit the durability and the useful life of the orthosis because these materials are prone to rapid and permanent shape deformation.[5]

For some individuals, extrinsic accommodative modifications are necessary to address a particular deformity. Examples of accommodative supplements are listed in Table 8.1.

Recent advancements in 3D printing processes involve the use of additive manufacturing technology utilizing various elastomers such as carbon elastomeric polyurethane to provide the most appropriate level of support for the given condition.[101] Current research is assessing best practices for 3D-printed materials that can improve durability and pressure relief and reduce sheering as well as minimize the time and labor intensive process of the fabrication traditional orthoses.[101,102]

Covering Materials

Once appropriate posts and supportive materials are attached to the shell of the orthosis, a covering material

Table 8.1 Accommodative Padding and Soft Tissue Supplements for Functional Foot Orthotics

Supplement	Description
Metatarsal mound	This is a dome-shaped addition in the form of a teardrop positioned with the apex just proximal to the metatarsal heads to support a collapsed transverse metatarsal arch. Often used to control symptoms of neuroma by reducing shearing of the metatarsals during the contact phase. Reduction of the shearing eliminates irritation to the interdigital nerves of the forefoot.
2–5 Bar	A pad of uniform thickness placed beneath the second through fifth metatarsal heads relieves pressure beneath the first metatarsal head during propulsion. It is used when a rigid plantarflexed first ray is present.
Metatarsal head cutout	This is a U-shaped pad positioned beneath a rigid plantarflexed metatarsal head to relieve pressure from a painful callosity. It is often used for hammertoe deformity.
Morton extension	This is an extension of the plastic shell, or the addition of an inlay made of dense material, beneath the shaft of the first metatarsal to the sulcus of the hallux. It is often used for a dorsiflexed first ray or Morton toe.
Heel cushion	This is placed in the heel cup of the orthosis to enhance heel cushioning and shock absorption. It is often made of the soft tissue–supplementing material Poron (Rodgers Co., Rogers, Connecticut) or a viscoelastic polymer. It is used when irritation or atrophy of the infracalcaneal fat pad is present or for a calcaneal stress fracture.
Forefoot extension	A soft tissue–supplementing material, such as Poron, is added to the distal end of the orthotic shell to cushion the metatarsal heads or as a base for other forefoot inlays.
Scaphoid pad	This is a material of soft to medium density placed beneath the medial longitudinal arch to decelerate pronatory forces.

is applied to provide an interface with the skin of the foot. Vinyl is a commonly used orthosis-covering material. Spenco (Spenco Medical Corporation, Waco, Texas) and various other fabric-covered neoprene materials are resistant to shearing and enhance shock absorption. They are often chosen as covering materials for certain sport orthoses when shear forces are expected to be high or for occupational situations that demand prolonged standing on hard surfaces.

Managing Rearfoot Deformity

In a well-aligned foot, 4 to 6 degrees of STJ pronation occur during the stance phase of gait. In rearfoot varus, more than 6 degrees of STJ pronation are present. A fully compensated rearfoot varus deformity of 10 degrees pronates at the STJ 10 degrees during gait to lower the medial condyle of the calcaneus to the ground, but only 6 degrees of this pronation are considered excessive.

The appropriate orthotic design for rearfoot varus is a medial post or medial wedge. Complete orthotic correction is difficult to achieve and quite uncomfortable for the individual wearing the orthosis. Because of this, the initial goal is often to create an orthosis that provides 50% correction of a rearfoot deformity. For example, to correct the excessive 6 degrees of pronation, a medial rearfoot post or wedge of 3 degrees would be applied to the orthosis.

If an individual with a rearfoot varus deformity of 10 degrees is uncompensated to −5 degrees of calcaneal eversion, a medial or varus wedge of 3 degrees is not effective because the STJ would reach its end-range eversion motion (−5 degrees) before the orthosis provided support. To manage uncompensated rearfoot deformity effectively, the varus wedge must be large enough to prevent the STJ from reaching its end ROM. In this example, a larger medial rearfoot varus post or wedge of at least 5 degrees is necessary. When the rearfoot is aggressively posted (more than 3 or 4 degrees of varus posting), the distal medial aspect of the orthosis shell loses contact with the ground, as if a forefoot varus deformity were present. In these circumstances, a medial forefoot post is used to counteract the induced apparent forefoot varus.

Managing Forefoot Deformity

For forefoot varus deformities, a medial (varus) wedge or post is indicated. For forefoot valgus deformities, lateral (valgus) posts or wedges are used. Forefoot deformities can be corrected through intrinsic plaster modifications or extrinsic posting. For an orthosis to be accurately balanced so that it does not wobble, a forefoot deformity must be corrected to its fullest extent (e.g., an 8-degree forefoot varus deformity requires an 8-degree medial wedge or post).

The addition of a large extrinsic post to the distal end of the orthotic shell often creates problems with shoe fit. One possible solution is to correct large forefoot deformities with a combination of intrinsic and extrinsic techniques. In this example, a 4-degree medial intrinsic plaster platform and a 4-degree extrinsic medial forefoot post or wedge would provide the desired correction without bulkiness. For individuals with a forefoot varus deformity of 10 degrees or more, a semipronated or pronated negative cast can reduce the forefoot deformity to a more manageable degree.[91]

Plantarflexion of the first ray is managed according to the level of flexibility of the deformity. A fully flexible plantarflexed first ray deformity does not require orthotic intervention. A semirigid or rigid plantarflexed first ray deformity requires the addition of a metatarsal (second through fifth) bar inlay. The thickness of the inlay is determined by how far below the first metatarsal head lies relative to the plane of the remaining metatarsal heads. The orthotic intervention for patients with a rigid plantarflexed first ray and forefoot varus is an extended medial forefoot wedge. The forefoot post is modified with a cutout to accommodate the dropped first metatarsal head position. In some cases, a small forefoot varus deformity combined with a large, rigidly plantarflexed first ray deformity results in a functional forefoot valgus (see Fig. 8.14).

Orthotic Checkout and Troubleshooting

Delivery of an orthosis includes evaluation of its fit, comfort, and mechanical alignment. The orthotic shell should end just proximal to the metatarsal heads. The width is evaluated to ensure that normal first ray plantarflexion and propulsion are not compromised. The position of the orthosis within the shoe is also evaluated; its volume, impact on heel height, points of excessive pressure, and tendency to cause pistoning during gait are considered. On initial fitting, many individuals report that the orthosis feels slightly strange or unusual. However, the orthosis should not cause undue discomfort. Fit and mechanical functioning of the orthosis are evaluated in standing and walking.

Patient education in appropriate break-in protocols and wearing schedules is an important component of orthotic delivery. A new orthosis is usually worn for 2 hours on day 1, 4 hours on day 2, 6 hours on day 3, and so forth, until the individual is able to wear the orthosis comfortably all day. A follow-up visit is scheduled after the orthosis has been worn for at least 2 weeks. By this time, the patient should feel comfortable with the orthosis for normal activities of daily living. Thereafter, progressively increased use of the orthosis for all activities, including sport and occupational use, should be well tolerated. Adjustments are occasionally necessary to optimize patient comfort and mechanical alignment.

BIOPSYCHOSOCIAL CONSIDERATIONS

Deschamps and collegues[11] emphasize the importance of moving beyond the sole focus on the biomechanical aspect of foot orthoses to consider the psychosocial contributions to chronic foot pain and the success of interventions. Recent research provides evidence that kinesiophobia, pain catastrophizing, fear avoidance, depression, and anxiety are more common in those with foot and ankle pain compared to those without foot pain.[12] Use of screening tools such as the Orebro Musculoskeletal Pain Questionnaire Short Form[103] or the Fear Avoidance Components Scale[10] may provide important information to assess the need of additional psychosocial interventions to enhance patient outcomes with orthotic intervention. Additionally, Huang and collegues[104] note the importance of including exercise as an intervention rather than relying on passive interventions, such as orthoses, alone. The meta-analysis found that short foot exercises were significantly effective at improving foot drop in individuals with flexible flatfoot. Additional research focusing on biopsychosocial impacts of foot pain on intervention outcomes is important to further identify those individuals that may be most receptive to orthotic intervention and those that may need additional multifactorial approaches to care.

Controversy With Root's Paradigm

Much discussion on the basic components of Root's theory has occurred in the past decades.[42,55,105–112] Root's theory is founded on "normal" foot structure and the concept of the STN position: the point of maximal congruence in the articulation of the talus and navicular.[8,16,32,65] STN position supposedly (1) minimizes stress to the surrounding joints and ligaments, (2) is the most efficient position regarding muscle function and attenuation of the impact forces at IC, and (3) represents the point at which the foot converts from a mobile adapter to a rigid lever.[8,46,65] According to Root's traditional theory, normal foot alignment occurs just before TSt during gait, when the STJ is in the neutral position and the MTJ is fully locked.[8]

The major criticisms of Root's paradigm raise concerns about the reliability of measurement of the STN position, the STN position during the gait cycle, and criteria for "normal" foot alignment.[42,45,66,111,113]

RELIABILITY OF MEASUREMENT

When considering available evidence about the reliability of foot measurements and the STN position, although acceptable levels of intrarater reliability exist,[43,44,51,53,114] interrater reliability of foot measurements and the STN position is low.[42,105,107,111] Diamond and colleagues[115] and Cook and colleagues[114] found that interrater reliability can be improved with training. McPoil and Hunt[116] noted that considerable confusion exists regarding the definition and measurement of STN position. They suggested that Root's STN position may misinterpret the work by Wright and colleagues,[117] who referenced relaxed standing position, not STN neutral, as the basis of their work. To further add to the confusion, the definition of STN position used in some reliability studies was not identical to Root's methods.[111] Based on the review of reliability studies, McPoil and Hunt[116] suggested that physical therapists are not able to agree on the position and motion of the STJ.

SUBTALAR POSITION IN STANCE

According to Root, ideal foot alignment occurs just before TSt during gait, when the STJ is in the neutral position and the MTJ is fully locked.[8,118] In a study of rearfoot motion of 51 healthy adults, McPoil and Cornwall[119] marked patients' lower leg and calcaneus with bisection lines and then filmed relative calcaneal and lower leg position while walking, while standing in a double-support relaxed standing, and while in the STN position. Their findings did not support Root's paradigm. They found that (1) the rearfoot is slightly inverted before IC, (2) the maximal rearfoot pronation was reached at the 37.9% point of stance phase, and (3) the neutral position of the rearfoot for the typical pattern of rearfoot motion should be the resting standing foot posture rather than STN position.[117] As a result, they suggested that the relaxed standing foot position rather than the STN position should be used during casting.[117]

Yang et al.[120] utilized biplanar radiographs and 3D modeling to assess tibiotalar and subtalar coupled motion during an overground walking task in 40 healthy ankles. They found that from IC through the first 30% of stance, tibiotalar plantarflexion is coupled with relative subtalar eversion. During the push-off phase, they found tibiotalar plantarflexion to be coupled with subtalar inversion. No significant differences were seen between males and females in this coupling motion. Munsch and colleagues[121] further analyzed the collected data to assess subtalar motion coupled with tibiofemoral rotation. They found that males achieved STN at MSt while females moved toward STN but remained in a relative subtalar inverted position. During push-off females experienced subtalar inversion coupled with tibiofemoral internal rotation and adduction, while males experienced subtalar inversion and tibiofemoral internal rotation without corresponding adduction. These differences in STJ position throughout gait in healthy individuals warrant additional studies to determine how coupled motion may be impacted by varied resting calcaneal positions and in affected populations.

CRITERIA FOR NORMAL ALIGNMENT

Root described deviations from normal foot alignment as intrinsic foot deformities, which can lead to aberrant lower extremity function and musculoskeletal pathological conditions.[8,65] Root and colleagues[118] defined three criteria for normal foot and ankle alignment in the loaded STN position: (1) a bisection of the lower leg being in parallel to the bisection of the calcaneus, (2) the plane of the metatarsal heads being perpendicular to the bisection of the calcaneus, and (3) the distal third of the lower leg being perpendicular to the floor. In an examination of forefoot to rearfoot relations of 120 healthy asymptomatic individuals, Garbalosa and colleagues[52] found that only 4.58% of the 234 feet studied exhibited normal criteria, 86.67% had forefoot varus, and 7.75% had forefoot valgus. Jarvis and colleagues[45] examined 100 symptom-free individuals and found that all feet had at least two deformities based on Root's criteria; however, these deformities were not associated with kinematic deficits. Of the feet examined, 97% demonstrated calcaneal inversion in neutral calcaneal stance and 76% were shown to have forefoot varus. These findings suggest that the "deformities" may not be deformities after all but instead are variations of normal alignment that do not translate into dynamic movement issues in need of correction. The evidence from these studies suggests that an "ideal" foot may be based on a questionable theoretical concept.

Foot Type and Lower Extremity Biomechanics

A question that has been the focus of recent research focuses on the relation between various foot types and the amount of pronation during gait. In 2002 Ball and Afheldt[111] first suggested that attempts to justify static classification of foot type schemes as a means of predicting dynamic joint function have had mixed results. In a recent study of 1090 US Military Academy cadets, Song et al.[122] concurred when they found that a planus foot posture does not always correspond with foot function. In the study center of pressure excursion was not greatest in those with flatfoot and instead was greater in those with a more flexible foot. The authors found that black participants were significantly more likely to have pes planus (91.7% vs. 73.4%) with a lower arch height index and increased malleolar valgus index but not have more foot pronation during gait; however, Asian participants had a more flexible arch and demonstrated significantly more pronatory motion with gait. In addition, females demonstrated more overpronation compared to males without any noted different in arch height index. According to Sanchis-Sales and Sancho-Bru,[123] extremes of foot type, either highly pronated or highly supinated feet demonstrate more dynamic stiffness during the propulsion phase of gait, with highly pronated greater than highly supinated, which may contribute to the development of injuries. Resende and colleagues[124] examined the relation between foot pronation and biomechanics of the ankle, knee and hip during gait. In the study they found that inducing foot pronation through the use of a laterally wedged sandal caused changes in segmental foot flexibility and reduced foot lever arm efficiency as well as compromised sagittal plane knee function; however, they found no change in sagittal plan biomechanics at the hip.

Foot Type and Lower Extremity Overuse Injuries

A number of published studies have provided conflicting evidence on the relation between foot type and lower extremity injuries.[125] Many researchers have reported an association between abnormal alignment of the foot and lower extremity and occurrence of lower extremity injuries. Perez-Morcillo and associates[126] demonstrated in a recent case-control study of 600 runners that the presence of either a highly supinated or highly pronated foot posture, according to the FPI, was significantly associated with the development of injury in recreational runners. Individuals with a highly supinated posture had an injury odds ratio of 76.87 while a highly pronated posture increased the odds ratio by 20.02 when compared to a neutral foot posture. The odds ratio of injury for those individuals whose feet were classified as generally supinated or pronated as compared to neutral was 42.3 and 4.80, respectively. Gross and colleagues[127] examined the relationship between forefoot and rearfoot varus alignment to hip conditions in 385 older adults. Older adults with more forefoot varus were 1.8 times more likely to have ipsilateral hip pain, 1.9 times more likely to have hip pain or tenderness, and 5.1 times more likely to have undergone total hip replacement when compared with older adults with less forefoot varus. There was not a significant relationship between older adults with rearfoot varus and hip conditions. In a cross-sectional study of rearfoot posture and foot pressure in medial tibial stress syndrome (MTSS), Kinoshita and colleagues[128] measured the leg-heel angle in 18 athletes with MTSS and 15 control subjects. They reported no difference between groups in the leg-heel angle (measuring rearfoot eversion) during unilateral stance; however, during gait the mean maximum leg-heel angle was 15.7 degrees in the MTSS group compared to 11.2 degrees in the control group indicating more rearfoot eversion. The two groups were not significantly different at heel strike, but results were significantly higher in the MTSS group at heel-off. Paths of pressure were also different between groups with the MTSS group exhibiting higher pressures under the medial metatarsals as well as a more medially aligned linear path.

Some reports do not support the relation between foot type and lower extremity injury. Donatelli and colleagues[129] reported no statistically significant relations among static or dynamic foot posture and injury status in professional baseball players. In a recent systematic review and meta-analysis, Hollander and collegues[130] reported that MLA height contributes to the biomechanics of the lower limb in running with runners with high arches demonstrating more leg stiffness and runners with low arches demonstrating more eversion at the rearfoot. However, they suggest that future well-controlled studies are necessary to definitively link the biomechanical changes to the development of overuse injuries.

FOOT STRIKE PATTERN DURING RUNNING AND LOWER EXTREMITY BIOMECHANICS

The current literature describes three foot strike patterns that are predominant when running: rearfoot, midfoot, and forefoot. Rearfoot striking occurs when the heel contacts the surface first. During midfoot striking simultaneously the heel and ball of the foot contact the ground first, and forefoot striking happens when runners land on the ball of their foot first.[131–133]

How the foot contacts the ground affects lower extremity joint moments and causes different kinematics of the lower extremity and contrasting kinetics.[133] Ruder and colleagues[134] examined tibial shock differences in 222 marathon runners with forefoot, midfoot, and rearfoot strike patterns. Runners with a forefoot strike pattern had significantly less tibial shock on impact than those with either a midfoot or rearfoot strike pattern. Huang and colleagues,[135] studied the effect of modifying multiple components of running including foot strike region, step rate, and trunk positioning while measuring the impact load in 19 healthy male runners. They found that forefoot strike combined with 10% increase in step rate produces the lowest load at impact while rearfoot loading with anterior trunk lean produces the highest impact.

FOOT STRIKE PATTERN DURING RUNNING AND LOWER EXTREMITY INJURIES

Habitual foot strike pattern may affect common lower extremity injuries during running. Mazzone and colleagues[136] studied the effect of altering foot strike patterns on chronic knee pain due to running among 16 military service members. Significant improvements in Lower Extremity Functional Scale scores and Numerical Pain Rating Scales scores were found after seven training sessions to adopt a nonrearfoot strike pattern. A cross-sectional study of recreational runners by Fukusawa and collegues[137] found no difference between foot strike pattern in the 60 participants with anterior knee pain and 62 participants without anterior knee pain. Both groups presented with over 90% of runners demonstrating a rearfoot strike pattern. In a randomized control trial (RCT), Chan and colleagues[138] examined 320 novice runners to determine the effect of running training on injury reduction rates. The runners in the retraining group participated in 2 weeks of treadmill training with visual feedback to encourage them to "run softer." While the examiners did not explicitly ask participants to shift the foot strike to a nonrearfoot strike pattern the act of decreasing GRFs required a shift forward in landing strategies. After 12-month follow-up, the retraining group had a 16% injury occurrence rate with primarily Achilles and calf injuries whereas the nonretraining group had a 38% injury rate with more reports of plantar fasciopathy and patellofemoral pain (PFP) suggesting that foot strike patterns may effect both rate of injury and types of injuries.

Orthoses and Lower Extremity Function

Overpronation has been implicated as a cause of many overuse injuries. Traditionally, a foot orthosis is used to help control abnormal foot functioning during the stance phase by controlling excessive STJ motion, decelerating pronation, and allowing the STJ to function closer to its neutral position during stance.[80–82] Literature regarding the efficacy of foot orthoses in controlling lower extremity and foot biomechanics is growing.[4,139,140] An RCT of 306 naval recruits conducted by Bonanno and colleagues[141] reported that there is evidence for the use of foot orthoses to prevent lower limb overuse conditions.

EFFECT ON REARFOOT BIOMECHANICS

The use of foot orthoses is based on the premise that control of frontal plane rearfoot motion in stance provides a means of controlling pronation of the foot. In a systematic review and meta-analysis conducted by Desmyterre and colleges[142] medially posted orthoses, either medial forefoot or both medial forefoot and rearfoot, better controlled rearfoot eversion in adults with flexible flatfoot while arch supports and neutral rearfoot posting did not control for rearfoot eversion. They report a 2-degree decrease in rearfoot eversion with the use of medial posted orthoses. Mo and colleagues[143] examined the impact of custom foot orthoses on lower extremity mechanics of 13 female runners with excess pronation. The runners performed trials under three conditions: with a custom plaster molded orthosis, with 3D-printed orthosis, and without the orthoses. The runners displayed a significant reduction in maximum rearfoot eversion angle in both the traditional orthoses and 3D-printed orthoses and comfort while wearing both types of orthoses. These findings that an orthosis is able to reposition the rearfoot concur with earlier studies examining the effects of orthoses on rearfoot mechanics.[97,144]

Desmyterre and colleagues[145] also examined the effects of utilizing 3D-printed orthoses and postings in 15 individuals with normal foot posture. Individuals ambulated for 3 minutes under five conditions: (1) shod, (2) with flexible orthosis, (3) medial posted flexible orthosis, (4) mediolateral posted flexible orthosis, and (5) rigid orthosis. Increasing the rigidity of the 3D-printed orthosis significantly decreased rearfoot eversion and increased rearfoot abduction throughout the stance phase of gait. The addition of postings to the flexible orthoses contributed to improved control of rearfoot eversion as compared to flexible orthotic alone. Although rearfoot mechanics appear to be altered by foot orthoses, further investigation into the mechanisms responsible for these effects is needed.

EFFECT ON LOWER LIMB BIOMECHANICS

Foot orthoses influence lower extremity kinematics and kinetics as well as rearfoot mechanics. In a systematic review and meta-analysis, Hajizadeh and colleagues[146] reported that medial postings produce decreased peak ankle eversion moments while lateral postings increase peak ankle eversion, abduction, dorsiflexion, and mediolateral GRF as well as decrease peak knee adduction moment. A systematic review by Martinez-Rico and collegues[147] considered the effect of frontal plane wedges on plantar pressures. Center of pressure shifted laterally with lateral wedges and medially with medial wedges. Included studies looking at changes in vertical GRFs were inconclusive.

Braga and collegues[148] examined the response to a 7-degree medial wedge at the forefoot and rearfoot in 19 runners with pronated and varus feet. Significant differences in lower limb biomechanics were found between the wedged and flat conditions. While wearing the medial wedge insoles participants demonstrated significantly less transverse plane motion at the knee and hip during stance. In the frontal plane participants demonstrated reduced ankle eversion, increased knee ROM, and decreased hip adduction in stance. In addition, the reduced inversion moment reflects decreased need for the tibialis anterior and posterior to eccentrically control pronation.

Costa and collegues[149] studied 16 participants with pronated feet during walking and running tasks utilizing arch supports with medial heel wedging at 0, 3, 6, and 9 degrees. Ankle eversion angle decreased with the wedged conditions during walking and in running with the 6- and 9-degree wedges during early stance, although this reversed during propulsion. Ankle eversion moment decreased with walking and with running with both the 6- and 9-degree wedges. Adductor moment at the knee increased during all conditions. During walking, adduction angle decreased but adduction moment increased with the 6- and 9-degree wedges. Findings supported a potential dose-response to increasing the angle of inclination of the wedges.

Sinclair[150] investigated the effects of the addition of 5-degree medial and lateral wedges in 19 healthy male runners. Participants were examined as they ran on a treadmill at 4 m/s. Peak knee adduction increased significantly in the medially wedged condition as compared to the laterally wedged condition and patellofemoral peak force increased significantly with both the medial and lateral conditions.

In a systematic review, Moisan and collegues[151] examined the effects of foot orthotics on functional tasks such as jumping, landing, squatting, and stair climbing. During both stair ascent and descent tasks, medial wedged foot orthotics provided control of pronation at the foot and ankle. Smaller effect sizes were seen at the knee and hip with reports of decreased hip adduction and decreased knee internal rotation during stair climbing. During jumping and landing tasks fewer significant effects were seen at the foot and ankle suggesting that higher load activities may impact outcomes.

Although evidence supports the fact that foot orthoses can and do influence lower extremity kinematics and kinetics, the variability of individual responses makes it difficult to determine exactly which biomechanical effects will occur. This variability also makes it difficult to forecast who is likely to benefit from orthotic intervention. Efficacy of foot orthoses is not solely the result of altered rearfoot kinematics, as proposed by Root. The contribution of the neuromuscular system to the effect of orthotic intervention is now being considered.

EFFECT OF THE NEUROMUSCULAR SYSTEM

Nigg and colleagues,[152] citing problems in previous studies (e.g., small skeletal changes produced by orthotic use, minimal decrease in impact forces, and nonsystematic effects caused by individual variability), proposed that mechanisms involving the neuromuscular system contribute to the way that foot orthoses alter lower extremity function. They were especially interested in sensitivity of the foot and pressure distribution on the foot surface, noting that (1) the foot has many sensory receptors to detect forces and deformations acting on it, (2) the sensors detected input signals into the foot with patient-specific thresholds, and (3) individuals with similar sensitivity thresholds seem to respond to their movement patterns in a similar way. They suggested that force signals from the floor were filtered by the shoe, the orthosis, and finally by the plantar surface of the foot, which then transferred the filtered information to the central nervous system. The central nervous system, in turn, prompted dynamic responses in the lower extremity on the basis of patient-specific conditions. Comfort of the orthosis is an important consideration; a comfortable orthosis is likely to minimize muscular work during walking. According to Nigg and colleagues,[152] an optimal orthosis would reduce muscle activity, feel comfortable, and improve musculoskeletal and neuromuscular performance in walking.

Based on his analysis of the role of impact forces on foot function in gait, Nigg[153] proposed a new paradigm focusing on locomotor systems and strategies for impact and movement control. The dynamic systems model of motor control suggests that locomotor systems keep general kinematic and kinetic situations similar for any given task. Nigg suggests that a muscle tuning reaction occurs to cause forces that affect muscle activation before ground contact, and that muscle adaptation (to ensure a constant joint movement pattern) affects muscle activation during ground contact. The interplay of the realignment of the skeleton and locomotor system muscle tuning affects joint and tendon loading and, in turn, fatigue, comfort, work, and performance. In a scoping review of sensory facilitation via foot orthoses, Robb and collegues[154] proposed an expansion of Niggs' neuromotor paradigm. The authors noted that the cutaneous reflex loop helps to modulate motor neuron pool excitability which in turn enhances efficacy of movement. To facilitate these effects, the foot orthoses should maintain full contact with the sole of the foot and may include textured or vibratory surfaces to provide an additive effect.

Electromyographic and Imaging Evidence

Cherni and colleagues[155] studied 19 individuals with asymptomatic flexible flatfeet using no orthosis, a custom 3D-printed flexible orthosis, a flexible orthosis with additional medial posting, and a custom 3D-printed rigid orthosis. After a 2-week period of familiarization with each orthoses, the authors analyzed the effects of each condition during 5-minute treadmill walking tasks on lower extremity electromyography, center of pressure as well as plantar pressure. Muscles studied included the anterior tibialis, medial gastrocnemius, soleus, and fibularis longus. No significant differences were found in EMG data between conditions and minimal changes in center of pressure were found. Plantar pressures were impacted by foot orthoses primarily in the midfoot region with peak pressure, mean pressure, and contact area increasing. The addition of the rigid orthosis and posting on the flexible orthosis enhanced the effects.

Kristanto and colleagues[156] examined electromyographic activity of the tibialis anterior and fibularis longus during standing in nine rice farmers with asymptomatic pronated feet in four conditions: no orthotic on rigid surface, customized medial wedge orthotic on rigid surface, no orthotic on muddy surface, and customized medial wedge orthotic on muddy surface. Rice farming requires standing in muddy surfaces for extended periods of time and complaints of foot and ankle pain as well as knee pain are common. Surface electromyographic activity data of the muscles was collected while the individuals stood for 1 minute in each of the varied conditions. During the muddy surface component an increase in both anterior tibialis and fibularis longus activity was seen as compared to the rigid surface measurements. With the addition of corrective insoles tibialis anterior activity decrease while fibularis longus activity increased in both the rigid and muddy conditions.

Reeves and colleagues[157] conducted a systematic review of 31 articles regarding the effect of footwear, taping, and foot orthoses on electromyographic activity. Eight of the included studies specifically examined foot orthoses. With the addition of orthotics, posterior tibialis activity was found to be decreased in early stance while fibularis longus activity increased during late stance. No significant effects were seen at the tibialis anterior. The authors report the need for additional studies specific to activity of the posterior tibialis as fewer studies have included these results due to the need for an indwelling EMG.

In another systematic review, Moisan and colleagues[151] examined the effects of foot orthoses on the muscle activity during functional tasks. During high impact activities, no significant changes in EMG activity were seen with the addition of foot orthoses.

Robb and colleagues[154] considered sensory input and electromyographic activity in a scoping review of current literature. They suggest inconsistency in research methods contributes to the lack of consistent findings in EMG research and highlight the need for future studies to include sensory components as this may impact electromyographic output.

Balance and Postural Control

If neuromuscular systems play a role in the effectiveness of orthoses, changes in balance and posture control would be anticipated with their use. Chang and collegues[158] examined the effects of 4-degree rearfoot medial wedge orthoses in 25 college baseball players with chronic ankle instability and 24 without ankle instability. Center of pressure displacement significantly improved during single leg standing balance with eyes closed for both groups with the addition of the medial wedge. In addition, dynamic balance, utilizing a repeated single leg hop test, improved significantly with the addition of the medial wedge in the chronic ankle instability group. The researchers propose that tactile and proprioceptive feedback from the foot orthoses enhanced the balance effects. In contrast, Hertel and colleagues[159] found that six different orthotic interventions (shoe only; molded Aquaplast orthoses [Aquaplast Thermoplastics, Wyckoff, New Jersey]; orthoses in the neutral, medially posted, and laterally posted positions; and a prefabricated, rigid, laterally posted heel wedge) did not influence postural sway in 15 patients with unilateral ankle sprains while they performed unilateral standing. None of the orthotic conditions decreased frontal or sagittal postural sway compared with shoes alone.

Gross and colleagues[160] have documented that placement of foot orthoses in the shoes of older adults can affect improvement in static and dynamic balance. Thirteen older adults over the age of 65 years who reported at least one inexplicable fall during the past year participated in the study. Participants were tested for tandem stance, one-leg stance, tandem gait, and alternating step tests during preintervention and postintervention sessions. Improvements in balance performance were seen immediately after foot orthoses were placed in the older adults' shoes in all tests except tandem gait. Although participants reported tandem gait as being the most challenging task, their balance also improved with this performance measure. They took more than three times the number of steps in the postintervention session when compared with their baseline performance.

Recent research has focused on the addition of textures to plantar surface of foot orthoses to enhance sensory cutaneous input. Robb and colleagues[161] compared the addition of a textured platform surface to a smooth surface during a perturbated gait termination activity in 30 young barefoot adults. In the study the participants repeatedly walked five steps on the platform with unexpected perturbations (medial, lateral, anterior, and posterior) occurring. With the texturized condition, participants had earlier onset and cessation responses in the upper leg musculature including the rectus femoris, vastus lateralis, vastus medialis, biceps femoris, and semitendinosus indicating earlier self-correction of the balance perturbation. In a study of seven individuals with Parkinson disease, Robb and colleagues[162] examined the effects of prefabricated heat-molded textured orthoses on dynamic balance and 180-degree turning. Participants were examined on three occasions over a period of 5 weeks in three conditions: shoes only, shoe with nontextured foot orthosis, and shoe with textured foot orthosis. The authors importantly noted a slight increase, although nonsignificant, in instability with initial placement of the foot orthotics. Additionally gait and turning were slowed initially. These finding may alert the clinician that an initial addition of foot orthoses may acutely present slight negative impacts to balance in individuals with Parkinson disease. However, after becoming accustomed to the orthoses, participants' dynamic balance was significantly improved with greater improvements in the textured orthoses condition.

Olmsted and Hertel[163] found that foot orthoses differentially benefit those with various foot types. They assessed static and dynamic postural control in 30 patients grouped by rectus, planus, or cavus foot type. Patients wore custom-molded, semirigid foot orthoses for 2 weeks between baseline and posttest measurement. Improvement in reach occurred in three of eight directions on the Star Excursion Balance Test in those with cavus foot type. Patients with cavus foot type also demonstrated a decreased center of pressure velocity in static stance.

Rome and Brown[164] examined postural sway in 50 patients identified as pronators (per the FPI) in a randomized clinical trial. Patients were assigned either to a control or an orthotic group. The orthotic group wore prefabricated, high-density ethyl vinyl acetate orthoses with low-density ethyl vinyl acetate rearfoot wedging for 4 weeks.

At 4 weeks, medial-lateral sway decreased in the orthotic group; however, no differences in anterior-posterior sway or mean balance occurred between the groups. Collectively, these studies suggest that orthoses do affect electromyographic activity, balance, and postural control. Health professionals may be better able to identify those most likely to benefit from orthotic intervention if measures of postural control and neuromuscular function are incorporated along with the assessment of lower extremity and foot skeletal alignment.

Management of Overuse Injuries

Although the specific biomechanical and neurological effects of foot orthoses on walking and running are not completely understood, orthoses can and do reduce symptoms and improve function. Although current evidence does not include many randomized, controlled clinical trials, the available evidence does support efficacy of orthotic intervention in the management of lower extremity injuries.

PAIN ASSOCIATED WITH FOOT DEFORMITY

A systematic review conducted by Dars and colleagues[165] examined the effect of foot orthoses on foot pain (and other factors) in children with flexible pes planus. Three of the five included studies that assessed pain showed significant decrease in pain with the use of foot orthoses. Hsieh et al.[166] performed an RCT of the effects of a customized foot orthosis in 52 children with painful flexible flatfoot. Participants in the intervention group received a custom-molded orthosis from the STN position. Participants were instructed to slowly increase wear time from 1 hour to 5–10 hours/day. After 12 weeks, the intervention group reported significant improvements in health-related quality of life, pain, and basic mobility. Arias-Martin[2] conducted a systematic review of customized orthoses in foot pain in varied foot conditions. Significant improvements in pain were seen in patients with rheumatoid arthritis, hallux valgus, and metatarsalgia.

KNEE OSTEOARTHRITIS

Ishii and colleagues[167] studied the effect of lateral wedge orthoses on extrusion of the medial meniscus in individuals with early and late osteoarthritis (OA) of the knee as well as a control group without OA. All participants wore a 7-mm lateral wedged orthosis for 3 months. Medial meniscus extrusion was measured by ultrasound at baseline and 3 months. Pain ratings on the Visual Analog Scale (VAS) decreased significantly from baseline in both the early and late OA groups. Average pain scores at baseline in the late OA group were 58.9, while at follow-up pain scores decreased to 37.5 in this group. Medial meniscus extrusion in weight bearing decreased significantly in the early OA group and was unchanged in the late OA group. Lateral wedge insoles are purported to impact the knee adduction moment, thereby impacting pain levels. In contrast, Zhang et al.[168] performed a meta-analysis on the use of lateral wedge insoles on medial knee pain and found no significant improvements in function or pain. Bartsch and collegues[169] recently suggested that careful selection of participants is necessary to distinguish those with OA that will benefit from lateral wedged inserts. They examined 20 participants with medial OA and found that those with more limited frontal plane hindfoot movement may be more appropriate for lateral wedge insert placement.

PATELLOFEMORAL PAIN SYNDROME

The roll of foot orthoses in management of PFP was analyzed in a 2019 clinical practice guideline.[170] The authors recommend prefabricated but not custom foot orthoses in the short-term management of PFP in individuals with excess foot pronation (measured by midfoot width mobility of at least 1.1 cm). The guideline cautions that the foot orthoses should be used in conjunction with exercise. In a 2019 consensus statement, Collins et al.[171] recommended the use of prefabricated foot orthoses as a component of treatment for the short-term management of PFP. However, they do not recommend custom orthoses.

Matthews and colleagues[172] reported the amount of foot pronation (measured by midfoot width mobility) should not be taken into consideration when selecting between prefabricated foot orthoses or hip exercise interventions in the management of PFP. Participants placed in the foot orthoses group received six physical therapy visits over 6 weeks to adjust the orthotic and review the foot exercise program to be completed at home twice per day. The hip exercise group attended a physical therapy supervised exercise program three times per week for 4 weeks. At 12 weeks they found no significant difference in success rates between participants receiving the foot orthoses and foot exercise program (48%) or hip exercises only (50%). Midfoot width mobility did not significantly impact success rates in either group. Previous research[11] suggested that individuals with PFP that also exhibit greater foot mobility might benefit most from foot orthoses.

Mølegard and colleagues[173] conducted a study in individuals with both PFP and excessive calcaneal eversion (greater than 6 degrees). The intervention group received a 12-week intervention of customized foot orthoses, twice weekly foot exercises (supervised by a physical therapist once per week), and thrice weekly unsupervised knee exercise program (supplemented with patellar taping and manual therapy to the knee for three visits). The control group received knee interventions only. The intervention group received custom orthotics designed to decrease pronation during loading using medial arch posting and/or heel posting. STN position in conjunction with comfort of the orthoses were emphasized in fitting. Participants were instructed to gradually increase wear of orthoses from 2 hours/day until a full working day was tolerated. Results revealed significantly decreased pain levels at 4 months. Knee Injury and Osteoarthritis Outcome Scores improved by an average of 8.9 points in the combined foot and ankle treatment group; however, at 12 months there was no difference between the groups.

Tan et al.[174] studied the impact on aging and foot mobility in 194 individuals with PFP as this may influence effectiveness of foot orthoses in this population. This study analyzed both midfoot height mobility and midfoot width mobility in three age cohorts: 18 to 29, 30 to 39, and 40 to 50 years. Mobility was calculated by determining the difference in the measures in non–weight-bearing and weight-bearing positions. Significant differences were found in the midfoot height mobility but not midfoot width mobility between all cohorts. Overall foot mobility magnitude was then calculated by incorporating data between the two measurements. Significant differences were seen between the youngest and oldest cohorts. Additional research would be beneficial in older populations.

Tan et al.[175] additionally assessed the biomechanical effects of prefabricated foot orthoses on 21 individuals aged 50 to 75 years with PFP. Participants walked 12 m on a level surface and while ascending and descending stairs. Participants walked in three conditions: with their normal shoes, with a sham insert, and with the intervention orthoses in random order. Both the sham and intervention orthoses were constructed of the same ethylene-vinyl acetate material with an identical synthetic cover. The intervention orthoses additionally provided arch support and a 6-degree varus wedge. A motion capture system was used to collect kinematic data. The use of the interventional orthoses was found to decrease both peak dorsiflexion angle and peak dorsiflexion moment compared to both a sham orthoses and shod conditions while performing over ground-level walking. No kinematic changes were seen with ascending stairs, but a decreased peak dorsiflexion moment was seen on stair descent. No significant kinematic changes were seen at the knee or hip in either the level walking or stair conditions. There were no significant effects in reports of pain in any condition.

PLANTAR FASCIOPATHY

The use of foot orthoses in the management of plantar fasciopathy has also been examined. A study by Harutaichun and colleagues[112] compared foot kinematics during gait in three different conditions: shod, orthotic wedging customized by using the traditional Root assessment method, and orthotic wedging utilizing the newer Monaghan assessment method in 35 individuals with plantar fasciitis. Participants were analyzed utilizing a 3D motion analysis system assessing kinematics of the lower limb and foot in each of the three randomized conditions. There was a significant improvement in comfort rating in the orthosis produced by the Root method compared to the shod condition, but no significant difference in comfort between the Root produced orthoses and the Monaghan orthoses. Both the Root assessment method and Monaghan assessment method produced orthoses that appropriately controlled pronation and diminished lengthening of the plantar fascia during the stance phase of gait.

Morrissey and colleagues[176] developed a best practice guide that sought to determine appropriate interventions by incorporating an analysis of systematic reviews and utilizing expert opinion and patient recommendations concerning effective timelines to initiate the interventions. This guide recommends a stepped approach to care. A trial of antipronation taping, plantar fascial stretching, and patient education are the core recommendations for the initial 6-week period. If no positive response is seen, the addition of extracorporeal shockwave therapy is recommended. At 12 weeks the addition of custom foot orthoses is recommended for those individuals that have not yet shown optimal improvement. The study noted that prefabricated orthoses are not recommended. The best practice guide highlights that the RCTs did not include patient education with the orthotic management. Failing to include patient education in load management, prognosis expectations, comorbidity management, and optimal footwear along with the orthotic intervention could prove detrimental to outcomes.

Bishop and colleagues[1] examined the use of custom foot orthoses on first step pain, average 24-hour pain, and plantar fascia thickness. Data were collected at baseline, 4 weeks, and 12 weeks. Diagnosis of plantar fasciopathy was confirmed by palpation, VAS scoring and ultrasound. Sixty participants were allocated to one of three groups: a control group using their own shoes and a sham insole, a shoe group receiving a new pair of athletic shoes, and an intervention group receiving a new pair of athletic shoes and a customized foot orthosis. Participants were instructed not to wear other shoes during the 12-week trial. At 12 weeks the custom orthosis group had significantly less first step pain than both the sham insole control group and the new shoes group. Average 24-hour pain was significantly less at 12 weeks in both the custom orthosis and new shoe group compared to the control group. Plantar fascia thickness, as determined by ultrasound, was significantly decreased at 12 weeks in the custom orthotic group only.

Recent research has focused on how to predict which individuals with plantar fasciopathy will benefit from the application of custom foot orthoses. Wu and colleagues[177] worked to identify a novel clinical prediction rule for the use of foot orthoses in heel pain. The study examined 74 patients with plantar heel pain. All 74 patients received antipronation taping for 1 week followed by the use of a customized foot orthosis for 6 months. The researchers identified five potential predictors that will need to be studied further in RCTs. The five predictors include a decrease in reported heel pain by 1.5 points out of 10 after the antipronation taping procedure and plantar flexion strength of involved side at least equal to uninvolved side. Additional predictors included three different ROM measures: greater than 54-degree ankle plantarflexion, greater than 45-degree hip external rotation, and less than 39-degree hip internal rotation. Participants with at least three of the five predictors had an 89% success rate.

LOW BACK PAIN

Castro-Mendez and collegues[178] examined the effects of custom-made foot orthoses compared to a placebo orthosis in 101 patients with nonspecific chronic low back pain and foot pronation in at least one lower extremity. The pronated foot position was determined by a score of 6+ or greater on the FPI. Patients completed both the Oswestry Disability Index Questionnaire (ODI) as well as the VAS at baseline and after wearing foot orthoses 8 hours per day for 4 weeks. All participants' feet were molded using the plaster casting technique. The control group received flat orthoses while the experimental group received custom orthoses of polypropylene with a polyethylene foam cover. At 4 weeks, the custom foot orthoses group reported a significant reduction in symptoms of chronic low back pain. Significant improvements in both ODI and VAS scores were observed in the experimental group only.

Rannisto and collegues[179] explored the use of custom foot orthoses in 34 meat packing workers with at least 5-mm leg-length discrepancy and low back pain. Individuals were randomized into the intervention group receiving custom insoles correcting the leg-length discrepancy by 70% while the control group received insoles without a correction. The participants were followed over 12 months. Those receiving the correction insoles reported significantly less low back pain and sciatic pain. Additionally, the intervention group had significantly decreased likelihood of taking sick leave and improved physical functioning as measured by the RAND-36.

Tarrade et al.[180] also looked at workers involved in prolonged standing in their repeated measures study. The study analyzed 34 production line workers with foot pain wearing customized 3D-printed orthoses. The workers included in the study had varied foot pathologies including metatarsalgia, plantar fasciitis, and heal spurs. A number of significant improvements were seen during the 3-week intervention including decreased plantar pressures, decreased leg discomfort, and improved postural stability.

Yazdani and colleagues[181] found that hyperpronated foot positioning (+10 or more on the FPI) modifies function of lumbopelvic musculature with delays in muscle activation and increased muscle guarding which potentially contribute to the development of low back pain.

Case Example 8.1 **Individual With Rearfoot and Forefoot Dysfunction**

M.L. is an active 50-year-old female who recently began to train for a local 10-km race. She is referred by her family physician for evaluation and intervention because of thickened and painful plantar callus under the second and fourth metatarsal heads and on the lateral surface of the hallux in both feet. The discomfort has increased to a point where she is unable to complete the distances she needs to run to prepare for the upcoming race.

M.L. is 5 feet, 5 inches tall and weighs 132 lb. In relaxed standing, no leg-length discrepancy is apparent, although both patellae are rotated inward, slight hyperextension and recurvatum at the knee is present (left more than right), and both feet are markedly pronated.

The following values are recorded in the non–weight-bearing and weight-bearing examinations:

Non–Weight-Bearing Examination Component	Left	Right
Rearfoot STN position	6-degree varus	7-degree varus
Calcaneus inversion	18 degrees	22 degrees
Calcaneus eversion	12 degrees	14 degrees
Ankle dorsiflexion	9 degrees	7 degrees
Rearfoot dorsiflexion	2 degrees	0 degrees
Forefoot STN position	Mild valgus	Moderate valgus
Locking mechanism	Fair	Poor
First ray	Slightly plantarflexed	Slightly plantarflexed
Hallux dorsiflexion	75 degrees	80 degrees
Medial longitudinal arch	Medium height	Medium height

STN, Subtalar neutral.

Weight-Bearing Examination Component	Left	Right
Calcaneal/floor alignment	Eversion	Eversion
Tibiofibular position	40 degrees	37 degrees
Navicular drop (STN to relaxed calcaneal stance)	10 mm	12 mm
Navicular position (Feiss)	Slightly below	Moderately below
Toe sign	2.5 toes visible	3 toes visible
Femoral torsion	14 degrees	16 degrees
Tibial torsion	25 degrees	27 degrees

STN, Subtalar neutral.

QUESTIONS TO CONSIDER

- What are the normative values for non–weight-bearing range of motion in the rearfoot (STN position, calcaneal inversion and eversion, dorsiflexion) and forefoot (STN position, midtarsal joint dorsiflexion, first ray position, and mobility)?
- What rearfoot and forefoot deformities do M.L.'s examination findings suggest?
- What are normal findings for the closed-chain static weight-bearing examination?
- How should the findings for M.L.'s weight-bearing examination be interpreted?
- How do the findings of M.L.'s non–weight-bearing and weight-bearing examinations relate to each other? Which deformities are compensated versus uncompensated?

Case Example 8.2 Individual With Rearfoot and Forefoot Dysfunction

M.L. wants to continue training for her upcoming race without increasing her pain and further damaging soft tissue in her feet. An appropriate prescription is being created for her on the basis of the findings of her examination and the principles of orthotic design.

EXAMINATION FINDINGS

Relaxed standing: no apparent leg-length discrepancy, both patellae rotated inward, slight hype knee (left more than right), marked pronation of both feet.

Non–Weight-Bearing Examination Component	Left	Right
Rearfoot STN position	6-degree varus	7-degree varus
Calcaneus inversion	18 degrees	22 degrees
Calcaneus eversion	12 degrees	14 degrees
Ankle dorsiflexion	9 degrees	7 degrees
Rearfoot dorsiflexion	2 degrees	0 degrees
Forefoot STN position	Mild valgus	Moderate valgus
Locking mechanism	Fair	Poor
First ray	Slightly plantarflexed	Slightly plantarflexed
Hallux dorsiflexion	75 degrees	80 degrees
Medial longitudinal arch	Medium height	Medium height

STN, Subtalar neutral.

Weight-Bearing Examination Component	Left	Right
Calcaneal/floor alignment	Eversion	Eversion
Tibiofibular position	40 degrees	37 degrees
Navicular drop (STN to relaxed calcaneal stance)	10 mm	12 mm
Navicular position (Feiss)	Slightly below	Moderately below
Toe sign	2.5 toes visible	3 toes visible
Femoral torsion	14 degrees	16 degrees
Tibial torsion	25 degrees	27 degrees

STN, Subtalar neutral.

QUESTIONS TO CONSIDER

- What are the primary short-term and long-term goals of orthotic intervention for M.L.? Are the therapeutic goals for orthotic intervention similar to or different from M.L.'s goals? How quickly will the orthosis have an impact on the level of pain and function?
- What options should be considered in addressing her forefoot deformity in each foot? What type of posting (intrinsic vs. extrinsic, medial vs. lateral) is most appropriate? How much of a wedge or post should be recommended? Why? How might the recommendations for each foot be similar or different?
- What options should be considered in addressing the rearfoot deformity in each foot? What type of posting (intrinsic vs. extrinsic, medial vs. lateral) would be most appropriate? How much of a wedge or post should be recommended? Why? How might the recommendations for each foot be similar or different?
- What type of materials would be most appropriate to use in her orthosis? Why?
- Are fabricating orthoses for both her running shoes and her usual daily footwear advisable? Why or why not?
- What type of wearing schedule should be recommended? Should she alter her training schedule or expectations about participating in the upcoming race? Why or why not?
- How frequently should M.L. be followed up during this episode of care? How should the outcomes of orthotic intervention be assessed?

In a systemic review and meta-analysis, Kong and colleagues[182] reported that there is moderate evidence to support the use of custom-made foot orthoses in the management of chronic low back pain. Improvements were seen in both pain scores and disability scores with custom orthotic use. Foot structure and type, orthotic materials, posting methods, and fabrication methods must be considered in determining who is likely to respond to orthotic intervention and in comparing the effectiveness of various orthotic interventions.

Summary

Root's theory remains a pivotal cornerstone in foot biomechanics and orthotic intervention research. Although some aspects of Root's theory have faced scrutiny, his work is undeniably important and serves as the foundation for many of the studies that explore the influence of the foot on lower extremity biomechanics and overuse injuries. Root's contributions have paved the way for investigating various foot types, correlations between foot posture and kinematic deficits, and biomechanical factors contributing to lower extremity pain, dysfunctions, and injuries.

Traditionally, researchers primarily focused on biomechanical components that impact the efficacy of orthotic interventions. However, the current literature expands on Root's work by exploring a broader range of factors that may influence outcomes. This emerging evidence suggests that the efficacy of foot orthotic interventions can be influenced not only by biomechanics but also by psychosocial factors.

Advancements in technology and modern examination tools have played a crucial role in enhancing the understanding of lower extremity function and foot orthoses' effectiveness. These advancements have enabled researchers and clinicians to delve deeper into the complexities of foot biomechanics and orthotic interventions.

Despite foot orthoses being a common intervention, additional research is still needed to provide clinicians with more confidence in prescribing orthoses based on their likely outcomes. A comprehensive understanding of the interactions between various factors influencing foot orthotics will help clinicians make more informed decisions about which type of orthotic intervention is best suited for each patient's unique circumstances.

The effectiveness of biomechanical foot orthoses depends on a number of factors. An understanding of causes and effects of aberrant foot motion on pathological conditions of the foot is essential in determining the appropriate orthosis prescription and plan of care. Clinicians who do not carefully consider biomechanical principles and other factors that contribute to clinical signs and symptoms are likely to prescribe an ineffective or inappropriate orthosis. Information gathered from all three components of the biomechanical examination (non–weight-bearing, static weight-bearing, and dynamic gait assessment) is critical for orthotic design and prescription.

Historically, the principles and design of the Root functional orthosis and the biomechanical foot orthosis have had consistently effective clinical results. Root's model demands a keen understanding of foot biomechanics, careful prescription, and advanced fabrication skills. With this understanding and attention to detail, the end result may be a lightweight, durable, cost-effective foot orthosis that substantially reduces the detrimental effects of aberrant foot motion.

References

The complete listing of the References are available in the accompanying enhanced eBook version included with the print purchase of this textbook. Visit Elsevier eBooks+ (eBooks.Health.Elsevier.com) to access this content.

9 Principles of Lower Extremity Orthoses

ERIC FOLMAR, HEATHER JENNINGS, AND LUKE L. BRISBIN

LEARNING OBJECTIVES

On completion of this chapter, the reader will be able to do the following:

1. Define the functional objectives (reasons) that an ankle-foot orthosis (AFO), knee-ankle-foot orthosis (KAFO), or hip-knee-ankle-foot orthosis (HKAFO) would be prescribed for persons with mobility dysfunction.
2. Explain the evaluative process used to determine appropriate prescription for individuals requiring a lower extremity orthosis.
3. Describe the biomechanical control systems for foot, ankle, knee, and/or hip designed into an AFO, a KAFO, or an HKAFO.
4. Describe how each type of lower extremity orthosis is designed to enhance achievement of stance phase stability, swing limb clearance, limb prepositioning, adequate step length, and efficiency of gait.
5. Describe how each of the most commonly prescribed AFO, KAFO, and HKAFO designs affect transition through the rockers of stance and swing phase of gait.
6. Compare and contrast the indications and limitations of prefabricated, custom-fit, and custom-molded lower extremity orthoses.
7. Apply knowledge of normal and pathologic gait, assessment of impairment, and functional potential in the selection of an appropriate lower extremity orthosis for patients with neuromuscular impairments.
8. Identify effective strategies for donning/doffing the orthosis, gait and mobility training, and orthotic maintenance for children and adults using lower extremity orthoses.
9. Select appropriate outcome measures to evaluate effectiveness of orthotic intervention and gait training for persons using lower extremity orthoses.

There are many factors to consider when selecting a lower extremity orthosis for individuals with musculoskeletal or neuromuscular dysfunction who have difficulty with mobility and walking. An orthosis may be designed to substitute for impaired muscle performance in the presence of weakness to improve foot clearance in the swing phase of gait.[1] An orthosis may be used to provide stance phase stability and support to enhance alignment of limb segments when there is structural instability of one or more lower extremity joints. An orthosis may be designed to limit joint motion or unload forces during weight bearing to allow healing after surgery or prevent injury to vulnerable joints.[2] For persons with impaired motor control and abnormal tone, orthoses may enhance mobility by minimizing the impact of abnormal movement associated with hypertonicity by positioning limb segments for optimal function.[3] Alternatively, an orthosis may be used to minimize the risk of development of bony deformity and contracture associated with long-standing hypertonicity, especially in growing children.[4] Given the many different reasons an orthosis might be prescribed, there is no "one size fits all" option: Health professionals must clearly define what they want an orthosis to accomplish, consider its practicality and cost, and sort through the many options available to select the design and components that will best meet the patient's needs and goals.

This chapter systematically reviews the design and the pros and cons of AFOs, KAFOs, and HKAFOs as a means to improve mobility and function for children and adults with neuromuscular dysfunction. We will start with a quick review of the gait cycle and its "rockers" as a foundation for understanding how an orthosis can provide stance-phase stability or enhance swing-phase mobility. Then we will compare and contrast the various AFO designs, discuss contemporary KAFO components and design, explore traditional HKAFOs and their uses, and finally consider orthotic options for reciprocal gait for patients with significant neuromuscular disease or disability. We will apply our growing understanding of lower extremity orthoses in problem-based cases for children and adults with cerebral palsy, and weakness due to spinal cord compression, multiple sclerosis, diabetic amyotrophy, and Guillain-Barré syndrome.

What Type of Orthosis Is Best?

When an individual with neuromuscular or musculoskeletal dysfunction has difficulty with mobility and walking, decisions about orthotic options are best made by collaborative interaction within the framework of an interdisciplinary team.[5] Members of this team include the person who will be using the orthosis, his or her family members or caregivers, any physicians involved in his or her care (e.g., a neurologist, orthopedist, or physiatrist), the physical and occupational therapists who are likely to be involved in functional training, and the orthotist who will design, fabricate, deliver, and maintain the orthosis. The combined knowledge and skills of all members of the team ensures that the prescription will best match orthotic design to the patient's functional needs (Table 9.1). If the team is not able to gather in one place as decisions are being made, there must be effective strategies for communication in place so that each team member can contribute his or her unique perspective about why an orthosis is indicated and how the orthosis will facilitate the individual's functional ability.

Physical therapists examine the patient to provide information about muscle performance and motor control, range of motion, alignment of the limbs, and the gait cycle, with attention to both primary impairments and the compensation strategies the individual uses while walking, as well as how the orthosis might impact biomechanically on other daily motor tasks (e.g., a child's ability to get up and down from the floor).[6] Physicians bring to the team an understanding of the specific disease or disorder the patient is dealing with, including the condition's natural history and likely prognosis, types of secondary musculoskeletal problems that are commonly encountered, and any cognitive, developmental, or multisystem involvement that may be associated with the disease.[7] Family members and the individual needing the orthosis are concerned with practical issues, such as who will be responsible for applying (donning) or removing (doffing) the device and the ease with which this can be accomplished, as well as information about the types of activities that the individual wants to be involved in while using the orthosis (lifestyle and leisure activities).[8] The orthotist uses knowledge of materials and biomechanics, information provided by team and family members, and results of the individual's physical examination to design and fabricate the orthosis that will best address the mobility problem that needs to be solved.[6]

Table 9.1 Components of the Preorthotic Prescription Examination Organized by ICF Categories

ICF Category	Domain		Concerns
Body structure and function	Joint integrity and stability		Ligamentous instability, joint deformity
	Range of motion		Soft tissue contracture, joint deformity
	Limb length and alignment		Rotational deformity, unequal limb length
	Muscle length		Fixed versus modifiable contracture
	Overall flexibility		Ability to don/doff; impact of orthosis on trunk, back
	Motor control		Quality of voluntary motion
	Muscle tone		Flaccidity, hypotonicity, hypertonicity, fluctuating tone
	Muscle performance		Strength, power, endurance
	Involuntary movement		Impact on tolerance of orthosis
	Coordination		Ability to don/doff
	Somatosensory function		Ability to detect skin irritation/damage
	Perceptual function		Ability to don/doff
	Upper extremity function		Ability to don/doff
	Postural control, balance		Ability to don/doff
	Visual function		Ability to perform skin checks, don/doff
	Cognitive function		Understanding of how to use orthosis
	Cardiovascular endurance		Ability to functionally use orthosis
Activity level	Gait analysis	Observational	Primary gait problems and compensations
		Kinematic	Primary gait problems and compensations
		Kinetic	Impact of orthosis on moment throughout gait cycle
		Energetics	Impact of orthosis on physical work of walking
		Assistive device	Safe function with orthosis and assistive device
		Various surfaces	Impact of resistance, unstable surface on gait
	Transitions	Sit to/from stand	Preparing to walk and returning to seated position
		To/from floor	Activities on the floor (especially for children/play)
		Managing falls	How to protect self and recover from fall
		Inclines/stairs	Degree of mobility in home and public environment
	Activities of daily living	Donning/doffing	Will assistance be necessary? Who will provide help?
		Self-care	How will orthosis impact on self-care ability?
		Toileting	Will orthosis need to be removed to use the bathroom?
		Dressing	Ability to manage clothes and shoes
Participation level	Home		Ability to take part in family activities, roles
	School		Mobility in classroom, hallways, outside play areas
	Work		Mobility in entrance, workspace, common areas
	Leisure		Mobility over surfaces, use of tools/devices
	Transportation		Ability to drive, use public transportation

ICF, The World Health Organization's International Classification of Functioning, Disability and Health.

The team must not overlook the significant contribution of the individual and caregiver in the prescription process. The use of an orthosis enhances, as well as constrains, lower limb function; for example, it requires considerable adjustment on the part of the person who will be wearing the orthosis. An understanding of the individual's or the caregiver's expectations about what the orthosis will accomplish is a key component of orthotic prescription and training. Discussion and education about what an orthosis will and will not do for the wearer can minimize potential mismatch of expectation versus actual outcome. Acceptance and functional use of the orthosis depend on just how well it meets identified needs and goals, as well as the cost of its use in terms of inconvenience and disruption of lifestyle.[9]

Careful consideration of the individual's diagnosis is also critical when selecting materials and designing the orthosis. Questions that the team should consider during the decision-making process include: Can we reasonably expect that an individual's musculoskeletal or neuromuscular status is stable and likely to remain the same over time? Does the disease typically have a progressive course, such that decline in function is anticipated over time? Or, as in the case of traumatic injury, will the person's condition and functional ability improve with time as healing occurs? What can be expected in terms of muscle function and strength, range of motion and joint function, and functional mobility and gait over time? How might growth and developmental status influence future orthotic needs? All of these must be accounted for in the design of the orthosis.

The selection of any orthotic device must include careful consideration of four factors:

1. The indications that the orthosis may be useful to the individual (i.e., the match between the person's characteristics and needs and what the orthosis will provide).
2. The *advantages* or positive outcomes expected when using the orthosis (i.e., how it will improve mobility and gait, influence tone, or protect a limb or body segment).
3. Any disadvantages or *concessions* that may be associated with its use (i.e., the ways in which it may complicate daily activity, mobility, or preferred activities; the energy cost associated with its use; the relative expense of the device).
4. The circumstances or characteristics of the individual that make use of the device detrimental or *contraindicated*.

Consideration of these four factors guides clinical decision-making when comparing and contrasting the various options for lower extremity orthoses. Characteristics of an ideal orthosis are summarized in Box 9.1.

To help an individual use the orthosis most effectively, the physical therapist must understand how the orthosis should fit with respect to its design (i.e., what are the optimal trim lines?) and force control systems (how does it act on the limb segments?) (Box 9.2). Every orthosis uses force applied to the limb to accomplish the goals of its design. An orthosis is most comfortable and effective when (Fig. 9.1):

1. The forces are distributed over large surface areas to minimize pressure on skin and soft tissue.
2. The forces are applied in such a way that a large moment arm reduces the amount of force needed to control the joint.
3. The sum of the primary force and opposing counterforces of each control system equals zero.

Box 9.1 Characteristics of an Ideal Orthosis

Function

- Meets the individual's mobility needs and goals
- Maximizes stance phase stability
- Minimizes abnormal alignment
- Minimally compromises swing clearance
- Effectively prepositions the limb for initial contact
- Is energy efficient with the individual's preferred assistive device

Comfort

- Can be worn for long periods without damaging skin or causing pain
- Can be easily donned and doffed (e.g., considering clothing, footwear, toileting)

Cosmesis

- Meets the individual's need to fit in with peers

Fabrication

- Can be made in the shortest period of time
- Uses a minimally complex design
- Has some degree of adjustability to enhance initial fitting
- For children, responds to growth or change over time
- Is durable: stands up to stresses/strains of daily activity

Cost

- Can be made with minimal initial cost and minimal cost for maintenance

Box 9.2 Principles Underlying Control Systems in Orthotic Design

1. Pressure = Force/Area
2. Torque = Force × Distance
3. Control direction of primary force and direction of counterforces
4. Equilibrium Σforces = 0

Determinants of Functional Gait

There are five factors that influence how well an individual is able to walk.[10] The first is *stance-phase stability*: The limb in contact with the ground must be stable enough to support body weight and respond to the ground reaction forces (GRFs) as the individual moves through stance phase. The second is *clearance in swing*: The advancing limb must clear the ground adequately during swing phase to minimize risk of stumbling and trips. Swing limb clearance is influenced by the ability to maintain a level pelvis by stance limb abductor muscles, as well as by action of the hip, knee flexors, and dorsiflexors of the swing limb as they relatively shorten the length of the swinging limb. The third is *swing-phase prepositioning*: By the end of swing, the foot about to contact the ground must be positioned for an effective initial contact and loading response as stance begins. The fourth is *adequate step length*: There must be adequate motor control and range of motion at the hip, knee, ankle, and forefoot of both limbs so that optimal step

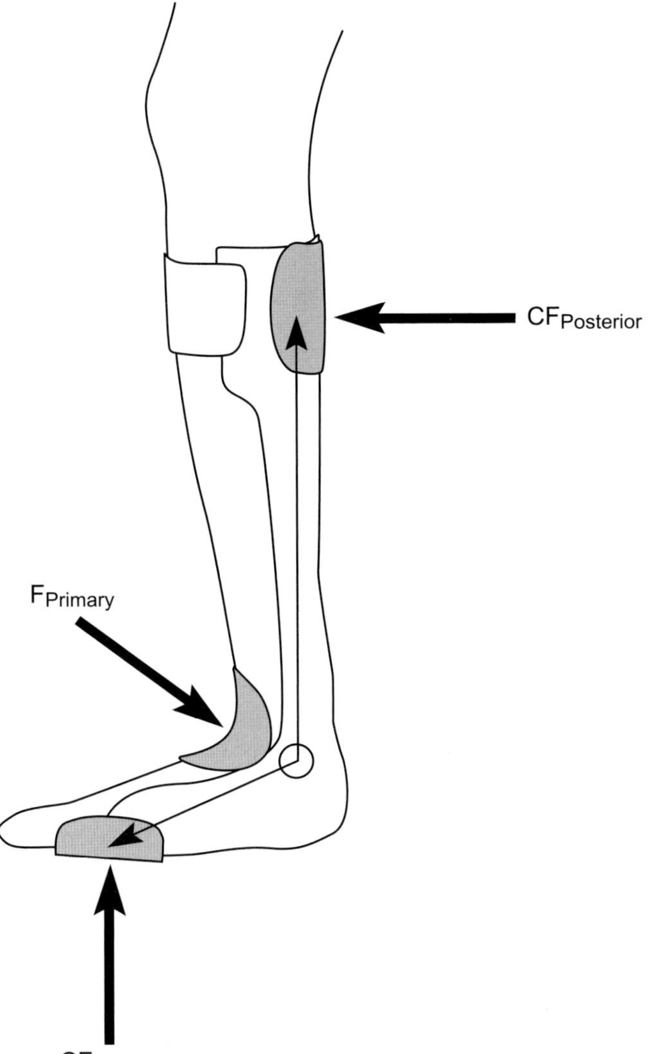

Fig. 9.1 Principles underlying the plantarflexion control system acting during swing phase in a rigid/solid ankle-foot orthosis. The large primary force ($F_{Primary}$) is applied in a posterior-inferior direction over a large surface area (stippled area) anterior to the axis of the ankle joint, usually by the shoe's closure or reinforced by webbing across the anterior ankle. The two counterforces, applied in an upward ($CF_{Plantar}$) and anterior ($CF_{Posterior}$) direction, also over a large surface area, far from the axis of the ankle joint, create an effective moment arm so that less force is required to achieve the desired stabilization. The sum of the primary *(large arrow)* and two opposing counterforces *(small arrows)* is zero in a well-balanced orthosis.

length can occur. The fifth is *energy conservation*: If there are problems with timing, muscle performance, coordination, or postural control during the gait cycle, the energy cost of walking rises substantially, and efficiency of ambulation is compromised.

If neuromuscular or musculoskeletal dysfunction substantially interferes with these determinants, functional ambulation may be an unrealistic goal without an appropriate orthosis. Refer to Chapter 5 for greater detail about characteristics of the normal and pathologic gait cycle.

Rockers of Stance Phase

Orthotists describe three transitional periods, or rockers, during stance phase of walking as the body progresses forward over the foot (Fig. 9.2).[11] During the *first (heel) rocker*, there is a controlled lowering of the foot from neutral ankle position at initial contact to a plantarflexed flat foot, as well as acceptance of body weight on the limb during loading response. When motor control and muscle performance is efficient, eccentric contraction of the quadriceps and anterior tibialis prevents "foot slap" and protects the knee as GRF is translated upward toward the knee. In the *second (ankle) rocker*, the tibia begins to rotate over the weight-bearing foot, from its initial 10 degrees of plantarflexion at the end of loading response, then through vertical into dorsiflexion as midstance is completed. Eccentric contraction of the gastrocnemius and soleus muscles "puts on the brakes" to control the speed of the forward progression of the tibia over the fixed foot throughout midstance. At the start of the *third (toe) rocker*, the forefoot has converted from its mobile adapter function of early stance to a rigid lever for an effective late stance, and the heel rises off the ground so that body weight has to roll over the first metatarsophalangeal joint through push-off in terminal stance. During fast walking and running, acceleration occurs as active contraction of the gastrocnemius-soleus complex propels the foot and leg into swing phase.

All lower extremity orthoses provide some degree of external stability to foot and ankle joints; as a result, the smooth transition through the rockers of stance phase is often compromised.[12] Disruption of forward progression during stance negatively impacts step length, cadence, and single-limb support time.[12] The optimal orthotic prescription must balance the need to provide external support with the possible compromise on forward progression and mobility: The orthotist strives to select an orthotic design that provides minimum necessary stability so that mobility will be the least compromised. In many instances, modifications of footwear, such as the addition of a cushion heel (which simulates controlled lowering of the foot in loading response) or a rocker bottom sole (which simulates forward progression of the tibia over the foot throughout midstance), can substitute to some degree for the mobility lost when external control is necessary.[13] The rehabilitation team must weigh the impact of stability provided by an orthosis on progression through stance and its impact on a patient's functional status: At times, compromise is unavoidable if the patient's functional deficits are to be addressed effectively.

Prefabricated, Custom Fit, or Custom Molded?

How does the team determine whether an individual would benefit from a relatively less expensive prefabricated orthosis versus a more costly (in both time and money) custom-molded orthosis designed specifically for the person? There are a number of factors to consider in making this decision.

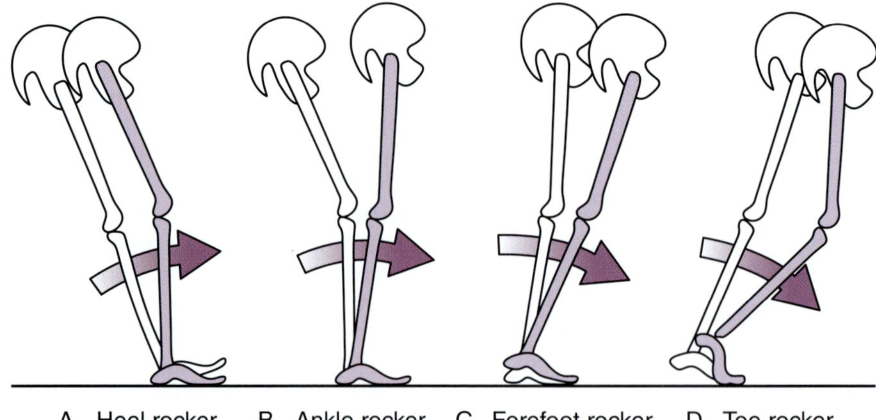

Fig. 9.2 Three transitional rocker periods occur as the body moves forward over the foot during stance. (A) During first rocker, the transition from swing into early stance, controlled lowering of the forefoot occurs, with a fulcrum at the heel. (B) During second rocker, controlled forward progression of the tibia over the foot occurs, with motion of the talocrural joint of the ankle. (C and D) In the third rocker, transition from stance toward swing occurs as the heel rises, with dorsiflexion of the metatarsophalangeal joints. (From Webster JB. Principles of normal and pathologic gait. In: Webster JB, ed. *Atlas of Orthoses and Assistive Devices*. Fifth ed. Elsevier Inc.; 2018:49–62 [chapter 4].)[11]

The effectiveness of an AFO is determined by the intimacy and consistency of its fit. Intimacy of contact between limb and orthosis is best achieved in custom-molded designs.

Mass-manufactured, prefabricated orthoses are available in a wide spectrum of orthotic designs, by shoe size, and made of a number of different materials. The degree to which they can be modified or adjusted to fit an individual varies; this may be problematic for persons with foot deformity, extremely wide or narrow feet, large calf muscles, sensory impairments, or variable limb volume. They are attractive to consumers because they are significantly less expensive than custom-fit or custom-molded orthoses. However, many rehabilitation professionals are not satisfied with the ability of a prefabricated orthosis to provide optimal external support and control of motion over time: Durability is directly related to the quality of material used and by the lack of intimate fit to an individual's limb. Even a minimal amount of pistoning or heel elevation within the orthosis during walking can lead to skin irritation or breakdown and, in the presence of hypertonicity, an increase of underlying abnormal extensor tone. Therapists may opt to use a trial run with prefabricated orthoses as an evaluative tool to determine which orthotic design might best meet the patient's needs during the time a custom orthotic is being prepared or when the patient's condition requires use of an orthosis for only a short time period or when the patient condition is unstable. Because prefabricated orthoses do not fit the foot intimately, they should be used with extreme caution in persons with neuropathic foot conditions whose ability to perceive soft tissue irritation and damage is compromised.[14–17]

Another alternative is a manufactured orthosis that is then custom fit using heating or relieving techniques or the application of additional materials to obtain as close a fit to the individual's foot and limb as possible. Custom-fit orthoses may be appropriate when change in functional status (either improvement or deterioration) is anticipated, such that the orthosis will need to be replaced or adjusted frequently.

Custom-molded orthoses provide the optimal control of the limb and, because of their intimate fit, are especially important for patients with impaired sensation, significant hypertonicity, or risk of progressive deformity associated with their condition. The orthotist constructs the orthosis around a rectified model of the person's limb, ensuring adequate pressure relief over vulnerable areas (i.e., bony prominences) and building in the desired stabilizing forces based on the orthotic prescription.[18] Refer to Chapter 6 for more details about the process of fabrication.

The only true contraindication of a custom-molded thermoplastic design is significantly fluctuating limb size associated with conditions that lead to edema of the braced extremity.[19] When limb size fluctuates, intimacy of custom-molded fit is lost: When the limb is at its lowest volume, excessive movement of the limb within the orthosis occurs, compromising orthotic control and increasing risk of skin irritation and damage. When the limb is significantly edematous, the AFO may become constricting, leading to pressure-related problems. For persons with congestive heart failure, advanced kidney disease on dialysis, or other conditions associated with unpredictable fluctuation in limb volume, the total contact of a custom-molded orthosis may be inappropriate, and a conventional double-upright orthotic design should be considered.

Appropriate Footwear

Whether the decision is to use a prefabricated, custom-fit, or custom-molded orthosis, the ultimate ability of the AFO to meet its therapeutic goals depends on the type and condition of the individual's footwear. Refer to Chapter 7 for more information about key characteristics of shoes worn with an orthosis. Recognition of the need to consider footwear is not always intuitive to the individual, caregivers, or health professionals working on improving the ability to ambulate. It may be necessary for the individual to wear a shoe that is one-half to a whole size larger to accommodate an orthosis; a shoe that is too short or too tight can interfere with the biomechanical function of the orthosis. Shoe closure of an Oxford-style or athletic shoe (whether tied with laces or closed with Velcro) often provides the diagonally directed force that stabilizes the calcaneus in the heel cup of the orthosis; if the calcaneus moves out of position during walking, the effectiveness of orthotic control is compromised. Loafer-type shoes and most sandals do not provide adequate stabilizing forces during the stance phase of gait. Although most thermoplastic AFO designs allow individuals to alternate among several pairs of shoes, changing heel heights dramatically alters the biomechanical function of the orthosis. The orthotist and therapist share responsibility for patient and family education about appropriate footwear, monitoring shoe condition to assess impact of wear and tear on its construction and stability, as well as ongoing evaluation of the effectiveness of the orthosis in meeting the individual's functional needs over time.

Ankle-Foot Orthoses

AFOs are, by far, the most frequently prescribed device used to control the lower extremity during each phase of the gait cycle for individuals with neuromuscular or musculoskeletal impairments that make walking difficult. It is important to note that the acronyms used to name lower extremity orthoses describe joints that are positioned within the orthosis. In reality, AFOs also effectively address stability of the knee joint (proximal to the orthosis) during stance.[20]

AFOs fall into two categories: *static orthoses* that prohibit motion in all planes at the ankle (e.g., solid AFO [SAFO], anterior floor reaction AFO, patellar tendon–bearing [PTB]/weight-relieving AFO). In contrast, *dynamic orthoses* allow some degree of sagittal plane motion at the ankle (e.g., posterior leaf spring [PLS] or spiral AFOs, articulating SAFOs). Whether static or dynamic, the primary goal of an AFO is to provide just enough external support for stability in stance and clearance in swing with minimal compromise of forward progression through the heel, ankle, and toe rockers of gait. The actions, indications, and contraindications for the various AFO designs are summarized in Table 9.2.

BIOMECHANICAL PRINCIPLES

The biomechanical principles of AFOs are founded on the functional anatomy of the ankle-foot complex. Dorsiflexion and plantarflexion of the ankle are multiplanar (i.e., movement occurs in all three planes of motion) as the talus rotates through the mortise of the ankle in both open chain movement and when the mortise moves over a relatively fixed (weight-bearing) talus in a closed chain movement.[21,22] The proximal surface of the mortise is shaped by the syndesmosis (fibrous articulation) between the distal tibia and fibula. The medial wall of the talocrural joint is formed by the medial malleolus, a downward extension of the tibia. The lateral wall, formed by the lateral malleolus of the fibula, is both longer and shifted posteriorly. Because of the shape of the articular surfaces of the talus in its mortise and the offset position of the malleoli, the axis of the ankle joint is slightly oblique, running in an anteromedial to posterolateral direction. As a result, dorsiflexion is accompanied by some degree of forefoot pronation and abduction along with hind foot valgus. Plantarflexion is accompanied by forefoot supination with adduction and hind foot varus. Note that during stance, movement occurs in a closed chain situation because the foot is fixed on the ground by weight-bearing forces, so that the mortise rolls over the head of the talus.

If an AFO has mechanical ankle joints, the axis of the mechanical joints should be aligned as closely as possible to the obliquely oriented anatomic axis of motion (Fig. 9.3). The mechanical joint heads are placed at approximately midline of the malleoli in the sagittal plane. This strategy reduces the likelihood of abnormal torque and shearing between the orthosis and limb as the individual wearing the orthosis walks. When there is incongruence between the anatomic and mechanical axes, excessive motion of the limb within the orthoses is likely, and action of the mechanical ankle joint is compromised.

Static Orthoses

Static AFOs are the most aggressive of the AFO designs in providing external support. They restrict ankle and foot motion in all three planes to provide significant stance-phase stability and swing limb clearance. However, because of their rigidity, these orthoses greatly compromise transitions through the first (heel), second (ankle), and, to less degree, third (toe) rockers of stance phase. Individuals using static AFOs do better functionally wearing a shoe with a cushion heel and rocker bottom to simulate these key transitions. The decision to recommend a static AFO should be made carefully, weighing the benefit of greater stability against the cost of lost mobility.

SOLID ANKLE-FOOT ORTHOSES

Characteristics

The SAFO, also known as a rigid AFO, is typically fabricated from relatively thick thermoplastic and aims to hold the ankle and foot in as close to biomechanically neutral position (zero degrees of ankle dorsiflexion, subtalar and calcaneal neutral, with a balanced forefoot) as possible given the individual's functional anatomy.[21] The anteroposterior trimline of the SAFO falls at or near the midline of the medial and lateral malleolus (Fig. 9.4). Medial and lateral corrugations may be incorporated into the shell of the orthosis to provide additional strength when hypertonicity or excessive weight creates loading forces that require a stronger orthosis. The proximal border is typically trimmed to fall 1½ inches below the apex of the head of the fibula for protection of the common peroneal nerve. The footplate is either trimmed just short of the plantar metatarsal heads or can be lengthened beyond the metatarsal distally into a toeplate if greater stability is required or hypertonicity is a concern.[4] Some orthotists recommend the addition of a tone-inhibiting bar if hypertonicity is severe. There is a tradeoff to consider if the footplate is lengthened: It is much easier to fit into and put on shoes with a shorter footplate; assistance may be necessary to don shoes when the SAFO has a full toeplate.

Table 9.2 Summary of Indications for, Impact on Gait of, and Contraindications for Commonly Prescribed Lower Extremity Orthoses

Type of Orthosis	Category	Actions	Indications	Contraindications	Options
UCBL orthosis	Static	Stabilize subtalar and tarsal joints in stance	Rearfoot valgus/varus Flexible pes planus	Rigid foot deformity	Thermoplastic Gillette modification
DAFO	Dynamic	Stabilize subtalar and tarsal joints in stance	Flexible pes planus Mild to moderate spastic diplegic or hemiplegic CP Hypotonic CP	Rigid foot deformity	Thermoplastic
Supramalleolar	Dynamic	Stabilize subtalar and tarsal joints in stance Preposition foot for IC by heel	Flexible pes planus Mild to moderate spastic diplegic or hemiplegic CP Hypotonic CP	Significant equinovarus hypertonicity	Thermoplastic
Posterior leaf spring	Dynamic	Assist limb clearance in swing Preposition foot for IC by heel	Dorsiflexion weakness, impaired motor control, LMN flaccid paralysis of dorsiflexors	Moderate-to-severe hypertonicity	Thermoplastic
Carbon graphite AFO	Dynamic	Assist limb clearance in swing preposition foot for IC by heel	Paralysis or impaired muscle performance of dorsiflexors	Moderate-to-severe hypertonicity	Custom or prefabricated
Neuro-orthoses	Dynamic	Assist limb clearance in swing Preposition foot for IC by heel	Dorsiflexion weakness or low tone	Flaccid paralysis Patient intolerance of electrical stimulation	Functional electrical stimulation
Articulating ankle	Dynamic	Assist limb clearance in swing Preposition foot for IC by heel Permit advancement of tibia (second rocker) in stance	Impaired motor control of ankle musculature Potential for recovery of neuromotor function	LMN paralysis (flaccidity) or hypotonicity as primary problem	Thermoplastic or metal double upright Dorsiflexion assist Plantarflexion stop Adjustable range into dorsiflexion can be incorporated Often requires shoe with cushion heel
SAFO	Static	Control ankle position throughout stance Provide stance phase stability via ankle-knee coupling Assist limb clearance in swing Preposition foot for IC by heel Distal trim line behind metatarsal heads or extended toeplate	Significant hypertonicity with seriously impaired motor control at ankle and knee	LMN paralysis (flaccidity) or hypotonicity as primary problem	Thermoplastic basis for KAFO and HKAFO Requires cushion heel and rocker bottom shoe
Tone-inhibiting AFO	Static	Control ankle position throughout stance Provide stance phase stability via ankle-knee coupling Typically extended toeplate	Significant hypertonicity with seriously impaired motor control	LMN paralysis (flaccidity) or hypotonicity as primary problem	Thermoplastic, Basis for KAFO and HKAFO Requires cushion heel and rocker bottom shoe
Anterior floor reaction AFO	Static	Provide stability in stance via ankle-knee coupling Control ankle position throughout stance	Weakness or impaired motor control at knee and ankle	Ligamentous insufficiency at the knee Genu recurvatum	Thermoplastic or carbon composite Custom made or custom fit
Weight-relieving AFO	Static	Protect lower leg and foot during stance by reducing weight-bearing forces.	Healing soft tissue, ligamentous, or bone injuries of the lower leg, ankle, or foot	Mechanical instability of the knee, or injury to proximal tibia Patient intolerance of PTB weight-bearing forces (rare)	Thermoplastic and metal hybrid Custom or prefabricated

AFO, Ankle-foot orthosis; *CP*, cerebral palsy; *DAFO*, dynamic ankle-foot orthosis; *IC*, initial contact; *HKAFO*, hip-knee-ankle-foot orthosis; *KAFO*, knee-ankle-foot orthosis; *LMN*, lower motor neuron; *PTB*, patellar tendon bearing; *SAFO*, solid AFO; *UCBL*, University of California Biomechanics Laboratory orthosis.

Indications

The SAFO design is often selected for individuals with moderate-to-severe hypertonicity where equinovarus significantly impairs the ability to walk. The SAFO may additionally be indicated in individuals with significant weakness in ankle dorsiflexion, with ligamentous injury, or with mild knee instability. It may also be used for persons with high or unpredictable fluctuating muscle tone (athetosis) to aid in improving stability during ambulation.[7] It may be recommended for persons with significant generalized lower extremity weakness or significant hypotonicity, providing external support as a substitute for impaired muscle performance that would otherwise prevent ambulation.[23] In these circumstances the SAFO is a substitute for severely impaired muscle activity or is aimed at providing structural support by limiting ankle joint movement. A custom-molded SAFO has also been used to protect the foot and ankle in the management of orthopedic conditions.[24] LMN paralysis (flaccidity) or hypotonicity as the primary concern would be a contraindication for this device.

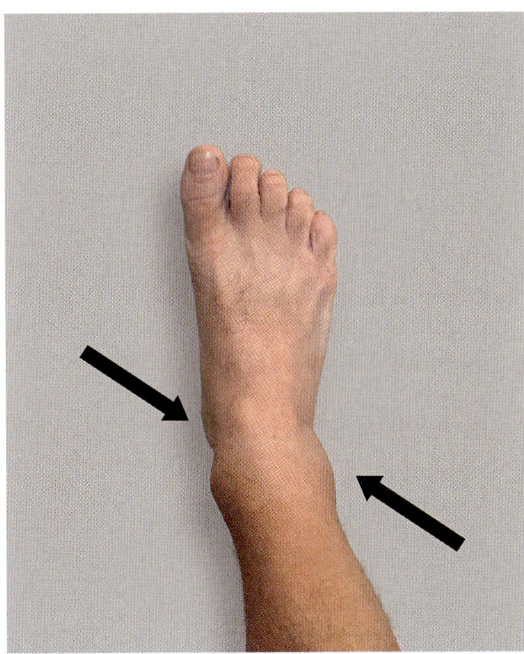

Fig. 9.3 Alignment of the mechanical ankle joint axes must reflect the degree of external rotation/tibial torsion that is present in the transverse plane.

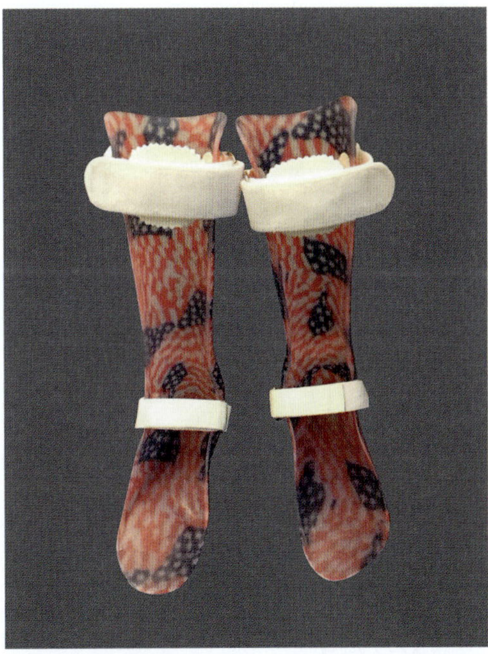

Fig. 9.4 Custom-molded, solid ankle-foot orthosis holds the ankle in as close to optimal static alignment as possible for a given patient. Mediolateral ankle stability is a result of trimlines at the midline of the malleoli. The crossed Velcro strap anterior to the ankle helps to position the rearfoot appropriately within the heel section of the orthosis.

Clinical Considerations

There are four distinct control systems incorporated into the SAFO design (Fig. 9.5). To resist plantarflexion during swing phase, there is a fulcrum force applied at the anterior ankle (by strapping or by the shoe's laces or Velcro closure) opposed by a distal counterforce upward under the metatarsal heads and a proximal counterforce at the posterior proximal surface of the AFO. To resist dorsiflexion during stance phase, there is an upward and inward compressive force at the posterior heel, opposed by a distal downward counterforce delivered by the shoe, and a proximal force applied by the anterior closure straps just below the knee. It is important to note that the locked ankle created by an AFO generates an extensor moment at the knee during stance. In this way, a SAFO can substitute for impaired motor control or muscle performance of knee extensors for persons with stroke, cerebral palsy, or other neuromotor dysfunction.

To resist varus and inversion of the foot, a medially directed force is applied just above and below the lateral malleolus, with laterally directed counterforces at the proximal medial tibia and the medial foot. To resist valgus and eversion of the foot, there is a laterally directed force applied above and below the medial malleolus, with medially directed counterforces just below the fibular head proximally and at the lateral foot distally.

The degree of control for the foot is also influenced by the position of the trim lines of the foot section. When there is midtarsal joint deformity with forefoot abduction or adduction to contend with, trim lines are adjusted to capture the shafts of the first and fifth metatarsals. If there is too much subtalar valgus, the height of the medial wall is increased, and a flange might be placed proximal to the medial malleolus. These strategies provide greater surface area for distribution of corrective forces applied by the orthosis so that the patient is more comfortable with the external stability it provides. If knee hyperextension at midstance is a problem for individuals with impaired motor control, the orthotist might fabricate the SAFO set in just a couple of degrees of ankle dorsiflexion, rather than neutral, to minimize excessive extension moment and preserve knee joint health over time. A Gillette modification can be added to the outer medial or lateral surface of the heel cup to influence excessive valgus or varus moment at the knee joint during stance. A medial or lateral post (similar to those used in a biomechanical foot orthosis) can be incorporated into the foot section to equalize forefoot to rearfoot relationships or to enhance biomechanical effects on the knee.

The SAFO biomechanically interferes with transitions through all three rockers of gait in stance phase because of the fixed ankle position inherent in the design and significantly reduces power generation in terminal stance.[7]

The orthosis prevents the controlled lowering of the foot that usually occurs in the ankle/first rocker during loading response. If the shoe does not have a compressive cushion heel to mimic controlled lowering, the orthosis propels the tibia rapidly to achieve foot-flat position. The individual wearing the orthosis needs some eccentric ability of the quadriceps to counteract the rapid knee flexion moment that accompanies the propulsive force of the SAFO acting on the tibia. This is especially true if the SAFO has been set in a few degrees of dorsiflexion to minimize risk of knee hyperextension in early stance.

The proximal anterior strapping used to hold the limb in the upper part of the SAFO acts with the fixed ankle position to prevent forward progression of the tibia over the weight-bearing foot during the second/ankle rocker that typically occurs during midstance. If the individual's shoe does not

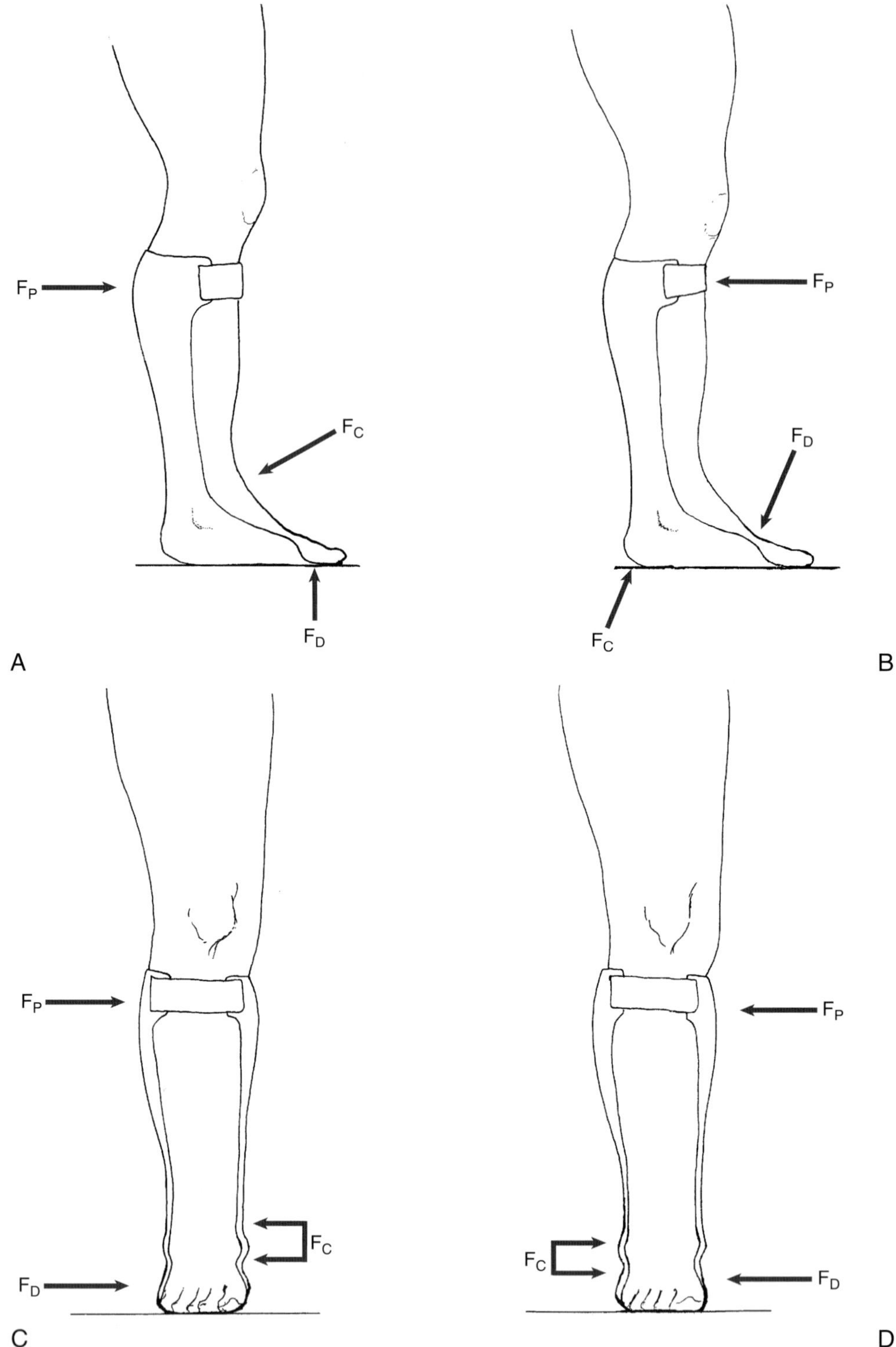

Fig. 9.5 The four force systems in a molded thermoplastic solid ankle-foot orthosis design. (A) Plantarflexion is controlled during swing phase by a proximal force *(F_P)* at the posterior calf band and a distal force at the metatarsal heads *(F_D)* that counter a centrally located stabilizing force *(F_C)* applied at the ankle by shoe closure. (B) For control of dorsiflexion during stance phase (i.e., forward progression of the tibia over the foot), F_P is applied at the proximal tibia by the anterior closure, F_D at the ventral metatarsal heads by the toe box of the shoe, and counterforce F_C at the heel, snugly fit in the orthosis. (C) The force system for eversion (valgus) locates F_D along the fifth metatarsal, F_P at the proximal lateral calf band, and F_C on either side of the malleolus. (D) To control inversion (varus) of the foot and ankle, F_D is applied by the distal medial wall of the orthosis against the first metatarsal, F_P at the proximal medial calf band, and F_0 at the distal lateral tibia and calcaneus/talus on either side of the lateral malleolus.

have rocker bottom characteristics, this check of forward momentum compromises effective preparation for push-off and transition from stance into swing phase and necessarily shortens stride length achieved by the swinging limb.

In nonpathologic gait, there are 60 degrees of extension at the hallux during the third, or toe, rocker of gait. For persons wearing a SAFO with a footplate that extends into a stiff toeplate, the third/toe rocker of the foot will certainly be limited. A shoe with rocker bottom characteristics can assist a smoother rollover when extension of the hallux is limited.

Advantages/Disadvantages

ANTERIOR FLOOR REACTION ANKLE-FOOT ORTHOSIS

Characteristics

An orthosis that has evolved from the basic SAFO design to better address impaired motor control of the knee and weakness of the quadriceps is the anterior floor reaction orthosis (FRO)[25] (Fig. 9.6A–D). In patients with cerebral palsy, the FRO have been shown to be effective in controlling advancement of the tibia over the foot during the second rocker phase of gait and improving knee extension during walking and standing. The FRO may also assist during swing phase of gait by providing a resistance to plantarflexion.[26] The FRO is fabricated to hold the ankle in a few degrees of plantarflexion. This restricts the ability of the tibia to roll forward over the foot in the second/ankle rocker of gait, creating an extensor moment that stabilizes the knee during stance (Fig. 9.7A–C). If stability is also needed in late stance phase, a stiff toeplate can be added to reinforce the extension moment at the knee. The FRO and SAFO use the same force systems to control foot and ankle position. Whether the FRO is fabricated in a single piece or as a SAFO with the addition of a thermoplastic anterior shell, padding is added where the FRO contacts the proximal surfaces of the tibia to make the extra extension force delivered by the orthosis more tolerable to the wearer.

Indications

The FRO is often used for children with neurologic conditions who demonstrate "crouch gait," who have paralysis, or who have weakness at the knee and ankle.[25] The FRO relies on a GRF vector that passes anterior to the anatomic knee joint. As knee and hip flexion contractures approach or exceed 10 degrees, the GRF vector nears or passes posterior to the anatomic knee joint and the FRO is less effective in stabilizing the knee during stance, though some studies have still shown a benefit despite hip, knee, and ankle contractures.[25,26] In patients prescribed FRO for crouch gait, the most improvements were noted in patients with lower functional status (slow walking speed, weak knee extensors, and weak ankle plantarflexors).[26] In children with a crouched gait pattern, FRO proved to be more effective in providing integrity of the ankle plantarflexion-knee extension couple compared to other orthotic devices.[27]

Clinical Considerations

Although the rigid control of ankle and knee enhances mechanical stability in stance, these external restrictions imposed by the FRO may compromise efficacy of postural responses. In those with balance impairment, an ambulatory assistive device (e.g., a cane, Lofstrand crutches, or rolling walker) may be needed for safety, especially if FROs are worn on both limbs. The FRO is contraindicated for persons with notable recurvatum during stance and those with cruciate ligament insufficiency; in these circumstances, the extra knee extension moment can further damage joint structure.

WEIGHT-RELIEVING ANKLE-FOOT ORTHOSES

Characteristics

The weight-relieving AFO, also known as PTB-AFO, incorporates the intimate fit and load-bearing characteristics of a PTB prosthetic socket into a SAFO or traditional metal double-upright AFO (discussed later) as a means of offloading or unloading weight-bearing forces during stance phase for individuals with a painful, unstable, or recently repaired ankle or foot.[28–30] The anterior shell of the AFO is modified to accept weight-bearing forces via the medial tibial flare and patellar tendon bar, along with total contact around the upper calf. As with a PTB prosthetic socket, the proximal portion of the PTB-AFO is set in approximately 10 degrees of knee flexion (with respect to vertical) to load some of the body weight onto the anterior shell at the medial tibial flare and patellar tendon bar during stance. This axial force is then transmitted to the ground through the medial and lateral walls of the thermoplastic orthosis, which may be reinforced with metal uprights or through the medial and lateral uprights of a traditional double-upright AFO.

Indications

This strategy of decreasing loading of the lower leg, ankle, and foot by shifting vertical ground reaction force to the anterior proximal tibia and calf effectively reduces axial loading of the ankle and foot during gait. This may be required in cases requiring decreased pressure to the foot and ankle, including ulcers, calcaneotomy, plantar skin graft or injury, severe foot or ankle trauma, and fractures.[28,31] Individuals wearing a weight-relieving AFO must have normal anatomic structure of the knee, adequate muscle performance and motor control of the quadriceps muscles for stability in early stance, and sufficient skin integrity to tolerate the loading forces applied by this orthotic design.

Clinical considerations

Individuals wearing a weight-relieving AFO must have normal anatomic structure of the knee, adequate muscle performance and motor control of the quadriceps muscles for stability in early stance, and sufficient skin integrity to tolerate the loading forces applied by this orthotic design.

Dynamic Orthoses

Dynamic orthoses allow some degree of sagittal plane motion at the ankle; many permit dorsiflexion during stance phase to facilitate the ankle rocker of gait but restrict plantarflexion during swing phase to facilitate swing limb clearance, incorporating some type of orthotic ankle joint. These dynamic orthoses are available in both thermoplastic and more traditional metal double-upright designs. These are reviewed in order from least restrictive to most supportive designs.

UNIVERSITY OF CALIFORNIA BIOMECHANICS LABORATORY ORTHOSIS

In the 1970s, researchers at the University of California Biomechanics Laboratory (UCBL) developed a custom-molded shoe insert, currently known as the *UCBL orthosis*,

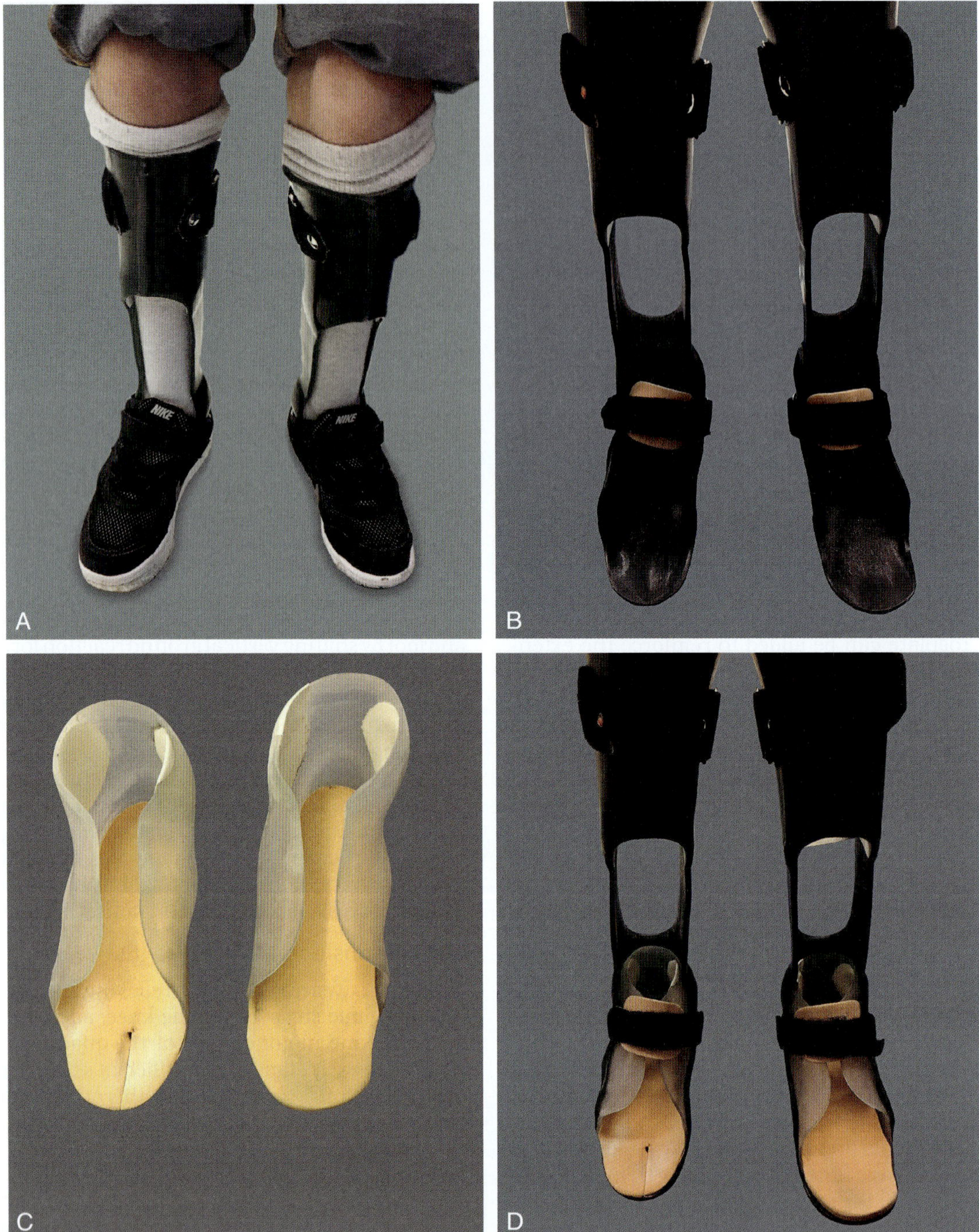

Fig. 9.6 (A and B) This floor reaction orthosis (FRO) was fabricated using carbon graphite and fiberglass in a thermosetting process because of the desire to provide maximum stiffness. The combination of a solid-ankle design and an anterior wall produces a knee extension moment at midstance and enhances stance phase stability. (C and D) This FRO has a solid supramalleolar orthosis that provides medial lateral joint stability to the ankle through the rigid design and custom fit.

as an orthotic intervention for subtalar joint instability. The UCBL controls flexible calcaneal deformities (rearfoot valgus or varus) and transverse plane deformities of the midtarsal joints (forefoot abduction or adduction) encapsulating the calcaneus and supporting the midfoot with high medial and lateral trim lines; it realigns the calcaneus, providing a more stable foundation for the articular surfaces of the talus, navicular, and cuboid bones in cases of instability.[32] The *Gillette modification*, an external post positioned either on the medial or lateral border of the heel cup, can be used to apply additional rotatory moments to the calcaneus during weight bearing. It is important to recognize that the UCBL orthosis acts primarily at subtalar and midfoot tarsal joints during weight bearing; it would not be appropriate for persons with swing-phase clearance issues, which require the trim line of the orthosis be placed above the ankle joint.

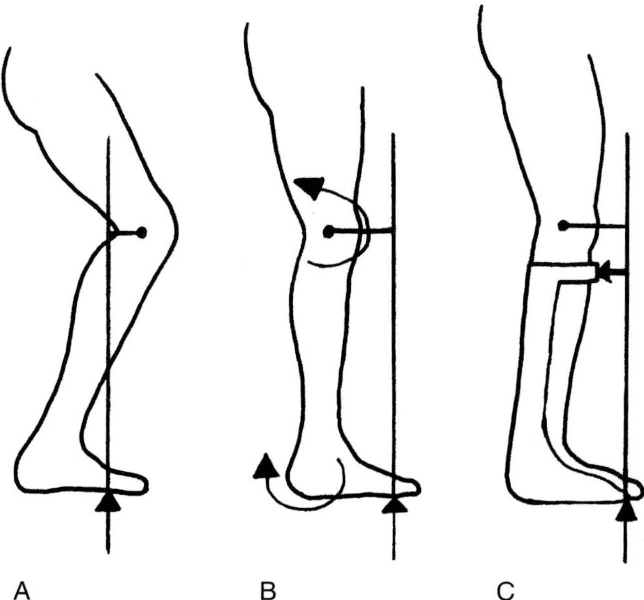

Fig. 9.7 (A) When a patient walks in a "crouch gait" pattern, the ground reaction force (GRF) vector passes behind the knee at midstance, creating a flexion moment at the knee, which must be counteracted to maintain upright position. (B) In normal gait, knee stability at midstance is assisted by a ground reaction moment as the body moves over the foot, and the GRF vector passes anterior to the knee. (C) The solid ankle-foot orthosis and the floor reaction orthotic designs use a fixed ankle position to harness the GRF, creating a large extension moment at the knee.

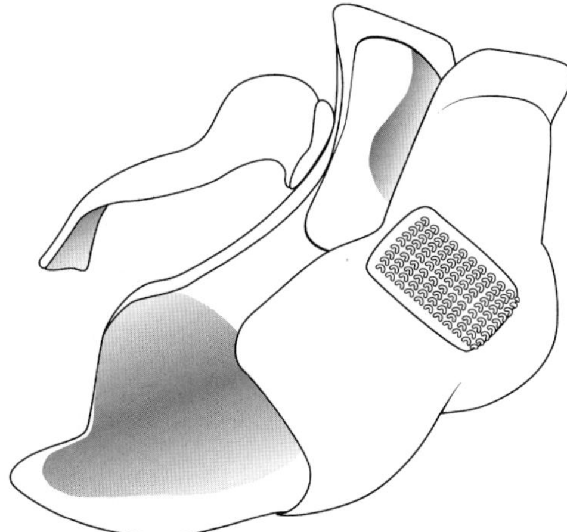

Fig. 9.8 The dynamic ankle-foot orthosis is a flexible polypropylene brace designed to optimize subtalar joint alignment through its supramalleolar design. (Reprinted with permission from Zablotny CM. Use of orthoses for the adult with neurological involvement. In: Nawoczenski DA, Epler ME, eds. *Orthotics in Functional Rehabilitation of the Lower Limb*. WB Saunders; 1997:229.)

SUPRAMALLEOLAR ORTHOSIS/DYNAMIC ANKLE-FOOT ORTHOSIS

Characteristics

The dynamic ankle-foot orthosis (DAFO), also described as a flexible supramalleolar orthosis (SMO), is a custom-molded orthosis that has evolved from the UCBL shoe insert to better address sagittal plane control of the ankle and foot during stance and to facilitate foot clearance in swing.[33]

Indications

Improved stability allows for a more stable base allowing for effective motor performance and postural control during standing and ambulation.

Clinical Considerations

Custom-molded from relatively thin thermoplastic, its proximal trim lines are just superior to the ankle joint, and its distal trim lines encase more of the forefoot than the UCBL (Fig. 9.8). This allows for improved control of the midfoot and forefoot, holding the foot in a more functional position. As compared to a solid AFO, the DAFO allows for graded amounts ankle motion in all planes, as well as graded foot motion and arch support to allow for improved balance reactions and weight distribution.[34]

HINGED THERMOPLASTIC ANKLE-FOOT ORTHOSIS

Characteristics

The thermoplastic hinged (articulating) ankle-foot orthosis (HAFO) allows sagittal plane motion at the ankle by incorporating a mechanical ankle joint between the foot and calf sections of the orthosis. This variation of the SAFO was designed primarily to allow the tibia to roll over the weight-bearing foot during stance, for a smooth ankle rocker, at the same time holding the foot in optimal alignment to control the impact of tone-related equinovarus forces throughout the gait cycle (Fig. 9.9). The shape, dimensions, and force control systems of the HAFO are almost exactly the same as those of a SAFO, except it has two separate pieces linked by an orthotic ankle joint rather than being a single, solid piece. The HAFO has a larger width at the ankle than the SAFO to accommodate the mechanical ankle joint.

Indications

Hinged AFOs can be fabricated to allow free motion at the ankle, to allow limited range of motion (i.e., allow dorsiflexion and stop plantarflexion, or the inverse), or to provide some assistance to dorsiflexion, depending on what orthotic ankle joint option motion best meets the individual's needs and maximizes the resources they bring to the task of walking.

Clinical Considerations

As compared with the SAFO, the HAFO also improves mobility in many functional activities, such as rising from the floor, ascending and descending stairs, and walking up or down inclines.[35,36] In children with cerebral palsy and in adults after stroke, these orthoses reduce energy cost of walking (compared with barefoot), as well as improve stride length, cadence, and walking speed.[37] There is some indication that HAFOs lessen the magnitude of abnormal muscle activation associated with spasticity in children with cerebral palsy.[38] HAFOs appear to reduce risk of falls in adults with long-standing hemiplegia after stroke, improve static postural control, and have less negative impact on dynamic postural control in standing than SAFOs.[39,40] However, for some children with moderate-to-severe spastic diplegic cerebral palsy, the mobility provided by a HAFO compromises stability in early stance, reinforcing crouch gait

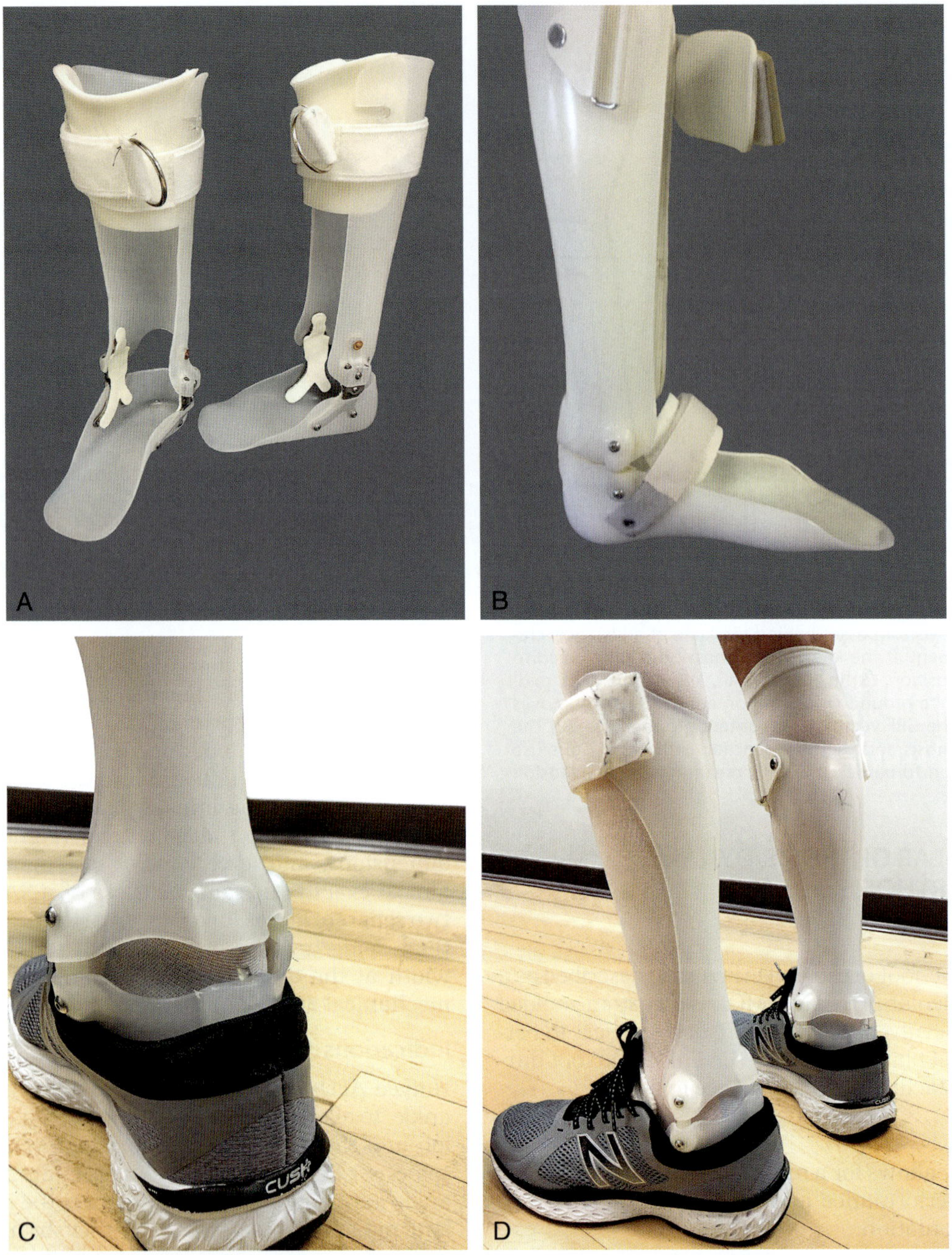

Fig. 9.9 (A) This hinged ankle-foot orthosis (HAFO), with compact double action ankle joint, allows forward motion of the tibia through the ankle rocker of stance phase and can be adjusted via springs or pins to allow more support or restriction. (B–D) This HAFO, with flexure ankle joints, has a built-in plantarflexion stop (when the posterior edges of the foot and calf section come into contact) and posterior strapping that can be adjusted to limit the amount of dorsiflexion available, based on the wearer's motor control and need for stability in stance.

pattern, reducing walking speed, and increasing energy cost as compared with a SAFO.[41]

A variety of mechanical thermoplastic joints are commercially available (Fig. 9.10A–C). Those with true articulations (e.g., the Oklahoma joint) have a single axis of motion that should be aligned as closely as possible to the anatomic ankle joint; other orthotic joints (e.g., the Gillette joint) are flexible and nonarticulating.

Traditional metal orthotic ankle joints have been incorporated into thermoplastic HAFOs as well; these designs are referred to as *hybrid orthoses*. Simple single-axis joints provide mediolateral stability without restriction of available dorsiflexion or plantarflexion; a motion stop can be

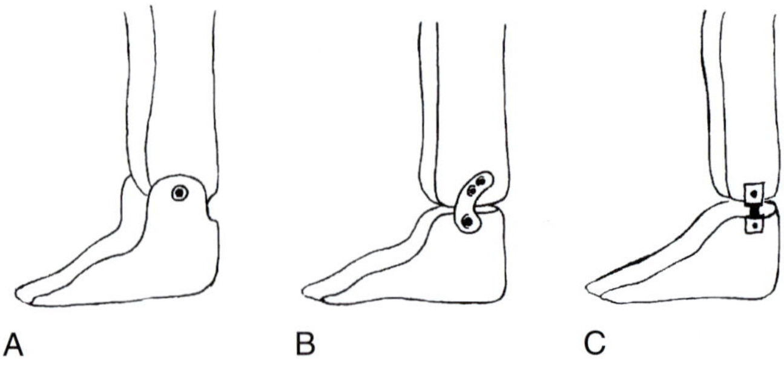

Fig. 9.10 Examples of thermoplastic ankle joints used in hinged ankle-foot orthosis. The overlap joint (A) and Oklahoma joint (B) are single-axis joints, whereas the flexible Gillette mechanism (C) allows movement into dorsiflexion and plantarflexion without an actual articulation.

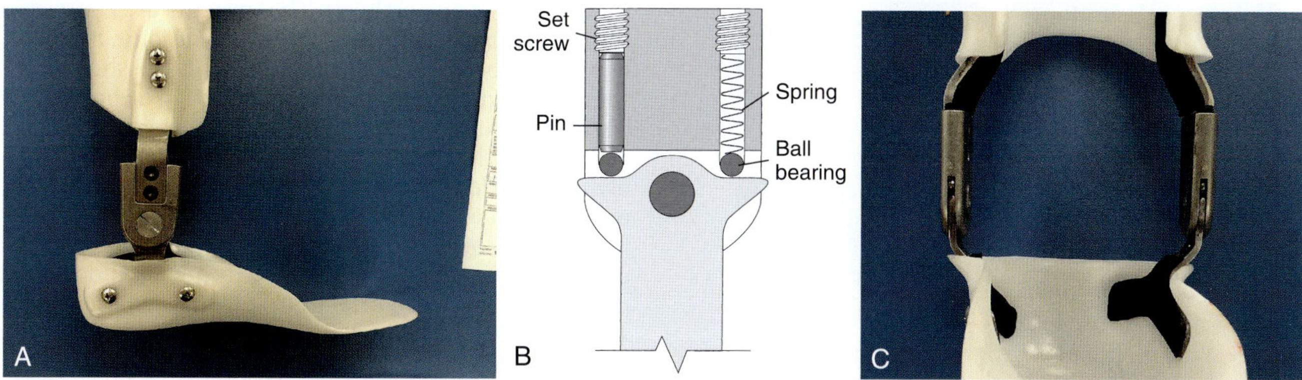

Fig. 9.11 (A) The double-action joint can be used in a conventional double-upright, metal ankle-foot orthosis and a thermoplastic-metal hybrid ankle-foot orthosis. Motion is assisted if a spring is compressed within the channel or can be blocked by placement of a steel pin within the channel. (B) The internal anatomy of the double adjustable ankle joint. Ankle joint mobility restrictions (e.g., plantarflexion stop) result from the locations of the pins in the anterior and posterior channels of the orthotic joint. A spring may occupy one of the channels, as depicted here, to assist motion (e.g., dorsiflexion assistance). The ball bearings allow the brace uprights to pivot with ease over the brace stirrup. The set screw can be adjusted to change the relative positions of the rods in each of the channels. (C) The hinged ankle joint can also exist with a duel-pin system to allow adjustment of the fixed angle and ankle range as the patient's functional status changes. The degree of limitation from the pins can be viewed anteriorly/posteriorly. (B, From Zablotny CM: Use of orthoses for the adult with neurological involvement. In: Nawoczenski DA, Epler ME, eds. *Orthotics in Functional Rehabilitation of the Lower Limb*. WB Saunders; 1997:227.)

incorporated if there is need to limit plantarflexion beyond neutral (for stability in early stance) or dorsiflexion (to limit weight bearing on the forefoot in later stance) as the individual's needs dictate. A bichannel adjustable ankle joint (also referred to as a *double-action ankle joint* or a *double Klenzak joint*) (Fig. 9.11) can be used to provide assistance and/or limit motion based on an individual's capabilities and needs for support. If motion assistance is desired, a coil spring is placed in the channel and a screw is used to adjust compression until the desired level of assistance is achieved. If motion is to be blocked, a solid steel pin is inserted instead of the spring to stop motion beyond a particular point in the range of motion. Because of its versatility and adjustability, the double-action ankle joint is often chosen when change in a patient's functional status (improvement or deterioration) is anticipated. Orthotic ankle joints allow the orthotist to adjust the available range of motion from none (as in a SAFO) through an array of limited anteroposterior stop settings. This would be an advantage when motor control around the ankle and knee is expected to improve over time, such as in individuals who are recovering from an acute stroke.

The HAFO allows free dorsiflexion; however, when motor control is compromised, such that additional support is needed during stance, the orthotist may choose to incorporate a mechanism, such as a check strap, to adjust the amount of dorsiflexion allowed (Fig. 9.9B–D). If the check strap is maximally tightened, the orthosis functions like a SAFO. The check strap can be loosened, lengthened, or elasticized as neuromotor control improves, allowing only as much forward progression of the tibia in the heel rocker as is safe and functional for the individual. This adaptation makes the HAFO versatile and useful when return of neuromotor control or function is anticipated.

It is important to note that a prerequisite for using this orthosis is at least 5 degrees of true ankle dorsiflexion, accomplished without compromise of subtalar or midtarsal joint position; for this reason, a HAFO may not be an appropriate choice for persons with severe spasticity that limits ankle motion or those with significant instability or malalignment of the midfoot.

POSTERIOR LEAF SPRING ANKLE-FOOT ORTHOSIS

Characteristics

The PLS is one of the groups of AFOs that provide dorsiflexion assistance. In contrast to the SAFO, medial and lateral trim lines are located well posterior to the midline of both malleoli so that the orthosis is flexible at the anatomic ankle joint (Fig. 9.12).[42] The degree of flexibility is determined by the thickness of the thermoplastic material used to construct the orthosis and width of the posterior upright in the distal third of the orthosis.[42] In custom-molded PLS orthoses, the orthotist tailors the stiffness of the orthosis using the trimline pattern that will best support the weight of the foot during swing, as well as the individual's needs for stability in stance.[42]

Indications

The PLS AFO is a dynamic thermoplastic AFO designed to accomplish two things:[43]

- Support the weight of the foot during swing phase as a means of enhancing swing limb clearance
- Assist with controlled lowering of the foot during loading response in stance as part of the first/heel rocker

Clinical Considerations

As initial contact occurs and loading response begins in the gait cycle, the flexible plastic of the PLS serves as a proxy for impaired or absent eccentric activity of the tibialis anterior muscle, slowing but not stopping the foot's descent toward the ground.[43] As stance phase continues, the flexible PSL allows the tibia to roll forward over the weight-bearing foot to accomplish a smooth ankle rocker of midstance to

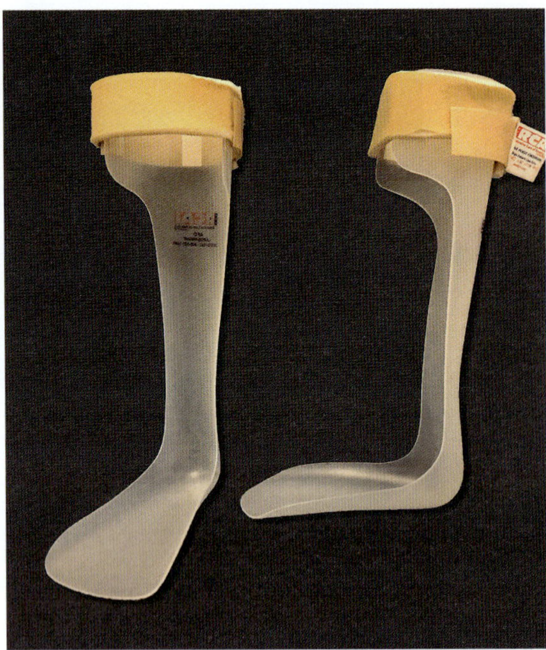

Fig. 9.12 The posterior position and arc of the trim lines at the ankle and the thickness of thermoplastic material used determine the degree of flexibility of the posterior leaf spring ankle-foot orthosis. This design assists with foot clearance by limiting plantarflexion during swing phase.

terminal stance. [43] As stance phase continues, the flexible PSL allows the tibia to roll forward over the weight-bearing foot to accomplish a smooth ankle rocker of midstance to terminal stance. As the foot leaves the ground in initial swing, the PLS is able to hold the ankle at the desired neutral 90-degree position, which assists swing clearance and keeps the toes elevated so that next initial contact will be made at the heel. PLS have demonstrated effectiveness in improving gait parameters and may help to improve push-off and reduce energy costs.[27]

Owing to its narrow posterior upright and relatively shallow heel cup, a PLS is not as effective in stabilizing the calcaneus and talus during stance as are the SAFO, DAFO, or UCBL designs. This makes it less effective in controlling mediolateral foot position, especially for persons with flexible deformities of the forefoot, midfoot, or rearfoot. In these circumstances the orthotist may opt to place medial and lateral trim lines somewhere between the midmalleolar position of a SAFO and the narrower PLS to provide additional stability. This modification is sometimes referred to as a *semisolid AFO*. The modification provides better control of ankle motion but at the cost of limiting mobility during the ankle rocker of gait.[44] Note that the flexibility of a PLS and a semisolid AFO makes them inappropriate for individuals with significant equinovarus or spasticity of the lower extremity: A high level of abnormal tone will overpower the control systems in these designs.

DOUBLE-UPRIGHT DORSIFLEXION-ASSIST ANKLE-FOOT ORTHOSIS

Characteristics

The conventional double-upright counterpart to the PLS uses a spring mechanism incorporated into the mechanical ankle joints of the orthosis. The uprights are connected to the distal stirrup at the mechanical ankle joint, and the stirrup is fixed between the heel and sole of the shoe. A coiled spring and small ball bearing are placed in a channel in the distal uprights that runs toward the posterior edge of the stirrup. Another option is the dual-channel *(double Klenzak)* orthotic ankle joint (see Fig. 9.11); by placing a spring in one channel and a rod in the other, this mechanical ankle joint can provide adjustable dorsiflexion assistance and plantarflexion stop (in persons with impaired dorsiflexion muscle performance) or plantarflexion assistance and dorsiflexion stop (for those with motor control or muscle performance impairment of the gastroc-soleus complex).[45]

Indications

Traditional or conventional double-upright orthoses are typically used when the individual who needs dorsiflexion assistance and plantarflexion control has a comorbid condition that causes fluctuation in limb size (edema), such as congestive heart failure or the need for kidney dialysis, which would compromise the intimate fit of a thermoplastic orthosis.[45]

Clinical Considerations

When the spring is compressed at initial contact and early loading response, it resists plantarflexion, allowing a controlled lowering of the foot to the floor, substituting for the heel rocker of early stance. Recoil of the spring when the foot is unloaded in preswing and initial swing assists dorsiflexion for swing-phase toe clearance.[41] The amount of dorsiflexion assist provided is determined by adjustment of a screw placed in the top of the channel to compress or decompress the spring further. The downside of the double-upright AFO is its less effective control of abnormal foot position and risk of skin irritation as the foot moves within the shoe. For persons with neuropathic foot conditions who are unable to directly perceive abnormal pressures and the discomfort of tissue stress, a custom-molded AFO that is intimately fit for the individual's foot would be the orthosis of choice unless significant fluctuating edema precludes this choice. To decrease the risk of skin irritation and maximize the coronal plane control of the double-upright AFO, a clinician may also consider use of a floating T-strap.[46] To decrease the risk of skin irritation and maximize the coronal plane control of the double-upright AFO, a clinician may also consider use of a floating T-strap.[46]

Carbon Fiber Spring Orthoses

Characteristics

Carbon fiber has been integrated into various AFO designs due to its lightweight and stiffness properties.[28] Typically, the carbon fiber material is integrated into the AFO design as either the primary structural material for the device, including the cuff and footplate, and/or as the posterior strut with other materials for cuff and footplate. Integration into the posterior strut is beneficial to the wearer as it allows for energy storage, typically during midstance as the tibia moves forward over the foot, and energy return, assisting with plantarflexion during transition from terminal stance to pre-swing.[47] Recent devices that integrate carbon fiber materials into their design include the Intrepid Dynamic Exoskeleton Orthosis (IDEO), ToeOff, WalkOn, Neuro Swing, and Chignon. The IDEO includes a carbon fiber footplate, cuff, and strut-like posterior spring. The ToeOff and WalkOn are both dorsiflexion-assist devices. The ToeOff consists of a carbon fiber footplate and anterior shin plate connected with a lateral carbon fiber strut. The WalkOn has a carbon fiber footplate and "medial to posterior" strut that connects to a posterior cuff just below the knee. The Neuro Swing has a carbon fiber footplate and anterior shin plate connected by lateral spring-hinged ankle joints. The Chigon has a carbon fiber cuff above the ankle and below the knee, joined together by steel articulations. The cuff above the ankle is connected to the footplate with elastic components that assist dorsiflexion and limit plantarflexion.[47]

The dual CFO, developed and tested primarily in Germany, is a modification of the traditional PLS design that cuts the PLS into a foot and calf section, then attaches overlapping carbon fiber springs (carbon fiber and Kevlar fibers impregnated with epoxy resin) between the sections (Fig. 9.13A and B).[48] Spring resistance is selected based on the individual's weight. This design aims not only to substitute for impaired or absent anterior compartment muscle activity but also to enhance the toe rocker of stance phase that is typically compromised by thermoplastic AFOs, and increasing the energy return for a more significant assist with push-off.[49]

There is a version of the CFO in which the carbon fiber spring is L shaped (see Fig. 9.13A and B) with its attachment to the foot component (a stiffer version of a supramalleolar DAFO) on the plantar surface rather than on the posterior heel.[50] The slight distance between the spring and posterior foot section acts as a dorsiflexion stop during stance, allowing some dorsiflexion for ankle rocker until the two surfaces come into contact. The proximal carbon fiber spring is fit into a slot in the posterior of a custom-molded section that resembles the upper half of a total contact prosthetic socket. A vertical slot drilled into the proximal spring allows it to slide up and down for several centimeters during stance phase to minimize potential skin friction. This CFO appears to enhance transition through both ankle and toe rockers of gait and to provide assistance for push-off.[28,50]

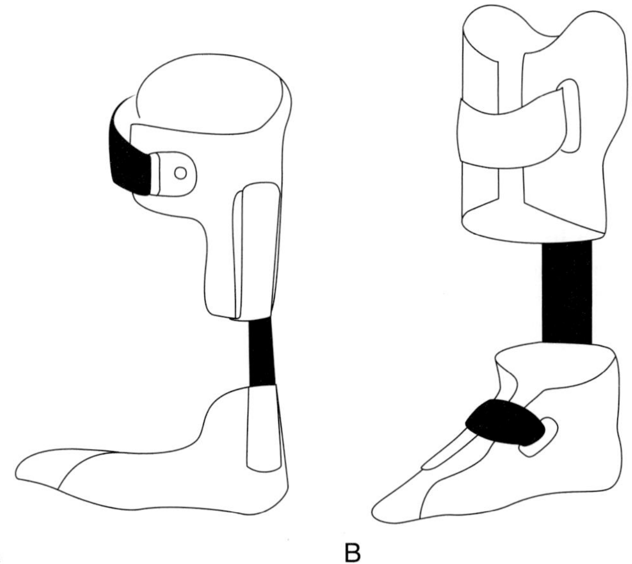

Fig. 9.13 (A) Note the carbon fiber springs inserted posteriorly between the foot and calf component of this carbon fiber orthosis. The springs provide dorsiflexion assistance for clearance in swing and prepositioning of the foot for initial contract, as well as preservation of the second and third rockers of stance phase. (B) The dual carbon fiber spring orthosis designed to provide assistance with plantarflexion/push-off for the transition from stance to swing for persons with weakness or paralysis of calf muscles/plantarflexors.

Indications

The CFO is primarily indicated for patients with impaired muscle function of dorsiflexor muscles limiting foot clearance during swing phase of gait and can contribute plantarflexion assist by releasing stored energy during toe-off phase of gait. Specific designs of CFOs have been shown to be most beneficial for certain patient populations. The IDEO was shown to be most beneficial for patients with lower extremity trauma to decrease pain and improve mobility.[47] The ToeOff improved gait parameters in patient's with cerebral palsy and hemophilia, and had high patient satisfaction in patients with peripheral neuropathy. The WalkOn improved kinematic patterns in patients with hemiplegia (best results when combined with botox injection) and cerebral palsy. The Neuro Swing resulted in improved energy cost in patients with cerebral palsy and improved ankle and knee kinematics in patients with various neurological disorders. The Chigon increased gait speed and gait kinematics in patients with hemiplegia.[47] As stated above, the CFO can also be structured to assist with increasing plantar flexion during toe-off. The CFO design has also been adapted to enhance walking ability of children with neuromuscular conditions that contribute to impaired or absent plantarflexor muscle performance.[50] Furthermore, in adults with various neurologic gait dysfunctions, switching from a noncarbon fiber AFO to a carbon fiber AFO promoted in increase in step length, decrease in tep-length differential, and improved gait velocity.[51]

Clinical Considerations

The carbon fiber spring AFO may be less commonly used due to higher costs and difficulty of construction. Maximizing an individual's energy return may require multiple fittings and remolding is not possible with carbon fiber materials. Computational analysis models have been created to assist in this process.[28,49] Carbon fiber designs have also been incorporated into a KAFO for children who require additional support or control at the knee and hip; more will be discussed in the "Knee-Ankle-Foot Orthosis Design Options" section.

Functional Neuromuscular Electrical Stimulation

Characteristics

Functional Neuromuscular Electrical Stimulation (FES) units (Table 9.3), also referred to as neuroprostheses, deliver electrical stimulation through surface electrodes to activate motor contractions to compensate for gait abnormalities, specifically the common peroneal nerve for ankle dorsiflexion.

FES units stimulate the peroneal nerve to assist with concentric dorsiflexion during swing limb advancement and may also be set to assist with eccentric lowering into plantar flexion during initial contact to weight acceptance phases of gait. The individual wears a cuff that is positioned snugly just below the knee, rather than an orthosis that must fit into the shoe (Fig. 9.14). The cuff holds a small stimulator

Table 9.3 Indications and Contraindications for Orthotic Knee Joint Designs

Desired Knee Control	Single-Axis Unlocked	Single-Axis Locked	Offset Unlocked	Offset Locked	Variable Position Locked
Stabilization of flail knee with use of knee extension moment and free knee joint motion	Contraindicated	Contraindicated	Indicated	Contraindicated	Contraindicated
Stabilization of flail knee without use of knee extension moment and free knee joint motion	Contraindicated	Indicated	Contraindicated	Indicated	Unnecessary
Control of genu recurvatum	Contraindicated	Indicated if orthosis will only be locked when ambulating	Indicated	Indicated when individual will lock knee intermittently	Contraindicated
Reduction of knee flexion contracture	Contraindicated	Lacks adjustability	Contraindicated	Lacks adjustability	Indicated
Control of genu valgum	Indicated	Indicated use of lock optional	Indicated	Indicated use of lock optional, unnecessary	
Control of genu varum	Indicated	Indicated use of lock optional	Indicated	Indicated use of lock optional, unnecessary	

Orthotic Knee Design columns: Single-Axis Unlocked, Single-Axis Locked, Offset Unlocked, Offset Locked, Variable Position Locked.

Modified from *Short Course in Orthotics and Prosthetics—Course Manual*. University of Texas, Southwestern Medical Center; 1993:8–22.

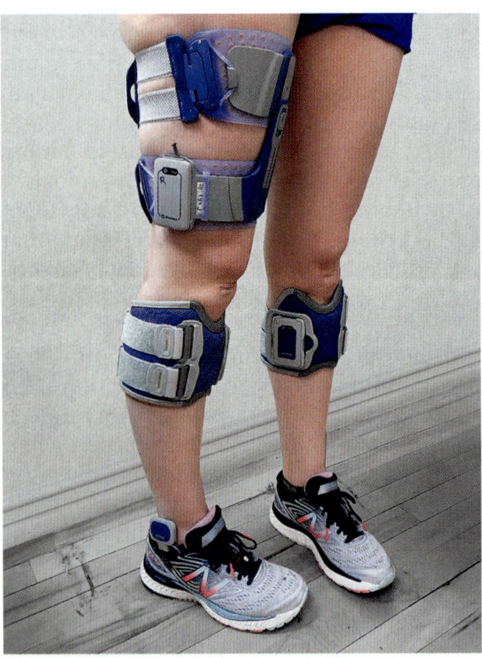

Fig. 9.14 The Bioness L300 System, as an example of a wearable functional electrical stimulation unit, is used to trigger muscle contraction during appropriate points in the gait cycle. The L300 system (photo R) triggers dorsiflexion during swing phase. The L300 + system (photo L) incorporates a thigh component that can stimulate the knee flexors or extensors during swing and/or stance phase to assist with stance stability or swing limb advancement.

medially with electrodes positioned laterally over motor end points of the peroneal nerve.[52] Depending on the model, appropriate timing of the FES for dorsiflexion activity is determined by a switch worn in the shoe, an inclinometer, or an accelerometer. Most use surface electrodes to deliver the stimulus for muscle contraction, although cuffless versions with surgically implantable electrodes are available.

Indications

Each of these devices must be adjusted to the individual's typical gait pattern. To be effective, all these devices require an intact and healthy peroneal nerve. They are not appropriate for people with peripheral nerve injury or neuropathy. Candidates who require range of motion restrictions that are associated with a contact support-based design should be excluded from consideration. FES systems are indicated when the clinician is seeking to increase swing limb clearance, reduce fall risk, improve balance, and increase gait symmetry.

Limitations that may lead to not selecting an FES system include peripheral neuropathy, sensory intolerance of the stimulation, knee buckling, plantar flexor spasticity ≥3 on the Modified Ashworth Scale, equinovarus, or genu recurvatum. Other considerations with these devices include cost of the device and electrode replacements, variable insurance coverage, and battery life.[53]

Manufacturers note that such devices are contraindicated in individuals with demand pacemakers or defibrillators, healing fractures, metal implants in the limb, or history of phlebitis; the unit should be used with caution in persons with varicose veins, inflammation in or around the knee, or sensory impairment. Although most devices are resistant to splashes, immersion in water during bathing or swimming or saturation while shoveling snow, for example, will damage the unit, rendering it nonfunctional.[53]

Three-Dimensional-Printed AFO

Technology has advanced over the last decade to introduce three-dimensional (3D)-printed AFOs. These devices required less skill and effort to manufacture and are more easily reproduced. This is because the modeling file can be easily stored and the automated software can apply preprogrammed template designs. Gait speed and stride length were comparable between conventional AFO and 3D-printed AFO when compared to no AFO. It should be noted that conventional AFOs were overall more effective than 3D-printed AFOs because the 3D material is more flexible, which may be a contributing factor to patients feeling more satisfied with the weight and ease of use.[54]

Commonly used materials for 3D printing include plastics, metals, resins, nylon, hydrogels, ceramics, and composite.[55] The variety of materials offer different advantages and disadvantages with regards to strength, eight, precision, and appearance.[55]

Commercially Available Dorsiflexion-Assisted Designs

Several manufacturers have developed carbon fiber orthoses to provide dorsiflexion assistance at the appropriate times in the gait cycle (e.g., Camp ToeOFF series, Allard USA, Rockaway, New Jersey; AFO Dynamic, Ossur Americas, Foothill Ranch, California; Matrix and Matrix Max, Prolaborthotics USA, Napa, California; WalkOn, Ottobock, Berlin, Germany; SpryStep, Townsend Thuasne USA, Bakersfield, California). In contrast to thermoplastic designs, many of these orthoses use a cushioned anterior shin or medial shank piece, held in place by strapping, that transitions into a medial upright and continues into a full footplate (Fig. 9.15A–C). These orthoses are designed to preposition the foot for heel strike at initial contact, substitute for impaired anterior compartment to allow controlled lowering of the foot into foot-flat position during the heel rocker of loading response, provide some medial lateral stability during stance while allowing forward progression of the tibia during the ankle rocker of stance phase, contribute to push-off in the transition from stance to swing, and support the weight of the foot for effective swing limb clearance.[56] Although there is some evidence that these dorsiflexion-assist designs have a positive impact on both the kinematics and energy cost of walking, there have been few published studies that directly compare them with traditional PLS orthoses or with articulating (hinged) thermoplastic AFOs or traditional metal double-upright AFOs with dorsiflexion-assist orthotic ankle joints.[56]

KNEE-ANKLE-FOOT ORTHOSIS

Characteristics

The KAFO metal and leather design was used during the 1950s to make ambulation possible for those recovering from polio.[57] However, the weight of the orthosis increased energy cost of ambulation significantly and ultimately made use of a wheelchair the preferred method of mobility for those requiring bilateral KAFOs to walk.[58] The development of the lighter-weight Craig-Scott orthosis in the 1970s, the advent of thermoplastic custom-fit or custom-molded components in the 1980s, and emergence of stance-control (SC) orthotic knee joints since 2000 have contributed to reduction in energy cost of ambulation with KAFOs; walking while wearing these orthoses has become more reasonable.[57] However, currently, many individuals decide that walking with bilateral KAFOs is too slow and requires too much effort to be truly functional for daily use.

Many KAFO designs use a SAFO or an HAFO as the distal component and one or more thermoplastic thigh bars or cuffs as proximal components, with metal uprights with a variety of orthotic knee joints to interconnect them.[58]

Indications

The rehabilitation team considers KAFOs only when stability during stance cannot be effectively provided by one of the AFO options.[59] KAFOs are often prescribed when, in addition to impairment of ankle control, there is the presence of (1) hyperextension or recurvatum that jeopardizes structural integrity of the knee joint[60] and/or (2) abnormal

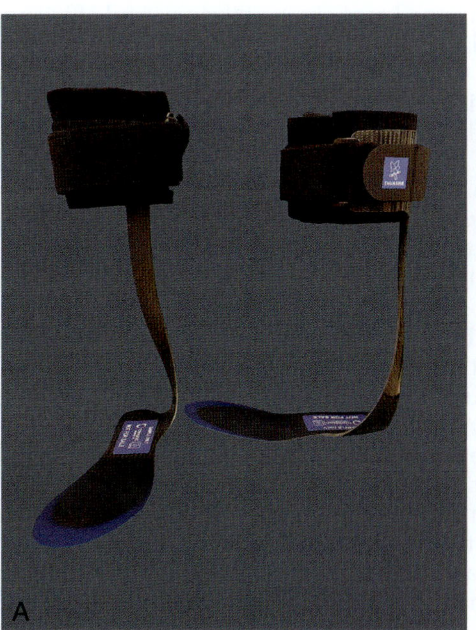

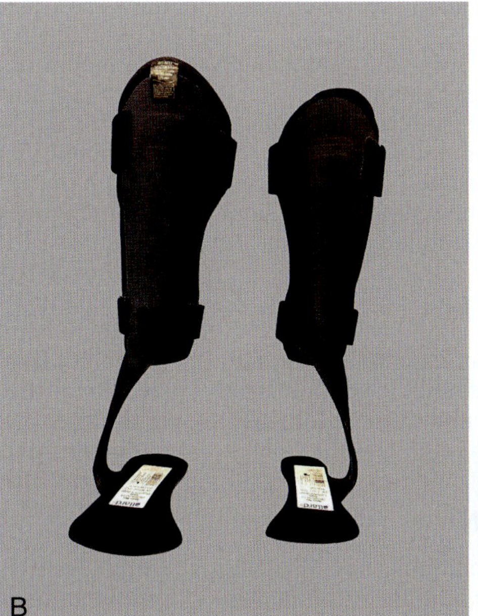

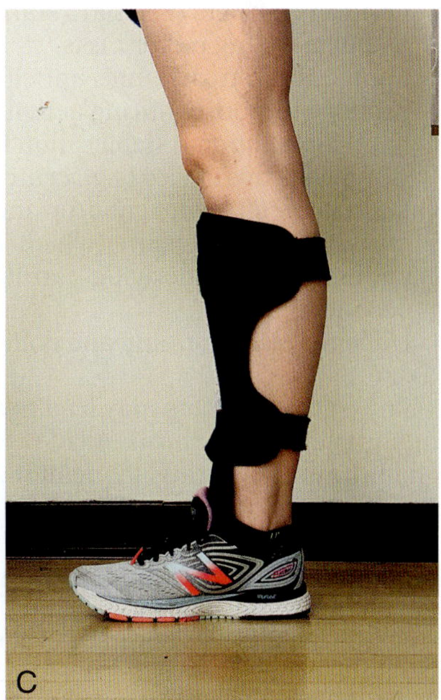

Fig. 9.15 Examples of a carbon fiber composite dorsiflexion assist ankle-foot orthosis used to substitute for activity of the anterior compartment of muscles of the lower leg. (A) Townsend SpryStep and (B *right* and C) Allard ToeOFF offer support primarily for ankle dorsiflexion. They may offer some mild knee support during stance. There are some carbon fiber ankle-foot orthoses designed with increased strength that may assist more with knee instability, such as Allard BlueRocker (B *left*), although not supportive enough to stabilize the moderately unstable stance knee.

or excessive varus or valgus angulation that occurs during weight bearing in stance phase.[58] If not recognized and addressed appropriately, both threaten joint function and structure during walking and, with repeated abnormal loading, increase risk of permanent damage to supporting structures within the knee and development of degenerative joint disease.[58] If not recognized and addressed appropriately, both threaten joint function and structure during walking and, with repeated abnormal loading, increase risk of permanent damage to supporting structures within the knee and development of degenerative joint disease.

Clinical Considerations

Challenges to knee-ankle-foot orthosis use

The key issues that must be addressed for safe ambulation with KAFOs are the same as those discussed earlier in the chapter for AFOs:[59]

- To provide stance-phase stability with minimal disruption of forward progression (especially through the ankle rocker of stance)
- To minimize disruption of swing limb clearance
- To prepare for an effective initial contact by holding the ankle in a neutral position

However, once the knee joint is encased in an orthosis, meeting these goals can be challenging, especially for persons who require bilateral KAFOs. These individuals typically have more proximal deficits in muscle performance, motor control, and postural control than those whose need for stability in stance and mobility in swing are addressed by any of the AFO designs.[61] These individuals typically have more proximal deficits in muscle performance, motor control, and postural control than those whose need for stability in stance and mobility in swing are addressed by any of the AFO designs.[61] Additional challenges that must be considered during the clinical decision-making process include:[61,62]

- Position transfers (i.e., sit to stand) can become complex and demanding motor tasks.
- Constraints on dynamic anticipatory and reactionary postural responses during activities in standing.
- Need for additional stabilization in the form of an ambulatory assistive device (e.g., crutches, walkers).
- Decreased efficiency and/or increased energy expenditure with movement (which may significantly limit patients with underlying cardiovascular conditions or deconditioning).
- Difficulty with donning and doffing.

Any of these factors may lead to an individual abandoning the use of the orthosis. All of these should be considered when the cost of fitting, fabrication, and training for KAFO use is factored in.[56,63]

KNEE FUNCTION AND ALIGNMENT

In early stance, under normal gait conditions, the GRF passes through the ankle, behind the knee, and through the hip, creating an external flexion moment at the knee (Fig. 9.16). To counteract this GRF-related flexion moment, the quadriceps muscles contract to prevent the knee from collapsing into further flexion, the hamstrings and hip abductors contract to stabilize hip position and maintain a level pelvis, and the gastrocnemius prepares to eccentrically control forward progression of the tibia.[57] This combination of muscle activity provides an internally generated knee extension moment that balances the external flexion moment at the knee generated by the GRF.[57] When musculoskeletal or neuromuscular impairment alters limb position or muscle activity at any lower extremity joint, the internal/external force system is no longer in equilibrium, and efficiency of walking and stability in stance will be compromised. The magnitude of disruption of the equilibrium between externally and internally generated moments determines whether the individual will be able to use his or her own resources (often in compensatory patterns or deviations) to address the imbalance or if an AFO or KAFO is necessary for functional walking. Consideration of the magnitude of disruption of this equilibrium helps the team to determine whether an AFO can effectively influence the position of the GRF as it crosses the knee or if instead a KAFO is needed to restore equilibrium. If there is evidence of ligamentous instability that threatens anteroposterior or medial lateral stability at the knee or markedly abnormal varus or valgus of the knee, a KAFO would clearly be indicated.

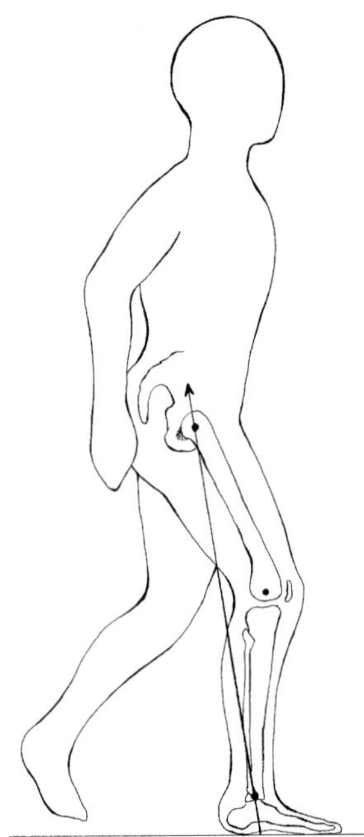

Fig. 9.16 The ground reaction force (GRF) passes through the ankle, behind the knee, and through the hip as loading response moves toward midstance, creating an external flexion moment at the knee. To achieve stability, muscle activity of the quadriceps, hamstrings, and gastrocnemius/soleus combine to create an internal extension moment to counterbalance the flexion moment of the GRF.

The evaluation process for KAFOs includes documentation of the individual's height and weight, the status of circulation and sensation in lower extremities, the condition and integrity of the skin, soft tissue density and bony prominences, as well as living, school, working, and leisure environments in which the KAFO is likely to be used. Specific attention is given to determination of available range of motion, ligamentous activity, fixed contractures, muscle performance, muscle and antigravity tone, leg length, and limb girth. The use of observational gait analysis, walking speed, other kinematic parameters, and, if appropriate, kinetic analysis, is used to document preorthotic gait pattern. The team synthesizes this information to make a recommendation. The orthotist selects appropriate materials and components then fabricates and fits the orthosis, adjusting as necessary. The physical therapist and individual begin the process of functional training, with adjustments being made to the orthoses as indicated.

Knee-Ankle-Foot Orthosis Design Options

KAFOs, much like the AFOs that form their distal component, can be made of primarily metal materials (e.g., steel, aluminum, titanium alloys, carbon fiber), thermoplastics, or as a hybrid combining both types of materials. Historically, the orthotic knee joints of a KAFO were locking or free swinging, but the development of stance-control knee units in the early 2000s showed the potential to change walking kinematics, function, and energy cost for individuals who use SC-KAFO for function or for exercise.[64–66] Although a KAFO does not directly control hip motion, if the individual wearing bilateral KAFOs is trained to stand with a forward pelvis, lumbar lordosis, and an extended trunk, the GRF at midstance will pass anterior to the knee and posterior to the hip, creating an extensor moment that will enhance stability. In this position, the Y ligaments of the hip are elongated, contributing to an internal stabilizing force at the hips as well. It should be noted that use of this strategy may, if used frequently over a long period of time, contribute to the development of degenerative joint disease of the lumbar spine and chronic low back pain.

Like any orthosis, KAFOs can both facilitate and challenge function. What works for one person may be inappropriate for another who has different physical or emotional characteristics or a different medical condition. For persons who want to walk using a KAFO, the orthotist must be even more thoughtful about durability and weight, matching the alignment of anatomic and orthotic joints, the impact of the forces used in each of the control system across all planes of motion, the ease of donning and doffing the device, the adjustability of the orthosis, the need for maintenance or replacement of worn-out components, and whether the orthosis will be comfortable and cosmetically acceptable to the person who will wear it. One study reports that among polio survivors, the most common explanations for discontinued use of KAFO devices included hinderance during daily activities, not reducing mobility problems, and an uncomfortable fit.[56]

CONVENTIONAL KNEE-ANKLE-FOOT ORTHOSES

During the early 1900s until the 1980s, most KAFOs were fabricated using a pair of uprights (stainless steel, titanium alloy, aluminum, or carbon composite) as a frame, leather-covered posterior thigh and calf cuffs that buckled across the anterior thigh and leg to secure the orthosis on the limb, a pair of single-axis locking orthotic knee joints, a pair of single-axis dorsiflexion assistance orthotic ankle joints with a plantarflexion stop, and metal stirrups that attached

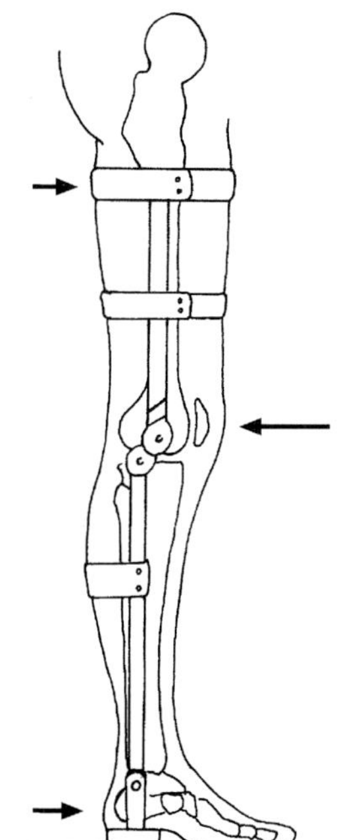

Fig. 9.17 Schematic diagram of the components and sagittal plane force system acting at the knee in a conventional knee-ankle-foot orthosis. The posteriorly directed force at the knee is counterbalanced by a pair of anteriorly directed forces at the posterior proximal thigh and posterior distal ankle.

between the heel and sole of the shoe (Fig. 9.17). At times, a leather anterior knee pad was added as an additional contact point for force application to stabilize the knee. These KAFOs were often worn over clothing during gait training and could later be worn under clothing if the individual so desired.

In most KAFO designs, a three-point pressure system is used to stabilize the knee in the sagittal plane to control flexion/extension: There is a single posteriorly directed force (applied by the anterior kneepad or by anterior thigh and calf straps, or both) and two anteriorly directed counterforces (applied by the posterior thigh band proximally and the shoe and posterior calf band distally) that keep the knee extended in stance. Typically, the knee joint may be unlocked manually to allow sagittal knee rotation for sitting.[57] There are two additional force systems acting in the frontal plane: one to control valgus and one to control varus at the knee. Typically, the knee joint may be unlocked manually to allow sagittal plane knee rotation for sitting.[57] There are two additional force systems acting in the frontal plane: one to control valgus and one to control varus at the knee. Given the less-than-intimate fit of a conventional KAFO at the knee, the efficacy of the varus and valgus systems is likely to be less than optimal. The advantages of conventional KAFOs include their durability and adjustability; however, they tend to be heavier and less cosmetically pleasing than thermoplastic versions. In addition, if porous leather is used to cover thigh cuffs, the absorption of bodily fluids may render their KAFO malodorous over time. The advantages and disadvantages and the indications and contraindications of conventional KAFOs are summarized in Box 9.3.[64]

The Craig-Scott orthosis, also known as a *double-bar hip-stabilizing orthosis*, is a lightweight variation of a traditional

Box 9.3 Advantages and Disadvantages of Conventional Knee-Ankle-Foot Orthoses

Advantages

- Strong
- Most durable
- Easily adjusted

Disadvantages

- Heavy
- Must be attached to shoe or shoe insert
- Less cosmetic
- Fewer contact points reduce control

Indications

- When maximum strength and durability are needed
- For individuals with significant obesity
- For individuals with uncontrolled or fluctuating edema (e.g., congestive heart failure, dialysis)
- Knee and/or hip contracture up to 20 degrees
- Unilateral or bilateral legs with paralysis

Contraindications

- When issues of energy expenditure make weight of the orthosis a factor
- When control of transverse plane motion is important
- Knee and/or hip contractures > 20 degrees
- Moderate-to-severe spasticity
- Hip abductors strength less than grade 3 (measured on 0–5 scale)

KAFO designed for persons with paraplegia after spinal cord injury (SCI). The goal of this KAFO design is to maximize stability in stance with the minimal amount of bracing possible. A single thigh band and anterior strap are positioned just below the ischial tuberosity at the level of the greater trochanter; a single calf band and support are positioned just below the knee. Persons without active hip control are stable in standing with hip hyperextension, exaggerated lumbar lordosis, and a backward leaning trunk; stability is augmented by the orthosis' dorsiflexion-assist ankle joints and offset locking knee joints. With this combination of orthotic design and exaggerated posture, the GRF passes just anterior to the knee and posterior to the hip so that little or no muscular activity to provide internally generated counterforce is necessary. Although a reciprocal gait pattern with Lofstrand crutches typically requires the ability to volitionally activate hip flexions and quadratus lumborum (hip hikers) to initiate a step, persons with thoracic level SCI can use Craig-Scott orthoses and Lofstrand crutches using a two-point swing-through gait pattern.[67] Although a reciprocal gait pattern with Lofstrand crutches typically requires the ability to volitionally activate hip flexions and quadratus lumborum (hip hikers) to initiate a step, persons with thoracic level SCI can use Craig-Scott orthoses and Lofstrand crutches using a two-point swing-through gait pattern.[67]

Conventional KAFOs are frequently used to preserve upright mobility for children with neuromuscular conditions (i.e., Duchenne muscular dystrophy).[68] A lightweight adjustable KAFO system that allows the orthotist to adjust the length of the uprights has been developed specifically for children, allowing for earlier implementation of the device and decreased device changes through childhood, which may allow for earlier adoption of a more efficient, energetic, and safe gait pattern and decreased required re-adaptation to changing devices.[69] One study reports that among polio survivors, the most common explanations for discontinued use of KAFO devices included hinderance during daily activities, not reducing mobility problems, and an uncomfortable fit.[69]

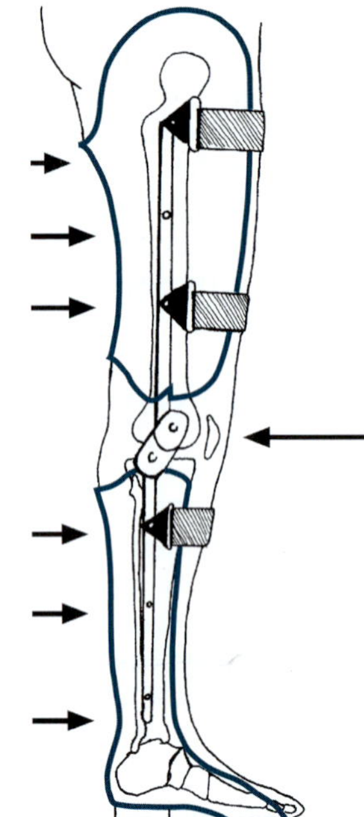

Fig. 9.18 Schematic diagram of the components and sagittal plane force systems that are necessary to control knee flexion/extension. Because the point of force application is distributed over the entire posterior surface of the intimately fitting orthotic shell, more precise and more comfortable control of the limb is possible.

THERMOPLASTIC KNEE-ANKLE-FOOT ORTHOSES

A *molded thermoplastic* KAFO (also known as a hybrid thermoplastic and metal orthosis) is designed to have an intimate fit so that it can be worn under clothing and fits within the patient's shoe (Fig. 9.18). The distal component (a SAFO or an HAFO) and the proximal thigh component are vacuum formed over a rectified positive model of the patient's limb. The proximal component often encases the thigh from greater trochanter to femoral condyles and is closed with a pair of anterior Velcro straps. Orthotic knee joints and metal uprights (sidebars) connect the proximal and distal shells. The intimate total contact fit of molded thermoplastic allows significantly more effective control of the limb.[64] The forces necessary for stabilization of the limb are distributed over a large surface area, reducing the possibility of discomfort or skin irritation.[64] The forces necessary for stabilization of the limb are distributed over a large surface area, reducing the possibility of discomfort or skin irritation. Such problems would arise only if the fit of the orthosis allows pistoning of the limb within the components while walking or if growth, weight gain, or edema makes the fit too snug, such that tissue is compressed and damaged while walking.

This design also controls the limb using a series of overlapping three-point force systems. Flexion/extension

Box 9.4 Advantages and Disadvantages of Thermoplastic Knee-Ankle-Foot Orthoses

Advantages

- Lightweight
- Interchangeability of shoes
- Greater cosmesis worn under clothing

Disadvantages

- Can be hot to wear

Indications

- Intimate/total contact fit makes maximum limb control possible
- When energy expenditure makes weight of the orthosis an issue
- When control of transverse plane motion is needed

Contraindications

- Intimacy of fit is difficult when the individual is significantly obese
- Intimacy of fit is compromised when the individual has uncontrolled or fluctuating edema

control in the sagittal plane is the same one used in a conventional KAFO, except that the posterior counterforces are distributed over a wider surface area. The intimate fit provides more precise control in both the frontal and transverse planes; this is particularly important when dealing with segmental deviations arising from transverse plane rotation related to abnormal tone or longitudinal rotational deformity.[58] The intimate fit provides more precise control in both the frontal and transverse planes; this is particularly important when dealing with segmental deviations arising from transverse plane rotation related to abnormal tone or longitudinal rotational deformity.[58] Control of rotation is better accomplished with the total contact thermoplastic KAFO as compared with the double-upright system of conventional KAFOs. However, this intimate fit is problematic for persons with medical conditions associated with fluctuating edema and changing limb volume (e.g., congestive heart failure, kidney dialysis), as well as those who cyclically gain and lose weight.

Like most thermoplastic AFOs, the use of different pairs of shoes (as long as heel height is constant) can also occur with thermoplastic KAFOs. However, one of the downsides of using thermoplastics is keeping cool while wearing them. As lightweight as they are, the large contact area inherent in thermoplastic KAFOs compromises dissipation of body heat; they may be uncomfortably warm. Advantages and disadvantages of thermoplastic KAFOs are summarized in Box 9.4.

CARBON COMPOSITE KNEE-ANKLE-FOOT ORTHOSES

Carbon composite materials have begun to be used in place of thermoplastics in KAFOs for persons with residual impairment for whom fatigue is a major concern, and for devices intended to have better cosmetic appeal (Fig. 9.19A and B). On average, because carbon composite KAFOs (CC-KAFOs) are as much as 30% lighter in weight than other materials, the energy cost of walking with CC-KAFOs may be up to 10% less (as measured by maximum volume of oxygen [VO_2 max] and physiologic cost index).[70,71] Advantages of CC-KAFOs include improved cosmetics, increased walking speed, improved kinetic characteristics of walking, and exceptional durability.[70,71] It is important to note that the cost of CC-KAFOs may be nearly double that of a custom-molded thermoplastic KAFO.[70–72] However, studies have also shown that patient satisfaction increases with use of SC-KAFO designs compared to older devices.[72] The only noted negative attributes have been related to excessive perspiration, skin irritation from the material, and inability to alter shape with circumferential limb changes.[72]

CONTROLLING THE ANKLE

The ankle joints used in KAFOs are the same as those that are available for AFOs: nonarticulating solid (rigid) designs that hold the ankle in a fixed position (i.e., SAFO) or hinged orthotic joints that allow dorsiflexion (for forward progression of the tibia over the foot in stance phase), block plantarflexion, provide dorsiflexion assistance (to enhance swing-phase clearance), or allow free dorsiflexion and plantarflexion within a specific range of motion.

The key question to consider in deciding which ankle control system is appropriate for a given individual is how orthotic control at the ankle and the GRF will impact knee function and forward progression during stance phase. If a locked ankle is necessary, the orthotist may opt to set the orthosis in several degrees of dorsiflexion to minimize compromise of forward progression and to allow the individual to achieve the stable hips-forward trunk-back stance position quickly (i.e., to achieve stability with the GRF passing anterior to the knee and posterior to the hip as soon as possible during stance). When ankle motion must be constrained to protect the joint, to control the impact of abnormal tone, or because of fixed deformity, the orthotist may use a rocker sole on the patient's shoe to simulate the normal rockers of gait. This strategy facilitates forward progression during stance by reducing the toe lever of the orthosis, improving the smoothness of the patient's gait, and reducing the likelihood of compensatory gait deviations.

An articulating or hinged orthotic ankle joint that allows some plantarflexion enhances the transition from initial contact to loading response (although the locked knee may compromise the shock absorption function of loading response). Similarly, a hinged orthotic ankle joint that permits movement into dorsiflexion during stance enhances forward progression of the body over the foot during stance, especially when the orthotic knee is also locked.

CONTROLLING THE KNEE

Historically, if a patient with motor control or muscle performance impairment was unable to keep the knee stable in stance and an AFO was not able to provide the necessary stability, the only option was a KAFO with knee joints that remained locked at all times while walking.[57] This created a challenge for limb advancement in swing and often resulted in compensatory patterns such as increased upper body lateral sway, vaulting of the contralateral leg, swing leg circumduction, swing leg excessive hip hiking, or lateral

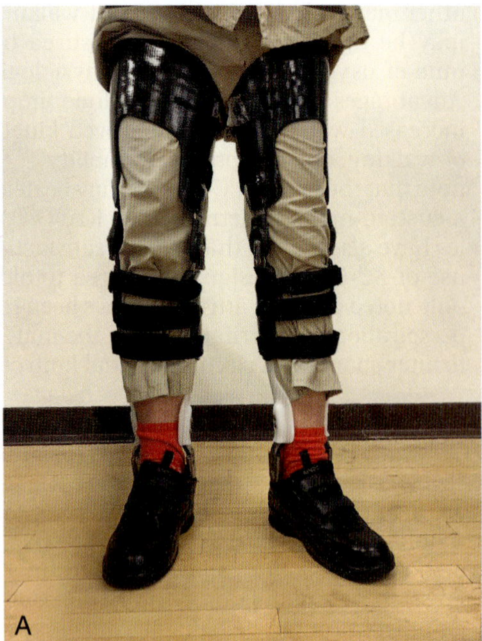

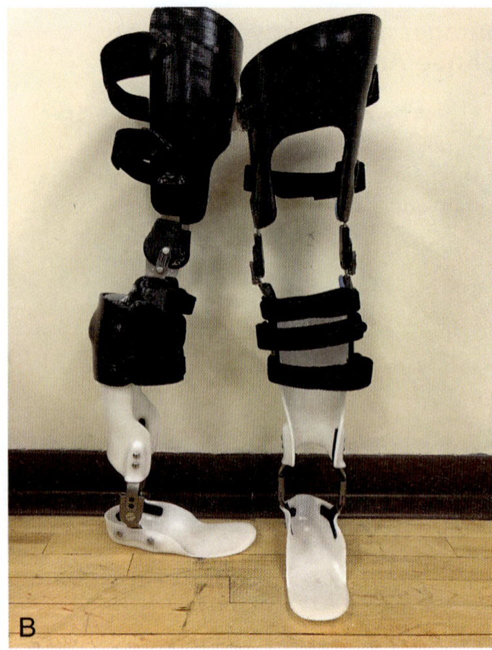

Fig. 9.19 (A and B) This carbon composite knee-ankle-foot orthosis has an anterior proximal shell with a posterior midshell and uses a stance-control knee unit and a foot component similar to that of a hinged ankle-foot orthosis.

leaning to the opposite side in an effort to clear the swinging leg.[66] Although compensatory strategies accomplished the goal of limb clearance, they also markedly increased the energy cost of walking and may lead to soft tissue and/or joint dysfunction in the lower back and hip.[66] Those who had functional motor control and muscle performance who required a KAFO to protect a mechanically unstable knee from extreme valgus or varus may be able to use unlocked single axis orthotic knee joints.

There are a number of options for orthotic knee joints that provide mechanical stability. The recent development of various SC-KAFO knee joints that allow free knee motion in swing but lock into extension during stance has had a significant impact on KAFO prescription and use.[66] A brief overview of the mechanical joints is provided, and the impact of SC-KAFOs is considered in more detail.[66] See Table 9.3 for a set of general guidelines for choosing the conventional orthotic knee joints based on the knee control they provide.

Single-Axis Knee Joints

The single-axis orthotic knee joint *(straight knee joint without drop lock or a free knee)* is essentially a simple hinge that allows full flexion and extension to neutral in the sagittal plane (most designs prevent hyperextension) while providing mediolateral stability (Fig. 9.20A). It is important that the medial and lateral orthotic joints be positioned at the approximate axis of the anatomic knee joint. Given the polycentric structure of the anatomic knee versus the single-axis structure of the orthotic knee joint, a small torque is likely, even if the single-axis orthotic joints are correctly positioned. For many persons using the orthosis, this is not problematic. This knee joint is appropriate for those who have sufficient muscle performance resource to achieve knee stability in stance but need a KAFO to minimize or prevent recurvatum, protect a structural (mediolateral) unstable knee, or prevent excessive varus or valgus in stance.

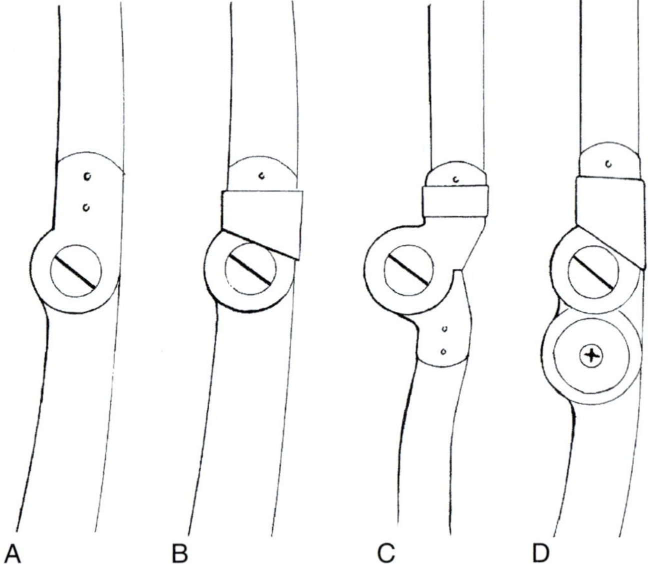

Fig. 9.20 Orthotic knee joints historically used in conventional and thermoplastic knee-ankle-foot orthoses. (A) A single-axis, or free, knee allows full flexion and extension while providing mediolateral and rotational stability to the knee joint. (B) A drop lock holds the knee in extension in standing, providing stability in all planes. It must be unlocked for knee flexion to occur when returning to sitting position. (C) Because the axis of the offset orthotic knee joint is positioned behind the anatomic knee axis, biomechanical stability of the orthosis is enhanced. It is available with and without a locking mechanism. (D) A variable-position, or adjustable, orthotic knee joint permits the orthotist to accommodate for changing range of motion or for fixed contracture at the knee.

Single-Axis Locking Knee

When a locking mechanism is added to maintain knee extension, the KAFO with a single-axis knee joint becomes rigidly stable in all planes. A locked knee has traditionally been used for those whose motor control or muscle performance deficits make them unable to control the knee effectively during stance phase, such that they need additional external stability to prevent knee flexion as body weight is transferred onto the limb during stance.[57]

The most used locking mechanism is a simple ring or drop that captures the halves of the orthotic joint when fully extended, blocking subsequent movement into flexion or hyperextension (see Fig. 9.20B). A small ball bearing in the upright holds the drop lock in position until the individual or caregiver purposefully unlocks the orthosis to allow for flexion. Optimally, there is a drop lock on both the medial and lateral uprights of the orthosis. Note that the knee must be fully extended for the lock to be engaged or disengaged; this can be challenging when transitioning between standing and sitting, especially for persons with limited hand function, significant lower extremity spasticity, or dependence on assistive devices when standing.[57]

An alternative lock that may be considered is a spring-loaded bail lock (also known as pawl or Swiss lock). The posterior bail connects the medial and lateral locks so that they can be locked or unlocked simultaneously. To unlock the KAFO when returning to sitting, the individual backs up against the edge of a seating surface (e.g., wheelchair, mat table, kitchen, or desk chair) and pushes the posterior bar into the seat to disengage the lock. This option is best used for persons with enough upper body strength and coordination to control the descent into sitting.[57] There is a risk that the lock will disengage if the bail behind the knee is inadvertently bumped, and a fall will occur.

Offset Knee Joint

The offset knee joint (also known as a *posteriorly offset, free knee*) is aligned with its axis posterior to the axis of the anatomic knee (see Fig. 9.20C). In early stance, during double support, the ground reaction passes nearer to the axis of the orthotic joint, reducing the magnitude of the external flexion moment that is acting to flex the limb. With forward progression toward midstance, the GRF moves anterior to the orthotic joint, creating an extensor force that mechanically augments stance phase stability during single-limb support.[57] However, to be effective, the alignment between ankle and knee must be finely tuned.[57] Transitions between sitting and standing become less problematic if the knee does not have to be unlocked. However, a drop lock or other locking mechanism can be added to stabilize the knee when the individual using the orthosis will be standing for long periods of time or when additional stability is advisable (e.g., when the patient is walking on uneven ground). An offset knee joint is often most suitable for those with lower motor neuron disease, hemiparesis that requires increased stability with greater force of moment arm into extension, or other causes for painful genu recurvatum (e.g., poliomyelitis, low thoracic upper lumbar SCI, hemiparesis with plantarflexion contracture).[73,74]

Polycentric Knee Joint

A polycentric knee joint more closely replicates the natural arthrokinematics of knee function which includes a degree of translation and rotation. Similar to the knee joints listed above, it provides stability in extension by maintaining anterior GRF. However, these joints tend to be more complex with several moving parts that may require more frequent maintenance.[57]

Variable Position Orthotic Knee Joint

The variable position locking orthotic knee joint *(ratchet lock, dial lock, adjustable locking knee joint, serrated knee lock)* (see Fig. 9.20D) is used for those who are unable to fully extend the knee during stance because of knee flexion contracture. The ratchet lock allows for free knee extension movement, and may not be appropriate for patients with knee instability into extension, or concerns for injury with repetitive knee hyperextension.[57] When there is a knee flexion contracture of more than 10 degrees, the GRF remains posterior to the anatomic knee joint during the stance phase, and it becomes significantly more difficult for those with weakness or motor control impairment to generate the necessary muscle force for stance stability. For these individuals, the variable position knee joint is locked in the most extended position possible, providing an external mechanical stability.[57] Allowing the knee to be locked in some degree of slight knee flexion during stance may facilitate energy-efficient walking, but does not change gait speed, cadence, or stride parameters compared to gait with knee locked in extension.[75]

Stance-Control Orthotic Knee Joints

The initial SC options for KAFO orthotic knee joints were intended for individuals with a history of poliomyelitis who were coping with ineffective quadriceps activity, as well as postpolio syndrome.[76] Use of SC-KAFO has been extended to persons with stroke, brain tumor, acquired brain injury, incomplete SCI, spinal degenerative diseases, muscular dystrophy, multiple sclerosis, myopathy, radicular and peripheral nerve injury, and polyneuropathy.[65] A variety of mechanisms (i.e., mechanical, hydraulic, or computer microchip electronic joints) are available (Fig. 9.21).[57] All are designed to lock the orthotic knee joint in extension at initial contract and during most of stance, while unlocking the knee on heel rise during the toe rocker in the transition from terminal stance to preswing.[57,66] Hydraulic, electronic, and powered superelastic SC orthotic joints add resistance to knee flexion when the limb is loaded in less than a fully extended position, which potentially improves function when the wearer is ascending stairs or walking on uneven surfaces.[57,66] Most SC orthotic knee joints are placed on the lateral upright of the KAFO.[65] Pneumatic orthotic knee joints to assist with knee extension during swing are also available, added onto the medial or lateral uprights of the KAFO. Many of the SC knee units can be incorporated into KAFOs based on metal uprights, thermoplastic thigh and AFO components, or laminated designs. Characteristics of some of the commercially available SC and swing assist knee units are summarized in Table 9.4. Additional SC-KAFO devices exist in the literature, including motor powered KAFO, Quasi-Passive Complaint SC-KAFO, Hydraulic SC-KAFO, Belt-Clamping Joint SC-KAFO, Spring actuated Dynamic KAFO, and Pneumatically powered KAFO; however, these are not as commercially available at this time.[57]

Most prescription guidelines for SC-KAFO indicate that the individual must demonstrate muscle strength of at least 3 of 5 on manual muscle testing at hip extensors and flexors,

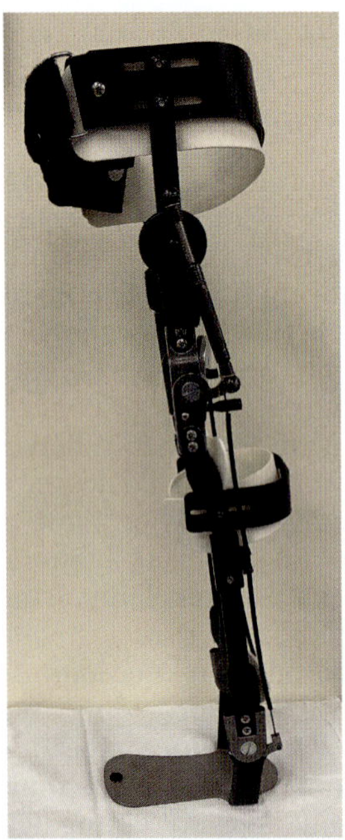

Fig. 9.21 The Becker UTX is a mechanical stance-control knee-ankle-foot orthosis: The knee unit contains a cable-driven ratchet that locks the knee as it extends in terminal swing in preparation for stance phase and unlocks it at terminal stance to allow knee flexion necessary for limb clearance during swing phase. Note the lightweight lateral upright medial cable, anterior padded cuffs, and velcro-closing posterior straps.

full extension of the anatomic knee joint, and ability to fully stabilized the torso and stand freely.[64] Contraindications for SC-KAFO use include fixed hip or knee flexion contracture >10 degrees, fixed plantarflexion contracture, significant spasticity, leg-length discrepancy greater than 6 inches (15 cm), valgus or varus deformity greater than 10 degrees, and excessive body weight (>275 lbs). Persons with cognitive impairment may not be able to comprehend how to safely use or maintain a SC-KAFO; SC options must be used with caution when cognitive ability and judgment are impaired.[64]

The positive impact of SC knee joints on kinematics of walking is well documented. In addition to improving self-selected walking speed, cadence, and stride length, use of these orthotic knee joint improves symmetry of gait, reduces compensatory movement, and allows safer management of inclines and obstacles when compared with KAFOs with locked knees.[64–66,76] When comparing a microprocessor-controlled knee (C-Brace) with a stance- controlled KAFO and locking KAFO, KAFO users showed improved static balance, dynamic balance, gait, speed, walking endurance, stair descent, self-reported falls, and ADLs with the microprocessor knee compared to SCO.[64–66,76–78] Persons who have used traditional KAFOs with locked knees for long periods before adopting SC designs benefit from additional functional training to be able to take full advantage of the mobility that a SC-KAFO provides, taking 3 to 6 months to adjust.[65,66] The few studies that have examined wearers' experience with SC-KAFOs indicate better acceptance and general satisfaction with the devices in terms of effectiveness in improving mobility, dependability, and performance of the device and enhancing the wearer's sense of well-being. The major concerns raised by wearers include ease of donning and doffing, weight of the orthosis, and cosmesis. While kinematics of gait and efficiency have been shown to improve with use of a SC-KAFO compared to older models, it is still unclear if this leads to changes in usability. Prior studies examined wearers' experience with SC-KAFOs and indicated better acceptance and general satisfaction with the devices in terms of effectiveness in improving mobility, dependability, and performance of the device and enhancing the wearer's sense of well-being.[79,80] However, recent reviews are less conclusive, with one study indicating that up to 50% of comments regarding KAFOs were negative[81] and another indicating that of 98 polio survivors prescribed custom-made KAFO, 24% discontinued use.[56] Specific to SC-KAFOs, this study also found that users of stance-control devices were more likely to discontinue use compared to those prescribed with locked KAFO.[79,80] This may have been due to selection criteria for SC-KAFO (subjects who may have had better walking ability without orthosis leading to limited gains with device use), as well as increased complexity of delivering and learning to walk with SC-KAFO.[56] Newer designs may have the potential to further improve patient satisfaction to increase usability and satisfaction.

MEDIALLY LINKED BILATERAL KNEE-ANKLE-FOOT ORTHOSIS DESIGNS

For persons with mid-to-low thoracic and lumbar SCI, several options have been developed to link a pair of conventional KAFOs in an effort to allow reciprocal gait without having to brace about the hip in a conventional HKAFO (Fig. 9.22). The Walkabout Orthosis, the Moorling Medial Linkage orthosis and the Primewalk orthosis each use a single-axis hinge between the two medial uprights of the KAFOs, and are most effective for individuals with some residual volitional hip flexion who have sufficient thoracolumbar spinal mobility, especially into lateral flexion.[82–84] In both of these systems, the linkage system limits abnormal abduction of the limbs during gait. Preparation for swing limb advancement begins with an exaggerated lateral lean for weight shift onto the stance limb; the wearer then initiates swing using residual hip hiking or hip flexion ability. When compared with reciprocal gait HKAFO (see later), medially linked KAFOs (MLOs) provided better ability (less assistance required) to accomplish sit-to-stand transitions, but walking speed tends to be slower, management of inclines more problematic, and performance on measures of balance somewhat less effective.[62] When compared to reciprocating gait orthoses, MLOs show improved independence with donning/doffing and improved cosmesis, but increased energy expenditure due to lack of support for the pelvis and trunk. In addition, persons with SCI who wore both devices over a 3-month period reported that both were useful for standing and there was no functional advantage of medially linked KAFOs over reciprocal gait HKAFOs in terms of mobility.[62] It has also been found that, when compared to all patients using the Walkabout device, patients with paraplegia were required to use increased compensatory pelvic rotation and increased arm movements to maintain balance, both of which increase energy requirements when walking.[85] Newer medially linked devices

Table 9.4 Stance-Control Knee-Ankle-Foot Orthosis Characteristics

Name	Manufacturer	Control System	Orthotic Components	Other Characteristics
Stance-control orthosis	Horton, Little Rock, Arkansas	Mechanical	Pushrod and cam system Thermoplastic stirrup at ankle causes pushrod to engage cam into friction ring to lock knee at initial contact, unloading in late stance repositions Pushrod to disengage cam from friction ring, allowing free knee flexion during swing	Dual uprights Three settings: locked, automatic, unlocked Lightweight but bulky May require larger shoe size to accommodate nested thermoplastic stirrup and AFO Most effective at constant walking speed and consistent stride length (not cadence responsive)
Free Walk	Ottobock Healthcare, Duderstadt, Germany	Mechanical	Cable-driven pawl lock system Spring-loaded pawl locks the knee when in full extension during stance Unit unlocks with dorsiflexion of ankle in late stance to allow free knee flexion during swing	Single lateral upright with medial cable Very light weight Requires full knee extension to engage the lock, although uprights can be contoured to accommodate up to 10 degrees of knee flexion contracture Requires at least 5 degrees of mobility at ankle Requires at least 3/5 hip flexion and extension strength for safe and effective use Not appropriate for those with varus >10 degrees
UTX	Becker Orthopedic	Mechanical		
Swing Phase Lock 2	Fillauer Chattanooga, Tennessee	Mechanical	Gravity-activated pendulum system with weighted pawl lock Weighted pawl causes knee to lock when hip flexion in late swing Moves thigh anterior to body in preparation for initial contact in late stance, when thigh is posterior to body, weight pawl moves to unlocking position	Dual-upright, with SC gravity system in lateral upright Swing control spring to control/assist knee extension during swing phase can be incorporated into medial knee unit No cables or pushrods Not effective on stairs, inclines, uneven ground Four settings controlled by a remote push button switch: manual lock, manual unlock, automatic, or free swing
E-Knee	Becker	Microchip	Electromechanical system with pressure-sensitive footplate that feeds information to microprocessor to engage/disengage locking mechanism	Dual-uprights Can be used with thermoplastic and laminated materials Lithium battery must be charged daily Provides locking in increments of 8 degrees at any angle of knee flexion at initial contract No minimum strength or ROM requirements
Load Response	Becker	Mechanical	Spiral torsional spring designed to mimic shock absorption during loading response	Locking mechanism responsive for 0 to 18 degrees of knee flexion at initial contract Not effective for persons with fixed knee flexion contracture or valgus 15 degrees
GX-Knee	Becker	Mechanical and pneumatic	Pneumatic spring on lateral joint provides assistance with knee extension during swing phase	Does not provide mechanical stability in stance phase Requires 4/5 hip flexion and extension strength for safe use
Full Stride	Becker	Mechanical	Cable-driven system	Requires full-knee extension to engage lock, although uprights can be contoured to accommodate knee flexion contracture Requires 5 degrees of ankle motion to achieve necessary cable excursion to operate locking mechanism
Safety Stride	Becker Orthopedic	Mechanical	Cable-driven system	Resists knee flexion in stance regardless of knee angle No minimum strength or ROM requirements GX swing assist system can be incorporated
Sensor Walk	Ottobock Healthcare	Electromechanical	Unidirectional wrap-spring clutch-actuated by pressure sensors in heel and forefoot and motion sensor at knee	Heavy-duty custom KAFO accommodates up to 15 degrees of knee flexion contracture Powered by lithium-ion battery Locks knee joint when footplate indicates a stumble
C-Brace	Ottobock Healthcare	Microprocessor	Microprocessor stance and swing control KAFO. Carbon fiber strut with integrated ankle moment sensor and monocentric microprocessor-controlled knee joint.	Allows for controlled walking on level ground, uneven ground, different velocities, and alternating ramp or stair descent. Knee angle sensor provides feedback on knee angle and angle velocity, extension and flexion dampening adjusted at 50 Hz frequency with ankle moment, knee ankle, knee angle velocity and temperature of hydraulic as input.

AFO, Ankle-foot orthosis; *KAFO*, knee-ankle-foot orthosis; *ROM*, range of motion; *SC*, stance control.

Modified from Operating instructions for the E-Mag and Free Walk orthosis. Ottobock, Germany. http://www.ottobock.com/cps/rde/xbcr/ob_com_en/im_646a214_gb_free_walk.pdf; Stance Control Overview Guide II, Becker Orthopedic. Troy, Michigan. http://www.beckerorthopedic.com/assets/pdf/stance:control.pdf; MO25-SPL Manual. Fillauer, Chattanooga, Tennessee. http://www.fillauer.com/Orthotics/SPL2.html; Yakimovich T, Lemaire ED, Kofman J. Engineering design review of stance-control knee-ankle-foot orthoses. *J Rehabil Res Dev*. 2009;46(2):257–267;[66] Probsting E, Kannenberg A, Zacharias B. Safety and walking ability of KAFO users with the C-Brace ORthotronic Mobility System, a new microprocessor stance and swing control orthosis. *Prostheti Orthot Int*. 2017;4(1):65–77.[78]

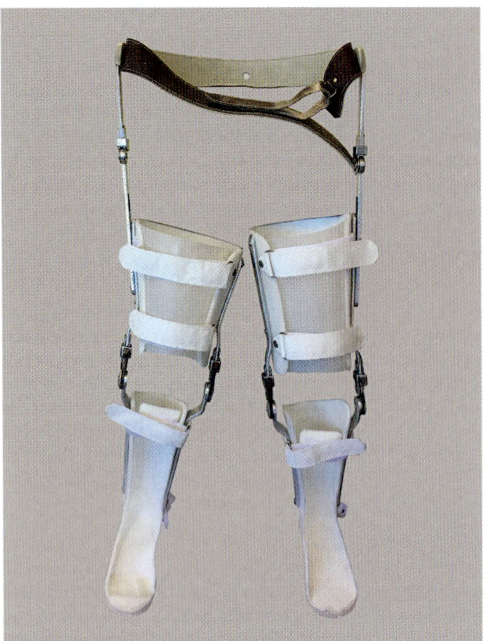

Fig. 9.22 Themoplastic hip-knee-ankle-foot orthoses (HKAFOs), typically lighter in weight than conventional HKAFOs, also have a pelvic band and orthotic hip and knee joints. Because they distribute forces over a wider thigh and calf band, an anterior knee stabilization pad may not be necessary. Many incorporate a solid or articulating ankle-foot orthosis design, fitting inside the shoe rather than in an external stirrup.

that increase congruency between anatomic and orthotic hip joints may help address the issues of increased energy demand and difficulty navigating sloped surfaces, as with other medially linked KAFOs.[62,85] Hybrid systems, consisting of medially linked KAFOs and FES, have also been used as an approach to improve the ability to walk for persons with SCI.[86] Though robotic-assisted devices may help with energy demand, they tend to be bulky, difficult to independently don, and increase applied forces on the limb, all of which may decrease utilization by the wearers.[62,87] Newer devices combining the medially linked KAFO design with robotic-assisted hip, knee, and ankle joints (such as the Wearable Power-Assist Locomotor-WPAL) may also improve the energy efficiency of walkers with SCI, but also require the use of a rolling walker to carry the battery and motor drivers of the device.[87]

KAFO Delivery and Functional Training

Once fabrication is completed, the orthotist inspects the KAFO to ensure that selected components work as intended, that finish work of plastic edges and metal components are effective, that the placement and contours are appropriate to the individual's limbs, and that orientation of the axis of the orthotic ankle and knee match anatomic joint axis. This initial fitting process not only identifies the fit of the orthosis in its intended functional upright and weight-bearing positions but also closely examines potential for soft tissue irritation in vulnerable areas of the person's skin. Length of the uprights and position and alignment of components are carefully inspected. The goal is a comfortable standing position with no discomfort or skin irritation. If minor problems are identified, the orthotist often makes simple adjustments of fit and alignment before functional training. The team then evaluates the ability of the orthosis to meet the functional goals of the orthotic prescription.

If the team determines that fit is acceptable and that orthotic goals (a combination of joint protection, structural stability, especially in stance, and functional mobility) have been met, functional training then begins. In most cases, especially if a patient is new to the use of an orthosis, a wearing schedule is developed, tailored to the patient's specific needs and physical condition, in which the patient gradually increases to full-time wear.

Whether the orthosis is of conventional KAFO design or is an SC-KAFO, physical therapy programs should include:

- Exercises to strengthen muscle groups and improve control of hip, knee, and core (trunk) musculature to maximize ability to use the device.
- Practice donning/doffing the device.
- Rising to standing and returning to sitting.
- Activities to facilitate anticipatory and reactionary postural control and balance.
- Gait training under various task-environment conditions.
- Practice on stairs, uneven surfaces, and inclines.
- Functional training in variety of environments.

Training should also focus on developing a clear understanding of the fit of the orthosis on the limb, proper adjustment of stabilizing straps, education about appropriate footwear, and management of the locking mechanisms and function of the knee unit. Wearers and their caregivers must understand the care and maintenance of the orthosis, which is a mechanical device with moving parts that requires regular cleaning and occasional lubrication of its mechanical parts.

Hip-Knee-Ankle-Foot Orthosis

INDICATIONS

There is much less evidence available in the clinical research literature to guide prescription and selection of HKAFOs than for selecting AFOs and KAFOs. Because HKAFOs encompass the hip, pelvis, and sometimes the trunk, they tend to be much more cumbersome to use, more challenging to don and doff, more expensive to fabricate, and require more maintenance than AFOs and KAFOs. HKAFOs only partially restore functional mobility, often with high energy cost. The additional control of joint motion achieved by moving proximally with a hip joint and pelvic band or an attached lumbosacral orthosis must be balanced against the practical challenges the wearer will face when using the device.

Persons who use HKAFOs for standing and for the limited mobility they provide typically have much more neuromotor system impairment than those who use AFOs and KAFOs. These orthoses are most often prescribed for children with neurologic involvement and individuals with SCI but may also be appropriate for those with progressive neuromuscular disorders—in effect, for any person for whom the ability to stand may not only enhance function for some functional tasks but also contribute to bone health, skin integrity, efficacy of digestion, urinary and bowel health, respiratory capacity, cardiovascular fitness and exercise response, and the psychological benefit that comes from being upright when interacting with peers.[88] Children, with their lower center of mass, may not be quite as concerned about the consequences of a fall, but for adults, upright standing in HKAFOs may be made more challenging by concerns about the potential to fall and related consequences.[89]

CLINICAL CONSIDERATIONS

As in the case of AFOs and KAFOs, HKAFOs can be fabricated with many different materials (e.g., metals, thermoplastics, carbon composites) and with orthotic ankle, knee, and hip components. Historically, during the years immediately following the polio epidemic until the mid-to-late 1980s, orthotists fabricated HKAFOs by adding a hip joint and pelvic band to conventional KAFOs. To better meet the developmental and educational needs of children with neurologic conditions, conventional HKAFO designs evolved into standing frames, parapodiums, and swivel walkers. Building on this, several HKAFOs specifically designed to mechanically facilitate reciprocal gait were developed to meet the needs of persons with SCI.

CONVENTIONAL HIP-KNEE-ANKLE-FOOT ORTHOSES

Fig. 9.22 illustrates the configuration of conventional HKAFOs. These devices are designed to hold both lower extremities in a stable extended position for upright standing; persons wearing this orthosis use either a hop-to gait with walkers or a swing-through gait with a pair of crutches for ambulation. Typically, HKAFOs require an assistive device to use upper extremity and trunk compensatory mechanisms to advance the orthosis. On rare occasions, a single HKAFO might be used for persons with neuromuscular or musculoskeletal impairment affecting one lower extremity. Even after the incorporation of lightweight thermoplastic or carbon composite materials, the energy cost of ambulation with conventional HKAFOs is significant and often functionally prohibitive.

The most distal component of the HKAFO is usually a solid or dorsiflexion assist articulating AFO. These are typically set in a few degrees of dorsiflexion to direct the tibia forward enough that the individual's weight line falls anterior to the knee and posterior to the hip when in a tripod standing position with crutches or a walker (Fig. 9.23A). Traditionally, the orthotic knee joint is locked into extension, although for persons with incomplete SCI capable of reciprocal gait, a SC knee joint might be considered. Thermoplastic thigh cuffs are effective in resisting torsional forces that would otherwise act on the limb in standing. A variety of commercially available orthotic hip joints include various single-axis designs that can be used in locked position, allow free motion when unlocked, or allow motion only within a limited range. The axis of motion (center) of the orthotic hip joint must be positioned just proximal and anterior to the greater trochanter to best match the anatomic axis of motion of the hip. Because orthotic hip joints are fixed to the pelvic band and to lateral uprights of the thigh section, they effectively restrict abduction/adduction and rotation of the limb as well. Single-axis hip joints meet the needs of most individuals who require HKAFOs to stand and to ambulate. There are also several types of dual-axis hip joints with separate mechanical control systems for flexion/extension and for abduction/adduction. The proximal pelvic band is positioned between the trochanter and iliac crest. The pelvic band provides solid support from a position slightly medial to the anterior superior iliac spines (ASIS) and around the posterior pelvis. The pelvic band can be fabricated from metal, laminated components, or thick thermoplastic and is typically closed anteriorly by a belt or webbing with a Velcro fastener.

For stability in standing, the individual typically stands in a tripod position, with crutch tips diagonally 12 to 18 inches forward and a slightly exaggerated lumbar lordosis. This position ensures that the individual's center of gravity (weight line) falls posterior to the hip joint, creating an extension moment at the hip, achieving stability by alignment. To achieve forward motion, the individual uses the "head-hips" principle with shoulder joints acting as a fulcrum (Fig. 9.23A–F). A quick forceful "pike" (chin tuck and forward inclination of the trunk) while pushing downward through the handles of the assistive device elevates the lower extremities from the ground. This is immediately followed by head, neck, and back extension to "throw" the lower extremities forward for the next initial contact. As soon as the feet contact the ground, the individual quickly advances the crutches to reach the stable "tripod" position once again.

To effectively use HKAFOs, hip and knee joints of the lower extremity must be flexible enough to be positioned in extension. Although exaggerated lumbar lordosis may compensate for mild hip flexion contracture in achieving upright position, over time and with repeated forceful loading of swing through gait, this lordosis will likely contribute to development of disabling low back pain. Prevention of flexion contracture or deformity of the hips and knees is a key component of physical therapy intervention, especially for growing children with neurologic conditions.

HIP GUIDANCE ORTHOSIS AND PARAWALKER

The hip guidance orthosis (HGO) and the Orthotic Research and Locomotor Assessment Unit (ORLAU) Parawalker allow individuals with impaired muscle performance (those unable to accomplish the lifting of body weight needed for swing through gait pattern with crutches) to "walk" with crutches with a lateral weight shift. The HGO and Parawalker require the use of an ambulatory assistive device; training usually begins in the parallel bars and progresses to over ground level surfaces using a rolling walker or bilateral Lofstrand crutches. The HGO orthotic hip joint is stable when weight is borne through the lower extremity during stance but allows a pendular swing of the unweighted extremity for swing clearance. This occurs because of the rigid support the HGO provides during single limb stance, keeping the limbs parallel in the coronal plane, which enhances swing limb clearance as the opposite limb advances.[90] In the original evaluation of the HGO prescribed for children with myelomeningocele, the

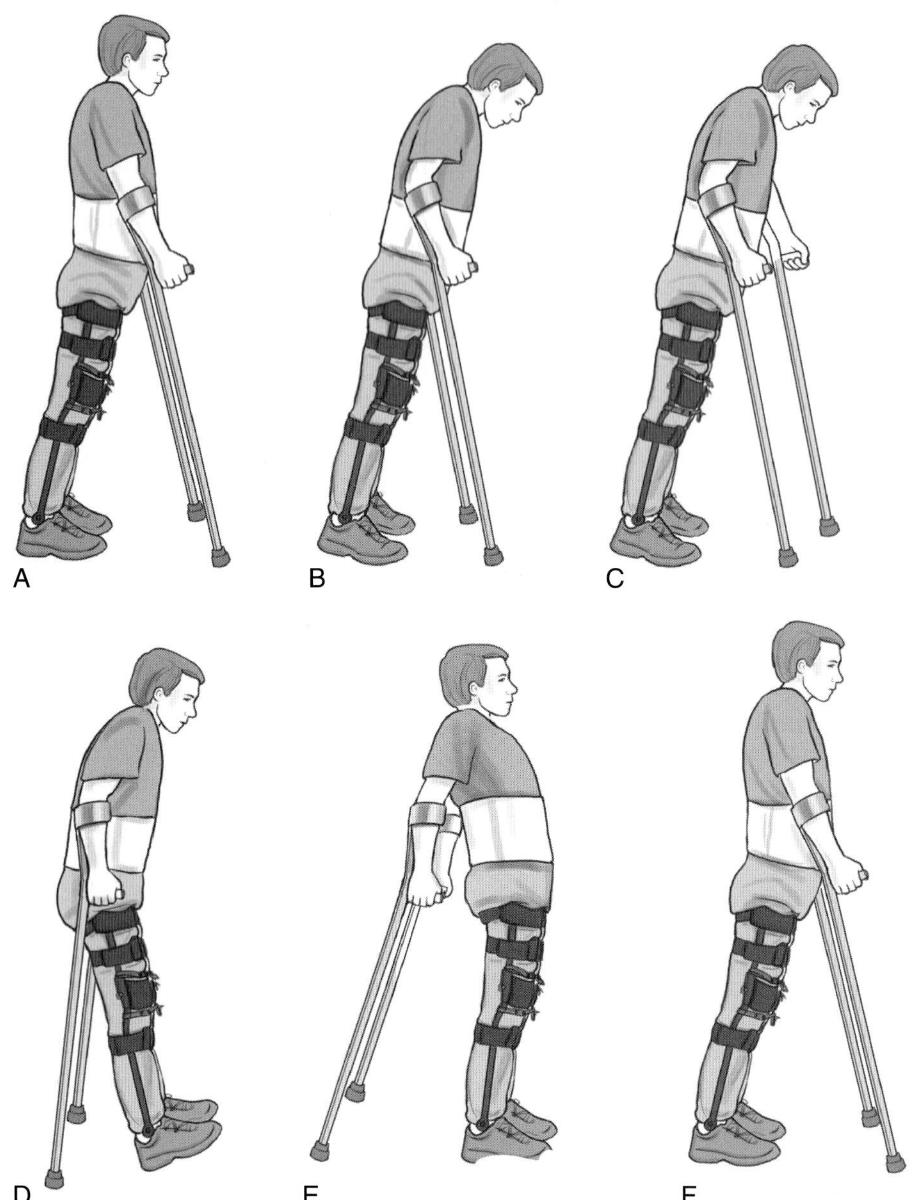

Fig. 9.23 Illustration of the head-hips principle in swing through gait using bilateral knee-ankle-foot orthoses and Lofstrand crutches, with shoulder joints acting as the fulcrum for movement. (A) Resting position is a stable hips forward, shoulders back posture, with a tripod formed by the individual's feet and the tips of the crutches. (B) Mobility is initiated with a quick and forceful chin tuck that (C) is combined with downward pressure through the crutches to unweight the feet. (D) A backward head movement then propels the lower body forward until (E) the hips are forward and shoulders are back to once again assume a stable inverted tripod position. Finally (F) the individual quickly propels off of the crutches to move them anteriorly to the stable starting position. (From Mulcahey MJ. Managemenr of the upper limb in individuals with tetraplegia. In: Sisto SA, Sliwinski MM, eds. *Spinal Cord Injuries: Management and Rehabilitation*. Mosby; 2009:388.)

ability to sit unsupported (hands free) for extended periods was the best predictor of successful use of the HGO.[91] The Parawalker, similar in design, provides more proximal support to the thorax and trunk (making it even more rigid) and uses a smaller orthotic hip joint. Because of its higher proximal trim line, the Parawalker can be used for standing and limited mobility (i.e., therapeutic walking) for persons with SCI at upper thoracic levels.[92–94]

RECIPROCAL GAIT ORTHOSES

The reciprocal gait orthosis (RGO), originally designed for children with myelomeningocele and currently used for adults with SCI, extends a pair of thermoplastic KAFOs upward to include a pelvis and thoracic bands; providing rigid stability for stance, it uses a cable-coupling system to provide hip joint motion for swing phase (Fig. 9.24).[95,96] Its dual cable system operates by reinforcing extension of the stance limb as the swing limb flexes forward when unloaded by lateral weight shift. This reciprocal dual cable also reduces risk of "jack-knifing" during ambulation by preventing both hips from flexing at the same time. Like the HGO and Parawalker, the RGO requires the person to use an assistive device (rolling walker, bilateral Lofstrand crutches, bilateral canes), relying on upper extremity motor control and muscle performance to a large degree to operate the

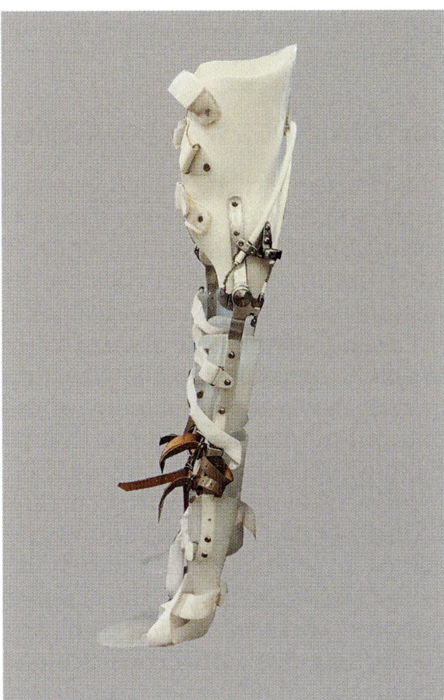

Fig. 9.24 The reciprocal gait orthosis uses a dual-cable system to couple flexion of one hip with extension of the other. This coupling assists forward progression of the swing limb while ensuring stability of the stance limb.

system. The advanced RGO (ARGO) is an adaptation of the design, using a single cable, and engineered to allow standing with unilateral or no upper extremity support.[97,98] A prototype for an adjustable AGRO has been described; this would provide opportunity for a trial of ambulation with ARGO during rehabilitation to assist decision-making about capacity to use the device before a custom ARGO is fabricated.[99] There is some evidence that persons with neuromuscular conditions who consistently use an RGO or ARGO for therapeutic walking are less likely to develop significant secondary complications (i.e., contractures, decubitus ulcers, and/or scoliosis) than those with similar conditions who do not.[100]

HYBRID ORTHOSES: FUNCTIONAL ELECTRICAL STIMULATION

The most recent investigations of reciprocal orthoses for persons with upper motor neuron SCI have added FES to HGO/Parawalker and RGO/ARGO designs.[101] SC orthotic knee joints (described in the section on KAFOs) have also been incorporated in hybrid RGO-FES systems to afford a more natural pattern of swing limb advancement.[102] The major benefit of hybrid RGO-FES systems appears to be in greater distance covered, lower energy cost (as measured by physiologic cost index), and somewhat faster walking speed.[99,101] It is important to note that, although such hybrid systems are promising, they do not fully restore the ability to walk at preinjury levels. Walking speeds with hybrid devices have been reported to be between 0.20 and 0.45 m/s, whereas limited community walking becomes possible when walking speed is greater than 0.6 m/s, and usual waking speed for healthy adults ranges from 1.0 to 1.3 m/s, depending on height.[101–103]

Implications for Rehabilitation

The costs and benefits need to be carefully weighed when considering whether an orthosis that would facilitate therapeutic reciprocal walking would be appropriate for an individual with paralysis. The individual and/or the caregivers must clearly understand that these devices cannot fully restore the ability to walk at what would be considered community level. They must explore and embrace the goals of therapeutic walking: enhancement of bone health, cardiovascular conditioning, and digestive and urinary health, among others. For many individuals, gaining the motor skills necessary for safe use of the device may require substantial time and effort; training times reported in the literature range from 45 to 80 hours over a period of weeks to months. They must be ready to adhere to stretching protocols to ensure sufficient range of motion at the hip, knee, and ankle so that the device will both fit and operate optimally. They must be prepared to work to improve muscle performance and postural control of trunk and upper extremities so that they can use the orthosis most effectively. They must be willing to maintain a stable weight so that the orthosis will fit over many months or years. They must have the postural control necessary to (eventually) don and doff the orthosis without substantial assistance. They must understand the design of the orthosis and the function of its components enough to recognize when maintenance, adjustment, or repair is necessary. This is quite a bit to commit to; it is often wise to have the person interested in pursuing use of such an orthosis interact with someone else who has successfully used one to get a clear sense of what is required and what the potential outcomes are.

Outcome Measures in Orthotic Rehabilitation

How do the healthcare team, the individual using an orthosis and their caregivers, and the payers of the healthcare system determine successful use of a lower extremity orthosis, whether it be as simple as a UCBL insert for a child with mild diplegic cerebral palsy, an adult using an articulating AFO, a person with postpolio syndrome using a SC-KAFO, or a person with SCI using an ARGO? Initial criteria to consider might include:

- Can the person don and doff the orthosis independently?
- Does the person understand how the orthosis should fit on the limb, and can the person recognize signs that fit may not be appropriate (especially for growing children and for adults with peripheral or central sensory impairment)?
- Can the person transition from sitting to standing and back to sitting safely, independently, and with reasonable effort?
- Does the person have sufficient postural control to use the device not only on level nonresistant surfaces (e.g., tile or wood floors) but also on other surfaces (e.g., carpet, grass, inclines, stairs), which are likely to be encountered in the course of daily life?
- Children often play on the floor, and adults are often concerned with risk of falls. Can the person transition from

the floor to standing safely, independently, and with reasonable effort? If not, can the person direct those who would offer assistance?
- Does the person know how to manage his or her body and assistive devices in case of a fall?
- Does the person understand the care and maintenance requirements of the device?

These questions, while ensuring that the individual is able to use the orthosis safely, do not sufficiently address the efficacy of the orthosis in enhancing the individual's ability to walk. Although observational gait analysis might allow the orthotist and physical therapist to evaluate changes in orthotic effects at each subphase of the gait cycle, this description of the quality of walking is not enough evidence to justify orthotic intervention. A variety of outcome measures must be used to address efficacy of an orthosis and the physical therapy intervention that facilitates its use.

WALKING SPEED

Probably the most robust indicator of the ability to walk is walking (gait) speed. Although technology can provide precise data about gait velocity, walking speed can be quickly and easily captured using a stopwatch over a known distance.[103,104] There is clear evidence for validity, reliability, and responsiveness of walking speed (measured over a 10-m distance), as well as information about typical walking performance values, correlations with fall risk, and criteria for limited versus full community ambulation ability for most of the medical diagnoses in which a lower extremity orthosis may be prescribed (stroke, SCI, cerebral palsy, traumatic brain injury, among others).[103,105] Documenting comfortable and maximum walking speed at intervals without and with the orthosis at time of delivery and change in walking speed over the course of physical therapy intervention, along with discussion of the change in walking speed with respect to age-base and disease-reference norms, provide powerful information about efficacy of intervention.

ENDURANCE DURING WALKING

The ability to sustain walking over a period is also a key outcome of orthotic and physical therapy intervention. The most frequently used measure of endurance while walking is the 6-minute walk test, in which the distance an individual walks during a 6-minute period is measured. Also valid is a 2-minute walking test. Orthotic devices such as AFO can have significant positive impact on ambulatory capacity in a variety of conditions.[106–108]

A self-report indicator of effort of physical activity that has also been used extensively in the clinical research literature is Rating of Perceived Exertion. In his original work, Borg presented a scale ranging from 6 (no effort) to 20 (maximum effort)[109]; a modified version, which uses a 1 to 10 scale (for adults) or color-coded schematic pictures of the face (for children and those with cognitive dysfunction), may be more interpretable for patients.[110,111] Improvements in walking endurance have been demonstrated across multiple patient populations with orthotic intervention. Specific device design or features are specific to the individual need, making superiority of one type over another difficult to assess.[53,106,112]

MOBILITY AND BALANCE WHILE WALKING

The ability to change direction and transition between surfaces (i.e., sit to stand) is also a key aspect of successful use of a lower extremity orthosis. During the TUG test, an individual must rise from a seated position, walk forward over a 3-m distance, turn around, walk back to the chair, and return to sitting, either at a usual pace or as quickly and safely as able.[113] Because most lower extremity orthoses constrain joint movement, and many of those who use them have neuromuscular impairments that place them at risk for falling, the TUG may provide a snapshot of dynamic postural control during walking with an orthosis. The TUG has been successfully used to assess functional status and predict outcomes in persons with a variety of neurologic and orthopedic conditions across the lifespan.[106,114] Self-reported measures, such as the Falls Efficacy Scale and Activities-Specific Balance Confidence Scale, can supplement performance-based outcomes to measure the change in a patient's fear of falling pre- and postbracing.[89,115–118]

Summary

This chapter explored the biomechanical design and component options of lower extremity orthoses used to facilitate the ability to walk for persons with a variety of neuromuscular impairments and at various ages and developmental stages of the life span. We discovered that no orthosis can make walking "normal," although an appropriate orthosis can make walking more functional and less energy costly. We currently can evaluate how an orthosis will impact each of the rockers of stance phase, as well as the ability to clear the limb during swing phase. We currently have ideas about how footwear, such as an athletic shoe that provides a cushion heel and a rocker bottom, may compensate if an orthosis limits forward progression over the foot during stance. We discovered that the selection of an appropriate orthosis involves input from many members of the rehabilitation team, not the least being the person who will wear the orthosis and his or her caregivers. We certainly gained an appreciation that there is no "one size fits all" when it comes to choosing an orthosis, but that orthotic prescription requires thoughtful deliberation about both the functional benefits and tradeoffs, as well as the financial cost of the device. We learned that using an orthosis effectively requires much more than simply putting it on; there must be adequate time filled with appropriately challenging activities so that motor practice can build skill, postural control, and endurance necessary for functional walking. Finally, we began to consider strategies to assess outcomes of orthotic and physical therapy interventions for persons who require an AFO, KAFO, or HKAFO to accomplish their mobility goals.

Acknowledgments

The authors recognize professional colleagues Robert S. Lin, CPO (Director of Pediatric Clinical Services and Academic

Programs, Hanger Orthopedic Group at the Connecticut Children's Medical Center, Hartford, Connecticut), Thomas V. DiBello, BS, CO (President, Dynamic Orthotics and Prosthetics, Inc., Houston, Texas), and James H. Campbell, PhD, CO (Director of Research and Development, Engineering and Technical Services, Becker Orthopedic, Troy, Michigan), whose excellent chapters on ankle-foot orthoses, knee-ankle-foot orthoses, and hip-knee-ankle-foot orthoses in the previous editions of this text provided a solid foundation for this integrative chapter.

Case Examples

Recommendations are intended as ideas and guides for the clinician, not an all-inclusive or complete answer.

Case Example 9.1

P.M. is a 7-year-old child with a primary diagnosis of spastic diplegic cerebral palsy. He is anxious to keep up with his nonimpaired peers at school, but his moderate "crouch gait" (despite using Lofstrand crutches as assistive devices) limits his mobility and endurance. He is referred by his neurologist for evaluation in the interdisciplinary "brace clinic" at the local children's medical center.

On physical examination, P.M. is found to have moderate tightness and soft tissue shortening of his plantar flexors, distal hamstrings, adductors, and hip flexors. Although he exhibits moderate extensor-pattern spasticity in both lower extremities, sagittal and coronal plane motions of his hip, knee, and ankle are within 10 degrees of normal. Structurally, he exhibits 25 degrees of femoral anteversion and 15 degrees of internal tibial torsion. However, upon barefoot weight bearing, his foot progression angles appear to be normal, at approximately 10 degrees external (outward) angle.

QUESTIONS TO CONSIDER

- What are the most likely gait problems in each subphase of gait that might be effectively addressed by an AFO?
- What musculoskeletal (alignment and flexibility) and neuromuscular (control) impairments or characteristics, as well as developmental issues, will have to be considered by the team as they sort through orthotic options for this child?
- Which of the orthotic options (static vs. dynamic) might you choose for this child? What are the possible benefits and tradeoffs of each?
- How might you assess if the orthosis chosen is accomplishing the desired outcomes?

RECOMMENDATIONS OF THE TEAM

Given the finding of dynamic pes planus and valgus deformity and the boy's propensity to crouch during stance, the team recommends bilateral polypropylene SAFO be custom molded for P.M. When P.M. receives his AFOs, he attends several sessions of outpatient gait training. His gait pattern demonstrates improved plantarflexion–knee extension couples, with virtually all of the preorthosis knee persistent knee flexion eliminated. Subtalar joint alignment is also improved, with an effective support of the medial longitudinal arch.

FOLLOW-UP CARE

Three weeks later, the patient's mother schedules a follow-up visit because, as she observes, "The AFO is causing P.M.'s feet to turn in." On this return visit, observational gait assessment reveals an apparent 30-degree internal (inward) foot progression bilaterally. This is causing difficulty with clearance of the advancing limb during swing phase. Examination of the fit and alignment of the AFOs reveals appropriate design and fit, with effective subtalar neutral position.

The team recommends computerized gait analysis to be performed to determine the underlying factors leading to this significant change in foot progression angle despite appropriately fit and designed SAFO. The team suspects that this altered foot progression angle is most likely the result of underlying musculoskeletal deformities (tibial torsion and femoral anteversion) unmasked when compensatory motion of the subtalar and midtarsal joints during stance is restricted by the AFOs. In effect, when foot alignment is well supported by the AFO, the effect of excessive tibial torsion and femoral anteversion during gait become more evident.

It is not possible for an AFO to effectively address or control gait problems arising from existing underlying transverse plane (rotational) deformity. The team and family begin to consider the possibility of femoral/tibial derotation osteotomy as a solution to the gait problems that have emerged.

Case Example 9.2

A 40-year-old male presented to the emergency department with severe shooting back pain radiating down both legs (right greater than left), weakness of the feet, saddle anesthesia, and urinary incontinence for 2 to 3 weeks with worsening over the past 4 days. Magnetic resonance imaging revealed multilevel degenerative disease with severe central canal stenosis at L2–L3 and L3–L4, thoracic spine spondylosis with severe stenosis, and spinal cord compression C3–C7. He underwent C3–C7 and L2–L5 laminectomies. The patient continues to exhibit persistent weakness and foot drop bilaterally postoperatively.

1. *Past medical history*: Remote history of motor vehicle accident with severe right knee trauma.
2. *Social history*: Patient lives with fiancé in second-floor apartment with one flight of outdoor stairs with a single railing to enter plus one flight of stairs without a railing to the third-floor bedroom and bathroom. Prior to injury, patient was independent with activities of daily living, instrumental activities of daily living, and mobility.
3. *Patient goals*: To walk. To return to his apartment. To resume his studies to complete his undergraduate degree including mobility on campus.

He is now admitted to the acute rehabilitation SCI unit for functional retraining. Present examination findings include:

Case Example 9.2 **Cont'd**

1. *Sensation:* Intact light touch, localization throughout bilateral lower extremities
2. *Proprioception:* Impaired right great toe and ankle. Intact left great toe and ankle.
3. *Integumentary*: Intact
4. *Range of motion:* Right ankle dorsiflexion (DF) to neutral. Left ankle DF −6 degrees.
5. *Strength MMT:* Hip grossly 2–3/5. Knee extension 4/5. Knee flexion 2/5. Ankle 0/5 in all planes except left plantarflexion 1/5.
6. *Gait:* 40 feet with bilateral Lofstrand crutches with excessive knee flexion during weight acceptance, hyperextension thrust at early-to-midstance transition, excessive knee extension and genu varus during midstance and terminal stance phase, excessive plantarflexion throughout swing phase causing reduced foot clearance, excessive forward pelvic rotation and hip hike bilaterally during swing phase, B Trendelenburg hip drop, with step lengths short with swing heel landing near stance toe.
   - What are the critical phases of gait where the patient's body structure/function impairments are evident?
   - Which of these gait abnormalities could be supported/reduced using an orthosis?
   - What are the positive outcomes expected when using an orthosis for this patient (i.e., how will it improve mobility and gait, influence tone, or protect a limb or body segment)?
   - How might you assess whether the orthosis chosen is accomplishing the desired outcomes?

TEAM RECOMMENDATIONS

Weakness is evident during *weight acceptance* as demonstrated by excessive knee flexion and again during midstance as hyperextension thrust is a compensation to lock the knee into a stable position due to the inability to effectively use strength to stabilize tibia advancement. Weakness is also negatively affecting *swing limb advancement* reflected in excessive plantarflexion and need for hip hike compensation.

An orthosis could stabilize the distal limb during stance, improving weight acceptance and reducing abnormal knee forces during forward progression. It could assist with functional shortening of the limb by limiting excessive plantarflexion, which could reduce the need for hip hiking and pelvic rotation compensations to clear the limb in swing.

An orthosis can be expected to reduce excessive biomechanical forces from abnormal foot and tibial position, as well as improve gait efficiency, reducing energy consumption and allowing further ambulation tolerance and greater independence.

Valid and highly recommended outcome measures for a patient with spinal cord injury that could be used to assess the patient's outcomes with the orthoses include the following: Walking Index for Spinal Cord Injury II (WISCI II), 10-meter walk test, Timed Up and Go, 6-minute walk test (Neuro EDGE SCI incomplete).

Case Example 9.3

An 81-year-old male presented to the hospital with weakness and was diagnosed with Guillain-Barré syndrome. He was treated with intravenous immunoglobulin/prednisone. His course was complicated by limb and bulbar weakness and aspiration pneumonia. He was transferred to an acute rehabilitation hospital for functional retraining.

Past medical history: Hypertension, hyperlipidemia, prostate cancer s/p prostatectomy, small left rotator cuff tear

Social history: Patient lives at home with wife in a two-level home plus basement. There are three steps to enter with a railing from the garage or three steps to enter the front entrance with no railing. The bedroom is located on the first floor as is the bathroom; however, the shower has a 6-inch lip to enter. There is one flight of 8 + 8 steps with railing to access the patient's second-floor home office. Prior to injury, the patient was independent with ADLs, IADLs, and mobility. He was playing tennis 3 days per week and bicycling during warm-weather months.

1. *Patient's goals*: To get in and out of bed independently. To walk. To negotiate stairs to his second-floor office. To return to tennis.

Present examination findings include:

1. *Sensation:* Absent to diminished throughout bilateral lower extremities
2. *Proprioception:* Absent at bilateral great toe and ankles
3. *Spasticity:* 0/4 (modified Ashworth Scale)
4. *Integumentary:* Intact
5. *Range of motion:* Hamstring muscle lengths limited to approx. 80 degrees bilaterally via straight leg raise.
6. *Strength MMT:* Right hip grossly 1/5. Left hip flexion 1/5 otherwise left hip 0/5. Bilateral knee extension 1/5. Bilateral hip flexion 2−/5. Right ankle DF 0/5. Left ankle DF 1/5. Bilateral ankle plantarflexion 1/5. Upper extremity strength is grossly 3/5 except hand function is limited to 2/5 bilaterally with impairments in fine motor control.
7. *Bed mobility:* Supine to sit with maximal assist of one person
8. *Transfers:* Sit to stand dependent via standing frame or maximal assist of two persons
   - What type of orthosis is most appropriate to consider for early standing and gait training with this patient?
   - What are the positive outcomes expected when using an orthosis for this patient (i.e., how will it improve mobility and gait, influence tone, or protect a limb or body segment)?
   - What are the expected disadvantages or tradeoffs that may be associated with use of an orthosis (i.e., the ways in which it may complicate daily activity, mobility, or preferred activities; the energy cost associated with its use; the relative expense of the device)?
   - What are the indications that the orthosis may be useful to the patient (i.e., the match between the person's characteristics and needs and what the orthosis will provide)?
   - Considering the prognosis for recovery with this patient, how might the patient's orthosis be progressed/changed as his motor control improves?

TEAM RECOMMENDATIONS

Prognostic indicators for patients with Guillain-Barré syndrome suggest that 80% are able to ambulate within 6 months and 84% are able to ambulate at 1 year. Therefore the SAFO can progress with the patient by adding a hinged or articulating ankle joint to allow tibial progression during stance or by cutting back the trim lines to lessen stability.

(Continued)

Case Example 9.3 **Cont'd**

Factors impacting the decision for early orthosis include significant muscle weakness, absent sensation and proprioception, and no tone present. Given lower extremity muscle strengths grossly in the absent (0) to poor (1) range, this patient will need a highly stable orthosis to maintain the ankle and knee in position to effectively stand. His upper extremities are also weak, limiting the patient's ability to rely on them for support in standing further, indicating the need for a highly stable brace. With no tone present, the patient will not be able to rely on tone to substitute for lack of strength. There do not need to be any considerations for a brace that will minimize spasticity. The absence of sensation and proprioception suggests that the brace must be well fitting to reduce pressure and shear forces that could occur during mobility.

Considerations for bracing selection could range from, at simplest, a custom-molded solid AFO to a more complex KAFO. In the interest of selecting the least restrictive prescriptive orthoses, a solid AFO would be an appropriate initial brace to provide stability to the ankle and knee by limiting tibia mobility, thus stabilizing the leg in standing.

A solid AFO will provide two primary patient benefits: stability in stance and assistance with clearance in swing.

The ankle ROM restrictions will provide distal stability to the limb in stance, limiting the degrees of freedom and allowing the patient and therapist to focus on proximal stability training at the core and trunk. The fixed ankle position will assist with swing limb clearance by limiting excessive plantarflexion during swing phase.

There may be increased caregiver burden for donning and doffing due to upper extremity weakness and impaired fine motor control.

The patient is unable to stand without an external standing device or two-person assist. Stabilizing the distal limb by orthoses may allow the patient increased standing tolerance and increased frequency of standing if it can be reduced to the assistance of a single caregiver.

Meythaler JM. Rehabilitation of Guillain-Barré syndrome. *Arch Phys Med Rehabil*. 1997;78(8):872–879; Rajabally YA, Uncini A. Outcome and its predictors in Guillain-Barré syndrome. *J Neurol Neurosurg Psychiatry*. 2012;83(7):711–718.

Case Example 9.4

A 70-year-old male presented to the hospital with left leg pain of 3 months' duration and weakness over the past several weeks due to diabetic amyotrophy now with worsening of right leg weakness.

1. *Past medical history*: Arteriosclerosis, diabetes mellitus, umbilical hernia (repaired), bradycardia
2. *Social history*: Patient lives with his wife in a two-story home with 15 steps to enter from the garage level to the first floor. He has an additional flight of stairs to the second floor, where his bedroom and full bathroom are. On the first floor are a small living area, couch, and bathroom with shower stall. Patient has been staying on the couch on the first floor due to 11 falls in the past month on stairs. A few months prior to presentation, patient was regularly hiking on weekends and working as a homeland security agent. One month prior to injury he began using a right short solid AFO due to foot drop and a cane. More recently he also began using a rolling walker.
3. *Patient goals*: To get his legs strong and to not have any more falls.

Present examination findings include:

1. *Sensation:* Absent light touch to bilateral feet, diminished light touch and localization throughout bilateral lower extremities distal to knee left worse than right.
2. *Proprioception:* Absent bilateral hallux. Diminished bilateral ankles.
3. *Integumentary:* Intact
4. *Range of motion:* Within functional limits but noted bilateral hamstring muscle length limitations.
5. *Strength MMT:* Left lower extremity grossly 2−/5 except knee extension 1/5.
6. Right hip flexion, adduction, and extension 4/5. Right hip abduction 3−/5. Right knee 3/5. Ankle dorsiflexion and plantarflexion 0/5.
7. *Gait:* 250 ft with rolling walker with minimal assistance except minimal- to-moderate assistance to recover when knees buckle. Patient wearing right personal short semi-solid AFO and left loaner Allard ToeOFF (carbon fiber) AFO. Gait is remarkable for left knee buckling when center of mass is anterior to the left foot during terminal stance, with similar but less severe presentation of right knee. Decreased left heel strike at initial contact, with absent foot clearance on left.

- Which of these gait abnormalities could be supported/reduced through the use of an orthosis?
- What are the positive outcomes expected when using an orthosis for this patient? (i.e., how will it improve mobility and gait, influence tone, or protect a limb or body segment).
- What are the expected disadvantages or tradeoffs that may be associated with use of an orthosis? (i.e., the ways in which it may complicate daily activity, mobility, or preferred activities; the energy cost associated with its use; the relative expense of the device)?
- Considering the prognosis for recovery with this patient, how might the patient's orthosis be progressed/changed as his motor control improves?

TEAM RECOMMENDATIONS

Given the patient's continued buckling with an AFO and his degree of weakness, a KAFO may be the most appropriate device to effectively assist with foot clearance and heel strike by stabilizing the ankle in near neutral while also providing limitations of tibial advancement and knee flexion during stance phase.

Use of an orthosis will allow control of knee and ankle joint range during weight bearing in stance phase. Limiting the range of both joints will prevent significant knee buckling, improving the patient's ability to ambulate safely, build confidence, and reduce fall risk.

Use of a KAFO is more complex for the patient to don and doff as part of activities of daily living. It is less cosmetically appealing compared with a less significant brace, such as an AFO. The brace will limit ROM during sitting tasks. The KAFO has more bulk and weight than an AFO, only which can increase energy demands during gait.

The prognosis for recovery of strength is fair to good for persons with diabetic amyotrophy; therefore as the patient's motor control improves, the KAFO can be progressed to an AFO, providing more degrees of freedom for movement, reduced energy demand, and a less cumbersome donning/doffing process.

Case Example 9.5

A 69-year-old male presented to outpatient rehabilitation clinic with gait abnormalities in the setting of multiple sclerosis.

1. *Past medical history*: Hypertension, neurogenic bladder, rotator cuff syndrome, dyslipidemia, low back pain, osteoarthritis of the knee
2. *Social history*: Patient lives with his wife in a two-level home with stair slide to access the second floor. He is able to ambulate independently with a rolling walker. He has a manual wheelchair for community distances but rarely uses it.
3. Patient goals: To walk better. To walk in the community more.

Present examination findings include:

1. *Sensation:* Present but diminished light touch and localization in bilateral lower extremities distal to the knee.
2. *Proprioception:* Present bilateral ankle and hallux.
3. *Integumentary:* Intact
4. *Range of motion:* Within functional limits except bilateral ankle dorsiflexion limited to neutral.
5. Spasticity: 1 + bilateral ankle plantarflexors; 1 + bilateral hip adductors via modified Ashworth Scale.
6. *Strength MMT:* Lower extremities are grossly 2 to 3/5 throughout via functional observation except bilateral ankle dorsiflexion 2−/5 and bilateral ankle plantarflexion 2/5. Unable to formally do a manual muscle test due to inability to isolate single plane movement during testing in setting of increased lower extremity tone.
7. *Gait:* 40 ft with rolling walker and close supervision. Gait is remarkable for bilateral excessive plantarflexion during swing phase resulting in toe drag throughout; bilateral hip adduction with narrow base of support; short step lengths bilaterally; limited knee flexion during midswing phase and excessive knee extension, even hyperextension during stance phase.
   - What are the critical phases of gait where the patient's body structure/function impairments are evident?
   - Which of these gait abnormalities could be supported/reduced through the use of an orthosis?
   - What are the positive outcomes expected when using an orthosis for this patient (i.e., how will it improve mobility and gait, influence tone, or protect a limb or body segment)?
   - What are the expected disadvantages or tradeoffs that may be associated with use of an orthosis (i.e., the ways in which it may complicate daily activity, mobility, or preferred activities; the energy cost associated with its use; the relative expense of the device)?
   - Considering this patient's diagnosis, how might the patient's orthosis be progressed/changed over time?

TEAM RECOMMENDATIONS

The patient's dorsiflexion weakness is evident during *swing limb advancement*. Plantarflexor spasticity may also be a contributing factor to the excessive plantarflexion seen during swing phase. Both of these body structure/function impairments result in a functionally long limb. Combined with weakness of the more proximal limb muscles and adductor tone, the patient has insufficient foot clearance.

Ankle dorsiflexion can be easily supported through the use of an orthosis. One option for this patient could be a neuroprosthesis such as Bioness 300 or WalkAid. Peripheral nerve integrity should be intact given the patient's diagnosis with an upper motor neuron disease process. Stimulation applied to the common peroneal nerve/anterior tibialis timed with swing phase can increase functional strength of ankle dorsiflexion and potentially reduce effects of antagonist spasticity. This will in effect make the limb shorter and easier to clear during swing, as well as provide a more normal heel strike at initial contact.

If adductor tone and proximal muscle weakness are limiting his ability to achieve hip and knee flexion during swing, a thigh component such as the Bioness L300 + can be added to the hamstring to cause knee flexion during swing phase, further shortening the limb and allowing improved swing limb advancement. It is important to note that hamstring flexion during swing phase is not normal muscle activity during gait, rather hamstrings would normally only be active eccentrically as the patient approaches terminal swing. In this case, the neuroprosthesis is being used as a compensatory strategy to reduce the energy associated with foot clearance and reduce risk of falls from inability to clear the limb.

Use of a neuroprosthesis will provide improved gait efficiency by reducing effort for swing limb advancement, reduce fall risk by improving limb clearance, and possibly provide functional strength recovery with continued stimulation use.

Neuroprostheses are associated with greater cost than more traditional bracing styles and therefore likely require a higher level of documentation of medical necessity and possibly greater advocacy on the part of the patient to obtain clinic/insurance coverage. In addition, the maintenance requirements are higher for battery life and electrode life, and some require the pad to be damp, which could require the patient to re-dampen midday.

The patient's cognition and sensation should be monitored over time. The use of a neuroprosthesis requires greater insight of the patient to ensure proper maintenance and wear and skin integrity checks. This patient has a degree of impaired sensation. This is not a contraindication for use of a neuroprosthesis but must be considered with other factors to ensure the patient maintains a healthy integumentary system. If the patient's sensation decreases, it will require greater cognitive awareness to monitor skin regularly. If the patient's cognition declines, he may require assistance from a caregiver for skin checks or require another type of brace if he cannot individually manage it.

References

The complete listing of the References are available in the accompanying enhanced eBook version included with the print purchase of this textbook. Visit Elsevier eBooks+ (eBooks.Health.Elsevier.com) to access this content.

10 Neurological and Neuromuscular Disease Implications for Orthotic Use

ARCO P. PAUL, BRENDAN MCNULTY, KEVIN K. CHUI, AND DONNA M. BOWERS

LEARNING OBJECTIVES

On completion of this chapter, the reader will be able to do the following:

1. Describe the contribution of the major components of the central nervous system (CNS) and the peripheral nervous system (PNS) to functional, goal-directed movement.
2. Describe the impact of CNS and PNS pathologies commonly encountered in physical therapy and their implications for orthotic practice.
3. Explain the interaction of muscle tone and muscle performance on goal-directed, functional movement.
4. Describe the characteristics of muscle tone in the CNS and PNS pathologies most commonly encountered in physical therapy and implications for orthotic practice.
5. Describe the contributions of various CNS and PNS components to, and key determinants of, effective movement control.
6. Describe the contributions of various CNS components to, and key determinants of, motor control during functional activity.
7. Discuss the roles of orthopedic and neurosurgical procedures, central and peripherally acting pharmacological agents, and various orthotic options for the management of hypertonicity.
8. Plan a strategy for examination and evaluation of persons with CNS and PNS dysfunction to determine the need for an orthosis or adaptive equipment to optimize functional movements.
9. Describe strategies for orthotic use to reduce the risk of developing secondary musculoskeletal impairments in persons with hypertonicity.
10. Describe strategies for orthotic and adaptive equipment use to support postural control in persons with hypotonicity.

Movement Impairment in Neurological and Neuromuscular Pathology

Pathologic conditions of the neuromuscular system may manifest in a complex array of clinical signs and symptoms. To select the most appropriate therapeutic interventions, be it exercise to promote neuroplasticity and neurorecovery, functional training, or the use of various orthoses and assistive devices to accommodate for functional problems, the clinician must understand the implications of a medical diagnosis and prognosis of the disease process, and the ways in which a neurologic condition has led to impairments in body structures or functions, activity limitations, or participation restrictions in an individual.[1,2] The personal and environmental context of a person's impairments, activity limitations, and desire to participate in chosen pursuits must also be accounted for in deciding a course of physical therapy interventions, including the use of orthotics.

Health professionals use a number of organizational strategies as frameworks for decision-making during rehabilitation of individuals with pathologic conditions leading to neuromuscular dysfunction. Many neurologists use a medical differential diagnosis process of localization to determine whether the lesion is located within the central nervous system (CNS) or involves structures of the peripheral nervous system (PNS) or the muscle itself.[3] They do this by triangulating evidence gathered through focused patient histories, which leads to examination of tone, deep tendon reflexes, observation of patterns of movement, postural control, and specific types of involuntary movement.[3–5] They may also interpret results of special diagnostic tests such as nerve conduction studies, electromyography, computed tomography (CT), and magnetic resonance imaging.[6,7] These tests might pinpoint areas of denervation, ischemia, hemorrhage, or demyelination and help health professionals arrive at a medical diagnosis.

In collaboration with neurologists, rehabilitation professionals are most interested in the functional consequences associated with the various neuromotor conditions. They examine the ways in which the underlying neurologic condition affects cognitive function, sensory and motor systems, balance and coordination, and overall movement patterns during functional tasks.[8,9] Rehabilitation professionals are not only concerned about function at the present time but also consider the long-term impact of neuromotor impairment on the person's posture and movement abilities, including the changing needs in older adults with progressive conditions and growing children.[10,11]

This chapter considers the ways that key components of the CNS and PNS contribute to functional movement. We explore the concepts of muscle tone and muscle performance, considering how their interaction influences an individual's ability to move. We investigate how abnormalities of tone resulting from CNS and PNS pathologic conditions are described in clinical practice. We consider the determinants of postural control and of coordination and how CNS and PNS pathologic conditions might lead to impairments of balance and movement. We provide an overview of the ways commonly encountered CNS pathologic conditions impact muscle tone, muscle performance, postural control, movement, and coordination as a way of understanding how an orthosis or adaptive equipment might help improve an individual's ability to walk and use their arms/hands for functional movement to participate in meaningful activities and roles. We consider how the physical therapy examination contributes to the determination of a need for an orthosis or adaptive equipment. We also explore the clinical decision-making process by asking key questions about how an orthosis might help (or hinder) function. Finally, we apply what we have learned using five clinical cases to develop orthotic prescriptions.

Differential Diagnosis: Where Is the Problem?

Most neurological and neuromuscular diseases affect either the CNS or the PNS; only a few diseases, such as amyotrophic lateral sclerosis, affect both CNS and PNS. Diseases of the CNS and of the PNS may both contribute to motor or sensory impairment; however, there are patterns and characteristics of dysfunction that are unique to each. Selection of the appropriate orthosis, seating/wheelchair system, or other assistive devices is facilitated when the therapist, orthotist, members of the rehabilitation team, patient, and patient's family understand the typical patterns of functional loss and consequences of the disease process of the neurological subsystem that is affected.

THE CENTRAL NERVOUS SYSTEM

The CNS is the body's "central processing unit" and is responsible for giving us the ability to think, feel, and move. It also controls vital autonomic and physiologic functions that are important for maintaining life, helps us learn new information and skills, and processes our memories. Readers are encouraged to refer to a recent neuroanatomy or neuropathology textbook to refresh their understanding of CNS structure and function.[12] Knowledge of the roles of various CNS structures and their interactions is especially important for understanding the perceptual, postural control, coordination, and overall motor control systems[13] and is foundational for evidenced-based clinical decision-making when considering orthoses for individuals with neurologic dysfunction.

Some diseases affect a single CNS system or region (e.g., Parkinson disease affects basal ganglia's role of regulating voluntary movements; a lacunar stroke in the internal capsule may interrupt motor transmission only within the pyramidal/corticospinal system) leading to a specific array of signs/symptoms characteristic of that system or region. Other pathologic conditions disrupt function across several systems: a thromboembolic stroke in the proximal left middle cerebral artery may disrupt voluntary movement and sensation of the right side of the body, as well as communication and vision. Several exacerbations of multiple sclerosis may lead to plaque formation in the cerebral peduncles/pyramidal system, cerebellum, and spinal cord pathways, in which case it would be important to sort through the various types of impairments to select the most appropriate therapeutic or orthotic intervention for the individual.

Pyramidal System

The pyramidal system, specifically the lateral corticospinal and the corticobrainstem tracts, is responsible for the execution of voluntary movement.[14] The cell bodies of pyramidal neurons are located in the postcentral gyrus/primary motor cortex. The motor cortex (Brodmann area 4) in the left cerebral hemisphere influences primarily the right side of the body (face, trunk, and extremities); the right cortex influences the left side of the body. The axons of pyramidal neurons form the corticobulbar and corticospinal tracts, projecting toward alpha (α) motor neurons in cranial nerve nuclei and anterior horn of the spinal cord. To reach their destination, these axons descend through the genu and posterior limb of the internal capsule, the cerebral peduncles, the basilar pons, the pyramids of the medulla, and finally the opposite lateral funiculus of the spinal cord. A lesion at any point in the pyramidal system has the potential to disrupt voluntary movement. The degree of disruption varies with the extent and functional salience of the structures that are damaged, manifested on a continuum from mild weakness (paresis) to the inability to voluntarily initiate movement (paralysis).[14]

Immediately following insult or injury of the pyramidal system, during a period of neurogenic shock, there may be substantially diminished muscle tone and sluggish or absent deep tendon reflexes.[14] As inflammation from the initial insult subsides, severely damaged neurons degenerate and are resorbed, while minimally damaged neurons may repair themselves and resume function.[15,16] The more neurons that are destroyed, the greater the likelihood that hypertonicity will develop over time due to the altered balance of descending input of pyramidal (corticospinal) and extrapyramidal (reticulospinal, vestibulospinal, rubrospinal) tracts.[14] As the recovery period continues, individuals may begin to move in abnormal synergy patterns whenever voluntary movement is attempted.[17,18] When the damage to the system is less extensive, individuals may eventually recover some or all voluntary motor control; the more extensive the damage to the system, the more likely there will be residual motor impairment.[15,18]

Extrapyramidal System

The extrapyramidal system is made up of several subcortical structures and spinal pathways that influence motor planning, organize patterns of movement from among the many possible movement strategies, and make automatic feedforward (in anticipation of movement) and feedback adjustments (in response to sensations generated as movement occurs) during performance of functional tasks.[14,19] The motor planning system is a series of neural loops interconnecting the motor, premotor, and accessory motor cortices in the frontal lobes; the nuclei of the functional basal ganglia (caudate, putamen, globus pallidus, substantia nigra, subthalamus); and several nuclei of the thalamus. Damage to motor planning areas can lead to apraxia, the inability to effectively sequence components of a functional task and to understand the nature of a task and the way to use a tool in performance of the task.[20] Damage to basal ganglia structures can lead to muscle tone disruptions causing involuntary hypokinetic or hyperkinetic movement problems.[21] If there is damage to the caudate and putamen (also called the *corpus striatum*), underlying muscle tone may fluctuate unpredictably leading to involuntary writhing (athetosis) or dance-like (chorea) movement problems.[22] Damage to the subthalamic nuclei can lead to forceful, often disruptive, involuntary movement of the extremities (ballism) that interrupts purposeful activity.[22] Damage to the substantia nigra characteristically leads to resting tremor, rigidity of axial and appendicular musculature (hypertonicity in all directions), and bradykinesia (difficulty initiating movement, slow movement with limited excursion during functional tasks), which are most commonly seen in persons with Parkinson disease.[21] Motor impairments resulting from damage to the thalamic nuclei are less well understood but may contribute to less efficient motor planning, for example, by decreasing reaction times when initiating movements.[23]

The extrapyramidal pathways include the rubrospinal tract, the reticulospinal tracts, the tectospinal tract, and the vestibulospinal tracts.[19] The reticulospinal tracts, originating in the lower pons and medulla, are thought to provide feedforward adjustments for postural control and gross functional locomotion movements by influencing muscle tone of the proximal antigravity muscles.[14,19] The vestibulospinal tracts receive information about head movements from the vestibular system, and also help to maintain balance by influencing activity in the neck and proximal axial muscles.[14,19] The tectospinal tracts, originating in the collicular nuclei of the dorsal midbrain, also contribute to balance by controlling head and upper extremity movements based on incoming visual and auditory information.[19]

Coordination Systems

The coordination, or error-control, system is composed of several sensory and motor control components that dynamically interact with each other to provide smooth functional movements.[24–27] In anticipation of movement, motor planning information is shared between the cortical motor areas, the cerebellum via pontine nuclei, and the basal ganglia. Based on memory of past experiences of the intended movement, the cerebellum sends feedforward "prediction" of the consequence of the plan to the motor cortical areas via the thalamus and to the brainstem motor nuclei. The motor plan is then updated and sent down to the spinal motor neurons for execution of the motor task. Feedback information is generated during movement from the various peripheral somatosensory receptors (muscle spindles, cutaneous receptors) and sent to the cerebellum via the spinocerebellar pathways. The cerebellum compares this incoming sensory information to the "predicted" plan, and if an "error" is detected between the "intended" and actual movement consequences, it sends feedback adjustments to the motor cortical and brainstem centers to refine movements for improved coordination.[24,25] The role of the cerebellum in movement control is to act as a "comparator" and "callibrator" that constantly judges if the movement occurs as planned and if the outcome of the movement was as intended.

Somatosensory and Perceptual Systems

The somatosensory system is composed of a set of ascending pathways, each carrying specific sensory modalities from the spinal cord and brainstem to the thalamus, postcentral gyrus of the cerebral cortex, reticular formation, or cerebellum. The anterolateral (spinothalamic) system carries exteroceptive information nociceptors that monitor protective senses against injury (e.g., pain, temperature, irritation to skin and soft tissue).[19,28,29] This tract originates in the dorsal horn (substantia gelatinosa) of the spinal cord and the spinal trigeminal nucleus, crosses the midline of the neuraxis to ascend in the lateral funiculus of the spinal cord to the contralateral ventral posterior thalamus, and then continues to the postcentral gyrus. The dorsal column/medial lemniscus carries information from encapsulated receptors that monitor light touch and proprioceptive senses to track body movements.[28–30] This tract ascends from the spinal cord to reach the nuclei gracilis and cuneatus in the medulla of the brainstem, then crosses midline to ascend to the contralateral ventral posterior thalamus and on to the postcentral gyrus. The postcentral gyrus (somatosensory cortex) is organized as a homunculus, with each region of the body represented in a specific area.[19,28] Sensation from the lower extremities (lumbosacral spinal cord) is located at the top of the gyrus near the sagittal fissure. Moving downward toward the lateral fissure, the next area represented is the trunk (thoracic spinal cord), followed by upper extremities and head (cervical spinal cord), and finally face, mouth, and esophagus (trigeminal nuclei) just above the lateral fissure.[28] A lesion in one of the ascending pathways may result in a discrete area of numbness or loss of conscious proprioception in one area of the body; a lesion on the somatosensory cortex can lead to more profound, multimodality impairment on the opposite side of the body.

Although sensory information is logged in at the postcentral gyrus, the location of the somatosensory cortex, interpretation and integration of this information occurs in the somatoperceptual system in the parietal and temporal association areas.[30,31] These association areas further process the incoming sensory inputs in complex ways to give meaning to the sensations that are generated as people move and function in their environments. This is how people perceive and understand the relationships among their various extremities and trunk (body schema), as well as their relationship to and position within our physical environment. Lesions in these association areas often lead to conditions where patients are unable to perceive objects, events, or their own body parts in the affected space (neglect, agnosia), even though the sensory pathways are intact.[30,32]

Visual and Visual Perceptual Systems

The visual system begins with processing of information gathered by the rods and cones in the multiple layers of specialized neurons in the retina, located in the posterior chamber of the eye. Axons from retinal ganglion cells are gathered into the optic nerve, which carries information from that eye toward the brain. At the optic chiasm there is reorganization of visual information, such that all information from the left visual field (from both eyes) continues in the right optic tract, and that from the right field continues in the left tract. This information is relayed, through the lateral geniculate body of the thalamus, via the optic radiations, to the primary visual cortex on either side of the calcarine fissure of the midsagittal occipital lobe.[33–35] Damage to the retina or optic nerve results in loss of vision from that eye. Damage to the optic chiasm typically leads to a narrowing of the peripheral visual field (bitemporal hemianopsia). A lesion in one of the optic tracts or radiations leads to the loss of part or all the opposite visual field (homonymous hemianopsia). Damage to the visual cortex can result in cortical blindness, in which visual reflexes may be intact but vision is impaired.[34,35]

Visual information and its environmental context is further interpreted and perceived through complex communication between the various visual association areas that are spread out in the frontal, temporal, parietal, and occipital lobes.[35,36] Specific details about the environment, especially about speed and direction of moving objects with respect to the self and of the individual with respect to a relatively stationary environment, are important to perceive for appropriate functional movements depending on the task.[37] Interconnections between the frontal, parietal, and occipital association areas serve to integrate visual, somatic/kinesthetic perception, and memory to provide important input for motor planning and motor learning systems.[35,38]

Effective visual information processing is founded on three interactive dimensions: visual spatial orientation, visual perceptual skills, and visual motor skills.[39] Developmentally, visual spatial orientation includes spatial concepts used to understand the environment, the body, and the interaction between the body and environment that are part of functional activity (e.g., determining location or direction with respect to self, as well as respect to other objects or persons encountered as people act in their environment). Visual analysis skills allow people to discriminate and analyze visually presented information, identify and focus on key characteristics or features of what people see, use mental imagery and visual recall, and respond or perceive a whole when presented with representative parts. The visual motor system links what is seen to how the eyes, head, and body move, allowing one to use visual information processing skills during skilled, purposeful activities. This also provides the foundation for movements requiring eye-hand coordination, both large upper extremity movements such as throwing, and fine movement skills such as typing or manipulation of objects.[25]

Executive Function and Motivation

The ability to problem solve, consider alternatives, plan and organize, understand conceptual relationships, multitask, set priorities, and delay gratification, as well as the initial components of learning, are functions of the frontal association areas of the forebrain.[40,41] These dimensions of cognitive function are often described by the phrase *higher executive function*. Quantitative and other analytical skills are thought to be primarily housed in the frontal association areas of the left hemisphere, while intuitive understanding and creativity may be more concentrated in the right hemisphere. Most people tap the resources available in both hemispheres (via interconnections through the corpus callosum) during daily life, although some may fall toward one end or another of the analytical–intuitive continuum. Individuals with acquired brain injury involving frontal lobes often exhibit subtle deficits that have a significant impact on their ability to function in complex environments, as well as under conditions of high task demand; difficulty in these areas certainly compromises functional efficiency and quality of life.[42,43]

The neuroanatomical structures that contribute to the motivational system include the nuclei and tracts of the limbic system, prefrontal cortex, and temporal lobes; all play major roles in managing emotions, concentration, learning, and memory.[41,44] The motivational system not only has an important impact on emotional aspects of behavior but also influences autonomic/physiological function, efficacy of learning, interpretation of sensations, and preparation for movement (Fig. 10.1).[45] Dimensions of limbic function that influence motivation and the ability to manage challenges and frustration include body image, self-concept, and self-worth as related to social roles and expectations, as well as the perceived relevance or importance (based on reward or on threat) of an activity or situation.[46,47] The structures of the limbic system play a crucial role as motivators and repositories of memory, influencing readiness to move or act.[48] This system helps individuals predict movement needs in various situaons by drawing on past experiences, considering both the physical and emotional dimensions of the environment.[49]

Consciousness and Homeostasis

The ability to be alert and oriented when functioning in a complex environment is the purview of the consciousness system and is a function of interaction of the brainstem's reticular formation, the filtering system of thalamic nuclei, and the thinking and problem solving that occur in the association areas of the telencephalon, especially in the frontal lobes.[50,51] The reticular-activating system, located in the inferior mesencephalon and upper pons of the brainstem, is responsible for regulating the sleep-wake cycles and level of alertness.[51] The thalamus and the reticular formation help people habituate to repetitive sensory stimuli while they focus on the type of sensory information that is most relevant to the task at hand.[52] The frontal association areas are known to provide cognitive flexibility and fluid decision-making ability to generate appropriate adaptive behavior depending on the environmental, social, and motivational contexts.[53] Alteration in quality and level of consciousness and behavior are indicators of evolving problems within the CNS.[54] Increasing intracranial pressure, the result of an expanding mass or inflammatory response following trauma or ischemia in the CNS, may be initially manifest by confusion and impairment in cognitive functions (lethargy, memory, and attention problems), but may progress to more severe states of altered consciousness, including wakeful unresponsiveness (sometimes described as vegetative state) or even coma, if brainstem structures keep getting compressed due to herniation of nearby lobes.[55]

Homeostasis and the ability to respond to physiological stressors are functions of the components of the autonomic nervous system.[56] The nuclei of the hypothalamus serve as the command center for parasympathetic and sympathetic nervous system activity via projections to parasympathetic cranial nerve nuclei in the brainstem, the sympathetic centers of the intermediate horn in the thoracic spinal cord, and

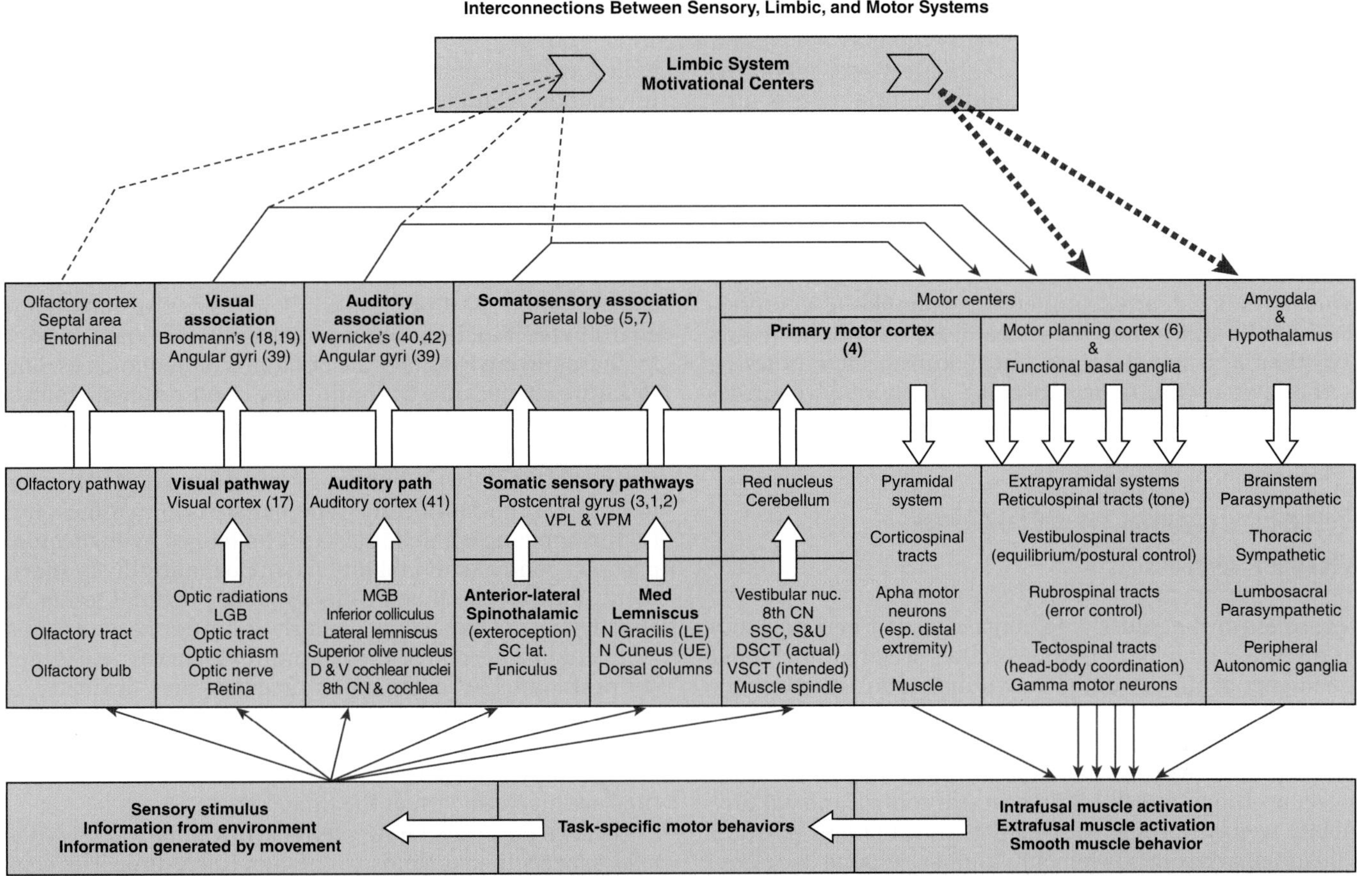

Fig. 10.1 A conceptual model of the interactions and interconnections among sensory, limbic, and motor systems that influence functional movement. *CN*, Cranial nerve; *D*, dorsal; *DSCT*, dorsal spinocerebellar tract; *N Cuneus*, nucleus cuneus; *N Gracilis*, nucleus gracilis; *S&U*, saccule & utricle DB; *SC lat*, spinal cord lateral; *SSC*, somatosensory cortex; *V*, ventral; *VPL*, ventral posterolateral nucleus; *VPM*, ventral posteromedial nucleus; *VSCT*, ventral spinocerebellar tract.

the parasympathetic centers in the lumbosacral spinal cord. The hypothalamus has extensive interconnections with the limbic system, bridging physiological and emotional/psychological aspects of behavior and activity.[57] The hypothalamus also integrates neural-endocrine function through interconnections with the pituitary gland. Clearly, this relatively small area of forebrain plays a substantial integrative role in physiological function of the human body. Damage or dysfunction to this area therefore has significant impact on physiological stability and stress response.

PERIPHERAL NERVOUS SYSTEM

The PNS serves two primary functions: to collect information about the body and the environment and to activate muscles during functional activities. Afferent neurons collect data from the various sensory receptors distributed throughout the body and transport this information to the spinal cord and brainstem (sensory cranial nerves) for initial interpretation and distribution to CNS centers and structures that use sensory information in the performance of their various specialized roles.[58] The interpretation process can have a direct impact on motor behavior at the spinal cord level (e.g., deep tendon reflex) or along any synapse point in the subsequent ascending pathway (e.g., righting and equilibrium responses) as sensory information is transported toward its final destination within the CNS.[59] Efferent neurons (also described as lower motor neurons or, more specifically, α and γ motor neurons) carry signals from the pyramidal (voluntary motor) and extrapyramidal (supportive motor) systems to extrafusal/striated and intrafusal (within muscle spindle) muscle fibers that direct functional movement by executing the CNS's motor plan.[19,60,61]

The cell bodies of these α and γ motor neurons live in the anterior horn of the spinal cord and in cranial nerve somatic motor nuclei. In the spinal cord, α and γ axons project through the ventral root, are gathered into the motor component of a spinal nerve, and (in cervical and lumbosacral segments) are reorganized in a plexus before continuing toward the targeted muscle as part of a peripheral nerve. In the brainstem, α and γ axons project to target muscles via motor cranial nerves (oculomotor, III; trochlear, IV; motor trigeminal, V; abducens, VI; facial, VII; glossopharyngeal, IX; spinal accessory, XI; hypoglossal, XII).[33,59,62] When α and γ axons reach their target set of muscle fibers (motor unit), a specialized synapse—the neuromuscular junction—triggers muscular contraction.[63]

Pathologic conditions of the PNS can be classified by considering two factors: the modalities affected (only sensory, only motor, or a combination of both) and the anatomical location of the problem (at the level of the sensory receptor, along the neuron itself, in the dorsal root ganglion, in the anterior horn, at the neuromuscular junction, or in the muscle itself).[64,65] Poliomyelitis is the classic example of an anterior horn cell disease; Guillain-Barré syndrome is a demyelinating infectious autoimmune neuropathy that impairs transmission of electrical impulses over the length of motor and sensory nerves. The polyneuropathy of diabetes (affecting motor, sensory, and autonomic fibers) is the classic example of a metabolic neuropathy. Radiculopathies (e.g., sciatica) result from compression or irritation at the level of the nerve root, while entrapment syndromes (e.g., carpal tunnel) are examples of compression neuropathies over the more distal peripheral nerve. Myasthenia gravis, tetanus, and botulism alter function at the level of the neuromuscular junction. Myopathies and muscular dystrophies are examples of primary muscle diseases.[65]

Determinants of Effective Movement

Regardless of the underlying neurological or neuromuscular disease, rehabilitation professionals seek to understand the impact of the condition on an individual's motor control (ability to initiate, guide, sustain, and terminate movement) by determining the underlying effects on muscle tone and muscle performance (strength, power, endurance, speed, accuracy, and fluidity); postural control and balance (ability to stay upright, to anticipate how to make postural adjustment during movement, and to respond to unexpected perturbations); and coordination to move effectively during goal-directed, functional movement necessary for daily life.

MUSCLE TONE AND MUSCLE PERFORMANCE

Effectiveness of purposeful movement is determined by the interaction of underlying muscle tone and muscle performance. *Muscle tone* can be conceptualized as the interplay of compliance and stiffness of muscle, as influenced by the CNS. Ideally the CNS can set the neuromotor system to be *stiff* enough to align and support the body in functional antigravity positions (e.g., provide sufficient baseline postural tone). At the same time, it allows the system to be *compliant* enough in the limbs and trunk to carry out smooth and coordinated functional movement and effectively respond to changing environmental conditions or demands as daily tasks are carried out.[66,67] In the tone continuum of stiffness to compliancy, the interplay of stiffness and compliance is optimal at the center, such that motor performance is well supported (Fig. 10.2, horizontal continuum). At the low-tone end of the continuum, where there is low stiffness and high compliance, individuals are challenged by inadequate postural control and inability to support antigravity movement, and by the inability to support proximal joints for effective use of limbs, particularly in antigravity motions. At the high-tone end of the continuum, where there is high stiffness and low compliance, freedom and flexibility of movement are compromised. Among individuals, postural tone varies with level of consciousness, level of energy or fatigue, and perceived importance (salience) of the tasks they are involved with at the time.[26,68]

Effective purposeful movement occurs when *muscle performance* meets the demands of the movement task. The components of muscle performance are the ability to (1) produce sufficient force (strength); (2) produce at the rate of contraction required for the task at hand (speed); (3) sustain the

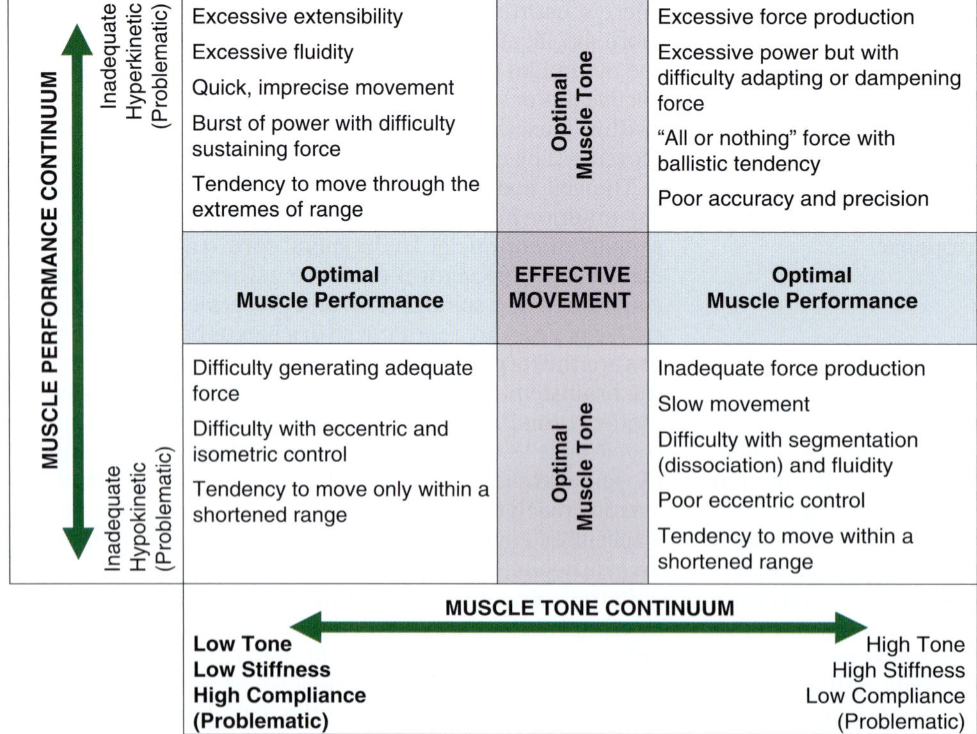

Fig. 10.2 A conceptual model of the interrelationship of muscle tone and muscle performance as they interact to influence functional movement. The muscle tone ranges from excessively compliant (easily extensible on passive movement) to excessively stiff (resistant to passive movement). The muscle performance continuum ranges from hypokinetic (exhibiting minimal movement during task activity) to hyperkinetic (exhibiting excessive movement during task activity). Movement is most effective at the intersection of optimal muscle tone (with balanced stiffness and compliance) and optimal muscle performance (with appropriate force production and adaptability of speed and power).

concentric, holding/isometric, or eccentric contraction necessary to meet task demands (muscle endurance); (4) ramp up or dampen force production in response to task demands (accuracy and power); and (5) coordinate mobility and stability of body segments to complete the task (fluidity).[69] Muscle performance can also be conceptualized as having a continuum with optimal control of its components around the center and inadequate control on either side: hypokinesis (little movement) at one extreme and hyperkinesis (excessive movement) at the other (see Fig. 10.2, muscle performance continuum).

While muscle tone and muscle performance are distinct contributors to movement, they are certainly interactive.[70,71] Movement is most effective and efficient when an individual's resources fall within the center of each continuum. A problem with muscle tone, muscle performance, or a combination of both leads to abnormal and less effective and efficient movement. Consider what will happen if there is a combination of low-tone and inadequate hypokinetic muscle performance: individuals will have difficulty with postural control and proximal support for limb movement, force production, power, and eccentric and isometric control, such that movement will tend to occur in shortened ranges and for short periods of time (less sustainability of contraction/endurance). For example, an infant with Down syndrome (characterized by low-tone) struggles to sustain adequate support of the shoulder girdle in prone on elbows to lift one arm to reach for a toy (hypokinesis).

In the presence of low-tone and hyperkinetic muscle performance, movement is fast but imprecise, with bursts of power that cannot be sustained. For example, a toddler with Down syndrome (with low tone) who is beginning to walk takes rapid and inconsistent steps (hyperkinesis). In contrast, in the presence of high-tone and hypokinetic muscle performance, movement is slow and stiff, with inadequate force production, compromised segmentation, impaired eccentric control (difficulty letting go), and constrained range. For example, an individual with Parkinson disease takes short steps and has little reciprocal arm swing when walking.

In the presence of high-tone and hyperkinetic muscle performance, there tends to be "all or nothing" force production, with somewhat ballistic and inaccurate movement occurring between the extremes of ranges. For example, a child with spastic quadriplegic cerebral palsy (CP) rising from sitting to standing often employs rapid mass extension (lower extremity and trunk), compromising his or her ability to move toward flexion to effectively rise; the child would also have difficulty lowering back into sitting without collapsing. Although muscle performance, especially the ability to generate force, does tend to decline with aging, the impact of inactivity is even more profound; all aspects of muscle performance can improve with appropriate training, even in the very old.[72–74]

Traditionally, an individual's muscle tone has been described clinically as hypertonic or spastic, rigid, hypotonic or low, flaccid, or fluctuating.

Hypertonus and Spasticity

Hypertonus is a term used to describe muscles that are excessively stiff or overly biased toward supporting antigravity function. Spasticity is a type of hypertonus that typically occurs when there is damage to one or more CNS structures of the pyramidal motor system and is encountered as a component of many neuromuscular pathologies.[26,75–79] Decrements in underlying tone and muscle performance, in bipedal humans with impairment of the pyramidal system, most often occur in a *decorticate* pattern: the upper extremity is typically biased toward flexion, such that the limb can be easily moved into flexion but not into extension (decreased compliance of flexors). The lower extremity is biased toward extension, such that the impaired compliance of extensors makes movement into flexion difficult (Fig. 10.3). In persons with severe acquired brain injury, entire groups of muscles could become hypertonic and lead to abnormal posturing depending on the location of lesion. In decorticate posturing, flexor muscles in the upper extremities and extensor muscles in the lower extremities could become hypertonic, which reflects the loss of cortical control with motor patterns similar to those seen in a cortical stroke. In decerebrate posturing, the extensors of both the upper and lower extremities could become hypertonic, reflecting injury at the superior border of the pons, resulting in the loss of inhibitory control of the cortex and basal ganglia. A progression from decorticate to decerebrate posturing in the acute phase of care is seen as a negative sign, as lower levels of the brain are affected. Both decorticate and decerebrate conditions are unidirectional in nature; there is an increase of muscle stiffness and resistance to passive elongation (impaired compliance) in one group of muscles (agonists) with relatively normal functioning of opposing muscle groups (antagonists).

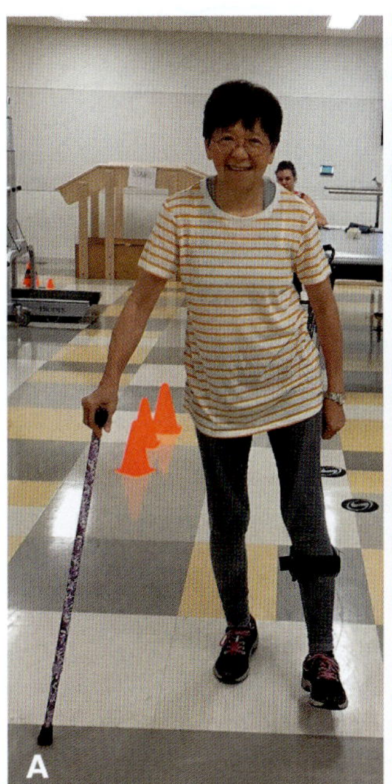

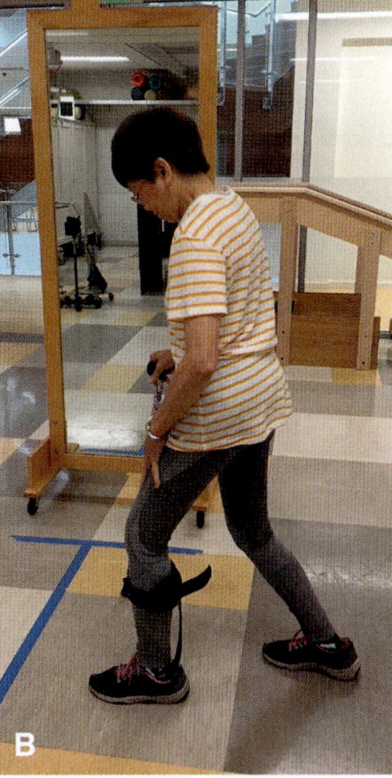

Fig. 10.3 Hypertonicity following cerebrovascular accident. (A) The extensor pattern hypertonus in the affected lower extremity precludes swing-limb shortening normally accomplished by hip and knee flexion; instead, the individual uses an abnormal strategy such as pelvic retraction and hip hiking to advance the involved limb; swing is assisted by the ankle-foot orthosis (AFO) to prevent plantarflexion at the ankle. (B) The affected upper extremity shows a flexed posture. Although the extensor bias in the lower extremity may cause hyperextension at the knee, the AFO provides a counter force to allow knee flexion.

Spasticity is a velocity-dependent phenomenon. Under conditions of rapid passive elongation, spastic muscle groups "fight back" with increased stiffness, a result of a hypersensitive deep tendon reflex loop (Fig. 10.4). Another aspect of spasticity is the clasp-knife response, in which the spastic limb "gives" after an initial period of resisting passive

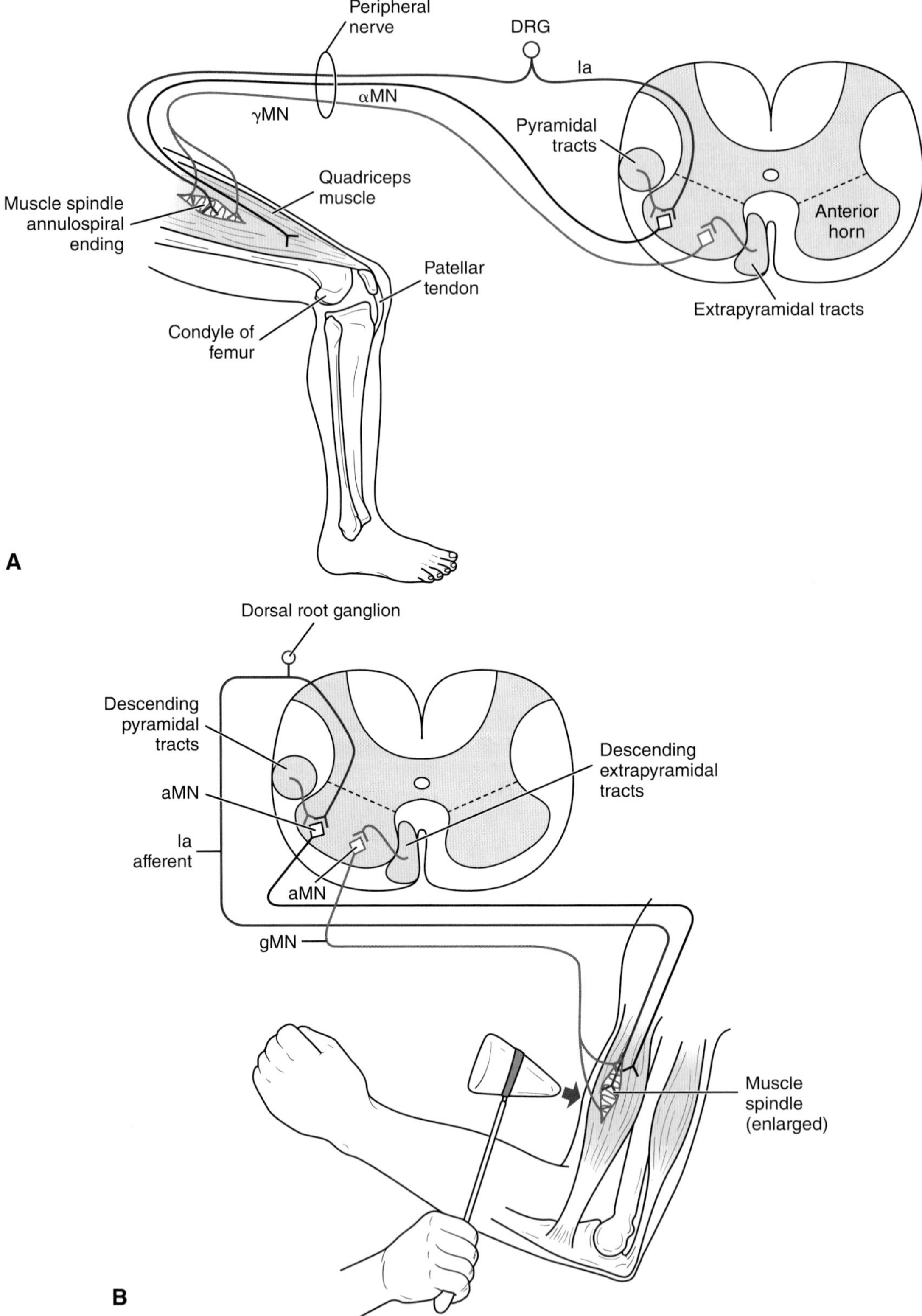

Fig. 10.4 Diagram of the deep tendon reflex loop: stimulation of the annulospiral receptor within muscle spindle of the quadriceps (A) and biceps brachii (B) (via "tap" on the patellar tendon with a reflex hammer) activates 1a afferent neurons, which in turn assist motor neurons in the anterior horn of the spinal cord. These motor neurons project to extrafusal muscle fibers in the quadriceps, which contract, predictably, as a reflex response. Sensitivity of muscle spindle (threshold for stimulation) is influenced by extrapyramidal input, reaching γ motor neurons (*γMNs*) in the anterior horn, which project to intrafusal muscle fibers within the muscle spindle itself. *aMN*, Alpha motor neuron; *DRG*, dorsal root ganglion; *gMN*, gamma motor neuron.

movement in the way a pocket knife initially resists opening when near its initially closed position but then becomes more compliant once moved past a threshold position as it is opened. Growing evidence indicates that the stiffness encountered during passive movement has both neurological (spasticity) and musculoskeletal (changes in muscle and associated soft tissue) components that combine to increase the risk of contracture development.[80,81]

Given the unidirectional nature of severe hypertonus, it is common for persons with severe hypertonus to develop chronic atypical postures. The limb or body segment assumes an end-range position the limb would not normally be able to assume (e.g., equinovarus with marked supination in an individual with severe acquired brain injury, equinovalgus with marked pronation in a child with CP).[80,82] If persistent, these fixed postures are associated with a significant likelihood of secondary contracture development.

Hypertonicity is also associated with deficits in muscle performance, most notably diminished strength (force production); diminished ability to produce power (force production with increased speed); diminished ability to effectively isolate limb and body segments (segmentation); diminished excursions of movements within joints (i.e., moving within a limited range of motion [ROM]); and inefficiency with altering force production or timing of contractions to meet changing (fluid) demands of tasks (accuracy and functionality).[83–85] Muscle performance deficits can contribute to an imbalance of forces around a joint that leads to habitual abnormal patterns of movement. These habitual patterns are often biomechanically inefficient and, over time, contribute to the development of secondary musculoskeletal impairments such as adaptive shortening or lengthening of muscles and malalignment of joints.[78] Strengthening exercises can have a positive impact on function, even in the presence of hypertonicity.[83,85,86] Orthotics and adaptive equipment play a crucial role in positioning and supporting trunk, limbs, and joints to prevent or minimize development of contractures in individuals with hypertonicity.

Rigidity

Individuals with Parkinson disease and related neurological disorders often demonstrate varying levels of rigidity: a bidirectional, co-contracting hypertonicity in which there is resistance to passive movement of both agonistic and antagonistic muscle groups.[21,87] Co-contraction of flexor and extensor muscles of the limbs and trunk creates a bidirectional stiffness that interferes with functional movement. Rigidity is often accompanied by slowness in initiating movement (bradykinesia), decreased excursion of active ROM, and altered resting postures of the limbs and trunk (Fig. 10.5). The rigidity of Parkinson disease can be overridden under certain environmental conditions: Persons with moderate-to-severe disease can suddenly run reciprocally if they perceive danger to themselves or a loved one; once this initial limbic response has dissipated, they will resume a stooped and rigid posture, with difficulty initiating voluntary movement, limited active ROM, and bradykinesia. Because rigidity creates a situation of excessive stability of the trunk and limbs, orthoses may not always have a beneficial effect in the functional mobility of individuals with Parkinson disease.[88]

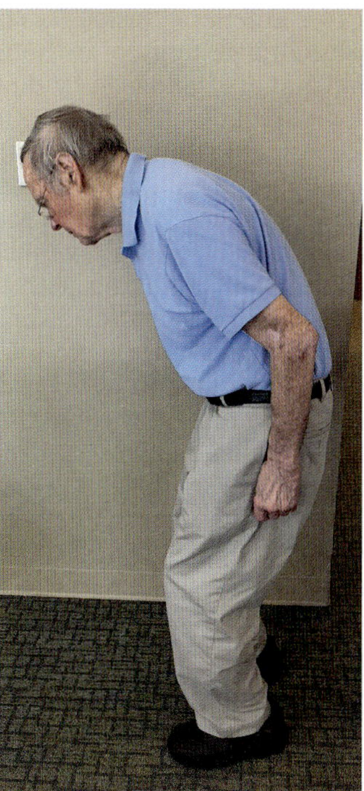

Fig. 10.5 A person with Parkinson disease showing typical standing posture; note the forward head, kyphotic and forward flexed trunk, and flexion at hip and knees. The upper extremities are held in protraction with flexion. The altered position of the body's center of mass, when combined with rigidity and bradykinesia, significantly decreases the efficacy of anticipatory postural responses during ambulation, as well as a response to perturbation.

Hypotonus

Hypotonus is defined as a decrease in skeletal muscle tone leading to decreased resistance to passive stretching.[89] As a result, hypotonic muscles do not produce adequate force during contraction or support upright posture against gravity. In children, hypotonia can arise from abnormal function within the CNS (approximately 75%) or from problems with peripheral structures (peripheral nerve and motor units, neuromuscular junction, the muscle itself, or unknown etiology).[90] Hypotonia can be congenital (seen as "floppy" infants), transient (e.g., in preterm infants) or part of the clinical presentation of CP, Down syndrome, and other genetic disorders, as well as autism spectrum disorders.[90–95]

Hypotonic muscles are considerably more compliant on rapid passive elongation (i.e., less resistant to passive stretch) than muscles with typical tone, as well as those with hypertonus/spasticity. Because their postural muscles are less stiff, individuals with hypotonicity often have difficulty when assuming and sustaining antigravity positions.[96] To compensate for their reduced postural tone, individuals with hypotonicity may maintain postural alignment by relying on ligaments and connective tissue within joint capsule and muscle to sustain upright posture. With overreliance on ligaments in extreme ends of range, further degradation to joint structures often occurs. Additionally, individuals may rely on the upper extremities for postural support, such as a child who uses arms to aid in floor sitting or an adult who holds onto a table when standing. This reliance on upper extremities diminishes the ability to use those extremities for functional tasks. This has implications for seating and standing systems, or orthotic use to provide external support that will allow individuals to use their upper limbs for play, work, and daily activities[90] (Fig. 10.6).

In addition to postural control dysfunction, individuals with hypotonia often have difficulty with coordination of movements. This may be due to the decreased efficacy of afferent information collected by a lax muscle spindle during movement execution.[90] Children with hypotonia often have impaired control of movements at midrange of muscle length, suggesting that kinesthetic information is not being used efficiently to guide movement or that the ability to regulate force production throughout movements is compromised. In either case, muscle performance is notably less efficient, especially in activities that require eccentric control (e.g., controlled lowering of the body from a standing position to sitting on the floor).[78,90] Individuals with hypotonia have difficulty regulating force production and collaboration between agonists and antagonists is not well coordinated.[89]

Immediately after an acute CNS insult or injury, there is often a period of neurogenic shock in which the motor system appears to shut down temporarily, with apparent loss of voluntary movement (paralysis) and markedly diminished or absent deep tendon reflex responses.[97–99] This phenomenon is observed following cervical or thoracic spinal cord injury and early on following significant stroke. During this period, individuals with extreme levels of hypotonus are sometimes (erroneously) described as having flaccid paralysis. Most individuals with acute CNS dysfunction will, within days to weeks, begin to show some evidence of returning muscle tone; over time, many develop hyperactive responses to deep tendon reflex testing and other signs of hypertonicity.[98] If they continue to have difficulty activating muscles voluntarily for efficient functional movement, these individuals are described as demonstrating spastic paralysis. Orthotics can be used to support joints in individuals with hypotonia to minimize degradation. For example, a child with hypotonia may use bilateral supramalleolar orthotics to provide improved postural support of the foot and ankle.[100]

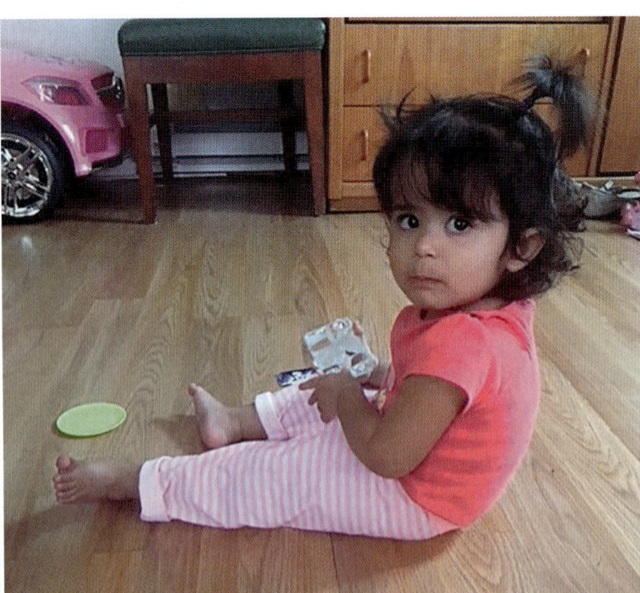

Fig. 10.6 Postural control is often inefficient in children (and adults) with hypotonicity or low tone. This 18-month-old child has insufficient muscle tone to maintain her trunk in an upright position; note the curvature of the thoracic and lumbar spine, with weight bearing on the sacrum (sacral sitting with kyphosis). This leads to shortening of the hamstrings over time, note right knee flexion.

Flaccidity

The term *flaccidity* is best used to describe muscles that cannot be activated because of interruption of transmission or connection between lower motor neurons and the muscles they innervate.[19,59] True flaccidity is accompanied by significant atrophy of muscle tissue, well beyond the loss of muscle mass associated with inactivity; this is the result of loss of tonic influence of lower motor neurons on which muscle health is based.[101]

The flaccid paralysis seen in persons with myelomeningocele (spina bifida) occurs because incomplete closure of the neural tube during the early embryonic period (soon after conception) prevents interconnection between the primitive spinal cord and neighboring somites that will eventually develop into muscles of the extremities.[102] The flaccid paralysis observed in persons with cauda equina-level spinal cord injury is the result of damage to axons of α and γ motor neurons as they travel together as ventral roots to their respective spinal foramina to exit the spinal column as a spinal nerve.[103] After acute poliomyelitis, the loss of a portion of a muscle's lower motor neurons leads to marked weakness; the loss of the majority of a muscle's lower motor neurons results in flaccid paralysis.[59] In Guillain-Barré syndrome, the increasing weakness and flaccid paralysis seen in the early stages of the disease are the result of demyelination of the neuron's axons as they travel toward the muscle in a peripheral nerve.[104] After injection with botulinum toxin, muscle tone and strength are compromised because of the toxin's interference with transmitter release from the presynaptic component of the neuromuscular junction.[105] Orthotics and adaptive equipment play a critical role in providing antigravity support for upright positioning and locomotion in individuals with flaccidity. Additionally, orthotics are used to prevent contracture in joints with unbalanced muscle activity. This allows individuals to participate in desired activities in the home, school, or community. For example, a child with a thoracic-level myelomeningocele may require adaptive seating for school, while a child with lumbar-level myelomeningocele may require orthotics for lower extremity support for ambulation, and a positioning device to prevent contractures of the hip adductors.[100]

Athetosis and Chorea

Athetosis is a term used to describe involuntary slow, writhing, purposeless movements, and is commonly seen in children with dyskinetic CP.[21] It is known to affect both distal and proximal muscles, making fine motor control and postural stability very difficult. It is thought to occur due to unpredictable fluctuations in muscle tone as a result of damage to basal ganglia and thalamus.[21,83,106] The etiology of athetosis is not well understood, but it is frequently attributed to hypoxic-ischemic injuries, hemorrhages and developmental malformations of the CNS occurring in the vulnerable brain of preterm or even full-term infants.[78] Another closely related involuntary movement problem resulting from such injuries is chorea, which is seen as abrupt, jerky movements in the limbs.[21] Chorea can also develop into involuntary "dance-like" movement patterns, commonly seen in Huntington disease, a genetic degenerative disease of the basal ganglia.[107] Individuals with dyskinetic syndrome often show combined choreoathetoid complex movement problems, resulting in lack of motor control and postural stability. They tend to compensate for postural instability by assuming end-range positions, relying on mechanical stability of joints during functional activity. Although less common than spasticity or hypertonicity, choreoathetosis can have a significant (and often more pronounced) impact on activities of daily living.[83,108] Individuals with choreoathetosis are less likely to develop joint contracture than those with long-standing hypertonicity, but they are more likely to develop secondary musculoskeletal complications that compromise stability of joints, a result of extreme posturing, imbalance of forces across joint structures, and the need to stabilize in habitual postural alignment patterns for function.[109] Orthotic usage in individuals with athetosis must be evaluated carefully to consider the balance of supportive versus restrictive influences of the device.

POSTURAL CONTROL

Postural control has three key dimensions: (1) *steady-state postural control* is defined as the ability to control the location of the body's center of mass (COM) within the area defined by the base of support (BOS) under predictable, quasi-static conditions, and this includes the ability to adapt motor behavior to meet the demands of different task and environmental conditions; (2) *anticipatory postural control* is the ability to generate postural adjustments prior to the onset of and during voluntary movement for the purpose of either countering an upcoming postural disturbance due to voluntary movement or realigning the body's COM prior to changing the base of support, and this includes the ability to adapt motor behavior to meet the demands of different task and environmental conditions; and (3) *reactive postural control* is the ability to respond to an unexpected sensory input (from perturbation originating external to the body or secondarily to an internally generated movement) that signals a need for a unanticipated response to ensure successful maintenance of postural control, and this includes the ability to adapt motor behavior to meet the demands of different task and environmental conditions.[110] One has functional postural control if the COM can be maintained within one's BOS under a wide range of task demands and environmental conditions. This requires some level of ability across the triad of steady-state, anticipatory, and reactive control.

The key interactive CNS systems involved in postural control include extrapyramidal and pyramidal motor systems; visual and visual perceptual systems; conscious (dorsal column/medial lemniscal) and unconscious (spinocerebellar) somatosensory systems; the vestibular system; and the cerebellar feedback/feedforward systems.[111] Clinical measures used to assess efficacy of steady-state postural control include timing of sitting or standing activities and measures of center of pressure excursion in quiet standing.[112] The Clinical Test of Sensory Interaction and Balance sorts out the contribution of visual, vestibular, and proprioceptive systems' contribution to balance, as well as the individual's ability to select the most relevant sensory input when there is conflicting information collected among these systems.[111,113]

Measures of anticipatory postural control consider how far the individual is willing to shift his or her COM toward the edge of his or her sway envelope during voluntary movements.[114,115] Clinically, anticipatory postural control is often quantified by measuring reaching distance in various postures, or by measuring stability during transitional movements.[116–118] Measures of reactive postural control consider the individual's response to unexpected perturbations (e.g., when pushed or displaced by an external force, when tripping/slipping in conditions of high environmental demand).[117–119] Although these three dimensions of postural control are interrelated, competence in one does not necessarily ensure effective responses in the others.[120]

Many individuals with neuromuscular disorders demonstrate inefficiency or disruption of one or more of the postural control subsystems.[121] An individual with mild-to-moderate hypertonicity or spasticity often has difficulty with anticipatory and reactive postural control, especially in high task demand situations within a complex or unpredictable open environment.[122,123] Difficulty with muscle performance, such as impairment of control of force production or the imbalance of forces acting across a joint, might constrain anticipatory postural control in preparation for functional tasks such as reaching or stepping. Impairment of the ability to segment trunk from limb or to individually control joints within a limb may affect the individual's ability to react to perturbations in a timely or consistent manner.[123] Individuals with hypotonicity also exhibit deficits in more than one postural control subsystem. They often have difficulty with sustaining effective postural alignment in antigravity positions such as sitting and standing.[90] They are likely to demonstrate patterns of postural malalignment such as excessive lumbar lordosis and thoracic kyphosis. Because of difficulty with muscle force production (especially in midrange of movement), individuals with hypotonia also have difficulty with anticipatory postural control.[124] A lack of on-demand motor control contributes to difficulty moving within one's postural sway envelope; this may be observed as a tendency to stay in one posture for long periods of time, with infrequent alterations in position during tasks.[124] Inability to activate postural muscles in anticipation of voluntary arm movements has been reported in children and adults with Down syndrome.[125] Reactive postural control is also impaired in such conditions. Children with Down syndrome have been shown to exhibit delayed activation of proximal muscles leading to sequencing problems between proximal and distal synergistic muscles following platform perturbations.[125] They are also shown to have delayed onset of protective postural responses to perturbations as compared to typically developing children.[125]

MOVEMENT AND COORDINATION

Many functional activities require us to move or transport the entire body (e.g., mobility or locomotion) or a segment of the body (e.g., using one's upper extremity to bring a cup toward the mouth to take a drink) through space. The locomotion task that receives much attention in rehabilitation settings is bipedal ambulation—the ability to walk. For full functional ability, individuals must be able to manage a variety of additional locomotion tasks: running, skipping, jumping, and hopping. To fully understand an individual's functional ability, therapists and orthotists must also consider the environmental context in which ambulation is occurring.[126] What are the physical characteristics of the surface on which the individual needs to be able to walk or traverse? Is it level, unpredictably uneven, slippery or frictional, or structurally unstable? Is the ambulation task occurring where lighting is adequate for visual data collection about environmental conditions? Does it involve manipulation of some type of object (e.g., an ambulatory assistive device, a school backpack, shopping bags, suitcases)? Is it occurring in a familiar and predictable environment (e.g., at home) or in a more unpredictable and challenging open environment such as a busy school, supermarket, mall, or other public space? The task demands of locomotion in complex and challenging environments create more demand on the CNS structures involved in motor control (perceptual-motor function, motor planning, cerebellar error control), as well as on the musculoskeletal effectors (muscles and tendons, joints, ligaments, and bones) that enact the motor plan necessary for successful completion of the task that relies on body transport. Individuals with neurological and neuromuscular system problems related to muscle tone, muscle performance, and postural control are typically less efficient, less adaptable, and more prone to fall when walking, especially if there are competing task demands and the environment is complex and challenging.[127]

The use of a limb segment can also be defined by the nature of the task and the circumstances in which the movement is performed. Upper extremity functional tasks can involve one or more components: reaching, grasping, releasing, manipulating, or any combination of these four purposes.[25] Upper extremity tasks can also be defined by considering the function to be accomplished by the movement: grooming, dressing, meal preparation, self-care, or writing. Many upper extremity mobility tasks are founded on effective postural control (e.g., making appropriate anticipatory postural adjustments as the COM shifts while throwing, lifting, lowering, or catching an object).[25] Complex mobility tasks require simultaneous locomotion and segmented use of extremities (e.g., reaching for the doorknob while ascending the steps toward the front door, throwing or catching a ball while running during a football or baseball game). For individuals with neurological and neuromuscular system dysfunction, the ability to safely and efficiently perform complex mobility tasks is often compromised due to abnormal muscle tone, impaired muscle performance, and poor postural control.[127]

Coordination can be thought of as the efficacy of execution of the movement necessary to complete a task. A well-coordinated movement requires effective simultaneous control of many different dimensions of movement: the accuracy of a movement's direction and trajectory; the timing, sequencing, and precision of muscle activation; the rate and amplitude of force production; the interaction of agonistic and antagonistic muscle groups; the ability to select and manage the type of contraction (concentric, isometric, or eccentric) necessary for the task; and the ability to anticipate and respond to environmental demands during movement.[128] Coordination can be examined by considering the individual's ability to initiate movement, sustain movement during the task or activity, and terminate movement according to task demands.[112]

For movement and coordination to be functional, one must have muscle performance that is flexible/adaptable to varying demands.[129] Mobility or transport tasks cannot be performed independently (safely) unless the individual is able to (1) transition into and out of precursor positions (e.g., getting up from the floor into a standing position, rising from a chair); (2) initiate or begin the activity (e.g., take the first step); (3) sustain the activity (control forward progression with repeated steps); (4) change direction as environmental conditions demand (e.g., step over or avoid an obstacle); (5) modulate speed as environmental conditions demand (e.g., increase gait speed when crossing the street); and (6) safely and effectively stop or terminate the motion, returning to a precursor condition or position (quiet standing, return to sitting).[129]

For individuals with neuromuscular disorders who have difficulty with muscle performance, abnormal tone, or impaired postural control, coordination of functional movement can be compromised in several ways. To complete a movement task, the individual might rely on abnormal patterns of movement with additional effort and energy cost.[130] Many individuals with hypertonicity initiate movement with strong bursts of muscle contractions but have difficulty sustaining muscle activity and force of contraction through the full ROM necessary to perform a functional movement.[127] Deficits in timing and sequencing of muscle contractions, as well as difficulty with dissociation of limb and body segments, also contribute to difficulty with performance of functional tasks.[131] An adult with hemiplegia following a cerebrovascular accident may be able to initiate a reach toward an object but not be able to bring the arm all the way to the target.[132] The same individual may have difficulty with timing and segmentation, leading to inability to open the hand before reaching the target in preparation for grasping the object.[133] The muscle performance of many children with CP is compromised by inappropriate sequencing of muscle contractions when activation of synergists and antagonists happens simultaneously.[127] Conversely, an individual with hypotonus who has difficulty with stabilization often moves quickly with diminished accuracy and coordination.[112]

The following tables provide an overview of incidence/prevalence, etiology and risk factors, clinical presentation, and impact on muscle tone, muscle performance, postural control, and movement for the most common pathologies that might indicate use of an orthosis: stroke (Table 10.1), CP (Table 10.2), spina bifida (Table 10.3), multiple sclerosis (MS) (Table 10.4), and spinal cord injury (SCI) (Table 10.5).

When considering an upper or lower extremity orthosis or an adaptive equipment system to support the trunk for individuals with neurological or neuromuscular dysfunction, the rehabilitation team must clearly define what they hope the orthosis will accomplish and consider the needs of the individual and family. Goals for orthosis and adaptive equipment usage include provision of stability for trunk, limb segment, or specific joint for postural control;

Table 10.1 Stroke

Also known as	Brain attack, cerebrovascular accident
Incidence	Approximately 795,000/year in the United States[a]
	~ 610,000 are first attacks.
	~185,000 are recurrent attacks
Prevalence	2.7% of total US population have had stroke[a]
	Prevalence of stroke by age and sex:
	20–39 years: Males = 0.3%, Females = 0.6%
	40–59 years: Males = 1.8%, Females = 2.4%
	60–79 years: Males = 6.5%, Females = 6.1%
	80+ years: Males = 13.8%, Females = 14.9%
Etiology and Risk Factors	
Ischemic stroke (87%)	
Thrombus	Hypertension, high blood cholesterol and other lipids, diabetes, overweight and obesity, smoking/tobacco use, nutrition, physical inactivity, family history/genetics, chronic kidney disease, sleep apnea, psychosocial factors
Embolism	Disorders of heart rhythm (e.g., atrial fibrillation), atherosclerosis in carotid/vertebral arterial systems; previous embolic stroke
Hemorrhagic stroke (10%)	
Intracranial hemorrhage	Uncontrolled hypertension, ruptured aneurysm
Stroke syndromes (By artery)	
Middle cerebral (most common)	Contralateral hemiparesis/hemiplegia, lower face, UE > LE
	Contralateral sensory loss of lower face, UE > LE
	Contralateral homonymous hemianopia (optic tract)
	Possible dysarthria and dysphagia
	R hemisphere: visual spatial or somatic perceptual impairment
	L hemisphere: communication impairment (various aphasias)
Lenticulo-striate (lacunar MCA)	Contralateral hemiparesis/hemiplegia, lower face, UE = LE
	Cortical functions (perception, communication) intact
Anterior cerebral	Contralateral hemiparesis/hemiplegia LE > UE
	Sensation often intact or only mildly impaired (contralateral)
	Incontinence
	"Alien hand" syndrome (involuntary/unintended movement)
	Motor (nonfluent/Broca) aphasia may occur
Posterior cerebral	Contralateral homonymous hemianopsia (optic radiations)
	Visual inattention
	L hemisphere: alexia (unable to read), with ability to write preserved
Thalamogeniculate (lacunar PCA)	Contralateral sensory loss, often severe
	Sensory ataxia (uncoordinated movement due to lack of proprioception)
	Thalamic pain and hyperpathia syndrome
Basilar (complete)	Loss of consciousness, comaHigh mortality
Superior cerebellar	Ipsilateral ataxia, falling to side of lesion
	Intention tremor
	Contralateral loss of pain temperature sensation from body
	Contralateral loss of proprioception
	Ipsilateral Horner syndrome (meiosis, ptosis, anhidrosis)
Anterior-inferior cerebellar	Ipsilateral facial paralysis (both upper and lower face)
	Ipsilateral loss of pain and temperature of entire face
	Contralateral loss of pain and temperature from body
	Loss of taste sensation, loss of corneal reflex, ipsilateral hearing loss, nystagmus, vertigo, nausea
	Ataxia and incoordination of limb movement
	Ipsilateral Horner syndrome (meiosis, ptosis, anhidrosis)
Vertebral	Contralateral loss of pain, temperature sensation from body
Posterior-inferior cerebellar (Wallenberg syndrome) (lateral medullary syndrome)	Ipsilateral loss of pain and temperature sensation from face
	Ipsilateral Horner syndrome (meiosis, ptosis, anhidrosis)
	Dysphonia, dysphagia, dysarthria, diminished gag reflex
	Nystagmus, diplopia, vertigo, nausea
	Ipsiversive falling (toward side of lesion), incoordination, ataxia

(Continued)

Table 10.1 Stroke—cont'd

Prognosis	Ischemic: severity depends on site of occlusion within arterial tree and the size of the area that is without blood flow Embolic: risk of recurrence is higher than in thrombosis; risk of hemorrhage at site of embolism Hemorrhagic: highest morbidity and mortality Static event, with evolving symptoms in weeks/months following initial damage, due to initial inflammatory response and subsequent tissue remodeling/healing
Muscle tone	Initial hypotonus (sometimes appearing to be flaccid) due to neurogenic shock. Some individuals remain hypotonic, most develop various levels of hypertonus in weeks/months following event. Hyperactive deep tendon reflexes evolve over time
Muscle performance	Upper extremity often biased toward flexion, with lower extremity biased toward extension. Impaired force production, speed and power, eccentric/isometric control, accuracy, and fluidity
Postural control	Frequently impaired, especially if lesion included gray matter of R hemisphere, with perceptual dysfunction
Mobility and coordination	Asymmetry in ability to use trunk, limbs during functional activity; tendency to move in abnormal "synergy" (flexion UE, extension LE). Frequently require AFO and ambulatory device

[a]Virani SS, Alonso A, Benjamin EJ, et al. Heart disease and stroke statistics-2020 update. *Circulation*. 2020;141(9).
AFO, Ankle-foot orthosis; *L*, left; *LE*, lower extremity; *MCA*, middle cerebral artery; *PCA*, posterior cerebral artery; *R*, right; *UE*, upper extremity.

Table 10.2 Cerebral Palsy

Prevalence in the United States	About 1 in every 345 children born in the United States.[a]
Prevalence in developed countries worldwide	1-4 per 1000 live births.[a]
Etiology	Abnormal development of the brain or damage that can happen before birth, during birth, within a month after birth, or during the first years of a child's life, while the brain is still developing.[a]
Risk factors	Low birth weight, premature birth, multiple births, assisted reproductive technology, infections during pregnancy, jaundice and kernicterus, medical conditions of mother, birth complications.[a]
Classification of CP	
Spastic CP[a]	
■ Spastic diplegia	Lower extremities affected more than upper extremities.
■ Spastic hemiplegia	Unilateral upper and lower extremities.
■ Spastic quadriplegia	All four extremities.
Most common type of CP, affects about 80% of people with CP[a]	Involvement of motor cortex and sensorimotor cortical tracts (gray and white matter). Spasticity and hyperreflexia contribute to impaired posture and movement.
Dyskinetic CP (also includes athetoid, choreoathetoid, and dystonic cerebral palsies)[a]	Involvement of the basal ganglia. Contributes to atypical posture and involuntary and sometimes stereotypical movement.
Ataxic CP[a]	Involvement of the cerebellum. Contributes to instability and altered posture, uncoordinated and imprecise movements.
Mixed CP[a]	Elements of spasticity and dyskinesia.
Gross Motor Function Classification System[b]	Standard for describing motor disability in children with cerebral palsy. Includes Levels I through V in children between 6th and 12th birthday and children between 12th and 18th birthday.
Children Between 6th and 12th Birthdays	Level I Walk at home, school, outdoors, and in the community. Can navigate stairs. Can run and jump. Difficulty with speed, balance, and coordination. Level II Walk in most settings and navigate stairs with railing. May have difficulty with long distances, uneven terrain, inclines, obstacles, or crowded spaces. May need physical assistance, handheld mobility device, or wheeled mobility for long distances. Minimal ability to run and jump. May need adaptations for recreational activities. Level III Walk with a handheld mobility device in indoor settings, navigate stairs with rail and assistance. Use wheeled mobility for long distances. Need adaptations for recreational activities. Level IV Mobility requires physical assistance or powered mobility in most settings. Require adaptive seating and body support walker for home and school activities. For community activities, require transportation in manual or powered wheelchair. Level V Require transportation in manual wheelchair, adaptive seating and standing systems. Require full assist for transfers and self-care.

Table 10.2 Cerebral Palsy—cont'd

Children Between 12th and 18th Birthdays	Level I
	Walk at home, school, outdoors, and in the community. Can navigate stairs and curbs. Can run and jump. Difficulty with speed, balance, and coordination.
	Level II
	Walk in most settings; environmental factors and personal preference influence mobility choices. May require handheld mobility device for safety and assistance or rail for stairs. May use wheeled mobility for long distances in community. May need adaptations for sports and recreational activities.
	Level III
	Walk with handheld mobility device; need assistance or rail for stairs. Need physical assistance or upper extremity support for transfers. At school may use self-propelled manual wheelchair or powered mobility. In community are transported in manual chair or powered mobility.
	Level IV
	Use wheeled mobility in most settings. Physical assist required (one to two persons) for transfers. Indoors may walk with assistance or body support walker. Outdoors are transported in manual chair or powered mobility.
	Level V
	Transported in manual chair in all settings. Require adaptive seating and standing systems. Self-mobility is severely limited even with assistive technology.

[a]Centers for Disease Control and Prevention. *Cerebral palsy*. https://www.cdc.gov/. Published February 23, 2023. https://www.cdc.gov/ncbddd/cp/index.html.
[b]Palisano RJ, Rosenbaum P, Bartlett D, Livingston MH. Content validity of the expanded and revised Gross Motor Function Classification System. *Dev Med Child Neurol*. 2008;50(10):744–750.

Table 10.3 Spina Bifida

Prevalence	About 1 in every 2,758 births in the United States. Hispanic females have the highest rate of having a child affected by spina bifida (3.80 per 10,000 live births), when compared with non-Hispanic White (3.09 per 10,000 live births) and non-Hispanic Black females (2.73 per 10,000 live births).[a]
Etiology	Unknown; genetics and environmental factors may play role.[a]
Risk factors	Folic acid deficiency in early pregnancy.[a]Prescription and over-the-counter drugs, vitamins, and dietary or herbal supplements (e.g., use of valproic acid for seizure management during pregnancy).[a,b]Maternal diabetes or obesity.[a]Overheating of body (when using hot tub or sauna).[a]High fever early in pregnancy.[a]
Types of Spina Bifida[a]	
Occulta	The mildest type of spina bifida. Abnormal formation of lumbar or sacral vertebrae, with intact spinal cord and spinal nerves, and full skin coverage. This usually does not cause any disabilities.
Meningocele	Vertebral defect such that meninges and cerebrospinal fluid protrude but spinal cord, cauda equina, and spinal nerves remain within the spinal column. Vertebral defect may or may not be covered by skin. Often associated with minor to mild impairment of motor and sensory function.
Myelomeningocele	The most serious type of spina bifida. The meninges and incompletely closed spinal cord protrude; associated with lower motor neuron dysfunction (flaccid paralysis) and complete sensory loss below level of lesion; may have spasticity of muscles innervated by spinal nerves just proximal to level of lesion. Urinary and fecal incontinence common, risk of neuropathic wounds high; risk of osteoporosis of lower extremities high.
Prognosis	Incomplete closure of neural tube soon after conception; leading to flaccid paralysis and total sensory impairment of all structures innervated at and below level of lesion. May be concurrent with hydrocephalus, often managed by ventriculoperitoneal shunt. Associated with multiple secondary musculoskeletal deformities including hip dysplasia, hip dislocation, knee valgus or varus, rearfoot valgus, forefoot equinovarus, scoliosis and kyphosis, osteoporosis, overuse injuries of upper extremities.[c]Static, nonprogressive condition; however postural impairments and decreasing levels of mobility occur with aging, particularly in adolescence and young adulthood.Depending on level of lesion, voluntary bladder and bowel control may also be impaired or absent.
Muscle Tone	Typically flaccid paralysis below the segmental level of the lesion.[d] Some may have spasticity associated with central nervous system impairments.
Mobility	Ranges from bipedal ambulation to wheeled mobility and may change depending on setting and mobility needs. Ambulation distances typically assessed by home, school, or community needs. Orthoses range from ankle/foot orthotic to reciprocating gait orthoses (hip/knee/ankle/foot orthotic). May or may not need assistive device. Wheeled mobility often needed for long distances including school and community venues. Evaluation criteria to determine feasibility for ambulation and/or wheelchair mobility[d]: Household distances —evaluate for endurance; effectiveness of transfers; directionality; management of obstacles including doors; thresholds; efficiency/speed; safety; accessibility to all rooms/areas of house. School distances—evaluate for endurance; effectiveness of transfers; stairs; curbs; ramps; indoor and outdoor surfaces; management of obstacles including classroom furniture, cafeteria furniture; doors and thresholds; efficiency/speed; safety; accessibility to all rooms/areas of school including bathrooms, special classrooms such as auditoriums, stages, art rooms, computer rooms, gymnasium, and playground. Community distances—evaluate for endurance and sufficient speed for public places including medical offices, stores; entertainment and recreational venues; parks and outdoor spaces; effectiveness of transfers; stairs, curbs, and ramps; indoor and outdoor surfaces; management of obstacles including structures, furniture, and people; efficiency/speed; safety; accessibility to all areas of public buildings including bathrooms, lobbies, and parking areas.

[a]Centers for Disease Control and Prevention. *Spina bifida*. Available at: https://www.cdc.gov/. Published October 17, 2022. https://www.cdc.gov/ncbddd/spinabifida/index.html.
[b]Hughes A, Greene NDE, Copp AJ, Galea GL. Valproic acid disrupts the biomechanics of late spinal neural tube closure in mouse embryos. *Mech Develop*. 2018;149:20–26.
[c]Conklin MJ, Kishan S, Nanayakkara CB, Rosenfeld SR. Orthopedic guidelines for the care of people with spina bifida. In: Brei T, Castillo H, Castillo J, eds. *J Pediatr Rehabil Med*. 2020;13(4):629–635.
[d]Gober J, Thomas SP, Gater DR. Pediatric spina bifida and spinal cord injury. *J Personal Med*. 2022;12(6):985.

Table 10.4 Multiple Sclerosis

Incidence	About 10,000 new cases of MS diagnosed yearly in the United States.[a]
Prevalence	About 1,000,000 in the United States, and more than 2.8 million worldwide.[a,b]
Etiology	Unknown; CNS demyelinating disease possibly from a combination of genes that are exposed to some trigger in the environment.[b]
Risk factors	Abnormal immune response causing inflammation and damage to CNS myelin. Occur more frequently in areas farther from the equator. Low vitamin D levels. Smoking. Obesity in childhood and adolescence, particularly in females. Many viral and bacterial infections, particularly measles, human herpes virus-6 and Epstein-Barr virus.[b]
Classifications of multiple sclerosis (MS)[b]	
Clinically isolated syndrome (CIS)	An individual experiences a clinically isolated syndrome (CIS): a single neurologic episode that lasts at least 24 hours, with symptoms including vision problems, vertigo, sensory loss in face, weakness in arms and legs, balance and coordination problems, bladder problems.
Relapsing remitting (RRMS), the most common disease course, with 85% of cases	Cycle of relapses/exacerbations (new signs/symptoms) followed by partial to complete recovery/remissions during which there is no apparent worsening of the disease process.
Secondary progressive (SPMS)	Individuals diagnosed with RRMS who eventually go on to have a secondary progressive course, in which neurologic function worsens progressively or disability accumulates over time.
Primary progressive (PPMS)	Individuals in which neurologic function worsens or disability accumulates as soon as symptoms appear, without early relapses or remissions.
Prognosis	Unpredictable exacerbations result from inflammation and destruction of myelin around pathways within the CNS. Residual impairments are the consequence of slowed transmission of neural impulses across plaques interrupting connections between CNS structures. May impact on any subsystem within CNS (voluntary motor, postural control, coordination, memory, perception, sensation). Definitive diagnosis made if there have been at least two different episodes of impairment, involving two different neurological subsystems, affecting two different parts of the body, at two different periods of time. Variable course, with many different types of impairment accruing over time with repeated exacerbations. Typically, onset of initial symptoms in young and mid-adulthood. Often diagnosis by exclusion; when neurological signs/symptoms cannot be attributed to other disease processes.
Muscle tone	Varies, depending on location and size of residual plaque. Some individuals may exhibit normal tone and deep tendon reflexes, in the presences of perceptual, postural, or coordination impairment. Others may demonstrate hypertonus and hyperactive reflexes is various muscles. Others may have hypotonus and impaired muscle performance.
Muscle performance	Varies, depending on the location of MS plaque. If in pyramidal system, may have weakness, impaired muscle endurance, poor eccentric control, among others. If in cerebellar systems, may demonstrate ataxia, intention tremor, among others.
Postural control	Postural control and equilibrium responses may be impaired due to a combination of pyramidal and/or extrapyramidal motor system impairment, sensory impairment or somatosensory, spinocerebellar, or visual pathways, or damage of major integrative while matter structures such as the corpus callosum, or medial longitudinal fasciculus.
Mobility	Mobility and locomotion may be impaired, along with postural control, depending on location of lesion. Some individuals with impaired muscle performance benefit from AFOs (for support and positioning of lower extremity in gait) associated with weakness or hypertonicity. Many choose to use ambulatory aides and assistive devices for function and safety. Some with significant multisystem impairment benefit from seating and wheeled mobility systems.

[a]American Brain Foundation. *Multiple sclerosis*. https://www.americanbrainfoundation.org/. Published 2023. https://www.americanbrainfoundation.org/diseases/multiple-sclerosis/.
[b]National Multiple Sclerosis Society. https://www.nationalmssociety.org/. Published 2023.
AFO, Ankle-foot orthosis; *CNS*, central nervous system.

Table 10.5 Spinal Cord Injury

Incidence	About 18,000 new cases diagnosed every year in the United States, approximately 54 cases per one million people.[a]
Prevalence	Approximately 302,000 persons, with a range from 255,000 to 383,000 persons.[a]
Etiology	Usually traumatic (e.g., vehicle crashes [37.6%], falls [31.5%], violence - primarily gunshot wounds [15.4%], sports/recreation activities [8.3%]), sometimes infectious (e.g., transverse myelitis) or ischemic (e.g., complication of abdominal aortic aneurysm repair).[a]
Risk factors	Young age, male gender (~78%), drunk driving, participation in extreme sports, all-terrain vehicle accidents, military injury.
Spinal cord injury (SCI) syndromes	
Complete SCI[a]	Quadriplegia (cervical cord injury) or paraplegia (thoracic cord injury) with spastic paralysis.
Complete quadriplegia 12.5%Complete paraplegia 19.8%	Consequence of compression, contusion, or ischemia of spinal cord as a result of vertebral fracture or dislocation sustained in fall, collision, diving, gunshot wound, or other high-impact event. Exacerbated by resultant inflammatory process. Spinal cord below level of lesion survives but is disconnected from brain and brainstem, only able to operate reflexively (e.g., neurogenic bladder and bowel function).

Table 10.5 Spinal Cord Injury—cont'd

Incomplete SCI[a] Incomplete quadriplegia 47.1% Incomplete paraplegia 20.1%	Similar mechanism of injury but with sparing of one or more areas of spinal cord such that there is some volitional motor function and sensation along with more typical UMN (for cervical and thoracic vertebral lesions) or LMNs (for lumbosacral vertebral lesions) (e.g., central cord syndrome: upper extremity involvement > lower extremity involvement, often with preserved volitional bladder and bowel function). Becoming more common with advances in emergency care on newly injured persons.
Cauda equina syndrome	Paraplegia consequence of compression, contusion of lumbosacral nerve roots (cauda equina) within the lower spinal canal, resulting in flaccid paralysis and sensory loss below the level of lesion.
Prognosis	Improved emergency and acute medical management often result in incomplete lesion, with varying combinations of return of function and spastic paralysis. Lengths of stay in the hospital acute care unit have declined from 24 days in the 1970s to 12 days since 2015. Rehabilitation lengths of stay have also declined from 98 days in the 1970s to 31 days since 2015.[a]
Muscle tone	Initial hypotonicity during period of neurogenic shock. Many develop significant hypertonicity/spasticity in the months after injury; some may have muscle spasm needing pharmacological intervention. Sudden increase in resting tone may signal unrecognized skin irritation, bladder distention or infection, or bowel impaction. At risk of secondary musculoskeletal deformity (contracture) due to long-standing abnormal tone and limited mobility.
Muscle performance	Impaired with reflexive activity. Flaccid, areflexic paralysis during initial spinal shock period, with gradual transition to spasticity with hyperreflexia over weeks and months. Muscles that remain innervated are often initially weak; but are likely responsive to interventions to enhance force production, muscle endurance, power.
Postural control	Varies from minimal to significantly impaired, depending on location and severity of lesion. Sitting trunk control may or may be present depending on level of lesion. Paralysis of the lower extremities limit standing ability without orthotic support.
Mobility	May temporarily use spinal orthosis (CO, CTO, TLSO) until surgical stabilization of damaged vertebrae is well healed. Often require seating and wheelchair systems for mobility. Persons with cervical-level lesions may require upper extremity splints and adaptive equipment for activities of daily living, or resting splints or orthoses to manage abnormal tone and prevent contracture. Persons with low thoracic and lumbosacral lesions may use AFO, KAFO, or HKAFO along with assistive device (rolling walker, crutches) for ambulation, either as part of rehabilitation or of fitness program; energy cost of ambulation for community distances often high enough to be impractical.

[a]Data from National Spinal Cord Injury Statistical Center, University of Alabama at Birmingham. *Traumatic Spinal Cord Injury Facts and Figures at a Glance.* https://www.nscisc.uab.edu/. Published 2023. https://www.nscisc.uab.edu/public/Facts%20and%20Figures%202023%20-%20Final.pdf.
UMN, Upper motor neuron; *LMN*, lower motor neuron; *CO*, cervical orthosis; *CTO*, cervical thoracic orthosis; *TLSO*, thoraco-lumbo-sacral orthosis; *AFO*, ankle-foot orthosis; *KAFO*, knee-ankle-foot orthosis; *HKAFO*, hip-knee-ankle-foot orthosis.

provision of stability for improved efficiency of movement; reduction of the influence of hypertonicity/spasticity on movement; minimization/prevention of the development of contractures; and increasing participation in desired activities of the individual. There is no perfect orthosis or adaptive equipment piece that will address all dimensions of movement dysfunction; there are always trade-offs that must be taken into account.

Management of Neuromuscular Impairments

Effective care of persons with movement dysfunction secondary to neurological and neuromuscular pathologies requires collaboration of health professionals from many disciplines: neurologists, orthopedist, physiatrists, physical and occupational therapists, and orthotists, among others.[134–137] Physicians and surgeons manage spasticity and correct orthopedic deformity with medication and surgery. Nurses are involved in wellness care, as well as medical and surgical management. Rehabilitation professionals facilitate return of function after an acute event and provide functional training and postoperative rehabilitation for individuals across the spectrum of neurological and neuromuscular pathologies. Orthotists contribute their knowledge of orthotic options to improve gait and function. The multidisciplinary approach leads to greater satisfaction with care and less risk of abandonment of orthoses and assistive devices by the person for which they were made.[138]

MEDICAL AND SURGICAL CARE

Medical management of CNS dysfunction often includes prescription of pharmacological agents. Physicians can select from a range of centrally acting tone-inhibiting medications (e.g., baclofen) or pharmacological interventions that target lower motor neurons, peripheral nerves, or muscle (e.g., botulinum toxin injection, intrathecal baclofen) for individuals with significant hypertonicity.[139–145] Knowledge of the effects of medications and the most effective prescription to delay progression and reduce exacerbations of MS continue to develop with disease-modifying therapies. Other MS medications attempt to manage symptoms rather than the disease itself, although many are been found to be no more effective than placebo.[146–152] Many individuals with CNS disorders also must cope with seizure management; many antiepileptic drugs affect arousal and ability to learn.[153,154] It is important for physical therapists and orthotists to be aware of the potential impact of neuroactive medications on an individual's ability to concentrate and learn, overall health status, and neuromotor control.[155] A summary of pharmacological agents used in the management of spasticity, neuropathic pain, and seizures resulting from various neurological and neuromuscular disorders is presented in Table 10.6.

Table 10.6 Pharmacological Interventions for Individuals With Neurological and Neuromuscular System Impairments

Trade Names	Generic Name (Class)	Administration	Indications	Adverse Effects
MANAGEMENT OF DYSTONIA AND CENTRAL NERVOUS SYSTEM–RELATED SPASM[a]				
NeuroBloc Myobloc	Botulinum B toxin (neurotoxin)	Intramuscular	Facial spasm, spasmodic torticollis, blepharospasm	Pain at injection site, ptosis, eye irritation, weakness of neck muscles, dysphagia, dry mouth, heartburn
MANAGEMENT OF HYPERTONICITY, CLONUS, AND TICS[a]				
Botox Dysport	Botulinum A toxin (neurotoxin)	Intramuscular or perineural injection, intrathecal	Chronic severe spasticity or dystonia	Pain or bruising at injection site, muscle weakness, tiredness, drowsiness, nausea, anxiety
Catapres	Clonidine (antihypertensive)	Oral or transdermal	Spasticity in MS	Dry mouth, gastrointestinal disturbances, fatigue, headache, nervousness, insomnia, skin irritation (transdermal)
Ceberclon Klonopin Rivotril Valpax	Clonazepam (benzodiazepine)	Oral	Spasticity in CP, dystonic, chorea, akathisia (also for seizures, panic attacks)	Sedation, dizziness, unsteadiness, incoordination, memory problems, muscle or joint pain, blurred vision, frequent urination
Dantrium	Dantrolene sodium (skeletal muscle relaxant)	Oral or injection	Chronic severe spasticity of UMN origin	Drowsiness, dizziness, generalized weakness, malaise, fatigue, nervousness, headache
Ethanol	Ethyl alcohol (neurotoxin)	Intramuscular or perineural injection	Severe spasticity, with serial casting follow-up	Neuritis, hyperesthesia, or paresthesia
Lioresal	Baclofen (skeletal muscle relaxant)	Oral, injection, or intrathecal	Chronic severe spasticity for conditions including SCI, ABI, MS; not effective in CP	Sedation, confusion, hypotension, dizziness, ataxia, headache, tremor, nystagmus, paresthesia, diaphoresis, muscular pain or weakness, insomnia, behavioral changes
Neurontin	Gabapentin	Oral	Adjunct to other antispasticity medications for SCI and MS	Drowsiness, dizziness, ataxia, fatigue, nystagmus, nervousness, tremor, diplopia, memory impairment
Phenol	Phenol	Intramuscular or perineural injection	Severe lower limb spasticity (with serial casting follow-up) pain control	Damage to other neural structures
Robaxin	Methocarbamol	Oral or injection	Short-term relief of muscle spasm or spasticity	Sedation, drowsiness, lightheadedness, fatigue, dizziness, nausea, restlessness
Valium	Diazepam	Oral or injection	Short-term relief of muscle spasm or spasticity	Sedation, drowsiness, fatigue, ataxia, confusion, depression, diplopia, dysarthria, tremor
Zanaflex Sirdalud	Tizanidine (skeletal muscle relaxant)	Oral	Spasticity from MS or SCI	Sedation, drowsiness, fatigue, dizziness, mild weakness, nausea, hypotension, GI irritation
MANAGEMENT OF DYSESTHESIA/NEUROPATHIC PAIN[b]				
Carbatrol Epitol Tegretol Dilantin Neurontin Zonegran Norpramin	Carbamazepine Phenytoin Gabapentin Zonisamide Desipramine (anticonvulsants)	Oral	Trigeminal neuralgia, pelvic pain, intense episodic/lancinating/burning pain, pins/needles, cramping, dysesthetic extremity pain, tonic spasms, other neurogenic pain, nocturnal spasms	See Seizure Medications
Adapin Sinequan Triadapin Zonalon Elavil Imavate Janimine Tofranil Vivactil	Doxepin Amitriptyline Imipramine Protriptyline (tricyclic antidepressants)	Oral	Chronic neurogenic pain (e.g., dysesthetic extremity pain such as burning, tingling)	Drowsiness, blurred vision, dizziness, GI and urinary disturbances, tachycardia, hypotension, weight gain, fatigue, headache
MANAGEMENT OF SEIZURES[c]				
Amytal	Amobarbital (barbiturate)	Intravenous	Status epilepticus	Sedation, nystagmus, ataxia, vitamin K and folate deficiency
Ativan	Lorazepam (benzodiazepine)	Intravenous	Status epilepticus	Sedation, ataxia, changes in behavior

Table 10.6 Pharmacological Interventions for Individuals With Neurological and Neuromuscular System Impairments—cont'd

Trade Names	Generic Name (Class)	Administration	Indications	Adverse Effects
Atretol Convline Epitol Macrepan Tegretol	Carbamazepine (iminostilbene)	Oral	Complex partial seizures, tonic-clonic seizures, trigeminal neuralgia, bipolar disorder	Ataxia, diplopia, drowsiness, fatigue, dizziness, vertigo, tremor, headache, nausea, dry mouth, anorexia, agitation, rashes photosensitivity, heart failure
Celontin	Methsuximide (succinimide)	Oral	Alternative to ethosuximide for absence seizures	Nausea, vomiting, headache, dizziness, fatigue, lethargy, dyskinesia, bradykinesia
Cerebyx	Fosphenytoin (hydantoin)	Intravenous	Status epilepticus	GI irritation, confusion, sedation, dizziness, headache, nystagmus, ataxia, dysarthria
Depacon	Sodium valproate (carboxylic acid)	Oral or injection	All types of seizures	Ataxia, tremor, sedation, nausea, vomiting, hyperactivity weakness, incoordination, risk of hepatotoxicity
Depakene	Valproic acid (carboxylic acid)	Oral	Absence seizures, as adjunct for other seizure types	Nausea, sedation, ataxia headache nystagmus, diplopia, asterixis, dysarthria, dizziness, incoordination, depression, hyperactivity, weakness, risk of hepatotoxicity
Depakote	Divalproex sodium (carboxylic acid)	Oral	Complex partial seizures, absence seizures, as adjunct for other seizure types	Headache, asthenia, nausea, somnolence, tremor, dizziness diplopia, risk of hepatotoxicity
Diamox	Acetazolamide (sulfonamide)	Oral	Absence seizures, myoclonic seizures	Drowsiness, dizziness
Dilantin Diphen Diphentoin Dyantoin Phenytex	Phenytoin (hydantoin)	Oral or injection	Status epilepticus, tonic-clonic seizures, simple complex seizures	Ataxia, slurred speech, confusion, insomnia, nervousness, hypotension, nystagmus diplopia, nausea, vomiting
Felbatol	Felbamate (second generation)	Oral	Partial seizures, absence seizures Used for severe seizure disorders unresponsive to other medications	Aplastic anemia, liver failure, insomnia, headache, dizziness, loss of appetite, nausea, vomiting
Gabitril	Tiagabine (second generation)	Oral	Partial seizures	Generalized weakness, dizziness, tiredness, nervousness, tremor, distractibility, emotional lability
Keppra	Levetiracetam (second generation)	Oral	Adjunct for partial seizures in adults	Sedation, dizziness, generalized weakness
Klonopin Rivotril	Clonazepam (benzodiazepine)	Oral or injection	Myoclonic seizures, absence seizures, kinetic seizures	Drowsiness, dizziness, ataxia, dyskinesia, irritability, disturbances of coordination, slurred speech, diplopia, nystagmus, thirst
Lamictal	Lamotrigine (second generation)	Oral	Partial seizures, tonic-clonic seizures	Dizziness, headache, ataxia, drowsiness, incoordination, insomnia, tremors, depression, anxiety, diplopia, blurred vision, GI disturbances, agitation, confusion, rash
Luminol Solfoton	Phenobarbital (barbiturate)	Oral or injection	Status epilepticus, all seizure types except absence seizures	Drowsiness, lethargy, agitation, confusion, ataxia, hallucination, bradycardia, hypotension, nausea
Mebaral	Mephobarbital (barbiturate)	Oral	Tonic-clonic seizures, simple and complex partial seizures	Drowsiness, sedation, nystagmus, ataxia, folate and vitamin K deficiency
Mesantoin	Mephenytoin (hydantoin)	Oral	Partial seizures, tonic-clonic seizures used if Dilantin is not effective	Similar to Dilantin, but more toxic
Milontin	Phensuximide (succinimide)	Oral	Alternative to Zarontin for absence seizures	Nausea, vomiting, headache, dizziness, fatigue, lethargy, bradykinesia, dyskinesia
Mysoline	Primidone (barbiturate)	Oral	All seizure types except absence seizures, essential tremor	Ataxia, vertigo, drowsiness, depression, inattention, headache, nausea, visual disturbances
Nembutal	Pentobarbital (barbiturate)	Intravenous	Tonic-clonic seizures, simple and complex partial seizures	Sedation, nystagmus, ataxia, vitamin K and folate deficiency
Neurontin	Gabapentin (second generation)	Oral	Partial seizures in adults and children older than 3 years, neuropathic pain	Drowsiness, dizziness, ataxia, fatigue, nystagmus, nervousness, tremor, diplopia, memory impairment

(Continued)

Table 10.6 Pharmacological Interventions for Individuals With Neurological and Neuromuscular System Impairments—cont'd

Trade Names	Generic Name (Class)	Administration	Indications	Adverse Effects
Peganone	Ethotoin (hydantion)	Oral	Tonic-clonic seizures; used if Dilantin is not effective	Similar to Dilantin, but more toxic
Seconal	Secobarbital (barbiturate)	Intravenous	Tonic-clonic seizures, partial seizures	Sedation, nystagmus, vitamin K and folate deficiency
Topamax	Topiramate (second generation)	Oral	Partial seizures, adjunct to tonic-clonic seizures	Ataxia, confusion, dizziness, fatigue, paresthesia, emotional lability, confusion, diplopia, nausea
Thosutin Zarontin	Ethosuximide (succinimide)	Oral	Absence seizures	Drowsiness, headache, fatigue, dizziness, ataxia, euphoria, depression, myopia, nausea, anorexia
Tranxene	Clorazepate (benzodiazepine)	Oral	Adjunct for partial seizures	Sedation, ataxia, changes in behavior
Trileptal	Oxcarbazepine (iminostilbene)	Oral	Partial seizures, tonic-clonic seizures	Ataxia, drowsiness, nausea, dizziness, headache, agitation, memory impairment, asthenia, ataxia, confusion, tremor, nystagmus
Valium Valrelease	Diazepam (benzodiazepine)	Injection	Status epilepticus, severe recurrent seizures	Drowsiness, fatigue, ataxia, confusion, depression, dysarthria, syncope, tremor, vertigo
Zonegran	Zonisamide (second generation)	Oral	Adjunct for partial seizures in adults	Sedation, ataxia, loss of appetite, fatigue

[a]Skeletal muscle relaxants. In: *Pharmacology in Rehabilitation*. Updated Fifth ed. FA Davis Company; 2022:173–194.
[b]Bates D, Schultheis BC, Hanes MC, et al. A comprehensive algorithm for management of neuropathic pain. *Pain Med*. 2019;20(suppl_1):S2–S12.
[c]Antiepileptic drugs. In: *Pharmacology in Rehabilitation*. Updated fifth ed. FA Davis Company; 2022:113–128.
ABI, Acquired brain injury; *CP*, cerebral palsy; *GI*, gastrointestinal; *MS*, multiple sclerosis; *NMJ*, neuromuscular junction; *SCI*, spinal cord injury; *UMN*, upper motor neuron.

Alternatively, physicians may recommend various neurosurgical procedures and orthopedic surgeries to correct deformity, improve flexibility, or reduce level of abnormal tone, with the goal of enhancing mobility and improving performance of functional tasks. Neurectomy and neurotomy, for example, may be used to manage severe equinovarus and upper extremity spasticity after stroke and for children with CP.[156,157] Selective dorsal rhizotomy (SDR) effectively reduces problematic hypertonicity for children with CP but does not seem to reduce the future risk of developing deformity or improve functional mobility, which would then require orthopedic surgery.[158] Unlike SDR, neurectomies allow for more focal spasticity management as well as sparing of sensory nerves.[156] Intrathecal baclofen (ITB) pumps have been used as a strategy to manage severe spasticity in persons with traumatic brain injury, stroke, SCI, MS, and CP.[159–163] Intrathecal pumps have shown a low rate of adverse reactions and high acceptance rate.[139] Botulinum toxin A (BoNT-A) is another common spasticity intervention with validated use in populations including CP, stroke, SCI, and MS. BoNT-A[140,143 145,164] can be applied focally via intramuscular injection impairing acetylcholine transmission at local neuromuscular junctions.[144,165] Other available oral antispasticity medications include benzodiazepines, alpha-adrenergic agonists (tizanidine, clonidine), dantrolene sodium, and gabapentine.[166] An algorithm for treating disabling spasticity in adults using BoNT-A and/or ITB in conjunction with physical rehabilitation and orthotic devices was developed through expert consensus amongst a group of European spasticity specialists that included neurologists, physical medicine and rehabilitation physicians, physical therapists, neurosurgeons, and specialist nurses (Fig. 10.7).[139]

Despite pharmacological and positioning interventions, musculoskeletal deformities can still develop, particularly in the growing child. Surgical interventions are used to correct musculoskeletal defaults of the spine and limbs, realign joints for better mechanical advantage, improve ease of caregiving and hygiene management, promote cosmesis, or reduce and prevent pain. Tendon lengthenings or transfers are commonly used to correct contractures and provide greater functional ROM to improve the ability to walk in children with CP.[167–172] Tendon lengthening or tenotomy can also be used to reduce deformities such as equinovarus following SCI or stroke.[173–175] Derotation osteotomies are another option that have traditionally been used to improve or correct deformity and improve walking ability in children with CP.[176–179] Because children with CP and acquired brain injury who have significant hypertonicity are at risk for developing neuromuscular scoliosis (NMS), various spinal surgeries are used to improve spinal alignment and reduce pelvic obliquity, although postsurgical complication rate is high.[180–183] Surgical interventions for NMS most consistently improve seated stability with potential benefits in gastrointestinal function, back pain, cardiopulmonary function, and functional transfers.[184–186] Growing rods may be used to accommodate expected growth with aging while correcting NMS. Traditional growing rods require repeated surgery under anesthesia while newer magnetically controlled growing rods allow for noninvasive outpatient adjustments.[181,187,188] Rather than subject children with CP to multiple surgeries over time, many centers perform multiple procedures at the same time and utilize a dual-surgeon approach.[189–195] To achieve maximum benefit, rehabilitation is a necessary component following any of these surgeries.[196–198]

Individuals with significant spasticity are commonly managed with a combination of these strategies to most effectively diminish the impairment, improve the

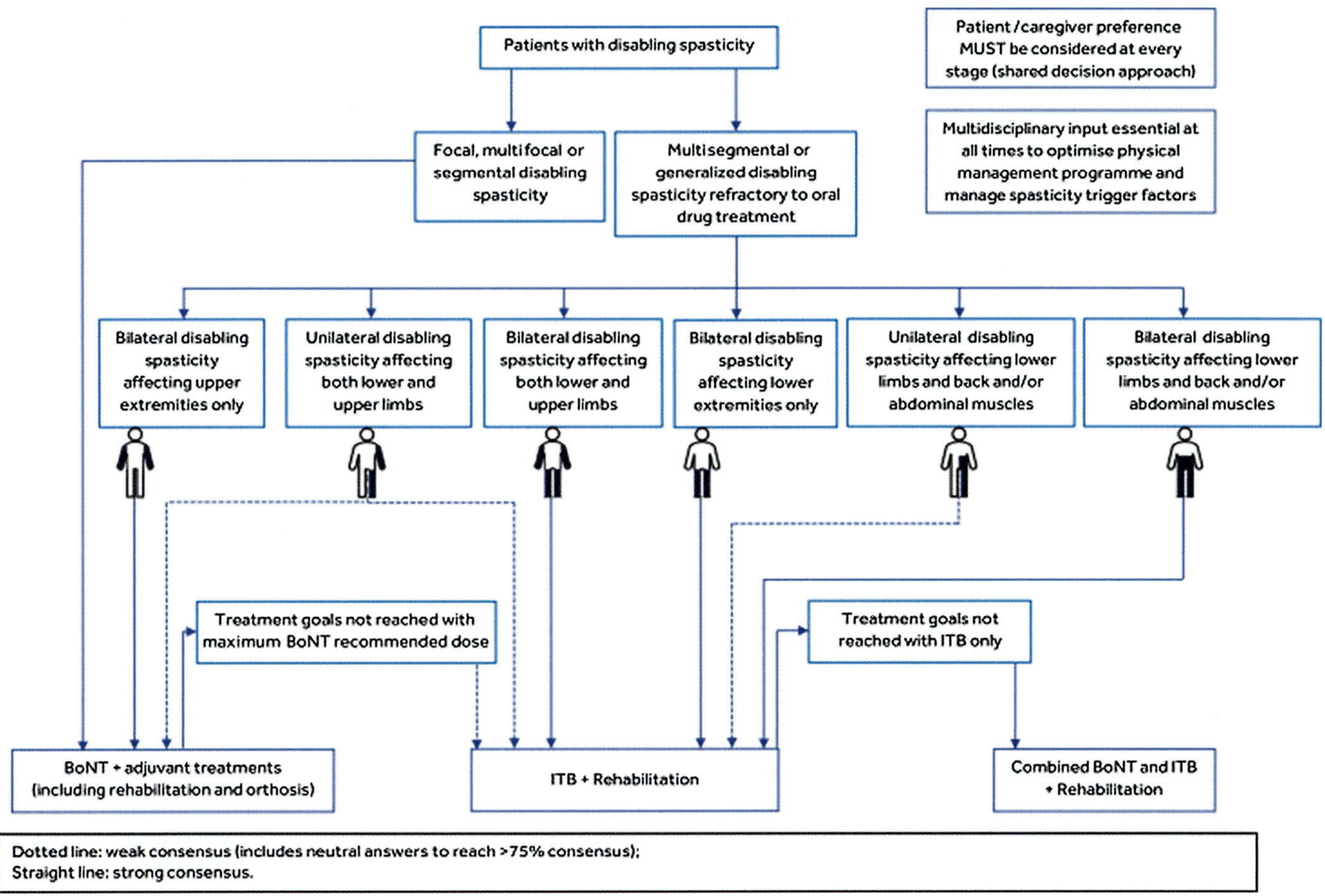

Fig. 10.7 Algorithm developed by a European expert panel for the management of adult patients with disabling spasticity. *BoNT-A*, Botulinum toxin A; *ITB*, intrathecal baclofen. Courtesy Biering-Sørensen B, Stevenson V, Bensmail D, et al. European expert consensus on improving patient selection for the management of disabling spasticity with intrathecal baclofen and/or botulinum toxin type A. *J Rehabil Med*. 2022;54:jrm00241.

functional ability, and help them participate in activities that are important to them.[199–201] Increasingly, instrumented gait analysis is being used to inform clinical decision-making in selecting the most appropriate intervention or combination of interventions for ambulatory individuals with functional limitation secondary to neuromuscular pathologies and their associated secondary impairments.[202–204]

REHABILITATION

Rehabilitation professionals use a variety of examination strategies to determine the nature and extent of dysfunction across systems that are associated with a particular pathological condition. The components of a complete evaluation when considering orthotic or equipment decisions include asking specific history questions; a biomechanical analysis of the limb(s)/segment(s); and examination of neuromotor status, motor control, functional movement ability, integumentary integrity, sensory processing, cognitive function, and psychosocial factors. See Table 10.7 for an example.[205] The physical therapist evaluates this information to (1) determine an appropriate movement-related physical therapy diagnosis, (2) predict potential outcomes (prognosis), and (3) structure an appropriate plan of care.[205,206]

Physical therapists use adaptive equipment, orthoses, and seating as key components of an effective plan of care for persons with neuromotor/neurosensory system dysfunction.[207–212] Consideration of the use of an orthotic or other equipment must be made in the context of the patient's activity needs/desires and participation in life activities that contribute to quality of life.[213]

Orthoses are used to:

1. Align or position limb segments to enhance voluntary limb movement and improve function (e.g., an ankle-foot orthosis [AFO] to provide prepositioning of the foot during swing-limb advancement and stability during the stance phase of gait).
2. Minimize the influence of abnormal tone on posture and movement (tone-inhibiting designs).
3. Provide individuals with a variety of comfortable and safe positions in which they can sleep, eat, travel, work, or play.
4. Promote joint alignment and minimize risk of contracture development and other secondary musculoskeletal sequelae (especially in growing children).
5. Protect a limb following orthopedic surgery performed to correct deformity or instability.
6. Enhance alignment following pharmacological intervention with botulinum toxin.
7. Provide alternative methods for mobility.

Table 10.7 Elements of a Physical Therapy Examination in Consideration for Prescription/Use of Orthoses, Adaptive Equipment, or Serial Casting

Examination Element	Examination Strategies	Implications for Orthosis, Equipment, or Cast
Chief complaint: What is the *MOVEMENT PROBLEM* that brings the individual to physical therapy?	Interview of individual and caregivers	Ambulation/gait dysfunction—consider need for LE orthosis. Reach, grasp, manipulation dysfunction—consider need for UE orthosis.
History of current illness, past medical history: How did the *MOVEMENT PROBLEM* develop or evolve? Explore duration of the presenting problem; previous and concurrent pharmacological management; previous and concurrent orthopedic or neurosurgical management; previous orthotic management; current health status; comorbidities and their management	Review of medical record Interview with individual and caregivers Consultation with clinical colleagues	Consider what strategies are currently working or not. Consider combination of strategies that might be possible. For example, hypertonicity reduction medication coupled with an orthosis.
Biomechanical evaluation: ROM, flexibility (especially of multijoint muscles), muscle length, alignment of joints, pelvis, and spine, torsional/rotational deformity of hip, femur, tibia	Goniometric measurement; evaluation of muscle length (e.g., Thomas test, straight-leg raise); integrity of ligaments and supportive structures; radiograph; inclinometer	Consider strategies for contracture management. For example, Botox injection followed by serial casting or orthosis. If contracture may be "permanent" or severe, consider accommodation needs for positioning. For example, heel wedge to accommodate fixed plantarflexion contracture.
Postural alignment in sitting and standing	Spatial relationships of head, upper trunk/limb girdle, mid trunk, lower trunk/pelvic girdle, extremity symmetry	Consider seating or standing adaptations and/or seating/standing systems.
Anthropomorphic characteristics	Height, weight, limb length, limb girth, body mass	Implications for sizing.
Neuromotor status: Muscle tone (compliance vs. stiffness) Deep tendon reflex testing Antigravity stiffness/postural tone Involuntary movement	Resistance to passive movement at various speeds Palpation tone scales (e.g., modified Ashworth), descriptive category (hypertonic/spastic, rigid, hypotonic, fluctuating, flaccid) amplitude of response, pattern of response (distal-proximal), symmetry of response	Consider strategies and combination of strategies to manage hypertonicity.
Motor control: Recruitment/adaptation of contractions Segmentation of limbs, joints within a limb	Ability to move between concentric, eccentric, and holding contractions during functional activity Ability to initiate, sustain, and terminate contraction and movement. Influence of abnormal synergy or abnormal developmental reflexes	Determine if trunk or extremities require positioning or orthosis to provide control (minimize tonal influence, support body structure).
Muscle performance: Strength Speed/power Accuracy Timing Fluidity Muscle endurance Relationship of agonist/antagonist	Observation of antigravity movement Manual muscle testing, dynamometer Isokinetic testing Description: hypokinetic, functional, hyperkinetic Control for concentric, eccentric, isometric contractions, repetitions to test endurance	Consider postural support requirements for UE tasks; trunk and LE support requirements for LE tasks.
Postural control	Static balance tests (e.g., timed single limb stance) Anticipatory balance tests (e.g., reach distances, ability to change direction) Reactionary balance test: perturbation	Consider postural support requirements for UE tasks; trunk and LE support requirements for LE tasks.
Functional movement ability, functional task abilities ADL	Ability to adapt movement strategies in different environmental conditions and to different task demands. Observation of movement during task Self-report of individual or caregiver Various ADL scales Ability to don/doff orthosis	Consider orthoses to improve efficiency, effectiveness of movement. Consider equipment that may assist in task completion.
Dexterity, coordination, agility	Observation of performance during functional activity Special tests Developmental scales and profiles	Consider orthoses to improve efficiency, effectiveness of movement.

Table 10.7 Elements of a Physical Therapy Examination in Consideration for Prescription/Use of Orthoses, Adaptive Equipment, or Serial Casting—cont'd

Examination Element	Examination Strategies	Implications for Orthosis, Equipment, or Cast
Transitional movements and transfers To/from floor Sit to stand Bathroom transfers Car transfers	Assistance required Level of difficulty Task analysis to identify where in movement difficulty occurs and contributors to difficulty	Consider LE orthosis for standing and movement needs; consider seating needs, wheelchair usage. Consider mechanical lift needs.
Mobility and locomotion	Observational gait analysis, with and without orthosis Gait speed, other kinematic measures Use of assistive devices Level of assistance required Gait lab kinetic measures (moments, torques, force plate, activity via video, and EMG analysis)	Consider orthosis needs for gait cycle impairments. Consider assistive device needs.
UE function and use of hands	Observation during various fine and gross UE motor tasks	Consider UE orthosis needs.
Cardiovascular endurance	Heart rate, blood pressure, oxygen saturation during activity Ratings of perceived exertion during tasks 6-Minute walk test Fatigue scales	Consider orthosis for efficiency, to decrease energy expenditure.
Environmental assessment (home, work, school, leisure)	Environmental safety checklists Interview with individual and caregivers about characteristics of environments in which individual must function	Consider environmental adaptations.
Integumentary integrity Skin condition	Inspection for neuropathic, dysvascular, or traumatic wounds Document callus and scarring Document pressure sensitive areas Document protective sensation, insensate weight-bearing areas	Consider protection of vulnerable areas; consider custom fit to minimize/prevent wound development.
Sensory organization and processing Sensory integrity	Adequacy of vision (acuity, peripheral vision, tracking, visual field loss) Screening for exteroception, proprioception ability Document insensate areas, especially of hands/feet Document paresthesia and dysesthesia	Consider protection of vulnerable areas; consider custom fit to minimize/prevent wound development.
Perceptual function Visual spatial perception Awareness of position in space Awareness of body parts	Observation of movement during functional tasks Developmental tests, measures Special perceptual tests, measures	Consider workstation, home adaptations.
Cognitive function: Ability to learn and remember Ability to problem solve Motivation Distractibility/focus Ability to manage frustration, uncertainty	Reports of teachers, clinicians; neuropsychological testing; observation when presented with challenge; self-report of individual and caregivers	Consider ability to manage orthosis, cleaning and maintenance of devices. Consider ability to don/doff orthosis. Consider ability to know if fit feels wrong and ability to seek appropriate assistance.
Communication	Adequacy of hearing and auditory processing; Ability to understand language; Ability to use language; oral-motor function (dysarthria); Impact of position on voice	Consider ability to understand and follow instructions for proper fit, wearing schedules.
Psychosocial factors Desired participation in leisure or play activities, school or work-related activities. Family and caregiver Quality of life	Typical activities and roles: demands and barriers encountered for activities. Availability and capacity of others to assist with respect to use of orthosis Self-efficacy scales Patient/caregiver satisfaction with orthosis/device	Consider use of orthosis, adaptive equipment for different environments. Consider training of caregiver if needed.

ADL, Activities of daily living; *EMG*, electromyography; *LE*, lower extremity; *ROM*, range of motion; *UE*, upper extremity.
Truman H, Nair P. Orthotics: evaluation, intervention, and prescription. In: Lazaro RT, Reina-Guerra SG, Quiben M. *Umphred's Neurological Rehabilitation*. Seventh ed. Elsevier; 2020:930–946.

The risk for developing secondary musculoskeletal impairments is high in the presence of hypertonicity.[214–217] Passive stretching programs alone are generally ineffective as a management strategy for reducing risk for contracture development.[218,219] Prolonged positioning for several hours a day is a critical adjunct to stretching.[220–222] Adaptive equipment can be used to provide structural alignment for prolonged periods of time to maintain extensibility of muscles, decrease the effect of muscle imbalance across joints, and provide postural support, particularly to increase effectiveness in daily activities such as feeding and play.[223–226] An adaptive seating system, for example, would provide upright postural support for sitting; maintain spinal alignment and pelvic positioning; support optimal hip, knee, and ankle positions; and promote the best position for upper extremity function.[223–225] Positioning devices for supported standing are often used to maintain extensibility of muscles, to promote bone mineral density through weight bearing, and to promote musculoskeletal development such as acetabular depth in a developing child with hypertonicity (Fig. 10.8).[227–229] Increased benefits may be seen with standing frames incorporating dynamic movement.[230] Other examples of positioning devices include prone, supine, and sidelyer systems; bathing and toileting seating systems; and a variety of mobility alternatives such as gait trainers.[231–233] Although there are many options for adaptive equipment designed to assist function and caregiving for persons with neurological and neuromuscular dysfunction, knowledge about options and limitations in funding limit access for many who might otherwise benefit from such devices.[234–236]

Serial corrective casts have long been used as a primary intervention for individuals with significant hypertonus to provide a prolonged elongation of soft tissue over a long time period. They increase the length of a contracted muscle and its supportive tissues and reset the threshold for response to stretch reflex.[237,238] Some splints or dynamic orthoses are used primarily at night to provide 8 or more hours of stretch on a regular basis; others can be worn during daily activities to provide a longer period of stretch (Fig. 10.9).[142,239–241] More recently, serial casting and dynamic splinting have been used in conjunction with pharmacological interventions for the management of spasticity in both children and adults with severe hypertonicity.[242,243] Although the pharmacological agent may reduce the degree of spasticity in hypertonic muscles, concomitant shortening of the muscles and tendons must be addressed while the neurological

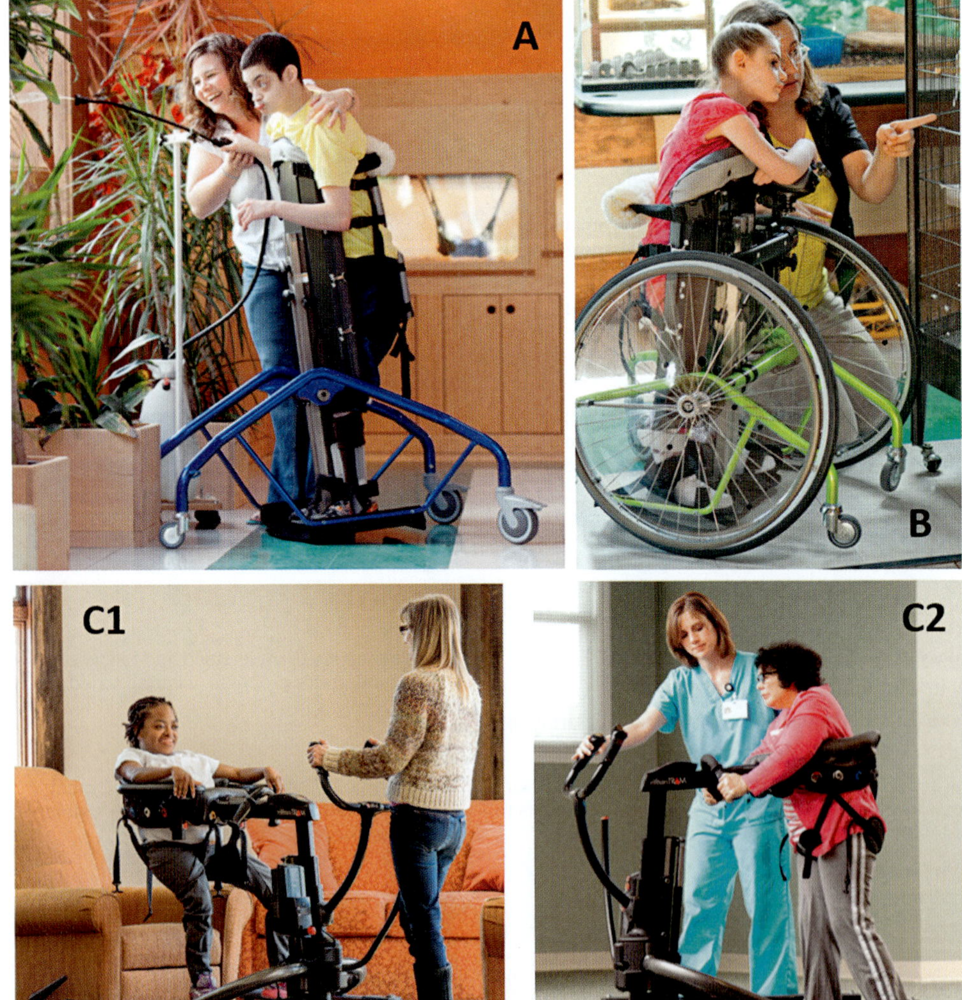

Fig. 10.8 Examples of adaptive equipment to assist with standing, transfers, and mobility in the presence of impairment of muscle tone, muscle performance, postural control, or difficulty with movement and coordination. (A) Mobile stander. (B) Mobile stander with large wheels. (C) Transfer and mobility device illustrated for functional transfers (C1) and assisted ambulation (C2). Courtesy Rifton Equipment https://www.rifton.com).

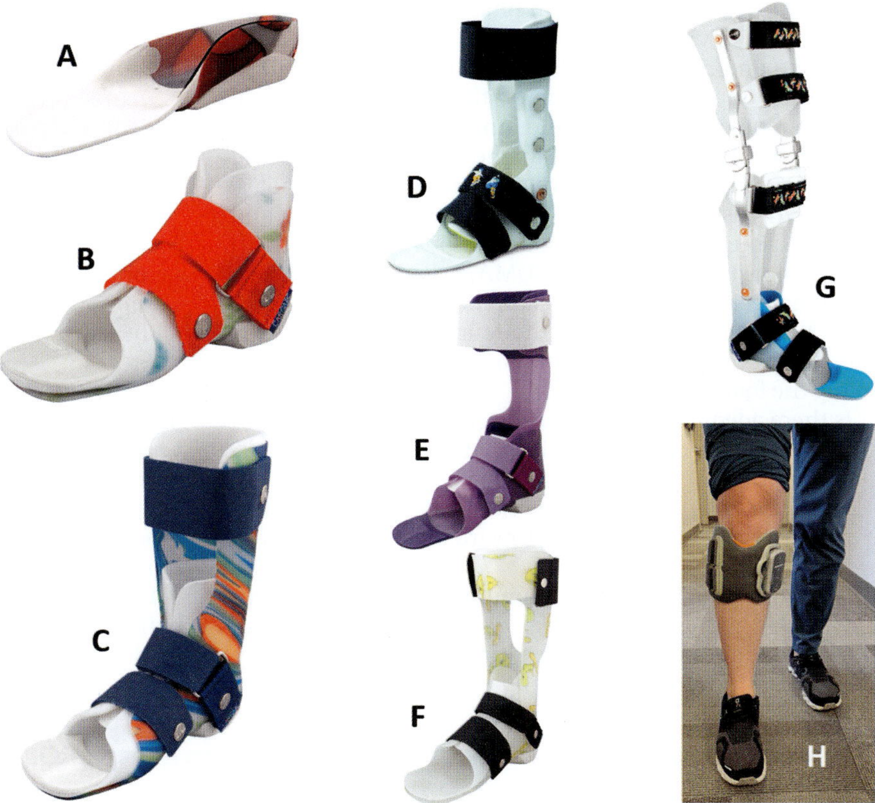

Fig. 10.9 Examples of various orthosis. (A) Custom-molded foot orthosis for moderate foot pronation and associated gait instability. (B) Supramalleolar orthosis for excessive foot pronation and/or supination along with hypotonus and sensory problems. (C) Solid ankle-foot orthosis (AFO) to provide maximal stability (but limited mobility) for severe hypertonus, foot drop, weak dorsiflexion and/or plantarflexion, medial/lateral instability of ankle/foot, and mild knee instability. (D) Articulating AFO with plantarflexion stop for toe walking and moderate knee hyperextension. (E) Posterior leaf spring AFO for moderate plantarflexor hypertonus, ankle/foot instability, and knee hyperextension in the presence of some motor control. (F) Floor reaction AFO for crouch gait to prevent knee buckling. (G) Knee-ankle-foot orthosis for higher-level paraplegia with medial/lateral knee and ankle instability, quadriceps weakness and knee hyperextension. (H) L300 Go functional electrical stimulation system to stimulate dorsiflexors to dynamically clear foot precisely during swing phase of gait cycle. A–G, Custom DAFO: "DAFO® images courtesy of Cascade Dafo, Inc." H, Courtesy student volunteer, DPT program, Radford University Carilion, Roanoke, Virginia.

influence is altered, as should concomitant deficits in other dimensions of muscle performance and motor control.[142] Several physical agent modalities have also been shown to have some effect on reducing spasticity, including focal or whole body vibration,[244–247] dry needling or acupuncture,[248–252] extracorporeal shockwave,[253–257] electrical stimulation[258–264] and transcranial magnetic stimulation,[265–268] although the evidence for long-lasting effects is limited.

SELECTING THE APPROPRIATE ORTHOSIS

Rehabilitation professionals play an active role in deciding what type of orthosis would be most appropriate for an individual with neuromuscular impairment. A number of factors contribute to the decision-making process; the collective wisdom of physical and occupational therapists, orthotists, physicians, family, and the patient who might benefit from orthotic intervention is necessary for appropriate and effective casting or orthotic intervention.[208,269,270]

The primary goal of orthotic or adaptive equipment prescription is to select the device and components that will best improve function, given the individual's pathologic condition and prognosis, desired activities, and participation needs, both in the immediate situation and over time. To do this, the cast, splint, or orthosis might provide external support, control or limit ROM, optimally position a limb for function, reduce the risk of secondary musculoskeletal complications, or provide a base for adaptive equipment that would make function more efficient. What evidence is available to support clinical decision-making with respect to orthotic prescription? Although many professionals rely on expertise gained by working with persons with neuromotor impairment over years of clinical practice, a growing number of articles on orthotic design for particular patient populations in the rehabilitation and orthotic research literature are available to guide decision-making not only for individuals with hypertonicity but also for those with SCI, myelomeningocele, and muscular dystrophy.[271–273] Evaluation of the effectiveness of the orthotic intervention is becoming increasingly important in clinical decision-making. Several articles related to specific outcome measures for effectiveness of orthotic use and patient satisfaction have recently been published.[274–281]

This chapter has discussed general orthotic and adaptive equipment usage; however, lower extremity orthotics are often a significant component of physical therapy practice, particularly for ambulation and gait dysfunction. When the primary goal of orthotic intervention is to improve safety and functionality during ambulation, it is imperative to identify where in the gait cycle abnormal tone or muscle performance is impaired (refer to Chapter 5 for more information on critical events in each subphase of gait, as well as detailed information about strategies to examine gait). Systematic consideration of a series of questions can help identify where within the gait cycle (considering both stance and swing phases) problems occur.[280,281]

Rehabilitation professions must recognize that no orthosis will fully normalize gait for persons with neurologically based gait difficulties. Whenever an external device is placed on a limb, it is likely to solve one problem while at the same time creating other constraints on limb function. The therapist, orthotist, and patient collectively problem solve during the orthotic prescription phase to prioritize the difficulties the individual is having during gait and then select the design and components that will allow the person to be most functional while walking, with the least additional constraint on other mobility and functional tasks.

The rehabilitation team at Rancho Los Amigos National Rehabilitation Center has developed an algorithm that is particularly useful in guiding clinical decision-making and sorting through possible orthotic options for adults with neuromotor impairment (ROADMAP: Recommendations for Orthotic Assessment, Decision-Making, and Prescription).[282] When considering orthotic interventions for persons having difficulty with ambulation, this team suggests asking the following questions:

1. Is there adequate ROM in the lower extremities to appropriately align or position limb segments in each subphase of gait?
2. Does the individual have the motivation and cognitive resources necessary to work toward meeting the goal of ambulation?
3. Does the individual have enough endurance (cardiovascular and cardiopulmonary resources) to be able to functionally ambulate? If endurance is not currently sufficient, might it be improved by a concurrent conditioning program?
4. Does the individual have adequate upper extremity, trunk, and lower extremity strength; power; motor control; and postural control for ambulation (with an appropriate assistive device, if necessary)? If these dimensions of movement are not currently sufficient, might they be improved with concurrent rehabilitation intervention?
5. Is there sufficient awareness of lower limb position (proprioception, kinesthesia) for controlled forward progression in gait? If not, might alternative sensory strategies be learned or used to substitute for limb position sense?

If the answers to most of these questions are "yes," the individual is considered to be a candidate for orthotic intervention. The next determinant is knee control and strength: If the individual has antigravity knee extension with the ability to respond to some resistance (manual muscle testing grade of 3+ strength), even if there is impaired proprioception in the involved limb, then an AFO may be appropriate. If there is impairment of strength or of proprioception (or both), then the team is more likely to recommend a knee-ankle-foot orthosis. Box 10.1 is an example of a decision

Box 10.1 Decision Tree for Orthotic Options Based on Rancho ROADMAP Algorithm

Is a KAFO Indicated?

- Is there at least antigravity with some resistance (MMT 3+/5 strength) in quadriceps bilaterally?
- Is proprioception intact bilaterally?

If yes: continue with the assessment for ankle-foot orthosis (AFO).

If no: KAFO may improve gait—continue assessment process.

Which KAFO Components Are the Most Appropriate?

- Is there at least antigravity with some resistance (MMT 3+/5 strength) in one lower extremity?
- Is proprioception intact in at least one lower extremity?

If no: consider trial of bilateral KAFOs or a reciprocal gait orthosis.

If yes: unilateral KAFO may be indicated—continue assessment to determine if knee locking mechanism is necessary.

Can the Knee Be Fully Extended, Without Pain, During Stance?

If no: consider KAFO with knee lock.

If yes: consider KAFO with variable knee mechanism and continue assessment.

Is There at Effective Active Control of Knee Extension During Stance?

If no: consider stance control knee mechanism.

If yes: consider free motion knee mechanism. Continue with AFO decision tree to determine appropriate ankle control strategy.

Is an AFO Indicated?

- Is there impairment of ankle strength?
- Is there impairment of proprioception?
- Is there hypertonicity of plantarflexors?
- Is there a combination of all of the above?

If no: may not require lower extremity orthosis.

If yes: lower extremity orthosis may improve gait—continue assessment process.

Which AFO Design and Components Are the Best Option?

- Does impaired strength hamper foot position in stance or swing?
- Does impaired proprioception hamper foot placement in stance or swing?
- Does hypertonicity/spasticity hamper foot position in stance or swing?

If no: consider adjustable articulating ankle joint (allows full DF and PF).

If yes: consider limiting or blocking ankle motion and continue assessment process.

Is There More Than Minimal Impairment of Static and Dynamic Postural Control in Standing?

- Is there significant spasticity?
- Is proprioception significantly impaired?

If no: consider adjustable articulating ankle joint that blocks PF beyond neutral ankle position and continue assessment.

If yes: consider solid ankle AFO or adjustable articulating ankle that is fully locked (consider rocker bottom shoe).

- Is there also plantarflexion strength ≤ MMT 4 in standing?
- Is there also excessive knee flexion and dorsiflexion during stance?
- Is there also excessive plantarflexion with knee hyperextension during stance?

If no: consider adjustable articulating ankle joint with PF stop, and continue assessment.

If yes: consider adjustable articulating ankle joint with PF stop and limited DF excursion, and continue assessment.

- Is there also dorsiflexion strength ≤4 in standing?

If no: consider adjustable articulating ankle with PF stop, limited DF excursion instance, no DF assist necessary.

If yes: consider adjustable articulating ankle with PF stop, limited DF excursion, and DF assist for effective swing phase.

DF, Dorsiflexion; *KAFO*, knee-ankle-foot orthosis; *MMT*, manual muscle testing; *PF*, plantarflexion.

tree used to guide the selection of components based on the ROADMAP algorithm.

AFO selection for persons with CP requires a nuanced assessment of strength, range of motion, and knee and ankle mechanics to compensate for weakness, control movement, and prevent deformity.[283] Several common gait patterns can develop with CP, including equinus, apparent equinus, jump gait, and crouch gait, and each requires different interventions.[283] Equinus refers to continuous excessive plantarflexion through stance and swing phase while maintaining knee and hip extension and commonly results in recurvatum of the knee, while apparent equinus incorporates compensatory hip and knee flexion. In jump gait, excessive plantarflexion is present with compensatory dorsiflexion at the midfoot with incomplete hip and knee extension during stance phase. Crouch gait involves ankle dorsiflexion with excessive knee and hip flexion. Wright and DiBello have provided some recommendations for orthotic interventions for such gait deviations in CP, as outlined in Table 10.8.[283] When used appropriately, AFOs have been shown to improve gait speed, cadence, dorsiflexion at initial contact, function of calf muscles, and ambulatory endurance.[284–286]

Another orthotic intervention is functional electrical stimulation (FES), which has been used to dynamically stimulate appropriate muscles at the right time to compensate for foot drop or impaired dorsiflexion for individuals with stroke, SCI, MS, CP, and brain injuries.[287] A Clinical Practice Guideline from the Academy of Neurologic Physical Therapy has provided recommendations for using AFOs or FES to improve lower extremity motor control following acute or chronic stroke resulting in poststroke hemiplegia.[288] They recommended assessing the various types of beneficial effects of using AFO or FES on patients. An immediate orthotic effect would mean improvements in mobility immediately after donning the device without any additional training or period of use. A training effect refers to mobility improvements seen with the device donned after a period of training with it. A therapeutic effect would show mobility improvements without a device donned after a period of training with it. Overall, they recommended using AFO or FES for improving gait speed, dynamic balance, walking endurance, muscle activation, gait kinematics, overall mobility, and quality of life, but not for improving plantarflexor spasticity. However, since various types of AFO (prefabricated, articulating, custom-fit) and FES (Bioness, WalkAide, Odstock) devices are available in the market, clinical decisions need to made regarding the device type, the timing of application, the duration of training with it, and long-term follow plans for optimal outcomes.[100,289] It is critically important that the individual who will use the orthosis and caregivers, as appropriate, are actively involved in the decision-making process. To make an informed decision, the person needing an orthosis must understand both the benefits and constraints associated with the orthotic designs and components being considered. He or she must be able to consider the range of orthotic options, as well as medical/surgical intervention and additional rehabilitation interventions that might affect his or her ability to walk. The entire team must consider what the individual who will be wearing the orthosis wants to accomplish, as well as the preferences he or she might have in terms of

Table 10.8 A Summary of Gait Pattern, Recommended AFO Interventions, and Considerations in Cerebral Palsy

Gait Pattern	Orthosis Options	Goals of Orthosis	Keys to Success
Equinus	Articulating AFO PLS AFO Solid AFO	■ Provide swing phase clearance ■ Allow ankle dorsiflexion as available	■ Evaluation of ankle dorsiflexion ROM with midfoot position considered ■ Strong soft tissue support to the midfoot within the AFO
Jump	PLS AFO Solid AFO	■ Provide swing phase clearance ■ Accommodate existing plantarflexion contracture ■ Minimize/eliminate compensatory dorsiflexion at the midfoot ■ Reestablish function of the PF_KE couple	■ Evaluation of ankle dorsiflexion ROM with midfoot position considered ■ Strong soft tissue support to the midfoot within the AFO ■ Proper alignment of the AFO within the footwear ■ Adequate stiffness to increase knee extension
Apparent equinus	Solid AFO FR-AFO	■ Provide swing phase clearance ■ May reestablish heel-first initial contact ■ Restrict unwanted/excessive tibial progression ■ Reestablish function of the PF-KE couple	■ Consideration of severity of spasticity ■ Proper alignment of the AFO within the footwear ■ Complementary interventions ■ Adequate stiffness to increase knee extension
Crouch	FR-AFO	■ Minimize demand on the quadriceps through reestablishment of the PF-KE ■ Prevent further progression of lever arm dysfunction	■ Evaluation of ankle dorsiflexion ROM with midfoot position considered ■ Consideration of orthopedics for transverse plane bony deformity ■ Strong soft tissue support to the midfoot within the AFO ■ Proper alignment of the AFO within the footwear ■ Adequate stiffness to increase knee extension ■ Complementary interventions

AFO, Ankle-foot orthosis; *PLS*, posterior leaf spring; *FR*, floor reaction; *PF-KE*, plantarflexion-knee extension.
Adapted from Wright E, DiBello SA. Principles of ankle-foot orthosis prescription in ambulatory bilateral cerebral palsy. *Phys Med Rehabil Clin N Am.* 2020;31(1):69–89.

ease of donning/doffing, wearing schedule, and cosmesis of the device being recommended. Beginning with a trial orthosis, perhaps a prefabricated or multiadjustable version would be helpful before finalizing the orthotic prescription, especially if it is unclear whether ambulation will eventually be possible. Certainly, most individuals with neuromuscular conditions that compromise their ability to walk benefit from a chance to experience what ambulation with an orthosis requires, given their individual constellation of impairments. Some may decide that using orthoses and an appropriate assistive device for functional ambulation throughout the day meets their mobility needs. Others may opt to use a wheelchair for primary mobility and reserve the use of orthoses to exercise bouts aimed at building cardiovascular endurance, since the energy cost of walking with knee-ankle-foot orthoses or hip-knee-ankle-foot orthoses are relatively high. Some may decide that orthotic intervention will not meet their needs and pursue other avenues to address mobility and endurance issues. Once a decision is made and the orthosis or adaptive equipment has been procured, education and practice are key components to successful adoption and usage of the device. The patient and the family/caregiver need specific training for each device including don/doff, putting patient into or out of the device, visual inspection for proper fit, and wear/use schedules. Additionally, training must include the assessment of skin integrity after use. Following trial, usage, and time for practice with the device for a period of time, the rehabilitation team must assess the patient/family/caregiver satisfaction with the product. Education, time, and practice with the product are the best indicators of long-term usage with functional benefits.[274,290,291]

Summary

This chapter reviewed several factors that influence the need for orthotics and adaptive equipment usage in the presence of neurological and neuromuscular disorders. The factors discussed include the functions and roles of structures and systems in both the CNS and the PNS; the impairments that are likely to occur when particular structures or systems are damaged by injury or disease process; abnormalities of tone and muscle performance; influence of impaired motor control on an individual's ability to move effectively and efficiently (including ambulation); the likelihood of developing secondary musculoskeletal impairments; and some of the pharmacological and surgical options available to manage hypertonicity and correct deformity that may develop over time. Strategies to determine gait impairments in an individual with various neuromotor impairments were explored, as well as the orthotic options that might best address those limitations the individual faces. This chapter provided a strong foundation for physical therapy examination and considerations for orthotic/equipment prescription. Next, the reader should consider physical therapy interventions that follow orthotic acquisition. The following case examples provide an opportunity for readers to focus on wearing, using, and caring for the prescribed orthosis, including (1) strategies to enhance motor learning when a new ambulatory aid (orthosis and/or assistive device) is introduced, (2) practice using the device under various environmental conditions (surfaces, obstacles, people moving within the environment), and (3) the ability to use the orthosis and ambulatory assistive device during functional activities, beyond walking, at comfortable gait speed.

Case Example 10.1 **A Young Child With Spastic Diplegic Cerebral Palsy**

T.H. is a 4-year-old child who was born prematurely at 32 weeks' gestation and was diagnosed with spastic diplegic cerebral palsy (CP) at 10 months of age. She is being evaluated for potential botulinum A injection as a strategy to manage significant extensor hypertonicity that is increasingly limiting her ability to ambulate as she grows. At present she uses bilateral articulating ankle-foot orthoses with a plantarflexion stop and a posterior rolling walker for locomotion at home and at preschool. Her articulating orthoses allow her to move into some dorsiflexion as she transitions to and from the floor during play. She has difficulty pushing to stand from half-kneel secondary to poor force production of hip and knee extensors. Muscle endurance is impaired, contributing to a crouch gait position, especially as she tires after a full day of activity. She falls frequently when she tries to run. She has been monitored in a CP clinic at the regional children's hospital; the team is concerned that she is developing rotational deformity of the lower extremities, as well as plantarflexion contracture and forefoot deformity due to her long-standing hypertonicity.

QUESTIONS TO CONSIDER

- In which subphases of the gait cycle is function or safety compromised when T.H. ambulates without her orthoses?
- In what way does T.H.'s hypertonicity contribute to her difficulty with floor mobility and ambulation?
- In what ways does T.H.'s inadequate muscle performance contribute to her difficulty with floor mobility and ambulation? What are the most likely dimensions of muscle performance that are impaired, given her diagnosis of spastic diplegia?
- Are there primary or secondary musculoskeletal impairments that are influencing her function and safety during ambulation? How do her age and future growth influence her risk for developing secondary impairments?
- Given her constellation of impairments, how can ambulation become more efficient and effective?
- What orthotic options (design, components) are available to address T.H.'s impairment of locomotion and related functional limitations? What are the pros and cons of each?
- What alternative or concurrent medical (surgical/pharmacological) interventions might assist improvement in safety and function for T.H.?
- What additional rehabilitation interventions might assist improvement in function and safety for T.H.?
- How do you anticipate T.H.'s orthotic needs might change as she develops and grows?
- What outcome measures are appropriate to assess efficacy of orthotic, therapeutic, pharmacological, or surgical intervention for T.H.?

Case Example 10.2 **A Child With Spastic Quadriplegic Cerebral Palsy**

J.T. is an 11-year-old boy with significant spastic quadriplegic cerebral palsy (CP) who is in the midst of a preadolescent growth spurt. He currently uses a custom seating system in a wheelchair for assisted mobility at school and in the community. At home he divides his time between an adaptive seating system and using a ceiling-mounted tracking system for assisted standing and mobility. J.T.'s mom reports that it is becoming increasingly difficult to transfer him in and out of the chair and help him with self-care activities because of upper extremity flexor tightness, increasing hip and knee flexion contractures, plantarflexion tightness, and his growing size.

In addition, when supine, J.T.'s resting position is becoming more obviously "windswept," with excessive right hip external rotation and excessive left hip internal rotation, causing a pelvic obliquity and rotation in his spine. He receives physical therapy at school several times each week to help him with functional abilities in the classroom and around school, with additional outpatient visits focusing on improving postural control and muscle performance. Both of his therapists are becoming concerned about his increasing limitation in range of motion, as well as the risk for increasing hip rotational deformity and spinal deformity as he grows. His outpatient therapist accompanies J.T. and his mother to the CP orthotics clinic at the regional children's medical center to explore the possibility of functional bracing or dynamic orthoses, or both, to manage the musculoskeletal complications that are developing because of his spasticity. They also have questions about surgical and pharmacological intervention.

QUESTIONS TO CONSIDER

- In what way does J.T.'s hypertonicity contribute to his difficulty with mobility/locomotion and other functional activities?
- In what ways does J.T.'s impaired muscle performance contribute to his difficulty with functional activities?
- In what ways does J.T.'s impaired postural control contribute to his difficulty with locomotion/ambulation? What are the most likely dimensions of his impairment in postural control, given his diagnosis of spastic quadriplegic CP?
- Are any primary or secondary musculoskeletal impairments influencing J.T.'s function and safety during mobility and transfer tasks?
- Given his constellation of impairments, what compensatory strategies is J.T. likely to use to accomplish his functional tasks at school and at home?
- Which of J.T.'s anticipated or observed impairments are remediable? Which will require accommodation?
- What orthotic options (design, components) are available to address J.T.'s impairments and functional limitations? What are the pros and cons of each?
- What adaptive equipment options are available to address J.T.'s impairments and functional limitations? What are the pros and cons of each?
- Given the pelvic obliquity and spinal rotation, what secondary musculoskeletal complications need to be monitored as J.T. grows? How might these concerns be addressed by seating or orthoses?
- What alternative or concurrent medical (surgical/pharmacological) interventions might assist improvement in safety and function for J.T.?
- What additional rehabilitation interventions might assist improvement in function and safety for J.T.?
- How do you anticipate J.T.'s orthotic and equipment needs might change as he develops and grows?
- What outcome measures are appropriate to assess efficacy of orthotic, equipment, therapeutic, pharmacological, or surgical intervention for J.T.?

Case Example 10.3 **A Young Adult With Acquired Brain Injury and Decerebrate Pattern Hypertonicity**

G.P. is a 17-year-old girl who sustained significant closed-head injury in a motor vehicle accident 3 weeks ago. She was admitted to the brain injury unit at the regional rehabilitation hospital earlier this week. Now functioning at a Rancho Los Amigos Cognitive Level 5 (confused and inappropriate), G.P. exhibits significant decorticate posturing whenever she attempts to move volitionally (right greater than left). She has marked limitations in passive range of motion at the elbow and wrist, as well as equinovarus at the ankle, both of which are limiting her ability to stand and effectively propel her wheelchair. While sitting, she falls when she tries to throw a ball to her therapist. Her gait is characterized by large range ballistic extensor thrust throughout stance, which impedes forward progression. She is most focused and responsive to intervention when involved in ambulation-oriented activities. Currently, her hypertonicity is being managed with oral baclofen (Lioresal). However, her therapists are concerned that contracture formation continues. During rehabilitation rounds, the physiatrist, neurologists, and therapists agree that a trial of serial casting should be added to her regimen to enhance her rehabilitation.

QUESTIONS TO CONSIDER

- In which subphases of the gait cycle is function or safety compromised when G.P. attempts to ambulate?
- In what way does G.P.'s hypertonicity contribute to her difficulty with postural control and locomotion/ambulation?
- In what ways does G.P.'s impaired muscle performance contribute to her difficulty with postural control and locomotion/ambulation? What are the most likely dimensions of her impairment in muscle performance, given her diagnosis of acquired brain injury?
- Are any primary or secondary musculoskeletal impairments influencing her function and safety during ambulation? What do you think is likely to develop as she recovers from her head injury?
- Given her constellation of impairments, what compensatory strategies is G.P. likely to use to accomplish the task of locomotion?
- Which of G.P.'s anticipated or observed impairments are remediable? Which will require accommodation?
- What orthotic options (design, components) are available to address G.P.'s impairment of locomotion and related functional limitations? What are the pros and cons of each?
- What orthotic options (design, components) are available to address G.P.'s impairment of specific joints? What are the pros and cons of each?
- What alternative or concurrent medical (surgical/pharmacological) interventions might assist improvement in safety and function for G.P.?
- What additional rehabilitation interventions might assist improvement in function and safety for G.P.?
- How do you anticipate G.P.'s orthotic needs might change as she recovers over the next year?
- What outcome measures are appropriate to assess efficacy of orthotic, therapeutic, pharmacological, or surgical intervention for G.P.?

Case Example 10.4 Two Individuals With Recent Stroke

You work in the short-term rehabilitation unit associated with the regional tertiary care hospital in your area. This week two gentlemen recovering from stroke sustained 3 days ago were admitted to the unit for a short stay in preparation for discharge home. Both indicate that their primary goals at this time are to be able to walk functional distances within their homes, manage stairs to enter/leave the house, and get to bedrooms on the second floor. You anticipate that they will receive intensive rehabilitation services for 5 to 8 days, with home care for follow-up after discharge.

M.O., 73 years old with a history of hypertension, mild chronic obstructive pulmonary disease, and an uncomplicated myocardial infarction 2 years ago, has been diagnosed with a lacunar infarct within the left posterior limb of internal capsule. On passive motion, he has been given modified Ashworth scores of 3 in his right upper extremity and 2 in his right lower extremity. When asked to bend his knee (when supine), he demonstrates difficulty initiating flexion, and when he finally begins to move, his ankle, knee, and hip move in a mass-flexion pattern; he is unable to isolate limb segments. When asked to slowly lower his leg to the bed, he "shoots" into a full lower extremity synergy pattern. He rises from sitting to standing with verbal and tactile cueing, somewhat asymmetrically, relying on his left extremities. Once upright, he can shift his center of mass to the midline, holding an effective upright posture, but feels unsteady when shifted beyond midline to the right. With encouragement and facilitation, he can shift weight toward his right in preparation for swing-limb advancement of the left lower extremity, and he is pleased to have taken a few steps, however short, in the parallel bars. Before his infarct, he was an avid golfer and enjoyed bowling. He is fearful that he will never be able to resume these activities.

E.B. is a 64-year-old recently retired car mechanic with an 8-year history of diabetes mellitus previously controlled by diet and oral medications who has required insulin since his stroke. Magnetic resonance imaging indicates probable occlusion in the right posteroinferior branch of the middle cerebral artery, with ischemia and resultant inflammation in the parietal lobe. Because E.B. has been afraid of hospitals for most of his life, he resisted seeking medical care as his symptoms began, arriving at the emergency department 12 hours after the onset of hemiplegia. He currently displays a heavy, hypotonic, somewhat edematous left upper extremity. He is unusually unconcerned about the fact that he has had a stroke and tells you that he should be able to function "well enough" when he returns home to his familiar environment. On examination, he demonstrates homonymous hemianopsia, especially of the lower left visual field, and impaired kinesthetic awareness of his left extremities. You observe that he appears to be unaware when his lower upper extremity slips off the tray table of his wheelchair and his fingers become entangled in the spokes of the wheel as he propels forward using his right leg. When assisted to standing in the parallel bars, he does not seem to be accurately aware of his upright position, requiring moderate assistance to keep him from falling to the left. When asked to try to walk forward a few paces, he repeatedly advances his right lower extremity, even when prompted to consider the position and activity of his lower left extremity.

QUESTIONS TO CONSIDER

- In what ways are the stroke-related impairments observed in these two gentlemen similar or different? How can you explain these differences?
- In what subphases of the gait cycle is function or safety compromised when each of these gentleman attempts to ambulate?
- In what way does each gentleman's abnormal tone contribute to his difficulty with postural control and locomotion/ambulation?
- In what ways does each gentleman's impaired muscle performance contribute to his difficulty with postural control and locomotion/ambulation? What are the most likely dimensions of each male's impairment in muscle performance, given his etiologic condition and location of stroke?
- Are any primary or secondary musculoskeletal impairments influencing each male's function and safety during ambulation? How does each male's age and concomitant medical conditions influence his risk for developing secondary impairments?
- Given each gentleman's constellation of impairments, what compensatory strategies are likely to be used to accomplish the task of locomotion in each male?
- Which of each gentleman's anticipated or observed impairments are remediable? Which will require accommodation?
- What orthotic options are available to address each gentleman's impairment of locomotion and related functional limitations? What are the pros and cons of each?
- What alternative or concurrent medical (surgical/pharmacological) interventions might help improve in safety and function for each individual?
- What additional rehabilitation interventions might help improve function and safety for M.O. and E.B.?
- How do you anticipate each gentleman's orthotic needs, which might change as he recovers from central nervous system damage?
- What outcome measures are appropriate to assess the efficacy of orthotic, therapeutic, pharmacological, or surgical intervention for each gentleman?

Case Example 10.5 A Young Adult With Incomplete Spinal Cord Injury

Z.C. is a 23-year-old male who sustained an incomplete C7 spinal cord injury 3 weeks ago when he lost control and crash-landed during a failed acrobatic stunt during a half-pipe snowboard competition at a local ski resort. After being stabilized on site, he was quickly airlifted to a regional spinal cord injury/trauma center. Methylprednisolone was administered within 1.5 hours of injury, and his cervical fractures were repaired by fusion (C5–T1) the day after injury; he now wears a Miami J cervical orthosis. He was admitted to your rehabilitation center 5 days ago. He demonstrates no activity of triceps brachii bilaterally but reports dysesthesia in the C7 and C8 dermatomes and can point his index finger on the left. He is aware of lower limb position in space and can activate toe flexors and extensors, plantarflexors, knee extensors, and

Case Example 10.5 A Young Adult With Incomplete Spinal Cord Injury

hip flexors and abductors at 2+/5 levels of strength. Deep tendon reflex at the Achilles heel is brisk bilaterally, whereas more proximal lower extremity reflexes are diminished. He demonstrates positive Babinski reflex bilaterally. Biceps and wrist extensor deep tendon reflexes, initially diminished, are now rated 2+; the triceps reflex, initially diminished, is now quite brisk. He requires moderate assistance of 1 to come to sitting from supine but can hold a static posture in sitting, demonstrating a limited sway envelope when attempting to shift his weight anteriorly, posteriorly, and mediolaterally. He requires moderate assistance of 1 to rise from seated in his wheelchair to a standing position in the parallel bars. He is determined to "walk" out of the facility on discharge, which is anticipated after 3 more weeks of rehabilitation.

QUESTIONS TO CONSIDER

- Given Z.C.'s history and present point in recovery from spinal cord injury, what is the anticipated prognosis concerning his functional performance and ability to ambulate?
- In what subphases of the gait cycle is function or safety likely to be compromised when Z.C. attempts to ambulate?
- In what way does Z.C.'s abnormal tone contribute to his difficulty with postural control and locomotion/ambulation? What strategies would be useful in documenting/assessing the severity and type of his abnormal tone?
- In what ways does Z.C.'s impaired muscle performance contribute to his difficulty with postural control and locomotion/ambulation? What are the most likely dimensions of his impairment in muscle performance, given his etiologic condition and level of injury?
- Are any primary or secondary musculoskeletal impairments likely to influence Z.C.'s function and safety during ambulation? How do Z.C.'s age and concomitant medical conditions influence his risk for developing secondary impairments?
- Given Z.C.'s constellation of impairments, what compensatory strategies is he likely to use to accomplish the task of locomotion?
- Which of Z.C.'s anticipated or observed impairments are remediable? Which will require accommodation?
- What orthotic options (design, components) are available to address Z.C.'s difficulty with locomotion and related functional limitations? What are the pros and cons of each?
- What alternative or concurrent medical (surgical/pharmacological) interventions might assist improvement in safety and function?
- What additional rehabilitation interventions might assist improvement in function and safety for Z.C.?
- How do you anticipate Z.C.'s orthotic needs might change as he recovers from his spinal cord injury?
- What outcome measures are appropriate to assess the efficacy of orthotic, therapeutic, pharmacological, or surgical intervention for Z.C.?

Case Example 10.6 A Middle-Aged Adult With Chronic Stroke

A.T. is a 57-year-old male presenting to your outpatient clinic who suffered a left middle cerebral artery stroke 2 years prior, which has resulted in right foot drop and diminished right upper extremity dexterity. He ambulates with a cane for short distances in the community, but has difficulty on inclines and uneven surfaces and has had three falls in the last year. He reports he does not walk more than 500 feet at a time due to fatigue. He avoids stairs due to apprehension. On observation, a steppage gait pattern is noted for adequate right toe clearance during the swing phase. His wife still works and is available to provide assistance and transportation only in the evenings. He would like to know what options are available to allow him to navigate in the community more effectively and reduce fall risk.

QUESTIONS TO CONSIDER

- What orthotic interventions may benefit A.T. in improving walking endurance and dynamic balance?
- What factors must be considered regarding ability to utilize a recommended orthotic during training and daily activities?
- How likely is an orthotic to benefit A.T. given the elapsed time passed since the initial incident?
- Which complaints and mobility challenges can A.T. expect to improve with proper orthotic use?
- What length of training and use should A.T. anticipate prior to mobility benefits being noted?
- Which outcome measures would be appropriate for baseline assessment and monitoring progress?

References

The complete listing of the References are available in the accompanying enhanced eBook version included with the print purchase of this textbook. Visit Elsevier eBooks+ (eBooks.Health.Elsevier.com) to access this content.

11 Orthoses for Knee Dysfunction

S. TYLER SHULTZ

LEARNING OBJECTIVES

On completion of this chapter, the reader will be able to do the following:

1. Describe the various types and classifications of knee orthoses.
2. Appreciate normal knee function.
3. Identify common knee conditions for which bracing is a component of conservative intervention.
4. Compare and contrast the purposes, indications, and limitations of prophylactic, functional, and rehabilitative knee orthoses.
5. Apply current research evidence to clinical decision-making with regard to knee bracing as an intervention, including biomechanical and functional implications.
6. Provide clinical rationale for utilizing knee orthoses as an intervention for impairments at the tibiofemoral and patellofemoral joints.

Introduction

Knee orthoses are used as a common intervention in orthopedic and physical therapy practice, not only for the treatment of knee impairments, but also for injury prevention. The clinical goals of using knee orthoses include pain reduction, joint protection, functional or recreational improvement, and injury prevention. The effectiveness of bracing to meet these clinical goals by providing joint unloading, external stability, or patellofemoral tracking is not universally accepted by clinicians and does not have high-level evidence.[1] Additionally, patients may find knee braces to be uncomfortable, ineffective, or cumbersome, which negatively impact brace effectiveness.[2]

Knee orthoses can be organized by their intended function: prophylactic, functional, and rehabilitative knee braces. Prophylactic knee orthoses (PKOs) are designed and used to protect athletes from sustaining debilitating injuries, usually ligamentous, without inhibiting overall knee function and mobility.[3] Prophylactic knee bracing continues to be used despite inconclusive and at times, conflicting evidence supporting brace ability to protect the user from injury[1,4] Clinically, PKOs tend to be used with individuals who are deemed to be at high risk for knee injury based on their chosen sport and individual history of previous knee dysfunction. Functional knee orthoses (FKOs) attempt to provide external support and biomechanical stability to the joint following a knee injury.[3] FKOs can be further categorized based on impairment or limitation in the knee structure with which they are intended to help. FKOs that are designed for individuals who have ligamentous instability, for example, provide external support that would limit the same knee motion as the ligament. These braces can also serve a rehabilitative function, as seen with patients who have suffered anterior cruciate ligament (ACL) rupture and have undergone surgical repair. Furthermore, rehabilitative braces function to provide protection and progressive range of motion (ROM) to the joint (Fig. 11.1). Rehabilitative braces include unloading braces and patellofemoral braces. These braces are used to decrease joint load across the tibiofemoral and patellofemoral joints and reduce pain in the arthritic joint. Orthoses for patellofemoral disorders are rehabilitative braces that often attempt to correct patellar tracking (Fig. 11.2). Each of these different types of braces can be custom-designed for patients or prefabricated. This chapter will describe in further detail the design, function, effectiveness, and clinical decision-making involved with the use of these knee orthoses.

In order for a clinician to select and prescribe the appropriate knee orthoses for a patient, a patient-centered approach must be used. The clinician needs to understand the purpose for bracing and have an underlying mastery of normal knee structure and function. For example, the knee brace prescribed to an individual following a tear of the ACL would be different than the brace used to treat medial knee osteoarthritis (OA). The implications of a pathologic condition of the knee, as well as the functional goals of braces, will be presented. Indications for bracing in the management of patients with knee injury and dysfunction are also discussed.

Anatomy of the Knee

The articulations at the tibiofemoral joint and the patellofemoral joint form the knee complex. An understanding of the anatomy and biomechanics of each respective joint is critical in knowing the potential stresses and implications of pathologic conditions of the knee that can occur at the knee complex.

THE TIBIOFEMORAL JOINT

The knee joint is a hinge-like articulation between the medial and lateral condyles of the femur and the medial and lateral tibial plateau (Fig. 11.3). Because of the shape and asymmetry of the condyles, the instantaneous axis of knee flexion/extension motion changes through the

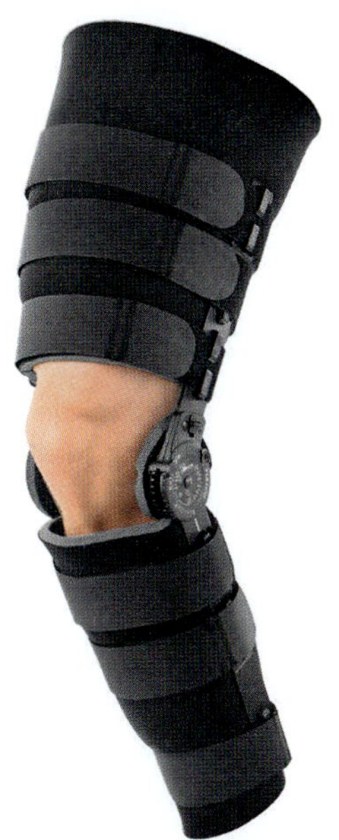

Fig. 11.1 Example of a common style of postoperative brace. Notice the longer areas of support to the thigh and calf areas. The sidebars are connected with a hinge that allows for limiting or progressing range of motion available at the joint. (Courtesy Breg. Retrieved from: https://www.breg.com/wp-content/uploads/product_images/Post_Op.png.)

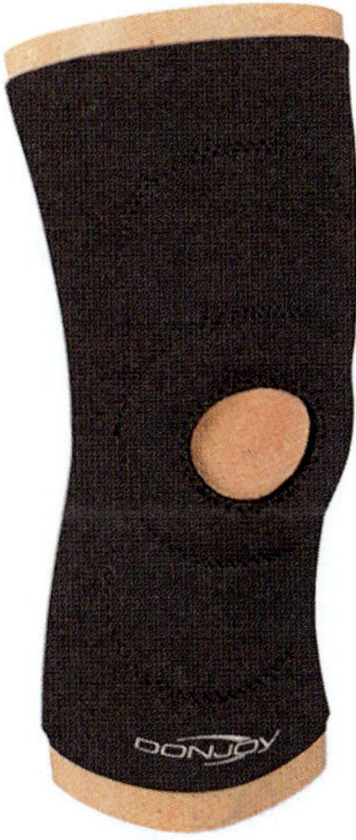

Fig. 11.2 Example of an open patella neoprene knee sleeve. (Courtesy DonJoy.)

arc of motion. As the knee moves from extension to flexion, the instant center pathway moves posteriorly.[5] In open chain movements (non–weight-bearing activities), the tibia rotates around the femoral condyles. In closed-chain movements (weight-bearing activities), an anatomical locking mechanism is present in the final degrees of extension as the longer medial femoral condyle rotates medially on the articular surfaces of the tibia. Consequently, if the instant center of pathway changes, it will alter the optimal joint mechanics and therefore result in abnormal knee stressors. The alignment between an adducted femur and relatively upright tibia creates a vulnerability to valgus stress in many weight-bearing activities. The capsule that encases the knee joint is reinforced by the collagen-rich medial and lateral retinaculum. The medial and lateral menisci rest on the tibial plateau. They are fibrocartilaginous, nearly ring-shaped disks that are flexibly attached around the edges of the tibial plateau (see Fig. 11.3). These menisci increase the concavity of the tibial articular surface, enhancing congruency of articulation with the femoral condyles to facilitate normal gliding and distribute weight-bearing forces within the knee during gait and other loading activities.[6] The menisci also play an important role in nutrition and lubrication of the articular surfaces of the knee joint.

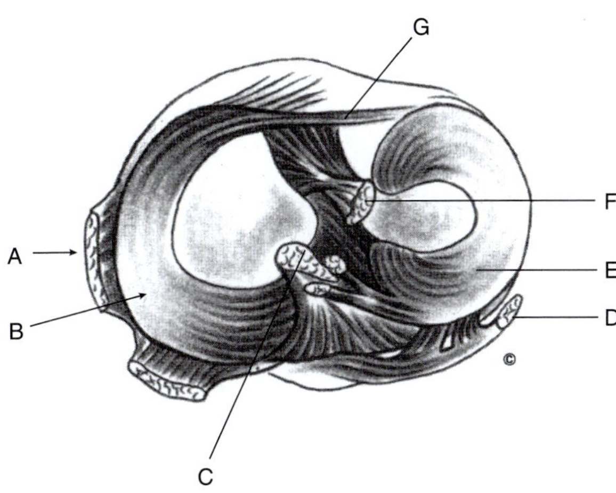

Fig. 11.3 In this view of the surface of the tibia, we can identify the medial collateral ligament (A), the C-shaped medial meniscus on the large medial tibial plateau (B), the posterior cruciate ligament with the accessory anterior and posterior meniscofemoral ligaments (C), the tendon of the popliteus muscle (D), the circular lateral meniscus on the smaller lateral tibial plateau (E), the anterior cruciate ligament as it twists toward the inside of the lateral femoral condyle (F), and the transverse ligament (G). (From Greenfield BH. *Rehabilitation of the Knee: A Problem Solving Approach*. FA Davis; 1993.)

Stability to the tibiofemoral joint is provided by sets of ligaments. The medial (tibial) collateral ligament (MCL) and the lateral (fibular) collateral ligament (LCL) are extrinsic ligaments. The collateral ligaments counter valgus and varus forces that act on the knee. In addition, two intrinsic ligaments of the tibiofemoral joint, the ACL and the posterior cruciate ligaments (PCLs), check translatory forces that displace the tibia on the femur. The location of attachments makes each of these ligaments most effective at particular points in the knee's normal arc of motion.[6] Additionally, contraction of the quadriceps and knee flexor muscle groups produce compressive forces that help stabilize the knee. Muscles of the hip and lower leg also make contributions to the mechanics of the femur and tibia, respectively, which impact the movements of the knee complex.

Medial Collateral Ligament

The MCL is a strong, flat membranous band that overlays the middle portion of the medial joint capsule (Fig. 11.4). It is most effective in counteracting valgus stressors when the knee is slightly flexed to fully extended. Approximately 8 to 10 cm in length, it originates at the medial epicondyle of the femur and attaches to the medial surface of the tibial plateau. The MCL can be subdivided into a set of oblique posterior fibers and anterior parallel fibers.

A bundle of meniscotibial fibers, also known as the *posterior oblique ligament*, runs deep to the MCL, from the femur to the midperipheral margin of the medial meniscus and

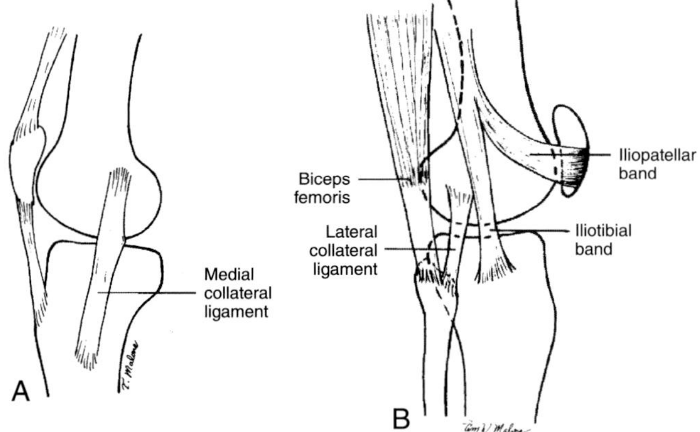

Fig. 11.4 (A) A medial view of the right knee showing structures that provide medial support to the right knee. (B) A lateral view of the right knee illustrating structures that give lateral support to the knee. (Reprinted with permission from Levangie PK, Norkin CC. The knee. In: *Joint Structure and Function: A Comprehensive Analysis.* Third ed. FA Davis; 2017.)

toward the tibia. These fibers connect the medial meniscus to the tibia and help form the semimembranosus corner of the medial knee. Additionally, the medial patellar retinacular fibers play a reinforcing role.[7]

Lateral Collateral Ligament and Iliotibial Band

The LCL resists varus stressors and lateral rotation of the tibia and is most effective when the knee is slightly flexed. The LCL runs from the lateral femoral condyle (the back part of the outer tuberosity of the femur) to the proximal lateral aspect of the fibular head (see Fig. 11.4). The tendon of the popliteus muscle and the external articular vessels and nerves pass beneath this ligament.

Another lateral structure that acts on the knee complex is the iliotibial band (ITB). The ITB is positioned slightly anterior to the LCL and is taut in all ranges of knee motion. Its lateral position allows it to stabilize against varus forces along with the LCL.

Anterior Cruciate Ligament

The ACL runs at an oblique angle between the articular surfaces of the knee joint and prevents forward shift and excessive medial rotation of the tibia as the knee moves toward extension (Fig. 11.5). The ACL attaches to the tibia in a fossa just anterior and lateral to the anterior tibial spine and to the femur in a fossa on the posteromedial surface of the lateral femoral condyle. The ACL's tibial attachment is somewhat wider and stronger than its femoral attachment. Some authors divide the fasciculi that make up the broad, somewhat flat ACL into two or three distinct bundles. The ligament's anteromedial band, with fibers running from the anteromedial tibia to the proximal femoral attachment, is most taut in flexion and relatively lax in extension. The posterolateral bulk (PLB), which begins at the posterolateral tibial attachment, is most taut in extension and relatively lax in flexion. An intermediate bundle of transitional fibers between the anteromedial band and PLB tends to tighten when the knee moves through the midranges of motion. This arrangement of fibers ensures tension in the ACL throughout the entire range of knee motion. The ACL is most vulnerable to injury when the femur rotates internally

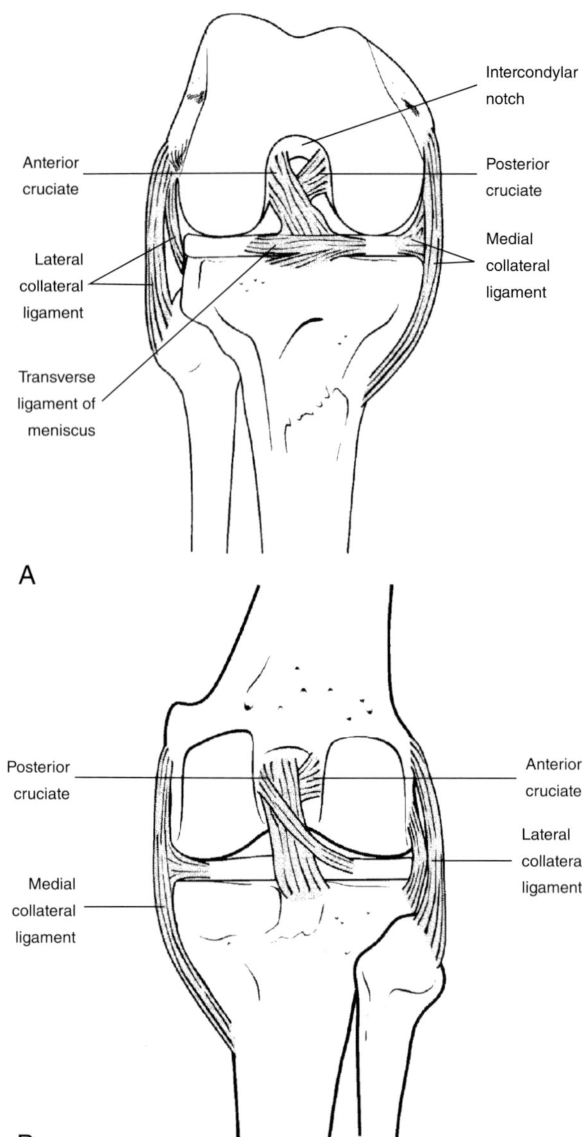

Fig. 11.5 (A) Anterior view of the tibiofemoral joint in 90 degrees of knee flexion showing the menisci and the ligamentous structures that stabilize the knee. (B) Posterior view of the knee in extension. (Reprinted with permission from Antich TJ. Orthoses for the knee; the tibiofemoral joint. In: Nawoczenski DA, Epler ME, eds. *Orthotics in Functional Rehabilitation of the Lower Limb.* Saunders; 1997.)

on the tibia when the knee is flexed and the foot is fixed on the ground during weight-bearing activities.

Posterior Cruciate Ligament

The PCL restrains posterior displacement of the tibia in its articulation with the femur, especially as the knee moves toward full extension.[6] The PCL is shorter and less oblique in orientation than the ACL; it is the strongest and most resistant ligament of the knee. PCL fibers run from a slight depression between articular surfaces on the posterior tibia to the posterolateral surface of the medial femoral condyle (see Figs. 11.3 and 11.5). Like the ACL, the PCL can be divided into anterior and posterior segments. The larger anterior medial band is most taut between 80 and 90 degrees of flexion and is relatively lax in extension. The smaller PLB travels somewhat obliquely across the joint, becoming taut as the knee moves into extension. The PCL plays a role in the locking mechanism of the knee as tension in the ligament produces lateral (external) rotation of the tibia on the femur in the final degrees of knee extension. The PCL may also assist the collateral ligaments when varus or valgus stressors are applied to the knee.[6]

Coursing along with fibers from the MCL is the meniscofemoral ligament, which stretches between the posterior horn of the lateral meniscus and the lateral surface of the medial femoral condyle. The anterior meniscofemoral band (ligament of Humphry) runs along the medial anterior surface of the PCL and may be up to one-third of its diameter. The posterior meniscofemoral band (ligament of Wrisberg) lies posterior to the PCL and may be as much as one half its diameter. The meniscofemoral ligaments pull the lateral meniscus forward during flexion of the weight-bearing knee to maintain as much articular congruency as possible with the lateral femoral condyle.

POSTEROLATERAL CORNER OF THE KNEE

The lateral meniscus is somewhat more mobile than the medial meniscus because of the anatomy of the posterolateral corner of the knee. The arcuate complex and posterolateral corner run from the styloid process of the fibula, joining the posterior oblique ligament on the posterior aspect of the femur and tibia. The arcuate ligament is firmly attached to the underlying popliteus muscle and tendon. The tendon of the popliteus muscle separates the deep joint capsule from the rim of the lateral meniscus.

PATELLOFEMORAL JOINT

The *patella*, a sesamoid bone embedded in the tendon of the quadriceps femoris, is an integral part of the extensor mechanism of the knee. The patella functions as an anatomical pulley, increasing the knee extension moment created by contraction of the quadriceps femoris by as much as 50%. It also guides the forces generated by the quadriceps femoris to the patellar ligament, protects deeper knee joint anatomy, protects the quadriceps tendon from frictional forces, and increases the compressive forces to which the extensor mechanisms can be subjected.[6]

Although the anterior surface of the patella is convex, the posterior surface has three distinct anatomical areas: a lateral, medial, and odd facet. The lateral and medial facets are separated by a vertical ridge. The odd facet articulates with the medial condyle at the end range of knee extension (Fig. 11.6). The posterior patellar surface is covered with hyaline articular cartilage, except for the distal apex, which is roughened for the attachment of the patellar tendon. Pressure between the patella and trochlear groove of the femur increases substantially as the knee flexes. During knee flexion, the patella moves in a complex but consistent three-dimensional (3D) pattern of multiplanar rotation, tilting, and shift relative to the femur.

The stability of the patella is derived from the patellofemoral joint's static structural characteristics and dynamic (muscular) control. Static stability is a product of the anatomy of the patella—the depth of the intercondylar groove, and the prominent and longer lateral condyle of the femur.

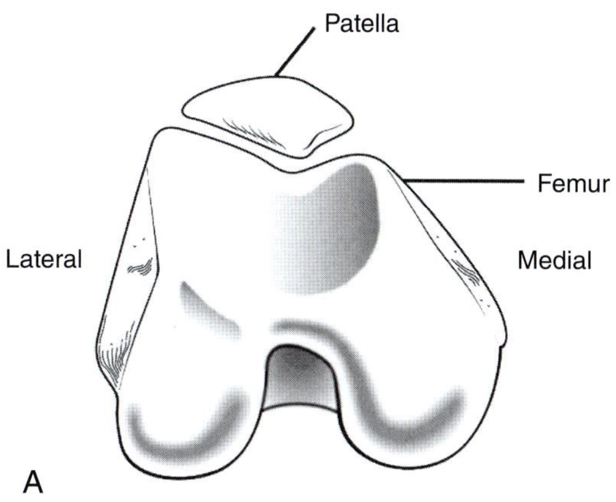

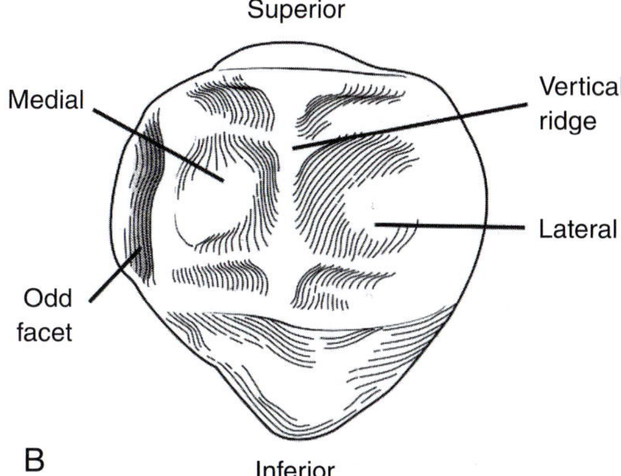

Fig. 11.6 (A) The normal position of the patella in the intercondylar groove of the distal femur. (B) Underside of the patella with its three facets and vertical ridge. (Reprinted with permission from Belyea BC. Orthoses for the knee: the patellofemoral joint. In: Nawoczenski DA, Epler ME, eds. *Orthotics in Functional Rehabilitation of the Lower Limb*. Saunders; 1997.)

Wiberg[8] divides the patellofemoral joint into six types based on the size and shape of facets (Table 11.1). The depth of the patellar trochlea and the facet pattern are important in patellar stability.

Dynamic stability of the patellofemoral joint is derived primarily from activity of the quadriceps femoris as well as from the tensile properties of the patellar ligament (Fig. 11.7). The four components of the quadriceps muscle act together to pull the patella obliquely upward along the shaft of the femur, whereas the patellar ligament anchors it almost straight downward along the anatomical axis of

Table 11.1 Classification of Patellar Types, Listed From Most to Least Stable

Patellar Type	Description
I	Equal medial and lateral facets, both slightly concave
II	Small medial facet, both facets slightly concave
II/III	Small, flat medial facet
III	Small, slightly convex medial facet
IV	Very small, steeply sloped medial facet with medial ridge
V (Jagerhut)	No medial facet, no central ridge

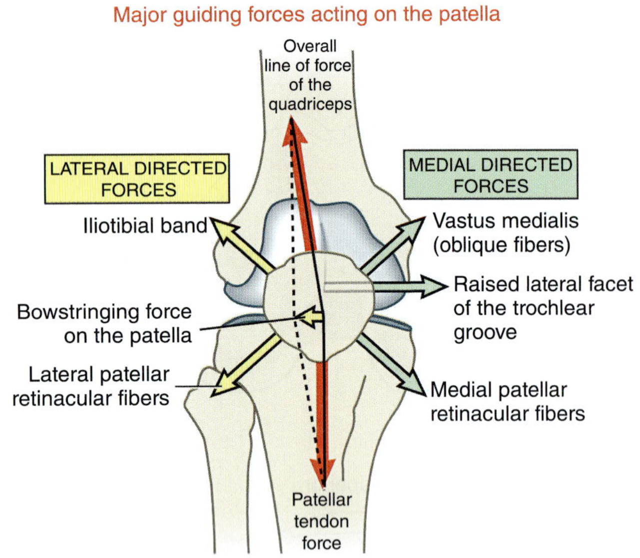

Fig. 11.7 A schematic diagram of structures that act on the patella. (Reprinted with permission from Neumann DA. *Kinesiology of the Musculoskeletal System: Foundations for Rehabilitation*. Third ed. Mosby Elsevier, 2017.)

the lower leg. The tibial tubercle is typically located at least 6 degrees lateral to the mechanical axis of the femur.

Because the structure of the patellofemoral articulation and the muscular/ligamentous forces that act on the patella are complex, patellar dynamics involve much more than simple cephalocaudal repositioning as the knee is flexed or extended. Patellar movements, with the execption of flexion, are influenced by the rotation of the tibia and the dynamic stabilization of the muscles that act on the patella.

Biomechanics of Knee Motion

Although it is beyond the scope of this chapter to comprehensively cover the biomechanics of knee motion, it is important to have a basic foundation of knee biomechanics to understand the use of knee orthoses as an intervention for pathologic conditions of the knee. Evaluating and managing injuries of the knee requires an in-depth understanding of the biomechanical characteristics of the knee joint. The *kinematics of the knee* describe its motion in terms of the type and location and the magnitude and direction of the motion. The *kinetics of the knee* describe the forces that act on the knee, causing movement.[6] Kinetic forces are classified as either external forces that work on the body (e.g., gravity) or as internal body-generated forces (e.g., friction, tensile strength of soft tissue structures, muscle contraction).

Motion in the tibiofemoral joint can be best understood by separating the motion into its physiological and accessory components. Physiological motion can be controlled consciously, most often through voluntary contraction of muscle. Osteokinematic (bone movement) and arthrokinematic (joint surface motion) are examples of physiological motion. Accessory motion occurs without conscious control and cannot be reproduced voluntarily. Joint play, which is elicited by passive movement during examination of a joint, is an example of an accessory motion. The magnitude and type of accessory motion possible are determined by the characteristics of a particular articulation and the properties of the tissues that surround it. The arthrokinematics of the tibiofemoral joint will vary depending on whether the lower extremity is in a weight-bearing or loaded position. For example, with tibial-femoral extension the tibia moves anteriorly relative to the femur, and with femoral-tibia extension the femoral condyles slide from anterior to posterior, while rolling anteriorly.[7]

One of the important accessory component motions of the tibiofemoral joint is its *screw home* or locking mechanism. In the final degrees of knee extension, the tibia continues to rotate around the large articular surface of the medial femoral condyle. This motion cannot be prevented or changed by volitional effort; it is entirely the result of the configuration of the articular surfaces. When the knee is flexed to or beyond 90 degrees, however, conscious activation of muscles can produce physiological (osteokinematic) external (lateral) or internal (medial) rotation of the tibia on the femur.

Three osteokinematic motions are possible at the tibiofemoral joint. Knee flexion/extension occurs in the sagittal plane around an axis in the frontal plane (x-axis). Internal/external rotation of the tibia on the femur (or vice versa) occurs in the transverse plane around a longitudinal axis (y-axis). Abduction and adduction occur in the frontal plane around a horizontal axis (z-axis). The arthrokinematic movements of the tibiofemoral joint are rolling, gliding, and sliding (Fig. 11.8). It is important to note that the roll-glide ratio is not constant during tibiofemoral joint motion: Approximately 1:2 in early flexion, the roll-glide ratio becomes almost 1:4 in late flexion. Rolling and gliding occur primarily on the posterior portion of the femoral condyles. In the first 15 to 20 degrees of flexion, a true rolling motion of the femoral condyles occurs in concert with the tibial plateau. As the magnitude of flexion increases, the femur begins to glide posteriorly on the tibia. Gliding becomes more significant as flexion increases.

From a kinematic standpoint, the ACL and PCL operate as a true gear mechanism controlling the roll-glide motion of the tibiofemoral joint. With rupture of either or both of the cruciate ligaments, the gear mechanism becomes ineffective, and the arthrokinematic motion is altered. In an ACL-deficient knee, the femur is able to roll beyond the posterior half of the tibial plateau, increasing the likelihood of damage or tear of the posterior horn of the medial or lateral meniscus.

Because the knee has characteristics of a hinge joint and an arthrodial joint, two types of motion (translatory and rotatory) can occur in each plane of motion (sagittal, frontal/coronal, transverse). For this reason, knee motion is described as having six degrees of freedom. The three translatory motions of the knee include anteroposterior translation, mediolateral translation, and compression-distraction motion. The three rotatory motions occur in flexion/extension, varus/valgus, and internal (medial)/external (lateral) rotation.[6]

Knee Orthoses Components

Commercially available knee orthoses are comprised of different components, depending on the purpose of the brace

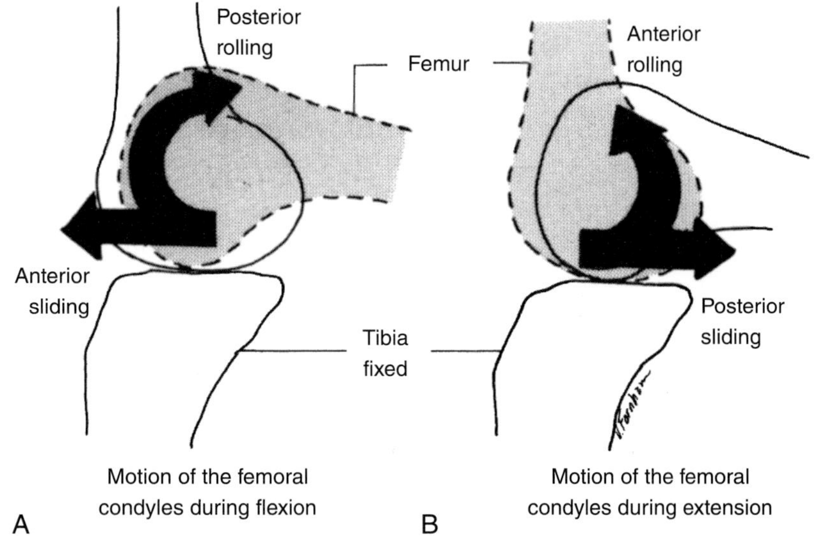

Fig. 11.8 Diagram of femoral motion on a fixed tibia. (A) As the knee flexes, the femoral condyles roll posteriorly *(curved arrow)* while gliding/sliding forward *(straight arrow)*. (B) As the knee extends, the condyles roll forward *(curved arrow)* while gliding posteriorly *(straight arrow)*. (From Hartigan E, Lewek M, Snyder-Mackler L. The knee. In: Levangie PK, Norkin CC, eds. *Joint Structure and Function: A Comprehensive Analysis*. Fifth ed. David, 2011:355.)

(Fig. 11.9). Braces to unload or protect the joint will likely have some type of sidebar support and connect with either a freely moving hinge or one that can be set to limit knee ROM (see Fig. 11.1). Sidebars can be constructed of plastic, metal, or a composite material. Sidebars attempt to prevent varus and valgus motion at the joint. Straps are provided to help secure the brace to the lower extremity, often utilizing hook-and-loop closure. Other orthoses may include components that rest on the anterior or posterior aspect of the lower leg to limit anterior or posterior translation of the tibia, an important treatment consideration following cruciate ligament injury.

Prophylactic Knee Orthoses

Knee injuries are extremely common and are some of the most severe sporting injuries.[9] Additionally, knee pain is second to the lumbar spine as the most commonly reported area of of pain in the body.[9] Among knee injuries in athletes, soft tissue injury to knee ligaments are of particular concern. Ligamentous injury often results in extensive lost playing time and cost due to surgical repair and rehabilitation. PKOs are knee braces that are designed to mitigate or altogether prevent soft tissue injury, usually ligamentous, to the healthy knee (Fig. 11.10). However, the use of these braces for injury prevention purposes continues to be debated in scientific literature.[4,10]

PKOs are nonadhesive devices that are external to the joint itself. Usually worn by athletes, these braces are designed to prevent injury to the soft tissue structures of the knee from contact or noncontact injuries. It is important to note that there is significant variation in brace design among manufacturers, but the basic goal of ligament protection remains the same despite design. To prevent injury to the MCL or LCL, a brace would need to limit the amount of valgus or varus force, respectively, that the joint receives. For ACL protection, the PKO needs to limit anterior tibial translation forces.

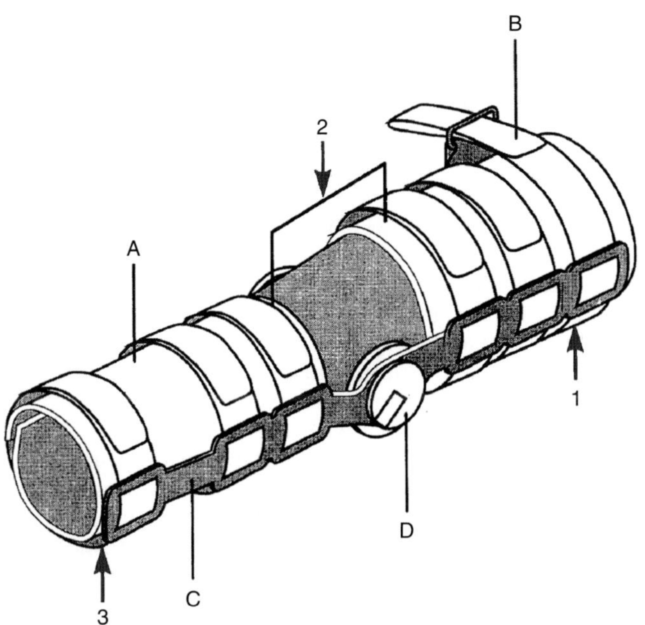

Fig. 11.9 The components of most commercially available rehabilitation knee orthoses include an open cell foam interface that encases the calf and thigh (A); a nonelastic adjustable Velcro strap for closures (B); lightweight metal, composite, or plastic sidebars (C); and single-axis or polycentric hinge that can be locked or adjusted to allow or restrict motion (D) within the therapeutically desired range of motion. The force systems of these orthoses apply a pair of anteriorly directed forces at the proximal posterior thigh (1) and distal posterior calf (3), against a posteriorly directed force (2) applied over or on either side of the patella. Varus and valgus stressors are resisted by the sidebars. (Reprinted with permission from Redford JB, Basmajian JV, Trautman P. Lower limb orthoses. In: *Orthotics: Clinical Practice and Rehabilitation Technology*. Churchill Livingstone, 1995:195–230.)

For clinicians, understanding the design and intended purpose of a brace in conjunction with the physical demands of the athlete's sport is critical to prescribing an appropriate PKO.

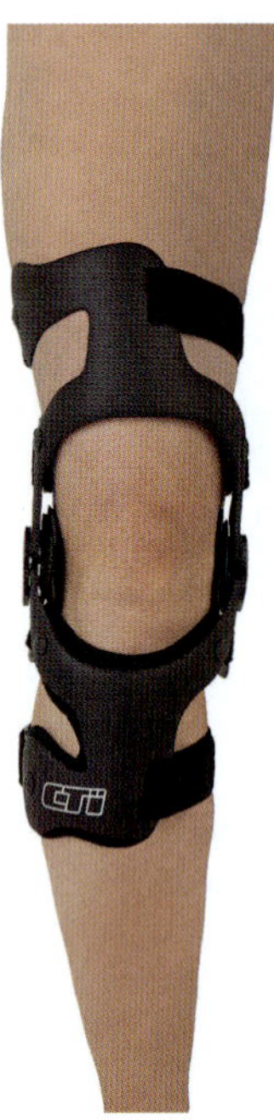

Fig. 11.10 CTi Custom Knee Brace from Ossur. Example of a custom fit prophylactic knee orthoses. This brace is custom fabricated for a more precise fit. This brace can be further individualized based on the physical activity requirements of the patient. (© Össur.)

BIOMECHANICAL IMPLICATIONS

The application of a PKO can have effects on joint kinetics and kinematics, proprioception of the knee joint, as well as muscle activation, limb stiffness, and athletic performance. Specific brace design may have an impact on any or all of these factors in a healthy knee.[11]

Noncontact ligamentous knee injuries often occur when an athlete makes a cutting maneuver or lands on a hard surface after jumping, such as with a basketball rebound. Moon et al.[12] examined the effects of simulating a jump landing on lower-extremity joint kinetics among healthy athletes with and without prophylactic bracing. The results indicate that PKOs reduced the joint's maximum flexion angle, abduction angle, and adduction moment. However, the estimated ACL load and shear force on the knee joint during the drop landings was unaffected by brace use. Based on these findings, bracing was found to have no negative impact on athletic performance, which corroborates past research that examined the effects of brace use on overall athletic performance. This study does not support the use of PKOs to reduce the risk of ACL injury during drop landings in athletes.

Bodendorfer et al.[13] performed a comprehensive study to examine the effects of PKOs on an athlete's cutting ability by examining their performance on common tests (vertical drop, single-leg squat, Y-excursion, and cutting). Findings from this study suggest that the PKO does have an effect on the outcome of these tests. Similarly to the study completed by Moon et al.,[12] there was a significant reduction in the knee flexion angle and abduction during drop landings. During the other dynamic test conditions, PKOs were found to produce significant reductions in hip internal rotation, knee flexion, and knee abduction when compared to a no-brace control. The tests selected by the authors of this study represent a broader picture as to how PKOs affect neuromuscular control. The reductions in hip internal rotation, knee flexion, and knee abduction did not affect the cutting agility, indicating no decrease in neuromuscular control from using a PKO. Furthermore, those reductions may offer some protective benefit against noncontact ACL injury.[12,13]

One proposed model for how PKOs can provide stability to the knee is by altering lower limb muscle stiffness. Knee stiffness is influenced by the force through the joint in relation to how much flexion occurs during a jump, hop, or landing. The effect of PKOs on leg stiffness during single-leg hopping activities has also been examined.[14] Athletes with increased stiffness demonstrate decreased knee flexion during these high-force maneuvers.[15] When considering different frequencies of hopping activities, PKOs showed no difference in leg stiffness when compared to not wearing a PKO or a neoprene knee sleeve. These findings are relevant to knee injury prevention, specifically ACL injuries. Athletes who demonstrate increased knee stiffness seem to be at an increased risk of noncontact ACL injuries.[15] The connection between lower limb muscle stiffness and ligament protection is not well understood at this time.

Prill et al.[16] examined the effects of the use of a PKO, a neoprene knee sleeve, and no brace on the coordination of subjects during a battery of dynamic lower-extremity tests. Impaired coordination during these movements may predispose an athlete to a lower-extremity injury. The findings from this study suggest that there is no significant effect on coordination of movement by the use of either a neoprene knee sleeve or a PKO. Therefore there is no expected disadvantage of using a PKO on coordination during dynamic sport- related activities, such as cutting agility and 40-yard dash times.[16,17]

Baltaci et al.[11] found that across five different types of PKOs, maximal muscle force was enhanced through the use of a PKO. Similarly, PKOs with knee extension support have been shown to increase force production and improve dynamic balance.[18] It is believed that the reduction in ROM produced by these braces allowed for an increase in maximal force production.

The effect of PKOs on neuromuscular control of the muscles that act as agonists and antagonist to the ACL has also been examined.[19] Primarily, the quadriceps and gastrocnemius act as ACL antagonists and can contribute to ACL tears through anterior translation, while the hamstrings and soleus act as ACL agonists, supporting the ACL.[19] The use of a PKO during regular walking and perturbed walking and its effect on neuromuscular control was examined by Haddara et al.[19] Findings from this research suggest that PKOs that limit both knee hyperextension and varus/valgus motion have the ability to alter the neuromuscular patterns around the knee. These alterations resulted in a decrease in the maximum force produced by the quadriceps, thereby offering some protective effect on the ACL. It is important to note that these findings are dependent on the brace design, and cannot be universally applied to all PKOs. This study is of particular value, as past research has focused on muscle force production during isolated movements, such as knee flexion or extension, but not during an unexpected perturbation, similar to what an athlete might encounter.[11,20]

EVIDENCE OF EFFECTIVENESS

When considering the use of a PKO in a healthy patient population, it is important to consider that there is no published data available on the role of bracing in preventing ligamentous injury in healthy knees.[21] As previously discussed, the effects these braces have on joint kinematics, coordination, and muscle performance should not hinder a healthy athlete's performance, so any additional ligamentous protection gained from brace use would be beneficial. The use of bracing has been advocated in athletes who are determined to be at high risk for ligamentous knee injury or in those individuals who are ACL-deficient or have ACL-reconstructed knees.

Approximately 70% of ACL ruptures are due to noncontact injuries.[22] Intrinsic risk factors for noncontact ACL injury include a narrow intercondylar notch, weak ACL, generalized joint laxity, lower-extremity alignment, and sex—with females being more at risk than males.[23] Extrinsic risk factors include quadriceps and hamstring strength imbalances, altered neuromuscular control, and the athlete's playing style and surface.[23] In a systematic review by Bodendorfer et al.,[24] several factors for identifying at-risk population are identified: being between the ages of 13 and 18 years, and participating in pivoting and jumping sports (basketball, football, soccer, and skiing among others). In a recent systematic review conducted by Mokhtarmanand et al.[21] support the use of PKOs in individuals who are susceptible to ACL rupture. The findings suggest PKOs can be advantageous for athletes, even without a prior history of knee injury, who participate in sports that require speed and agility. This population may benefit from prophylactic bracing as the intrinisic risk factors cannot be altered.[21] In individuals who are ACL deficient, bracing may be an effective way to prevent further injury that could be sustained for extra anterior tibial translation.[21,24] Bracing following ACL reconstruction and its efficacy is further discussed later in the chapter.

The remaining (30%) of ACL ruptures are due to contact injuries, which typically occur when external impact is made to the knee joint when it is in a nearly fully extended position, combined with some element of valgus and tibial rotation moments.[22,25] The effectiveness of PKOs on protecting the joint during an impact is not well understand, and requires the consideration of multiple variables, such as force and direct of external impact, that are not easily replicated in research. An in vitro study examining the protective effects of PKOs support this notion, finding that the direction and height of the impact on the braced knee can have a positive, negative, or neutral effect on knee joint protection.[25]

Potential negative effects of PKO use are not fully understood or well documented in the scientific literature. However, healthy patients who wear PKOs may develop an increased sense of security due to subjective increases in proprioception and comfort.[21] This sense of security may be false, as the ability for these braces to prevent injury in healthy individuals is not fully understood.

RECOMMENDATIONS

There is currently a lack of current research to suggest that PKOs significantly reduce knee function or reduce contact-related ligamentous injury risk. In a normal healthy population, PKO use is not warranted based on the available literature at this time. However, in those individuals identified as high risk for ACL injury, bracing may offer a viable way to reduce injury risk, particularly noncontact injuries to the ACL, and should be recommended. Clinicians should recognize individuals who are high risk and prescribe an appropriate PKO in an effort to mitigate injury risk, specifically to the ACL.

Orthoses for Anterior Cruciate Ligament Insufficiency

ACL and PCL function to provide stabilization of the knee joint in multiple directions. The ACL attaches superiorly to the femur on the posterior medial aspect of the lateral condyle. Distally, the ACL attaches anteriorly and laterally to the intercondylar notch of the tibia. The primary role of the ACL is to limit anterior translation of the tibia on the femur, and the PCL functions to limit posterior translation of the tibia on the femur.[26] Additionally, the ACL provides some stability in the transverse and frontal planes, limiting both tibial rotation and abduction.[26] Besides these mechanical functions, the ACL also plays an important role in knee joint proprioception.[27] The critical function of the cruciate ligaments from a mechanical and proprioceptive perspective is complex, and beyond the scope of this chapter. However, a basic understanding of the joint mechanics is necessary to appreciate the design and function of orthoses, as well as prescribing appropriate devices to individuals with ACL injury.

As discussed previously in this chapter, the purpose of a PKO is to prevent injury to the soft tissue structures of the knee from contact or noncontact injuries. In the event that an injury to the ligamentous support structures of the knee does occur, an FKO is often prescribed (Fig. 11.11A). The purpose of an FKO is to provide the mechanical stabilization that is usually provided by intact support structures. For example, a patient who has suffered an ACL rupture may be provided with a brace to prevent anterior translation of the tibia. Utilizing an FKO can serve two main purposes: First, it may be used to protect the joint from further injury that may occur due to the lack of ligamentous support. The chronic instability and altered kinematics may lead to increased injury risk of other ligaments, the meniscus, or the articular cartilage.[7,27] Secondly, an FKO can be used to protect a surgical repair of a ligament or other support structure in the knee during rehabilitation and return to sport phases.

ACL INSUFFICIENCY

ACL injuries are the most common ligamentous knee injuries, and account for approximately 50% of all injuries to the knee.[21,28,29] Nearly 70% of ACL injuries are deemed to be "noncontact" injuries.[12] Due to the complex role of the ACL in mechanical stabilization and proprioception, individuals who are ACL deficient often report symptoms of instability and "giving way" in the knee. Although many individuals elect to undergo surgical repair of the ACL, there is a subset of the population that is able to return to previous levels of function without an intact ACL. This group is collectively

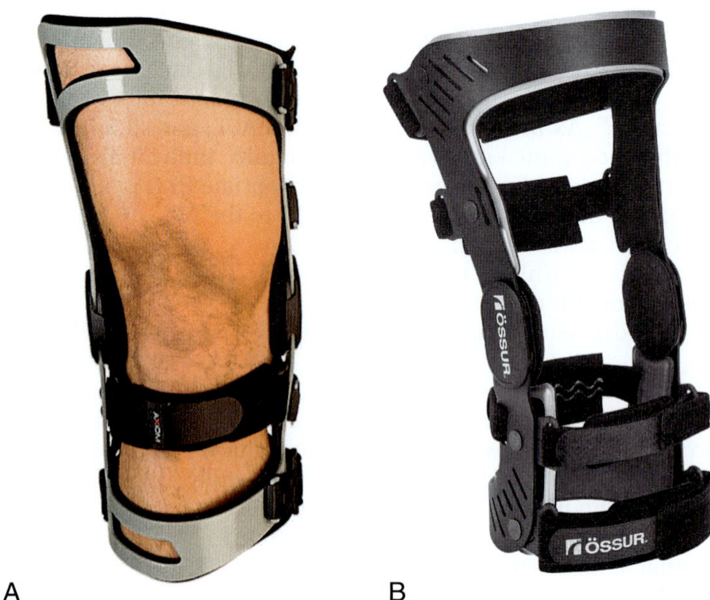

Fig. 11.11 (A) Axiom Elite Ligament Knee Brace by Breg. Example of a knee brace that could be used for either prophylactic purposes or following collateral ligament repair. The rigid metal frame and dual hinges provide support and protection. (B) Rebound ACL Brace by Ossur. Example of a knee brace that is used for nonsurgical treatment of anterior cruciate ligament (ACL) rupture or following surgery for ACL reconstruction. (A, Courtesy Breg. Retrieved from: https://www.breg.com/wp-content/uploads/product_images/Axiom_Elite_Standard_Straight-001-705x705.png. B, © Össur.)

known as "copers," whereas those with continued reports of instability are deemed noncopers. FKO use in copers would serve the purpose of protecting the joint from further injury by providing an external mechanical force to the joint to replicate the normal function of the ACL (see Fig. 11.11B). Several studies have explored the ability of an FKO to replicate those normal functions.

Biomechanical Implications

Focke et al.[27] examined the effects of an orthosis on the arthrokinematics of the ACL-deficient knee during regular walking and 180-degree cutting activities, which were then challenged with a laterally tilting plate. The authors found both a soft and a rigid brace were successful in reducing the maximum valgus angle of the knee as compared to a no-brace condition. The rigid brace outperformed the soft brace with regards to limiting knee extension and increasing transverse plane ROM and peak internal rotation angle. The authors note that these biomechanical changes of the rigid brace may cause unphysiological loading of the knee cartilage, and a soft brace may be enough to limit detrimental positions of the ACL-deficient knee without unnecessary loading.

Jalali et al.[29] utilized CT imaging of the knee to examine the knee arthrokinematics of the ACL-deficient knee during lunge activities. In this study, the braces used were custom fabricated but were characteristic of an FKO. No significant differences were reported for anterior tibial translation in braced and unbraced conditions. This lack of findings is significant as often the purpose of an FKO is to provide the anterior stability of the knee lost by ACL rupture. Additionally, one might assume that a custom fabricated FKO would be superior in providing this support as compared to an off-the-shelf brace.

Ghadikolaee et al.[30] examined the effect of custom FKOs to reduce anterior tibial translation in individuals who are ACL deficient during walking. The researchers found the brace was not able to reduce anterior tibial translation or normalize vertical GRFs, as they could not provide enough force on the proximal tibia. This is consistent with prior research by Pierrat et al.,[31] which examined the ability of prefabricated FKOs to reduce anterior tibial translation in individuals who are ACL deficient. They found that at a low force, which resulted in low anterior displacement, an FKO can replace the mechanical role of the ACL.[31] However, they determined that an FKO cannot fully replace the role of the ACL, as braces generally reach a firm "stop" in a linear manner, whereas the intact ACL increases stiffness as load increases in a nonlinear manner. It is likely that these braces are not effective for higher knee loads or activities that produce higher levels of anterior tibial displacement, although further research is necessary.

Functional Implications

Noveas et al.[32] studied the effect of ACL deficiency and anterolateral ligament deficiency on postural control. They reported a significant difference in overall postural stability between injured and noninjured knees, as well as in patients with isolated ACL injury, with injured knees having worse postural control. Lehmann et al.[33] also found decreased postural control in ACL-deficient athletes during static and dynamic activities. Palm et al.[34] examined the effect of a commercial knee sleeve, which consisted mainly of a compressive sleeve with patellar pads, on postural control. After application of the sleeve, the authors noted an increase in overall postural stability by nearly 22%, finding that this increased postural control to a level similar to that of the uninjured knee. Clinically, a bulkier FKO is often used to manage patients who have isolated ACL deficiency. In healthy knees, the addition of an FKO brace only improves postural control in patients who also demonstrate quadriceps weakness.[18] The results of these studies indicate that a simple sleeve can improve the overall postural control in these individuals and may be sufficient when compared with bulkier FKOs.

Mortaza et al.[35] examined the effect that FKOs have on the isokinetic muscle performance and functional performance in individuals who have ACL-deficient knees. Functional tests included single-leg crossover hopping distance and vertical jump height. The results indicated that FKO use did not have any positive or negative effect on knee performance in either of the examined groups. However, small effects of the brace on peak knee extension torque and power were measured. The authors conclude that although not statistically significant, these findings have rehabilitation implications in reducing muscle function asymmetry during the rehabilitation process.

Recommendations

Although these studies demonstrate that an FKO does not limit the anterior tibial translation that often causes a feeling of joint instability, they may still be helpful by increasing postural stability and proprioception.[32–34] Additionally, they may also be helpful for low-load activities or when limiting tibial rotation to avoid further injury is the main goal of use.[30,31] It is important to remember an FKO cannot match the nonlinear stiffening exhibited by the healthy ACL as demand is increased.[31] Therefore it is important for the clinician to consider the use of FKOs in the rehabilitation of ACL-deficient individuals. For example, if an individual is planning to undergo ACL repair, and the goal is to limit the subjective feeling of instability, a brace may be useful to improve postural stability. In the preoperative ACL patient, a simple sleeve can often provide this support without the bulkiness of a traditional FKO.[27,34] In those individuals who elect to not have surgery to repair the ACL, bracing can provide support for low-level activities, but likely not enough external support for high-loading activities. There is limited to no evidence available to compare the short- or long-term outcomes of rehabilitation programs versus orthoses use in ACL-deficient individuals.

POSTOPERATIVE ACL RECONSTRUCTION

Immediately after surgery for ACL reconstruction, it is common practice to provide bracing to protect the quadriceps-inhibited knee from a sudden flexion moment in weight bearing.[36,37] For this reason many surgeons opt to prescribe an FKO for the purpose of protecting the surgical repair from rerupture and to prevent meniscal injury.[38] Over the course of rehabilitation, bracing may serve the additional purpose of providing more stability as the patient progresses to return to sport training. Despite being common practice, FKO use during the rehabilitation phase following ACL repair has become more controversial as more information is gathered about the effect bracing has on the ACL-reconstructed knee.[36,39–41]

Biomechanical Implications

There is a significant lack of recent evidence to suggest that FKOs are able to protect a surgically repaired ACL, both in the short and long term. This has served as driving force for newer braces to be developed, in an attempt to provide some degree of protection. Tomescu et al.[38] examined the effect of an FKO that utilizes a dynamic tensioning system to provide more protection of a repaired ACL. The dynamic tensioning system serves to apply an angle-dependent anteriorly directed force on the posterior femur, reducing stress on the repaired ACL. The results suggest that a brace with a dynamic tensioning system was able to reduce the peak and average strain on the ACL. However, it is important to consider that there is extremely limited research on dynamic tensioning braces.

LaPrade et al.[42] examined the differences between dynamic and static braces on the posteriorly directed forces from the brace on the proximal tibia during open- and closed-chain knee movements in healthy individuals. Dynamic braces were found to be superior to static braces, most closely matching physiological ACL function. As previously reported, the ACL stiffens in a nonlinear way during active knee ROM, and dynamic bracing attempts to match this phenomenon.[31]

Hanzilikova et al.[43] examined the impact that a soft, proprioceptive knee brace would have on knee stability following ACL reconstruction through the use of 3D kinematic modeling. Researchers found that the proprioceptive brace was most effective in reducing transverse plan motion at the knee during dynamic activities such as pivoting and jumping when compared to the same activities performed without the brace. Additionally, subjects reported that the dynamic activities were easier to perform with the proprioceptive brace on. This can be especially important as some individuals post ACL reconstruction report feelings of rotary instability.

Moon et al.[12] examined shear forces through the ACL during drop landings. The researchers compared shear forces with a brace, a knee sleeve, and no-brace conditions. Findings indicate that while the brace and sleeve both prevented some flexion movement, neither were able to reduce the ACL force when compared to the no-brace condition.

In a high-quality systematic review conducted by Yang et al.,[41] compiled findings suggest that overall knee function, stability, and Visual Analog Scale pain scores were not impacted by the use of a knee brace after ACL reconstruction. The authors examined functional outcome measures as well as side-to-side differences with static and dynamic tests. Despite findings from individual studies that show promising advancements, the consensus viewpoint is that an FKO cannot replicate the function of a healthy ACL, nor provide biomechanical protection.

Role in Rehabilitation

Common impairments following ACL reconstruction include pain, effusion, muscle weakness, and ROM loss, among others. The use of bracing during the rehabilitation phase following ACL repair is generally not supported in the literature to address these impairments.[44] Recent high-quality studies have found that the use of bracing following ACL reconstruction is largely unnecessary. Di Miceli et al.[45] found that bracing following ACL repair had a negative influence on long-term functional outcomes, especially when combined with delayed weight bearing. The authors postulate that brace use may provoke muscle atrophy, loss of extension ROM, and increased fatiguability, which result in poorer long-term outcomes.

A systematic review by Glattke et al.[44] found that postoperative bracing in this population does not improve any limb asymmetry that may exist. The authors found that there were no positive effects on rehabilitation from brace use. The findings were further supported by Knapik et al.[36] that bracing did not decrease strain on the ACL or offer protection of graft integrity. A large-scale systematic review of clinical practice guidelines by Andrade et al.[39] again supports the notion that bracing has little to no positive effect on this population. The sum findings of multiple clinical practice guidelines on the topic recommend against functional bracing in the postoperative rehabilitation period.

Despite these findings, there may be patients who would benefit from brace use. One such population is those with kinesiophobia or fear of reinjury.[46,47] Harput et al.[46] found that bracing provided a reduction in kinesiophobia, allowing patients to have improved knee function and return to preinjury levels when compared with kinesiology taping or no-brace conditions. A systematic review by Lowe et al.[47] suggests using a brace following ACL reconstruction after return to sport for ligament protection and to reduce kinesiophobia. It is the role of the clinician to recognize those individuals who demonstrate kinesiophobia and may benefit from complementary brace use in addition to comprehensive rehabilitation following ACL reconstruction.

Although the findings of recent research suggest bracing after ACL reconstruction is unnecessary, it remains commonplace for patients and surgeons to utilize braces following surgery. However, clinical practice guidelines routinely favor the use of joint mobilization, strength training, and neuromuscular rehabilitation as recommended interventions.[39] Comprehensive rehabilitation without a brace can indirectly prevent reinjury and is generally a cheaper method.[48] It remains the job of the rehabilitation team to appropriately prescribe exercises and activities that result in the intended healing, without reliance on external bracing. Weaning patients from brace use requires careful consideration of the patients' function, kinesiophobia level, and patient confidence. This decision should always be made with the collaboration of the patient and the surgeon.

Once the patient has successfully completed a comprehensive rehabilitation program and is ready to return to sport, functional bracing may once again be utilized. Peebles et al.[49] found that hop distance symmetry and plantar loading symmetry are both improved while wearing a functional knee brace during the return to sport phase of rehabilitation. Dickerson et al.[50] found that the use of an FKO during the return to sport phase did not have any negative affects on athlete agility or vertical jump height, and may offer some protective benefit.

A review by Lang et al.[51] found that brace use for the first 6 to 12 months following return to sport can increase the athlete's confidence. The systematic review by Lowe et al.[47] arrived at a similar conclusion, suggesting brace use for 6 to 12 months following return to sport to decrease kinesiophobia and improve patient confidence, allowing for return to previous level of competition.

Preventing reinjury to the ACL once an athlete returns to play is another goal of rehabilitation. The review by Lowe et al.[47] found limited evidence to suggest bracing decreases the rate of reinjury. However, individuals who participate in high-risk activities would benefit from brace use to reduce reinjury rates, with similar anticipated benefits of wearing an PKO. However, a systematic review by Marois et al.[40] found that using a knee brace during return to sport does not reduce the rate of reinjury for the first 18 months following surgery.

Recommendations

High-quality studies suggest there is limited to no benefit to routine FKO use in the postoperative rehabilitation phase for patients undergoing ACL reconstruction.[39,40,44,48] Patients with kinesiophobia after surgery, those who participate in high-risk sports, or adolescent athletes may benefit the most by using bracing after surgical repair.[46,47] Given the increasingly high rates of surgical success and continued surgical innovation, there is generally no conclusive scientific evidence to support the routine use of an FKO following ACL repair, especially when patients complete a comprehensive rehabilitation program.[39,40]

Orthoses for Osteoarthritis

In healthy tibiofemoral and patellofemoral joints, the articular surfaces are covered in articular cartilage. The role of the articular cartilage is to provide for smooth movement of the knee by reducing friction and providing even force distribution across joint surfaces. Articular cartilage by nature is both avascular and aneural in adult humans. This cartilage is composed of a complex matrix of water, chondrocytes, and proteoglycans.[26] OA is characterized by a disruption or alteration of the cartilage matrix, usually resulting in surface fibrillation, fissures, and eventual removal of cartilage from the underlying bone.[26] OA is a common source of knee pain and discomfort and is associated with high rates of disability. The development and progression of OA is multifactorial, and there are multiple models that outline the development and progression of the disease that are beyond the context of this chapter.

OA that develops in either the tibiofemoral or patellofemoral joint causes considerable pain and disability and imposes a major economic burden on those affected and society as a whole.[52,53] The inability of the cartilage to sustain loads and distribute forces in the tibiofemoral joint often results in degradation of the cartilage and a reduction of joint space, known as collapse, in one or more compartments of the knee. This breakdown can cause pain and swelling, with unicompartmental collapse causing a change in the alignment of the joint.[54] OA that affects the medial compartment of the tibiofemoral joint may cause an increase in genu varus alignment, whereas lateral collapse may cause an increase in genu valgus alignment. Patients with knee OA report joint pain and demonstrate ROM loss. These symptoms are typically exacerbated in weight-bearing activities, such as the stance phase of gait, negotiating stairs, or getting up from sitting. Conservative interventions such as exercise, bracing, injections, or medications are commonly used in managing knee OA, with total or unicompartmental

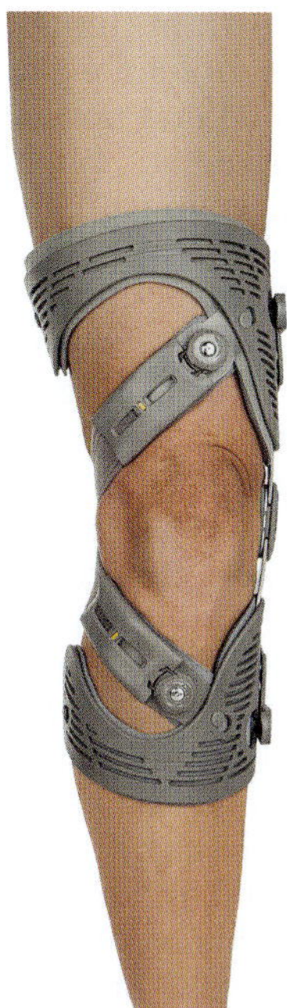

Fig. 11.12 Ossur unloader one brace. This is an example of a medial unloading brace used in the treatment of moderate-to-severe osteoarthritis of the knee. The location of the hinge, sidebars, and straps provide leverage to unload a single compartment in the knee. (© Össur.)

joint arthroplasty utilized when symptoms cannot be managed with conservative interventions.

Braces have been designed to help alleviate these symptoms, as well to address inappropriate joint loading as a result of unicompartmental collapse. Unloading braces are designed for this specific purpose, and consist of external stays, hinges, and straps (Fig. 11.12). As with PKOs and FKOs, they can be used off-the-shelf or custom made for a specific individual. They aim to decrease the compressive load, or "unload" the surface, and restore joint alignment.[54–56] They can be used to address varus or valgus alignments. Valgus unloading braces used to reduce the load on the medial compartment are more common, as medial compartment OA with varus alignment is the most common type of unicompartmental knee OA. The use of these braces has become more popular as clinicians and patients attempt to reduce pain and avoid or prolong the need for joint arthroplasty. In contrast to unloading bracing, some clinicians opt for soft brace use, especially for those patients with mild-to-moderate OA.[57] Based on the current research, the Osteoarthritis Research Society International guidelines for managing knee OA recommends against brace use due to poor quality evidence.[58] The American College of Rheumatology and Arthritis Foundation recommend bracing for patient with OA, which are severely impacted by the disease, including those with ambulation difficulty or use of an assistive device.[52] It is also recognized that bracing for OA is inconvenient and burdensome.[52] Some of the inconsistency with regards to brace prescription recommendations may be explained by the highly individualized nature of the presentation and progression of OA, as well as the lack of long-term controlled research and the variety of braces available.

BIOMECHANICAL IMPLICATIONS

The ability for valgus bracing to provide this desired unloading effect by increasing joint space has long been unclear, and the focus of much research and clinical debate.[53,55] Nagai et al.[56] compared medial joint space in patients with knee OA during walking with the use of biplanar radiographs. The results of this research showed a significant increase in joint space while using the unloading brace. However, there were no differences found in the GRFs experienced at the knee for either condition. Subjectively the participants in this study reported less pain with brace use. The researchers attribute the decrease in reported pain to the increase in joint space provided by the brace. Additionally, joint space increases with the use an offloading was confirmed with fluoroscopic examination during gait, which is consistent with nonarthritic joints.[59] Use of imaging is recommended to objectively evaluate the impact bracing may have on cartilage and joint space.[60] However, this research was not able to identify individuals who would respond well to bracing or what prescriptive criteria should include. In the patellofemoral joint, bracing has been shown to alter the patellar position and loads during weight-bearing activities.[61] Patellofemoral joint OA is further discussed in the section "Patellofemoral Osteoarthritis".

It is important to consider that the unloading effect of bracing that provides for increased joint space and reduced cartilage compression may come at a cost. The use of bracing on arthritic knees has been shown to alter the loading patterns of the contralateral knee and hip, which may cause degeneration in these joints as well.[53]

Instability of the tibiofemoral joint in patients with OA can result in altered muscle activation patterns as the muscles attempt to dynamically stabilize the joint. However, this change in muscle activation patterns may also increase the joint load, ultimately becoming counterproductive. Hall et al.[55] examined the effects an unloader brace would have on tibiofemoral contact forces and the contributions of knee muscles to those forces in a healthy population. The results suggest that there is a slight increase in the contribution of muscle to the medial compartment loading when wearing a brace. Brandon et al.[61] performed a similar study utilizing subjects with knee OA. The findings suggest that the braced condition reduced medial joint loading by approximately 10%, with having only minimal effect on muscle electromyography (EMG) activity surround the knee. Hart et al.[62] produced a similar finding on muscle EMG in patients with lateral OA and a varus unloading brace. These findings suggest that an unloading brace may provide for minimal mechanical stability in those with knee OA but does not have a similar effect in those with healthy joints. New or novel designs of unloading braces need further examination to determine their effects on muscle activation and strength.

The varus alignment that develops as a result of medial compartment collapse changes the force distribution within the tibiofemoral joint. Due to this malalignment, the ground reaction forces (GRFs) experienced during ambulation are shifted medially; this shift is known as the knee adduction moment (KAM) and results in increased load in the medial tibiofemoral compartment.[63] A significant reduction in KAM through the use of an unloading brace has been described in previous biomechanical studies among individuals with OA.[64–66] Reduction of the KAM is one of the proposed mechanisms of action described by Brandon et al.,[67] as the unloader brace provides an abduction moment to the knee. Similarly, there is evidence to suggest that small changes in KAM can be achieved through the use of a neoprene knee sleeve in individuals with early OA, providing some relief of symptoms.[68] It is unclear how a flexible knee sleeve would compare to a more rigid unloading brace to reduce KAM. A systematic review found that large reductions in KAM lead to larger improvements in pain, function, and nonsurgical interventions.[63] When combined with lateral wedging insoles, valgus bracing was found to have a positive effect on KAM and enhanced effectiveness of the knee orthoses.[69] A systematic review with meta-analysis supports these findings, that the addition of a laterally wedged insole in conjunction with a valgus brace can provide positing improvements in pain and function in patients with medial compartment OA.[70]

EVIDENCE OF EFFECTIVENESS

In many cases the biomechanical changes that come from unloader brace use as described by Pereira et al.[63] translate into pain reduction for patients with knee OA. With decreased pain, conservative intervention approaches can then focus on addressing other impairments and improving overall function. Soft braces may provide for pain reduction and improved function in those individuals with mild OA; however, an unloading brace is likely to be required in individuals with joint deformity[68,71] (Fig. 11.13).

Meta-analysis of randomized trials supports the ability of both soft and unloading braces to reduce pain and improve overall function.[57,72] A systematic review by Gohal et al.[73] found that valgus unloader braces are an effective treatment for reducing pain in this population. Despite the pain-reducing effects of unloading braces, the long-term use is not well understood and not advocated in the available literature.[72,74] A systematic review found that valgus bracing is effective in improving quality of life and reducing pain during activities of daily living in patients with knee OA.[74] The long-term effects are mainly limited to the bulkiness and inconvenience of wearing the brace.[74] Perhaps one reason bracing shows limited long-term improvements is the progressive nature of OA.

Subjective studies about pain reduction through the use of unloading braces indicate that the braces provide for adequate joint support, improved pain management, and improved freedom of movement.[75] Improvements in pain and function have been attributed to unloading braces across multiple studies.[75–78] Braces that provide for a decrease in pain and improvement in patient function allow for patients to maintain a healthy activity level and to increase overall physical health.

Aside from the beneficial treatment effect of these braces, like all treatments, they do not come without potential side effects. Negative side effects of brace use are not commonly researched and are occasionally reported when present. Potential side effects include small reductions in available active ROM and skin irritation from poorly fitting braces. As a general rule with knee orthoses, brace fit can be improved with the use of a custom brace versus an off-the-shelf model. Another possible limitation to effectiveness is patient adherence to brace usage and brace cost.[76,79] Unloading braces in particular tend to be larger and bulkier than smaller sleeves, which may limit a patient's ability to effectively don and doff the brace. There is no clear prescriptive criteria for the use of bracing in OA either, which may present a limitation in providing braces to appropriate patients.

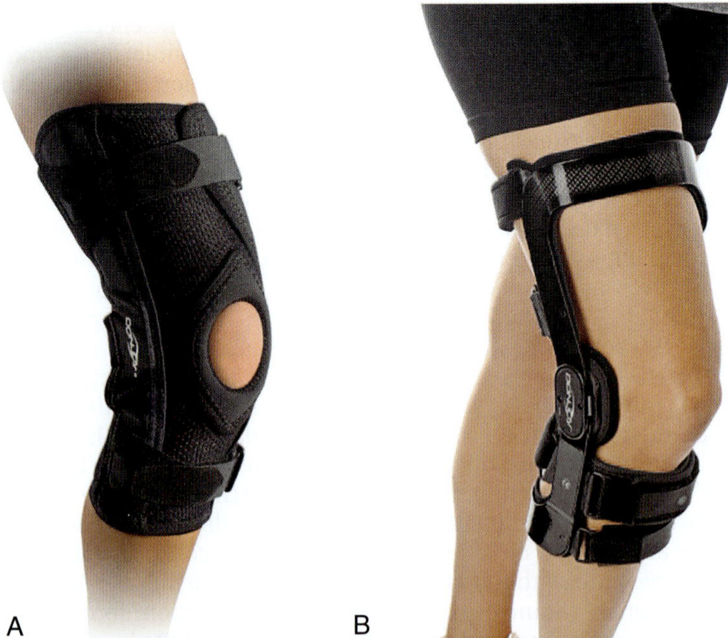

Fig. 11.13 (A) Hinged knee brace with straps produced by DonJoy. This brace provides moderate compression with increased support from dual-hinged sidebars. This brace would be appropriate for patients with mild-to-moderate osteoarthritis (OA). (B) OA Fullforce Knee Brace by DonJoy. Notice the longer lateral support on the femoral component of the brace. When combined with straps and hinges, this brace unloads the medial aspect of the knee. (A, Courtesy of DonJoy; B, Courtesy DJO Global. Retrieved from: https://www.djoglobal.com/sites/default/files/styles/product_large/public/11-1578_OAFullforce_hires.jpg?itok=ubXIPAFS.)

RECOMMENDATIONS

Recent research suggests that unloading braces can alter tibiofemoral and patellofemoral joint positions, both statically and dynamically.[56,59,61] Unloading braces are also effective in increasing joint space and decreasing compression through the arthritic portions of the knee joint without sacrificing muscle strength.[53,55,56,59] Additionally, both unloader and soft braces reduce the KAM force experienced during gait, which distributes forces more uniformly in the joint, thereby reducing pain.[61] These biomechanical changes result in decreased pain and improved function, specifically gait parameters. These improvements result in increased quality of life and confidence in patients with knee OA.[74] Additionally, these improvements may prolong the time to total knee replacement surgery.[80,81] Further research is needed to examine the effects that new brace designs to the market have on biomechanics, pain, and function among this patient population over the long term.[82] The majority of these recent studies focus on relatively short-term effects of brace use. Due to the chronic and progressive nature of OA, it would be beneficial to examine the long-term effects of brace use.

Conservative intervention continues to be the first line of treatment for patients with knee OA. Physical therapy, exercise, weight reduction, bracing, and anti-inflammatory medications are among the most common conservative interventions.[52,58,83,84] Guided exercise programs carry an Osteoarthritis Research International recommendation level of 1B and bracing is not recommended based on best evidence.[58] Despite the inconclusive opinion from the Osteoarthritis Research International recommendations, the addition of a brace to these interventions may prove to be useful, but more long-term randomized studies and decision-making tools for clinicians are necessary.[81,85] Identifying which patients will benefit from the addition of bracing to a conservative program can be difficult for many practitioners and may present as a barrier to brace use. Establishment of an industry-wide validated model of brace implementation would prove to be greatly beneficial.[85] However, clinicians may be able to match patient impairments with the known biomechanical effects of certain braces to produce a desired treatment effect. As a general rule, those with a passively correctable varus or valgus deformity as a result of unicompartmental OA are ideal patients for unloader brace use. The decision to implement a brace should be made in as a shared decision between the practitioner and patient, considering the patient's comorbidities, values, and likelihood of adherence to brace use.[52,86] In those patients with mild or early OA, a soft brace may be an effective treatment.[57]

Orthoses for Patellofemoral Disorders

It is important to consider the contributions of the patellofemoral joint to both normal tibiofemoral joint motion and painful conditions of the knee. The patella is a sesamoid bone positioned in the tendon of the quadriceps femoris. On its posterior, it has two large facets medially and laterally, and a small odd facet on the medial aspect.[26] These facets articulate with the medial and lateral femoral condyles during flexion and extension movements of the knee, respectively. When the knee is extended and the quadriceps relaxed, there is relatively little contact between the patella and the femur. Normal alignment finds the patella positioned just laterally to the femoral trochlear notch at rest.[26] Under normal conditions the patella functions to increase the moment arm of the quadriceps tendon, therefore the patella is critical to normal function of the quadriceps muscle and tibiofemoral joint.[26] During tibiofemoral flexion, the patella glides distally on the femur. At the same time the patellofemoral joint surface experiences an increase in compressive force.[26] During knee extension, the patella glides superiorly on the femur. In addition to superior and inferior translation, there is movement of the patella medially and laterally, as well as tilting and rotation during tibiofemoral flexion and extension.[26] The term "patellar tracking" is often used to describe this complex set of motions that occurs at the patellofemoral joint. Compressive force at the patellofemoral joint is also affected by other factors besides tibiofemoral joint angle, such as weight bearing or external loading. Abnormal knee function and pain have been hypothesized to be caused by problems with static or dynamic patellofemoral alignment, tracking, and force distribution across the joint surface or a combination thereof. Models that explain normal and abnormal patellofemoral joint motion and force distribution are far more complex, however, and are beyond the scope of this chapter. Having knowledge regarding normal function is important to understanding the purpose of patellofemoral orthoses.

Patellofemoral orthoses, like other knee braces, are a form of conservative treatment that are frequently used in conjunction with other nonoperative measures. They function to reduce the pain experienced in the anterior knee and retropatellar area in individuals with patellofemoral pain syndrome (PFPS) or patellofemoral OA by modifying patellar position.[87,88] Designs of orthoses for this purpose are highly variable and range from simple straps to knee sleeves to full patellar support braces (see Figs. 11.2 and 11.14). Patellofemoral braces are generally less bulky than tibiofemoral counterparts, yet the design of these braces are highly variable.[88] There are significant differences in prescriptive criteria and little consensus among healthcare professionals regarding the use of these orthoses for long-term reduction in symptoms.[89–92]

PATELLOFEMORAL OSTEOARTHRITIS

OA that affects the patellofemoral joint can be a significant cause for anterior and retropatellar pain. Due to the compressive nature of the patellofemoral joint, patellofemoral OA tends to be a particularly painful condition. Bracing in this population is thought to decrease contact stress across the patellofemoral joint by encouraging proper alignment or tracking, thereby reducing painful compression by reducing patellofemoral joint forces.[90] Restoring normal forces across a larger surface area on the facets of the posterior patella may reduce focal stress through any one area that has degenerative changes. It is common for tibiofemoral and patellofemoral OA to occur in simultaneously. Newly developed tricompartmental braces (TCOs) are being investigated to determine the effects on global knee OA.[61,93]

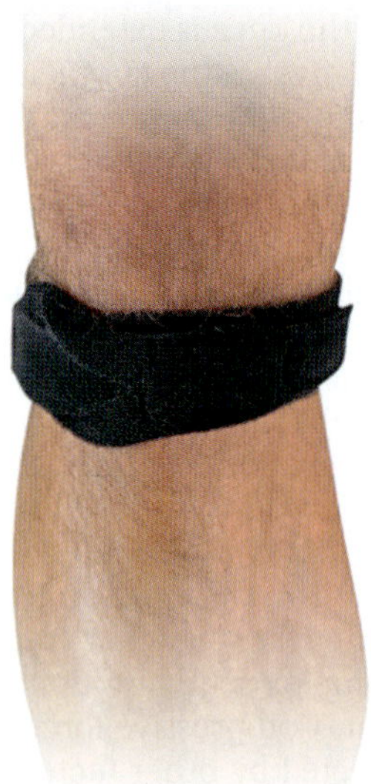

Fig. 11.14 Patella strap by DonJoy. Example of a compressive strap worn directly over the patellar tendon. (Courtesy DJO Global. Retrieved from: https://www.djoglobal.com/sites/default/files/styles/product_large/public/images/products/patella-front.jpg?itok=ukUDqXKI.)

Unlike bulky FKOs or other tibiofemoral braces, knee sleeves used in this population are typically soft and can be worn underneath long pants.

Biomechanical Implications

Weakness of the quadriceps is a common impairment that is observed in individuals with OA of the knee. In a recent systematic review, Callaghan et al.[89] summarized the effect of wearing a knee brace on quadriceps strength in individuals who have patellofemoral OA. This study utilized an off-the-shelf knee sleeve, which allowed full ROM of the knee. This type of brace is commonly used in the treatment of PFPS and for general knee joint support. After 6 and 12 weeks, no difference in maximum voluntary contraction or reduction in quadriceps inhibition was found, meaning the use of the brace did not reduce the strength, but increased the activation of the quadriceps. This study also reports the improvement of patellar position following a trial of brace wearing.

Correcting improper patellar tracking or position may also be a goal in the treatment of patellofemoral OA in an effort to manage symptoms.[90] In a small-scale study (n = 15), patella position and patellofemoral joint space were measured using magnetic resonance imaging in patients with patellofemoral OA and compared against individually matched asymptomatic controls.[94] The results of this study showed that in individuals with patellofemoral OA, there was a 27% greater lateral displacement of the patella and 12-degree larger lateral patellar tilt. Bracing aimed at reducing this excessive displacement and tilt of the patella should be beneficial in reducing patient reported pain. A study by Zhang et al.[95] examined the effect that bracing would have on improving symptoms in relation to patellar alignment. The authors found that bracing improved patellar position, but those individuals with the greatest amount of displacement were less likely to benefit from bracing. This is likely due to the ability of the brace to increase the contact area between the posterior patella and femoral trochlea, thereby distributing force in a more even manner. A single study investigating the newly described TCO devices have found reductions in joint loads by 30% to 50% across all structures.[61]

Although promising, these studies were conducted in a static position, which reduces the clinician's ability to apply the results to more dynamic functional activities that are often impaired, such as ambulation. It is also noted that malalignment of the patella in isolation may not be sufficient to cause pain, and is likely the result of the progression of OA.[95]

Conservative Management

Isolated bracing in this population has been found to produce nonsignificant improvements in function, as measured by the Knee Osteoarthritis Outcome Score, and participant reported pain.[89,90,95] Conservative interventions that are recommended in this population include physical therapy, patient education, weight loss, and cold therapy.[90]

The TCO device shows more promising results, but the available evidence is extremely limited. In a single retrospective analysis of the TCO brace, Budarick et al.[93] (2021) found improvements in function, as indicated by an increase in Lower Extremity Functional Scale scores and a reduction in pain levels. Participants in this study also improved their physical activity by approximately 60%, which could aid in other conservative approaches such as weight loss.

When combining conservative management approaches, the clinician may elect to recommend a brace in conjunction with these effective interventions. Outcomes suggest that patients can expect a short-term improvement in symptoms through this combined approach, but the long-term outcomes are not well understood at this time.[89,90] When compared to neoprene knee sleeves, the combination of patellofemoral orthosis had superior outcomes at 1 year.[87]

It is important to note that the limited efficacy of bracing in this population is also seen with pharmaceutical and surgical interventions as well. A systematic review by Macri et al.[96] found that most pharmaceutical and surgical interventions for patellofemoral OA have not undergone sufficient investigation to warrant their routine use.

Recommendations

OA affecting the patellofemoral joint frequently results in pain and decreased function in affected individuals. Conservative management of a multidisciplinary nature has been shown to improve these outcomes in both short- and long-term follow-up studies.[89,90,95] The effects of the addition of a brace to conservative management is not well understood. Current literature suggests that brace use will not reduce quadriceps strength but can improve inhibition, and can change the static position of the patella.[89,94,95] No large-scale negative effects of brace use have been reported in the recent literature. Bracing for patients with patellofemoral OA may be used to complement a conservative multidisciplinary approach to improve pain and function. Newly developed TCO braces for multicompartmental OA need additional investigation to determine effectiveness.

These recommendations agree with the 2019 American College of Rheumatology/Arthritis Foundation Guidelines, which provide conditional recommendation for the use of bracing in this population.[52] Conditions for successful bracing may include impairments with ambulation, joint stability, or pain.[52]

PATELLOFEMORAL PAIN SYNDROME

PFPS is a global term used to describe pain that occurs in the anterior patellar or retropatellar areas. Symptoms in the area are generally worsened during prolonged sitting, ascending and descending stairs, walking down slopes, athletic activities, squatting, or kneeling.[97–99] The repetitive nature of these activities contributes to the onset of symptoms. PFPS is a common disorder of the knee, affecting 10% to 20% of the general population, with females, especially athletic females, being more commonly affected.[100,101 88,89] Due to the complex nature of normal patellar function and anatomic variation, it is likely that there is a wide variety of biomechanical reasons that patellar tracking becomes abnormal and painful.[98] Despite the exact etiology of PFPS being unclear, the basic premise of PFPS is that abnormal movement of the patella in the femoral trochlear results in altered force distribution and pain in the joint.[97,98,101] When possible, identifying the underlying cause of altered tracking would be beneficial for directing conservative treatment, including orthoses use, for those with PFPS. For example, if a patient demonstrates excessive lateral tracking of the patella, a brace designed to apply a medially directed force may be used to keep the patella situated in the femoral trochlea. As patients with patellofemoral pain often demonstrate alterations in the normal tracking of the patella, and the goal of patellar bracing is to correct these biomechanical abnormalities and reinforce proper mechanics,[88] additional conservative treatment might include quadriceps strengthening, stretching of lateral thigh and knee structures, and avoidance of painful activities. A review of conservative management alone and in combination with orthoses use is provided later in this chapter.

Biomechanical Implications

Patellar strapping is commonly used to control pain in individuals with PFPS related to patellar tendinopathy.[88] The patellar strap is a small brace that places additional force on the patellar tendon in an attempt to decrease tensile stress of the tendon itself.[9,88,102] In a systematic review by Sisk and Fredericson,[88] the authors reviewed the benefits of patellar strapping among subjects with patellar tendinopathy. Findings suggest that patellar strapping reduces quadriceps activation, increases knee proprioception, and reduces pain with low likelihood of negative effects. These positive findings are also reported by Sprouse et al.,[102] which assign an evidence rating of "B" to the use of patellar straps. However, high-powered studies are lacking in this area which could provide additional guidance regarding patients who would benefit from patellar strapping or braces that include patellar straps.

Individuals with PFPS are frequently prescribed a knee sleeve or a soft knee brace for management of symptoms. These prefabricated braces are also available over the counter for individuals choosing to self-manage their PFPS. The review by Sprouse et al.[102] also reported on the effectiveness of soft braces for the management of PFPS. Findings suggest that a brace is more effective than a soft-neoprene sleeve at correcting faculty patellar mechanics. Regardless of bracing or sleeve use, most benefit on pain and function is seen in the short-term timeframe.

Priore et al.[103] compared brace usage to minimal intervention to examine the effects of brace use on kinesophobia in subjects with patellofemoral pain. The results of this study suggest that subjects experienced decreased kinesiophobia with brace use at both a 2- and 6-week follow-up timeframe. However, the authors note that the benefit of brace use on kinesophobia should be used to facilitate exercise therapy in this population, and not used in isolation. These results suggest a psychological impact of brace use.

Conservative Management

Effective exercise interventions should target the underlying impairments found to contribute to patellofemoral pain. Commonly, targeted strengthening of the quadriceps, hip extensors, and hip abductors are utilized.[9,99,101,104] Limiting patellofemoral loading during exercise interventions is advocated. Other frequently used interventions include muscle stretching of the hamstrings, hip flexors, quadriceps, triceps surae, and ITB.[101] Patient education of the nature of PFPS, avoidance of aggravating activities, and indications for brace use should also be included.[99]

Exercise therapy should be the front-line treatment for PFPS, and clinicians should consider bracing as an adjunctive treatment.[88,105] A clinical practice guideline published for physical therapists gives an evidence grade of "A" for combined interventions to manage PFPS, with exercise therapy as the critical component.[105] As a stand-alone therapy, brace use was given an evidence grade of "B."[105] The American Society of Pain and Neuroscience published a scoping review on the management of knee pain, including PFPS.[9] The authors concluded that bracing for PFPS should be performed only during pain-provoking activities, and have a lower quality recommendation in isolation as compared to physical therapy.[9] In a Cochrane review by Smith et al.,[100] the authors conclude that there is very low-quality evidence that using a knee orthosis in combination with physical therapy may not reduce pain.

Recommendations

The overall low quality of available evidence shows the need for improved and continued research methodology to help guide clinicians' utilization of orthoses for PFPS and patellar tendinopathy. Additionally, it makes the task of prescribing such an orthosis challenging. PFPS and patellar tendinopathy should initially be managed with conservative intervention, which is individually tailored to the impairments of the patient and may include the use of a patellofemoral orthosis, especially for short-term improvements in pain and function, or when kinesiophobia is present. When used, orthoses should be used in conjunction with selected exercise and behavior modification interventions.[9,102,105]

Summary

This chapter reviewed the normal structure and function of the tibiofemoral and patellofemoral joints and the common pathologic conditions that affect these joints. The different categories of orthoses for the knee complex are prophylactic orthoses, functional orthoses, and rehabilitation orthoses. Emphasis was placed on unloading knee orthoses and patellofemoral orthoses as a subcategory of rehabilitation orthoses. A review of the literature was presented. Although there continues to be debate among the research and clinicians regarding the use of these orthoses, improvements in the quality and strength of recommended orthoses has improved compared with previous orthoses. Identifying appropriate patients who would benefit from brace use is key to brace prescription. Interprofessional communication among the patient's healthcare team, with input from the patient, is essential. This chapter discussed the application of the current research to allow the clinician to make the best possible decision for their patient's care. It is important for clinicians to continue to view knee orthosis use in a complementary sense to other conservative interventions, such as a comprehensive evidence-based rehabilitation program. The intent of this chapter was to provide clinicians with the ability to evaluate the design and the intended treatment effects of a given knee orthosis and for appropriate application in the clinical setting. This chapter also highlighted evidence in current research, including gaps in present knowledge. These gaps include the long-term effects of knee orthosis use and effects of new or novel brace design with the hopes of encouraging participation in ongoing research on the topic.

References

The complete listing of the References are available in the accompanying enhanced eBook version included with the print purchase of this textbook. Visit Elsevier eBooks+ (eBooks.Health.Elsevier.com) to access this content.

12 Orthoses in Orthopedic Care and Trauma*

AMANDA KNOWLES

LEARNING OBJECTIVES

On completion of this chapter, the reader will be able to do the following:

1. Review the characteristics of normal bone structure and function across the lifespan.
2. Describe the most common musculoskeletal injuries that occur at various points in the lifespan.
3. Identify orthotic interventions for congenital and growth-related musculoskeletal impairments.
4. Classify fracture of bone by type and severity and describe the interventions most often used by orthopedists and orthopedic surgeons on the basis of fracture type.
5. Discuss the different orthotic options for fracture management: joint immobilization, fracture bracing, and external stabilization in common orthopedic injuries to the extremities.
6. Delineate the roles of healthcare team members in the rehabilitation and orthotic management of individuals with congenital and acquired musculoskeletal impairment.

Orthoses play a significant role in orthopedic and rehabilitative care of individuals with many different types of musculoskeletal pathologic conditions and impairments. Dysfunction of the musculoskeletal system can be the result of congenital or developmental disorders or can be acquired as a result of overuse injury, systemic disease, infection, neoplasm, or trauma at any point in the lifespan. This chapter focuses on the use of orthoses to manage congenital and developmental musculoskeletal problems in children and fractures of long bones of the lower extremity.

The understanding of how orthoses are helpful in the care of those with musculoskeletal impairments is founded on knowledge of the development and physiology of musculoskeletal tissues (bone, cartilage, ligaments, menisci, muscles, and their tendons or aponeuroses); the kinesiological relationships among these tissues; and an understanding of how these tissues remodel in response to physical stressors (forces).[1,2] This chapter begins with an overview of the anatomy of bone, its growth and remodeling, and the principles behind the rehabilitation (examination and intervention) of persons with disorders of bone. Then the authors look specifically at disorders of the hip joint and orthotic/orthopedic strategies for limb fractures.

Bone Structure and Function

In anatomy classes and texts, students learn that the mature adult human skeleton is composed of 206 bones (Fig. 12.1), ranging from the long bones of the extremities, the block-like vertebrae of the spine, the encasing protective ribs and skull, and the multiarticulating carpals and tarsals of the wrist and ankles that enable positioning of the hands and feet for functional activities.[3,4] Bony prominences formed during development from the force of muscle contraction at tendinous origins and insertions are identified.[1] Students scrutinize articular surfaces to understand how joints move, consider the hyaline cartilage that protects the joint from repeated loading and shear during activity, and learn to examine the ligaments that maintain alignment for normal joint function. From a skeletal model or examination of bone specimens in anatomy laboratory, it is not intuitively apparent that living bone is a dynamic and metabolically active tissue serving multiple purposes and physiological roles.[5] These include storage and homeostasis of calcium, phosphate, magnesium, sodium, and carbonate (via ongoing osteoblastic and osteoclastic activity in conjunction with kidney function); production of erythrocytes, granular leukocytes, and platelets in the marrow; physical growth and development (by responsiveness to the pituitary hormones at the epiphyseal plate); provision of a protective and functional frame for the organs of the thorax and abdomen (how would people breathe without ribs?); and body weight support when the body is either at rest or in motion during functional activities.[6]

Bone is a dense, regular, connective tissue derived from embryonic mesoderm. It contains a combination of specialized cells (osteoblasts, osteocytes, osteoclasts) embedded in a matrix of minerals (70%), protein (22%), and water (8%). The many bones of the human body can be described as long or short tubular bone (e.g., the femur, tibia, metatarsals, phalanges), flat bone (e.g., the pelvis or skull), irregular bone (e.g., the tarsals and carpals), sesamoid bone embedded within tendons (e.g., patella), or accessory bones (e.g., ossicles of the middle ear). Alternatively, they can be classified as primarily cortical (dense) or cancellous (trabecular) bone on the basis of the density and arrangement of their components. Long bones are subdivided into regions, each of which has its own blood supply (Fig. 12.2). The diaphysis (shaft) is supplied by one or more nutrient arteries that penetrate the layers of the bony cortex, dividing into central longitudinal arteries within the marrow cavity. The flared metaphyses serve as an area of transition from cortical to cancellous bone and are supplied by separate metaphyseal arterioles. The epiphyses are metabolically active areas

*The authors extend appreciation to William J. Barringer, Melvin L. Stills, Joshua L. Carter, and Mark Charlson, whose work in prior editions provided the foundation for this chapter.

of cancellous bone with supportive trabeculae, with an extensive capillary network derived from epiphyseal arteries. The epiphysis is actively remodeled over the lifespan in response to weight bearing and muscle contraction during activity.[7] In childhood and adolescence, before skeletal maturation, the bony metaphyses and epiphyses are connected by cartilaginous epiphyseal (growth) plate, which calcifies and fuses throughout various periods of development. The periosteum is a layer of less dense, vascularized connective tissue that overlies and protects the external surface of all bone and houses osteoblastic cells necessary for bone deposition and growth. The periosteum is replaced by articular (hyaline) cartilage within the joint capsule. The endosteum, a thin connective tissue lining of the marrow cavity of

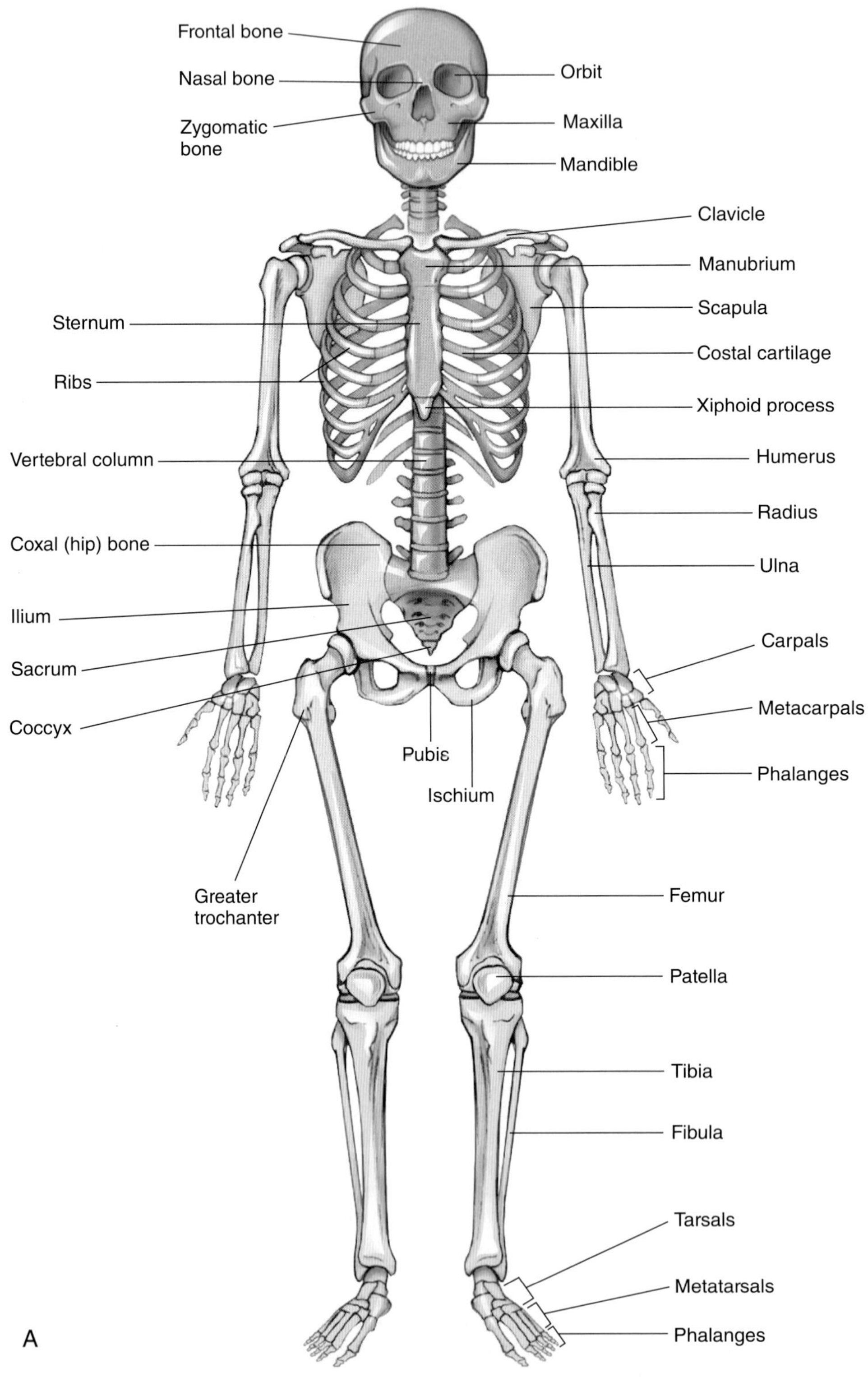

Fig. 12.1 The bones of the human skeleton. (A) Anterior view.

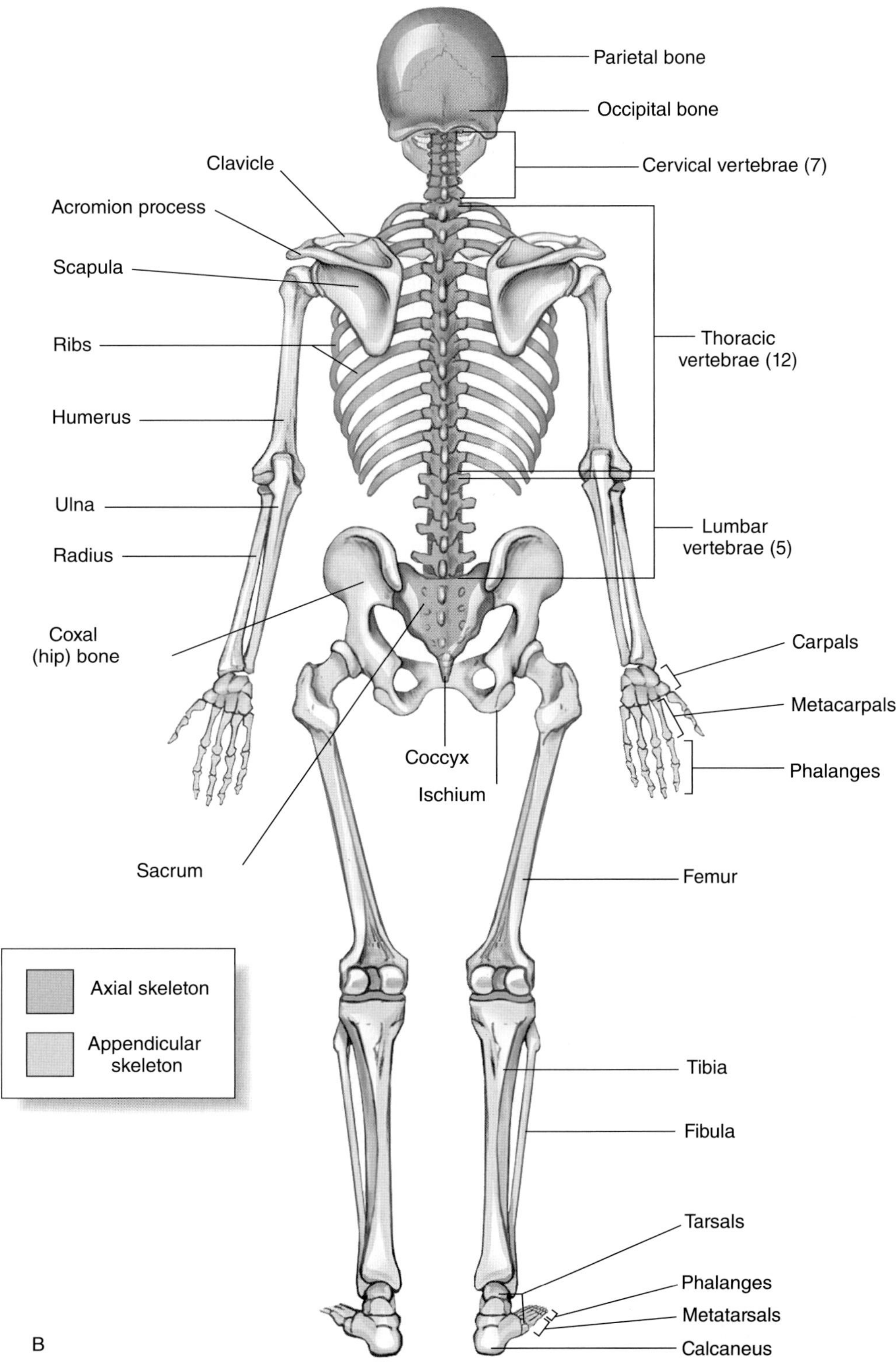

Fig. 12.1, cont'd (B) Posterior view. (From Thibodeau GA, Patton KT. *Anatomy and Physiology*. Fifth ed. Mosby; 2003.)

long bones and the internal spaces of cancellous bone of the marrow space, also houses osteoblasts. Both linings are active as part of osteogenesis during growth and fracture healing.

Cortical bone is the most highly mineralized type of bone found in the shafts (diaphyses) of the long bones of the body and serves as the outer protective layer of the metaphysis and epiphysis of tubular bone, as well as the external layers of flat, irregular, and sesamoid bones. Most of the bones in the human skeleton (80%–85%) are primarily cortical with cancellous/trabecular bone in the metaphyseal and epiphyseal region. A cross-section of a long tubular bone reveals three layers of cortical bone: the inner or endosteal region next to the marrow cavity, the metabolic intracortical or haversian region with its haversian canals surrounded by concentric layered rings (osteons) and Volkmann canals containing a perpendicularly arranged anastomosing capillary network, and the dense outer periosteal region (Fig. 12.3).

Cancellous (trabecular) bone with its honeycomb or spongy appearance is much more metabolically active and much less mineralized than cortical bone. Cancellous bone is composed of branching bony spicules (trabeculae) arranged in interconnecting lamellae to form a framework for weight bearing (Fig. 12.4A). In the vertebral bodies, for example, trabeculae are arranged in an interconnecting horizontal and vertical network oriented perpendicular to the lines of weight-bearing stress into a boxlike shape (see Fig. 12.4B). In contrast, trabeculae in the proximal femur form an archlike structure to support weight-bearing forces between the hip joint and femoral shaft. In living bone, cavities between trabeculae are filled with bone marrow. When bone becomes osteoporotic, the cavities enlarge due to loss of bone mass.

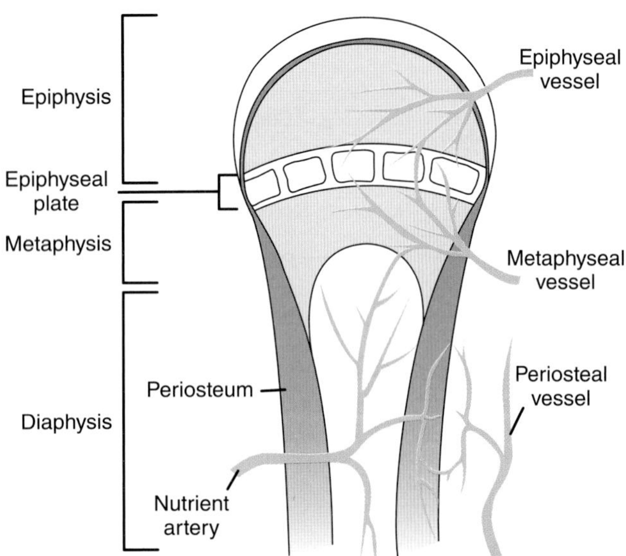

Fig. 12.2 Diagram of the regions (epiphysis, epiphyseal plate, metaphysis, and diaphysis) of a long bone and their arterial vascular supply. (Modified from Lundon K. *Orthopedic Rehabilitation Science, Principles for Clinical Management of Bone*. Butterworth-Heinemann; 2000.)

Three types of cells are embedded within the various compartments of bone. *Osteoblasts*, bone building cells, synthesize and secrete the organic matrix of bone (osteoid) that mineralizes as bone matures. They are located under periosteum and endosteum and are active in times of bone growth and repair. *Osteocytes* are matured and inactive osteoblasts that have become embedded within bone matrix. Osteocytes remain connected to active osteoblasts via long dendritic processes running through the canaliculi (small channels) within the bone matrix. Both osteoblasts and osteocytes are responsive to circulating growth hormones, growth factors, and cytokines, as well as mechanical stressors and fluid flow within the bone itself.[8,9] Osteocytes are thought to be involved in mineral exchange, detection of strain and fatigue, and control of mechanically induced remodeling.[10] *Osteoclasts*, derived from precursor cells in bone marrow, are macrophage-like cells that can move throughout bone to resorb bone by releasing minerals from the matrix and removing damaged organic components of bone.[11,12]

The epiphyses of long bones, the vertebrae, and large flat bones house nociceptors and mechanoreceptors and a network of afferent sensory neurons that contribute to exteroceptive (primarily pain) pathways.[13] The periosteum has a particularly rich neural network with branches that continue along with penetrating nutrient arteries into the haversian canals into the diaphysis.

Bone Growth and Remodeling Over the Lifespan

During childhood and adolescence, growth occurs through the process of modeling, in which bones increase in length and diameter and are reshaped until the epiphyseal plates calcify and skeletal maturity is achieved (typically in mid-adolescence for females and early adulthood for males).[14] In adulthood, bone health is maintained by the ongoing process of remodeling, in which there is a balance and coupling between osteoblastic deposition of new bone substance

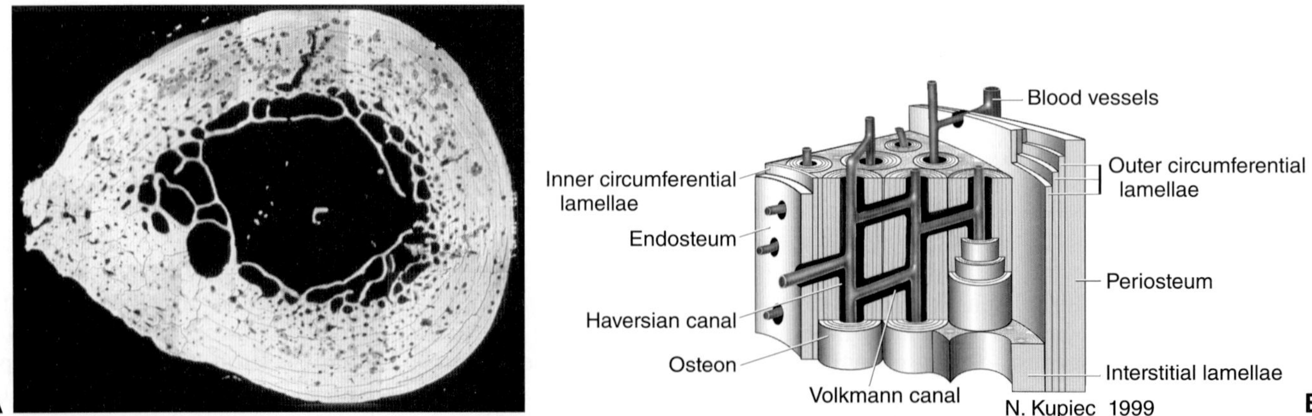

Fig. 12.3 (A) A cross-section through the diaphysis of a long bone, with the external periosteal layer, the middle haversian/intracortical layer, the inner endosteal layer, and the marrow cavity. (B) Diagram of a cross-section through the diaphysis of a long bone. (From Lundon K. *Orthopedic Rehabilitation Science: Principles for Clinical Management of Bone*. Butterworth-Heinemann; 2000.)

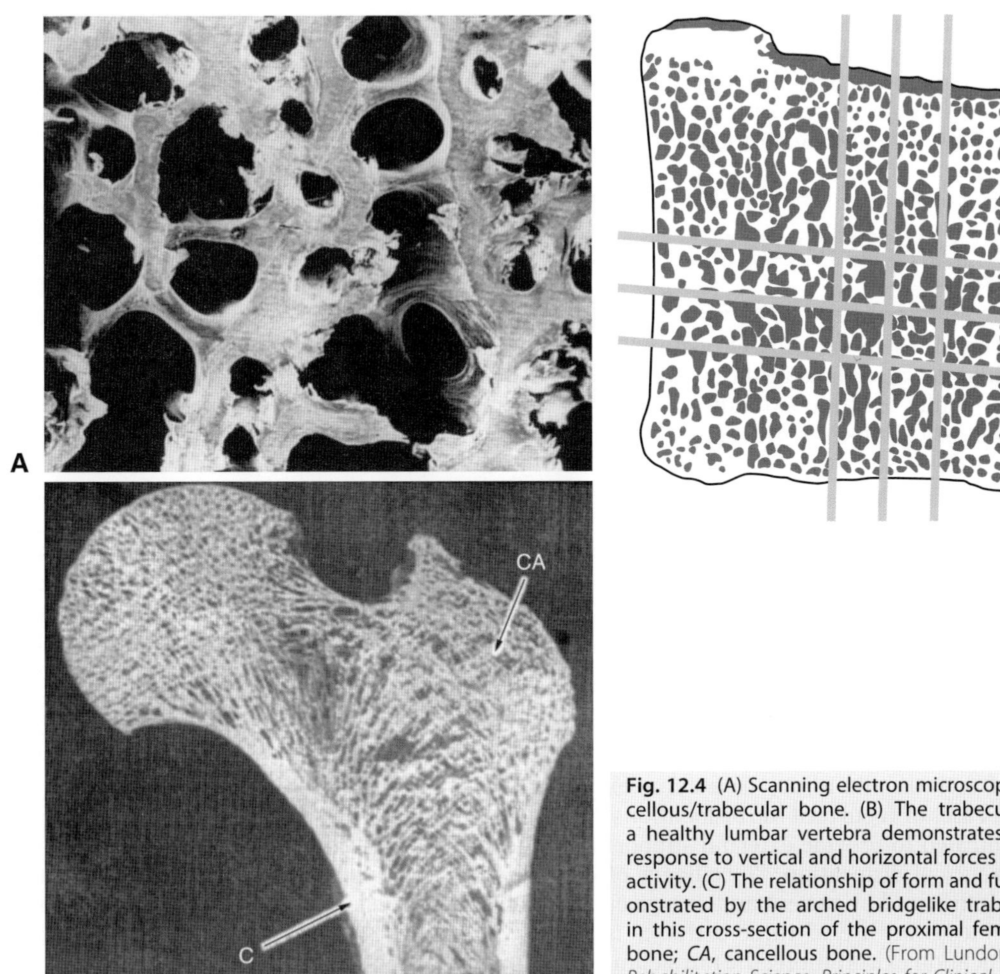

Fig. 12.4 (A) Scanning electron microscope view of cancellous/trabecular bone. (B) The trabecular pattern in a healthy lumbar vertebra demonstrates bone tissue's response to vertical and horizontal forces during upright activity. (C) The relationship of form and function is demonstrated by the arched bridgelike trabecular pattern in this cross-section of the proximal femur. *C*, Cortical bone; *CA*, cancellous bone. (From Lundon K. *Orthopedic Rehabilitation Science: Principles for Clinical Management of Bone*. Butterworth-Heinemann; 2000.)

and osteoclastic resorption of existing bone.[15] This ongoing process of turnover means that the internal architecture of living bone is actively restructured and replaced at a rate of approximately 5% per year in cortical bone and up to 20% per year in cancellous bone.[5] The rate of bone formation, resorption, and turnover is influenced by both systemic hormones and other substances (e.g., parathyroid hormone, calcitonin, vitamin D from the kidney, growth hormone, adrenocorticosteroids, estrogen, progesterone, androgens); local cell–derived growth factors; and availability of essential nutrients (calcium, fluoride, vitamin A, vitamin D, and vitamin E).[16–18] These substances, along with blood or urinary levels of certain enzymes active during turnover and metabolites of bone resorption, are monitored as biomarkers to track progression of bone diseases associated with high rates of bone resorption (e.g., Paget disease, osteoporosis, hyperparathyroidism) and to determine efficacy of medical-pharmaceutical interventions for these diseases.[19–21]

In the prenatal period and in infancy, the flat bones of the skull develop as the fetal mesenchyme that forms the periosteum begins to ossify (intramembranous ossification). Most long bones, as well as the vertebrae and pelvis, develop from a cartilaginous framework or template. In this process of endochondral bone formation, cartilage cells mature and eventually ossify.[7] During childhood and adolescence, bones grow in both length and diameter and are dynamically modeled toward their mature configurations.[22] During puberty, accumulation of bone mass accelerates; by the end of puberty, as much as 90% of mature bone mass is established.[23] For young children with abnormal skeletal development, orthoses attempt to capitalize on the dynamic modeling process, applying external forces to influence bone shape and length.[24] For approximately 15 years following puberty, after closure of the epiphyseal plates of the long bones, bone mass continues to increase—a process described as *consolidation*.[22] Sex differences in peak bone mass have been well documented: average peak bone mass in females is approximately 20% less than that of males. Early in the midlife period, both males and females enter a period of gradual endochondral bone loss that appears to be genetically determined; the rate of bone loss is also influenced by hormonal status, nutrition, smoking and alcohol use, and activity level.[25–28] It is estimated that males will lose between 15% and 40% of cancellous bone mass and 5% to 15% of cortical bone mass over their lifetime. In females, menopause accelerates the rate of bone loss; there may be up to a 50% decrease from peak cancellous bone mass and 30% decrease in cortical bone mass over their lifetimes.[29] Significant loss of bone mass is associated with increasing vulnerability to fracture, especially among postmenopausal females.

Orthoses in the Management of Hip Dysfunction

Hip orthoses are important in the management of hip disorders in infants and children, as well as in the postsurgical care of children and adults. An understanding of the designs of and indications for various hip orthoses is essential for physicians and rehabilitation professionals working with individuals who have orthopedic problems of the pelvis, hip joint, or proximal femur. For children with developmental dysplasia of the hip (DDH) or Legg-Calvé-Perthes disease (LCPD), hip orthoses are the primary intervention for prevention of future deformity and disability. Hip orthoses are essential elements of postoperative care and rehabilitation programs for children with musculoskeletal and neuromuscular conditions who have had surgical intervention for bony deformity or soft tissue contracture. Hip orthoses can also be major postoperative interventions for adults who have had repair of a traumatic injury or a complex total hip arthroplasty. In cases of recurrent hip dislocations, hip orthoses may be indicated to provide external support to prevent future occurrence of dislocation. The efficacy of orthotic intervention is influenced by patient and caregiver adherence: The key to successful use of these orthoses is clear, and open communication exists among the physician, therapist, orthotist, and family concerning the primary goals of the orthosis, its proper application and wearing schedule, and the possible difficulties that may be encountered. Positive healthcare outcomes and happy patients and families are contingent on the ability of the healthcare team to communicate.

WHEN ARE HIP ORTHOSES INDICATED?

Most nontraumatic hip joint dysfunction or pathology occurs either in childhood or in late adult life and is frequently related to one or more of the four following factors:

1. Inadequate or ineffective development of the acetabulum and head of the femur in infancy
2. Avascular necrosis of the femoral head associated with inadequate blood supply during childhood
3. Loss of cartilage and abnormal bone deposition associated with osteoarthritis
4. Loss of bone strength and density in osteoporosis

Orthotic intervention is an important component in the orthopedic management of many of these conditions. Most often, hip orthoses are used to protect or position the hip joint by limiting motion within a desirable range of flexion/extension and abduction/adduction. It is important to note that hip orthoses alone are not effective in controlling internal/external rotation of the hip joint. If precise rotational control is desired, the feet must be included in a hip-knee-ankle-foot orthosis (HKAFO).

HIP STRUCTURE AND FUNCTION

The hip (coxofemoral) joint is a synovial joint formed by the concave socketlike acetabulum of the pelvis and the rounded ball-like head of the femur (Fig. 12.5). Because of the unique bony structure of the hip joint, movement is possible in all three planes of motion: flexion/extension in the sagittal plane, abduction/adduction in the frontal plane, and internal/external rotation in the transverse plane. Most functional activities blend movement of the femur on the pelvis (or of the pelvis on the femur) across all three planes of motion.

The hip joint has two important functions. First, it must support the weight of the head, arms, and trunk during functional activities (e.g., erect sitting and standing, walking, running, stair climbing, and transitional movements in activities of daily living). Second, it must effectively transmit forces from the pelvis to the lower extremities during quiet standing, gait, and other closed chain activities.[30]

The acetabulum is formed at the convergence of the pubis, ischium, and ilium. Its primary orientation is in the vertical, facing laterally, but it also has a slight inferior inclination and an anteverted, or anterior-facing, tilt. Developmentally, the depth of the acetabulum is dynamically shaped by motion of the head of the femur during leg movement and weight bearing. The acetabulum is not fully ossified until late adolescence or early young adulthood. The articular surface of the acetabulum is a horseshoe-shaped, hyaline cartilage–covered area around its anterior, superior, and posterior edges. A space along the inferior edge, called the acetabular notch, is nonarticular,

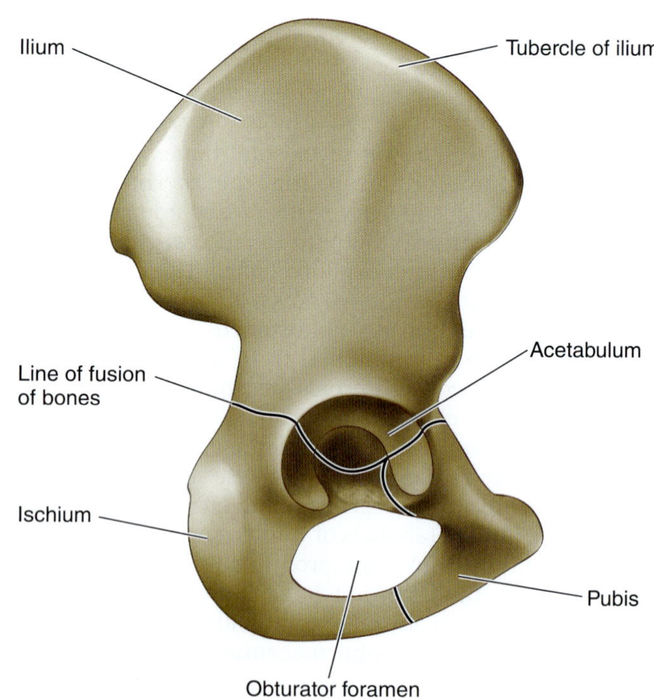

Fig. 12.5 Anatomy of the hip. (From Berry DJ, Lieberman JR. *Surgery of the Hip*. Vol. 2, Sec VII–XII. Elsevier; 2013.)

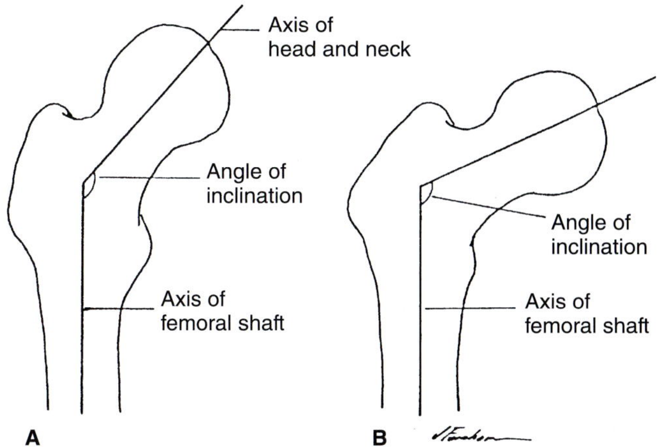

Fig. 12.6 (A) Normal angle of inclination between the neck and shaft of the femur is 125 degrees in adults. A pathological increase in the angle of inclination is called *coxa valga*, and a pathological decrease in the angle of inclination (B) is called *coxa vara*. (From Levangie PK. The hip complex. In: Norkin CC, Levangie PK, eds. *Joint Structure and Function: A Comprehensive Analysis*. Second ed. FA Davis; 1992:305.)

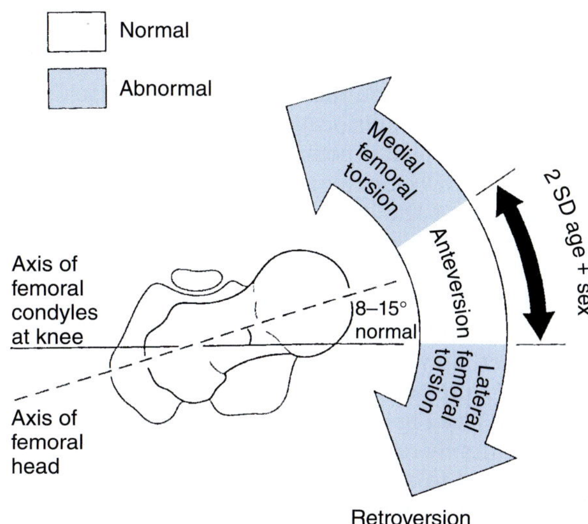

Fig. 12.7 Normal relationship between the axis of the femoral neck and the axis of the femoral condyles (viewed as if looking down the center of the femoral shaft) is between 8 and 15 degrees. Excessive anteversion leads to medial (internal) femoral torsion. Insufficient angulation, retroversion, is associated with lateral (external) femoral torsion. *SD*, Standard deviation. (From Staheli LT. Medical femoral torsion. *Orthop Clin North Am*. 1980;11:40.)

has no cartilage covering, and is spanned by the transverse acetabular ligament. The acetabular labrum is a fibrocartilaginous ring that encircles the exterior perimeter of the acetabulum, increasing joint depth and concavity. The center of the acetabulum, the acetabular fossa, contains fibroelastic fat and the ligamentum teres, and is covered by synovial membrane.

The femoral components of the hip joint include the femoral head, the femoral neck, and the greater and lesser trochanters. The spherical articular surface of the femoral head is covered with hyaline cartilage. Because the femoral head is larger and somewhat differently shaped than the acetabulum, some portion of its articular surface is exposed in any position of the hip joint. The femur and acetabulum are most congruent when positioned in a combination of flexion, abduction, and external rotation. The proximal femur, composed primarily of trabecular bone, is designed to withstand significant loading while also permitting movement through large excursions of range of motion. The orientation of the femoral head and neck in the frontal plane, with respect to the shaft of the femur, is described as its angle of inclination (Fig. 12.6).

In infancy the angle of inclination may be as much as 150 degrees but decreases during normal development to approximately 125 degrees in mid-adulthood and to 120 degrees in later life.[31] The orientation of the proximal femur to the shaft and condyles in the transverse plane, called the *angle of anteversion*, is also a key determinant of hip joint function (Fig. 12.7). Anteversion may be as much as 40 degrees at birth, decreasing during normal development to approximately 15 degrees in adulthood.[31] These two angulations determine how well the femoral head is seated within the acetabulum and, in effect, the biomechanical stability of the hip joint. The functional stability of the hip joint is supported by a strong fibrous joint capsule and by the iliofemoral, ischiofemoral, and pubofemoral ligaments. Fibers of the capsule and ligaments are somewhat obliquely oriented, becoming most taut when the hip is in an extended position.

INFANTS AND CHILDREN WITH DEVELOPMENTAL DYSPLASIA OF THE HIP

DDH is the current terminology for a condition previously called *congenital dislocation of the hip*. This new term includes a variety of congenital hip pathologies including dysplasia, subluxation, and dislocation. This terminology is preferred because it includes those infants with normal physical examination at birth who are later found to have a subluxed or dislocated hip, in addition to those who are immediately identified as having hip pathologies.[32–34]

INCIDENCE AND ETIOLOGY OF DEVELOPMENTAL DYSPLASIA OF THE HIP

Incidence of instability of the hip due to DDH ranges from as low as 1 per 1000 to as high as 34 per 1000 with most of these classified as hip subluxation (9.2/1000), followed by true dislocation (1.3/1000) and dislocatable hips (1.2/1000).[33,35] Commonly, female, family history, and breech presentation are reported as risk factors for DDH.[36–38] A higher incidence of DDH is also found among newborns with other musculoskeletal abnormalities including torticollis, metatarsus varus, clubfoot, or other unusual syndromes.[36,37,39] Other factors have been identified in late presenting DDH. Late presenting DDH is defined as a diagnosis after 3 months of age. In late presenting DDH, a history of swaddling and cephalic presentation were found to have increased risk of DDH. Cephalic presentation incidence was attributed to a decrease in monitoring due to normal birth presentation. With late presenting DDH, the likelihood of irreducible hip dislocations is high.[40]

At birth the acetabulum is quite shallow, covering less than half of the femoral head. In addition, the joint capsule is loose and elastic. These two factors make the neonate hip relatively unstable and susceptible to subluxation and dislocation. Normal development of the hip joint in the first year of life is a function of the stresses and strains placed on the femoral head and acetabulum during movement. In the presence of subluxation or dislocation, modeling of the acetabulum and femoral head is compromised. The most common clinical signs of DDH include asymmetry of the gluteal folds, unequal length of the femur bone (Galeazzi sign), dislocation of the hip with adduction (Barlow maneuver), and repositioning of the femur into the acetabulum with abduction associated with an audible "click" or "clunk" (Ortolani sign; Fig. 12.8).[41] On clinical examination, a "clunk" (Ortolani sign) felt when upward pressure is applied at the level of the greater trochanter on the newborn or infant's flexed and abducted hip (see Fig. 12.8) indicates that a dislocated hip has been manually reduced.[42] The goal of orthotic management in DDH is to achieve optimal seating of the femoral head within the acetabulum while permitting the kicking movements that assist shaping of the acetabulum and femoral head for stability of the hip joint.[43,44] This is best achieved if the child is routinely positioned in flexion and abduction at the hip. If DDH is recognized early and appropriate intervention is initiated, the hip joint is likely to develop normally. If unrecognized and untreated, DDH often leads to significant deformity of the hip as the child grows, resulting in compromised mobility and other functional limitations.

EARLY ORTHOTIC MANAGEMENT OF DEVELOPMENTAL DYSPLASIA OF THE HIP: BIRTH TO 6 MONTHS

In 1958 Professor Arnold Pavlik of Czechoslovakia described an orthosis for the treatment of dysplasia, subluxation, and dislocation of the hip.[45,46] The orthosis he developed, the Pavlik harness, relies on hip flexion and abduction to stabilize the hip at risk. Although a multitude of braces and orthoses have been used historically in the treatment of hip instability, including hip spica casts, the Frejka pillow, the Craig splint, the Ilfeld splint, and the von Rosen splint, the Pavlik harness has become widely accepted as a mainstay for the initial treatment for the unstable hip in neonates from birth to 6 months of age.

At first glance, the Pavlik harness seems a confusing collection of webbing, hook-and-loop material, padding, and straps. In reality, this dynamic orthosis (Fig. 12.9) has three major components:

1. A shoulder and chest harness that provides a proximal anchor for the device
2. A pair of booties and stirrups used as the distal attachment
3. Anterior and posterior leg straps between chest harness and booties used to position the hip joint optimally

The anterior strap allows flexion but limits extension, whereas the posterior strap allows abduction but limits adduction. The child is free to move into flexion and abduction, the motions that are most likely to assist functional shaping of the acetabulum in the months after birth.[45–47] To be effective, however, the fit of the harness must be accurately adjusted for the growing infant and the orthosis must be properly applied. The family/caregiver must be involved in an intensive education program when the newborn is being fit with the Pavlik harness. Nurses, physical and occupational therapists, pediatricians, and orthopedic residents who work with newborns also need to understand the function and fit of this important orthosis. The guidelines for

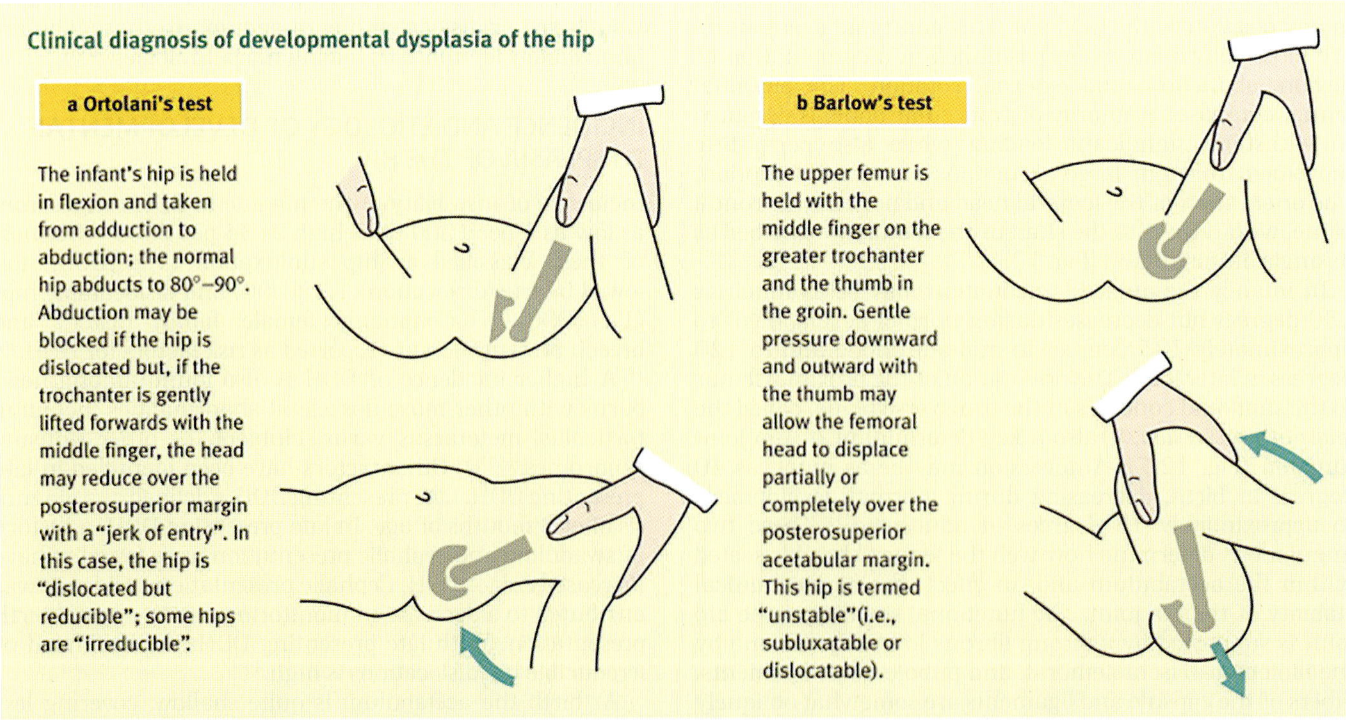

Fig. 12.8 Clinical diagnosis of developmental dysplasia of the hip. (From Campion JC, Benson M. Developmental dysplasia of the hip. *Surgery*. 2007;25(4): 176–180, Copyright © 2007 Elsevier Ltd.)

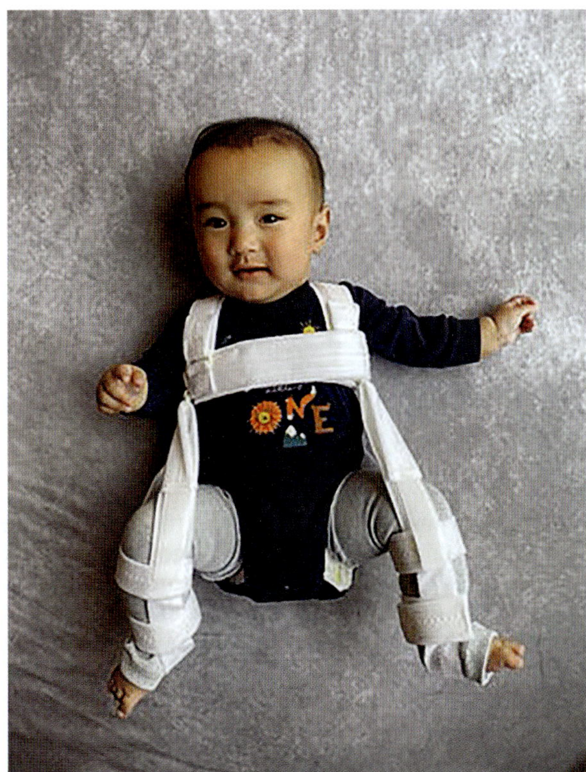

Fig. 12.9 Pavlik harness. A Pavlik harness positions the infant's lower extremities in hip flexion and abduction in an effort to position the femoral head optimally within the acetabulum, assisting normal bony development of the hip joint. The anterior leg straps allow hip flexion but limit hip extension; the posterior flaps allow abduction but limit adduction. (Courtesy Rhino Pediatric Orthopedic Designs, Inc.)

properly fitting a Pavlik harness include the following key points[43,48]:

1. The shoulder straps cross in the back to prevent the orthosis from sliding off the infant's shoulders.
2. The chest strap is fit around the thorax at the infant's nipple line.
3. The proximal calf strap on the bootie is fit just distal to the knee joint.
4. The anterior leg straps are attached to the chest strap at the anterior axillary line.
5. The posterior leg straps are attached to the chest strap just over the infant's scapulae.

In a correctly fit orthosis, the lower extremity is positioned in 100 to 120 degrees of hip flexion, as indicated by the physician's evaluation and recommendation. The limbs are also positioned in 30 to 40 degrees of hip abduction. The distance between the infant's thighs (when the hips are moved passively into adduction) should be no more than 8 to 10 cm. In a well-fit orthosis, extension and adduction are limited, whereas flexion and abduction are freely permitted: The infant is able to kick actively within this restricted range while wearing the orthosis. This position and movement encourage elongation of adductor contractures, which in turn assists in the reduction of the hip and enhances acetabular development. Three common problems indicate that the fit of the harness requires adjustment[43,49]:

1. If the leg straps are adjusted too tightly, the infant cannot kick actively.
2. If the anterior straps are positioned too far medially on the chest strap, the limb is positioned in excessive adduction rather than the desired abduction.
3. If the calf strap is positioned too far distally on the lower leg, it does not position the limb in the desired amount of hip flexion.

Optimal outcomes in infants with DDH are associated with early aggressive intervention of the unstable hip using the Pavlik harness.[50,51] Families and healthcare professionals must seek proper orthopedic care to avoid misdiagnosis and mistreatment. One of the most common misdiagnoses is mistaking dislocation for subluxation and implementing a triple- or double-diapering strategy for intervention. Although this strategy does position the infant's hip in some degree of flexion and abduction, bulky diapers alone are insufficient for reducing dislocation.

Initially, most infants wear the Pavlik harness 24 hours a day. The parents can be permitted to remove the harness for bathing, at the discretion of the orthopedist. Importantly, especially early in treatment, the fit and function of the orthosis must be reevaluated frequently to ensure proper position in the orthosis. The many straps of the Pavlik harness can be confusing to even the most caring of families. The proper donning and doffing sequence should be thoroughly explained and demonstrated to the family. Additional strategies to enhance optimal reduction of the hip such as prone sleeping should be encouraged.

Families must be instructed in proper skin care and in bathing the newborn or infant wearing the orthosis. Initially, they may be advised to use diapers, but not any type of shirt, under the orthosis. The importance of keeping regularly scheduled recheck appointments for effective monitoring of hip position and refitting of the orthosis as the infant grows cannot be overstressed to the parents or caregivers.[51–53] Missed appointments often result in less than optimal positioning of the femoral head with respect to the acetabulum, a less than satisfactory outcome of early intervention, and the necessity of more invasive treatment procedures as the child grows.

As a general rule, the length of treatment in the harness is equal to the child's age when a stable hip reduction is achieved plus an additional 3 months. Thus if a stable reduction is achieved at 4 months of age, the total treatment time would be 7 months. Over time, when hip development is progressing as desired, the wearing schedule can be decreased to night and naptime wear. This often welcomed change in wearing time can begin as early as 3 months of age if x-ray, ultrasound, and physical examination demonstrate the desired bone development. When the orthopedist determines that the hip is normal according to radiographs and ultrasound and is satisfied with the clinical examination, the orthosis can be discontinued. If development of the hip is slow or the infant undergoes rapid growth, it may be advisable to continue the treatment with another type of hip abduction orthosis designed for older and larger babies, to maintain the position of flexion and abduction for a longer period of time.

MANAGEMENT OF DEVELOPMENTAL DYSPLASIA OF THE HIP: AGE 6 MONTHS AND OLDER

For older infants and toddlers (4–18 months) whose DDH was unrecognized or inadequately managed early in infancy, intervention is often much more aggressive and may include an abduction brace, traction, open or closed reduction, and hip spica casting.[33,54–56] For infants who are growing quickly or whose bone development has been slow, an alternative to the Pavlik harness is necessary. After the age of 6 months, especially as the infant begins to pull into standing in preparation for walking, the Pavlik harness can no longer provide the desired positioning for reduction. Often, the infant is simply too large to fit into the harness. By this time, families who have been compliant with harness application and wearing have grown to dislike it and are ready for other forms of intervention.

A custom-fit prefabricated thermoplastic hip abduction orthosis is often the next step in orthotic management of DDH. This orthosis consists of a plastic frame with waist section and thigh cuffs, waterproof foam liner, and hook-and-loop material closures. The static version is fixed at 90 degrees of hip flexion and 120 degrees of hip abduction (Fig. 12.10). An adjustable joint can be incorporated into the abduction bar; however, hip flexion is maintained at 90 degrees. This orthosis appears to be static, but the child is able to move within the thigh sections while the safe zone for continued management of hip position is maintained.

Many families view the hip abduction orthosis as an improvement over the Pavlik harness: The caregivers and the infant are free from cumbersome straps, the orthosis is easily removed and reapplied for diaper changing and hygiene, and the orthosis itself is waterproof and easier to keep clean. Parents and caregivers can hold the infant without struggling with straps, and the baby is able to sit comfortably for feeding and play.

Because most hip abduction orthoses are prefabricated, the knowledge and skills of an orthotist are necessary to ensure a proper custom fit for each child. To determine what the necessary modifications are, the orthotist evaluates three areas:

1. The length of the thigh cuffs. Thigh cuffs are trimmed proximal to the popliteal fossae. Cuffs that are too long can lead to neurovascular compromise if the child prefers to sleep in a supine position, as the risk of compression of the legs against the distal edge of the cuffs is present.
2. The width of the anterior opening of the waist component. Although the plastic is flexible, the opening may need to be enlarged for heavy or large-framed infants.
3. The foam padding of the thigh and waist components. All edges must be smooth to avoid skin irritation or breakdown, and the circumference of the padding should fit without undue tightness.

Modifications may require reheating or trimming of the plastic or foam padding. Usually this fitting takes place in the orthotist's office or the clinic setting, where the necessary tools are readily available. Once the fit is evaluated and modified as appropriate for the individual child, the parents or caregivers are instructed in proper donning/doffing and orthotic care.

The static hip abduction orthosis is used in either of two ways. First, the orthosis may be a continuation of the course of treatment established by the Pavlik harness, as determined by the orthopedist's evaluation of the child's hip. As a continuation of treatment, the orthosis can be worn day and night; most often, however, it is reserved for nighttime use while the child is sleeping.[41,43,54] The use of the orthosis at night is believed to assist development of acetabular growth cartilage. If the orthosis is worn consistently for several months and evidence of effective reduction and reshaping of the joint is present, it is less likely that more aggressive forms of treatment will be necessary as the child grows.

The second application for the hip abduction orthosis is for follow-up management for children with DDH who require an orthopedic intervention such as traction, surgical reduction, or casting. In this case the orthosis provides external stability to the hip during the postoperative weeks and months, while the baby regains range of motion and continues to grow and progress through the stages of motor development. This extra stability reduces parental and physician concern about dislocation and other undesired outcomes of the orthopedic procedure.

The static hip abduction orthosis has obvious advantages over plaster or synthetic hip spica casts, including greater ease in diaper hygiene and bathing, and is often welcomed by families as a positive next step in treatment. Fitting requires the knowledge and skills of an orthotist familiar with proper fitting techniques and who can manage potentially irritable babies just freed from a confining hip spica cast.

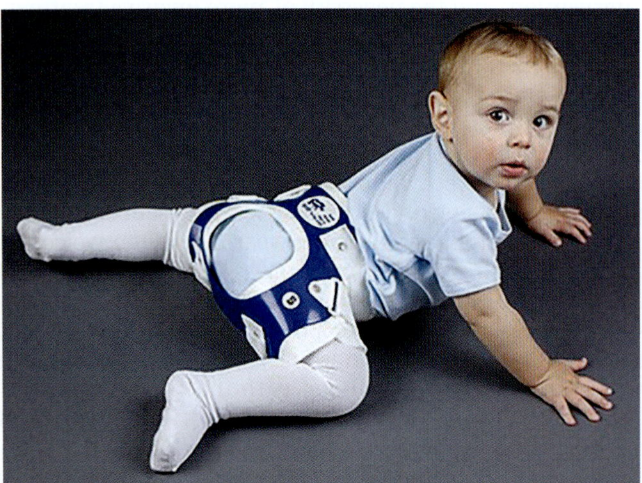

Fig. 12.10 Rhino hip abduction orthosis. A posterior view of a static hip abduction orthosis that positions the infant in 90 degrees of hip flexion and 120 degrees of hip abduction. (Courtesy Rhino Pediatric Orthopedic Designs, Inc.)

GOALS OF ORTHOTIC INTERVENTION FOR CHILDREN WITH DEVELOPMENTAL DYSPLASIA OF THE HIP

To be effective, orthotic intervention for DDH must have a set of clearly described treatment objectives against which success can be measured. The components necessary for effective orthotic interventions for children with DDH include the following:

1. Clearly presented verbal, hands-on, and written instructions for the child's family or caregivers, with an additional goal of minimizing stress in an already stressful situation.
2. Effective communication among members of the healthcare team about the appropriate use and potential pitfalls of the orthosis. This often includes education about the orthosis provided by the orthotist and careful monitoring of family compliance and coping by all members of the team (orthotists, orthopedists, pediatricians, therapists, nurses, and other health professionals who may be involved in the case).
3. Safe and effective hip reduction to minimize the necessity of more aggressive casting or surgery. This requires proper orthotic fit and adjustment, as well as consistency in wearing schedules.

The ultimate goal is to facilitate normal development of the hip joint, providing the child with a pain-free, stable, functional hip that will last throughout his or her lifetime.

COMPLICATIONS OF ORTHOTIC MANAGEMENT OF DEVELOPMENTAL DYSPLASIA OF THE HIP

In most cases the Pavlik harness, perhaps followed by abduction orthosis use as the child grows, is a successful intervention for DDH. A small percentage of infants with DDH managed by the Pavlik harness (<8%) develop complications, the most serious of which is avascular necrosis of the femoral head, which may be caused by overtightening the posterior straps to force a position of abduction.[33,52–59] Children who have complications differ from those without complications in a number of ways. They tend to have larger acetabular angles (>35 degrees) and less total coverage of the femoral head within the acetabulum (<20%) on radiography or ultrasound, have an irreducible dislocation at initiation of orthotic intervention, have delayed diagnosis and intervention (older than 3 months of age), and have not demonstrated a prior ossific nucleus on radiograph or ultrasound.[52,53,57,60] A concern of continued research into the development of DDH screening protocols is the overscreening and overtreatment, which is leading to a rise in avascular necrosis development.[36]

ORTHOTIC MANAGEMENT OF LEGG-CALVÉ-PERTHES DISEASE

LCPD is a pathologic condition of the hip that affects otherwise healthy school-aged children. Although the clinical signs and symptoms of LCPD, as they differ from tuberculosis involving the hip, were first described by Arthur T. Legg in 1910,[61] the etiology of this condition is not clearly understood and its treatment and orthopedic management continue to be controversial. The hallmark of LCPD is a flattening of the femoral head, thought to be a result of an avascular necrosis insult. Left untreated, LCPD leads to permanent deformity and eventual osteoarthritis in the adult hip. The disease is four times as common in boys between the ages of 4 and 8 years old as in girls, although outcomes in girls tend to be less satisfactory.[62–64] LCPD generally involves only one hip; only approximately 12% of cases are bilateral. It is rare within the Black population. Exposure to smoking in utero, obesity, low socioeconomic status, and repetitive high-impact activities have also been considered as risk factors with the development of LCPD.[65–68] Several options for orthotic management of LCPD have evolved. All are designed to help maintain a spherical femoral head and normal acetabulum.

Etiology of Legg-Calvé-Perthes Disease

The etiology of LCPD remains controversial more than 100 years after it was first described. Most researchers believe that LCPD is a result of some event or condition that compromises blood flow to the femoral head and leads to avascular necrosis. The exact mechanism that triggers this compromise is unknown. Some theories focus on an acute trauma that damages the vascular system of the femoral head, whereas others suggest that repeated episodes of a transient synovitis may compromise blood flow.[63,69,70] Another theory suggests an abnormality of thrombolysis in children who develop LCPD.[71] A genetic predisposition to delayed bone age that exposes vessels to high rates of compression as they pass through cartilage to the bony head has also been suggested.[69] Although the exact etiology of LCPD remains a mystery, it is certainly linked to episodes of avascular necrosis in the femoral head. The goal of intervention in children with LCPD is to assist revascularization of the femoral head and to restore normal anatomical shape and alignment of the hip joint.

Evaluation and Intervention for Legg-Calvé-Perthes Disease

LCPD should be suspected in children with one or more of the following signs or symptoms[72,73]:

1. A noticeable limp, often with a positive Trendelenburg sign
2. Pain in the hip, groin, knee, or a combination of these locations
3. Loss of range of motion of the hip joint

When these symptoms are present, radiographic, ultrasound, or magnetic resonance imaging studies of the hip are used to discriminate between LCPD (Fig. 12.11) and

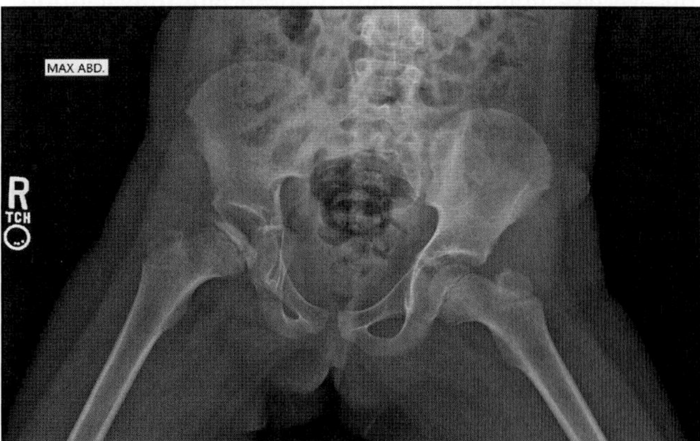

Fig. 12.11 Legg-Calvé-Perthes disease (LCPD) photograph of x-ray. A radiograph of a child with LCPD comparing the shape and density of the head of the femur and of the capital epiphysis on the normal *(right side of image)* and affected *(left side of image)* right hip.

other hip disorders (e.g., slipped capital femoral epiphysis, fracture, rheumatic disease, infection).[74] These studies are used by the orthopedist to determine severity and progression of the disease, considering the stage of the disease, the shape of the femoral head, the degree of congruence with the acetabulum, and the length and angle of the femoral neck.[75,76] A variety of classification systems have been developed to rate severity of involvements. The Catterall system describes four groups on the basis of the location of involvement and identifies four "head at risk" signs for the orthopedist or radiologist to focus on in interpreting radiographs.[77] Studies of the interrater and concurrent reliability of the Catterall systems have not all been positive.[78–80] The Salter-Thompson system rates severity of involvement on the basis of the location and extent of subchondral fracture that may be observed early in the disease process.[81,82] The Herring system examines the condition of the lateral pillar of the femoral head on radiographs.[74,80,83] Refer to texts on orthopedic conditions in pediatrics for further information about classification.[69,70] LCPD is a self-limiting process that often resolves in 1 to 3 years. The disease progresses through three stages:

1. Necrotic stage: avascular necrosis
2. Fragmentation stage: resorption of damaged bone
3. Healing/reparative stage: revascularization, reossification, and bony remodeling

Factors that influence the eventual outcome of the disease include age at onset, severity of damage to the femoral head and epiphysis, and quality of congruency of the acetabulum and femoral head.[63,64,69,70]

Because the disease process is self-limiting, the optimal intervention strategy is controversial. The three most commonly used avenues of treatment for LCPD are observation, surgical intervention, and conservative orthotic management. Decisions about treatment are often guided by age of the child, extent of femoral head deformity, and severity of incongruency between the femoral head and acetabulum.[69,70,84] More recent data suggest that patients younger than 6 years of age at the time of disease onset are best managed nonsurgically, whereas the treatment for patients older than 8 years may involve surgery and is less well defined.[85]

For children with minimal bony deformity, observation and exercise may be the most appropriate intervention.[86] Because the child is likely to continue to limp until sufficient revascularization and remodeling have occurred (which may require several years), parents may be uneasy, preferring instead a more aggressive intervention. Parents are reassured when close clinical follow-up is performed, with periodic reexamination by x-ray evaluation to monitor progression of the disease process.

Surgical intervention is based on the principle of containment, optimally positioning the femoral head within the acetabulum. Proximal femoral derotation osteotomy is used to decompress and center the femoral head within the acetabulum for more functional weight bearing in an extended position.[87,88] A pelvic osteotomy, which repositions the acetabulum over the femoral head, is sometimes necessary when a significantly enlarged or subluxed femoral head cannot be effectively repositioned by femoral derotation osteotomy.[89,90] Shelf arthroplasty to reshape the acetabulum to better accept the femoral head has also been used as an intervention.[91–93] The outcome of surgery is likely to be most positive for children who have full hip range of motion preoperatively. Parents must understand the goals and risks of the surgical procedure and must be actively involved in postoperative rehabilitation efforts.

The goal of conservative orthotic management of LCPD is similar to that of surgical intervention: to contain the femoral head within the acetabulum during the active stages of the disease process so that optimal remodeling can occur.[44,93] Much debate has taken place concerning whether surgery or orthotic intervention is most efficacious. If both are viable methods of treatment, the end result should be the same: a well-shaped femoral head and pain-free hip. Comparing the efficacy of surgical versus orthotic management of LCPD is challenging because of relatively low incidence as well as differences in study design and definition of control for variables such as age of onset, duration of the disease, gender, and inadequate interobserver reliability of classification systems.[94,95] Although two reports published in 1992 question the efficacy of orthotic treatment,[96,97] other studies advocate orthotic treatment even in severe cases of the disease. Because studies have reported success, as well as lack of success for all three types of intervention (noncontainment/observation, surgery, and the use of orthoses), the most appropriate management of LCPD has not been clearly determined.

Orthotic Management in Legg-Calvé-Perthes Disease

Currently the most commonly used orthosis in the nonoperative management of LCPD is the Atlanta/Scottish-Rite hip abduction orthosis (Fig. 12.12). The design of this orthosis allows the child to walk and be involved in other functional activities while containing the femoral head in the acetabulum with abduction of the hips.[98–100] The Atlanta/Scottish-Rite orthosis has three components: a pelvic band, a pair of single-axis hip joints, and a pair of thigh cuffs. An abduction bar may also be included, interconnecting the

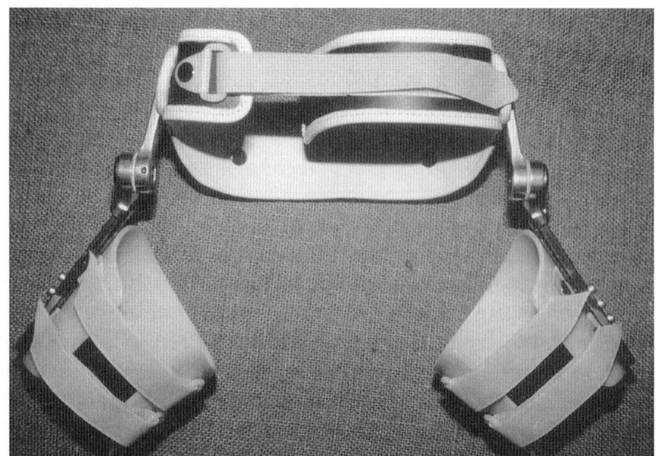

Fig. 12.12 An Atlanta/Scottish-Rite hip abduction orthosis used in the conservative management of Legg-Calve-Perthes disease. This orthosis has three components: the pelvic band, the free-motion hip joints, and thigh cuffs. This orthosis has an abduction bar to provide increased stability and maintains desired position of abduction.

thigh cuffs with a ball-and-socket joint as an interface. This orthosis holds each hip in approximately 45 degrees of hip abduction, permits flexion and extension of the hip, and can be worn over clothing. While in the orthosis, the hips are abducted and flexed but the patient has no limitation in knee range of motion and therefore can sit or walk without difficulty. The orthosis is not designed to control internal rotation of the hip. This type of orthosis is most effective if the child who is wearing it has close to normal range of motion at the hip joint. Limitations in range of motion cause the child to stand asymmetrically in the orthosis, which effectively reduces the amount of abduction and containment of the femoral head.

Historically (in the 1960s and 1970s), a number of other orthoses were developed on the basis of the principles of containment of the femoral head. The Toronto orthosis (Fig. 12.13A) and the Newington orthosis (Fig. 12.13B) hold both limbs in 45 degrees of abduction with internal rotation but, unlike the Atlanta/Scottish-Rite orthosis, require the use of crutches for safe mobility.[101,102] These orthoses are cumbersome to wear and significantly affect the ease of daily function. Because the efficacy of the Atlanta Scottish-Rite orthosis is as high as or higher than the efficacy of the Toronto and Newington orthoses, the latter two orthoses are not commonly used in current management of children with LCPD.[44,103] In addition, orthoses like an "A-frame" may be used after several weeks of Petrie casting, another nonsurgical treatment option enforcing hip abduction.[85] The use of the "A-frame" device with daily ROM exercises has been found to be successful following adductor tenotomy and abduction casting for improving spherical congruency of the femoral head.

If the disease process progresses and the hip begins to lose additional range of motion, the orthotist may be the first to recognize this problem. The parents may bring the child to the clinic for an orthotic adjustment because the thigh cuffs have become uncomfortable. If loss of additional range of motion is noticed by parents or by therapists who are working with the child, an immediate referral to the orthotic clinic or physician is necessary. The Atlanta/Scottish-Rite orthosis is not designed to increase range of motion; its primary function is to hold the hips in abduction comfortably. Using the orthosis to restore range of motion defeats the purpose of the orthotic design and compromises treatment principles.

Communication among the orthopedist, orthotist, therapist, and family is essential. Parents must understand that this is a demanding form of treatment. Typically, the orthosis is worn continually for 12 to 18 months. Once radiographic evidence of femoral head reossification is seen, time in the orthosis is gradually reduced.

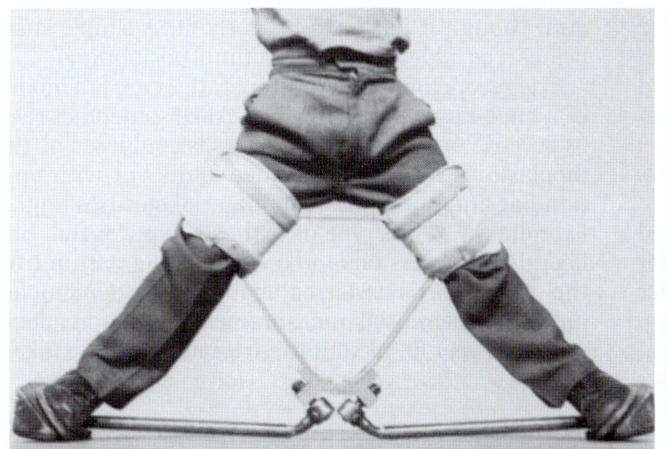

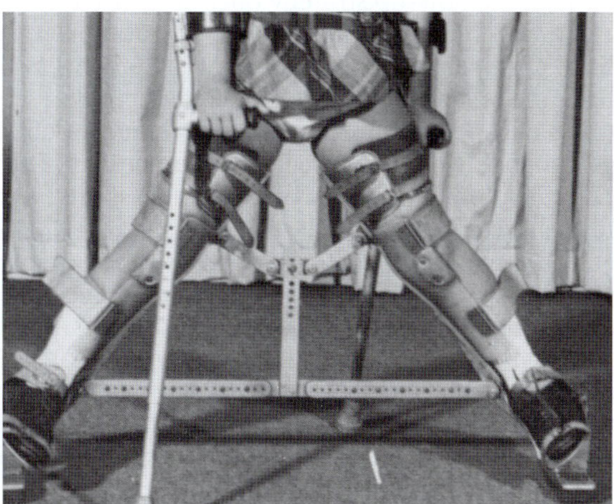

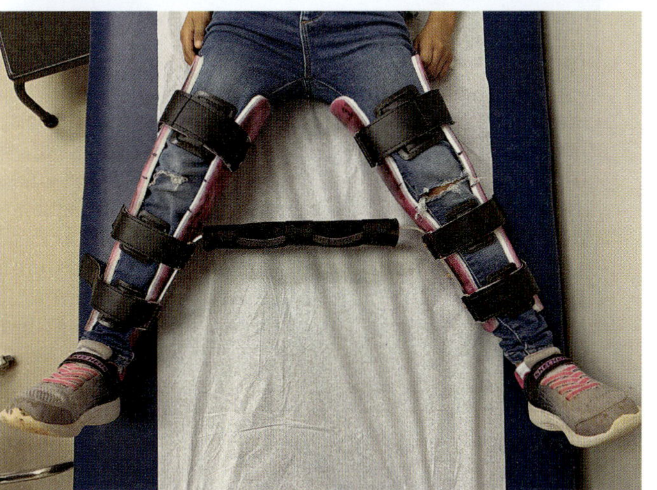

Fig. 12.13 Earlier designs for hip abduction knee-ankle-foot orthoses used to manage Legg-Calvé-Perthes disease. The Toronto hip-knee-ankle-foot orthosis (A) and Newington orthoses (B) were more cumbersome to don and to function with than the Atlanta/Scottish-Rite hip abduction orthoses. (C) Contemporary designs combine thermoplastic, foam, and aluminum bar stock to create a lower profile orthosis. (From Goldberg B, Hsu JH, eds. *Atlas of Orthotics and Assistive Devices.* Third ed. Mosby; 1997.)

Absolute compliance with the wearing schedule is necessary for maximum effectiveness: a well-designed and well-fit orthosis can only work if it is being used. The first few days and weeks in the orthosis are often stressful for the parent and the child. With the hips held in an abducted position, routine tasks including walking may require assistance until the child learns effective adaptive strategies. Physical therapists may work with the child on crutch-walking techniques on level surfaces, stairs, inclines, and uneven surfaces. They may make suggestions for adaptation of the home and school environments so that sitting and transitions from flooring, chairs, and standing quickly become manageable. If family education and support efforts are effective and enable parents and children to weather this difficult initial stage in orthotic management well, the likelihood of compliance in the remaining months of intervention is significantly enhanced. Expectations for continued care and follow-up, including adjustments following growth and increases in range of motion, should be conveyed to family and caregivers to ensure success.

PEDIATRIC POSTOPERATIVE CARE

Numerous musculoskeletal and neuromuscular conditions, in addition to LCPD and developmental dysplasia, may necessitate surgical intervention for children with hip and lower extremity dysfunction or deformity. Orthoses that control hip and leg position are often used in the weeks and months after surgery as an alternative to traditional plaster casts or as a follow-up strategy once casts are removed. Although a cast may be applied in the operating room for immediate postoperative care, orthoses are often fit soon afterward and effectively shorten the time that a child spends in a cast. Hip orthoses are used when immobilization and support will be required for a long period of time, when complications arise, or when a child's special needs demand their use.

One of the major benefits of an orthosis (as compared with a plaster cast) is in regard to hygiene, especially for children who have not yet developed consistent bladder and bowel control. Additional benefits of postoperative hip orthoses include the following:

1. Being much lighter than traditional casts, hip orthoses reduce the burden of care for parents and caregivers who must lift or carry the child.
2. Hip orthoses can be removed for inspection of surgical wounds and for bathing and skin care.
3. Hip orthoses can be removed for physical therapy, range of motion, mobilization, strengthening, or other appropriate interventions.
4. Thermoplastic orthoses using closed cell foam are water resistant; therefore residues of perspiration or urine can be easily cleaned and sanitized with warm soap and water.
5. A well-fit orthosis is less likely to cause skin irritation or breakdown and, unlike a cast, can often be adjusted if areas of impingement develop.
6. The position and amount of abduction can be easily adjusted by the orthotist.
7. A hip orthosis can be custom designed for a patient with complicated needs, especially those who have had multiple surgical procedures.

Postoperative Hip Orthoses

Two basic designs are available for children's postoperative orthoses. The first is composed of thigh cuffs that fit between the knee and hip joint, an abduction bar, and hook-and-loop material closures (Fig. 12.14). This orthosis can be fabricated from measurements taken before surgery and fit with no delay as soon as the cast is removed. It can also be fit in lieu of a cast if the surgical procedure was minor or when static positioning of the hip is required. This type of orthosis is commonly used after adductor release or varus osteotomy with adductor release or for the management of a septic hip. A postoperative hip orthosis is most often used for extended periods of nighttime-only wear but in some circumstances can also be worn during the day.[104] In many clinics this orthosis is used after hip procedures in children with cerebral palsy.

Parents and caregivers find the postoperative hip orthosis a welcome relief from a cast. Despite its simple appearance, families should be given special instructions about how the orthosis is worn and cared for. These orthoses typically will have a closed cell foam inner liner that can be cleaned to ensure proper hygiene. It can be worn over clothing or pajamas or next to the skin if necessary. It should not cause skin irritation or discomfort on either side of the hip joint. If the patient experiences any hip joint pain, the orthotist should consult with the orthopedist to determine if the angle of abduction can be safely adjusted. Attempts to excessively abduct the hip can cause pain and reduce compliance. Occasionally, this orthosis may be difficult to keep in place even though it has been properly fit. A simple suspension belt can be added to ensure optimal positioning.

The second option for postoperative care is a modification of a knee-ankle-foot orthosis (KAFO) sometimes referred to as a Petrie orthosis. This orthosis is composed of two thermoplastic KAFOs without knee joints but with an abduction bar and hook-and-loop material closures (Fig. 12.15). Fabrication of this type of orthosis requires that plaster or fiberglass impressions to be taken along with a tracing of the orthopedist's preferred abduction angle: Simple length and circumferential measurements are not adequate to ensure proper fit. Ideally, these impressions are taken at the

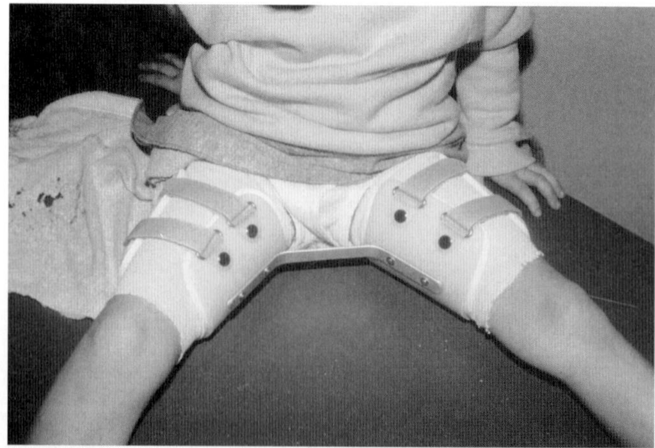

Fig. 12.14 A postoperative hip abduction orthosis has two components: a pair of thigh cuffs held in position by an abduction bar.

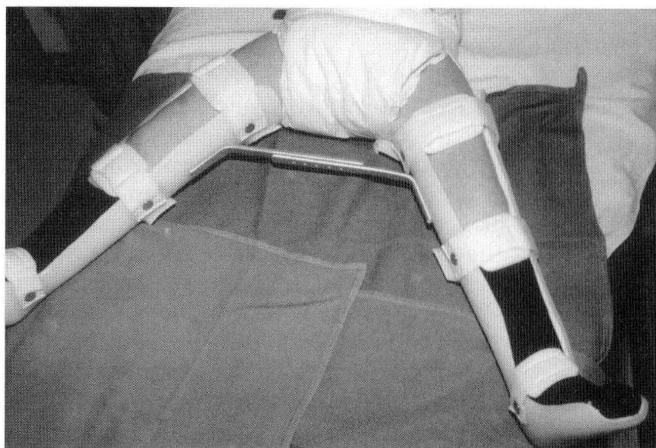

Fig. 12.15 Petrie orthosis. For postoperative management of children after extensive bony and soft tissue surgery, knee-ankle-foot orthoses with the addition of an abduction bar are often used subsequent to cast removal. Rotation of the hip is well controlled by the intimate fit of the orthosis, including the ankle-foot complex. When precise control of the hip is necessary, the postoperative hip abduction orthosis encompasses the pelvis as well.

first postoperative cast change. The orthosis is then fabricated, and fitting occurs during the next clinic appointment. Taking the impressions before surgery is not advisable. Postoperatively, each joint will be at a new angle, compromising the fit of the orthosis based on preoperative impressions. This type of orthosis is recommended for patients who have had bony procedures around the hip, as well as extensive soft tissue procedures such as hamstring or heel cord release, which require protection in the early stages of healing. This orthosis is often used for children with cerebral palsy, myelomeningocele, or Legg-Calve-Perthes Disease. In some circumstances, when more precise control of the hip joint is desirable, the orthosis can be extended upward to include the pelvis.

Because of the intimate fit of this orthosis, parents and caregivers must be given careful education concerning proper fit and cleaning. Especially important is a careful inspection of the posterior aspect of the calcaneus: This area is vulnerable to skin breakdown from prolonged pressure and may be overlooked during skin checks that focus on the healing surgical wounds. Because the foam lining and thermoplastic material do not breathe, perspiration cannot effectively evaporate. The orthosis should be removed periodically for cleaning to minimize the risk of skin maceration or infection from microorganisms that thrive in warm moist environments.

The postoperative orthosis has proven useful in the overall orthopedic management of children with musculoskeletal or neuromuscular diseases. The orthosis is an effective substitute for heavy casts, especially when skin irritation and incontinence are concerns. The postoperative hip orthosis helps ensure healing in the optimal joint position and reduces the likelihood of recurrence of the deformity that prompted surgical intervention.

MANAGEMENT OF THE ADULT HIP

Orthotic intervention for the hip in the adult population is limited, focusing on two groups of patients. Hip orthoses are most commonly used as postsurgical and postcast care of adult patients who have sustained a complex hip or proximal femoral fracture from a traumatic event such as a motor vehicle accident, industrial accident, or fall. In some circumstances a hip orthosis can be used for older adults after a total hip procedure, revision of a total hip, or fracture associated with total hip arthroplasty.[105,106] Although injury that affects the hip can occur at any point in the lifespan, most adults with trauma-related fractures who are managed with hip orthoses are young and middle aged, and many of those who are undergoing a new or revised total joint arthroplasty are 65 years or older. As the number of older adults increases in the US population, so will the number of hip fractures. One estimate suggests that as many as 512,000 hip fractures will occur in the United States by the year 2040.[107]

In both of these circumstances, stabilization of the orthopedic injury and rehabilitation planning are important issues. Patients with this type of injury of the hip often require extensive physical therapy programs. Clinicians must understand age-related pathophysiological changes that affect the healing musculoskeletal system, the impact and detrimental effects of prolonged bed rest, and the optimal point at which an orthosis should be integrated into the overall treatment plan.

Total Hip Arthroplasty

Although a hip orthosis is usually not indicated in most simple, elective total hip arthroplasties, in some circumstances this orthosis can assist healing and rehabilitation. Hip orthoses can be used for patients with significant osteoporosis in whom femoral fracture occurs during total joint surgery or for those who require emergency total joint replacement as a result of trauma. Hip orthoses are also used for patients who are undergoing revision of a total hip replacement as a consequence of recurrent dislocation or of aseptic loosening of the femoral component. If control of rotation is desired, an HKAFO can be prescribed to provide additional support and protection to healing structures.

Most HKAFOs have a pelvic band and belt and an adjustable hip joint that can be locked or can allow free motion or limit motion within a specific range (Fig. 12.16). An adjustable anterior panel can be added to the thigh section if a fracture has occurred during the surgical procedure and requires additional protection. The knee joint can also be locked, free motion, or adjustable for specific ranges of motion, depending on the patient's need. The ankle-foot orthosis (AFO) component is necessary to provide maximum control of unwanted rotation of the hip.

Typically, HKAFOs are custom fabricated on the basis of an impression of the patient's limb. This increases the likelihood of an optimal fit and allows customization of the orthosis to meet the specific needs of the patient. If this approach is not amenable to certain healthcare environments, prefabricated custom-fit HKAFOs and hip orthoses are available as alternatives to custom-molded orthoses.[106] These orthoses are fabricated from components that are then custom fit on the basis of the patient's limb measurements. Most postoperative hip orthoses are designed to limit flexion and adduction of the hip joint. They try to prevent dislocation by supporting the optimal position of the hip joint within a safe range of motion and by providing a kinesthetic reminder when patients attempt to move beyond these ranges.[106] Many of

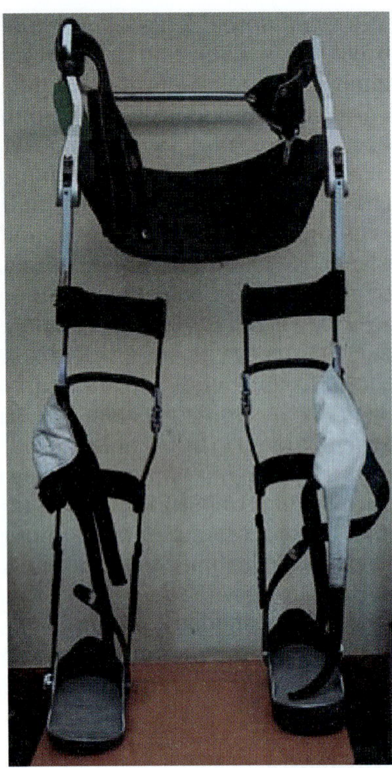

Fig. 12.16 Lateral view of a hip-knee-ankle-foot orthosis, prescribed for postoperative management after a complex total hip arthroplasty. Note the pelvic band, free hip joint, supportive thigh cuff, and free-knee joint. The ankle-foot orthosis component is necessary for effective control of rotary forces through the femur and hip joint. (From Luqmani R, Robb J, Porter D, et al. *Textbook of Orthopaedics, Trauma, and Rheumatology*. Second ed. Mosby; 2013.)

the prefabricated hip orthoses that are commercially available are unable to provide maximum control of rotation because they do not encompass the foot. Careful evaluation of the patient is required to determine which alternative is most appropriate. In both cases, the orthosis is worn whenever the patient is out of bed and, in some instances, while the patient is in bed as well. The orthosis is usually worn for at least 8 weeks after total hip revision.

Because lower extremity orthoses add weight to a lower extremity that is already compromised, orthotists must be sensitive to the selection of lightweight materials and components. This is especially true for older patients, who may have limited endurance because of cardiac or respiratory disease. Although the initial orthosis may restrict joint motion to provide external stability to a vulnerable hip joint, the orthotic hip, knee, and ankle joints can be adjusted to meet the patient's needs as the rehabilitation program progresses. Hip orthoses and HKAFOs may be important adjuncts for rehabilitation in the following ways:

1. A well-fit hip orthosis provides protection against dislocation in patients who are predisposed to this problem.
2. Hip orthoses protect and support healing fracture sites, often allowing earlier mobility and gait training than would otherwise be possible.
3. Early and safe weight bearing for older patients with dislocation or fracture reduces the risk of secondary complications associated with prolonged bed rest or immobility.
4. The orthotic hip, knee, and ankle joints can be adjusted to restrict or permit motion to match the patient's specific needs at initial fitting and as the treatment program progresses.

Following surgical intervention after fracture or total joint arthroplasty, the focus of the rehabilitation program shifts to mobility training, strengthening, flexibility, and endurance. The decision to recommend a hip orthosis is individual, influenced by the severity of the musculoskeletal problem, the patient's particular circumstances, and the experience and preferences of the health professionals involved in postoperative care. Few definitive guidelines or documentation are available concerning the efficacy of hip orthoses in the postoperative management of hip fracture or arthroplasty. An orthosis is best used to augment the goals of rehabilitation, including the return to preoperative ambulatory status, safe and protected weight bearing during ADLs, facilitation of union of the fracture site, and ultimately return to presurgical social and self-care independence.

Patients who have had recurrent hip dislocations are another population who may benefit from a hip abduction orthosis. In these patients, there may be a ligamentous laxity that has developed due to history of dislocations with or without an incidence of hip replacement. Surgical intervention may not be indicated in these situations, although the external stabilization of a hip abduction orthosis may help allow a limited range of motion. Range of motion limitations are directed by the treating physician in opposing motions that contributed to the dislocation. Utilizing hip abduction orthoses in these situations will provide external stabilization and allow for return to daily activity with kinesthetic reminder of limitations on hip joint motion. Patients will wear this orthosis at all times and will be directed to work with a physical therapist for strengthening of hip muscles once sufficient healing of hip joint has taken place.

Posttrauma Care

The other group of individuals who may benefit from hip orthoses are those who have experienced traumatic fractures of the femur, hip, or pelvis as a result of motor vehicle accidents, industrial accidents, or falls from great heights. Most of these patients are fit with their orthosis after stabilization of the fracture with internal fixation. The HKAFO is similar in design to the orthosis described for older patients after hip fracture or arthroplasty. Depending on the need for external support and stability, the hip joint can be locked to prevent flexion and extension or may allow motion within a limited range. For some patients, it may be necessary to incorporate a lumbosacral spinal orthosis to achieve the desired control of pelvic and hip motion. The AFO component provides control of hip rotation in the transverse plane.

When complete immobilization is warranted after orthopedic trauma of the lower spine, pelvis, and hip, a custom-molded thermoplastic version of a hip spica cast can be fabricated. This hip orthosis has anterior and posterior components, extending from the mid- to lower thoracic trunk to just above the femoral condyles of the fractured extremity and to the groin of the intact extremity. This design provides maximum stability and can be used in lieu of or after casting. The position of the lower extremity within the orthosis is determined by the type and extent of the surgical repair. When the patient is lying in the supine position, the anterior component can be removed for skin inspection and personal care.

Similarly, the posterior component can be removed when the patient is prone. This is an advantage for patients with open wounds or difficulty with continence and is especially appreciated if immobilization will be required for an extended period.

Many patients who are recovering from musculoskeletal trauma involving the pelvis and hip joint require physical therapy for gait and mobility training after surgery and an intensive rehabilitation program to regain preinjury muscle strength, range of motion, and functional status. The orthopedic surgeon and therapists, as well as the patient and family, must clearly understand the advantages provided and the mobility limitations imposed by postsurgical hip orthoses. An optimal orthosis can assist rehabilitation if fabricated with lightweight but durable components that can be adjusted as the patient progresses, while meeting the individual patient's need for stability or supported mobility of the hip. An appropriate hip orthosis also enhances early mobility and protected weight bearing, reducing the risk of loss of function related to bed rest and deconditioning.

Fracture Management

A fracture occurs when there is disruption in the continuity of bone.[108] Fractures are common consequences of trauma from falls, sports, work-related injuries, motor vehicle accidents, or violence.[109–111] Many disorders and diseases (e.g., osteopenia, malnutrition, paralysis, osteoporosis) and medications (e.g., corticosteroids), as well as primary or metastatic malignancies of bone, increase vulnerability to fracture.[112,113] Habitual activity level over the lifespan, health habits (e.g., smoking), and gender and age (e.g., bone density and menopausal status) influence bone density and, subsequently, the risk of fracture during daily activity.[114–117] Orthopedic intervention for fractures is dictated by the severity of the fracture, as well as etiology. Simple fractures, those with minimal fragmentation or displacement, are often managed with closed reduction followed by initial management in a plaster or fiberglass splint to provide stabilization, while allowing for swelling, and then a period of immobilization in a plaster or fiberglass cast or a custom-fit, prefabricated fracture orthosis until bony union is achieved.[118] More complex fractures, those with multiple fragments or significant displacement, often require open (surgical) reduction with internal fixation (ORIF; with plates, screws, or wires), prosthetic replacement (arthroplasty), or stabilization in an external rigging or fixator until there has been sufficient bony healing.[119]

The care provided to individuals recovering from a fracture is founded on understanding the mechanism of injury, fracture classification, and process of bone repair and healing.[120,121] The orthopedic surgeon and orthotist choose from a variety of casts, cast braces, splints, and fracture orthoses to provide the most effective fracture management strategy for each patient on the basis of the fracture type and location, degree of reduction, skin condition, mobility needs, and likelihood of compliance. Geographical and personal preferences regarding design, device selection, and treatment influence the choice of fracture management strategy, as do the training and experience of the health professionals involved. Few strategies for immobilization can provide 100% rigid fixation. Absolute immobilization is only possible with direct skeletal attachment. A variety of factors influence the quality of fit and function of any cast, cast brace, splint, or fracture orthosis. Each device has the potential to contribute to a successful result but only if used appropriately, with absolute attention to detail by each of the treatment team members.

MECHANISMS OF FRACTURE HEALING

Three distinct stages of physiological fracture healing occur: inflammation, repair, and remodeling.[121] Fracture damages bone, its periosteum, nutrient vessels, marrow, and often surrounding soft tissue and muscle. Disruption of vascular supply leads to ischemia and necrosis of bone cells and other injured tissues. These damaged tissues release inflammatory mediators into intracellular space, triggering an inflammatory response: A shift in plasma from capillary to intracellular space leads to significant edema. Migration of polymorphonuclear leukocytes, macrophages, and lymphocytes to the injured area is the first step in clearing necrosis. A hematoma forms; in a simple nondisplaced fracture on the shaft of a long bone, this hematoma provides the initial reconnection of edges of the fracture (Fig. 12.17A). In more complex fractures, the process of reducing the fracture to align bony fragments further irritates tissues, augmenting the inflammatory response that is the first necessary step in fracture healing. This initial inflammatory response to fracture can last 5 or more days, depending on the severity of injury and extent of tissue disruption.

The next stage of healing is the repair stage, a period of cell migration, proliferation, and granulation. The combination of chemotactic factors and bone matrix proteins released by damaged bone and during inflammation triggers the initiation of bony repair. The hematoma organizes into a fibrin "scaffold," and cells within the hematoma begin to release growth factors and other proteins that trigger cell migration and proliferation of osteoblasts from the periosteum and endosteum, as well as synthesis of a fracture callus matrix for bony repair (see Fig. 12.17B and C).[122] Initially the pH of the area around the fracture is acidic, and the fracture callus is primarily cartilaginous. As the repair stage progresses, the pH becomes more alkaline, creating an environment that enhances activity of the alkaline phosphatase enzyme, and subsequently mineralization of the cartilage of the fracture callus into woven bone tissue (see Fig. 12.17D). The deposition of new cartilage within the callus is accompanied by both endochondral and intramembranous ossification. Clinical union of the fracture during the repair stage can last up to 3 months postinjury (hence the need for long periods of immobilization).

The final stage of healing is the remodeling stage, during which the new bone woven within the callus is reshaped into the more mature lamellae of long bone and excess callus resorbed. During this phase, osteoclasts are active to reshape trabeculae and lamellae along the lines of weight-bearing forces. The process of maturation of the callus into a fully repaired bone can last a year or more, especially in complex fractures, whether managed by casting or ORIF. Factors that influence the duration of the remodeling stage include age, severity of injury, nutritional status, concurrent chronic illness, and medication use (especially corticosteroids).[123]

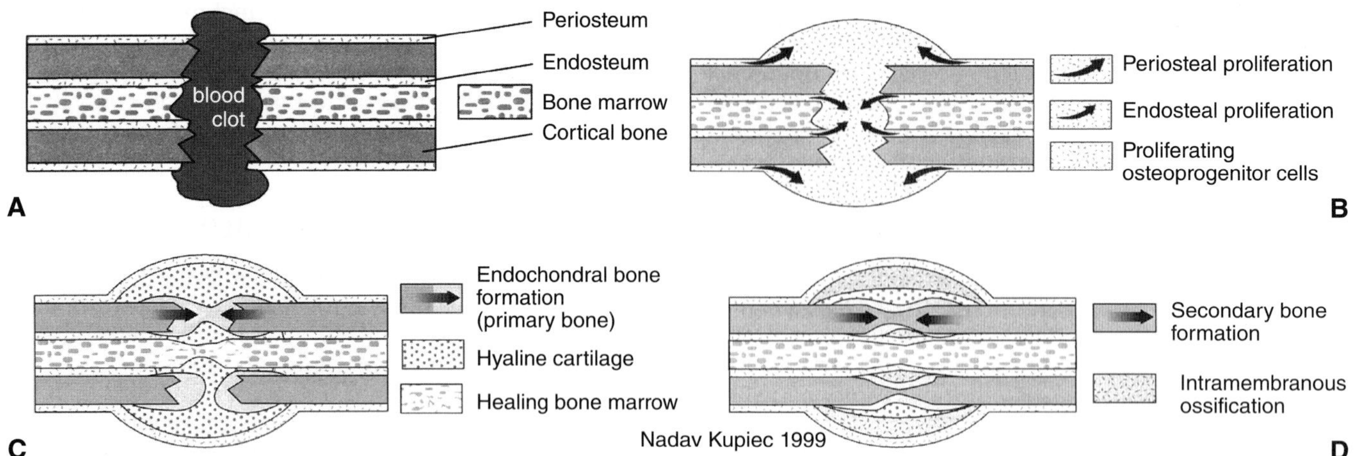

Fig. 12.17 Healing and repair of a long bone fracture. (A) Disruption of blood vessels in the bone, marrow, periosteum, and surrounding tissue at the time of injury results in extravasation of blood at the fracture site and the formation of hematoma. (B) Initiation and development of the fracture callus. (C) Note the simultaneous occurrence of chondrogenesis, endochondral ossification, and intramembranous bone formation in different regions of the fracture site. (D) Union of a long bone fracture. (From Lundon K. *Orthopedic Rehabilitation Science: Principles for Clinical Management of Bone.* Butterworth-Heinemann; 2000.)

FRACTURE CLASSIFICATIONS

Fractures are classified as either open or closed injuries on the basis of the presence of an open communication between the fracture and the outside world through a disruption of the soft tissues and skin.[124] In a closed fracture, the soft tissue envelope of muscles and skin around the bone fracture site is completely intact. Although muscle around the fracture site may be significantly damaged, the intact skin provides a barrier that prevents bacterial invasion of the injured muscle or bone. When an open or compound fracture occurs, the soft tissue envelope has been violated: The wound leaves muscle and fractured bone open to the environment and susceptible to infection. In many cases, bone may actually protrude through the skin. Open injuries are orthopedic emergencies; patients are taken urgently to the operating room for debridement of the wound and fracture. Severely damaged or contaminated tissue is removed, and the wound is carefully cleaned in an effort to avoid infection and provide optimal circumstances for healing.[119] The fracture is then stabilized with a cast or surgical implant.

Gustilo and Anderson[124] have developed a classification system applied interoperatively that rates the severity of open or compound fractures. The least severe is a type I injury, in which a small wound with minimal soft tissue damage (1 cm) communicates with the fracture. The wound in a type II fracture is generally between 1 and 12 cm, and significant soft tissue injury may be present underneath the laceration or wound. In a more severe, type III injury, the wound diameter is often greater than 12 cm, there is considerable periosteal stripping, and barely enough muscle or skin is present to cover the injured or fractured bone adequately. Type III open fractures are subdivided into another three categories—A, B, and C—on the basis of whether the soft tissue can cover the bone and whether neurological or vascular involvement is present in association with the open fracture. It should be noted that more important than the size of the skin defect is the damage to soft tissues and periosteum in determining type. Therefore a 1-cm open hole in a crushed and comminuted fracture may well be classified as a type III.

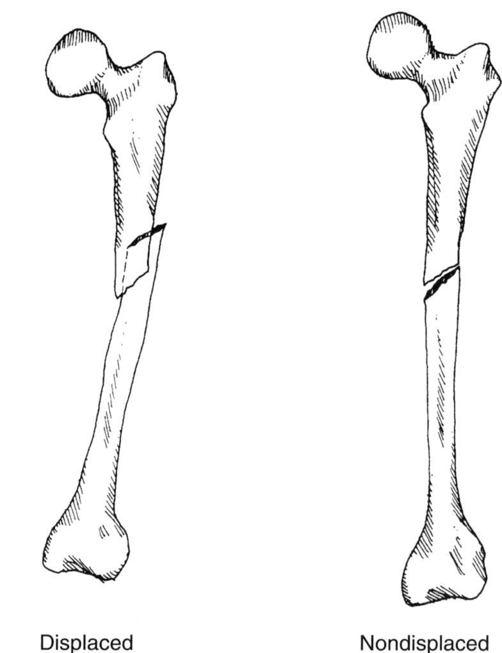

Fig. 12.18 Diagram of a displaced and nondisplaced fracture of the diaphysis of the femur. (From Gustilo RB. *The Fracture Classification Manual.* Mosby; 1991.)

The particular location and pattern of fracture determine whether the fracture is stable and can be effectively managed with a cast or brace, or unstable, requiring surgical intervention. A fracture with concurrent joint dislocation creates an extremely unstable condition, requiring surgical management of the fracture/dislocation and a long period of rehabilitation.

Fractures (whether closed or open) are described as displaced or nondisplaced on the basis of the degree of malalignment or overlap that is observed on a radiograph (Fig. 12.18). They are described as complete or incomplete, depending on whether the bone has fully transected. In children, a greenstick fracture is an incomplete oblique or spiral fracture that extends only partially through bone. Exact

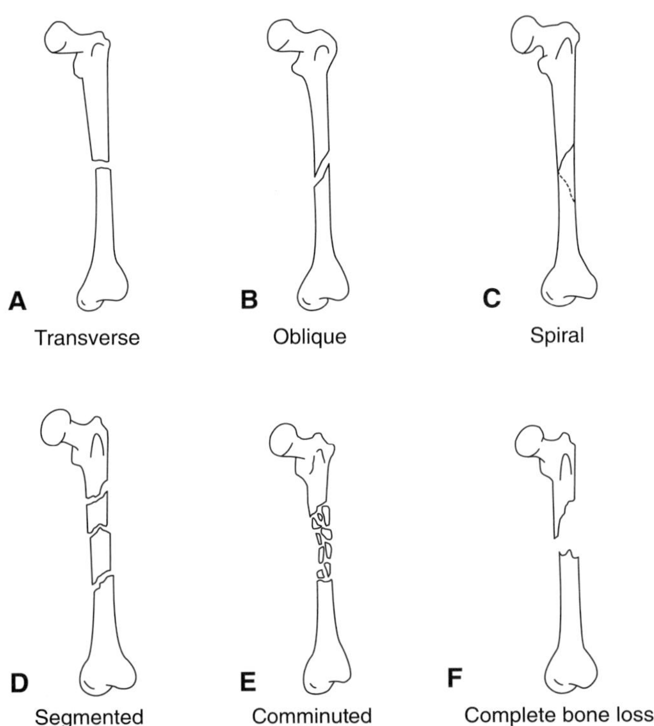

Fig. 12.19 Examples of types of long bone fractures illustrated in the diaphysis of the femur. A transverse fracture (A) is primarily perpendicular to the long axis of the bone, whereas an oblique fracture (B) diagonally transects the bone. A spiral fracture (C) is the result of a rotary force during injury. Segmental fractures (D) have one or more noncontinuous segments, whereas a comminuted fracture (E) has multiple small fragments. In cases of significant trauma, there may actually be loss of bone substance (F). (Modified from Gustilo RB. *The Fracture Classification Manual*. Mosby; 1991.)

location of the fracture is also important: Fractures of the diaphysis or metaphysis of a long cortical bone are extraarticular (Fig. 12.19), whereas those involving the epiphysis within the joint capsule are intraarticular. Intraarticular fractures, especially when displaced, have a high likelihood of causing posttraumatic arthritis, and often require surgical reconstruction of the joint surface.

Extraarticular fractures (Fig. 12.20A) can be transverse (mostly perpendicular to the axis of the bone), oblique (diagonal to the axis of the bone), or spiral (typically a result of torsional forces), depending on the direction of force contributing to the injury and the resulting alteration in bone configuration. When one or more substantive fragments are seen on the radiograph, the fracture is segmental; if there are multiple small fragments, the fracture is comminuted. In high-impact, complex fractures, there is often enough destruction of bone that there will be loss of bone length or substance. Fractures of the metaphysis are determined to be nondisplaced or displaced, simple, compressed, or comminuted (see Fig. 12.19). Before and during puberty (during times of rapid bone growth), there can be displacement of the proximal or distal epiphysis from the metaphysis through the cartilaginous epiphyseal plate (Fig. 12.21); the proximal (subcapital) epiphysis of the femur is particularly vulnerable.

Intraarticular fractures (Fig. 12.20B) are classified as linear, comminuted, impacted, or having a percent of bone loss (Fig. 12.22); complex intraarticular fractures involve both proximal and distal components of the joint (Fig. 12.23) and typically require ORIF.

In the proximal femur, fractures of the metaphysis are described as intertrochanteric fractures (extracapsular, linear or oblique, through or between the trochanters) or femoral neck fractures (intracapsular across the neck of the femur) or comminuted (with multiple fragments of neck and or trochanters; Fig. 12.24). These fractures fall into the category of hip fractures, and typically require ORIF or replacement with a femoral prosthesis (hemiarthroplasty) or even a total hip arthroplasty (Fig. 12.25). Fractures of

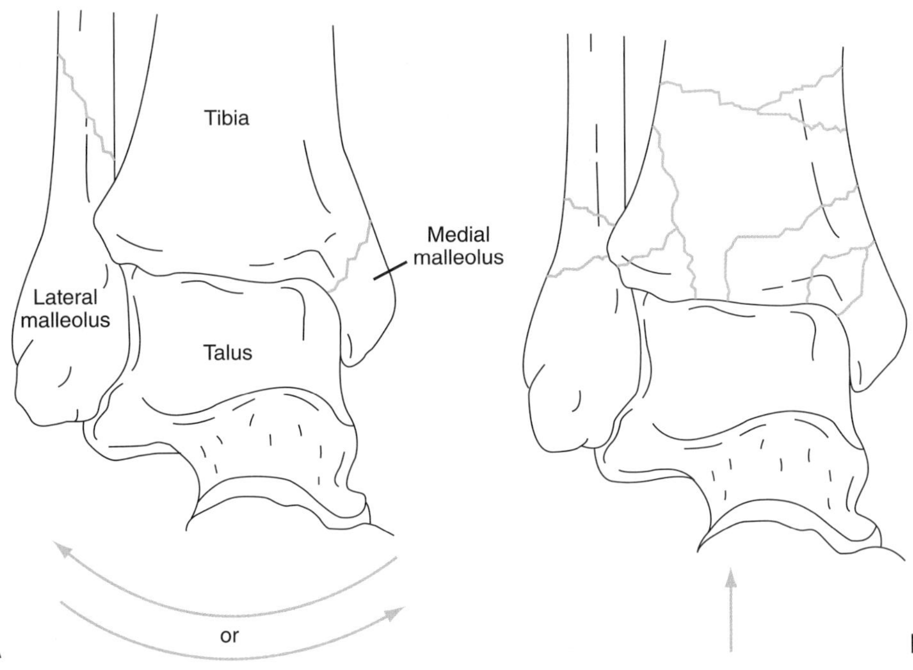

Fig. 12.20 (A) Extraarticular metaphyseal fracture of the malleoli of the tibia and fibula is often the result of rotational injuries. (B) Intraarticular fractures of the ankle mortis (also called *plafond* or *pylon fractures*) result from high-energy compressive injury. (Modified from Clark CR, Bonfiglio M, eds. *Orthopaedics: Essentials of Diagnosis and Treatment*. Churchill Livingstone; 1994.)

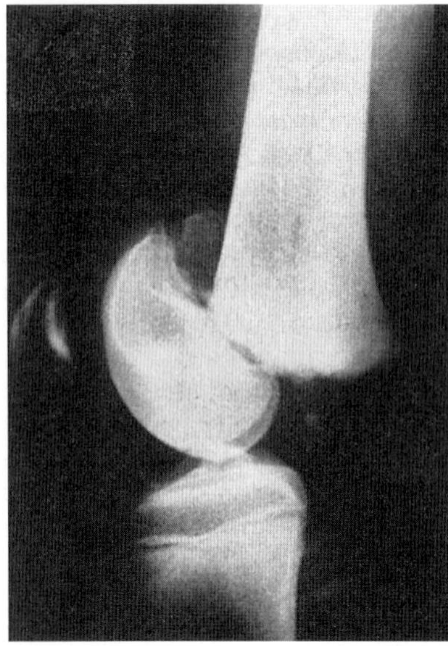

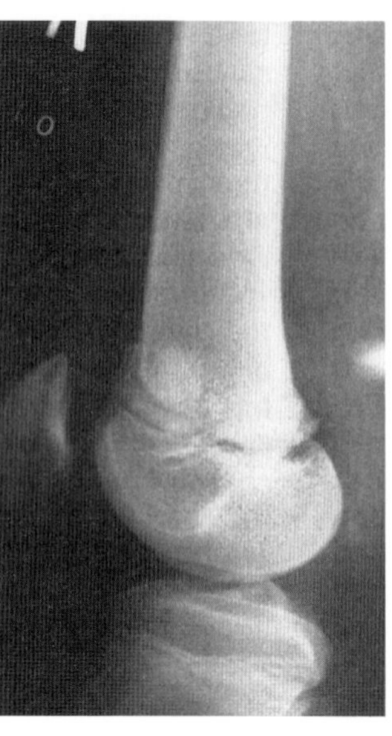

Fig. 12.21 Lateral view of an avulsed distal femoral condyle (A) before and (B) following closed reduction. (From Clark CR, Bonfiglio M, eds. *Orthopaedics: Essentials of Diagnosis and Treatment*. Churchill Livingstone; 1994.)

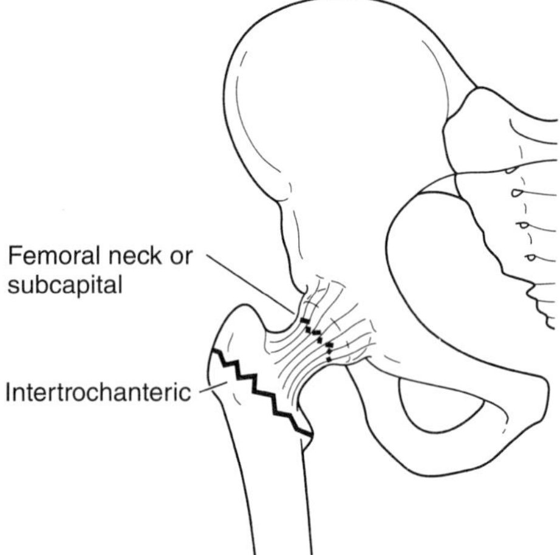

Fig. 12.22 Femoral neck fractures are intracapsular and traverse the blood supply to the femoral head. Intertrochanteric fractures spare the blood supply but are a greater risk for failure of fixation. (From Clark CR, Bonfiglio M, eds. *Orthopaedics: Essentials of Diagnosis and Treatment*. Churchill Livingstone; 1994.)

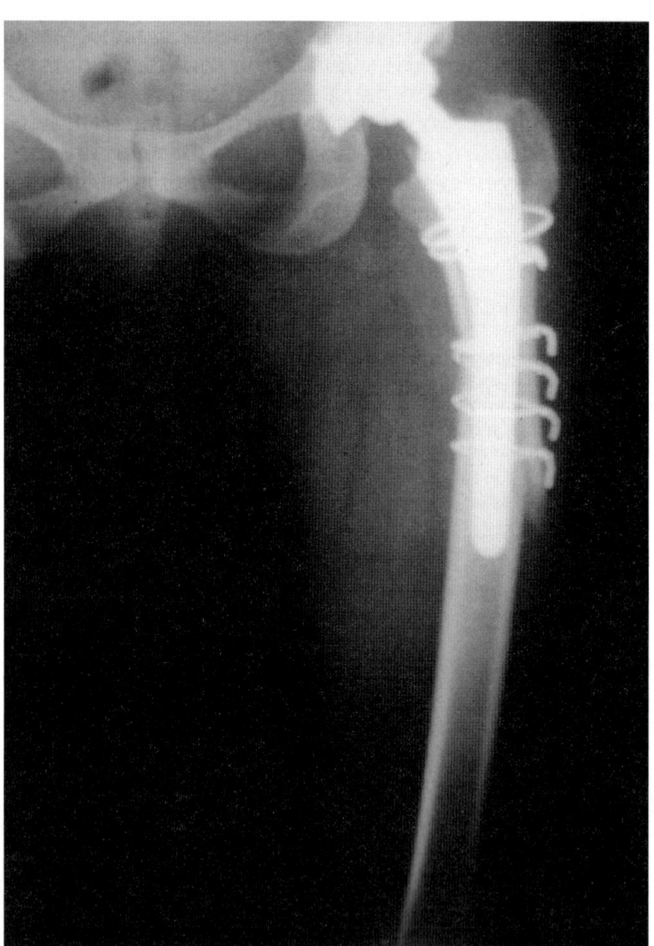

Fig. 12.23 A radiograph of a repaired complex fracture of the proximal femur with prosthetic total hip replacement and open reduction with internal fixation with circumferentially wrapped wires to stabilize a spiral fracture of the proximal femoral diaphysis.

the acetabulum are the result of either a longitudinal force through the femur into the pelvis or an upward oblique lateral force through the greater trochanter; if the hip happens to be adducted at the time of injury, this may lead to posterior dislocation (Fig. 12.26).

Fractures of the pelvis are classified as stable or unstable on the basis of the extent of damage that disrupts the circumferential integrity of the pelvis (Fig. 12.27). Persons with unstable fractures of the pelvis are at risk for life-threatening hemorrhage, as well as residual genitourinary or neurological complications, given the vessels, nerves, muscles, and organs that are housed within the pelvis.[125]

Fractures of irregularly shaped bones such as the tarsals and vertebrae tend to fall into three categories. Stress fractures result from repetitive loading of the bone, are often nondisplaced, and can disrupt either the inner scaffolding of the cancellous bone or the outer shell of cortical bone. Simple stress fractures typically heal well with immobilization; more complex stress fractures may require surgical stabilization. Pathological fractures occur when there is underlying disease (e.g., osteoporosis, Charcot osteopathy, neoplasm) that compromises bone density or metabolism. In pathological fractures the trabeculae are overwhelmed

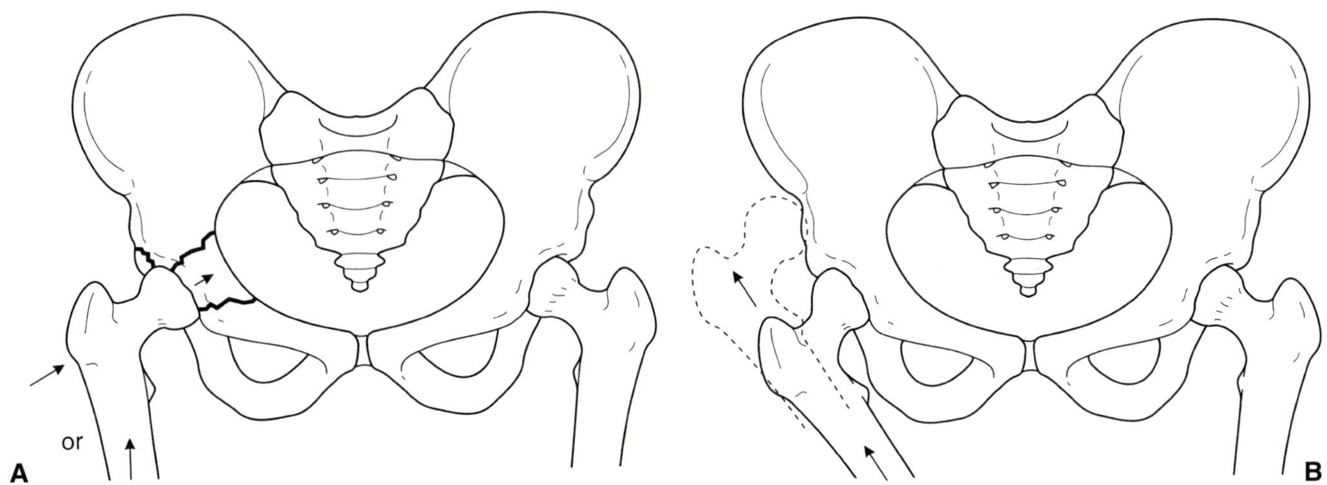

Fig. 12.24 (A) Acetabular fractures occur from a lateral blow over the greater trochanter or a proximally directed force transmitted up the length of the femur. (B) If the limb is injured with the hip in adduction and flexion, a posterior hip dislocation is likely. (From Clark CR, Bonfiglio M, eds. *Orthopaedics: Essentials of Diagnosis and Treatment*. Churchill Livingstone; 1994.)

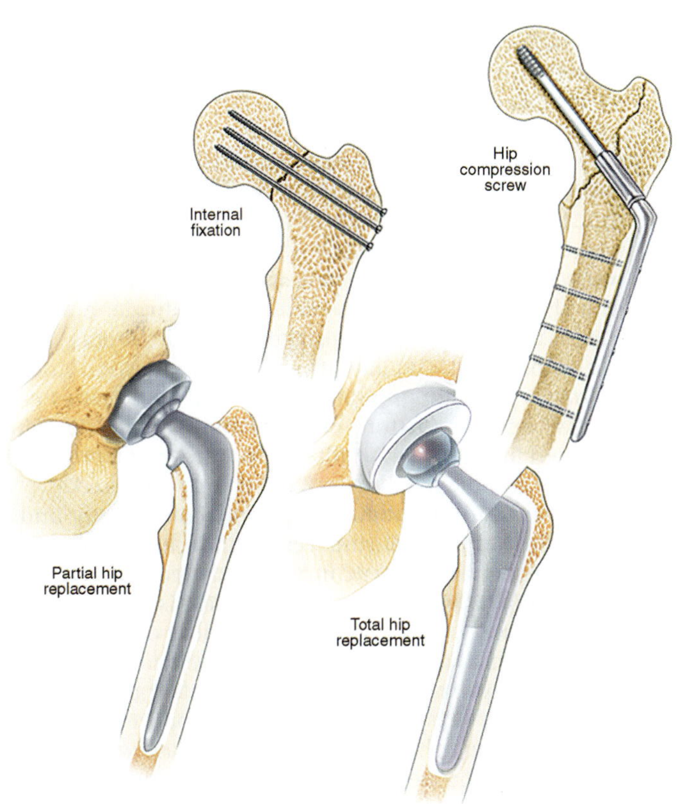

Fig. 12.25 Surgical management of femoral neck fractures. (Used with permission of Mayo Foundation for Medical Education and Research. All rights reserved.)

by the magnitude of force exerted through the bone, and the bone is compressed or fractured into fragments. Management of pathological fractures can be challenging, as bone healing is often compromised by the underlying disease process. Traumatic fractures are often comminuted; depending on severity, they may be managed by immobilization in a cast or orthosis, ORIF, or placement of an external fixation apparatus (Fig. 12.28).

CASTS AND SPLINTS

The primary goal of fracture management is to restore musculoskeletal limb function of the injured extremity with optimal anatomical alignment, functional muscle strength, sensory function, and pain-free joint range of motion. The most common methods used for immobilization of closed fractures include casts, splints, fracture orthoses, or a

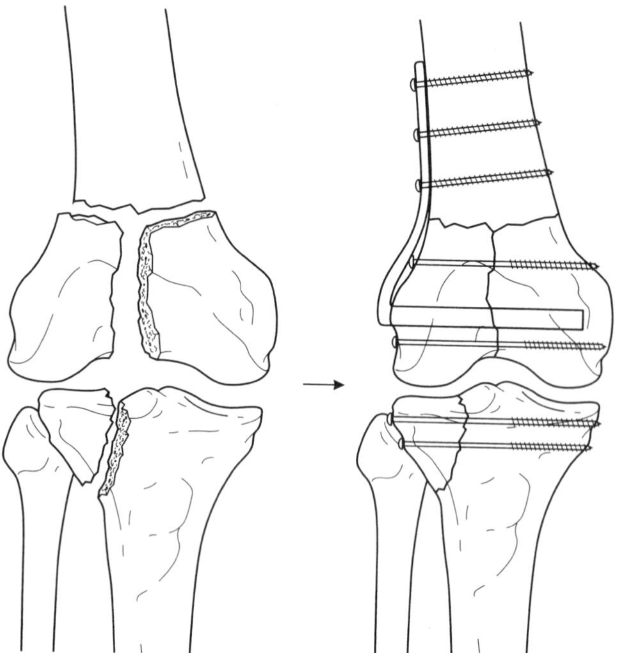

Fig. 12.26 Major intraarticular fractures of the distal femur and proximal tibia are typically managed by surgical open reduction with internal fixation using a combination of bone screws or nail and an external plate. (From Clark CR, Bonfiglio M, eds. *Orthopaedics: Essentials of Diagnosis and Treatment*. Churchill Livingstone; 1994.)

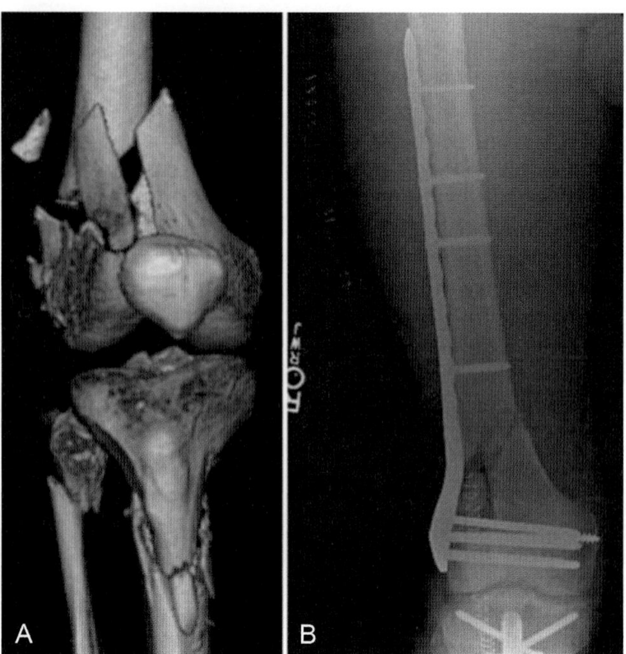

Fig. 12.28 Comminuted fracture of the femur with internal fixation. (A) Preoperative three-dimensional reconstruction of comminuted distal femur fracture. (B) Postoperative x-ray after surgery with lateral locked plate. (From Stancil R, Haidukewych GJ, Sassoon AA. Distal femur fractures. In: Scott WN, ed. *Insall & Scott Surgery of the Knee*. Sixth ed. Elsevier; 2018.)

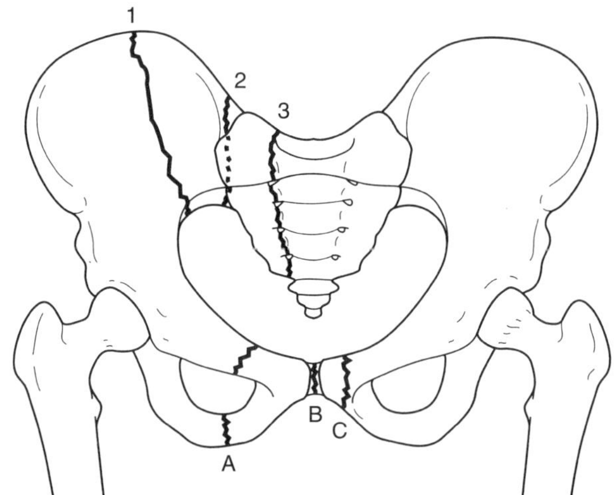

Fig. 12.27 Unstable pelvic fractures occur when pubic rami fractures *(A)*, symphysis disruption *(B)*, or pubic body fractures *(C)* are accompanied by fractures through the iliac wing *(1)*, sacroiliac joint *(2)*, or sacrum *(3)*. (From Clark CR, Bonfiglio M, eds. *Orthopaedics: Essentials of Diagnosis and Treatment*. Churchill Livingstone; 1994.)

hybrid cast-orthosis.[118,126] Immobilization may also be used after ORIF of open fractures.

In choosing the appropriate immobilization strategy for an individual's fracture, the orthopedist considers several issues. The first is the stability of the fracture site and how well a device will be able to maintain fracture reduction and achieve the desired anatomical result. The condition of the skin and soft tissue is also an important consideration, especially if wounds are present that must be accessed for proper care. Limb volume must be evaluated, especially if edema is present or anticipated: How will limb size change over time in the device? Length of immobilization time varies as well: Is the device designed for a short-term problem, or will protection of the limb be necessary for an extended period? Will the device need to be removed for hygiene or wound care? Can the limb be unprotected while sleeping or when not ambulating? Availability (time to application) may also influence decision- making. Casts and cast braces can be applied quickly. Custom orthoses need additional fabrication and fitting time; an alternative means of protection is often required while the device is being fabricated.

The individual's ability to comply consistently and reliably with weight-bearing restrictions and other aspects of fracture management must also be considered. Factors such as cognitive ability, emotional status, motivation, and physical ability, as well as the availability of assistance and environmental demands, influence the decision to provide additional external support. An unstable fracture managed by ORIF may not require additional support for those with sufficient strength and balance who have a clear understanding of the healing process. If the individual with a fracture cannot understand the need to protect the involved limb from excessive loading or is physically unable to do so, additional external support is essential. If compliance is questionable, the device of choice is usually a nonremovable cast or cast brace.

To effectively stabilize a fracture, the joints above and below the fracture site must be immobilized. The period of immobilization varies with fracture severity and location; in most cases the cast remains in place from 6 to 8 weeks or until a radiograph indicates that bone healing has progressed sufficiently for safe weight bearing and function.

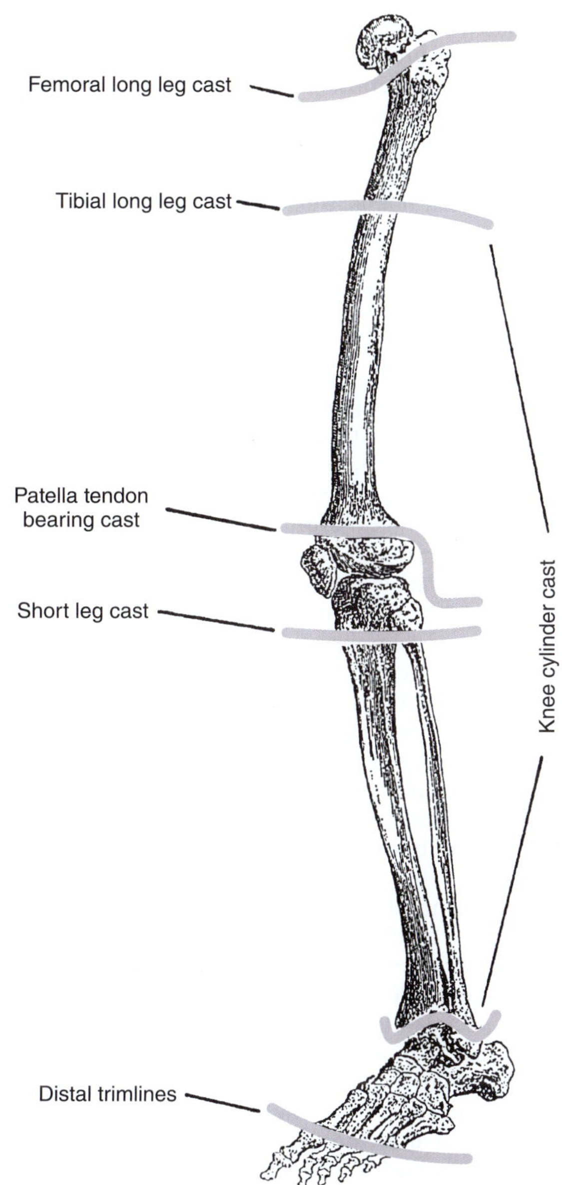

Fig. 12.29 Proximal and distal trimlines used in standard lower extremity casts. Typically, the joints above and below the fracture site are immobilized. Trimlines can be extended to provide better control and stabilization.

The time for immobilization is often less for children, due to their rapid healing response. Although immobilization is essential for effective bone healing, it also has significant consequences on other tissues: While in a cast, patients are likely to develop significant joint stiffness (contracture), as well as disuse atrophy and weakness of the muscles of the immobilized limb. Once the cast is removed, rehabilitation professionals are called on to help the patient regain preinjury muscle performance, flexibility, and range of motion.

A cast is a rigid, externally applied device that provides circumferential support to an injured body part.[107] Casts immobilize a body segment to maintain optimal skeletal alignment (Figs. 12.29 and 12.30). Once a cast has been applied, a radiograph can be used to assess the effectiveness of skeletal alignment. The cast may need to be modified, wedged, or replaced to improve alignment.[127]

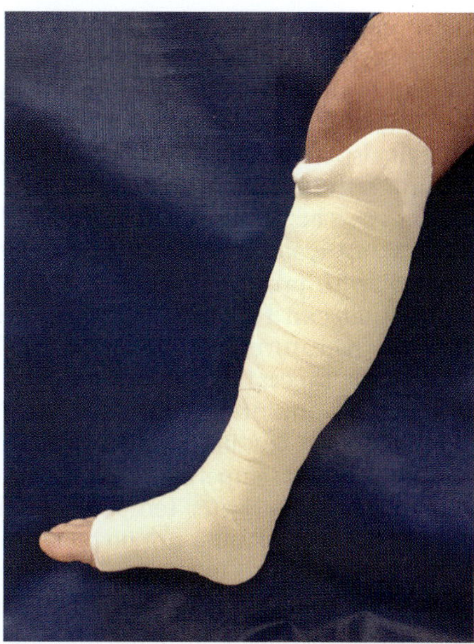

Fig. 12.30 Medial view of a patella tendon-bearing cast. (From Bruce Reider AB, Davies GJ, Provencher MT. *Orthopaedic Rehabilitation of the Athlete: Getting Back in the Game*. Elsevier; 2015.)

A splint is a temporary supportive device, usually fabricated from rigid materials, held in position on the fractured extremity with bandages or straps. Splints can be used for temporary immobilization before casting or surgical stabilization. They can be used to maintain fracture reduction while waiting for swelling to diminish or fracture blisters to clear or to provide comfort. The most commonly used splints include sugar tong splints (a long, У-shaped, padded plaster forearm splint named for its similarity to the tool used to pick up sugar cubes), short or long leg splints, thumb spica splints, ulnar or radial gutter splints, and coaptation splints.[116]

Casting and Splinting Materials

Before the 1800s, fracture casts were made from linen bandages soaked in beaten egg whites and lime. The modern era in fracture care began with the discovery of plaster of Paris (calcium sulfate), first used in the Turkish Empire as reported by Eaton in 1798.[128] Plaster of Paris was used in Europe in the early 19th century, and a Flemish surgeon (Mathijsen) is credited with combining the use of plaster of Paris and cloth bandages to form casts for the treatment of fractures in 1852.[127–129]

Plaster of Paris is created when heat is used to dehydrate gypsum. When water is added to plaster of Paris powder, the dehydration process is reversed, and crystals of gypsum are formed again. The new crystals interlock in a chemical exothermic (heat-producing) process.[130] The setting process is complete when heat is no longer being produced, although the cast remains wet to the touch until the excess water used in the process evaporates. Maximum cast strength is not reached until the plaster is completely dry. Drying time varies with the thickness of the cast, ambient humidity, and the type of plaster used. In most instances maximum cast strength is reached in approximately 24 hours.

Various types of plaster of Paris with different working characteristics are available. Manufacturers may add accelerators to the material that shorten the setting time: The limb has to be held still for less time while the plaster sets. Although this may be advantageous when a cast is applied to the limb of an anxious child or when an unstable fracture is cast, it also means that less working time is available to manipulate the extremity and optimally shape the cast. Setting time can be prolonged slightly if cold water is used. If warm or hot water is used to reduce setting time, care must be taken to protect the limb from injury from the higher heat that can be generated during the setting process.[127] Cast temperatures as high as 68.5°C have been reached with water temperatures of 40°C; burns can occur if cast temperature is maintained at 44°C for 6 hours or more.[131,132] To minimize any potential for burns in cast or splint application, room temperature tepid water (24°C) is recommended. If higher water temperatures have been used, the newly casted limb must not be placed on a pillow or other type of support that is likely to retain or reflect heat. Cast burns can also occur when insufficient padding has been placed between the plaster of Paris and the surface of the skin. Cast burns are avoidable if simple procedures are followed.

Cast strength is determined by three factors: the type of casting material used, the thickness of the cast, and the effectiveness of lamination among the layers of the cast material. The cloth mesh material that serves as the carrier for the plaster of Paris provides little strength for the cast. A plaster cast must be kept absolutely dry to prevent it from becoming soft and ineffective in immobilization.

The difficulties associated with the use of plaster of Paris have led to the development of newer and improved casting materials. Polyurethane-impregnated casting tapes have gained widespread popularity because of their superior strength, lightweight, shorter setting time, cleaner application, and low exothermic reaction. Polyurethane casts are also radiolucent, permitting x-ray evaluation of fracture site healing while the limb remains encased in the cast.

Polyurethane is a plastic material that can be impregnated into a fabric substrate. Although the polyurethane bonds the layers of substrate together, it is actually the substrate that determines the strength of the cast. A variety of substrate materials are available. The weave determines how elastic the material will be during cast application and how strong the cast will be when set. Cotton, polyester, fiberglass, polypropylene, and blends of these materials and others are used in synthetic casting tapes.[130,131,133,134]

Immersing the synthetic casting tape in room temperature water for 10 seconds begins a heat-producing exothermic reaction and causes the material to harden (polymerize). Setting is complete for most synthetic casting materials in 5 to 10 minutes. Because of this short setting time, the rolls of bandage material cannot be opened until they are ready to be applied as a cast. The application process requires skill and must move quickly to ensure adequate molding time. Unlike plaster of Paris, the plastic bandage does not need to be massaged to ensure proper lamination between the layers of material. Also unlike plaster of Paris, which can easily be washed from the hands or clothing, polyurethane is not easily removed: Adequate protective padding must be placed around the patient's limb and protective gloves worn to safeguard the applicator's hands. Polyurethane resin in its natural state is tacky. An additive may be incorporated into the casting tape to reduce its tackiness. In some cases the manufacturer provides special gloves with an antitacky additive to further minimize the tack.[130] The exothermic polymerization of polyurethane resin produces much less heat (44.9°C in 40°C water) than that of setting plaster of Paris. In addition, heat is quickly dissipated so that burns are much less likely to occur when synthetic materials are used. To further minimize the risk of burns, immersion of cast tape in room temperature water (24°C) is recommended.[127,131,135]

Cast Application

Stockinet is the first layer of a cast, applied over the skin, before any padding is added. The most common stockinet material is cotton. Synthetic materials such as polyester or polypropylene or Gore-Tex can be chosen in place of cotton because they do not retain water like cotton materials do. Stockinet also helps position dressings over wounds and provides extra circumferential control of soft tissue within the cast. Stockinet is folded over the proximal and distal edges to finish the cast (and prevents inadvertent removal of cast padding by a nonresponsible individual or a child).

Next, a layer of cast padding is added over the stockinet. A variety of materials are available to pad casts. Sheet cotton comes in various forms and is used to provide a barrier between the rigid walls of the cast and surface of the skin. Some cast materials have been elasticized for easier application and conformation, and others require more technique to ensure that they uniformly conform to the body part being casted.

Although synthetic cast tapes are not affected by water, cast padding or stockinet does retain water. The risk of skin maceration and breakdown is present if the inside of a cast remains damp for long periods of time. Some manufacturers market cast padding that reportedly permits exposure to water; however, manufacturer recommendations must be followed carefully.

The thickness of cast padding varies; ⅛ to ¼ inch is sufficient for most individuals. The goal is to protect bony prominences and soft tissue from the rigid walls of the cast while effectively immobilizing the fracture site. Soft tissue usually does well with a fairly thin, uniform two- or three-layer wrap. Extra padding is added to smooth and protect the irregular surfaces around bony prominences. Excessive padding reduces the ability of the cast to provide adequate immobilization. A well-molded cast that accurately follows the anatomical contours of the extremity requires less padding. Cast padding also provides a barrier so that the cast can be removed more easily when it needs to be changed or is no longer necessary.

Lower Extremity Casts

The short leg cast is used in the management of fractures involving the distal tibia or fibula, or both; the ankle joint; or the rear foot or midfoot. The foot is positioned in a functional neutral ankle position (90 degrees) or in slight dorsiflexion. This positioning prevents a plantar flexion contracture from developing by the time of cast removal. The foot can also be casted in a plantarflexed position to accommodate repair of an Achilles tendon rupture. The proximal trimline falls at the level of the tibial tubercle; the distal trimline usually encloses the metatarsal heads. The area around the fibular head is protected by adding extra cast padding to minimize the risk of compression of the peroneal nerve. A cast shoe should be used to protect the bottom of the cast if weight bearing is to be permitted.

For persons with midshaft fractures of the tibia, a patellar tendon-bearing (PTB) cast may be applied. This design incorporates a patellar tendon bar, which directs some of the limb loading force to the external shell of the cast, thus protecting the full length of the tibia against bending moments (see Fig. 12.30). This type of cast or orthosis is not effective, however, in reducing axial loading of the tibia or hind foot. The PTB is most often used when extra stability is desired for individuals who will be allowed some degree of weight-bearing activity. The cast is applied with the ankle maintained in neutral or slightly dorsiflexed position to minimize potential hyperextension moment at the knee in stance. Trimlines are similar to those used for a PTB transtibial prosthetic socket: at the midpatella (or sometimes suprapatella) anteriorly but trimmed and slightly flared posteriorly to permit knee flexion of at least 90 degrees. Proximally, the cast is well molded to the tibia in the area of the medial flare and around the patella.[136,137] Care must be taken to ensure that no pressure is placed on the peroneal nerve.

A knee cylinder cast is often applied when there have been fractures of the patella or surgical repair of the knee joint when the knee must be immobilized in full extension. To ensure the necessary stability for the knee joint, the proximal trimline encompasses the lower two-thirds of the thigh and the distal trimline the entire tibial segment to just above the malleoli. The cast can be applied using either plaster of Paris or synthetic casting tape. To limit the risk of pistoning when the person wearing the cast is standing or walking, the cast is carefully molded to fit the contours of the medial femoral condyle.

For closed fractures of the upper tibia, knee joint, or lower femur, a long leg cast provides the necessary stability for healing. Depending on the site of fracture and its relative stability, the limb is immobilized in nearly full extension or in a bent-knee position.[137] A straight-knee cast is usually applied with a slight (5-degree) knee flexion angle to enhance patient comfort. Bent-knee casts are usually chosen when non–weight bearing must be ensured during ambulation or to aid in controlling rotation of the tibia. With the relatively mobile arrangement of soft tissue that surrounds the femur, it is challenging to provide adequate immobilization, especially for persons who are particularly muscular or overweight. For this reason, control of rotational forces through the femur within a long leg cast is questionable. If the cast is being used to stabilize the tibia, the proximal trimline is at the junction of the middle and proximal third of the femur. If the cast is being used to stabilize the distal femur, the proximal trimline is at the level of the greater trochanter. Distally, the cast immobilizes the ankle and extends to a point just beyond the metatarsal heads. The fibular head should be well padded within the cast to minimize the risk of entrapment of the peroneal nerve.

A hip spica cast, which encases the hip and pelvis in addition to the lower extremity, is necessary for effective control of fractures of the proximal femur and of the hip joint[138] (Fig. 12.31). The hip spica cast is the primary method of treatment of femoral fractures in children under 5 years of

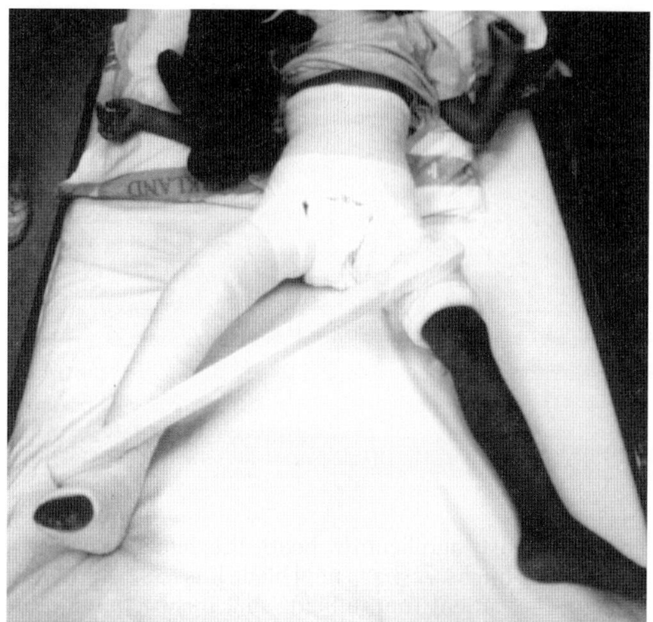

Fig. 12.31 This child has been placed in a 1½ hip spica cast to stabilize a fracture of the proximal femur. Note the opening for personal hygiene and the additional diagonal support bar incorporated between the short and long sections of the cast.

age and is used in adults when a prefabricated hip orthosis is not appropriate. Several variations of the hip spica cast are available. In a single hip spica cast, the plaster or synthetic cast material is anchored around the entire pelvis and lower trunk but immobilizes only the hip and knee of the involved side, allowing fairly unrestricted hip motion of the opposite limb. In a 1½ hip spica cast, the cast encases the entire lower extremity on the affected side, as well as the lower trunk, pelvis, and thigh on the uninvolved side. Usually the knee on the affected side is completely immobilized; however, an articulated knee joint can be incorporated if specific circumstances so dictate. In most instances, the hip joint of the affected limb is immobilized in 30 degrees of flexion and 30 degrees of abduction, and the perineal edges are trimmed back to allow for personal care and hygiene. The knee is usually positioned in 30 degrees of flexion. The proximal cast encases the lower to middle trunk (to the level of the costal margin or nipple line), depending on the amount of spinal immobilization required. The 1½ hip spica cast is often reinforced by the incorporation of a lightweight diagonal bar between the short and long extremity segments. Ambulation is possible but often quite challenging, requiring significant upper body strength to manage the adapted crutch-walking gait that the cast position makes necessary.

Cast Removal

A cast cutter or saw with a vibrating disk is used to cut the cast during cast removal. Modern cast cutter blades reciprocate back and forth approximately ⅛ inch in either direction. The vibrating blade easily cuts rigid materials such as metal, wood, plaster, or synthetic cast materials but does not cut through materials that are elastic or mobile. If used properly, a cast cutter does not cut skin. Incorrect or inappropriate use of a cast cutter can seriously cut or burn a patient. To reduce the risk of injury, the blade should not directly contact the patient's skin. Friction between the

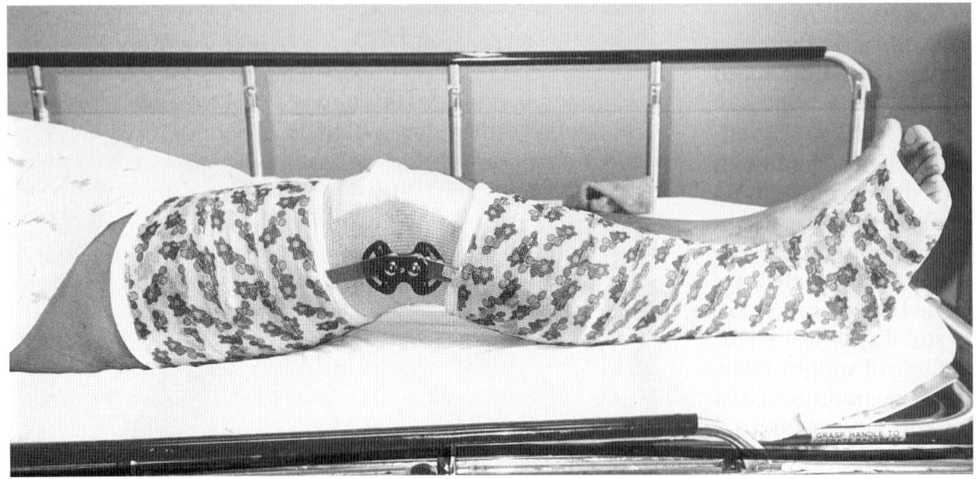

Fig. 12.32 A tibial cast brace with polycentric adjustable range of motion hinges. The patient has undergone an open reduction with internal fixation surgery after fracture of the tibial plateau. Note that synthetic cast tape is available in a wide variety of colors and patterns.

blade and cast significantly heats the blade, creating a potential for burns. A sharp new blade has less potential for burning the patient than a blade that has become dull or worn out. The noise of the cast cutter can be quite frightening to children or other particularly anxious patients. A careful explanation and a demonstration of the cast cutter's action are the first steps in the process of cast removal.

To remove a cast safely, the cutter is used in a repetitive in-out motion, to progressively open the cast, instead of sliding the blade through the cast. This strategy reduces the risk of a cut or burn on the patient's skin.[139] Safety strips may be incorporated into the cast at the time of application to allow for a safe path for the saw blade to penetrate through without damaging skin. These strips are especially important when friable liners like Gore-Tex are used under the cast. Safe technique involves the operator's thumb serving as a fulcrum on the cast as downward pressure is applied through the wrist. The thumb also controls the depth of the blade. Care is taken to avoid positioning the cast cutter in areas where skin is vulnerable: over a bony prominence or where significant edema or fragile healing skin is present. As the blade breaks through the inner wall of the cast, the sensation of reduced resistance to downward pressure as well as a change in sound occurs. Once an area of cast has been cut, the blade is repositioned farther along the cast and the process is repeated until the cast can be pried open completely. Bandage scissors are used to cut through padding and stockinet, and the limb is then extracted from the open cast. For infants and young children with small limbs, an alternative strategy can be used: a plaster of Paris cast can be removed by soaking it in water. This method works particularly well when a corrective clubfoot cast is removed from an infant's limb.

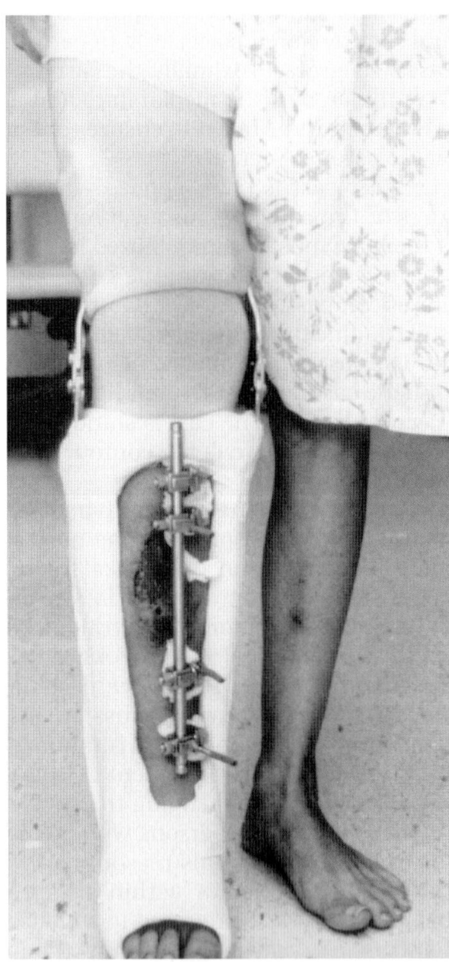

Fig. 12.33 This cast brace provides medial/lateral stability for a comminuted grade 3 open tibial fracture. The length of the tibia is being maintained by an external fixation device. The patient also sustained a closed femoral fracture, which has been supported by an intramedullary rod fixation. Because the proximal portion of the cast must not terminate near a fracture line, the femoral portion of the cast has been extended up to the level of the trochanter to avoid stress on the femoral fixation.

HYBRID CAST BRACES

Hybrid cast braces were first developed as a method of management of proximal tibial and distal femoral fractures near the knee just after World War I but then fell out of use until the mid-1960s (Fig. 12.32).[140–142] In some centers, the cast brace is the method of choice for the management of nondisplaced tibial plateau fractures. The cast brace is often used for additional support of fractures near the knee or of the femur that have been stabilized via ORIF surgery for external fixation (Fig. 12.33). This method is also used to control motion after knee ligament injury or reconstruction.

Cast braces incorporate orthotic components (e.g., hinge joints, range of motion locks) into a plaster or synthetic cast in an effort to provide additional stability to a healing limb.[143–151] The cast brace can be applied using either plaster of Paris or synthetic cast materials. Depending on the nature of the fracture and its stability, the orthotic knee joints incorporated into the cast brace may be chosen to provide limited, controlled, or free-knee range of motion. Because the anatomical center rotation of the knee moves in an arc centered over the femoral condyles, it is essential that the mechanical joints be carefully aligned with the anatomical knee joint to reduce the abnormal stress that occurs across the joint and fracture site.[152,153]

Many orthotists and orthopedic surgeons choose a polycentric orthotic knee joint because its motion more closely follows anatomical motion and reduces the torque-related stress that results from a single-axis mechanical joint. Palpating the condyles on a patient who has had recent trauma about the knee is difficult; the midpatella is a somewhat less precise alternative landmark for alignment. A properly placed polycentric metal joint will be proximal to the joint line and slightly posterior to the midline. Orthotic knee joints are positioned close to but not quite contacting skin. This is especially important medially, where contact between the knees during functional activity is likely.

Medial and lateral uprights are incorporated into the cast above and below the orthotic knee joint to provide protection against unwanted varus and valgus stress and to help control anteroposterior displacement of the tibia or femur.

The distal tibial cast holds the ankle in a neutral position and extends distally to encompass the metatarsal heads. The proximal trimline of the tibial cast is typically at the tibial tubercle, and the distal trimline of the femoral cast is an equal distance from the midpatella. Posteriorly, both tibial and femoral casts are trimmed to permit at least 90 degrees of knee flexion. If warranted, a slight varus or valgus stress can be applied at the time of cast brace application, or a varus/valgus strap can be added to aid in unloading a knee compartment. For persons with fractures of the upper tibia and knee, the proximal component encases the lower two-thirds of the femur. If fracture of the femur has occurred, the proximal component extends upward to the level of the greater trochanter. To be effective, careful molding of the proximal portion of the cast around the trochanter and medial wall is required. For fractures of the mid-to-upper femur, an orthotic hip joint and pelvic band must be added to ensure alignment and stability.

FRACTURE ORTHOSES

A custom-fabricated or custom-fit fracture orthosis is designed to maintain a body part in an optimal anatomical position, limit joint motion, and unload weight-bearing forces.[154–157] The major advantage of a fracture orthosis, as compared with a cast brace, is that the orthosis can be removed for wound or skin care. Fracture orthoses are fabricated from high-temperature thermoplastic materials. They are designed to provide total contact, circumferential control of a fracture while allowing the individual with a healing fracture to have functional mobility. Fracture stability is enhanced in two ways: by hydrostatic pressure forces created as the rigid walls of the orthosis compress soft tissue and muscles in the extremity and by the lever arm created by extension of the orthosis above and below the fracture site. Fracture orthoses do not entirely unload the lower extremity during weight bearing. If complete unloading or reduced loading is required to protect the fracture site, an appropriate assistive device (crutches or a walker) and a single limb gait pattern must be used.[149]

Two types of fracture orthoses are available: (1) those that are custom fabricated from a mold of the patient's limb and (2) prefabricated orthoses that are custom fit to match the patient's needs. Because of the wide variation in anatomical characteristics among individuals, it is not always possible to use a prefabricated orthosis. Likewise, because of anatomical similarities in the human skeleton, it is not always necessary to create a custom-fabricated device. In certain instances, an orthosis must be precisely fit to provide the desired stabilization of the fracture; in other cases, the orthosis must be heavily padded so that a precise fit is less important. The orthotic prescription must clearly designate the motions to be permitted and controlled, the corrective forces to be applied, and a precise diagnosis and description of the fracture.

Types of Fracture Orthoses

Fracture orthoses are named by the joints they encompass and the motion that they are designed to control. An AFO with an anterior shell is used to control ankle and distal tibia motion (Fig. 12.34). It encases the injured limb completely, limiting motion of the foot or ankle for patients with distal tibial or fibular fractures. The AFO fracture orthosis has two advantages: It can be removed for wound care and hygiene, and it can be worn with standard lace-up shoes if weight bearing is permitted. The application of a cushion heel and rocker sole may be necessary on the shoe to compensate for limited heel, ankle, and toe rocker motion during gait. Because total contact is essential, this thermoplastic

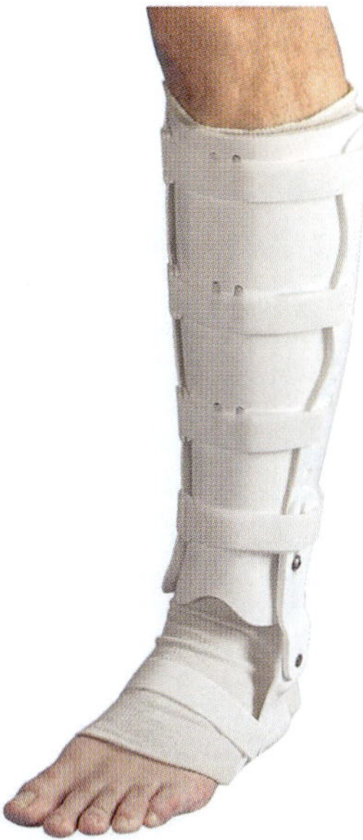

Fig. 12.34 Ankle-foot fracture orthosis with a patellar tendon-bearing design incorporated to protect the tibia for bending moments during weight bearing. This orthosis is typically utilized to encourage healing for fractures of the middle third of the tibia. This orthosis is typically with a shoe as orthosis has a low-profile footplate to prevent distal migration of orthosis. (Courtesy Alimed.)

orthosis is vacuum molded over a positive impression of the patient's limb. The anterior shell may be lined with soft-density foam to accommodate bony deformity or insufficient soft tissue. Perforated thermoplastic material is often used for the anterior section as a means of ventilation for patient comfort. The proximal anterior trimline is at the tibial tubercle. Adequate clearance must be provided for the head of the fibula and the peroneal nerve. The distal posterior section usually extends to just beyond the metatarsal heads on the plantar surface, whereas the anterior section is trimmed just proximally. A stocking or thin sock is worn to protect the skin and for comfort. The anterior section is held in place with a series of hook-and-loop material straps. Shoes must be worn if weight bearing is permitted.

A number of prefabricated short leg walkers are also commercially available; these devices are designed to substitute for a short leg cast and are intended to be removable by the patient. They are heavily padded and, if properly fit, provide excellent immobilization of the distal tibia, ankle, rear foot, and forefoot (Fig. 12.35). The various designs are similar, but manufacturers' instructions should be followed to maximize their effectiveness. The short leg walker's advantage is that it can be removed for wound and skin care. Its disadvantage may be slightly less effective immobilization. The ankle is positioned at a neutral (90-degree) angle. Some designs have an adjustable orthotic ankle joint that permits a controlled, limited range of motion, to assist forward progression during walking. The components of a short leg walker include a rigid foot piece that is attached to a pair of metal or thermoplastic uprights and a proximal cuff that helps to suspend a foam liner. Short leg walkers are manufactured in various styles and sizes. To ensure proper fit, the manufacturer's recommendations must be followed carefully.

The PTB fracture orthosis is the removable version of the PTB cast, providing significant protection from bending and rotatory torque for the tibia during weight-bearing activities. This thermoplastic orthosis is most often vacuum molded over a positive mold of the patient's limb for optimal total contact fit. Ankle position within the orthosis is often in slight dorsiflexion, once again to minimize hyperextension moment at the knee during the stance phase of gait. Trimlines are similar to those of an AFO with anterior shell, with the proximal trimline extending somewhat more proximally to the proximal pole of the patella anteriorly, medially, and laterally. The posterior trimline should permit free-knee flexion beyond 90 degrees. Hook-and-loop material straps are used to secure the anterior and posterior sections together. The anterior and the posterior sections can be hinged at the proximal edge for improved anteroposterior control.

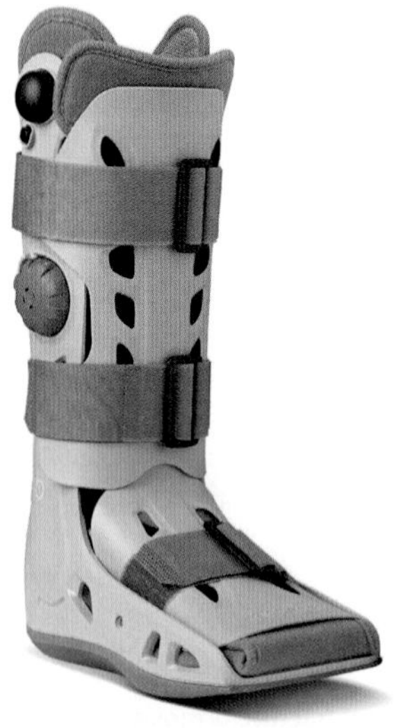

Fig. 12.35 An example of a commercially available short leg walker with a rocker bottom sole that can be used for individuals with Achilles tendon repair, stable healing fractures of the distal tibia/fibula, ankle, or foot, or with severe ankle sprains. (Courtesy DJO Global.)

The purpose of the knee-ankle-foot fracture orthosis is to provide long-term protection for fractures of the distal to middle femur or for fractures about the knee. This orthosis is often used as an alternative to a hybrid cast brace for persons who have had ORIF for fractures of the proximal tibia, knee, or distal femur. The orthosis is removable for wound care and personal hygiene and when protection is not required. Depending on the location of the fracture, the orthosis can be designed to limit range of motion or to permit full motion of the knee. Drop locks can be used to stabilize the knee in full extension during ambulation. The design of the orthosis also protects the knee from excessive mediolateral and anteroposterior shear stress during ambulation. If maximum stability is necessary, a solid-ankle design can be incorporated; if mobility of the ankle is desired, an articulated ankle joint with an appropriate motion stop mechanism can be used. The orthosis requires total contact within the femoral and tibial components. Proximal trimlines follow the anatomical contours of the proximal femur to the greater trochanter to provide femoral protection. To stabilize the knee or proximal tibia, encasement of the lower two-thirds of the femur is sufficient. The orthosis alone cannot effectively unload the femur, tibia, or foot; If axial unloading is desired, appropriate assistive devices (crutches or walker) must be used.

For individuals with proximal femoral fractures, a hip joint and pelvic band are often incorporated into a total contact KAFO (Fig. 12.36) in an effort to control motion and rotational forces through the femur. Depending on the patient's specific needs, hip flexion/extension motion can be restricted or free; abduction/adduction is usually restricted. The placement of the orthotic hip joint is approximately 1 cm anterior and 1 cm proximal to the tip of the greater trochanter in most adults. Knee and ankle motion can be free or limited, given the location and stability of the fracture. A variety of single-axis or polycentric orthotic hip joints can be incorporated. A pelvic belt is used to maintain the orthotic hip joint in proper functional position. The belt should fit midway between the crest of the ilium and the greater trochanter.

EXTERNAL FIXATION DEVICES

External fixation devices have evolved primarily to care for initial management of complex open or severely comminuted, unstable fractures that are most often the result of high-energy injury or multiple traumas (see Figs. 12.28 and 12.33).[158–162] In particular, external fixation is used for

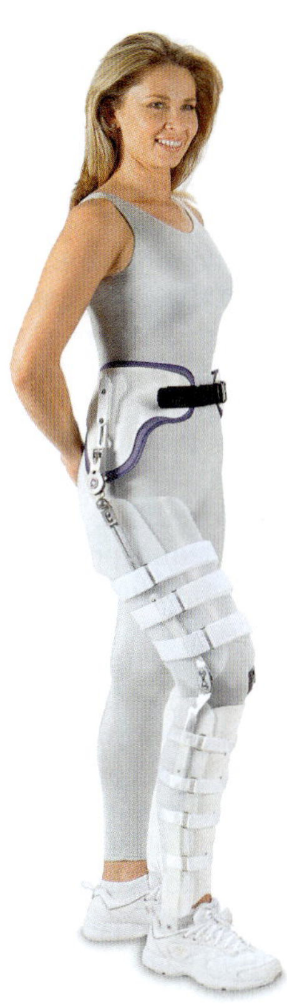

Fig. 12.36 A hip section has been utilized with this fracture knee-ankle-foot fracture orthosis to provide better control of hip abduction/adduction and rotation. This may be beneficial for complex injuries of lower extremity that may include a proximal femur fracture. Lateral stability from metal uprights helps to support femur in ambulation. Orthotic hip joints may be utilized to limit hip flexion and extension as well as adjust for abduction/adduction. (Courtesy Orthomerica Products.)

severe metaphyseal fractures, severe intraarticular fractures, when there has been nonunion, in cases of substantial bone loss with allograft, and for fractures in osteoporotic bone.[160,163] They are particularly useful when fracture disrupts pelvic stability.[164–166]

Pins are placed into bone on either side of the fracture and then clamped onto lightweight rods in an external frame. The external frame can be a single rod, a set of articulated rods that cross the joint axis, circumferential, or a combination of these options.[167–171] The goal is to provide optimal skeletal alignment while providing visual access to healing skin and muscle. The external fixator permits active range of motion of the joint above and below the fracture. It is removed when soft tissues have adequately healed and radiographs demonstrate healing of the fracture. Casts or orthoses can be used to provide immobilization after fixator removal to support and protect the fracture until healing is complete.

POSTFRACTURE MANAGEMENT AND POTENTIAL COMPLICATIONS

The postfracture issues and complications that are of concern to the managing physician and rehabilitation team include vascular injury, compartment syndrome, appropriate weight-bearing status, loss of reduction, delayed or nonunion, infection, implant failure (for ORIF), compression neuropathy, and skin breakdown. Each patient who presents to the emergency department with a fracture must be assessed for potential vascular injury and risk of developing compartment syndrome by careful physical examination. Whether a splint, cast, surgical ORIF, or placement of external fixators has been used to stabilize the fracture, the condition of the extremity must be monitored carefully by the physician, rehabilitation professional, patient, and family caregivers.

Fractures or dislocations around joints may have a concomitant arterial injury that can bruise or completely disrupt an artery, compromising or completely interrupting blood flow beyond the site of fracture.[172–174] This creates a grave situation: The physician has a window of less than 6 to 8 hours in which to restore blood supply and nutrition to the distal muscle and bone before significant tissue death occurs. The longer the period of ischemia, the greater the likelihood of delayed healing, infection, and necrosis. This is commonly seen in patients with blunt trauma due to the associated injuries, fractures, and dislocations. Severe damage may lead to amputation of injured limb.[175]

Compartment syndrome evolves when bleeding or inflammation exceeds the expansive capacity of semirigid muscle or soft tissue anatomical spaces (compartments) of the fractured limb.[176–178] Once interstitial pressure exceeds a critical level, blood vessels and muscles are compressed, and oxygen supply to the muscles is significantly compromised. Irreversible muscle or nerve damage occurs if compartment syndrome continues for longer than 6 to 8 hours. Presenting signs and symptoms include extreme pain and significant swelling of the extremity with taut skin. Passive motion of the fingers or toes causes excruciating pain. Compartment syndrome is considered a medical emergency: The treating physician must be notified immediately so that a fasciotomy can be performed to relieve excessive compartment pressures. All health professionals who are involved in the treatment of extremity trauma should be aware of the signs and symptoms of compartment syndrome. If unrecognized and untreated, compartment syndrome has devastating results.

One of the most important considerations for lower extremity fractures is weight-bearing status. A patient's weight-bearing status (full weight bearing, weight bearing as tolerated, partial weight bearing, toe-touch weight bearing, or non–weight bearing) is determined by the physician on the basis of the stability of the fracture and the immobilization method used. Once a patient is stable after an operation or a cast has been applied and is properly set, rehabilitation professionals work with the patient and family on mobility and gait training. The rehabilitation professional selects the appropriate assistive device for a patient's weight-bearing status, given the patient's physical and cognitive status and the characteristics of his or her usual living environment. Communicating quickly to the referring physician any signs of developing complications or difficulty with compliance that might put the fracture site at risk is important.

Loss of reduction of the fracture is a serious complication and can occur whether a splint, cast, ORIF, or external fixator has been used to realign and stabilize the limb.[168,178–180] A progressive angular deformity or abnormal position of the limb suggests loss of reduction and must be quickly reported to the managing physician. Even if reduction appears to be appropriate, inadequate immobilization within a splint or cast can lead to delayed union, nonunion (nonhealing), or malunion (healing in an abnormal position).

Any patient who has sustained an open fracture is at risk of developing infection of skin, deep tissue and muscle, or even bone. Both intravenous and local antibiotics are administered in the emergency department and operating room to minimize the likelihood of infection from contamination sustained at the time of injury.[181–185] Infections may also be iatrogenic.[182,186] An infection is a serious complication that requires aggressive antibiotic treatment or debridement, or both. If an infection occurs after ORIF, the implanted hardware may have to be removed and an external fixation device applied. For individuals with external fixation, the pins provide a tract for infectious organisms directly into bone.[187] Appropriate wound and pin care is essential to minimize the risk of infection.[188] Osteomyelitis, or infection of bone, is a serious situation that can result in deformity; joint destruction; and, in some circumstances, amputation.[188–191] Patients who have undergone ORIF are at risk of implant failure if repeated loading causes fatigue and ultimately exceeds the strength of the implant material and design.[192–194] Loosening or breakage of implanted screws, plates, or other devices also indicates excessive motion of the fracture site and increases the risk of delayed healing or nonunion. The patient's ability to function within weight-bearing limits established by the physician must be carefully assessed and monitored to reduce the risk of implant failure.

Complications also occur in patients whose fractures are managed by casting. The patient's neurovascular function is documented before cast application and carefully monitored while the cast is in place. In the distal lower extremity, the peroneal nerve is susceptible to prolonged pressure (compression-induced peroneal palsy) as it wraps around the head of the fibula.[118,195,196]

Complaints of edge pressure or toes being squeezed can be solved with cast modifications; however, excessive pressure and discomfort inside the cast often require removal and reapplication of a new cast.[197] On initial application, a cast is designed to have a snug but not tight fit. Signs of distal vascular compromise such as delayed capillary refill on compression of the nail bed suggest that the cast may be excessively tight.[118,197] It is not uncommon for cast fit to loosen over time as a result of several factors: initial edema resolves, compressive forces modify soft tissue composition, disuse atrophy occurs, and cast padding compresses over time. Fit must be carefully monitored over time: A loose cast provides less control of the skeleton, and fracture reduction may be lost. Pistoning of a loose cast on the extremity is likely to lead to skin breakdown and shear over bony prominences.

Casts applied postoperatively while the patient is anesthetized are usually univalved (split down the front) to accommodate postoperative swelling.[119] Excessive swelling is accompanied by significant pain. Limb elevation is the first defense against excessive swelling and pain; however, the cast can be opened further or bivalved to relieve extreme pressure.[3] The risk of compartment syndrome must always be considered: If the patient experiences significant pain on passive motion of the fingers or toes, the physician must be contacted immediately. Failure to recognize and appropriately treat a compartment syndrome results in muscle necrosis and possible loss of the limb.[176]

Occasionally, a window can be cut into a cast to inspect a wound or relieve a pressure area. If the limb is edematous, it is likely that soft tissue will begin to protrude through the window, resulting in additional skin irritation and breakdown. For this reason, any piece of cast that is removed to make a window must be reapplied and secured to the cast after modifications have been made.[197]

Patients with foot pain try to reposition the foot within the cast to make it more comfortable. Inappropriate plantar flexion of the foot within the cast creates excessive pressure on the posterior heel and dorsum of the foot. Discomfort can be reduced if the patient is able to push the relaxed foot gently downward while pulling the cast upward, as if pulling on a boot. If this fails to relieve pressure, the cast must be removed and reapplied.[197]

Foreign objects introduced into a cast are the most common cause of discomfort and pressure. In an attempt to relieve itching of dry skin, patients are sometimes tempted to insert coat hangers, rulers, sticks, pens, and similar objects into the cast to scratch the itchy areas. This strategy often leads to displacement of cast padding, creating lumps and bumps where smooth surface contact is essential. Objects can break off or become trapped within the cast as well. The best way to relieve itching is by tapping on the cast or blowing cool air into it.

Another common complication is skin maceration, which is the result of prolonged exposure to water or a moist environment within the cast. Although, ideally, a cast is kept completely dry, many become wet at some point after application. Plaster casts that become wet lose significant stability and must be replaced. Synthetic casts can be towel dried as much as possible and then further dried using a cool setting on a blower or hairdryer.

Summary

In this chapter the reader learned that orthoses play an important role in the management of traumatic (e.g., fracture) and developmental (e.g., DDH, LCPD) musculoskeletal conditions. Each member of the interdisciplinary rehabilitation team has a contribution to make to the care of individuals with pathologic conditions of the musculoskeletal system, as well as shared responsibility to monitor for changes in function and potential complications. Although many prefabricated orthoses are available, knowledge of appropriate fit, design, and dynamics of the orthoses is essential so that the device will most closely match the intention of intervention. Precise communication about the goals of the orthosis (e.g., to fully immobilize the limb or to allow joint motion within a restricted range), wearing schedule (e.g., all the time or during particular activities), and weight-bearing status while using the orthosis has a major impact on efficacy of the orthotic intervention. All team members participate in patient and family education about the orthosis and its purpose, maintenance and cleaning, signs that indicate problems, and strategies to put in place should problems arise.

References

The complete listing of the References are available in the accompanying enhanced eBook version included with the print purchase of this textbook. Visit Elsevier eBooks+ (eBooks.Health.Elsevier.com) to access this content.

13 Orthoses for Spinal Dysfunction*

THERESA E. LEAHY

LEARNING OBJECTIVES

On completion of this chapter, the reader will be able to do the following:

1. Identify the nomenclature for spinal orthoses.
2. Describe the basic structural and functional anatomy of the spine and its alignment.
3. Discuss the three-column concept of spine stability as it pertains to spine trauma.
4. Identify the types of injury and pathology for which spinal orthoses are used.
5. List the different types and functional use of spinal orthoses.
6. Anticipate the impact of wearing an orthosis on patient functioning.
7. Describe the potential complications associated with the use of spinal orthoses and methods of prevention.
8. Evaluate different areas of the spine as being amenable to bracing.
9. Discuss indications and contraindications for using spinal orthoses.
10. Describe basic pathophysiology of scoliosis and its implications.
11. Identify common braces used in the treatment of scoliosis.
12. Discuss the prescription process for a spinal orthoses.
13. Value the importance of a multidisciplinary team approach in treating disorders of the spine.

External orthoses are used to manage a variety of spinal conditions. The general purpose of a brace is to limit the motion of a spinal region, decreasing the amount of load applied to the region treated. Orthoses are most frequently used when there is concern that loading the spine may result in deformity (i.e., treating an unstable fracture); when the spine is compromised in a way that requires additional support for healing (i.e., postsurgical management or osteoporosis); when the patient is experiencing low back pain (LBP) that can be relieved by either limiting motion or increasing abdominal support; or there is existing spinal deformity such as scoliosis. Another major function of a spinal orthosis is to serve as a psychologic reminder to restrict trunk or neck motion or at least to encourage the patient to move cautiously.[1]

For spinal conditions, an orthosis is defined as an external device applied to the body to restrict motion in a particular body segment or spinal region. The American Academy of Orthopaedic Surgeons standardized the nomenclature used for describing orthoses in spinal management in 1973 and divided them broadly into five categories (Table 13.1)[2]:

- Sacroiliac
- Lumbosacral
- Thoracolumbosacral
- Cervical thoracic
- Cervical

Orthoses may also be classified by their rigidity (i.e., very rigid, semirigid, or flexible/elastic) or by a combination of their materials and whether they are prefabricated or custom-fit types. Traditional rigid spinal orthoses have been associated with problems such as discomfort, decreased compliance, atrophy of paraspinals, and reduced chest expansion.[3] Newer designs such as those utilizing three-dimensional (3D) printing, active braces, and robotics have been designed to mitigate those problems. Historically, orthoses have been named according to their inventor or city of invention. This chapter provides an overview of spinal anatomy and biomechanics as they apply to orthotic use, highlights tips to ensure optimal fit and avoid complications, and discusses each of the three major spinal regions that are amenable to orthotic management and the orthoses used in each region as well as the various types of pathology for which brace treatment is used. This chapter describes common spinal orthoses grouped by region (cervical, thoracic, and lumbosacral) and the clinical conditions that are most often assisted by the use of spinal orthoses.

Managing a patient who may benefit from a spinal orthosis requires an interdisciplinary team approach. Direct communication between the patient, physician, orthotist, nurse, physical therapist, and other rehabilitation personnel is necessary to ensure that the healthcare professionals, the patient, and caregivers all understand the rationale, limitations, and expected outcomes when the prescription and use of an orthosis is being planned. To avoid complications and promote optimal care, specific instructions must accompany the management of a spinal orthosis. Specific fitting, donning, and doffing instructions are available from the manufacturer with downloadable printouts online. Many also have posted videos. Rehabilitation professionals are responsible for designing therapeutic interventions that optimize function while also carefully observing the precautions and the treatment goals relevant to the management of persons using spinal orthoses. Understanding the design of and rationale for the orthosis being used is critical to the overall success of the program.

*The authors extend appreciation to Jeff Coppage and S. Elizabeth Ames, whose work in prior editions provided the foundation for this chapter.

Table 13.1 Nomenclature for Spinal Orthoses

Acronym	Name
RIGID THERMOPLASTIC OR METAL ORTHOSES OR BOTH	
SIO	Sacroiliac orthosis
LSO	Lumbosacral orthosis
TLSO	Thoracolumbosacral orthosis
CTLSO	Cervicothoracolumbosacral orthosis
CTO	Cervicothoracic orthosis
CO	Cervical orthosis
SOFT GARMENTS AND SUPPORTS	
SI belt	Sacroiliac belt
LS corset	Lumbosacral corset
DL corset	Dorsolumbar corset
Soft collar	Nonreinforced cervical collars made from foam or any low modulus material

Anatomy and Biomechanics

The spine consists of 7 cervical vertebrae, 12 thoracic vertebrae, 5 lumbar vertebrae, 5 sacral vertebrae, and 3 to 4 coccygeal segments. Load-sharing discs are interposed between adjacent vertebrae in the cervical, thoracic, and lumbar segments; in the sacral and coccygeal regions, the segments are fused. Two adjacent vertebrae and the intervertebral disc define the functional spinal unit (FSU). Multiple FSUs are combined in a superstructure capable of lateral bending, flexion, extension, and axial rotation. The various levels of the spine differ in their contribution to the spine's overall range of motion (ROM). In the cervical spine, the majority of motion in the sagittal plane (flexion/extension) occurs through Occiput–C2, C4–5, and C5–6.[4] The majority of axial rotation occurs at the level of C1–2 and is made possible by the unique anatomy of the atlantoaxial articulations. Lateral bending of the cervical spine is more evenly distributed, with the upper subaxial cervical spine contributing only slightly more than other regions. Sagittal motion in the thoracic spine increases in a cranial-to-caudal direction. The upper segments provide approximately 4 degrees at each level and the lower segments provide approximately 6 degrees, increasing to approximately 12 degrees per level at the thoracolumbar (TL) junction.[4] Axial rotation is greatest in the upper thoracic spine and gradually decreases caudally. Segmental contribution to lateral bending is fairly well distributed over the length of the thoracic spine. The lumbar spine contributes more flexion/extension but significantly less axial rotation. These regional differences in motion are related to anatomic differences, primarily articular process orientation, between the thoracic and lumbar vertebrae. The ligamentous structures of the spinal column play an important role in spinal kinematics by augmenting overall spinal stability while maintaining flexibility.

The normal spine is essentially vertical in the coronal plane but exhibits four curves in the sagittal plane. The terms *kyphosis* and *lordosis* are used to describe sagittal curves. *Kyphosis* refers to a curve in the sagittal plane with a posterior convexity (forward bend). The thoracic and sacral portions of the spine demonstrate kyphosis. The normal amount of thoracic kyphosis ranges from 20 to 50 degrees.[5] The term *lordosis* describes a curve in the sagittal plane with an anterior convexity (posterior bend). The cervical and lumbar portions of the spine demonstrate lordosis. The mean lordosis in the cervical spine is 35 to 40 degrees.[5–7] The normal range of lordosis in the lumbar spine is from 20 to 60 degrees.[5] Although multiple curves are present, an overall sagittal balance is maintained. The sagittal balance of the spine can be assessed using a plumb-line or gravity-line technique. In a normal balanced spine, a plumb line from the center of the C7 should fall ±2 cm from the sacral promontory in the sagittal plane.[8] These curves, as well as appropriate coronal and sagittal balance, allow for increased flexibility and shock-absorbing capacity while maintaining necessary stiffness and stability.[4]

The major load on the spine under normal physiologic conditions is axial. Axial loading causes compression of the vertebral column and its individual FSUs. The natural kyphotic and lordotic curves of the spine increase in magnitude, and components of individual FSUs (vertebrae and intervertebral discs) deform slightly in response to compression.[4] Soft tissue (ligaments and musculature) as well as bony architecture serve to limit the degree to which the gross architecture of the spine can be deformed, and the properties intrinsic to the vertebrae and intervertebral discs counter the effects of compressive forces. The spine must resist tension and shear forces in addition to axial loads. The properties of the spine conform to the Wolff law, which states that form follows function. Studies of the spine reveal that the spine as a whole can resist higher compressive loads than tension or shear forces.[4] Furthermore, segments of the spine that experience greater compressive loads have been found to be capable of withstanding higher loads before failure. Biomechanical studies demonstrate that the ability of the spine to withstand forces increases in a cephalocaudal direction, such that the lumbar spine, which must withstand the total weight of the body above it, has the greatest compressive strength.[9] The vertebral body (anterior column and anterior aspect of the middle column) provides the majority of this resistance to compression, which translates into increased overall stability in fractures in which the vertebral body is intact and a greater likelihood that bracing may not be necessary. This structure-function relationship is vital to understanding the rationale behind bracing and other treatments of back pain, spinal deformity, or spine injury.

The Three-Column Concept

An understanding of spinal injury and stability is vital to understanding the role played by bracing and various orthoses. The concept of the three-column spine was initially described by Denis[10] in 1984 and is widely used in defining spinal stability. Denis used the three-column model as a basis for his classification of traumatic spinal injuries. The three columns are the anterior, middle, and posterior columns (Fig. 13.1). The anterior column consists of the anterior aspect of the vertebral body, anterior annulus fibrosus, and anterior longitudinal ligament. The middle column includes the posterior longitudinal ligament, posterior annulus fibrosus, and posterior aspect of the vertebral body. The posterior column consists of the posterior vertebral arch as well as the supraspinous and interspinous

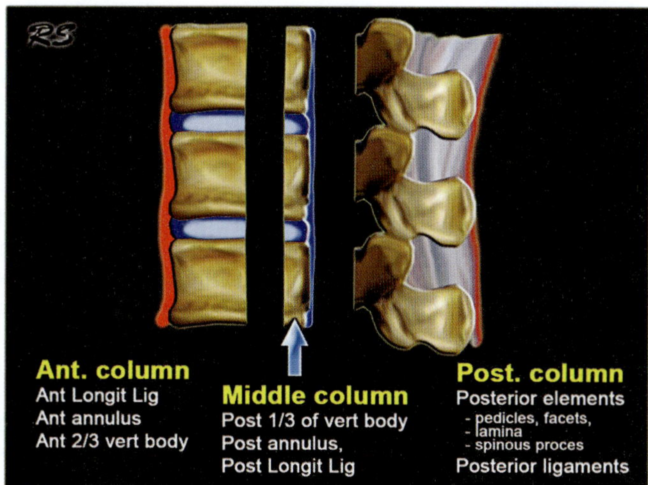

Fig. 13.1 The three-column concept (radiology assistant www.radiologyassistant.nl).

ligaments, facet joints, and ligamentum flavum. There is debate as to whether injury to the posterior column or the middle column is the main factor that destabilizes thoracolumbar spinal fractures.[4,11,12] The debate may be due to the portion of the middle column involved. A recent study concluded that the area of the vertebral body immediately in front of the spinal canal has very different fracture characteristics from that immediately in front of the pedicles.[13] The resulting proposed improvement to the three-column theory separates those two portions keeping the medial part in the middle column and including the part in front of the pedicles with the anterior column.[13] In any case, a combination of both middle and posterior columns results in a highly unstable spine. Compression fractures and burst fractures are the most common clinical entities where orthoses are considered. Denis defined these types of fractures using the three-column concept (Box 13.1).

Compression fractures are defined as failure and wedging of the anterior column and occur with axial forces combined with spinal flexion about an axis located in the middle column. The middle column remains intact, which provides stability and prevents retropulsion of bony fragments into the spinal canal. Some degree of partial failure of the posterior ligamentous structures may be present due to the tension forces of the initial forced flexion. Depending on the degree of anterior column failure, some compression fractures may undergo progressive collapse and lead to increasing posttraumatic kyphosis.[14] Compression fractures with >50% loss of vertebral body height are more likely to have instability due to associated posterior ligamentous involvement, which may result in progressive injury and kyphotic deformity because of the compressive forces conveyed by an upright posture.[4,14]

Burst fractures generally involve failure of the anterior and middle columns due to axial loading with or without additional moments, depending on the fracture pattern.[15] Although these fractures are defined as two-column involvement, there is frequently an associated greenstick fracture of the lamina (posterior column).[16] These injuries are referred to as *three-column burst fractures*. Involvement of the middle column is significant because it may lead to retropulsion of bony fragments in the spinal canal and subsequent spinal cord injury. Controversy exists regarding which burst fractures are "stable" and amenable to bracing and which require surgery. A recent randomized trial of hyperextension casting followed by brace management compared with operative management demonstrated that patients treated operatively experienced improved functionality more rapidly than those who were immobilized, but long-term outcomes in terms of deformity, chronic pain, and neurologic status were equivalent.[17]

Box 13.1 Classification System for Traumatic Fractures of the Thoracolumbar Spine

Compression Fractures (Denis Type 1)

Mechanism of Injury: Spinal Flexion With Compression

Subtype	I-A	Anterior fracture only
	I-B	Anterior fracture with lateral components

Burst Fractures (Denis Type II)

Mechanism of Injury: Spinal Compression With Flexion

Subtype	II-A	Fracture of both end plates or retropulsion, or both, of the posterior wall as a free fragment
	II-B	Fracture of the superior end plate, occasional retropulsion of inferior wall as a free fragment
	II-C	Fracture of the inferior end plate
	II-D	Burst fracture with rotational injury
	II-E	Burst fracture with lateral flexion injury

Seat Belt Injuries (Denis Type III)

Mechanism of Injury: Spinal Flexion With Distraction

Subtype	III-A	(Chance fracture) single segment, posterior or middle column opening
	III-B	(Slice fracture) single segment, posterior and middle column opening through soft and bony tissue
	III-C	Two segments, posterior and middle column opening through soft and bony tissue
	III-D	Two segments, posterior and middle column opening through soft tissue only

Fracture Dislocations (Denis Type IV)

Mechanism of Injury: Translation, Flexion, Rotation With Shear

Subtype	IV-A	Flexion and rotation injury with disruption through bone or intervertebral disc, or both
	IV-B	Due to shear (anterior-posterior or posterior-anterior) with fracture and dislocation of facet joints
	IV-C	Ligamentous injury to posterior and middle column, with failure (marked instability) of the anterior column
	IV-D	Oblique shear forces resulting in significant instability of involved segment (bone or disc)

Fit and Function of the Spinal Orthosis

All spinal orthoses have several common effects on the spinal region they treat. Their primary action is to reduce gross spinal motion, and the degree to which they accomplish this depends on both their materials and design. Secondary effects include the stabilization of individual FSUs, reducing the ROM of one vertebra relative to another. Spinal orthoses also apply closed chain forces designed to counter a deforming force, such as providing hyperextension to a fracture that is vulnerable in flexion. Finally, they reduce loads on the spine itself by preventing specific actions, such as bending and twisting to reduce stress on surgical implants. Each region of the spine has specific needs based on its predominant motions, loads, anatomic features, and physical condition.

The shape of a spinal orthotic, much like the natural shape of the spine, has an intimate relationship with its desired function. Braces often help to restore or exaggerate natural spinal structure. When thoracolumbar body casts were more commonplace in clinical practice, the casts were applied with patients positioned supine on a casting table with a belt under the lumbar spine such that they were casted in a position of hyperextension.[18] This hyperextension (hyperlordosis) has been used in many types of braces (i.e., Jewett and cruciform anterior spinal hyperextension [CASH] brace) because it removes or decreases the amount of flexion, which reduces compressive force on the fractured vertebral body and limits distraction of the posterior elements. Hyperextension braces achieve the intended positioning by using a three-point mold involving three points of applied force: one posteriorly and two anteriorly, with one located cephalad to the level of the posterior force and one caudal.[4] An analogy to this concept is if one were trying to break a pencil using two hands with the thumbs in the center and fingers located at either end. The resultant bending that would result is analogous to the intended effect of the three-point mold. The desired effect is prevention of the progressive kyphotic deformity associated with significant compression and burst fractures. Another example of three-point molding is seen in corrective braces used for the treatment of scoliosis except that the forces are directed in a coronal instead of a sagittal plane. It is imperative to ensure that the contour and fit of the brace promotes adequate alignment of the spine and avoids potential complications associated with forces applied to the body for long periods of time.

To be effective, an orthosis must have intimate contact with bony prominences, though opinions vary on the exact placement of points of pressure.[19] The biomechanical principles of bracing the spine itself can be understood in terms of the three-point model; in reality, however, using an orthosis to treat a human condition is subject to other variables. Compliance and the psychologic effects of bracing can be significant issues, including the development of a psychologic dependence on the orthosis.[19–24] The financial burden can be significant, with costs ranging from $35 to >$5000. Physical issues also apply, particularly in an increasingly obese population. The ability of a brace to apply appropriate forces, either stabilizing or corrective, depends on its ability to act on the structures of the spine. This, in turn, depends on the soft tissue envelope in the contact areas around the spine. Too little or too much pressures transmitted through soft tissues can result in significant physical complications including skin breakdown, loss or reduction of spinal alignment, pain due to the brace, weakening of the immobilized muscles, and soft tissue contractures.[3,23,25,26] The prescription and use of a spinal orthotic should always be governed by an appropriate monitoring system and rehabilitation program. Orthoses must be modified periodically, and a comfortable and appropriate fit is critical to preventing skin problems and ensuring compliance.

Compliance with brace wear is a significant clinical issue, particularly because the traditional rigid orthosis is specifically designed to restrict motion, which is neither an accommodating nor pleasant approach to therapy. Studies in adolescent patients with scoliosis wearing "smart braces" that can track wear time indicate compliance rates of 9% to 30%. Adults being treated with a thoracolumbar orthoses for osteoporotic fracture were found to have slightly better compliance, but still less than half of the prescribed time on average with females wearing the brace longer than males.[24] In the current healthcare environment, most patients with significant spinal conditions recover at home rather than in rehabilitation facilities. Orthosis designs that increase the difficulty of donning or doffing decrease patients' ability to use the brace effectively if they are not supervised and assisted daily. The only orthoses that ensure compliance are fiberglass casts, which are very rarely used today.

REGIONAL ORTHOSES

Cervical

The cervical spine is the most intuitively easy structure to consider bracing in that the bony occiput, mandible, sternum, and clavicles provide appropriate supporting structures. Unfortunately this advantage is offset by the limited surface area available for contact and the fact that the mandibles and clavicles are often in motion during normal activities. The complexity of the cervical soft tissues—vessels, airway, esophagus—is a disadvantage in that significant forces cannot be applied directly to the spine without significant visceral effects. Orthoses for the cervical spine can be limited to the subaxial spine itself—in the form of a cylinder that fits around the neck with a trim line at the occiput, mandible, and sternoclavicular structures—or it may extend proximally and distally (halo vest) or just distally onto the thoracic cage for additional control (cervicothoracic orthosis [CTO]).

Cervical orthoses may be used to improve head position and function for individuals with spinal muscle weakness, or to stabilize the cervical vertebral column after injury or surgery. The orthosis requirements for a person living with motor neuron disease (MND) are different than those needed for cervical immobilization. The Motor Neurone Disease Association offers several suggestions for head supports depending on the extent of weakness and the direction of loss of control[27] (Fig. 13.2). The Headmaster is a common choice to prevent head drop in early stages of amyotrophic lateral sclerosis (ALS) due to neck extensor weakness. The collar is low profile, light weight, able to be bent to customize fit, and the open front does not interfere with swallowing.

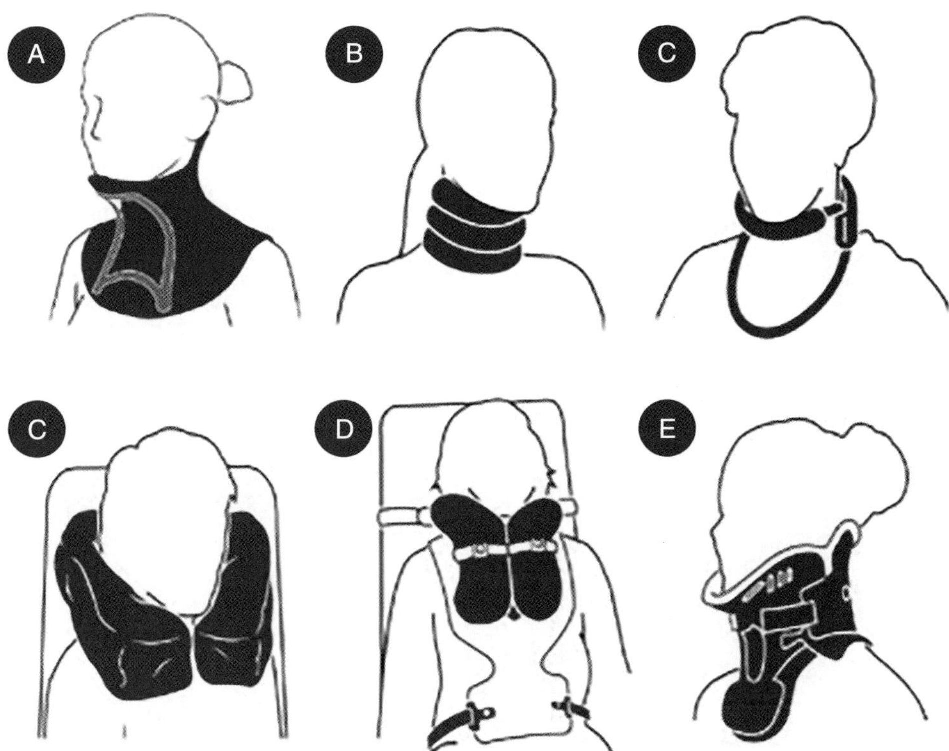

Fig. 13.2 Motor Neurone Disease Association–recommended collars. (A) HeadUp collar, (B) Hereford, (C) Headmaster, (D) Burnett vacuum neck and head supports, (E) Hensinger, and (F) Miami J cervical collar (MND Association | Fighting motor neurone disease).

It does not provide significant lateral support. The HeadUp collar was designed specifically for individuals with ALS and has been found to be a comfortable and useful support for people with other MNDs as well.[28] The orthosis consists of a cylindrical "sleeve" with supports that can be slipped in to pockets to provide control in specific areas around the neck as needed. In a multicenter trial, participants reported the device allowed freedom of head movement without loss of support and did not impede eating and swallowing. There were fewer reports of discomfort and pain compared to previously worn rigid collars. However, the HeadUp collar was found to be difficult to put on requiring an assistant.[28]

Cylindrical cervical braces limit a variable degree of motion, depending on the design, and primarily provide proprioceptive feedback as a reminder to limit the ROM of the neck.[1] Available choices are many, and this list is not exhaustive; commonly used choices include the soft collar, the Stifneck (Laerdal, Armonk, New York), the Philadelphia, the Miami J, and the NecLoc (Össur, Foothill Ranch, California) (Fig. 13.3).

Soft collars are composed of a piece of soft foam rubber covered with stockinette or another gentle fabric with a Velcro-type fastener. These tend to be the most comfortable of the available cervical collars but provide little stability to the cervical spine. A current systematic review and meta-analysis concluded that there was no significant difference in neck ROM for flexion/extension, side-bending and rotation when wearing a soft cervical collar compared to no collar.[29] Rigid collars were found to provide significantly more stability than the soft collar in sagittal plane and rotational movements.[29] Conversely, Miller et al.[30] analyzed differences in functional motion of the cervical spine between no collar, a soft collar, and a rigid collar during the performance of 15 different activities of daily living[a] (ADLs). The authors found that there was no significant difference in limitation of sagittal ROM between the soft and rigid collars during 13 of the 15 ADLs tested (significant differences were noted while reversing a car and sitting down in a chair). No significant differences were noted during lateral bending, and the difference in restriction of rotational movement was significant only while reversing a car. However, a study examining cervical ROM in 50 healthy adults performing cardinal plane and rotational neck movements while wearing no collar, a soft collar, or a neck brace did find differences between devices in the amount of motion allowed.[31] Whitcroft and colleagues found the soft cervical collar to reduce movement by an average of 17.4%, whereas the cervical brace reduced movement by 62.9%.[31] Differences between the two brace types were least in lateral bending. The authors concluded that a soft cervical collar is not sufficient after a whiplash injury when cervical immobilization is desired. The soft cervical orthosis is used primarily as a comfortable reminder to the patient to limit exaggerated neck movements and may be useful in cases of minor whiplash, cervical spondylosis, or as a postoperative adjunct

[a] ADLs tested include standing to sitting, backing up a car, putting on socks, tying shoelaces, reading a magazine in one's lap, cutting food with knife and fork and bringing food to the mouth, rising from a sitting position, washing hands in a standing position, shaving facial hair (males)/applying makeup (females), washing hair in shower, picking up object from floor (bending technique), picking up object from floor (squatting technique), walking, walking up stairs, walking down stairs.

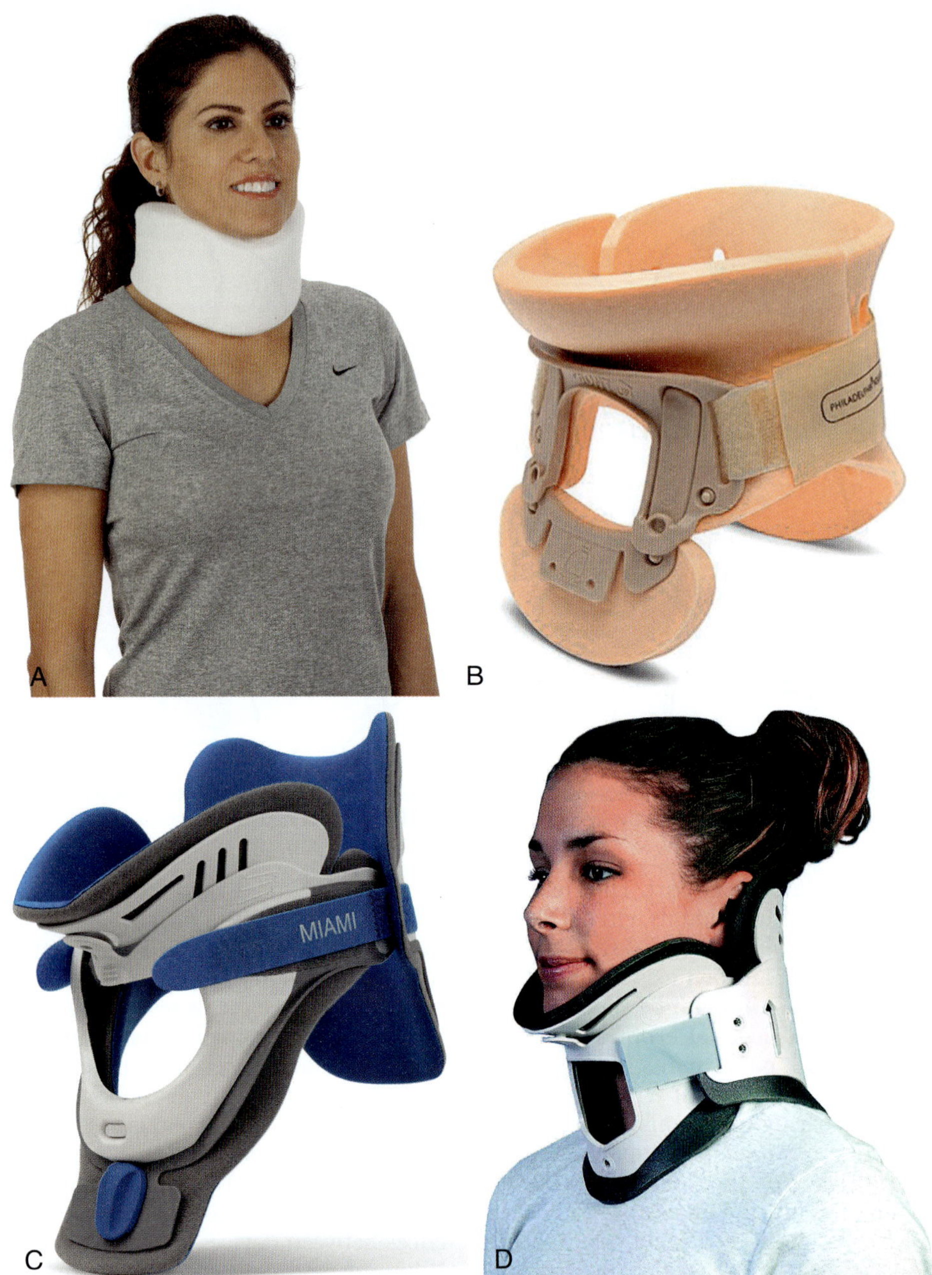

Fig. 13.3 (A) Soft collar. (B) Philadelphia collar. (C) Miami J collar. (D) NecLoc (© Össur).

with a stable spine.[32] Soft collars are generally considered to be inappropriate for use with an unstable cervical spine. A great deal more support is required in patients with injuries that compromise spinal stability. This prompted the development of the reinforced cervical collar, which is a commercially produced, prefabricated orthosis that combines some of the soft materials found in soft collars with a semirigid contoured plastic external frame. Many different types of reinforced collars are available, such as the Philadelphia, Aspen (Aspen Medical Products, Irvine, California), Miami J, NecLoc (Össur, Foothill Ranch, California), and Stifneck. Most reinforced collars have anterior and posterior shells with inner padding and trim; they close around the neck and fasten with Velcro-type fasteners. The collars are contoured such that they abut the sternum, clavicles, trapezius, and upper thoracic spine inferiorly and the mandible and occiput superiorly, which provides some degree of end-point control. Most have openings anteriorly to accommodate respiratory and ventilator equipment.

Although there are many similarities among the various cervical collars, studies have found significant differences in the degree to which the collars restrict the motion of the cervical spine. The ability of a cervical collar to provide cervical stability is very important in that approximately 3% to 25% of spinal cord injuries occur after the initial spinal injury.[33] Multiple studies have evaluated the various reinforced collars for their ability to promote cervical stability as well as to avoid complications. Askins and Eismont[33] studied five common reinforced cervical collars by using anteroposterior and lateral radiographs to assess the motion of the cervical spine in normal healthy volunteers. They found the NecLoc to be statistically superior with respect to the limitation of cervical motion in all planes, followed by the Miami J collar, as compared with Philadelphia and Aspen collars. Tescher et al. compared four collars (Aspen, Aspen Vista, Miami J, and Miami J Advanced) for cervical stability and tissue-interface pressure (TIP).[34] These researchers found the Aspen to be more restrictive than the Aspen Vista and Miami J but not significantly different from the Miami J Advanced. They report that, despite statistical difference between the collars, all provided restriction of cervical ROM, and they question the clinical significance of the differences. They further report that TIP increases for all collars with increasing patient body mass index and that the Miami J produced the lowest overall pressures.[34] The NecLoc and Miami J collars provide improved fit to increase stability and decrease pressure areas by sizing through phenotype (neck shape) rather than just small, medium, and large. The selection of an appropriate cervical orthosis must balance the need for stability with the potential for adverse effects. Wearing a rigid cervical collar has been associated with numerous complications including skin breakdown, eating and swallowing difficulties, increased intracranial pressure, peripheral nerve palsies, discomfort, sleep impediment, and difficulty with hygiene.[26,35–38] Wang et al. examined the rate of c-collar–related pressure injuries in the intensive care unit (ICU) over a 9-year period.[37] Time in the collar (6 days or more) and length of stay in the ICU were associated with skin breakdown. Interestingly, risk for pressure wound development increased with each repositioning episode. Investigators noted a drop in pressure ulcer development over the 9 years of data collection after the emergency responders changed to use of soft cervical collars rather than rigid to transport patients to the hospital.[37] In Australia, emergency medical personnel have switched to use of soft cervical collars for low-risk blunt trauma patients who are neurologically intact with potential for cervical spine injury.[32]

Investigators found a significant reduction in patient reports of neck and back pain, no skin issues, and reduced patient agitation when soft collars were used rather than rigid. The authors caution that much larger studies are needed to investigate secondary spinal injury rates between collar types. Randall et al. followed 45 patients who were discharged with a rigid cervical collar following blunt trauma with resultant neck pain, but with no new injury seen on imaging.[36] They discovered a high proportion of patients discontinued the collars due to one or more complications including: pain, skin irritation, and difficulty with talking, swallowing, and sleeping. They advise against sending a patient with negative imaging home with a rigid cervical collar. A higher prevalence of dysphagia and respiratory failure was found in patients wearing a hard collar compared to those who were not in a population of geriatric patients with traumatic brain injury and potential for spine injury in a hospital.[39] The authors noted that the patients with dysphagia demonstrated improvement with speech therapy. To optimize patient care, rehab professionals should verify need of a cervical orthosis, assure fit, be alert for signs of negative effects, and make appropriate referrals to help mitigate the problem.

While there is substantial evidence of injury related to use of a rigid cervical collar, the benefit of their use following surgery is not clear. Emerging evidence suggests that use of a rigid cervical collar after surgery or injury where the spine is stable may not improve outcomes. In a study of patients undergoing spinal fusion for degenerative conditions, no significant difference in fusion rates or complications was found between patients who were braced and those who were not.[40] Likewise, no difference in healing was found after odontoid fracture between elderly patients stabilized with a rigid or soft collar, but the soft collar was more comfortable.[41] A retrospective study of age- and sex-matched patients evaluated outcomes for a group who used hard cervical collars and those who wore none after undergoing posterior cervical laminectomy and instrumented fixation (PCLF) surgery.[42] Spinal stabilization was achieved during the surgery. There was no difference in pain or functional status between the groups at any of the follow-up time frames (1, 3, 6, and 12 months postoperative), although at 3 months the no-collar group demonstrated a higher quality of life rating. A 2022 systematic review and meta-analysis concluded that current evidence on the merits and risks for use of hard cervical collars is of low quality.[35] Further high-quality prospective studies are needed to generate clear guidelines for collar use following injury or surgery.

When cervical collars are used to provide spinal stability, optimizing fit may reduce negative impacts. Changing anthropometrics and soft tissue distribution with the aging process may contribute to the higher rate of complications with collar wearing in older adults.[43] Ladney et al. assessed the impact of five different cervical collars on optic nerve sheath diameter as a measure of increased intracranial pressure in healthy volunteers laying supine.[38] The greatest change occurred with the Philadelphia collar, a rigid collar with limited sizes, and the least with the Necklite, which is a moldable brace allowing for a more custom fit. 3D printing may hold future potential for personalized orthotic design and improved wearability. The process and outcomes for a single case were described by Xu et al. for a trauma patient who underwent a PCLF.[44] The resulting orthotic was reported to be affordable, comfortable to the patient, and very stable allowing <8 degrees of motion in all planes.

Braces that are required to immobilize the occipitocervical spine need fixation to the skull and significant rotational control. The most commonly used example is the halo vest (Fig. 13.4). Primary features include a ring anchored to the skull with skeletal pins and connected to a body jacket by four vertical uprights. Changes in material design and advances in plastics technology have allowed significant modifications to the halo vest—molded thermoplastic jackets, radiolucent rings and uprights, shaped rings open posteriorly for patient comfort while supine, and multidirectional adjustments in the connecting mechanisms—but the principles of fixation have remained the same. Six to eight transcranial pins provide secure proximal fixation (end-point control), and full contact support around the thorax and torso provides the distal fixation.

The ring of the halo is positioned 1 cm above the eyebrows and the tips of the ears, with care taken to keep the ring well clear of the skin surface. Four pins are inserted into the outer table of the skull with 6 to 8 lb/in of torque.[45] The anterior pins are placed at the equator (widest point) of the skull above the lateral third of the eyebrow to avoid the frontal sinus, supraorbital and supratrochlear nerves,

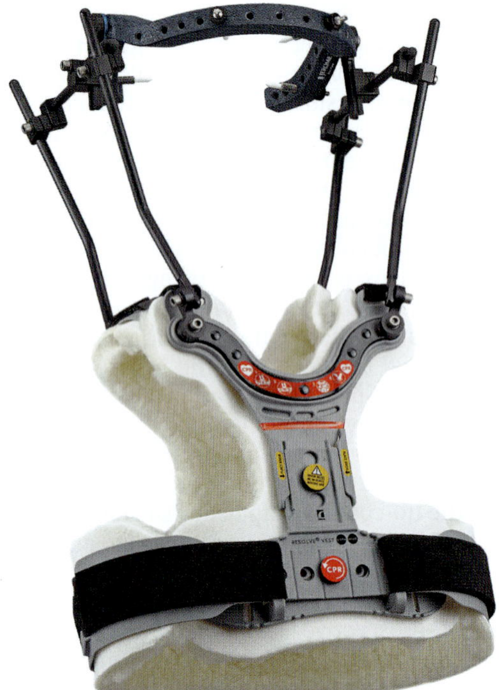

Fig. 13.4 Halo vest (© Össur).

and temporalis muscle. Posteriorly, pins are placed 1 to 2 cm posterior to the ear diagonally opposite the anterior pins. This provides secure fixation to allow for manipulation in flexion/extension and in translation.

The halo vest itself was originally a plaster cast that fit over the torso with a trim line at or slightly above the inferior costal margin of the last rib.[46] Advances in materials allow for bivalved thermoplastic shells that can be released with the patient supine to allow for hygiene, and some designs are fleece-lined. A four-pad halo vest that completely avoids the shoulder girdle has been proposed to avoid scapular movements transferring loads to the neck.[47,48] Two anterior and two posterior rods link the vest to the ring through a series of connectors. Modern connectors allow translation in multiple planes with the ability to lock them into position once reduction has been achieved.

Fixation with the halo vest may be used for the definitive treatment of cervical spine trauma, for fracture reduction and alignment prior to surgery, or for adjunctive postoperative stabilization.[49–52] Halo fixation (HF) is primarily used for upper cervical fractures, commonly odontoid and hangman types, but has been used for single or multiple fractures in other cervical spine locations as well.[53] It is commonly used for complex combined C1 and C2 fracture patterns where internal stabilization is not possible without extension to the occiput, which results in severe loss of motion.[54,55] It is used to provide additional stability after complex surgical reconstructions or noninstrumented fusion or wiring constructs after surgery at C1–2 and may be used to supplement instrumented fusions in situations with poor bone quality or significant instability, as in patients with osteoporosis or rheumatoid arthritis.[56] The halo is no longer used as frequently in subaxial (i.e., C3–C7) trauma due to advances in spinal instrumentation. It is still considered the treatment of choice for some types of fractures of the axis and in some flexion/compression injuries.[57,58] A fracture of the odontoid process at C2 is a common injury in older patients and historically has often been treated with a halo vest.[59–62] Currently the optimal treatment for these patients is controversial, with some authors reporting that simple collar immobilization provides equivalent results.[63] Others found equivalent outcomes when comparing HF to surgical fixation in terms of clinical outcomes, although the surgical group had a lower rate of pseudoarthrosis and higher patient satisfaction.[64] C2 is also a frequently injured vertebra in children. A 2021 systematic review found HF to be a successful intervention with high fusion rates for children with C2 vertebral injuries and atlantoaxial rotatory subluxation.[49] Similar to findings with adult and geriatric populations, unstable dislocation injuries were better treated with surgery. Stable atlas (C1) fractures are reported to achieve high fusion rates with conservative treatment in a halo, whereas fusion rates decline with unstable fractures.[65] In a retrospective sample of 53 patients, Shin et al. found a 71.4% success rate with unstable atlas fractures treated with halo immobilization.[66] Surgical internal fixation for unstable fractures resulted in 100% fusion rate with significant reduction, more favorable clinical outcomes, and a shorter healing time than those treated with HF. Conservative treatment with HF has been used for all ages from 1 year old to 90 years old. The average length of immobilization is 10 weeks but can be up to 16 weeks.[53] Close patient follow-up and monitoring is required during the halo treatment period.

Complications can occur with the use of a halo vest, including pressure sores, loss of reduction (particularly in injuries involving the posterior elements), pin infection and loosening, dysphagia, and cranial nerve palsies.[49–51,53,62,67,68] A retrospective review of 342 patients treated with HF after cervical spine injury revealed complications in 35%.[51] The most common occurrences were pin site infection and instability. All rehab team members should assure pin site hygiene. Therapists should regularly monitor neurologic function and report any decline, or subjective reports of movement, to the physician immediately. Incidence and severity of dysphagia due to halo-vest fixation has been suggested to be related to O-C2 angle and occurs more frequently in older patients.[68] Most available studies report a higher rate of complications in older patients. In a review of 53 patients with a mean age of 79.9 years, Horn and colleagues[69] recorded 31 complications in 22 patients. Serious complications included respiratory distress and dysphagia; these were the cause of death in 6 of eight patients who died within the treatment period and were thought to have some relation to the halo treatment. Modern halo vests should always have a wrench attached to the front for quick removal in case of a cardiac emergency. Significantly higher mortality has been reported in older patients treated with a halo compared with those treated with a cervical collar.[60,70] Daentzer and Florkemieier[71] performed a retrospective study of 29 patients divided into two groups based on age younger or older than 65 years and found that, although clinical and radiographic results were equivalent between the two groups, the interval to healing and rate of complications were higher in the older-than-65 age group. In contrast, a more recent review of 189 patient cases found the lowest rate of complications (33%) in the >60-year-old group compared to 63.3% in the <30-year-old group and 47.8% in the 31- to 60-year-old group.[53] Similar to previous studies, they did find that mortality rate, while small, was greater in the older population primarily due to cardiopulmonary complications.

Rehabilitation of the patient with a halo is challenging. The fixed head position affects the ability to use visual cues, and the weight of the vest and position of the head combine to change the patient's center of mass. Ambulatory patients in halo vests may exhibit a forward-flexion posture to accommodate this; a cane or walker may be required while the halo is in place, even for young neurologically intact patients. Likewise, there is a readjustment period after the halo has been removed, which may require postural reeducation as part of the rehabilitation strategy to prevent falls.

CERVICOTHORACIC AND THORACIC ORTHOSES

CTOs can be divided into two categories: those that use the thoracic spine to support treatment of a subaxial cervical spine or upper thoracic spine problem and those that support treatment at the upper cervical spine. Examples in the first category include thoracic extensions added to a cylindrical cervical orthosis (i.e., Extended Miami J) or an orthosis that utilizes pads on the chin and occiput to connect to the trunk with four stiff uprights or circumferential supports (i.e., Minerva). The Minerva brace (Fig. 13.5) is the most effective method for immobilizing C1–2 and has been shown to limit flexion/extension by approximately 79%, axial rotation by 88%, and lateral bending by 51%.[72] The cervicothoracic area is a particularly challenging area to immobilize in that it is a transitional area between the very mobile and lordotic cervical spine and the kyphotic thoracic spine. Little data exist in the literature regarding immobilization of the upper thoracic spine; for those conditions not requiring surgery, an extended cervical orthosis can be used.[73] The Minerva brace, Sternal Occipital Mandibular Immobilizer (SOMI) brace (Fig. 13.6), or a custom-molded CTO can be used for conditions extending as far caudally as T5. In general, increasing the length of the orthosis down the trunk enhances its capabilities.

The most common condition affecting the thoracic spine is the vertebral compression fracture (VCF). Approximately 700,000 VCFs occur each year, and it is estimated that 25% of American females will experience at least one VCF in their lifetimes.[74] Most patients will have a benign course, but up to 30% are significantly symptomatic and seek treatment for pain that limits function in either the short or long term.[74] Patients with multiple VCFs have been found to have significant decreases in trunk extension torque, spinal motion, functional reach, mobility skills, and walking distance compared with the normal age–matched population.[75] The goals for acute treatment of a nondisplaced VCF are aimed at pain relief and improved function. Bracing with a spinal orthosis may help reduce pain by limiting movement of bone fragments against one another.[74] A short period of rest and analgesics followed by gradual mobilization and physical therapy to reduce fear of falling may be needed along with the brace.[74] The type of orthosis used depends on the level of involvement. It might be an extended cervical orthosis, a CTO, or a thoracolumbar brace such as the CASH or Jewett.

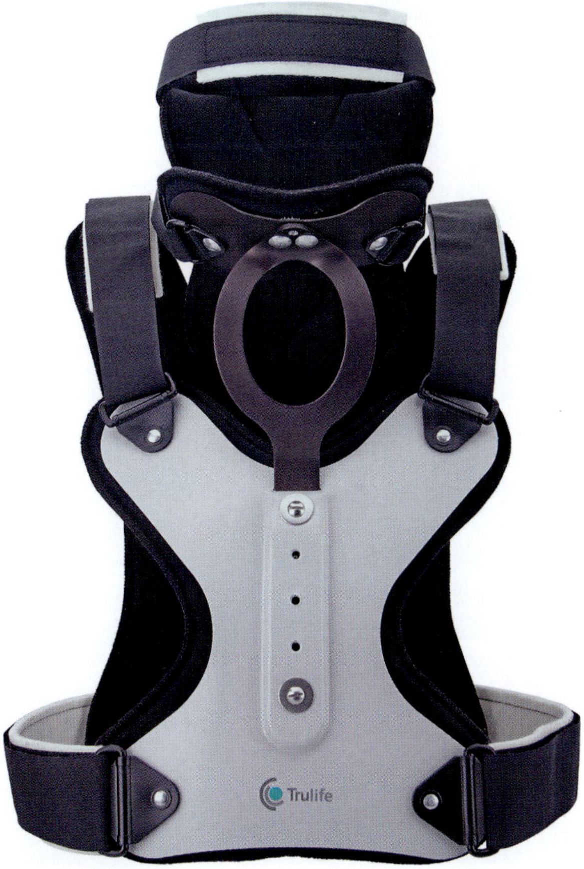

Fig. 13.5 Minerva brace (Otto Bock HealthCare LP, Austin, Texas).

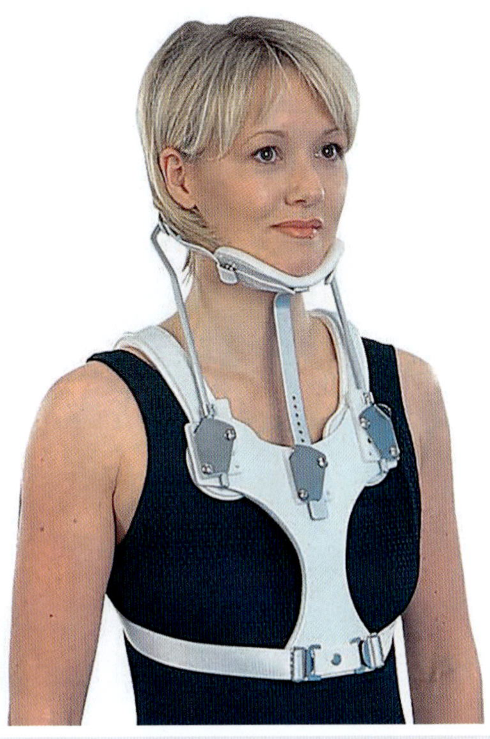

Fig. 13.6 SOMI brace. (Courtesy Trulife.)

THORACOLUMBAR

The thoracolumbar region is the most common region of the spine affected by VCF due to osteoporosis or traumatic fracture and the most likely region to benefit from orthotic support for the surgically treated spine. The integrity of the vertebral body is of primary importance to resisting compressive forces and axial loads, and this region is a transitional zone that should be neutral in alignment. Fractures involving the anterior body greatly decrease the spine's ability to withstand compressive load and tend to collapse into kyphosis, particularly if the posterior elements are also involved (i.e., a burst fracture). This results in displacement of the patient's sagittal balance, spinal deformity, pain, and, in the worst cases, neurologic deficit. Fractures of this area may be treated with orthoses or surgically, and there is some consensus in the literature for surgical management when the vertebral body is severely comminuted, the patient has a neurologic deficit, or the initial fracture alignment is unacceptable.[76,77] Advances in spinal instrumentation and techniques such as interbody support have improved the surgeon's ability to counteract kyphosis, but at the thoracolumbar junction this requires a combined thoracolumbar surgical approach through the thoracic and abdominal cavities, which carries significant morbidity. Surgeons often choose to use posterior spinal instrumentation alone in these cases. Posterior instrumentation is least effective in resisting kyphosis, so orthoses that reduce kyphotic forces on the thoracolumbar spine may be used to supplement internal fixation techniques.

When an orthosis is used for the management of a thoracolumbar fracture, the same principles apply. Optimal management includes a strategy to resist anterior flexion and therefore the development of a kyphotic deformity. Orthoses are best used for fractures from T10 to L2, although some types of orthoses can be adjusted to control up to T8. Several thoracolumbar hyperextension orthoses are designed to unload the anterior column.[1] The most common types are the Jewett brace (Fig. 13.7A) and the CASH brace (Fig. 13.7B). Both of these braces are available in prefabricated styles from various manufacturers. The Jewett orthosis has an aluminum frame anteriorly that is stabilized on the pubis, sternum, and lateral midline of the trunk against a posterior pad. The frame is open and is particularly suitable for patients with coexisting abdominal trauma or obesity. Trunk flexion is limited by a single three-point pressure system with posteriorly directed forces at the sternum and pubis opposing an anteriorly directed force applied by the posterior pad. Therefore it is contraindicated in patients with sternal fractures or an inability to tolerate direct pressure from the posterior pad. The goal of the Jewett is to prevent flexion while still allowing active

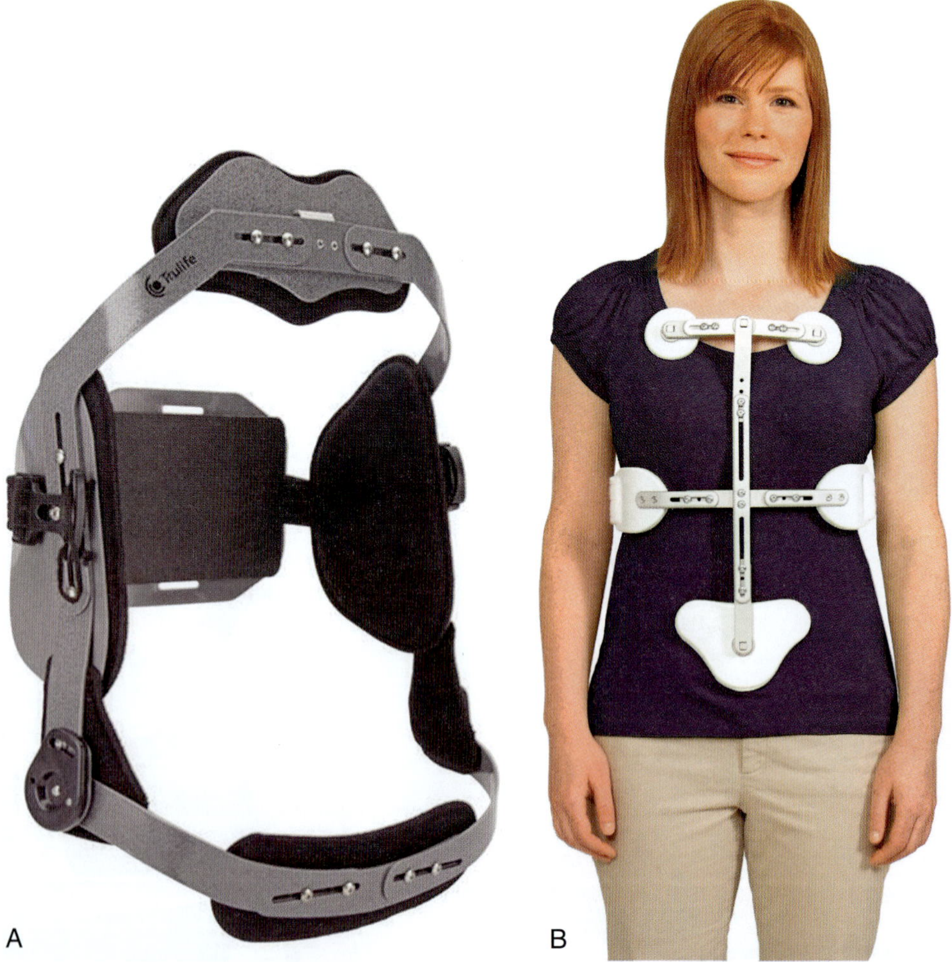

Fig. 13.7 (A) Jewett brace. (B) Cash brace (Otto Bock HealthCare LP, Austin, Texas).

hyperextension. The CASH brace uses the same three-point system. It has an adjustable-length anterior cross with sternal and pelvic pads at the end of the vertical bar and lateral pads on the horizontal bar. It also uses an anteriorly directed force provided by a posterior belt. Both the Jewett and CASH braces are options for those patients who cannot tolerate the constriction of a molded thermoplastic thoracolumbosacral orthosis (TLSO), but they are contraindicated in patients with injuries including significant three-column instability such as the thoracolumbar burst fracture.

The TLSO is the recommended treatment for significant fractures at the thoracolumbar junction that are being treated conservatively. TLSOs can be used to manage fractures from T6 to L4. Molded TLSOs provide total contact designed to restrict ROM in all planes. The superior trim lines of the TLSO are at the sternal notch and have an anteroinferior trim line at the groin; they are carefully shaped to envelop the pelvis, arching slightly laterally anteriorly to accommodate the thigh while sitting and trimmed low at the sacrococcygeal junction posteriorly. Patients frequently report uncomfortable pinching in the groin area when sitting. Providing supported seating with the back reclined slightly (10–15 degrees) reduces anterior pressure without negatively impacting swallowing and functional tasks. The superoposterior trim line falls just below the spine of the scapula. The custom molds are made of a ventilated thermoplastic, which may be lined with closed cell foam to increase comfort. They can be bivalved with side closures to facilitate donning and doffing and are generally worn over a light T-shirt for comfort and hygiene. Straps over the shoulders may increase the rigidity, particularly if a semiflexible or prefabricated model is chosen. TLSOs are also available in prefabricated models, although for maximum control of motion a custom mold is preferred. There is some controversy as to whether the made-to-measure or prefabricated orthoses fit and function as well as the custom-fabricated ones. A comparison of three types of braces (the semirigid Hohmann corset, the Jewett brace, and the TLSO) found similar levels of stability in the sagittal plane and rotational axis when used with healthy subjects performing voluntary tasks.[78] However, the rigidity of the softer braces was reduced when performing involuntary movements suggesting that the sensory feedback provided by the brace impacts motion restriction. Only the TLSO was found to provide significant rigidity in the sagittal plane during walking and sitting.[78]

Vertebral compression fractures (VCF) due to bone fragility are often treated with spinal orthoses, though evidence is mixed on use and efficacy. Moderate quality evidence to support use of spinal orthoses in patients 60 and older who are neurologically intact is reported in the literature.[79–81] Prost et al. suggest that conservative treatment with a back brace results in bone union for individuals with stable VCF with <20 degrees kyphosis and 25% loss in height with no neurologic changes.[79] They caution that spinal orthoses are not well tolerated in older patients. A 2021 systematic review by Kweh et al. concluded that bracing results in improvement in multiple domains including: reduced kyphotic deformity, improved strength, postural stability, and functional outcomes.[80] Similar findings were reported by Sanchez-Pinto-Pinto et al. in 2022 for patients wearing a dynamic hyperextension orthosis for as little as 2 hours/day for 6 months.[81] Furrer et al. also reported patient improvements overtime when treated nonoperatively with a hyperextension orthosis despite poor compliance.[24] Hidden sensors were used to determine actual wearing time of 2 to 9 hours a day when 15 hours was considered full compliance. Females were more compliant than males with an average wearing time of 6 hours/day versus 3; age and body mass index did not influence wearing behavior.[24] Authors of a 2023 systematic review concluded that although studies of different orthoses reported improvements in pain, function, and quality of life over time postinjury, these improvements were similar to patients treated without an orthosis.[82] Therefore no clear recommendations for spinal orthosis use with osteoporotic VCF could be made.[82] Further study is required to outline optimal general management strategies for using spinal orthoses in this population. There is general agreement that pharmaceutical treatment of osteoporosis along with physical therapy to improve core strength and balance during mobility is essential to help prevent new fractures.

LUMBOSACRAL

Immobilization of the lumbosacral spine presents a unique set of challenges. It is a transition zone between the highly mobile lordotic lumbar spine and the rigid sacropelvic structures; it has the largest absolute range of flexion/extension and bears the most load of any of the spinal regions. A rigid lumbosacral orthosis (LSO), which is simply a shorter version of the TLSO described earlier, is appropriate for bracing fractures at L2, L3, and L4; but the FSUs at L4–5 and L5–S1 require special treatment. Fidler and Plasmans[83] found that a unilateral thigh extension is necessary to effectively immobilize L4–5 and L5–S1. A thigh extension is generally a cuff attached by two longitudinal struts that have hinges, allowing a variable degree of flexion at the hip to facilitate toileting and sitting; generally it is set at allowing 20 to 30 degrees of flexion at a maximum. The mean percentage of motion allowed in the brace was 32% at L4–5 and 70% at L5–S1 in a brace without the extension; adding the extension resulted in an additional 15% to 30% reduction of motion[84] At best, restriction at the L5–S1 level still allows 40% of normal range. For this reason fractures at these levels are best treated with surgery (using an orthosis for postoperative support if necessary) if the treating physician desires to mobilize that patient during the healing period.

Up until the last few years, LSOs have commonly been used in the postoperative period. Advances in spinal instrumentation, with the advent of pedicle screws and interbody techniques, now allow many patients to go without bracing postoperatively. Pedicle screws connect the anterior load-bearing portion of the spine with a posterior construct by crossing the middle column and provide better limitation of motion and load sharing than previous hook/rod constructs. Interbody techniques place a block of bone between the vertebral bodies, either through placement by an intraabdominal approach or with hybrid approaches accessing the disc space from the posterior part of the spine. The placement of bone in the middle and anterior columns facilitates healing because increased surface area and favorable biomechanical conditions allow the bone graft to experience compression forces. The preponderance of recent evidence demonstrates equivalent outcomes in terms of pain and healing for individuals managed with or without a spinal orthosis following varying types of lumbar surgery.[85–88] Today postoperative bracing is reserved for patients who feel more comfortable with support (a lumbar corset) or those with poor bone quality or technical issues leading to concerns about healing or the stabilization provided by the instrumentation.

Patients with acute LBP may find the additional support and postural reminder of a lumbar corset helpful for pain reduction. Lumbar corsets are generally semirigid or flexible braces (Fig. 13.8A). Their function is to reduce gross trunk motion and increase intracavitary pressure in the abdomen by transmitting a three-point pressure system to the lumbar spine. They are designed to support the trunk in a neutral sagittal alignment and provide a kinesthetic reminder to limit motion. The lumbar corset has little resistance to gross body motion during sitting and standing.[89] Typically the anterior borders of the lumbosacral corset are superior to the symphysis pubis and inferior to the xiphoid process. The posterior borders extend between the sacrococcygeal junction of the pelvis and the inferior angle of the scapulae; some may incorporate shoulder straps. The Chairback Orthosis (Fig. 13.8B) is an lumbosacral corset with both a thoracic and a pelvic band connected by two paraspinal bars for optimized sagittal control. A pair of lateral bars can also be added for improved coronal control (the Knight orthosis).

The literature on the effectiveness of the corset is conflicting. In 2001 a systematic review of randomized controlled trial (RCT) and non-RCTs demonstrated no evidence that spinal orthoses were effective in the prevention or management of LBP.[90] An orthosis should be used in conjunction with a rehabilitation program focused on core strengthening and stabilization in these patients. A review published in 2022 examining the effectiveness of lumbar supports in managing LBP went further by distinguishing diagnosis and orthoses characteristics.[91] Pooled data revealed a positive effect only for orthoses that specifically addressed the biomechanical cause of patients' pain. No measurable effect was found where diagnosis or type of brace was unspecified.[91] These findings make clear the need for careful clinical examination and evaluation with prescription of an optimally fitting orthosis specific to individual needs. Landauer and Trieb present proposed nomenclature and orthoses descriptions as well as a treatment concept in chart form to help clinicians make orthosis choices.[91] Spinal orthoses have been found to have a deconditioning effect on the paraspinal muscles and trunk stabilizers. Electromyographic studies have found conflicting results, with some demonstrating a significant reduction in muscle activity in the brace and others finding either unchanged or increased activity.[92] An exercise regimen should be maintained when the clinical situation allows and the orthosis should be discontinued as soon as possible. Newer activating orthotic designs using exoskeletons or flexible support with muscle assistance during movement have been developed to help mitigate some of the complications of traditional rigid orthoses.[3,93,94] Evidence of their usefulness is not strong at this point and more research with well-designed RCTs is needed.

Cervicothoracolumbosacral Orthosis

Cases in which patients sustain multiple traumas to the cervical, thoracic, lumbar, and sacral segments of the spine may require the use of more complicated orthotic design. The cervicothoracolumbosacral orthosis (CTLSO) may be used to address the issues of stabilization and motion control involving multiple spinal segments. Use of CTLSOs is not limited to cases of multiple spinal segment trauma. It may also be employed pre- or postoperatively as a supplement to surgical procedures of the cervical spine requiring

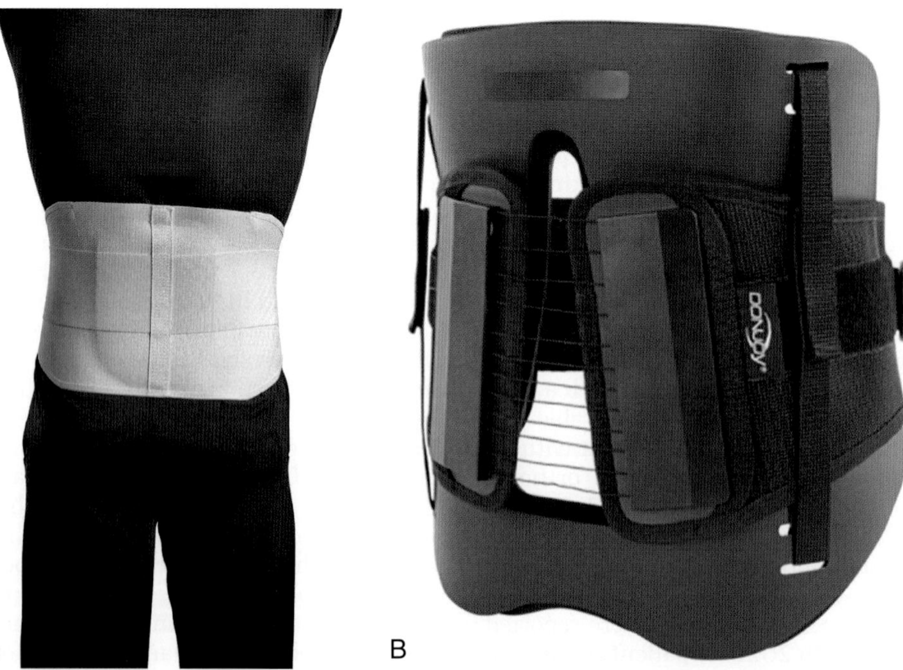

Fig. 13.8 (A) Lumbar corset (AliMed, Inc. www.alimed.com). (B) Chairback orthosis (DonJoy DJO Global http://djomerchandise.com/).

the level of control provided by a TLSO combined with a cervical component such as the Minerva collar or a SOMI proximal cervical component. Donning, doffing, and skincare issues for CTLSOs are consistent with those for CTOs and TLSOs.

Sacroiliac Joints

Estimates vary regarding the role that the sacroiliac (SI) joints play in the incidence of LBP. Estimates of LBP originating in the SI joints range between 22%[95,96] and 30%[97] of cases. The SI joints are vital links between the spinal column and the lower extremities.[98] They are the critical connection for the successful transference of upper body weight to the legs.[98] The etiology of SI joint pain covers a wide range, including rheumatoid arthritis, osteoarthritis, tumor, infection, pregnancy, and trauma.[99,100] An orthosis for the treatment of SI joint pain is the sacroiliac orthosis, also known as an SI or pelvic belt. The mechanism involved is a compressive or "squeezing" force across the pelvis that is transferred to the SI joints as a stabilizing force to reduce joint laxity, restrict motion, and thereby reduce pain.[98,101–103] Positioning of the SI belt during donning is key to the successful mitigation of pain related to the SI joint. The SI belt should be positioned and then tightened just proximal to the greater trochanters.[98,103,104] The position of the belt has been found to play a greater role in the reduction of SI joint laxity than the belt's tension.[105]

EMERGING TRENDS

Commonly reported complications of traditional rigid orthoses include: discomfort, decreased compliance, atrophy of paraspinal muscles, and restriction of chest expansion leading to chest infections.[3] Emerging technologies are producing orthoses such as exoskeletons and soft robotics proposed to support the spine and reduce pain while minimizing complications.[3,93] These new designs may have potential to reduce work-related injuries, and support osteoporotic spines, but much is yet to be worked out in manufacturing and safety standards before they are widely available for clinical research.[93] Several iterations of the Spinomed and Spinomed active orthosis (medi GmbH&Co. KG, Bayreuth, Germany) do have published research on efficacy and patient tolerance when worn by females ≥65 years with chronic back pain and chronic OVF.[22,106,107] An RCT with 96 participants compared wearing the activating spinal orthosis for 6 months to an exercise group and a control group.[106]

Improvements in back extensor strength and a reduction in pain were found in the orthotic group, though results did not differ significantly from the other two groups. A follow-up qualitative study revealed that the orthosis was well tolerated by the females.[22] A more recent 2022 RCT compared wearing a newer version of the orthosis to an untreated control group in a sample of 80 females ≥65 years old with kyphosis, back pain, and no OVF within the preceding 3 months.[107]

The "Spinomed active" comes in 36 standard sizes and six of the participants had custom-made orthoses. The posterior supportive splint was individually shaped to each participant to assure optimal fit and sensory input to activate spinal extensors. The participants in the orthotics group initially wore the device for 2 hours/day and increased to two 2- to 3 hour sessions/day. Researchers followed up with the participants with biweekly phone calls and adjustments were made to devices as needed by the orthopedic technician who originally fitted the orthosis. Results showed large and significant favorable effects for the orthotic group in back pain, disability, and kyphosis angle. Positive effects were also found for functional ability and trunk strength though they did not quite reach significance. No differences were noted for respiratory function and no adverse effects were reported.[107]

Synthesizing all the literature reviewed for the regional sections of this chapter, some recurring themes are evident. First, in order to be effective, orthosis must be designed to address the specific dysfunction the patient presents with and must be individually and properly fitted. Flexible orthoses seem to be better tolerated than rigid, and fewer hours of wearing per day than previously thought may allow positive benefits for pain and posture. Rigid orthoses may be needed to stabilize unstable spine segments. Patient education in wearing, donning, doffing, care, cleaning, purpose and potential adverse effects of the orthosis is critical to success. Follow-up by a member of the rehab team helps to improve compliance and identify potential problems early on. Putting all these tips in place will help to obtain the best result for each patient.

Scoliosis

Scoliosis is a general term that refers to a 3D spinal deformity characterized by coronal displacement of vertebral bodies away from the axis of gravity combined with abnormal vertebral rotation (Fig. 13.9). There are many types of scoliosis as well as many etiologies. Today, the only type of scoliosis that is typically and frequently managed with a spinal orthosis is the idiopathic curve. Adolescent idiopathic scoliosis (AIS) is the most common type of scoliosis and refers to a curvature and rotational deformity of the spine that develops with growth presenting in 10- to 18-year olds.[108] It can occur in the upper thoracic, thoracic, thoracolumbar, or lumbar spine, or some combination. There is often a primary curve (the curve with abnormal growth)

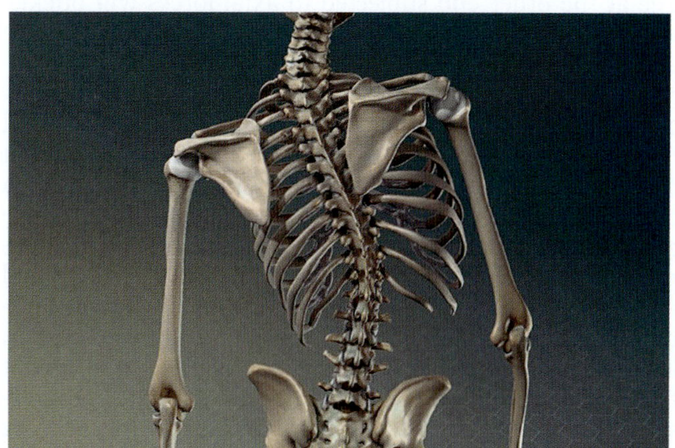

Fig. 13.9 Skeleton with scoliosis trunk shift (Dr. Spivak executivespine-surgery.com).

and a compensatory curve, which is a second region of the spine curving in the opposite direction to the primary curve to keep the head centered over the pelvis. The age of the child, the growth remaining, and the curve pattern all have implications for prognosis. Successful conservative management with a spinal brace is primarily associated with extent of initial in-brace correction and normalization of spinal curves.[109,110] Conversely, a large thoracic rotation is a negative prognostic indicator.[110]

PREVALENCE AND NATURAL HISTORY

Through frontal plane radiographs, the upper and lower end vertebra of the curve are identified and the Cobb angle is calculated from the orientation of these vertebrae. A wide range of prevalence (0.93%–12%) of mild scoliosis with Cobb angles >10 degrees has been reported for the general population with about equal incidence in males and females.[111] However, progression of AIS is more prevalent in females with the ratio of girls to boys progressing to 7:1 for curvatures above 30 degrees.[111] Large curvatures are associated with functional limitations, disability, health problems, and decreased quality of life in adulthood highlighting the need for intervention before skeletal maturity.[112,113]

The most important determinants of the likelihood of progression are those that reflect skeletal maturity: age, menarchal status, and the presence of mature growth centers on radiographs of the pelvis (Risser sign) or hand. The likelihood of progression determines the need for treatment; those at highest risk are those with a younger age at diagnosis, a curve that appears before the onset of menstruation, a double curve pattern, and a curve that is documented to change more than 5 degrees on serial radiographs taken at 6-month intervals. Curve magnitude and rotation are both correlated with increased progression rates.[8,114] This is the basis for the recommendation that curves >50 degrees in a growing child be treated surgically.

BIOMECHANICS

Curves progress when buckling loads change during growth, along with other hormonal and developmental factors. A straight, flexible column fixed at the base and free at the other end subjected to axial forces will buckle, which in the spine results in a combination of curvature and rotation. The loads at which these processes occur are related to the length and rigidity of the spine. The adolescent growth spurt results in a significant increase in spinal length and may result in increased flexibility as well, which contributes to the drastic increases in curve progression commonly observed during the adolescent years. As the curve progresses, a feedforward cycle is created. With curve progression, the spine is subjected to increasingly abnormal force vectors and deviates further from the normal anatomic alignment at which it is best equipped to resist such loading. Braces used for scoliosis are designed to interrupt this feedforward cycle. Efficacy of bracing to limit progression of high-risk curves was demonstrated by the Bracing in Adolescents with Idiopathic Scoliosis Trial.[115] This large, multicenter trial was stopped early due to clear benefit of bracing over observation.

There are three primary mechanisms by which an orthosis exerts forces on a developing spine: end-point control, curve correction, and transverse loading.[116–120] End-point control is the ability of the orthosis to constrain the spine. An example is the neck ring at the proximal end of the Milwaukee brace, which can control the position of the upper thoracic spine relative to the pelvis. Curve correction has the greatest effect because it stiffens the spine and reduces the curve, which in turn decreases the load on the spine and slows the rate of deformation. Transverse loading at the apex is the primary mode of correction within modern orthoses, but it begins to lose efficacy as the curves get larger.[118,119] Previously bracing was purported only to halt the progression of the curve until skeletal maturity or surgery. However, with new designs and more customized fit, partial curve correction is possible provided certain bracing and patient characteristics are fulfilled. There are some variations in the literature, but in general these are the most reported criteria for success. Patients should be skeletally immature with flexible curves of <50 degrees, and willing to be compliant with a wearing schedule of >20 hours/day. The brace should be designed to specifically address the individual's type of curve, immediate in-brace correction should be ≥50%, and a rigid type orthosis is used for larger curves. The brace will need to be worn until skeletal maturity (2–5 years) since flexible curves will regress back when the brace is removed.[117,121] For more details and assistance with decision-making for specific curve characteristics, the reader is directed to the most recent expert-derived guidelines published by the International Scientific Society on Scoliosis Orthopaedic and Rehabilitation Treatment (SOSORT).[111]

EVALUATION

The first step in evaluating a child with a spinal curvature is a thorough orthopedic history including age, growth patterns, family history of spinal problems, the age at which the curve was discovered, and any treatment that has previously been used. The primary goal of an orthosis in treating a scoliotic deformity is to control remaining spinal growth so that the spine reaches maturity with an acceptable curvature. There is no role for using an orthosis to prevent scoliosis, and at this time the evidence that bracing can ultimately reduce a curvature is still limited.[122,123] Scoliosis progresses as the spine grows, so an adolescent at the end of spinal growth has very little risk of progression, and there is no role for bracing a curve that has already reached a size where surgery is indicated.[115,118] Therefore it is critical to identify children with scoliosis at the early stages. A national screening program has been adopted in many countries for this purpose.

Physical examination and radiographs are used to measure the size, flexibility, and effects of each spinal curvature. The Scoliosis Research Society has adopted a set of terms and definitions to describe scoliosis as well as to describe the multitude of spinal conditions that can lead to scoliosis. Curves can be described either by etiology of the structural changes (Box 13.2) or by the spinal level of the anatomic apex of the curve. In a cervical scoliosis, the apex of the curve is at or between the vertebral body of C1 and C6. In a cervicothoracic curve, the apex is at C7, C8, or T1. A thoracic curve has an apex at or between T2 and T11. A thoracolumbar curve reaches its apex at the T12 or L1 vertebral body. A lumbar curve occurs at L2, L3, or L4, whereas a lumbosacral curve reaches its apex at L5 or S1. Numerous descriptive terms are also used in the diagnosis, evaluation, and management of scoliosis (Table 13.2). These standards and definitions are used throughout this chapter.

Scoliosis can also be described by etiology. A child or adolescent who develops scoliosis after relatively typical growth and development is diagnosed as having idiopathic scoliosis. An individual who develops scoliosis as a secondary complication of nervous system or muscle disease is described as having neuromuscular scoliosis. Clinical examination includes an assessment of the patient's posture, noting any

Box 13.2 Classification System for Idiopathic and Neuromuscular Structural Scoliosis

Idiopathic

Infantile (0–3 Years)

- Resolving
- Progressive

Juvenile (3–10 Years)
Adolescent (10–18 Years) Neuropathic

Neuromuscular

- Upper motor neuron
  - Cerebral palsy
  - Spinocerebellar degeneration
  - Friedreich ataxia
  - Charcot-Marie-Tooth disease
  - Roussy-Lévy disease
  - Syringomyelia
  - Spinal cord tumor
  - Spinal cord trauma
  - Other
- Lower motor neuron
  - Poliomyelitis
  - Other viral myelitides
  - Trauma
  - Spinal muscular atrophy
  - Werdnig-Hoffmann disease
  - Kugelberg-Welander disease
  - Myelomeningocele (paralytic)
  - Dysautonomia (Riley-Day syndrome)

Other

- Myopathic
- Arthrogryposis
- Muscular dystrophy
  - Duchenne (pseudohypertrophy)
  - Limb girdle
  - Fiber-type disproportion
- Congenital hypotonia
  - Myotonic dystrophica
  - Other

Table 13.2 Glossary and Definitions of Terms in Scoliosis

Term	Definition
Adolescent scoliosis	Spinal curvature presenting at or about the onset of puberty and before maturity.
Adult scoliosis	Spinal curvature that develops after skeletal maturity.
Angle of thoracic inclination	The angle between the horizontal plane and inclination plane across the posterior rib cage at the greatest prominence of a rib hump, assessed with the trunk flexed 90 degrees at the hips.
Apical vertebra	The most rotated vertebra in a curve; the most deviated vertebra from the vertical axis of the patient.
Body alignment 1. Alignment of the midpoint of the occiput over the sacrum in the same vertical plane as the shoulders over the hips. 2. In radiography, when the sum of the angular deviations of the spine in one direction is equal to that in the opposite direction (also described as balance or compensation).	
Café au lait spots	Light-brown, irregular areas of skin pigmentation; if they are sufficient in number and have smooth margins, they suggest neurofibromatosis.
Cobb angle or method	On radiograph, the uppermost and lowermost vertebrae in the curve are identified; a perpendicular line (curve measurement) is drawn from the transverse axes of these vertebrae, and the angle formed at their intersection (Cobb angle) measures the severity of the curve; if vertebral end plates are poorly visualized, a line through the bottom or top of the pedicles can be used.
Compensatory curve	A curve, which can be structural, above or below the major curve that tends to maintain normal body alignment.
Congenital scoliosis	Scoliosis due to congenitally anomalous vertebral development.
Double major scoliosis	Scoliosis with two structural curves.
Double thoracic curves	Two structural curves within the thoracic spine.

(*Continued*)

Table 13.2 Glossary and Definitions of Terms in Scoliosis—Cont'd

Term	Definition
End vertebra	
Fractional curve	Compensatory curve that is incomplete because it returns to the erect; its only horizontal vertebra is its caudad or cephalad one.
Full curve	Curve in which the only horizontal vertebra is at the apex.
Gibbus	Sharply angular kyphos.
Hyperkyphosis	Sagittal alignment of the thoracic spine in which more than the normal amount of kyphosis is present (a kyphos).
Hypokyphosis	Sagittal alignment of the thoracic spine in which less than the normal amount of kyphosis is present but not so severe as to be lordotic.
Hysterical scoliosis	Nonstructural deformity of the spine that develops as a manifestation of a conversion reaction.
Idiopathic scoliosis	Structural spinal curvature for which no cause is established.
Iliac epiphysis or apophysis	Epiphysis along the wing of an ilium.
Inclinometer	Instrument used to measure the angle of thoracic inclination or rib hump.
Infantile scoliosis	Spinal curvature that develops during the first 3 years of life.
Juvenile scoliosis	Spinal curvature that develops between the skeletal age of 3 years and the onset of puberty (10 years).
Kyphos	Change in alignment of a segment of the spine in the sagittal plane that increases the posterior convex angulation; an abnormally increased kyphosis.
Kyphoscoliosis	Spine with scoliosis and a true hyperkyphosis; a rotatory deformity with only apparent kyphosis should not be described by this term.
Kyphosing scoliosis	Scoliosis with marked rotation such that lateral bending of the rotated spine mimics kyphosis.
Lordoscoliosis	Scoliosis associated with an abnormal anterior angulation in the sagittal plane.
Major curve	Term used to designate the largest structural curve.
Minor curve	Term used to refer to the smallest curve, which is always more flexible than the major curve.
Nonstructural curve	Curve that has no structural component and that corrects or overcorrects on recumbent side-bending radiographs.
Pelvic obliquity	Deviation of the pelvis from the horizontal in the frontal plane; fixed pelvic obliquities can be attributable to contractures either above or below the pelvis.
Primary curve	First or earliest of several curves to appear if identifiable.
Risser sign	Rating system used to indicate skeletal maturity, based on degree of ossification of the iliac epiphysis.
Rotational prominence	In the forward-bending position, the thoracic prominence on one side is usually due to vertebral rotation, causing rib prominence; in the lumbar spine, the prominence is usually due to rotation of the lumbar vertebrae.
Skeletal age (bone age)	Age obtained by comparing an anteroposterior radiograph of the left hand and wrist with the standards of the Greulich and Pyle atlas.
Structural curve	Segment of the spine with a lateral curvature that lacks normal flexibility; radiographically, it is identified by the complete lack of a curve on a supine film or by the failure to demonstrate complete segmental mobility on supine side-bending films.
Vertebral end plates	Superior and inferior plates of cortical bone of the vertebral body adjacent to the intervertebral disc.
Vertebral growth plate	Cartilaginous surface covering the top and bottom of a vertebral body, which is responsible for linear growth of the vertebra.
Vertebral ring apophyses	Most reliable index of vertebral immaturity, seen best in lateral radiographs or in the lumbar region in side-bending anteroposterior views.

asymmetry in trunk alignment, shoulder height, scapular prominence, and pelvic rotation. Special attention is paid to the degree of thoracic kyphosis and lumbar lordosis as well as any tendency toward trunk shift to the right or left (spinal decompensation) (Fig. 13.10A). The Adams forward-bending test assesses the rotation of each curve by the degree of prominence over the apices, and the patient can be flexed laterally while bent forward to assess the degree of curve flexibility (Fig. 13.10B). Complete neurologic, skin, and cardiopulmonary examinations are then performed.

The timing of orthotic treatment is an important determinant of efficacy. The principles have remained the same regardless of the orthosis used. First, treatment should be initiated before skeletal maturity, when there is growth remaining, because bracing is effective only in a growing child; curves <20 degrees are generally observed and may be managed with physiotherapeutic scoliosis-specific exercises (PSSE), but once a curve is >20 degrees and/or demonstrates significant progression, bracing is initiated. Second, most braces should be worn full time, which has been variably described as somewhere between 18 and 24 hours/day.[111,117,124] The SOSORT guidelines recognize a "dose-response" and suggest the optimal number of hours may be individualized based on a number of factors including severity of curvature, age of the patient, and goal of treatment. Third, the brace should be worn until skeletal maturity. Last, there should be a weaning period accompanied by a rehabilitation program to rebuild muscle strength once skeletal maturity has been reached. A predictive model using in-brace correction and scoliometer measurements has been created to help identify those individuals who are likely to demonstrate progression of the curvature despite bracing.[125] This tool may be useful in management planning.

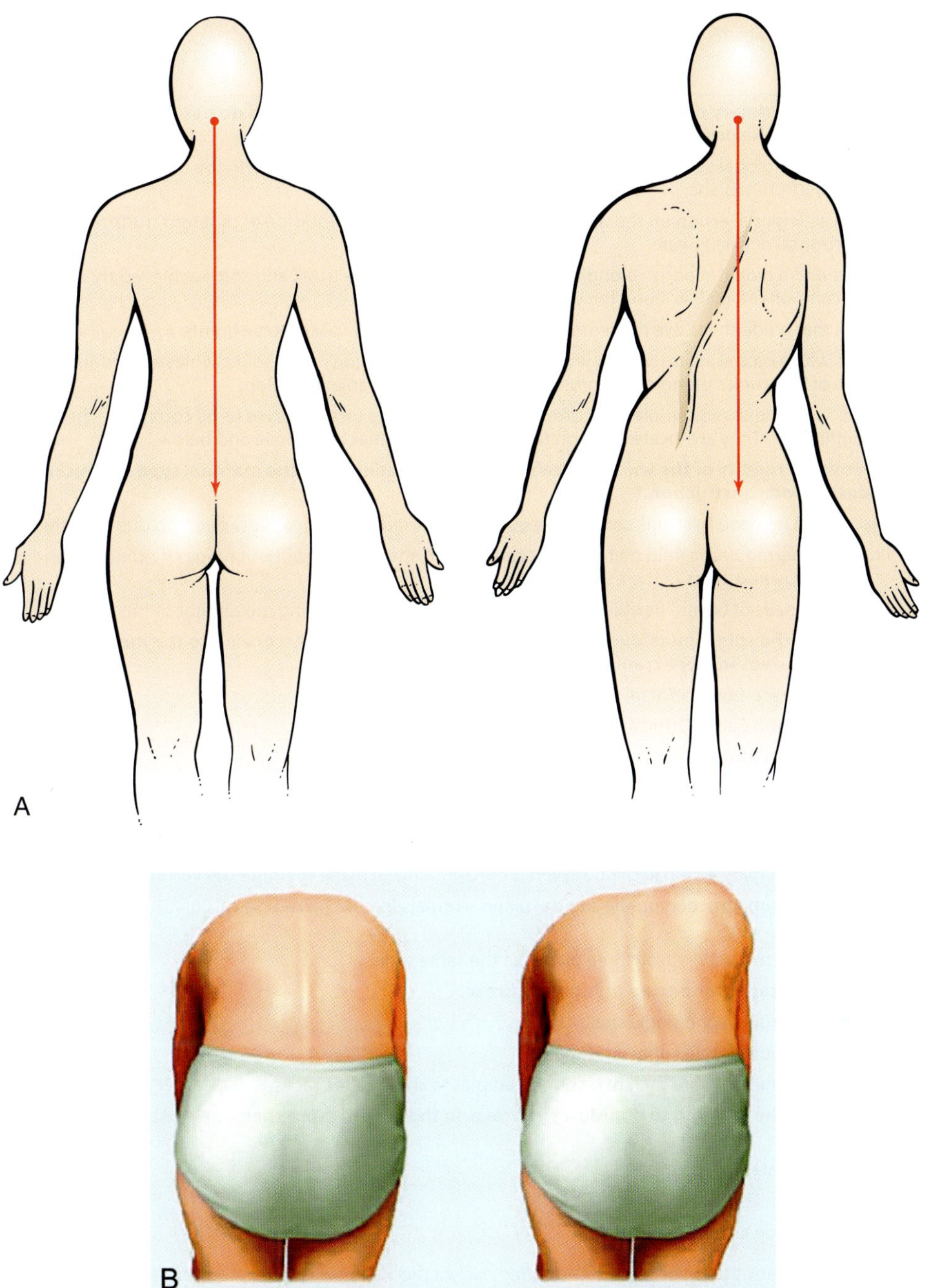

Fig. 13.10 (A) *Left*, normal skeletal alignment. *Right*, lateral trunk shift—scoliosis. (B) Adam's forward bend test. (A, From Schwartz M. *Textbook of Physical Diagnosis*. Seventh ed. Elsevier; 2014. B, Modified from Fine NF and Stokes OM. Clinical examination of the spine. *Surgery*. 2018;36(7):357–361.)

TYPES OF BRACES

There are varying reports on all aspects of scoliosis care in the literature, including brace efficacy, and few well-designed studies comparing outcomes between different braces. Negrini et al. suggest that one factor "impairing research and leading to clinical confusion in the field is the absence of a classification to understand differences and commonalities among braces."[126] Through an extensive qualitative research and consensus process involving the top experts from related professional societies around the world, definitions and a classification were published in 2022 for use in research, education, and clinical practice.[126]

See Table 13.3 for definitions of the terms used in the brace classification system. There are many different types of orthoses for scoliosis, with more under development. Braces have been generally described by the spinal region (CTLSO, TLSO, etc.) and by amount of rigidity. Very rigid braces are meant to stabilize and stop or reverse curve progression, whereas elastic or very flexible orthoses are meant to facilitate normal muscle activity and spinal movement during functional tasks. The new classification includes anatomy and rigidity as well as action, corrective plane, and construction. See Table 13.4 for classification of currently available braces. Widespread use of this classification system will enhance research and clinical decision-making. A

Table 13.3 The Definitions of the Terms Used in the Brace Classification System

Term	Definition
Primary action	**The overall primary mechanism of action of the brace. The terms used do not describe an exclusive biomechanical action but the prevalent one.**[a]
Bending	Braces with a global action of bending the trunk towards curve correction (in the direction of its convexity), mainly in the coronal/frontal plane.
Detorsion	Braces with global action on the whole spine through mutual derotation of different trunk regions, mainly in the transverse (horizontal or axial) plane.
Elongation	Braces with a global action in elongation/decompression of the trunk and spine achieved through distraction effect of cervical component, mainly along the vertical axis.
Movement	Braces that guide the active movement of the patient through specific constraints.
Push-up	Braces with a global action of elongation and localized detorsion of the spine achieved through three-dimensional compression of the trunk's pathological prominences in a caudo-cranial direction.
Three points	Braces with one or more triplets of corrective pressure forces on the curves to be corrected. They can be on a single plane or multiplanar. They are located one on the apex and the other two above and below.
Rigidity	**The overall rigidity of the whole brace's structure. It depends on the material type, its thickness, and the brace design and construction.***
Very rigid	Braces with (almost) full trunk coverage requiring hinges (or similar) to allow opening due to material rigidity.
Rigid	Braces of thermoplastic rigid material that can be deformed (opens without hinges if monocot) and multisegmented braces with uncovered areas of the trunk.
Elastic	Braces of elastic or (semi-) flexible plastic or multiple materials allowing movement of the trunk and spine.
Anatomy	**Regions of the spine (joint levels) where the orthosis is located. According to the mechanisms of action, they can also control curves in more cranial spine regions.**
CTLSO	Cervico-Thoraco-Lumbo-Sacral Orthosis.
TLSO	Thoraco-Lumbo-Sacral Orthosis.
LSO	Lumbo-Sacral Orthosis.
Primary corrective plane	**Main plane of action of the brace. In the case of two planes, the appropriate terms are combined.**
Frontal	Braces with primary action in the coronal/frontal plane to bring vertebral bodies toward the spinal midline.
Transverse	Braces with primary action in the transverse/horizontal/axial plane to rotate the vertebral bodies toward the spinal midline.
Sagittal	Braces with primary action on the sagittal plane, normalizing the physiological curvature of lumbar lordosis and/or thoracic kyphosis.
Three dimensional	Braces with direct action in all three planes at the same time.
Valves	**Pieces of material connected to form the brace.**
Monocot	Rigid braces built in one single shell.
Bivalve	Rigid braces built in two connected shells.
Multisegmented	Rigid braces built in more than two connected pieces and elastic braces.
Closure	**Location of the opening to don/doff the brace. In the case of more than one closure, the two appropriate terms are combined.**
Ventral	Braces with anterior closure.
Dorsal	Braces with posterior closure.
Lateral	Braces with side closure.

Participants accepted that the definitions are intuitive because of the current lack of precise knowledge of most braces' biomechanical effects on the trunk and spine. The primary authors' expertise provided these definitions, and the other experts' consensus formally accepted them.
[a]By definition, all braces act on the trunk three dimensionally. Consequently, each action or corrective plane of braces must be considered the primary, not exclusive.
Reproduced from Negrini S, Aulisa AG, Cerny P, et al. The classification of scoliosis braces developed by SOSORT with SRS, ISPO, and POSNA and approved by ESPRM. *Eur Spine J.* 2022;31:980–989.[126]

few of the more commonly used braces of different types are further discussed in this chapter.

Milwaukee Brace

The historic Milwaukee brace was developed by Blount and Schmidt in 1944. As a rigid CTLSO, it was initially employed as a postoperative modality but soon found a more important role. Since 1954 it has been used in the nonoperative treatment of idiopathic scoliosis.[127] The brace consists of a pelvic section, which helps to reduce lumbar lordosis, and an attached "superstructure." The superstructure consists of three metal uprights that are attached to a neck ring superiorly. It provides an end point of control to make the spine structurally more rigid and better aligned; it also provides a means of attachment for the spinal pads (Fig. 13.11). This style is considered a full-time brace and should be worn 23 hours a day. The initial design incorporated distraction; however, this has since been modified due to problems with malocclusion of the jaw. Temporomandibular joint disorders were found to be prevalent in adults who had completed treatment for AIS with the Milwaukee brace 23 years earlier.[128] Subsequent to the Milwaukee brace, various

Table 13.4 Classification of the Braces Currently Available and Published

Anatomy	Rigidity	Primary Action	Primary Corrective Plane	Construction	Closure	Brace Name
TLSO	Very Rigid	Detorsion	Frontal and Sagittal	Bivalve	Ventral	ART
		Push-Up	Three dimensional	Bivalve	Ventral	Sforzesco
	Rigid	Bending	Frontal	Monocot	Ventral	Charleston
						Providence
		Detorsion	Three dimensional	Monocot	Ventral	Chêneau
						Dynamic Derotating
						Rigo-Chêneau System
		Push-Up	Three-dimensional	Bivalve	Ventral	Sibilla
		Three point	Frontal	Monocot	Ventral	Wilmington
			Frontal and transverse	Monocot	Dorsal	Boston
			Sagittal	Monocot	Dorsal	TLI
			Three dimensional	Multisegmented	Ventral	Lyon
	Elastic	Movement	Frontal and Transverse	Multisegmented	Lateral	TriaC
			Three dimensional	Multisegmented	Frontal	Spinecor
CTLSO	Rigid	Elongation	Frontal and Sagittal	Multisegmented	Dorsal	Milwaukee
LSO	Rigid	Detorsion	Frontal and Transverse	Monocot	Ventral	PASB

ART, Asymmetric rigid three dimensional; *PASB*, progressive action short brace; *TLI*, thoracolumbar Lordotic Intervention; *TriaC*, three C, comfort, control, and cosmetics.

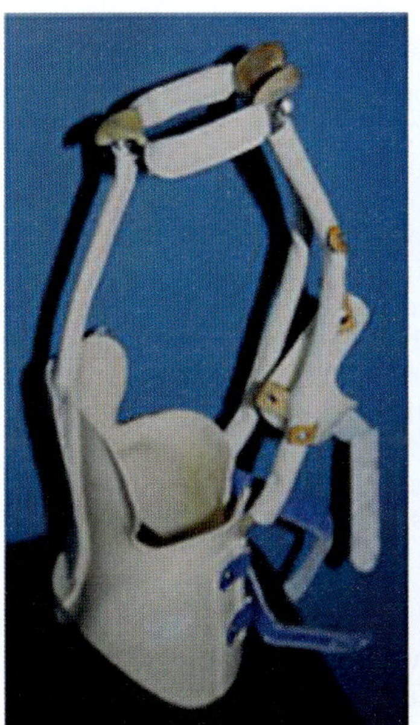

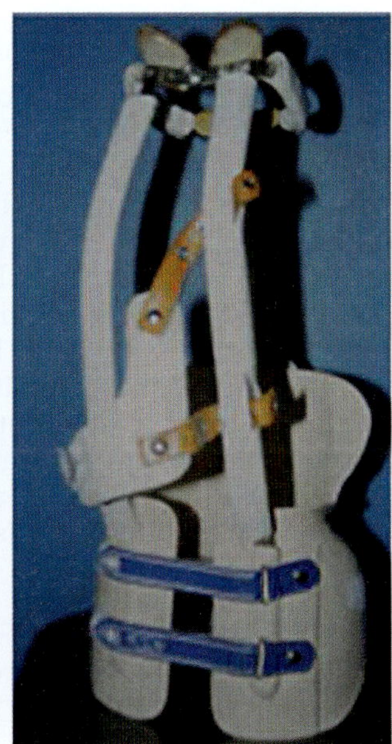

Fig. 13.11 Milwaukee brace. (From Palazzo C, Salihan F, Rivel M. Schuermann's disease: an update. *Jt Bone Spine*. 2013;81(3):209–214.)

low-profile TLSOs have been introduced. Most of these spinal orthoses are named for the city in which they were developed (e.g., Boston brace, Miami orthosis, Wilmington brace, Lyon brace). These spinal orthoses share one characteristic: all control the alignment of the thoracolumbosacral spine but have no superstructure. The Milwaukee brace is still used for upper thoracic and double curves, but is mentioned here primarily for its historic significance.[117] It requires a dedicated patient and family for compliance.

Boston Thoracolumbosacral Orthosis

In 1972, in response to patient concerns about the bulkiness and neck ring of the Milwaukee brace, Hall created a lower-profile modular TLSO, known as the *Boston brace*.[129] It is a rigid underarm TLSO that, with various modifications, has become the most prevalent type of orthosis used. The original Boston brace consisted of multiple modules that were fabricated in different sizes and could be combined to provide a custom-fitted brace that did not require as much time or expertise on the part of the orthotist.[129] The Boston brace has been determined to be effective in controlling progression of lower thoracic and upper lumbar curves, with maximum correction for curves with an apex between T6 and T9, provided the brace is worn for at least 18 hours/day.[130] Equivalent results have been found with the use of the original Boston brace or its related products compared with the Milwaukee brace, with the possible exception of use for high thoracic curves.[131] A new 3D-printed version has demonstrated good short-term outcomes for a sample of patients with AIS 1 year after being fitted.[132] Eighty-four percent of patients with a single curve and 69% with a double curve demonstrated no progression, or reduction of their curves. More time in brace was associated with improved results. A retrospective review followed 175 patients with Juvenile Idiopathic Scoliosis managed with the Boston brace to skeletal maturity.[121] Surgery was avoided in 33% of the children with minimal to no curve progression. Twelve of the 28 who avoided surgery actually improved spinal alignment >10 degrees. Boston braces are popular because of their low-profile and partially open design, which is comfortable and well tolerated.

NIGHTTIME BRACES

The requirement of having to wear a rigid brace all day, as with the Boston brace, negatively impacts the daily activities of adolescents and jeopardizes compliance with the treatment. Therefore hypercorrective nighttime braces have been developed that allow the young patient freedom during the day. The Charleston brace and the Providence nighttime brace (PNB) are two of the most common of this type.

One comparative study between the Boston and Charleston orthoses showed the Boston orthosis to be more effective in all curve patterns but the Charleston orthosis to have equal efficacy in 25- to 35-degree single thoracolumbar or lumbar curves.[133] In a comparison between the Boston brace and the PNB, no significant difference in curve progression was found between groups of adolescent females with AIS.[134] Both brace protocols were effective for lower thoracic and upper lumbar curves. The theoretical advantages of the nighttime orthoses in terms of body image and socialization issues are intuitive but have not been shown in rigorous studies; likewise, compliance problems are similar to those with other braces. A 2021 systematic review and meta-analysis comparing bracing concepts revealed that many of the bracing studies had high risk for bias.[135] Conclusions that could be drawn were that both the rigid full-time braces and the nighttime braces were on average 73% to 85% effective in preventing curve progression with no significant difference between types. Both of these approaches were found to be more successful than soft bracing, which on average was ~64% (55%–70%) effective.

SpineCor

In the early 1990s, the SpineCor brace was developed to prevent the complications associated with rigid bracing such as reduced breathability, bulkiness, and physical constraints resulting in muscle stiffness and atrophy. This flexible system uses elastic straps wrapped around the torso to apply 3D corrective forces as the individual moves.[120] The components of the brace include a pelvic base, two thigh bands, two crotch bands, a cotton bolero, and four to five corrective elastic bands that may be arranged in a number of different configurations depending on the specific deformity being treated. The pelvic base is a belt that includes three pieces of soft thermoplastic material. Fitting patients with the brace is done in a systematic fashion using supplementary computer software; a training course is offered to providers for education on proper fitting technique.

Coillard and Rivard, the developers of the SpineCor brace, published the initial clinical results in 2003.[136] They reported on the treatment results of 195 patients between 6 and 14 years of age with idiopathic scoliosis curves between 15 and 50 degrees and Risser stages 0 to 3. Success in their study was defined as either a correction or stabilization of about 5 degrees or more. Failure was defined as worsening of the curve by more than 5 degrees. The authors found that at 2 years of follow-up, there was an overall correction of >5 degrees in 55% of patients, curve stabilization in 38%, and worsening by >5 degrees in 7% of patients. This equates to 93% success at 2 years. At 4 years of follow-up, the probability of success was 0.88 to 0.92. Coillard and Rivard published results of the same prospective cohort again in 2007 using the Scoliosis Research Society scoliosis research inclusion criteria.[137] A total of 170 patients were included in the study. The authors reported that successful treatment was achieved in 59.4% of patients at the time of brace discontinuation, with 22.9% requiring fusion during the treatment period, at which point 1.2% of patients had curves exceeding 45 degrees at maturity. These initial results reported by the developers of the SpineCor brace were promising; however, further studies by independent investigators have yielded some conflicting results.

Weiss and Weiss[138] published the results of a small study that compared treatment with a SpineCor brace with TLSO bracing. The authors compared 12 SpineCor patients with 15 TLSO patients and found that the SpineCor patients with a starting Cobb angle of 21 degrees progressed an average of 10 degrees after 21 months of treatment versus 0.2 degrees in the TLSO patients who had a starting Cobb angle of 33 degrees. Wong and colleagues[139] compared 22 SpineCor patients with 21 TLSO patients and demonstrated that 68% of SpineCor patients maintained curve progression of ≤5 degrees compared with 95% of TLSO patients. Gammon and colleagues[140] compared 35 patients treated with a TLSO with 32 patients treated with the SpineCor brace and found no significant difference between the two outcomes with respect to progression of ≤5 degrees (60% in TLSO and 53% in SpineCor) or success in avoiding curve progression past 45 degrees (80% in TLSO and 72% in SpineCor). However, a retrospective study of 243 patients with AIS treated with either the SpineCor or the Boston brace revealed greater curve progression in the SpineCor group.[141] A higher percentage of patients in the SpineCor group had curve progression equal to or greater than 6 degrees (76% compared with 55% in the Boston brace group). Additionally the average curve progression was 14.7 degrees (±11.9 degrees) in the SpineCor group compared with 9.6 degrees (±13.7 degrees) in the Boston brace group.[141] Overall, it appears that rigid bracing is at least slightly more effective in controlling curve progression and curve correction than the flexible SpineCor system. Efficacy depends, in large part, on time in brace for both systems; physical comfort and cosmetic considerations impact compliance with wearing schedules. Literature addressing the impact of the SpineCor brace on comfort and cosmesis is scant. In their 2008 study comparing the SpineCor brace with TLSO bracing, Wong and colleagues administered a questionnaire at 3, 9, and 18 months of treatment to gain information about patient acceptance of the brace.[139] The only significant differences noted were problems with toileting (greater in the SpineCor group) and donning/doffing the orthosis (greater in the TLSO group).

EMERGING TRENDS

New developments such as wearable technology and computer-aided design (CAD) and manufacture (CAM) are quickly changing the landscape of brace treatment, which had been fairly stable for decades. Actuators are improving tension control in dynamic braces to counter the effects of immobility at the same time as rigid braces are improving correction potential through use of body scan technology.[142,143] One example of a new active corrective orthosis is the robotic spine exoskeleton RoSE developed by Columbia engineers and intended for full-time wear.[120] It is a big advancement in dynamic orthoses but may be limited in use at this time by need for power to run the actuators, as well by its size and weight.

The rigid Chêneau brace and its derivatives are manufactured using CAD and some with CAM.[122,142] Chêneau derivatives are asymmetrical trunk orthoses individually manufactured to produce the specific counter pressures for a particular patient's curve pattern. See Fig. 13.12 for an example. Named derivatives include Cheneau-Toulouse-Munster, Cheneau-Rigo, and Gensingen brace/GBW. Reported

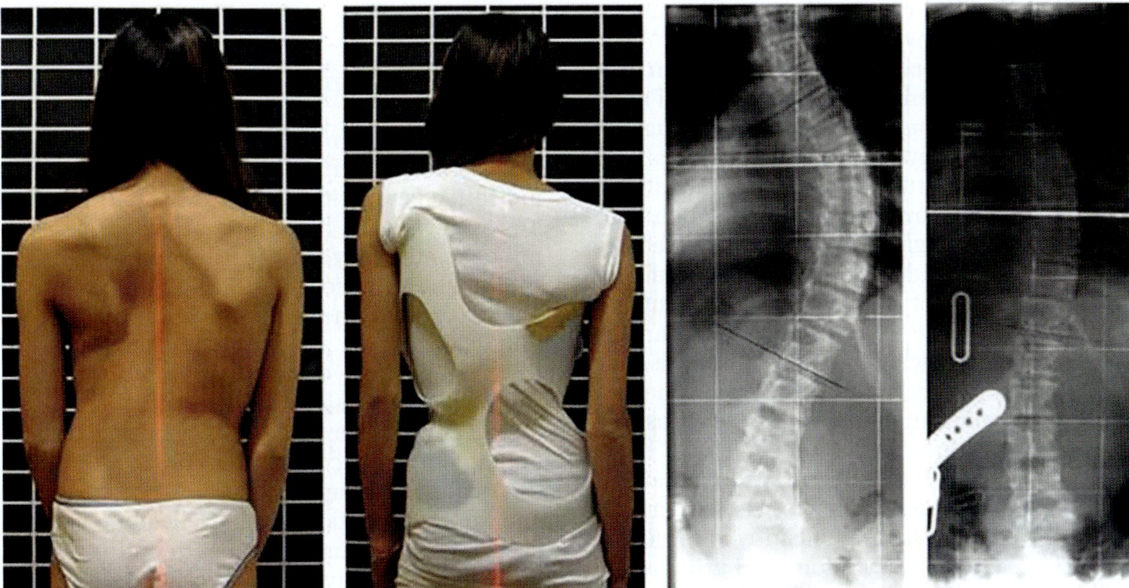

Fig. 13.12 Scoliosis patient in Chêneau brace correcting from 56 to 27 degrees Cobb (primary correction of 52%). Contributed by Wikimedia Commons, Weiss HR (CC by 2.0), https://creativecommons.org/licenses/by/2.0/

outcomes were derived with differing protocols with variable wearing times and length of treatment, as well as patient/curve-type selection.[122,142,144–147] Overall reported success rates with these braces (69%–93%) exceed previously published data for other types of TLSOs.[142,144,147] Chêneau-type hypercorrection braces have been found to be able to reduce large Cobb angles previously thought to require surgery (over 50 degrees), and completely correct smaller curves in skeletally immature adolescents.[142,147] Corrections were found to last, and in some cases to improve, 2 years after end of brace treatment.[142] Long-lasting improvement may be related to real structural change found in decreasing apical vertebral wedging.[122] Greater failure rates have been found for younger patients and higher thoracic curves.[144,146,147] Utilizing new technology, advancements in brace design are occurring rapidly; practitioners should keep an eye out for new developments and maintain open communication with orthotists and other team members.

Orthotic Prescription

An orthosis should initially improve the magnitude of the curve.[148] An orthosis that provides some correction theoretically decreases the load on the developing vertebrae, increasing the likelihood of long-term control of the deformity.[149] Over time the orthosis should be capable of preventing curve progression for long periods, frequently until the patient reaches skeletal maturity. Finally, an orthosis should be designed to be well tolerated and allow normal social and physical development; even then, compliance with brace wear is a significant issue for adolescents.[150–153] The effectiveness of an orthosis has been shown to be directly related to time spent in the brace, so the patient's willingness to wear the brace is of utmost importance.[154,155] "Smart braces" that measure compliance have demonstrated that even the most apparently compliant patient spends much less time in the brace than actually prescribed.[24,151,153,156,157]

The prescribing physician should specify the particular requirements for the orthosis based on the deformity, the goals of treatment, and his or her assessment of the likelihood for compliance. A team with physician, orthotist, or bioengineer should decide the exact type of brace, generally CTLSO or TLSO, with specifications of thoracic pad placement, lumbar pad placement, need for axillary slings, anterior gussets, trochanteric extensions, kyphosis pads, and the like depending on the type of deformity being treated. Computer-assisted design is useful in this process. Each pad requires a specified location, mediolateral orientation, and placement instructions. The choice between a CTLSO, TLSO, dynamic brace, or hypercorrection brace is dictated by the location of the curve, with high thoracic curves most effectively treated by the first. A TLSO has a much lower profile and is therefore more socially acceptable. The orthosis may be prefabricated and adjusted to fit or custom molded for patients who require additional adaptability.

The time in the orthosis is slowly increased over several weeks and then assessed both physically and radiographically by the prescribing physician. Specific pressure point relief and corrective pad adjustments may be required periodically because these patients are in a period of rapid spinal growth. For the youngest patients, multiple braces may be required before growth concludes.

Different goals are applied for patients with scoliosis of a neuromuscular origin such as cerebral palsy or muscular dystrophy. In these cases spinal bracing is frequently ineffective in significantly altering the progression of deformity but may still be useful when surgery is contraindicated.[158] Goals for the use of a spinal orthosis in such patients include maximizing sitting postural control, alleviation of pain, and facilitation of function and daily care.[158]

COMPLICATIONS

Complications with scoliosis orthoses are generally mild from a physical standpoint. Wearing a white cotton T-shirt under the brace can help reduce skin issues. However, bracing for AIS has also been associated with psychologic stress[159] and decreased pulmonary function.[160,161] Brace wearing in adolescents with AIS has been associated with increased anxiety.[162] Since compliance is a major factor in bracing success, efforts are being made to develop low-profile braces that may reduce wearer stress. A study of 63 adolescent patients demonstrated significantly lower stress levels when they were wearing the Cheneau light brace than when wearing their originally prescribed bulkier braces while obtaining equivalent correction in the brace.[159] A qualitative study of adolescents undergoing brace treatment revealed barriers to compliance included physical discomfort, cosmesis, and a lack of participation in the design and decision-making process.[23] To improve compliance adolescents' psychosocial needs should be addressed, as well as refinement of brace design. A meta-analysis of 237 patients with AIS determined that patients with thoracic curves who underwent preoperative brace treatment had significantly lower forced vital capacity and forced expiratory volume in 1 s than those who did not have bracing before surgery.[161] Finally, the successful use of bracing requires a supportive, constructive family and a similar relationship between healthcare team members and the adolescent.

FUTURE DIRECTIONS

The key to scoliosis treatment is to identify which children are likely to develop curve progression, avoiding bracing those with curves that will remain in the 25- to 35-degree range through their growth and therefore not require any intervention beyond scoliosis-specific exercises. Epidemiologic studies and skeletal maturity indicators have traditionally been used for this purpose and continue to be refined.[163] Recently genes that control the growth of scoliotic curves have been identified.[164–167] With this new information in combination with traditional methods, it may become possible to predict with a high degree of certainty which children will develop significant curves. Surgical treatments that harness asymmetric growth in the spine are also becoming available.[168–176] This combination of techniques may allow intervention before bracing becomes necessary. Meanwhile brace manufacturers are developing many new devices with the goals of decreasing deformity while increasing comfort, compliance, and chest expansion for pulmonary function.

Summary

Spinal orthoses are used to treat patients with a variety of spinal disorders ranging from LBP to complex spinal trauma and deformity. Selection of the appropriate orthosis for a specific patient is based on many factors, such as the indication for bracing and its severity, the age and body habitus of the patient, his or her willingness and ability to commit to a potentially long and difficult treatment course, and the patient's decisions after weighing the risks and benefits of orthotic treatment against other treatment modalities. These challenging treatment decisions are best managed by a multidisciplinary team comprising the treating physician, orthotist, physical and occupational therapists, and patient as well as his or her personal support network. Frequent follow-up and close communication between all members of the treatment team is essential to ensure thorough patient and family education, ensure adequate fit of the orthosis, evaluate for treatment efficacy, monitor for complications, and provide psychosocial support to the patient. Adequately addressing all of the issues surrounding orthotic treatment of spinal disease requires a thorough understanding of the natural history of the pathology being treated, the indications for bracing and use of specific braces, the mechanism of action of the orthosis, potential outcomes of the treatment, and potential complications and methods to minimize them. Comparative studies, long-term outcome analysis, and biomechanical studies have helped to promote understanding of and appropriate and effective use of spinal orthoses. Despite the large body of knowledge about these topics, there are still many unknowns surrounding spinal orthoses and their role in treating disorders of the spine. This chapter provides a brief overview of the basic functional anatomy of the spine, the fundamentals of spinal trauma and scoliosis, the various types of braces and their mechanisms of action and indications, and the potential complications. The ability to use spinal orthoses safely and effectively requires a comprehensive understanding of these topics.

References

The complete listing of the References are available in the accompanying enhanced eBook version included with the print purchase of this textbook. Visit Elsevier eBooks+ (eBooks.Health. Elsevier.com) to access this content.

14 Orthoses in the Management of Hand Dysfunction*

INGA WANG

LEARNING OBJECTIVES

On completion of this chapter, the reader will be able to do the following:

1. Define and differentiate between various terms related to orthoses, including articular and nonarticular orthoses.
2. Comprehend the different purposes of orthoses, such as immobilization, mobilization, and restriction, and recognize when each is appropriate.
3. Become familiar with various design descriptors, including choices of orthotic designs such as static orthoses, serial static orthoses, dynamic orthoses, and static progressive orthoses.
4. Understand key anatomy-related principles, such as the arches of the hand, palmar creases, and metacarpal length and mobility, as they relate to orthotic management.
5. Understand precautions related to soft tissues and the different stages of tissue healing. Recognize factors influencing tissue healing.
6. Grasp mechanical principles relevant to orthotic design, including levers, stress, angle of force application, and force application.
7. Familiarize oneself with various materials used in orthotic fabrication, including thermoplastic materials, and understand their handling and physical characteristics.
8. Gain an overview of the orthotic fabrication process, understanding the steps involved in creating orthotic devices for hand dysfunction.
9. Provide a brief description of the current trend in the design of hand orthoses.

Hand functions play a crucial role in activities of daily living (ADLs) and are essential for maintaining independence and quality of life.[1,2] Hands are utilized not only for self-care tasks like brushing teeth and using utensils but also for tool-use activities such as operating a vehicle, texting, and typing on a keyboard—critical for communication and work. Severe injuries, such as fractures, dislocations, or extensive soft tissue damage, along with disorders like rheumatoid arthritis or osteoarthritis, can lead to the loss of hand function. Neurological disorders such as stroke, spinal cord injury, and Parkinson disease can progressively impact hand function through various mechanisms, resulting in activity limitation and participation restrictions.

A therapist's skill in clinical intervention is crucial for optimizing hand use and significantly influencing overall function. An important tool available to therapists is the use of adaptive orthoses.[3–7] Strategically incorporating orthoses during specific phases of tissue healing, based on the patient's diagnosis, proves to be an effective complement to traditional therapy methods in restoring intended use to the affected extremity. In making treatment decisions, it is essential to consider a blend of knowledge, clinical experience, and patient-specific information, including diagnosis, general medical status, and any prescriptions from a qualified referral source. Clinicians should possess a strong understanding of the principles guiding the design and fabrication of orthoses, taking into account the unique characteristics of selected materials and models for intervention. The integration of these factors collectively contributes to facilitating the best possible therapeutic outcome for the patient.

This chapter explores orthotic management for hand dysfunction, covering essential concepts and practices. It begins by defining orthotic terms and discussing the purposes of interventions such as immobilization, mobilization, and restriction. Various orthotic designs are introduced, with a focus on anatomical principles, soft tissue precautions, and mechanical considerations. The chapter also touches on common hand disorders, provides orthotic examples, and concludes with a brief overview of the fabrication process, guiding practitioners in creating tailored orthotic devices for hand dysfunction. Lastly, the utilization of three-dimensional (3D) printing and sensor technology in the design of hand orthoses is described.

Nomenclature

The terms "splint," "brace," "support," and "orthosis" are often used interchangeably.[8] This can create confusion among medical providers, therapists, students, insurance companies, and device fabricators. While there is overlap in the usage of these terms, they can have distinct meanings in certain contexts. In general, a splint is a rigid or semirigid device used to support and immobilize injured or unstable body parts. A brace is a more comprehensive term that encompasses a variety of devices designed to support, control, or correct the function of a specific body part. Braces can be rigid or flexible and are often used for joints, muscles, or ligaments. The term "support" can include wraps, straps, or compression garments, and is a general term and refers to any device that helps maintain the stability of a body part. An orthosis is a broad term that encompasses any externally applied device used to provide support, correction, or

*The author extends appreciation to Brian J. Wilkinson, whose work in the prior edition provided substantial foundation for this chapter.

assistance in functions of the neuromuscular and skeletal system. Orthoses can include splints, braces, and other supportive devices. They are often custom made to address specific conditions or anatomical needs.

Classification Based on Splint Classification System

Hand orthoses can be classified based on various factors, including their purpose, design, and the materials used. The classification system could be traced back to 1989 when the American Society of Hand Therapists (ASHT) addressed issues related to splinting nomenclature through the establishment of a task force. This initiative led to the development of the ASHT Splint Classification System (SCS).[9,10] After research and debate, the ASHT-SCS divided splint/orthosis into "Articular" and "Nonarticular," which are further subdivided into "Location." Since articular splints involve joint movement so it has additional dimension on "Direction" of movement, which includes "Immobilisation, Mobilisation, and Restriction." The ASHT-SCS splint/orthosis classification system is outlined in Fig. 14.1.

ARTICULAR AND NONARTICULAR ORTHOSES

Overall, orthoses fall into two broad categories: *articular* and *nonarticular*. The primary distinction lies in whether the orthosis primarily involves joint structures (articular) or is focused on providing support to nonjoint structures (nonarticular). In other words, articular orthoses are those that cross one or more joints, while nonarticular orthoses do not cross a joint. Examples of articular orthoses include a wrist-finger orthosis and a dynamic elbow extension orthosis. On the other hand, a nonarticular humeral orthosis, used to stabilize the humerus, serves as an example of a nonarticular orthosis.

LOCATION

Location refers to the specific body part or articular surfaces included in the orthosis. The primary joint is considered the target joint, whereas the secondary joints are included for protection, stabilization, or comfort. When several primary joints are involved (e.g., crush injury to the hand), the description of the orthosis can be simplified by grouping all the involved joints together, such as in the descriptive terms *hand orthosis* or *digit orthosis*.

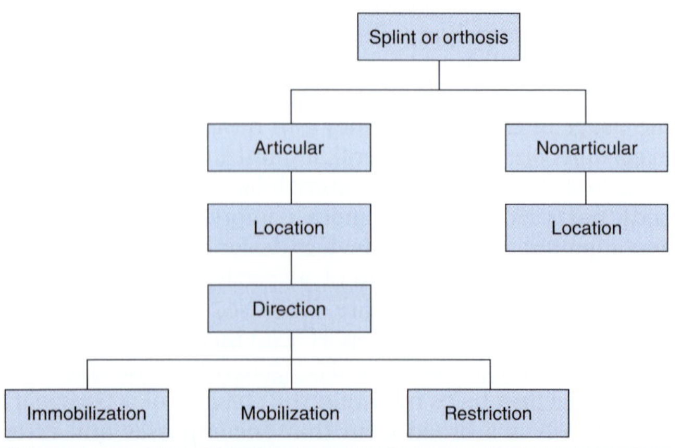

Fig. 14.1 The American Society of Hand Therapists Splint Classification System.

DIRECTION

Direction refers to the primary route of the force applied when the orthosis has been donned. This includes such terms as *flexion, extension, radial* or *ulnar deviation, supination, pronation, abduction*, and *adduction*. Information regarding direction is essential because it identifies the desired joint positioning of the orthosis. Specific notation of the direction is also necessary when fabricating a mobilization orthosis; accurate force application is essential to achieve the directional goal of joint or soft tissue mobility.

PURPOSE OF ORTHOSIS

The purpose or intent of the orthosis is the single most important aspect documented in the description. The purpose of the orthosis can be to (1) immobilize a structure (immobilization orthosis), (2) mobilize a tissue (mobilization orthosis), or (3) restrict a partial aspect of targeted joint motion (restriction orthosis).

Immobilization

The purpose of an *immobilization* orthosis is to place a structure in its anatomical or most comfortable resting position. Immobilization orthoses are among the most common and straightforward types, suitable for use in complex injuries as well. They aim to effectively restrain the joints they cross. An example of an immobilization orthosis is the proximal interphalangeal (PIP) immobilization orthosis (Fig. 14.2A) where the PIP joint is immobilized in a comfortable resting position, facilitating the healing of involved structures. This type is commonly employed for PIP ligament sprains.

Mobilization

Mobilization refers to moving or stretching specific soft tissues or joints to facilitate change.

The PIP flexion mobilization orthosis, for instance, stretches the PIP joint into flexion to address a PIP extension contracture using a static progressive approach (see Fig. 14.2B).

The benefits of using mobilization orthoses as a treatment modality have been well documented in the literature.[11–13] The effectiveness of mobilization does not rely on stretching tissue but rather on the facilitation of cell growth. The target tissue lengthens when the living cells of the contracted tissues are stimulated (by the application of force) to grow. This stimulation occurs when steady tension is applied through the orthosis over a specific period of time. The living cells recognize the tension applied and permit the older collagen cells to be actively absorbed and replaced with new collagen cells that are oriented in the direction of tension; this is a phenomenon known as *physiological creep*.[14–17] Tissue growth has been clearly demonstrated in cultures in which the elongation of certain body parts, such as the earlobes and lips, is popular. In these cultures, dowels are used to serially increase the diameter of the intended structure, slowly allowing expansion and accommodation of the tissue through new tension and diameter. Another common example includes the use of braces and retainers in the dental field to realign teeth over a period of time. In general, there are three choices

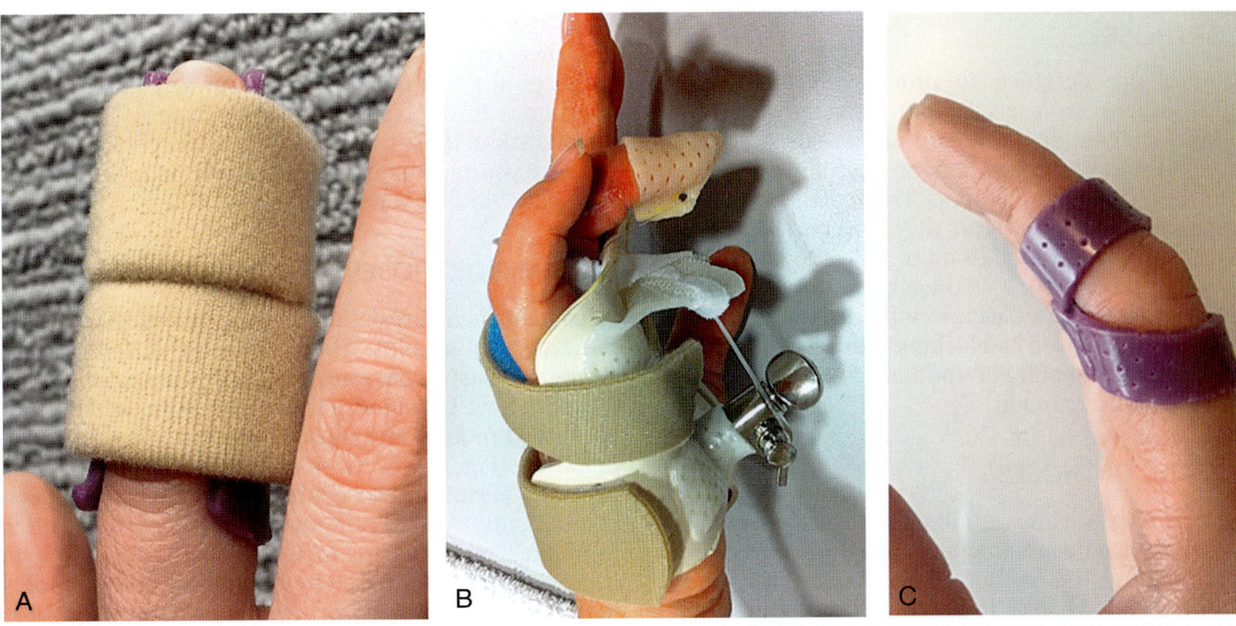

Fig. 14.2 Three different proximal interphalangeal (PIP) joint orthoses. (A) PIP immobilization orthosis. (B) PIP flexion mobilization orthosis. (C) PIP extension restriction orthosis.

of orthotic design aimed to mobilize tissue, including serial static, static progressive, and dynamic orthoses.

Restriction

Restriction orthoses restrict or block an aspect of targeted joint motion. Generally these are simple orthoses that are applied in a manner that seeks to limit motion. For example, within the boundaries of the PIP extension restriction orthosis, the PIP joint is restricted from full extension but allowed to flex fully (see Fig. 14.2C). This is commonly used for swan-neck deformities when the PIP joint tends to collapse into hyperextension. Nonetheless, therapists can construct static and dynamic orthoses or use forms of taping as types of restrictive orthoses because they can be made to restrict some portion of joint motion while allowing full, unrestricted motion in the opposite direction.

Naming Based on Medical Terms

In addition to the formal SCS classification naming system, orthoses may be named based on their function or the associated medical condition. For instance, the term "mallet finger orthosis" indicates that the orthopedic device is specifically designed to address the needs of individuals with mallet finger injuries. Similarly, the term "thumb spica splint" is crafted to describe a splint designed to immobilize and support the thumb and often the adjacent wrist area. The term "spica," derived from the Latin word for "spike," is used to characterize the design of a bandage or splint that encircles and stabilizes a joint.

Classification Based on Design Descriptors

The design descriptors are non-SCS nomenclature but are commonly used by the hand therapy and surgery community. Design descriptors are used to increase the clarity of a specific orthosis request and to provide detail in documentation to medical providers or reimbursement sources. The most commonly used descriptors are summarized in Box 14.1.

Box 14.1 Descriptors of Orthosis Designs

Digit based: Originates from the digit, allowing metacarpophalangeal joint motion
Hand based: Originates from the hand, allowing wrist motion
Thumb based: Originates from the thenar eminence or thumb, incorporating one or more joints of the thumb
Forearm based: Originates from the forearm, allowing elbow motion
Circumferential: Encompasses the entire circumference of the involved body part or limb segment
Gutter: Includes only the radial or ulnar portion of the limb
Radial: Incorporates the radial aspect of the limb
Ulnar: Incorporates the ulnar aspect of the limb
Dorsal: Traverses the dorsal (posterior) aspect of the hand, wrist, or forearm
Volar: Traverses the volar (palmar, anterior) aspect of the hand, wrist, or forearm
Anterior: Traverses the anterior aspect of the body part
Posterior: Traverses the posterior aspect of the body part

Classification Based on the Design and Functionality

The classification of orthoses into "*static, serial static, dynamic,* and *static progressive*" is based on the design and functionality of the orthotic devices. Each type serves specific purposes in addressing various musculoskeletal conditions and is classified as follows:

STATIC ORTHOSES

Static orthoses are designed to provide consistent and unchanging support to a specific joint or body part. They do not allow for dynamic movement and are used primarily for immobilization, stabilization, or maintaining a fixed position during the healing process. These orthoses have a rigid base, immobilizing the joints they traverse (Fig. 14.3). A static orthosis provides stabilization, protection, and support to a body segment such as the elbow, wrist, or finger. These orthoses can be used as a treatment adjunct in the form of an exercise device by blocking a distal or proximal joint to increase the mobility of another joint or to improve uninhibited tendon excursion.

SERIAL STATIC ORTHOSES

Serial static orthoses are a variation of static orthoses. They involve a series of adjustments or modifications over time to gradually change the position of a joint. This is done to address progressive changes in joint positioning or alignment during rehabilitation (Fig. 14.4). Tissue held in this end-range position should react and accommodate by stretching into the desired direction of correction. Serial static orthoses are often removed during therapy and exercise sessions so that the clinician and patient can work on the involved structures with interventions such as heat application, continuous ultrasound, joint mobilization, and range-of-motion (ROM) activities. The orthosis or cast is then remolded to maintain any gains achieved during the course of the therapy session. This design may provide greater patient compliance because of improved comfort and ensures that the targeted tissue is being continually stressed without the risk of the tissue rebounding (reverting back to original shortened state) on removal of the orthosis. Some therapists adopt a serial static approach in which the orthosis is worn continuously for several days and then removed in therapy. In other cases, using these orthoses at night may help preserve any gains made during the day through exercise and movement. Nonremovable serial static orthoses may also be a better choice for patients who are young, who have cognitive or behavioral issues, or who have variable tone and spasticity.

DYNAMIC ORTHOSES

Dynamic orthoses are designed to allow controlled and active movement of a joint. They use external forces, such as springs or elastic components, to assist or resist joint movement actively. Dynamic orthoses are often used to facilitate controlled motion and muscle strengthening during rehabilitation (Fig. 14.5). Most dynamic orthoses also have a base that permits the attachment of various outriggers and components, which can further advance their intended function. The mobilizing forces applied through a dynamic orthosis are elastic (stretchy) in nature and include such items as rubber bands, springs, or a wrapped elastic cord. The dynamic force applied is maintained as long as the elastic component can contract, even when the tissue reaches the end of its elastic boundary.

STATIC PROGRESSIVE ORTHOSES

Static progressive orthoses are a type of orthosis that provides a continuously increasing stretching force over time (Fig. 14.6).[11] They are commonly used to address conditions involving joint contractures or limited range of motion by applying a gradual, static stretch to improve flexibility and reduce stiffness. The goal is that the tissue will eventually accommodate to this position. The fabrication of a static progressive orthosis is similar to that of a dynamic orthosis, but the force applied is static or nonelastic. The mobilization force

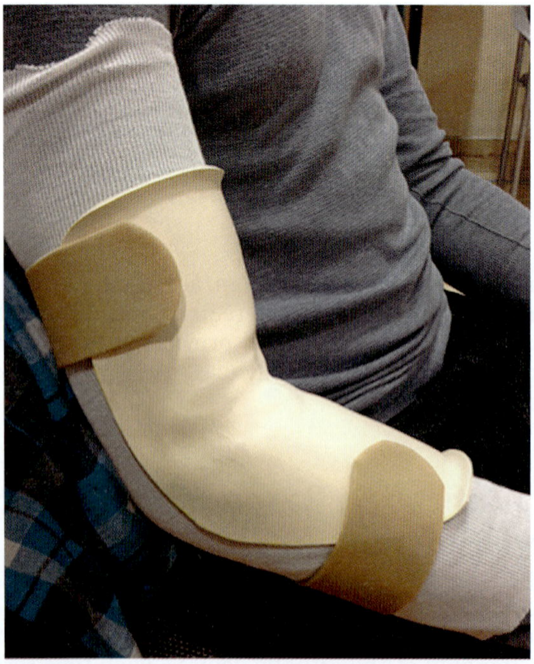

Fig. 14.3 Anterior elbow mobilization orthosis used to limit elbow flexion.

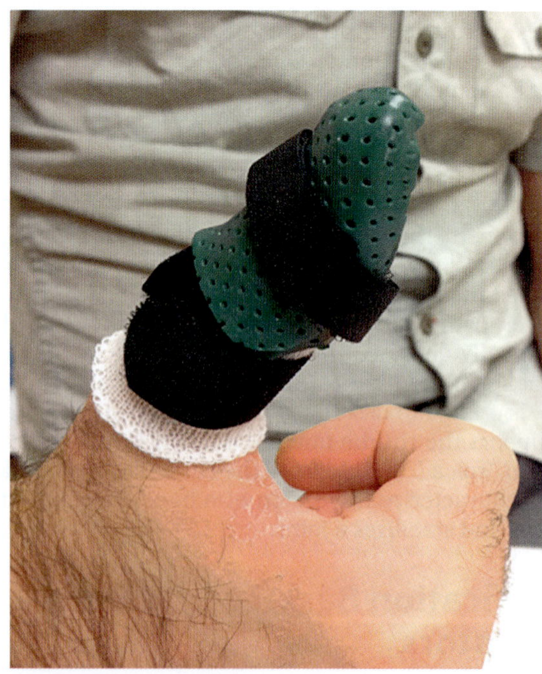

Fig. 14.4 Thumb interphalangeal extension mobilization orthosis designed to address a flexion contracture using a serial static approach.

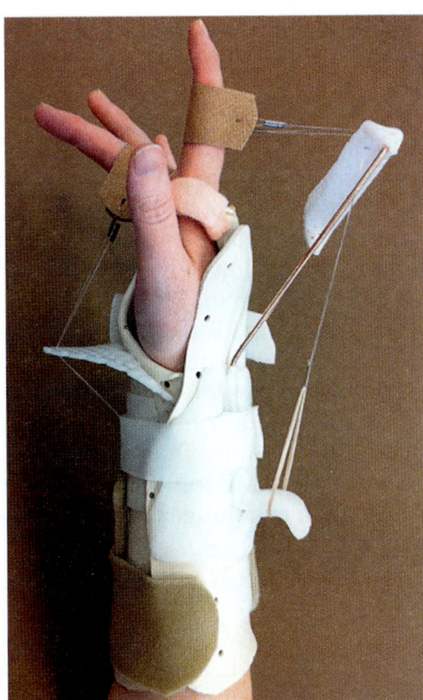

Fig. 14.5 Metacarpophalangeal extension mobilization orthosis using a rubber band to apply a dynamic force.

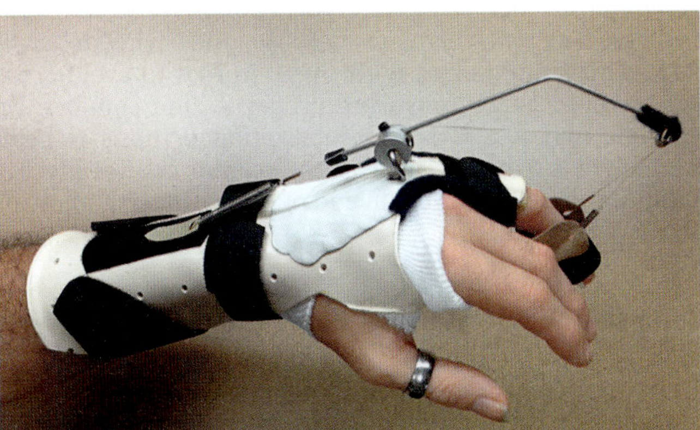

Fig. 14.6 Spring-loaded proximal interphalangeal extension mobilization orthosis using a static line and component to apply a static progressive force.

can be generated through static line, nonelastic strapping materials, hinges, turnbuckles, and various types of inelastic tape. When the desired joint position is achieved and the tension on the static progressive component is set, the orthosis will not continue to stress the tissue beyond its elastic limit. Force can be altered by the patient or therapist through progressive adjustments. Owing to the manner in which force is manipulated to facilitate tissue change, some patients may tolerate static progressive orthoses better than those that are dynamic. One reason may be that the joint position is constant while the tissue accommodates gently and gradually to the tension without the added influences of gravity and motion.[18]

Goals for Orthotic Intervention

The most essential objective for orthotic fabrication may not always be straightforward. There may also be multiple objectives for orthotic intervention as in a wrist and hand immobilization orthosis (resting hand orthosis) used on a patient with rheumatoid arthritis. The orthosis may be constructed to immobilize inflamed arthritic joints yet place the metacarpophalangeal (MP) joints serially in a gently extended and radially deviated position to minimize ulnar drift and periarticular deformity. Astute critical thinking is a necessary aspect of orthosis fabrication; multiple injuries, wound status, age, and lifestyle are a few of the key factors that must be taken into consideration. More skilled clinicians can appreciate that there can be several purposes for one orthosis; therefore creative problem solving must be used when orthotic devices for the more involved and complex injury are being fabricated.

IMMOBILIZATION ORTHOSES

Orthoses designed to hold or immobilize a joint or limb segment can be used to do the following:

- Stabilize and support injured or compromised joints.
- Immobilize a joint or body part.
- Place the injured structure in the anatomical or resting position.
- Provide symptom relief.
- Provide support and protection for soft tissue healing.
- Protect and position edematous structures.
- Provide postsurgical support and prevent unintended movement in the operated area.
- Improve and preserve joint alignment.
- Block and transfer both muscle and tendon forces.
- Influence a spastic muscle.
- Aid in maximizing functional use.

MOBILIZATION ORTHOSES

Orthoses designed to change or mobilize tissues or structures are used to do the following:

- Increase passive joint ROM
- Assist in muscle strengthening.
- Elongate soft tissue contractures, adhesions, and musculotendinous restrictions.
- Remodel preexisting, dense, mature scar tissue.
- Help individuals regain normal joint function after injuries, surgeries, or prolonged immobility.
- Provide dynamic support which allows for controlled movement.
- Provide indicated resistance for exercise.
- Realign or maintain joint and ligament profile.
- Substitute for weak or absent motion.
- Maintain reduction of an intraarticular fracture with preservation of joint mobility.

RESTRICTION ORTHOSES

Orthoses designed to restrict or limit motion may be used to do the following:

- Immobilize the joint during the initial stages of healing.
- Limit the ROM of a specific joint after nerve, tendon, bone or ligament injury or repair.
- Limit motion after integumentary injury or repair.
- Enhance joint stability by minimizing unwanted movements.

- Help with pain management by limiting movements that may exacerbate pain.
- Provide and improve joint stability and alignment.
- Assist in functional use of the hand.

Anatomy-Related Principles

Designing hand splints or orthoses involves considering various anatomy-related principles to ensure the device is effective and comfortable. Several key anatomy-related principles in designing hand splints or orthoses include arches of the hand, palmar creases, metacarpal length and mobility, joint axis alignment, thumb movement, antideformity and functional positioning, and soft tissue considerations.

ARCHES OF THE HAND

Three arches balance stability and mobility in the hand: the proximal transverse arch, distal transverse arch, and longitudinal arch (Fig. 14.7). The proximal transverse arch, anchored by the capitate as its keystone, is situated at the level of the distal carpus and remains relatively stable. In contrast, the distal transverse arch, with the head of the third metacarpal serving as its keystone, traverses all the metacarpal heads and exhibits greater mobility. The longitudinal arch, which extends from the wrist crease to the tip of either the middle or index finger, constitutes a carpometacarpo-phalangeal arch. During normal flexion, fingers point toward region of scaphoid.

This arch system is vital to positioning the hand in a manner that allows for normal function related to grasp and prehension. Incorporation of these arches within an orthosis is an essential tactic that promotes maximal function and allows for optimal comfort. Additionally, preservation of the arches helps to prevent undesired migration of the orthosis during use of the upper extremity.

The fixed proximal transverse arch is created by the configuration of the distal row of the carpal bones and the volar carpal ligament, which is inherently taut. This region is also referred to as the carpal tunnel, through which the long flexors and median nerve pass before they terminate in the hand. This secure structure provides mechanical advantage to the flexors, ultimately helping to maximize grasp function.

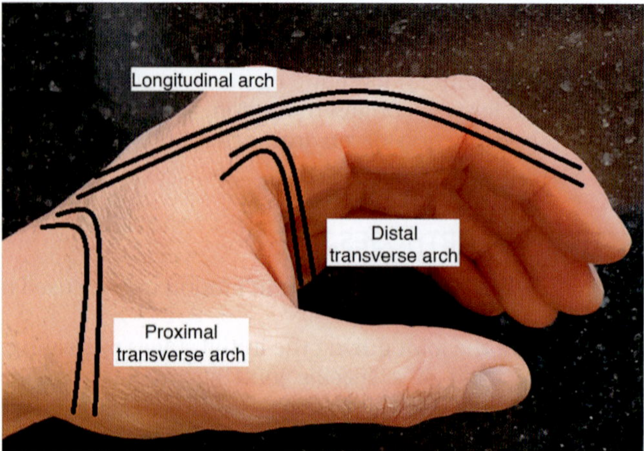

Fig. 14.7 Fixed proximal transverse arch, flexible distal transverse arch, and mobile longitudinal arch of the hand.

The mobile distal transverse arch is located at the level of the metacarpal heads. This arch is adaptive by the mobile fourth and fifth carpometacarpal (CMC) joints along the ulnar side of the hand as well as the highly mobile thumb trapeziometacarpal joint. The increased mobility of the peripheral digits further allows for better grasping ability.

The longitudinal arch spans the length from the metacarpal to the distal phalanx. A disruption of this arch commonly occurs in patients who have sustained an ulnar nerve injury, resulting in the loss of intrinsic muscle function. Because of interrupted motor input in the muscles associated with this innervation, the hand takes on an intrinsic minus position when the MP joints are hyperextended and the PIP and distal interphalangeal joints are flexed (claw-like deformity).

PALMAR CREASES

Palmar creases, also known as palmar flexion creases or lines, are epidermal flexure lines present on palmar surface of the hands (Fig. 14.8). These creases are formed during fetal development and remain relatively consistent across individuals. Those individuals who fabricate orthoses need to familiarize themselves with the location of these creases and how each one correlates with the underlying anatomy. The splint should align with these creases to avoid creating pressure points, ensuring proper fit and comfort. For example, when a wrist immobilization orthosis is being fabricated, the distal and proximal palmar creases must be left uninhibited by the distal end of the orthosis to allow for

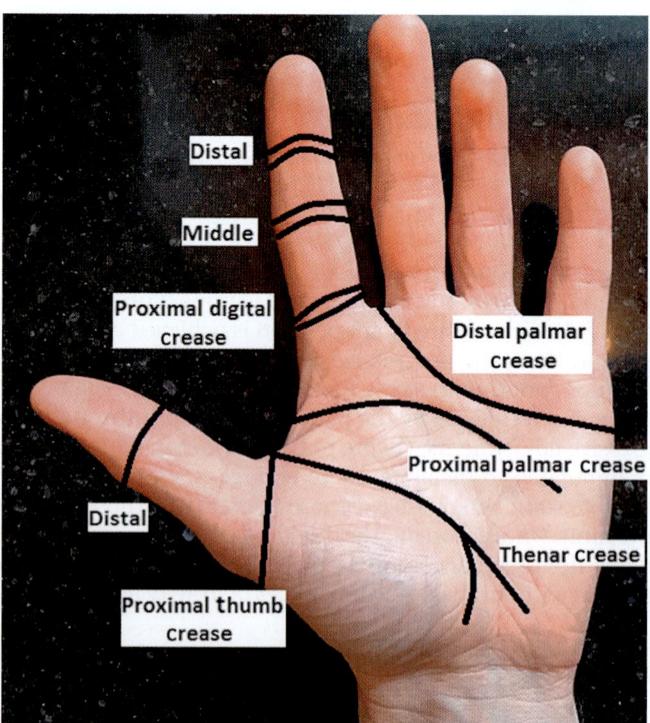

Fig. 14.8 The creases of the hand provide helpful landmarks during the process of fabricating an orthosis.

unrestricted ROM at the MP joints. However, care must be taken not to leave too much anatomy unsupported because the mechanical advantage of the orthosis can then be altered adversely.

METACARPAL LENGTH AND MOBILITY

Dual obliquity is a concept relating to the anatomy of the metacarpals. Because of the differing lengths of the metacarpals (radial side of hand longer than ulnar), an oblique angle is formed compared with the distal ends of the radius and ulna when an object is held in the hand (Fig. 14.9A). In addition, the object is angled in accordance with the distal transverse arch and the increasing mobility of the ulnar metacarpals (see Fig. 14.9B). This dual obliquity should be incorporated into an orthosis so that it provides a comfortable and functional structure that effectively resists migration.

JOINT AXIS ALIGNMENT

Ensure the orthosis aligns with the joint axes, promoting natural joint movement and preventing abnormal stresses. Proper alignment contributes to the comfort and functionality of the splint, promoting optimal therapeutic outcomes for the user. For instance, when designing a hand splint for conditions where the fingers need to flex while considering the scaphoid region, such as in certain cases of De Quervain tenosynovitis, it is crucial to align the splint with the natural flexion movement of the fingers while providing support to the wrist.

THUMB MOVEMENT

The thumb is crucial for hand function due to its unique anatomy and versatile movements, such as opposition, precision grasp, palmar pinch, tip pinch, lateral pinch, and power grip. Thumb orthoses should facilitate these movements while providing support and stability for functional activities.

ANTIDEFORMITY AND FUNCTIONAL POSITIONING

When the fabricator is deciding how to position the hand within an orthosis, many factors must be considered, including the patient's diagnosis, healing time frame, and goals of intervention. In addition to facilitating the healing of any affected tissues, being mindful of proper positioning within an orthosis can help to prevent future joint and soft tissue contractures.

The two most common positions described in the literature include the antideformity and functional position. See Fig. 14.10 for the general joint angles described for each position. In the functional position of the hand, the hand should be positioned with the wrist in 15 to 30 degrees of extension, the metacarpophalangeal (MCP) joints in 45 degrees of flexion, the PIP joints in 15 to 30 degrees of flexion, and the thumb abducted. This position optimizes finger flexor power. In the antideformity position of the hand, the hand should be positioned with the wrist in 15 to 30 degrees of extension, the MCP joints in 70 to 80 degrees of flexion, the IP joints fully extended, and the thumb abducted. This position preserves the hand's arch and places the MCP collateral ligaments in a maximal stretch position.

The antideformity position, commonly referred to as *safe position* in the clinical setting, considers the unique anatomic characteristics of the MP and PIP joints. The length of the collateral ligaments at the MP joint varies according to the position of the MP joint (Fig. 14.11). The collateral ligaments are slack with MP joint extension, whereas tension in the collateral ligaments increases with greater amounts of MP joint flexion. Placing these joints in flexion within an orthosis helps to prevent MP joint extension contractures (resulting in limited flexion postimmobilization). If the joints are placed in extension with resulting MP contractures, disruption of the longitudinal arch can greatly impair the patient's grasping ability.

Similarly, at the PIP joint level, the volar plate is placed on tension with PIP joint extension, whereas flexion at the PIP joint places the volar plate at risk for shortening

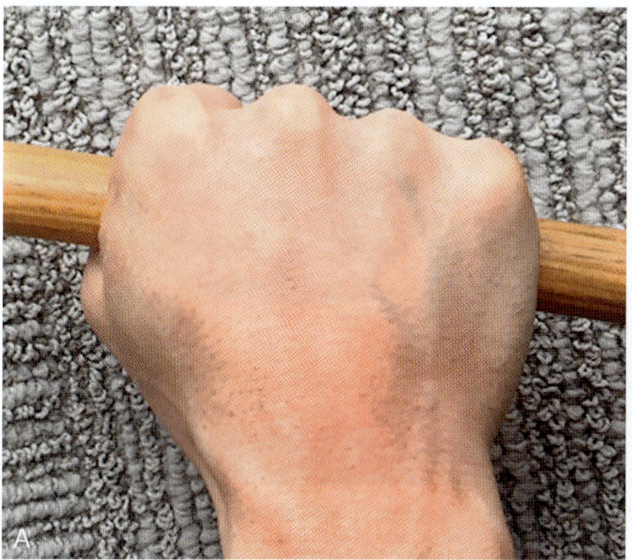

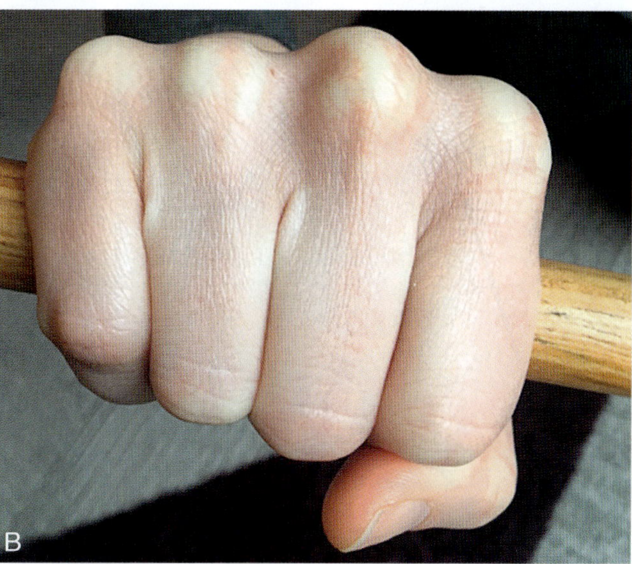

Fig. 14.9 The dual obliquity of the hand from the dorsal (A) and transverse (B) perspectives.

(see Fig. 14.11A and B). Shortening of the volar plate can result in debilitating PIP joint flexion contractures, which can significantly affect the ability not only to grasp but also release objects. Therefore careful positioning of the PIP joint in extension (as long as this is not contraindicated) is crucial to maintain the length of the volar plate tissue.

SOFT TISSUE CONSIDERATIONS

In the upper extremity, a number of areas exist where bony protuberances or superficial nerves are highly susceptible to compression from an orthosis (Box 14.2). If these areas are not accounted for during the fabrication process, the orthosis will likely become uncomfortable for the patient and there will be an increased potential for noncompliance. Special consideration must be given to patients with impaired sensation (those with peripheral nerve injury, neuropathy, nerve root compression, or central nervous system disorders). Those with limited or absent sensation do not have the normal ability to feel or detect areas of excess pressure; rather, they must rely on routine visual inspection to assess the integrity of both skin and soft tissue.

Because superficial bony prominences have minimal soft tissue coverage, they are especially vulnerable to compressive forces; excessive external pressure can place the tissue at risk for irritation and eventual breakdown (necrosis). Older adults may be at the greatest risk because they have minimal subcutaneous fat combined with extremely

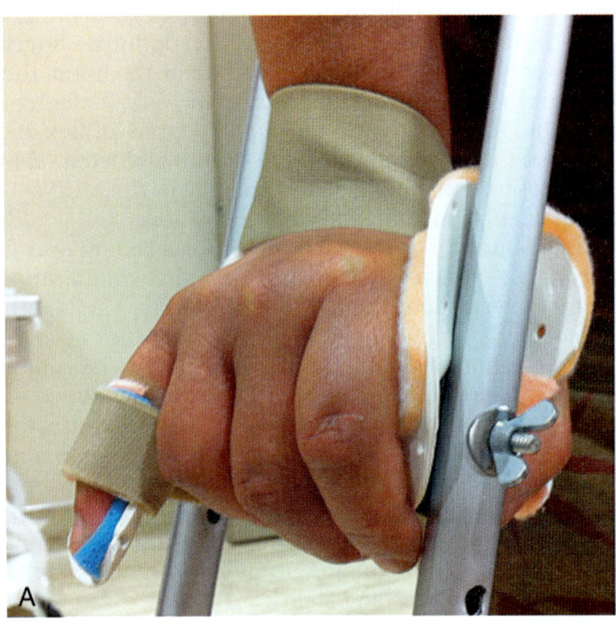

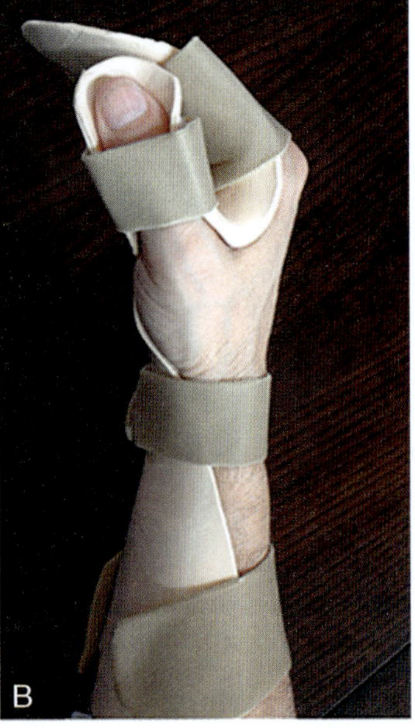

Fig. 14.10 The functional position of the hand (A) wrist in 15–30 degrees of extension, the MCP joints in 45 degrees of flexion, the proximal interphalangeal joints in 30 degrees of flexion, and the thumb abducted. This position optimizes finger flexor power. The antideformity position of the hand (B) places the wrist in 15–30 degrees of extension, the MCP joints in 70–80 degrees of flexion, the interphalangeal joints fully extended, and the thumb abducted. This position preserves the hand's arch and places the MCP collateral ligaments in a maximal stretch position.

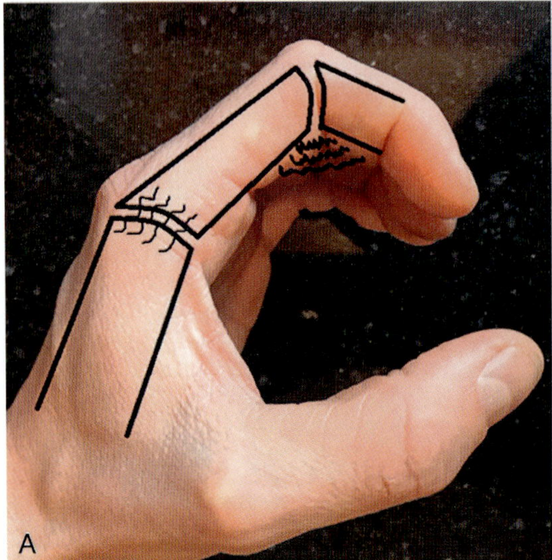

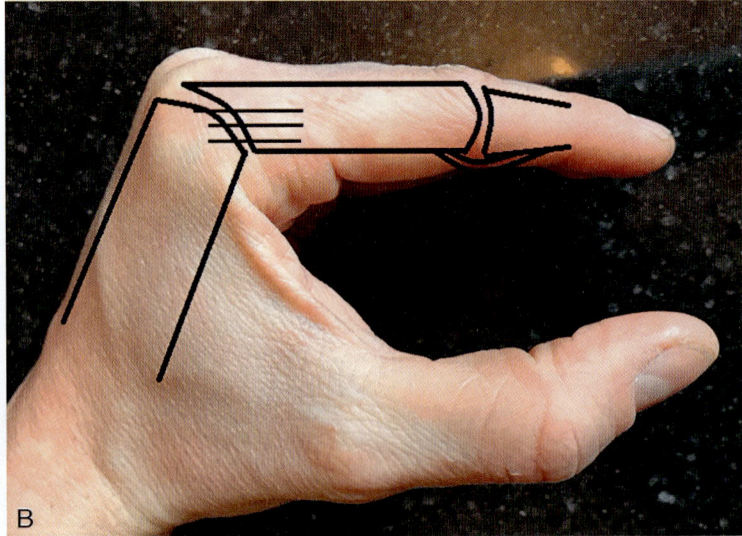

Fig. 14.11 Changes in the length of soft tissue associated with joint positioning. (A) Placing the metacarpophalangeal (MP) joint in extension will cause the MP collateral ligaments and the proximal interphalangeal (PIP) volar plate to become "slack" and at risk of becoming shortened over time. (B) Placing the MP joint in flexion elongates both the MP collateral ligaments and the volar plate of the PIP joint to minimize risk of shortening (contractures) of these structures.

fragile skin, making bony areas more susceptible to injury. If complications arise, patients may report pain, redness, and irritation over the bony area. To prevent such occurrences when they must be included in an orthosis, these at-risk bony areas can either be padded with foam/gel or flared away during the molding process (Fig. 14.12).

Therapists must also appreciate peripheral nerve anatomy and how orthoses and strapping may place excessive pressure over regions where nervous tissue becomes relatively superficial, potentially leading to unintended nerve compression. If this complication arises, patients may report pain, redness, paresthesia (tingling), and numbness in that nerve's distribution. Timely modification of the orthosis is therefore necessary to prevent long-term nerve irritation. Orthotic fabrication over positioned gel or the use of wider straps to disperse the pressure more evenly are two techniques that may be useful to limit this complication.

Also of note is the potential for compression of vascular structures when an orthosis is worn or an elasticized product is applied. Symptoms of vascular compromise—including color changes, temperature changes, pain, or a sensation of throbbing—should be dealt with in an immediate manner. The identification of these symptoms is especially important if any surgical reconstruction of vascular structures has been performed. Wide straps and slings to distribute pressure over greater surface areas along with the appropriate use of elasticized wraps can aid in preventing this problem. Most importantly, educating the patient regarding the potential signs and symptoms of bony and neurovascular compromise is key to preventing any long-term problems that may be created through the application of an orthosis.

Box 14.2 Superficial Structures Vulnerable to Pressure

Bony Prominences

- Olecranon process at the elbow.
- Lateral and medial epicondyles of the humerus.
- Ulnar and radial styloid processes at the wrist.
- Base of the first metacarpal.
- Dorsal thumb and digit metacarpophalangeal and interphalangeal joints.
- Pisiform bone.

Superficial Nerves

- Radial nerve at the radial groove of the humerus.
- Ulnar nerve at the cubital tunnel.
- Superficial branches of the ulnar and radial nerves at the distal forearm.
- Median nerve at the carpal tunnel.
- Digital nerves on the volar aspect of the digits.

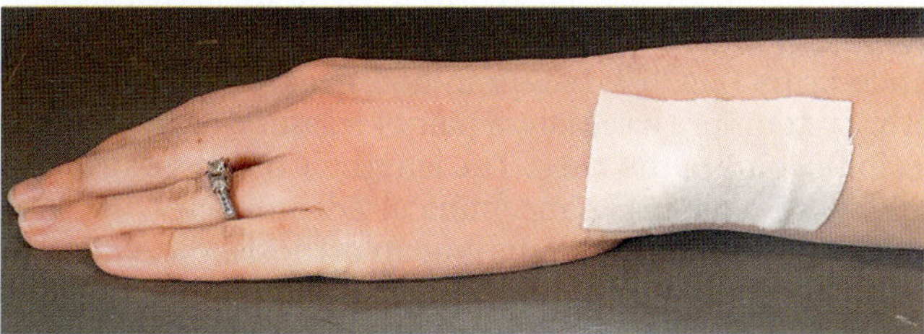

Fig. 14.12 Padding bony prominences, such as the ulnar styloid process, prior to molding an orthosis can decrease the risk of creating undesired areas of high pressure, thus reducing the potential for skin irritation or breakdown.

Tissue Healing

Different patients may progress through the stages of tissue healing at varying rates. Understanding these stages enables hand therapists to customize orthotics or splints based on the specific needs and progress of each patient.

STAGES OF TISSUE HEALING

The process of tissue healing involves a well-coordinated series of stages designed to repair and restore damaged tissues. Right after an injury, hemostasis acts as the initial response to tissue damage, which entails stopping the bleeding. This is accomplished through platelet aggregation, degranulation, and fibrin formation. Clotting factors are released at the wound site and coagulate with fibrin to form a blood clot. After hemostasis, the three main stages of tissue healing follow: the inflammatory phase, the proliferative phase (fibroplasia), and the remodeling phase (maturation) (Fig. 14.13).[19–21]

In the inflammatory phase, immune cells (neutrophils and macrophages) infiltrate to clear debris and pathogens. Inflammatory mediators, such as cytokines and growth factors, are released into the surroundings. Clinically, the tissue feels soft and boggy and is easy to mobilize. This stage typically lasts for 1 week or less. Rest is normally more important than exercise during the inflammatory stage, so immobilization orthoses are appropriate in the days immediately after tissue injury or surgery.

In the proliferative phase, new blood vessels form to supply nutrients and oxygen to the healing tissue (angiogenesis). Fibroblasts proliferate, and collagen deposition occurs, creating a structural framework (fibroplasia). Additionally,

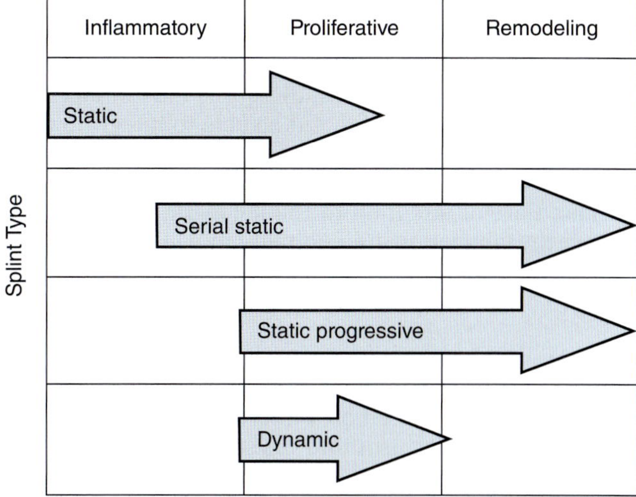

Fig. 14.13 An algorithm for the uses of various types of orthoses associated with the stages of normal tissue healing.

epithelial cells migrate and proliferate to cover the wound surface (epithelialization). The clinician begins to see and feel more tissue resistance (from scarring), although the tissue is still soft and movable despite inherent tension. This phase typically lasts from 1 to 6 weeks. Mobilization orthoses that gently stretch tissue can be effective during this time frame because they provide gentle stress that can facilitate tissue growth, resulting in tissue lengthening.

The final phase of tissue healing is known as the remodeling phase. During this stage, collagen undergoes organization as it remodels along lines of stress. Myofibroblasts cause the contraction of the wound site, reducing the size of the scar. The core aim of the remodeling stage is to achieve the maximum tensile strength through reorganization, degradation, and resynthesis of the extracellular matrix. Clinically, the tissues involved feel dense, hard, and inelastic. Tissues may actually shorten because of a decrease in elasticity; therefore stretching is a valuable tool to address undesirable contractures. Superficial scars also begin to soften during this stage. This stage begins as early as 6 weeks and can last up to 12 to 24 months. Serial static and static progressive approaches (or a combination of the two through day and night orthoses) to mobilize tissue during this phase are most appropriate.

FACTORS THAT INFLUENCE TISSUE HEALING

Tissue healing is influenced by various factors including age, sex, type of extent injury, stress, diabetes, obesity, medications, alcoholism, smoking, and nutrition.[22–26] For instance, tissue deprived of oxygen requires a longer healing time, directly impacting the necessary wearing time of an orthosis. Therapists should thoroughly discuss the patient's medical history and lifestyle habits to identify any factors that may potentially delay or impair tissue healing. Substances such as tobacco (nicotine) can detrimentally affect the body's healing capacity by diminishing blood flow and nutrition supplied to the tissue. Excessive alcohol intake can impair the immune system, leading to malnourishment and liver damage. Overall there are many varied factors that influence the rate of tissue healing (Box 14.3).

Box 14.3 Factor That Influence Tissue Healing

Common Factors

- Age
- Nutritional status
- Tobacco use
- Diabetes
- Edema
- Infection
- Rheumatoid arthritis

Less Common Factors

- Alcohol use
- Sickle cell disease
- Steroids
- Radiation therapy
- Peripheral vascular disease
- Raynaud disease
- Systemic lupus erythematosus

Mechanical Principles

Before fabricating an orthosis, therapists must understand basic mechanical principles and be able to integrate these details into the orthotic design and construction process. This section briefly reviews the most common principles to consider. Careful attention to the following principles will improve the fabrication, functionality, and fit of an orthosis.

LEVERS

Levers are rigid structures through which a force can be applied to produce rotational motion about a fixed axis. A lever system is composed of a fulcrum, or fixed axis, and two arms: the effort arm and resistance arm. The effort arm, also referred to as the force arm, is the segment of the lever between the fulcrum and the effort force that is attempting to impose action on a structure. In orthotic design, the fulcrum corresponds to the anatomic axis of the target joint, the effort arm is the segment of the orthosis that applies the effort force, and the resistance arm is the segment of the limb that resists the effort force. Ideally, the effort and resistance forces work in concert to create a balance of opposing torques about the fulcrum. However, cases occur in which the axis of rotation (fulcrum) has been impaired from disease or injury (e.g., fracture, rheumatoid arthritis), and achieving this desired equilibrium can be difficult.

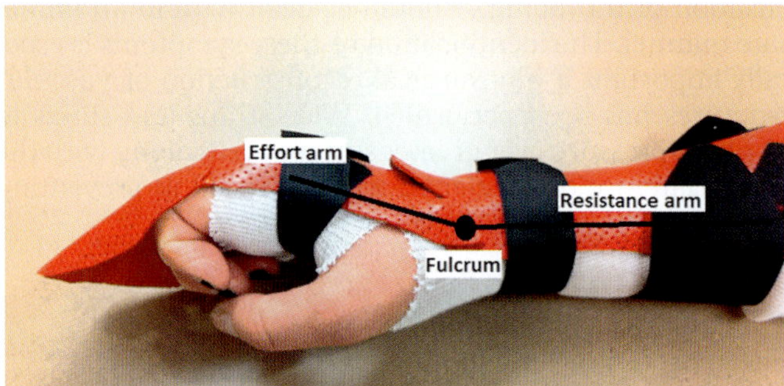

Fig. 14.14 The fulcrum of an orthosis is placed at the axis where joint motion occurs. The resistance arm is applied by the proximal segment of the orthosis, while the effort arm is applied by the distal segment of the orthosis.

Most orthoses are categorized as first-class levers, in which the fulcrum is located between the effort and resistance arms (Fig. 14.14). Common examples of first-class lever systems are a seesaw, a pair of scissors, or the atlanto-occipital joint in the neck. The length of the resistance arm greatly influences the mechanical advantage of the force applied. In the case of designing an orthosis, the effort arm can also influence mechanical advantage by how carefully it is molded around a body part.

Both the effort and resistance arms should be vigilantly formed by incorporating arches, clearing for creases, and allowing adequate surface area for the maximal distribution of created pressure. As forces actively influence a joint, a balance-counterbalance effect must occur. If the opposing force (effort arm) is not distributed well to counterbalance the distal forces (resistance arm), the orthosis may not rest adjacent to its designated body part. This condition may create high-pressure areas, shear stress, or an unproductive application of force. Clinicians can achieve mechanical advantage through careful application of orthotic principles and meticulous attention to detail while molding these devices. Clinically, orthoses tend to be most comfortable when they are well molded and adequate length and depth have been incorporated. Short, narrow, or shallow orthoses can cause increases in localized pressure and may add to overall discomfort.

STRESS

Stress can occur in various forms. The most common types that relate directly to orthoses are compression, shear, tension, bending, and torsion. Compressive stress (also referred to as pressure) is defined as force per unit area. In the process of creating and planning the design of an orthosis, therapists must understand the various forms of stress that can be produced by the external forces. For example, compression can be minimized by increasing the surface area (designing an orthosis base that is wider and longer) over which the force can be maximally distributed. Optimizing the conformity of materials to the shape of the body part can also serve to minimize any compressive stress that is created.

A number of factors can result in creating areas of high pressure. Narrow strap width, especially in conjunction with "shallow" orthoses, can produce high compressive stress on the supported soft tissue. The borders of an orthosis should lie flush with the skin surface traversed by the strap. The strap should not bridge the two borders of the orthosis; it should come in direct contact with the skin.

The slings used in mobilizing orthoses are another possible source of compression stress that should be considered, especially if edema or neurovascular issues are evident in the patient's extremity. Compression to the lateral, dorsal, or volar aspects of the digit can be avoided by using several techniques. One option involves attaching the orthosis line to each side of a sling (two pieces of line) and then joining the two pieces after they pass through the pulley. This design prevents the circumferential compression created when a single line is threaded through both ends of the sling. Alternatively, a custom-fabricated thermoplastic "pan" can be placed under the sling as a support. The digital pan disperses the compressive forces applied through the sling by lifting the borders away from the skin and increasing the surface area of force application (see Fig. 14.2B).

Shear stress results from a parallel force applied to a surface and produces a tendency for an object to either deform or slide along the surface. When a mobilization orthosis is being fabricated, the mobilizing force (which utilizes leverage through the proximal base of the orthosis) usually traverses the length of the orthosis and terminates distally at the body segment. If the proximal portion (base) of the orthosis is not adequately secured to the limb

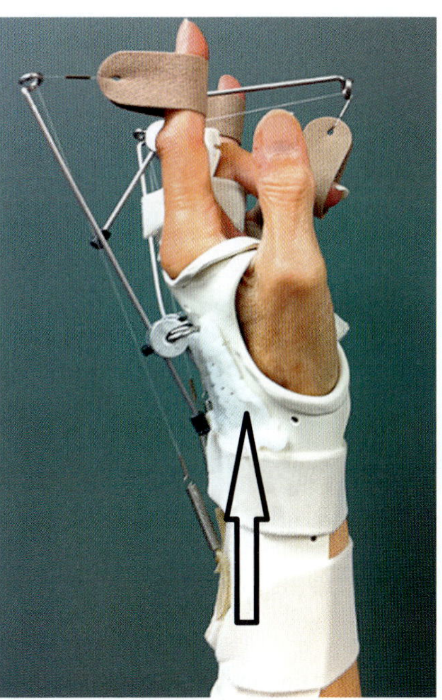

Fig. 14.15 When tension is applied to this proximal interphalangeal extension mobilization orthosis, shear stress is created as the proximal orthosis migrates distally on the forearm.

with appropriate strapping, there will be an undesirable migration or dragging and shearing of the proximal base over the skin when the mobilization force is applied distally (Fig. 14.15). Being careful to incorporate the arches of the hand as well as to procure a well-contoured orthosis during the molding process can help to prevent such migration. In some cases a nonskid material such Dycem foam tape (Dycem Technologies Limited, Bristol, England) or Moleskin (Consumer Health, Scranton, Pennsylvania) to line the orthosis can also help to keep the orthosis stable on the extremity.

ANGLE OF FORCE APPLICATION

The angle of force application is critical to the proper design and fabrication of mobilization orthoses. Ideally, the force should be applied at a 90-degree angle relative to the body segment being mobilized (Fig. 14.16) because this maximizes the therapeutic effect of the force being applied. With a pure 90 degrees orientation to the part being mobilized, there are virtually no forces disseminated in other directions (minimizing undesired compression or distraction). However, if the angle is not set at 90 degrees, a portion of the force is dissipated elsewhere, thus diminishing the therapeutic effect and causing potentially harmful compression or shear stress.

Clinically the use of custom-made or prefabricated line guides or pulleys can be helpful in achieving a 90-degree angle of force application. The therapist must view the orthosis from all angles to make sure the line of application is directed centrally over the segment and oriented properly in all planes. To improve flexion of the digits with a mobilization orthosis, the anatomic configuration of the hand requires the line of force application to converge toward the scaphoid. If this orientation is not incorporated

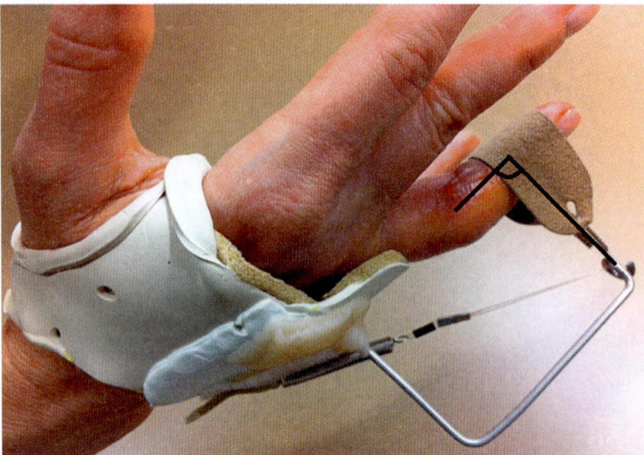

Fig. 14.16 Note the optimal 90-degree angle formed by the middle phalanx and the monofilament line in this proximal interphalangeal extension mobilization orthosis.

into the design of the orthosis, excessive stress will be placed on the digital joints, causing discomfort and potential harm. Occasionally a force applied in either a radial or ulnar direction is indicated, as with postoperative MP joint arthroplasties or sagittal band repairs. Except for special circumstances such as these, the line of application should be centrally located over the longitudinal axis of the bone being mobilized.

FORCE APPLICATION

When elastic force is being used to mobilize stiff structures, therapists must carefully consider the therapeutic objectives.[27,28] For example, there is a critical difference in achieving the goal of mobilizing a mature, dense joint contracture versus that of stabilizing the MP joints in extension after an MP joint arthroplasty. Both situations may require an elastic force. However, both the amount of force and the materials used to achieve these goals can vary considerably. The amount of force necessary to mobilize various tissues depends on such factors as individual tolerance, diagnosis, stage of tissue healing, chronicity of the problem, severity of contracture, density of contracture ("end feel"), patient's age, smoking, alcohol use, and other health-related issues. Ranges of 100 to 300 g have been suggested for mobilization of the small joints of the hand, whereas higher parameters (>350 g) may be more effective for larger structures. This 300-g threshold of force is based on what is tolerated per unit of surface area of the skin, not the tolerance of the contracted tissue to tension. In most cases, skin tolerance becomes the limiting factor in determining the appropriate quantity of tension, not the risk of injury to the specific targeted tissue. The therapist can almost always rely on the tissue's response to the tension to help determine the effectiveness of the mobilizing forces. Signs of too much stress include the onset of edema, skin blanching, vascular changes, impaired sensation, and exacerbated pain. The amount of time the force is applied is another factor to consider with mobilization orthoses.[29] In general, the goal is to provide a low load stress to the tissue over a long period of time.

Box 14.4 Distributors of Orthotic Fabrication Products

AliMed
297 High Street, Dedham, MA 02026
www.alimed.com
DeRoyal
200 Debusk Lane, Powell, TN 37849
www.deroyal.com
North Coast Medical
780 Jarvis Drive, Suite 100, Morgan Hill, CA 95037
www.ncmedical.com
Orfit Industries America
350 Jericho Turnpike, Suite 101, Jericho, NY 11753
www.orfit.com
Performance Health
28100 Torch Parkway, Suite 700, Warrenville, IL 60555
www.performancehealth.com
UE Tech
PO Box 2145, Edwards, CO 81632
www.uetech.com
WFR Corporation
30 Lawlins Park, Wyckoff, NJ 07481
www.reveals.com
3-Point Products
118 Log Canoe Circle, Stevensville, MD 21666
www.3pointproducts.com

Material and Equipment

Numerous companies market and distribute supplies for orthotic fabrication (Box 14.4); these include many types of thermoplastic materials, strapping, component systems, and other equipment. The best way to become educated regarding what is on the market is by spending time reviewing the catalogs/websites and contacting local sales representatives to request samples of desired materials. In addition, attending workshops on orthotic fabrication and hand therapy conferences can be a helpful means of gaining knowledge while providing opportunities to practice skills that can be used in the clinical setting.

THERMOPLASTIC MATERIALS

Low-temperature thermoplastics are most commonly used by therapists to fabricate custom orthoses. These materials are sold in sheets or precut designs and are softened in warm water prior to application to the intended body part. Once a low-temperature thermoplastic has been formed to the contour of the body, the material cools and hardens into shape. When fabricating a splint, therapists can select from a wide range of thermoplastic materials; this often creates confusion for novice practitioners who must choose which type to use for a specific case. The fabricator must have a sound understanding of the characteristics of the various thermoplastics to make an informed decision, taking into account the desired purpose of the orthosis as well as the patient's diagnosis. In addition to considering the patient's needs, therapists must consider other factors, including their own level of fabrication experience, the availability of materials, and any existing cost constraints.

Few studies have examined the characteristics of thermoplastic materials to categorize their differences.[30,31] However, a knowledge of the different categories of thermoplastic materials as well as their handling and physical characteristics can help therapists make more informed selections during the process of fabrication.

Handling Characteristics

Handling characteristics refer to the way a material behaves during the molding process. The three most important characteristics of orthosis materials that must be considered are conformability and resistance to stretch, memory, and bonding characteristics.

Conformability and Resistance to Stretch

The ability for a material to conform to a body part is related to its level of resistance to stretch (Fig. 14.17). A helpful system for organizing thermoplastic materials is to group them into categories according to their degree of resistance to stretch (Table 14.1). Materials with minimal resistance to stretch are highly conforming and may not be the best choice for novice fabricators. Reduced hands-on contact during the fabrication process is preferred because these types of materials tend to contour well without much guidance. In the clinic, high-stretch materials may be appropriate for a patient who has a high level of pain and would not tolerate an extensive hands-on molding process or for those orthoses in which achieving an intimate fit would be crucial to maximize comfort. Smaller orthoses that are more straightforward—such as those for a finger or hand—can be made more easily with these highly conforming materials. Regardless of the selected material, gravity-assisted positioning during the molding process is essential to achieving the proper shape.

Materials with maximal resistance to stretch are minimally conforming and inherently demand more hands-on work from the fabricator to obtain a better fit of the orthosis. Therapists with nominal experience in the fabrication of orthoses may do better with these materials because they tolerate more aggressive handling. These materials are appropriate when larger orthoses are being made, as in orthoses for the elbow or in situations in which fabrication against gravity is not an option (e.g., patients who are wheelchair bound). Because these materials do not contour with precision, they may be the best choice during fabrication over wound dressings in which the dimensions of the underlying material may be altered with each dressing change.

Memory

Memory refers to a material's ability to revert to its original shape once heated, ranging from 0% to 100% memory. Materials with this property are good choices for orthoses that must frequently be remolded, as when fabricating a serial static orthosis that must be reheated and reformed to the body part as ROM varies. Caution must be used when removing the orthosis from the body part after molding to ensure the material has cooled completely; otherwise the material may shrink to the point where proper fit is lost. Also, spot heating of thermoplastic orthoses is not advised, owing to the possibility of unintentionally altering regions adjacent to the targeted area.

Bonding

Bonding is the ability of a material to adhere to itself when heated fully. The presence of a protective coating, however, can prevent this occurrence. The coating allows two pieces of material to be pulled apart after the orthosis is formed, which can be particularly useful when a circumferential design is being applied, as around the thumb (Fig. 14.18). If bonding is desired, the coating must either be removed with solvent or disrupted by scratching the surface to allow for adherence; the latter is commonly required for attaching mobilization components. The coating may also make the orthosis easier to clean. Without a coating, the material may stick to a wound dressing, the patient's body hair, or itself. When material without a coating is being used, apply a barrier, such as a wet paper towel or a small quantity of hand lotion, between the two pieces to prevent unwanted adherence.

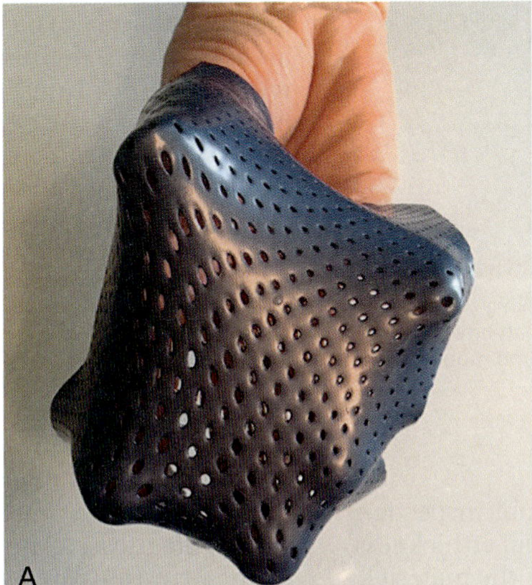

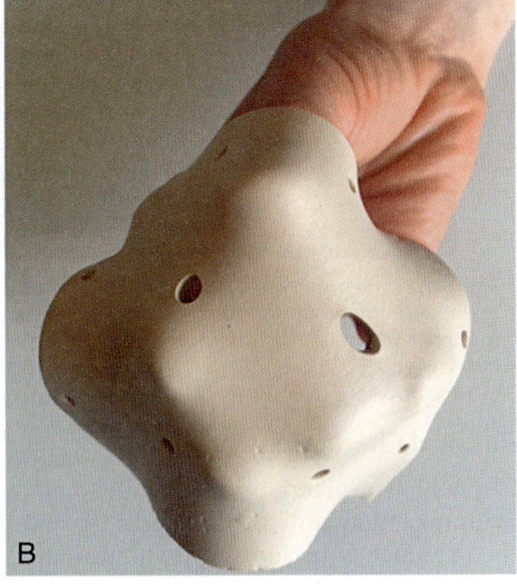

Fig. 14.17 The drape, or contouring quality of the material, placed over the hand on the left (A) illustrates a low resistance to stretch, whereas the less pliable material on the right (B) is more resistant to stretch.

Table 14.1 Characteristics of Thermoplastic Materials

	STRETCH RESISTANCE		
Company Name	**Minimum**	**Moderate**	**Maximal**
AliMed	Polyform	Orthoplast II	Ezeform
	Multiform	Polyflex II	Orthoplast
	Multiform Clear		
DeRoyal	LMB Drape	LMB Blend	
North Coast Medical	NCM Clinic	Encore	Omega Max
		NCM Preferred	Solaris
		NCM Vanilla	Omega Plus
		NCM Spectrum	Orfibrace
		Prism	Omega Black
Orfit Industries	Orficast	Orfilight	Orfit Eco
	OrfiCast More	Orfit Strips	Orfibrace NS
	Orfit NS	Orfit Colors NS	Orfit Classic Stiff
	Orfit Classic Soft	Orfit Flex NS	Dynasyst
	Aquafit NS Soft		Aquafit NS Stiff
	Tecnofit		
	Orfizip NS		
Performance Health	Polyform	Polyflex II	Ezeform
	Aquaplast ProDrape	Kay-Splint II	Aquaplast-T Resilient
		Aquaplast	Aquaplast-T Watercolors
		Watercolors	Synergy
		Tailorsplint	San-Splint
		Kay-Splint III	FabricForm
		Orthoplast II	
		CuraDrape	
WFR Corporation	Reveals XS	Reveals	Reveals LS
		Reveals colors	

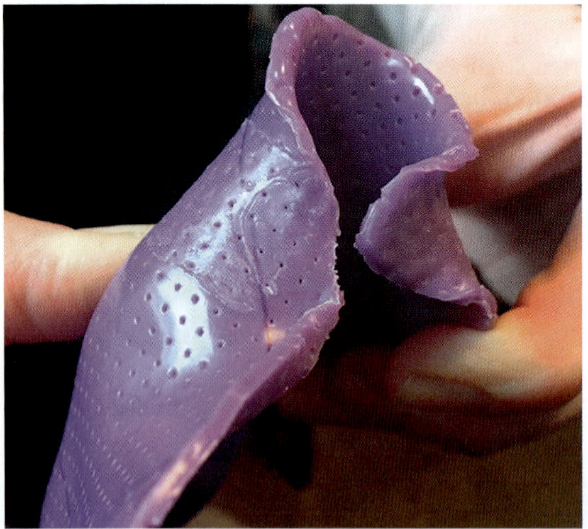

Fig. 14.18 The presence of coating on this material allows the circumferential segment around the thumb to be pulled apart after cooling to form a potential "trap door" on this wrist and thumb mobilization orthosis.

Physical Characteristics

Physical characteristics are evident on visual inspection. The most relevant ones include the material's thickness, the presence of perforations, and the color of the material.

Thickness

Low-temperature thermoplastics are available in a variety of thicknesses, including $\frac{1}{16}$, $\frac{3}{32}$, and $\frac{1}{8}$ inches. The appropriate thickness for an orthosis depends on the body segment, diagnosis, and required rigidity of the orthosis. For example, an elbow immobilization orthosis for a patient who sustained a fracture and underwent surgical fixation would best be made from a thicker $\frac{1}{8}$-inch material for a more rigid type of support. In another case, such as a hand-based thumb orthosis for an elderly patient with arthritis, it might be better to use a thinner $\frac{1}{16}$-inch material to achieve a light, compact type of support. The goal should be to provide the least bulky, lightest-weight orthosis possible that allows the device to perform its intended function optimally. Thinner materials are generally quicker to heat and faster to harden than their thicker counterparts.

Perforations

Thermoplastic materials with perforations allow for air exchange and produce a lighter-weight orthosis compared with those made with solid materials. Materials with a high density of perforations create an orthosis that is flexible (less rigid), which may not be appropriate for patients with specific diagnoses. Caution must be used to ensure the edges of the orthosis, derived from a thermoplastic sheet where the pattern is cut through its perforations, are smoothed to prevent unintended irritation of the patient's skin. This is commonly achieved with the use of a heat gun paired with manually rounding of the edges.

Colors

A wide array of colors are available, making the fabrication process even more creative. Providing choices in thermoplastic material and strap colors can improve compliance with orthosis use in all populations, most notably with pediatric clients. Issuing orthosis straps in a color other than white can also help patients to find orthoses that have been misplaced within bed linens. It is recommended to accept requests from patients during this aspect of the fabrication process to make them feel they have contributed to the construction of the orthosis and thus increase their personal acceptance of the need for wearing it.

Categories of Orthosis Materials

Thermoplastic materials can be categorized according to their chemical composition. This determines the way the material behaves during the fabrication process and affects how the completed orthosis functions. Thermoplastic materials may be made of plastics (e.g., Polyform [Performance Health, Warrenville, Illinois] or Multiform [AliMed, Dedham, Massachusetts]); rubber or rubber-like materials (e.g., Ezeform [Performance Health] or Orthoplast [AliMed]); combination plastic and rubber-like materials (e.g., Tailorsplint, PolyFlex II [Performance Health], or Encore [North Coast Medical, Morgan Hill, California]); and elastic materials (e.g., Aquaplast [Performance Health] or Reveal [WFR Corporation, Wyckoff, New Jersey]).

Plastic materials typically have a low resistance to stretch, allowing the completion of an orthosis that is highly contoured. Rubber or rubber-like materials are highly resistant to stretch but offer more control during the fabrication process. Combination plastic and rubber-like materials offer the blended advantages of each in terms of conformability and control during the molding process. Elastic materials possess memory and may be suitable for the novice orthosis fabricator who wishes to have the ability to remold the orthosis if necessary.

Orthoses may also be fabricated from alternative materials. These include lined materials (e.g., Silon-LTS [Performance Health], or Multiform Soft [Alimed]); mesh-type materials (e.g., X-Lite [Performance Health]); casting materials (e.g., plaster of Paris or QuickCast [Performance Health]); and soft materials (e.g., neoprene or Kinesio Tape [Performance Health]).

STRAPPING

Many different strapping systems are offered through distributors. The choice of appropriate strapping depends on the patient's diagnosis, the type of orthosis design, and the availability of the material in a manner very similar to the choice in selecting a thermoplastic material. Strapping is essential to properly secure the orthosis to the body part. If the strapping is not adequate, the orthosis can be uncomfortable or ineffective in achieving its desired goals. Generally adhesive hook-and-loop material (e.g., Velcro; Velcro USA, Manchester, New Hampshire) is applied to the orthosis base, and strapping material secures the segment within the orthosis. The most commonly used strapping mechanisms consist of traditional loop, foam, neoprene, or elasticized straps. In small areas where adhesive hooks may tend to pull off, rivets may be used to permanently secure the loop material to the thermoplastic pattern (Fig. 14.19).

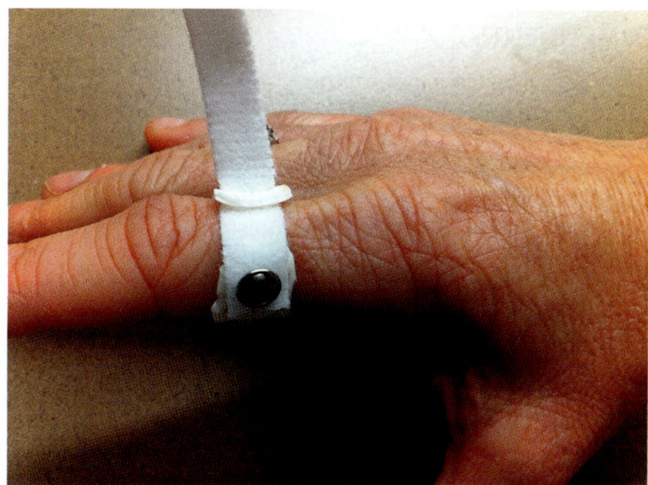

Fig. 14.19 A rivet can be applied to permanently secure strapping to the orthosis by forming holes in the thermoplastic material and in the strap with a hole punch; pliers are used to set the rivet in place.

Other adjuncts to strapping include D-rings that offer the ability to easily adjust the tension on the straps or circumferential wrapping (with an elasticized bandage) for those patients with significant edema. Straps should be wide and conforming so that they distribute pressure maximally but not wide to the point that they inhibit the ROM of adjacent joints. The patient should be educated in how to apply the straps tightly enough to secure the orthosis without compromising the neurovascular system.

PADDING AND LINING

Padding and lining products are available in a wide variety of thicknesses, textures, and materials. Therapists may use padding in specific regions during the orthotic fabrication process to accommodate bony prominences or superficial nerves. Ideally, the padding should be applied to the target area before molding the orthosis so that the modified device can contour to its adjusted proportions. Attaching the padding after the orthosis has been made can potentially cause a shift in pressure distribution and lead to problematic areas of high stress. Foam padding can also be adhered to straps at strategic places to improve joint position and to prevent migration of the orthosis.

Lining an orthosis with an adhesive product may be indicated in rare cases, such as when the patient has very fragile skin. Application of these adhesive liners should be done sparingly because of hygienic concerns; they are not easily cleaned or removed. As an alternative, disposable liners on the body part can be a way to improve comfort within an orthosis by placing a barrier between the skin and the thermoplastic material (see Fig. 14.19). Cotton and elasticized stockinettes are the most commonly used products in the clinic.

COMPONENTS

Component systems are an important element of mobilization orthoses. Rehabilitation catalogs help therapists stay abreast of what is available for their use. In general, outrigger systems are designed to help provide optimal force application to a body part. Ideally, these devices should be highly adjustable to allow the therapist to maintain the crucial 90-degree angle of force application. If the commercial systems are not accessible, therapists can fabricate equivalent prototypes using wire and scrap pieces of thermoplastic material. Four basic elements of an outrigger system are used in a digit mobilization orthosis: the proximal attachment device, the mobilization force, the pulley system, and finger slings (Fig. 14.20).

The proximal attachment device provides the means to secure the mobilization force to the orthosis. The mobilization force, whether it be static line (static progressive approach) or elastic (dynamic approach), traverses through a pulley system to maintain the desired 90-degree angle of force application. Distally, the force is imparted to the body part, in this case the finger, by a sling or loop.

Mobilization orthoses can be challenging to fabricate for a novice therapist. Learning through practice and obtaining feedback from more experienced colleagues are important ways to improve fabrication skills. Patients must consistently receive follow-up clinic visits to assess and modify the orthosis if a positive outcome is sought; these orthoses need frequent adjustments as the tissue responds to the stress applied by the device.

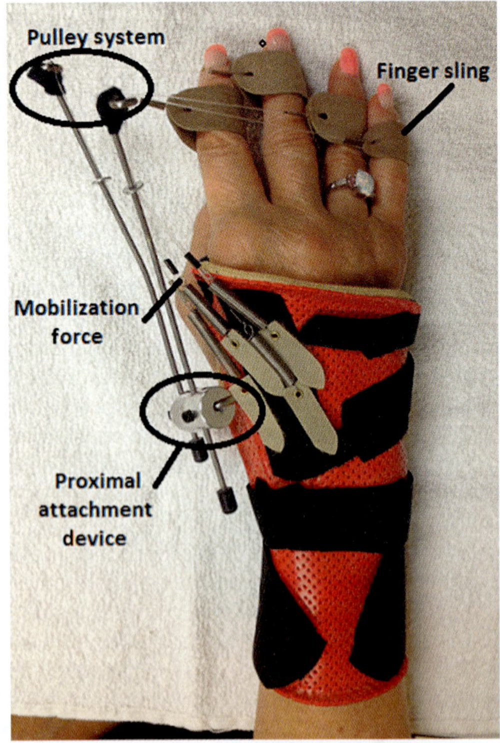

Fig. 14.20 Elements of this forearm-based metacarpophalangeal joint mobilization orthosis include a proximal attachment device, a mobilization force through a pulley system, and finger slings.

EQUIPMENT

Having access to quality tools in the clinic can help to make the orthotic fabrication process easier for the therapist. Sharp scissors designated solely for thermoplastic use are essential. If the scissors are used for all products, most notably adhesive products, the blades can retain the residue and make cutting the thermoplastic material difficult. Scissors with a nonstick, ceramic coating are available and are quite effective when cutting adhesive-backed products. Dull scissors do not provide a clean cut, which can lead to frustration and the creation of unsightly orthoses. Other tools that are helpful to keep on hand include a hole punch and a set of blunt-nose pliers for rivet application, a hand drill for creating holes or a series of perforations, and a heat gun to make minor adjustments to a formed orthosis.

Overview of the Orthotic Fabrication Process

A comprehensive prescription from the referral source is essential to implementing the appropriate orthotic application and optimizing the therapeutic effect of the device. In addition to the patient's name, the prescription must contain the following information:

- Diagnosis, including surgical procedures if applicable.
- Date of injury and any associated surgical procedure.
- Any precautions or contraindications that must be followed.
- Orthosis-related goals, including purpose, joint positions, and wearing schedule.

Having access to the relevant imaging such as radiographs as well as the patient's surgical report can help the therapist to gain a clear understanding of the tissues involved. As always, good communication with the referral source is essential in terms of gathering and sharing information regarding a patient's status.

After obtaining all critical information regarding the patient's diagnosis and the prescribed orders, the therapist should perform a comprehensive evaluation. This begins with a patient interview for gathering subjective information and continues with a review of systems and a detailed physical examination. The therapist uses the results of the history and examination to form a clinical judgment and establish a movement dysfunction diagnosis, including a list of impairments and functional limitations. From these problems, the therapist determines the prognosis for the fulfillment of functional goals and formulates an appropriate plan of care.

To prepare a comprehensive plan of care, therapists must use critical thinking skills to integrate their working knowledge with the information obtained from the referral source and the patient. The therapist has many modalities that can be used to treat the patient, only one of which is orthotic fabrication. Not all patients are appropriate for orthoses; determining if and when orthoses may be appropriate presents a consistent challenge for the therapist. Some patients may require orthoses initially whereas others may need one later in the process of their rehabilitation. An individualized approach is necessary to address each patient's unique needs.[32]

If an orthosis is indicated, the patient must be thoroughly educated regarding its proper use. This education must always include a written handout outlining the specifics of wear, care, and safety. The key points to stress include the following:

- Purpose of orthosis specific to the patient's diagnosis.
- Key indicators of potential adverse responses to the device and information about what to do if any occur.
- Expected functional limitations that might result from wearing the orthosis and suggestions of how to compensate for imposed limitations.
- Routine wearing schedule.
- Information about washing or cleaning the orthosis.
- Information or diagrams related to how to properly don and doff the orthosis (if applicable).
- Precautions and contraindications related to the patient's diagnosis and indicators of tissue tolerance (signs and symptoms of neurovascular compromise, soft tissue complication, or bony irritation).
- Avoidance of heat to prevent deformity of the orthotic structure.
- Contact information (the therapist's name and clinic phone number) with encouragement to reach out if any questions or problems arise with use.

Future Trends

3D-PRINTED SPLINTS

3D printed splints[34–40] offer several advantages in treating hand and finger disorders, providing innovative solutions in the field of orthopedics and rehabilitation. The utilization of 3D printing technology provides several benefits, including: (1) customization, (2) precision, (3) lightweight design, (4) breathability, (5) rapid prototyping, (6) cost-effective production, (7) incorporation of patient-specific features, and (8) involvement of users in the design process.

3D printing enables the creation of highly customized splints tailored to the specific anatomy of an individual's hand or finger. The digital nature of 3D printing allows for precise and accurate reproduction of complex geometries. When combined with a 3D surface scanner, 3D-printed splints allow for precise customization to match an individual's anatomical structure.

These splints can be designed with lightweight structures, enhancing patient comfort. The design flexibility of 3D printing also allows for the incorporation of ventilation or porous structures. Furthermore, 3D printing facilitates rapid prototyping, enabling healthcare providers to iterate and refine splint designs quickly based on patient feedback.

Once a digital design is established, 3D printing proves to be a cost-effective method for producing customized splints. This technology also allows for the incorporation of patient-specific features, such as integrating orthotic modifications or adapting the splint to accommodate specific deformities or conditions. In certain cases, users may actively participate in the design process, expressing their preferences and providing feedback. This collaborative approach can significantly enhance user satisfaction.

Several studies have demonstrated how the application of engineering concepts and emerging technologies could enhance outcomes for patients undergoing treatment for hand orthoses, including conditions. However, various aspects of 3D printing technology require further research to standardize procedures. Ongoing studies are investigating the mechanical properties of materials used in 3D-printed splints,[34,35,41–43] and evaluating the effectiveness of 3D-printed splints.[36–38,44,45]

SENSORISED HAND SPLINTS

With the advancement of sensor technology and artificial intelligence, it is evident that future hand splints may extend beyond being merely rigid thermoplastic devices. Sensorized hand splints have the potential to offer a means for monitoring and customizing personal care. Jones et al.[46] utilized a sensorized hand splint named HAILO, an instrumented splint designed for measuring the biomechanical effects of hand splinting and assessing interface loading characteristics for individuals with arthritis. In Weir et al.'s study,[47] temperature sensors were integrated into thermoplastic volar forearm splints.

Case Example 14.1 **A Patient With Osteoarthritis of the First Carpometacarpal Joint**

R.W. presents to the hand surgeon with a progressive, insidious onset of thumb pain near its base. Symptoms of aching and tenderness are exacerbated by activities such as turning keys, opening jars, holding open a book, and writing. Deformity from joint subluxation at the first carpometacarpal (CMC) joint with concurrent degenerative osteoarthritis (OA) is evident (Fig. 14.21). The patient also has a positive grind test; this involves the manual application of axial compressive force of the base of the first metacarpal into the trapezium (the test has a high specificity for CMC OA when crepitus and the reproduction of pain are present). R.W. receives a steroid injection into the CMC joint space to decrease localized inflammation and is given a prescription for hand therapy.

QUESTIONS TO CONSIDER

- Given this patient's current presentation, what additional tests and measures might be important to include in the evaluative process?
- What is an appropriate movement dysfunction–related diagnosis for this patient?
- What is a likely prognosis for this patient? What are the anticipated patient goals for intervention? What are suitable, realistic goals for rehabilitation? How long is it expected to take to achieve the goals collectively formulated by the patient and therapist?
- On the basis of the patient's goals and expectations as well as the therapist's understanding of the underlying disease process, what recommendations would be indicated for intervention at this point in time? What evidence from the current literature supports these recommendations? What should be prioritized from the list of possible interventions?
- What type of follow-up would be recommended? How might the goals and interventions change as the patient progresses through the stages of tissue healing? How would one assess the outcomes of any implemented interventions?

(Continued)

Case Example 14.1 A Patient With Osteoarthritis of the First Carpometacarpal Joint—Cont'd

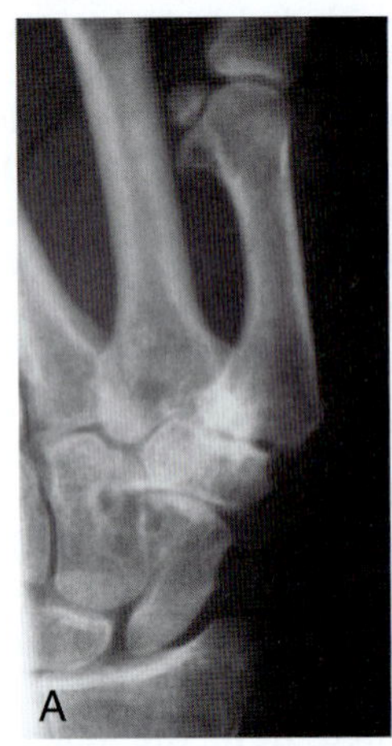
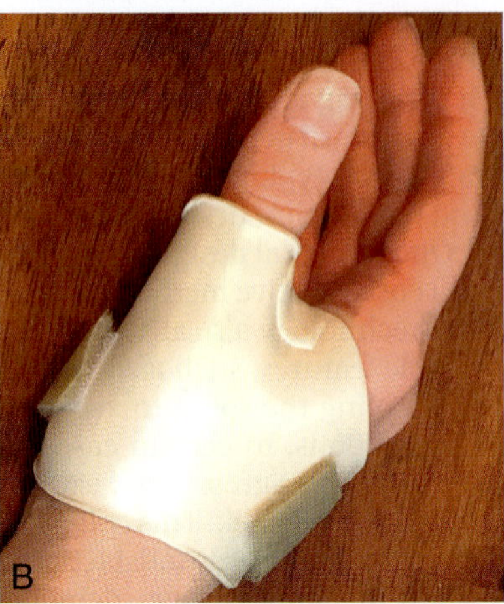
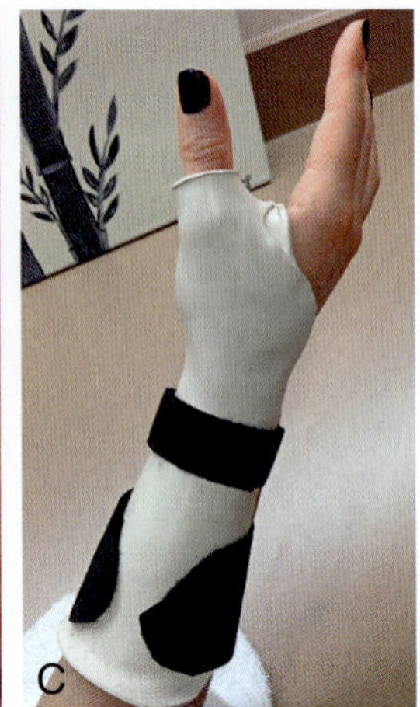
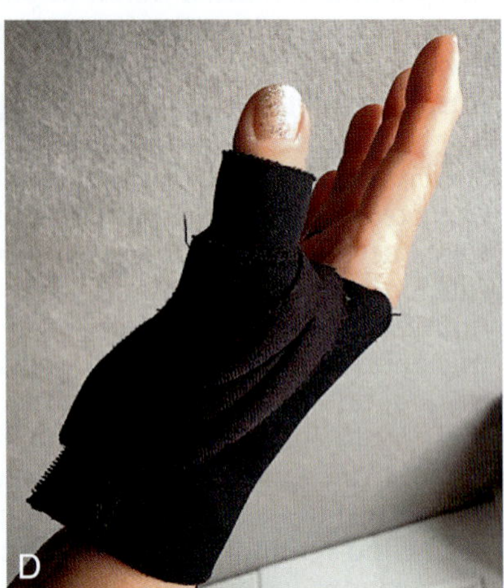

Fig. 14.21 (A) A radiograph indicating osteoarthritis at the carpometacarpal (CMC) joint of the thumb. (B) A custom thumb orthosis designed to reduce stress on the CMC joint during activities of daily living (ADLs). (C) After ligament reconstruction and arthroplasty, a forearm-based wrist and thumb immobilization orthosis is used during the proliferative stage of healing. (D) When adequate healing and fixation have occurred, the patient transitions into a neoprene orthosis to provide external support to the thumb during ADLs.

RECOMMENDATIONS FOR A PATIENT WITH OSTEOARTHRITIS OF THE FIRST CARPOMETACARPAL JOINT

A custom thumb orthosis is fabricated from a lightweight thermoplastic material (thickness: 1/16 inch) (see Fig. 14.21B). R.W. is instructed to use this device during daytime activities to decrease stress on the affected joint during functional tasks involving the thumb. The bulk of the skilled intervention is centered around education to allow the patient to adequately self-manage this chronic condition; the patient is thoroughly instructed in activity modification and joint protection principles. Some of the strategies include avoiding forceful, repetitive, and sustained pinching along with using pens and kitchen utensils with larger handles.

Despite these interventions, R.W. continues to have unmanaged symptoms and returns to the physician to discuss her medically related treatment options. R.W. undergoes a ligament reconstruction with tendon interposition (LRTI) arthroplasty, which includes a trapezium excision with a slip of the flexor carpi radialis interposed between the scaphoid and the first metacarpal. For the initial 3-week postoperative period after LRTI, in the inflammatory stage of healing during which tissue rest is indicated, a rigid cast is used to immobilize the treatment region. As healing progresses into the proliferative stage, around the 3-week period, the patient is placed in a removable forearm-based wrist/thumb immobilization orthosis that is removed for periodic ROM exercises (see Fig. 14.21C).

At approximately 6 weeks after surgery, as the healing continues to progress and no complications arise, the patient uses a prefabricated neoprene thumb orthosis to aid in the transition out of the rigid thermoplastic orthosis (see Fig. 14.21D). The neoprene material offers restrictive compression combining warmth and gentle support during functional tasks. At 12 weeks after surgery, the therapist encourages the weaning of all orthoses until they are fully discontinued and R.W. returns to normal activities without significant pain. Her comprehensive maintenance program includes therapeutic exercise centered on the recruitment of the first dorsal interosseous muscle to promote inherent stability of the first metacarpal during functional use.[33]

Case Example 14.2 A Patient With a Fracture of the Distal Radius

D.A. presents to the hand surgeon's office after a fall onto an outstretched hand (FOOSH). The radiograph reveals a comminuted fracture of the distal radius requiring surgical fixation. The surgeon performs an open reduction and internal fixation and implants a plate and screws for anatomic reinforcement (Fig. 14.22). At 5 days postsurgery, the patient is referred to hand therapy to receive a protective orthosis and initiate an early ROM program.

QUESTIONS TO CONSIDER

- Given this patient's current presentation, what additional tests and measures might be important to include in the evaluative process?
- What is an appropriate movement dysfunction–related diagnosis for this patient?
- What is a likely prognosis for this patient? What are the anticipated patient goals for intervention? What are suitable, realistic goals for rehabilitation? How long is it expected to take to achieve the goals collectively formulated by the patient and therapist?
- On the basis of the patient's goals and expectations as well as the therapist's understanding of the underlying disease process, what recommendations would be indicated for intervention at this point in time? What evidence from the current literature supports these recommendations? What should be prioritized from the list of possible interventions?

Case Example 14.2 **A Patient With a Fracture of the Distal Radius—Cont'd**

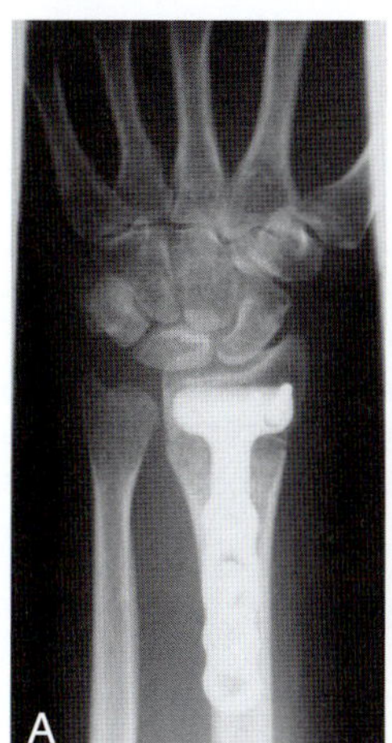
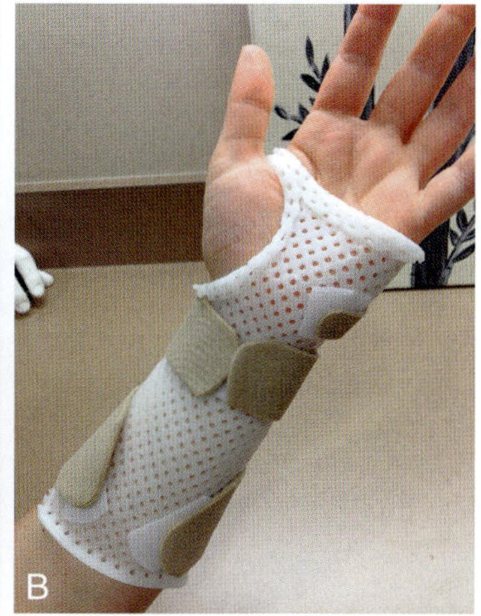
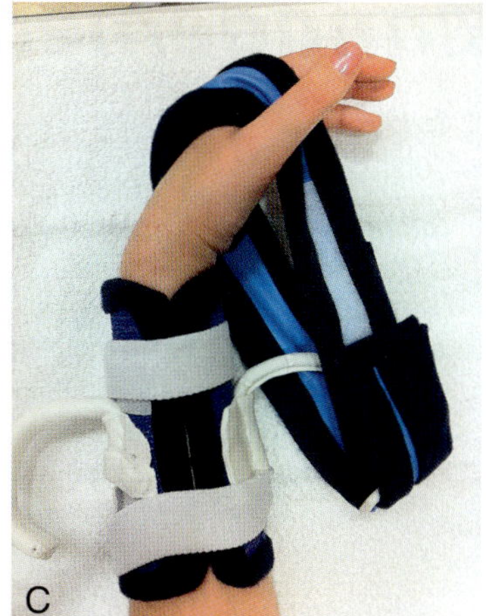
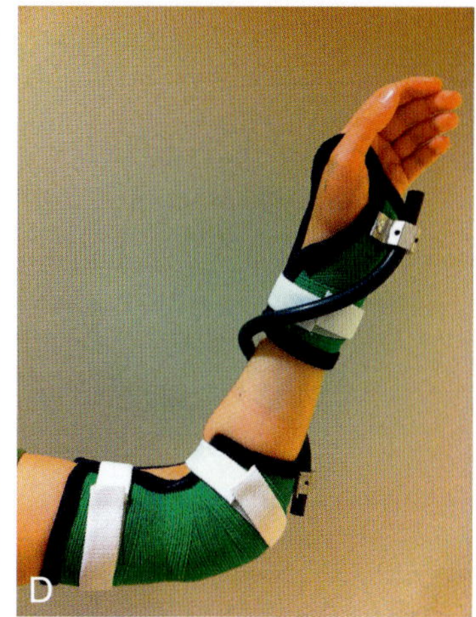

Fig. 14.22 (A) A radiograph of open reduction and internal fixation of a comminuted wrist fracture. (B) A forearm-based wrist immobilization orthosis used during the initial stages of healing. When adequate healing has occurred, a wrist flexion mobilization orthosis (C) and a forearm supination mobilization orthosis (D) are fabricated to help increase functional range of motion.

- What type of follow-up would be recommended? How might the goals and interventions change as the patient progresses through the stages of tissue healing? How would one assess the outcomes of any implemented interventions?
- Given the history of a FOOSH injury, is the patient at further risk for reinjury to the affected area of their upper extremity? Is there an underlying condition affecting the patient's balance that presents as a red flag for safety?

RECOMMENDATIONS FOR A PATIENT WITH OPEN REDUCTION AND INTERNAL FIXATION OF WRIST FRACTURE

A forearm-based wrist immobilization orthosis is fabricated with a ⅛-inch-thick material to obtain a rigid support to be used during the proliferative stage of healing (see Fig. 14.22B). D.A. is instructed to remove the orthosis six times a day for gentle ROM of the forearm, wrist, and digits. As expected, all forearm and wrist motions are significantly limited, and mild edema is localized to the area. During this phase, D.A. is encouraged to move the digits frequently between exercise sessions with the orthosis in place and to incorporate the hand in light ADLs.

At 4 weeks after surgery, because a radiograph has revealed adequate healing along with stable fixation provided by the plate and screws, the wrist orthosis is discontinued (except for heavy-resisted or repetitive activities) and therapy progresses with the addition of gentle passive ROM. All movements of the extremity improve except wrist flexion and forearm supination, which are significantly restricted during passive stretching. At 6 weeks, these limitations continue to be problematic and the physician recommends the addition of a wrist flexion mobilization orthosis (see Fig. 14.22C) and a forearm supination mobilization orthosis (see Fig. 14.22D).

The wrist flexion mobilization orthosis is fabricated with a delta cast material with a cloth sling to provide the mobilization force through a static progressive approach. This method is selected because of the high degree of stiffness present in the wrist. The supination mobilization orthosis is fabricated with a tubing mechanism to facilitate the stretching force. The patient is instructed to wear each device four times a day for 30 minutes, consistently increasing the passive stretch on the affected tissues as tolerated. The previously used wrist immobilization orthosis continues to be used at night as a serial static device and is remolded to position the wrist at maximal flexion; this aims to maintain the collective gains made during all waking hours.

After 4 weeks of consistent use, D.A. plateaus her active ROM at 55 degrees of wrist flexion and 70 degrees of supination, which is deemed to be functional and, because of the severity of the injury, also quite acceptable.

Summary

The fabrication of an orthosis is a commonly used intervention for clinicians who treat an impaired upper extremity. Gaining an appreciation for how different orthoses can be created for specific purposes aids in achieving maximal patient outcomes. This chapter reviewed many aspects of orthotic fabrication, including nomenclature, tissue healing, and anatomic and mechanical principles and provided an overview of the various products available to a qualified therapist. Through comprehensive study and practice, the fabrication and application of orthoses can be another tool used successfully in the clinic to benefit the patient, the therapist, and referring provider.

References

The complete listing of the References are available in the accompanying enhanced eBook version included with the print purchase of this textbook. Visit Elsevier eBooks+ (eBooks.Health.Elsevier.com) to access this content.

15 Orthoses in Burn Care: Splinting, Orthotics, and Prosthetics in the Management of Burns

JAMIE DYSON

LEARNING OBJECTIVES

On completion of this chapter, the reader will be able to do the following:

1. Identify the elements of burn injury that contribute to decision-making regarding applying splints, orthotics, and prosthetics.
2. Describe how wound care may affect splints, orthotics, and prosthetics use and application.
3. Discuss components of rehabilitation interventions that may incorporate or affect the use of splints, orthotics, and prosthetics.
4. Describe the use of splints and orthotics in caring for patients with burn injuries.
5. Describe the use of prosthetics for patients with amputations associated with burn injuries.

The rehabilitation of burn patients has two primary goals: maintain mobility and prevent and treat scars and contractures. Rehabilitation begins as soon as medically and surgically possible. As the survivability of major burns has increased, mobility and contracture management have become more challenging. Specific rehabilitation priorities change daily; however, these primary goals must be the foundation of all treatment plans.[1] Burn rehabilitation is vital to the patient's recovery and quality of life (QOL). The focus is on preserving and restoring mobility, activities of daily living (ADLs), limb positioning, splinting, and scar management.[2] Physical therapists (PTs) and occupational therapists are introduced to the burn patient early on in their course and continue to follow throughout their burn care journey. Hypertrophic scarring, scar contracture, heterotopic ossification (HO), loss of mobility, and pain are commonly part of the aftermath of a burn injury.[3,4]

Burn Injury

Approximately two million people suffer burn-related injuries every year in the United States. Of the total number of burn injuries, roughly 500,000 patients received medical evaluation and treatment. Approximately 40,000 patients required hospitalization for their burn injuries. Males account for most burn injury patients at 69%. The average age of burn injury patients is 32 years old. Children under age five account for 19% of burn injuries, while patients over 60 account for an additional 13%. Most burns (74%) involve less than 10% of the total body surface area (TBSA), which suggests that most burn injuries are relatively minor in terms of the affected area of the body. Nearly 80% of all burns are caused by flame or fire or by scalds, with scald injury occurring most in children younger than 5 years.[5] Various factors, including the burning agent's characteristics and temperature, the exposure duration, the injury's location, the presence of associated injuries, and the age and general health of the victim, determine the severity of a burn injury. These factors influence the potential complications, long-term effects, and the overall prognosis of burn injury. In addition, the cause of the injury, such as fire, hot liquids, chemicals, electricity, or radiation, can influence its severity. The depth of the burn refers to how far it has penetrated the layers of the skin. Deeper burns are generally more severe and require more extensive treatment. The percentage of the TBSA affected by the burn is essential in determining the severity. Burns involving a larger TBSA are typically more severe and can have systemic effects on the body. Burns on certain areas of the body, such as the face, eyes, ears, perineum, hands, and feet, are considered more critical due to their functional and cosmetic importance.[6,7]

The patient's preburn health status and any preexisting medical conditions can affect the severity and outcome of the burn injury. Certain factors, such as a compromised immune system, diabetes, or heart disease, can complicate healing. Burn injuries can be more severe for very young or elderly patients. Children and older adults tend to have less reserve and may experience more complications during rehabilitation. Additionally, associated trauma, smoke inhalation injury, and poor preinjury health status can further increase the severity of a burn injury. Understanding the nature of the burn injury, including the location and depth of the burn wound, is crucial for anticipating and addressing the potential challenges a patient may face during the rehabilitation process.[6,8]

CAUSES OF BURNS

Burns can have various causes and can be classified based on the source of injury. Thermal burns are the most common type of burn, as well as chemical burns, electrical burns, and radiation burns. Thermal burns from direct exposure to open flames from various sources such as fires, explosions, or flammable gases. Scalds due to contact with hot liquids or steam, such as boiling water, hot beverages, or cooking fluids. Touching hot surfaces like stoves, irons, heating appliances, or hot metals can also lead to thermal burns. Lastly, residential, industrial, or wildfires can cause severe thermal burns. Chemical burns due to contact with strong acids (e.g., sulfuric acid, hydrochloric acid) or alkalies (e.g., sodium hydroxide, potassium hydroxide). Mishandling or accidental contact with common household chemicals like bleach, drain cleaners, or pool chemicals can cause chemical burns. Working with hazardous chemicals in industries without proper safety precautions can also lead to chemical burns. Electrical burns can result from direct contact with sources, such as exposed wires, faulty electrical appliances, or lightning strikes. An electric arc or flash generated during electrical work or accidents can produce intense heat and cause burns. Radiation burns from prolonged exposure to ultraviolet radiation from the sun or tanning beds can result in sunburns. Accidental exposure to ionizing radiation sources like x-rays, nuclear radiation, or radioactive materials can also cause radiation burns. It is important to note that burns can also occur due to other causes, such as friction burns (caused by friction with rough surfaces), cold burns (caused by exposure to extreme cold), or electrical burns caused by internal sources like pacemakers or defibrillators.[6,9,10]

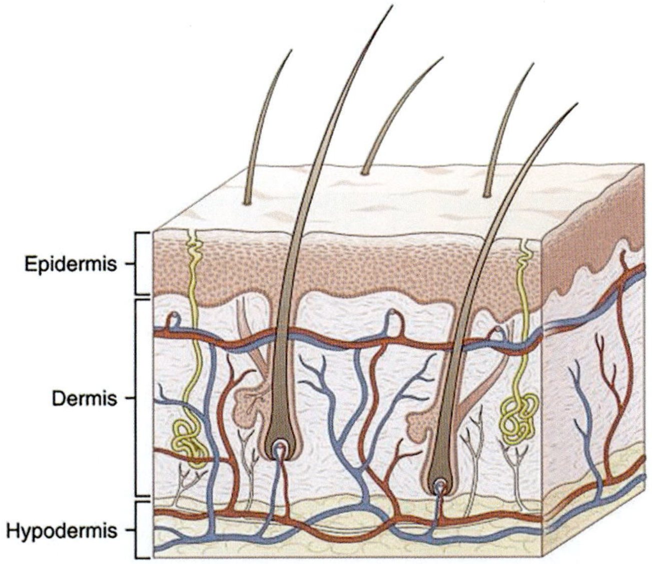

Fig. 15.1 The layers of the skin. (From Skirven TM, Osterman AL, Fedorczyk J, Amadio PC, Felder S, Shin EK. *Rehabilitation of the Hand and Upper Extremity*. Elsevier Health Sciences; 2020.)

BURN DEPTH

The depth of a burn is a crucial factor in classifying the burn and determining its healing prognosis. The degree of burn is determined through a comprehensive physical examination and knowledge of the anatomy of the epidermis (Fig. 15.1). However, the actual depth of the burn may not be immediately evident and may require operative excision for a definitive assessment. Therefore early clinical evaluation is essential not only for resuscitation purposes but also for determining the appropriate initial wound management (Fig. 15.2). First-degree burns (superficial) (Fig. 15.3) only affect the epidermis, the outermost layer of the skin. They are considered clinically benign since they do not form blisters or scars. Surgery is rarely required for their management. Second-degree burns (partial-thickness burns) extend into the dermis, the layer beneath the epidermis. Second-degree burns can be further classified into two types: superficial partial-thickness burns and deep partial-thickness burns. Superficial partial-thickness burns, which are hyperemic (red) and blanching in nature, are often accompanied by "weeping" or the release of fluid from the burn site (Fig. 15.4). Local wound care and topical therapies are usually sufficient for treating superficial partial-thickness burns. Deep partial-thickness burns appear drier and demonstrate a nonblanching pattern (Fig. 15.5). Surgical excision is often necessary to facilitate healing for deep partial-thickness burns. Third-degree burns (full-thickness burns) extend through the entire dermis and

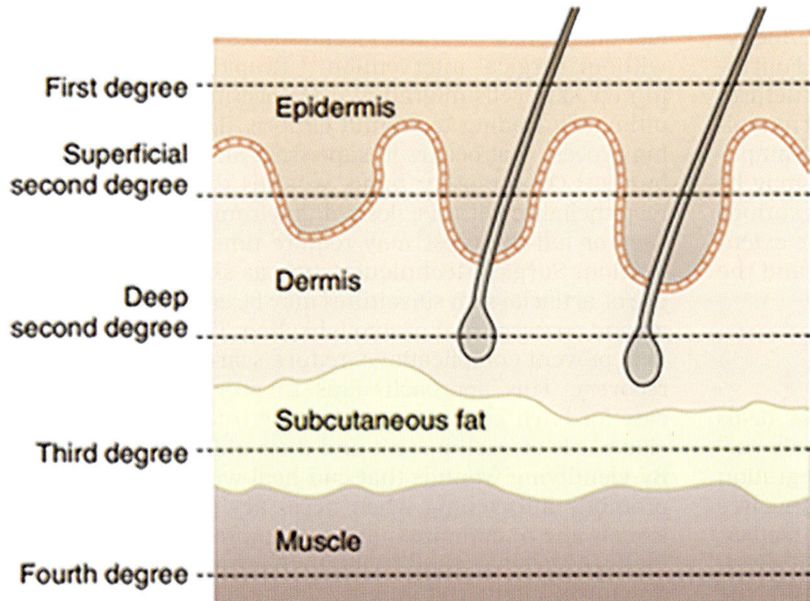

Fig. 15.2 Depths of a burn. First-degree burns are confined to the epidermis. Second-degree burns extend into the dermis (dermal burns). Third-degree burns are full thickness through the epidermis and dermis. Fourth-degree burns involve injury to underlying tissue structures such as muscle, tendons, and bone. (From Townsend CM, Beauchamp RD, Evers BM, et al., eds: *Sabiston Textbook of Surgery*. Nineteenth ed. Saunders; 2012.)

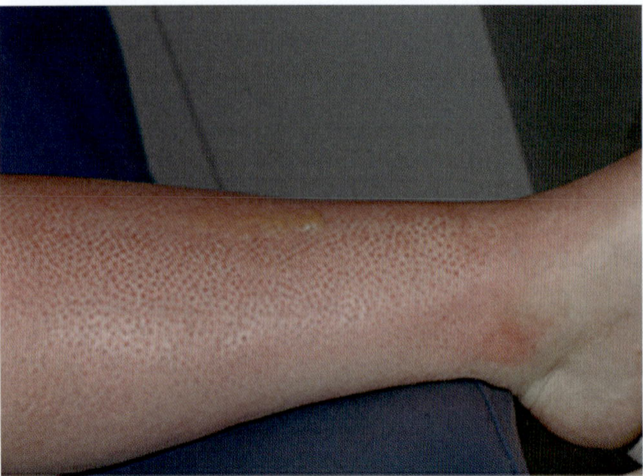

Fig. 15.3 **Patient with sunburn on the lower extremity (a superficial or first-degree burn).** (From Davis PJ, Cladis FP, Motoyama EK, eds. *Smith's Anesthesia for Infants and Children*. Eighth ed. Mosby; 2011.)

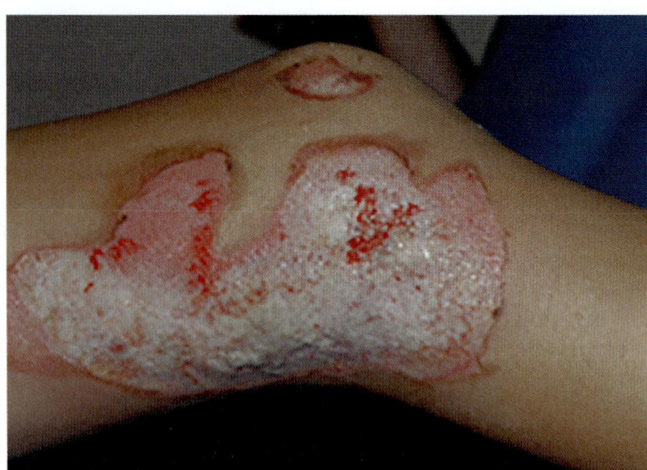

Fig. 15.5 **Partial-thickness injury extending beyond the subcutaneous layers (deep partial-thickness burn).** (From Davis PJ, Cladis FP, Motoyama EK, eds. *Smith's Anesthesia for Infants and Children*. Eighth ed. Mosby; 2011.)

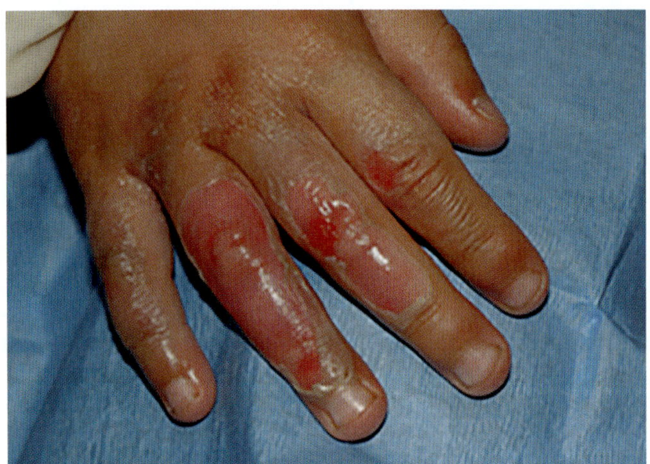

Fig. 15.4 **Partial-thickness injury of the hand (superficial second-degree burn).** (From Davis PJ, Cladis FP, Motoyama EK, eds. *Smith's Anesthesia for Infants and Children*. Eighth ed. Mosby; 2011.)

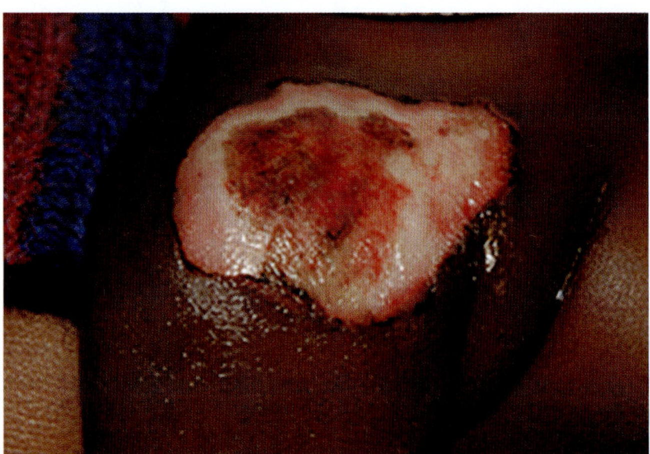

Fig. 15.6 **Full-thickness (third-degree) burn.** (From Davis PJ, Cladis FP, Motoyama EK, eds. *Smith's Anesthesia for Infants and Children*. Eighth ed. Mosby; 2011.)

reach the subcutaneous tissues. They may involve underlying structures such as muscle and bone (Fig. 15.6). Fourth-degree burns go even deeper and affect internal structures (Fig. 15.7). Both third-degree and fourth-degree burns typically require surgical intervention. In severe cases, amputation or removal of affected limbs or structures may be necessary.[5,11] The depth of the burn correlates with various factors, including the level of sensation present, the extent of excision required, the risk of wound infection, and the severity of scar formation.[11]

BURN SURGERY

Burn surgery is a specialized branch of surgery that deals with managing burn injuries. The priority is not only survival but also the overall QOL and successful reintegration of burn survivors into society. Optimal care now involves a comprehensive approach that considers various factors, including wound assessment and appropriate interventions. A crucial aspect of modern burn management is the identification of wounds that can successfully reepithelialize without surgical intervention.[12] Reepithelialization refers to new skin cells migrating and covering the wound bed, ultimately leading to wound closure. It is a natural healing process that occurs in superficial and partial-thickness burns.[13] On the other hand, wounds that are unlikely to reepithelialize within a desired timeframe or those that are deep or full-thickness may require timely operative intervention. Surgical techniques such as skin grafting or the use of artificial skin substitutes may be employed to achieve wound coverage and promote healing. These interventions help prevent complications, reduce scarring, and facilitate recovery. This approach aims to provide individualized care for burn patients, tailoring the treatment to the specific needs of each patient and their unique burn injuries. By identifying wounds that can heal without surgery and promptly intervening when necessary, healthcare professionals aim to optimize outcomes, improve the overall QOL for burn survivors, and facilitate their successful reintegration into society.[1,3–5,11,12]

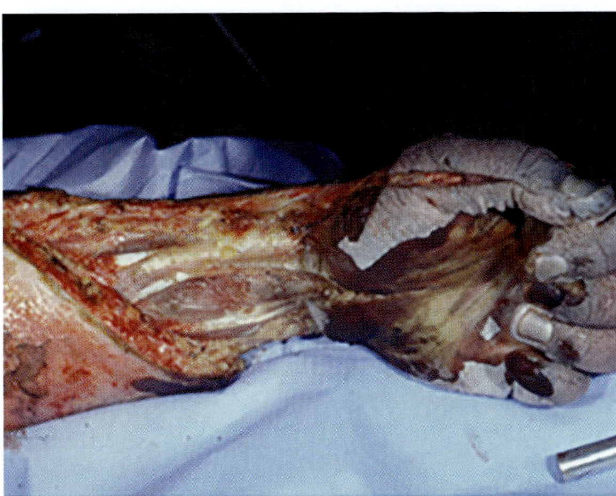

Fig. 15.7 Full-thickness injury with extensive tissue loss (fourth-degree burn). (From Davis PJ, Cladis FP, Motoyama EK, eds. *Smith's Anesthesia for Infants and Children*. Eighth ed. Mosby; 2011.)

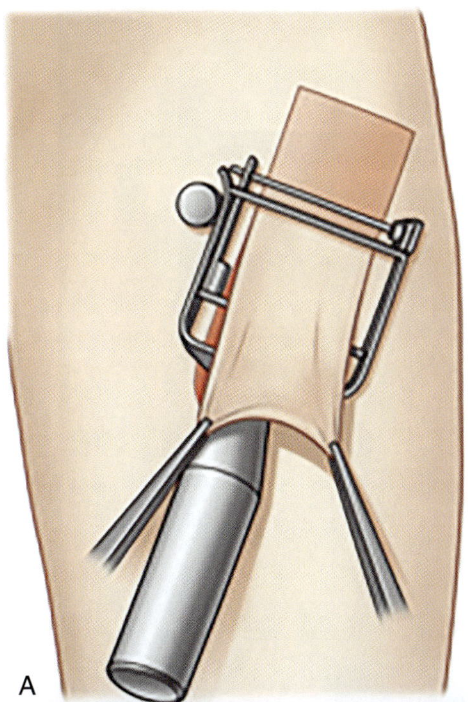

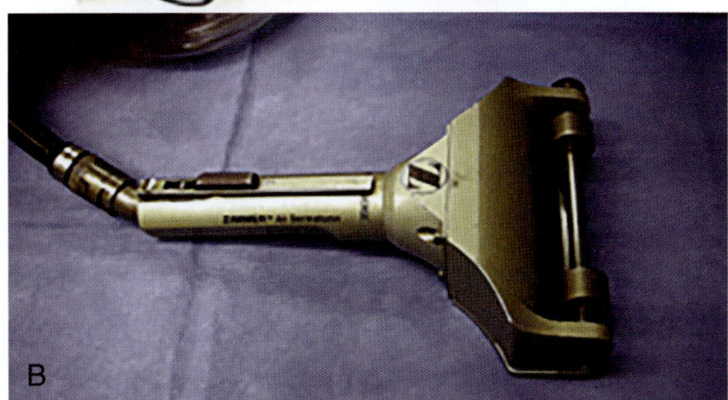

Fig. 15.8 (A) Split-thickness skin graft harvest using a powered dermatome at the thigh. (B) Donor skin is removed from an unburned area of skin through the use of a powered dermatome. (Revised from Orgill DP. Excision and skin grafting of thermal burns. *N Engl J Med*. 2009;360:893–901.)

Initial treatments and surgical interventions for burn patients involve wound debridement. Debridement consists of the removal of nonviable tissue, including necrotic tissue or eschar, from the wound bed. This process helps assess the wound, promote wound healing, and prepare the wound bed for further treatments, such as skin grafting.[4] Different debridement techniques can be employed, such as surgical debridement, mechanical debridement using a wet-to-dry dressing, enzymatic debridement using a daily application of ointment, autolytic debridement using occlusive dressings, or biological debridement where sterile larvae are applied to the wound. The healthcare provider will assess the situation and select the most appropriate debridement approach for each case.[1,3–5,11,12]

The most common procedure performed in burn surgery is skin grafting. Skin grafting involves taking healthy skin from another area of the patient's body and transplanting it onto the burned area, which helps to promote healing and prevent infection. Different types of skin grafts, including split-thickness grafts and full-thickness grafts, are selected based on the location and severity of the burn injury. An autograft involves using a patient's own skin and remains the primary method for wound closure in the field of burn care. Autografts can be performed as either split-thickness skin grafting (STSG) or full-thickness skin grafting (FTSG), each with its own characteristics and considerations. STSG involves harvesting a thin layer of skin that includes the epidermis and a portion of the dermis (Fig. 15.8A and B). The graft can be meshed to cover a larger area than the original donor skin (Fig. 15.9). This graft is then applied to the burn wound as a temporary covering (Fig. 15.10).[11] The advantage of STSG is that it leaves behind a portion of the dermis at the donor site, allowing for reepithelialization and healing of the donor area. Therefore this method is suitable for larger burn wounds where there is a need to cover a larger surface area. FTSG involves harvesting a graft that includes the entire thickness of the dermis. This graft is typically taken from an area with excess skin, such as the thigh or buttock, and requires subsequent primary closure at the donor site. FTSG provides a thicker and more durable graft, which is beneficial for areas requiring increased strength and contracture resistance.[5] However, FTSG is limited by the availability of appropriate donor sites and is typically used for smaller burn wounds or specific anatomical areas.[1,3,4,12–15]

While autografting is an effective method for wound closure, it is important to consider the potential drawbacks, particularly in the case of larger burn wounds. Autografting creates additional wounds at the donor site, adding to open wounds' TBSA (Fig. 15.11),[3,5] which can increase the patient's overall morbidity and affect their recovery. The size and location of the donor site must be carefully considered to minimize the impact on the patient's functional and cosmetic outcomes. Advancements have been made in alternative approaches to autografting, such as the use of skin substitutes or bioengineered grafts. These techniques aim to reduce the reliance on autografts and provide alternative options for wound closure (Box 15.1). However, autografting remains the gold standard and is widely used due to its effectiveness and ability to promote healing.[4,12,14]

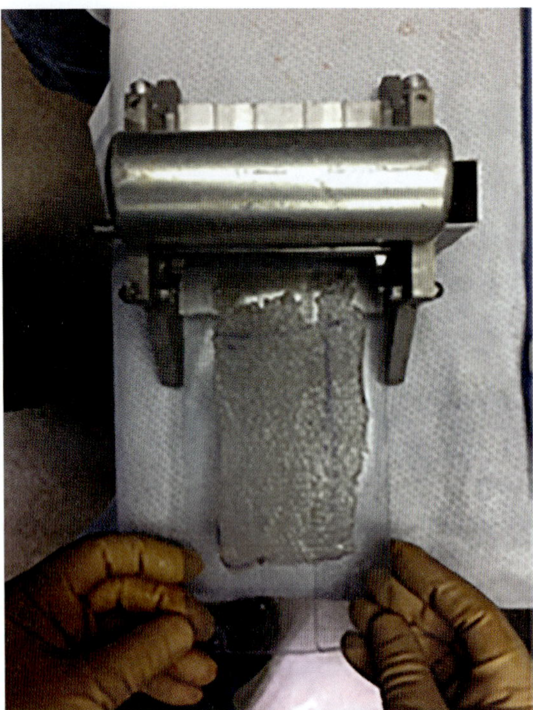

Fig. 15.9 A hand-crank powered mesher. (From Therattil PJ, Agag RL. Skin grafting. In: *Global Reconstructive Surgery*. Elsevier; 2019:60–65.)

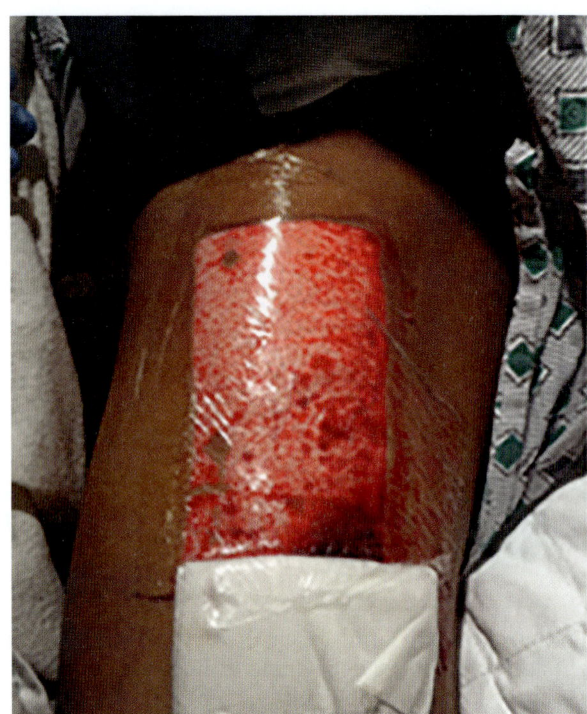

Fig. 15.11 Skin graft donor site. (From Therattil PJ, Agag RL. Skin grafting. In: *Global Reconstructive Surgery*. Elsevier; 2019:60–65.)

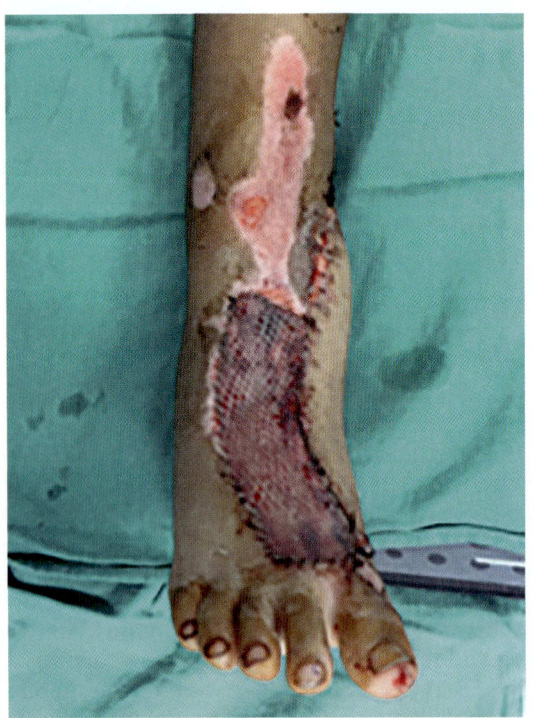

Fig. 15.10 A meshed split-thickness skin graft (meshing ratio 1:1.5) was used for coverage of the dorsal foot. (From Therattil PJ, Agag RL. Skin grafting. In: *Global Reconstructive Surgery*. Elsevier; 2019:60–65.)

After burn surgery, splinting is utilized as a part of the rehabilitation process to promote proper positioning, prevent contractures, and support the healing and functional recovery of the burned area. Splinting techniques can vary depending on the location and severity of the burn, as well as the specific needs of the patient. Splints are used to immobilize the affected area, reducing pain and preventing further damage. Splints maintain the proper positioning of joints and tissues to prevent contractures and deformities. Splints provide a physical barrier that protects the healing skin and tissues from friction, pressure, and trauma. In addition, splints provide support to weakened muscles and structures, aiding functional recovery. Splints should be designed to accommodate wound dressings and allow for regular dressing changes. Proper padding is essential to prevent pressure sores and ensure comfort. Regular monitoring of the splinted area is important to assess healing and skin condition and to adjust the splint as needed.[1,4,12–15]

BURN SIZE

Determining burn size involves the calculation of the percentage of TBSA. Accurate burn size estimation helps guide fluid resuscitation, determine the need for transfer to specialized burn centers, plan further management strategies, assess prognosis, and conduct research studies. Several methods are commonly used for estimating burned TBSA. The patient palm method relies on the patient's palm size, where the patient's palm, including fingers, is considered to be roughly 1% of their TBSA. Therefore the burned area can be estimated by comparing it to the size of the patient's palm. The rule of nines (Fig. 15.12) divides the body into regions, each representing a multiple of 9% of the TBSA. This method quickly estimates by assigning specific percentages to different body regions. However, it may not be as accurate for children due to variations in body proportions. The Lund and Browder chart (Fig. 15.13) is a more precise and accurate method that considers the changing proportions of body regions based on age. It divides the body

Box 15.1 **Types of Skin Grafts**

Type of Graft	Description	Type of Burn
Xenografts	Temporary wound coverage to assist with pain, protection from bacteria, and moisture control of the wound. The most used xenograft today is porcine derived.	Partial-thickness burns
Allograft	Cadaver skin that contains epidermis and some dermis used to assist with the preparation of the wound bed, decrease pain, and protect the tissue from the external environment. It is also used when there is limited donor site availability for autograft.	Full-thickness burns
Integra	Synthetic, permanent, acellular skin substitute created to help promote vascularization within the wound bed. It is a bilayer skin product that consists of an epithelial and silicone layer created from bovine tendon collagen.	Full-thickness burns
Apligraf	Bioengineered, cellular skin substitute that is created from foreskin-derived neonatal keratinocytes and bovine collagen.	Clean uninfected burns
Cultured epidermal autograft	A permanent skin substitute used to replace the epidermal layer of tissue. The process involves taking a skin biopsy of unburned skin and removing the dermis and subcutaneous tissue from the epidermis. Cells from the epidermis are then grown into new sheets of skin in a laboratory.	Used on burn patients with greater than 30% TBSA who do not have a large surface area of unburned skin that can be used to harvest skin grafts.

TBSA, Total body surface area.
Modified from Saraswat AB. Acute surgical management of the burn patient. *Surg Clin*. 2023;103(3):463–472.

into smaller regions and provides specific percentages for each area, considering the age-specific body proportions. Advancements in technology have introduced computerized methods for burn size estimation. Planimetry involves using computer software to trace the burn wound's outline and calculate the percentage of body surface area (BSA) involved. Three-dimensional photography and smartphone applications have also been developed, offering precise measurements by capturing the burn wound in three dimensions or utilizing specialized algorithms.[7,16–23]

LOCATION OF THE BURN

Burns involving the hands, feet, face, genitalia, perineum, and those that cross major joints can be challenging to manage and, according to the American Burn Association, should be transported to a burn center. Lasting damage to these areas can have a severe impact on patient outcomes. Impairments to the hands can affect grip and can therefore have harmful effects on the ability to work or handle ADLs. Burns of the feet or those that cross joints can severely limit mobility, while burns to the face can impair vision and the ability to eat and have an emotional impact due to altered appearance. Inhalation injuries often accompany injuries to the face. Burns to the genitalia and perineum can restrict patient autonomy, hindering urinary and sexual function or the ability to defecate. Special consideration should be given to burns that are completely circumferential around a part of the body, such as a limb or the trunk. Due to the tissues beneath the wound becoming edematous, circumferential wounds can cause increased pressure, resulting in compartment syndrome and leading to ischemia. The classic symptoms are the five "Ps": pain, pallor, paresthesia, pulselessness, and paralysis.[24]

Wound Care

Proper wound care, infection prevention, and timely medical interventions are crucial for optimizing burn wound healing and minimizing scar formation. Each burn injury is unique, and the healing process can vary depending on various factors, including the depth and extent of the burn, the location of the injury, and individual patient factors. Infection is a common complication that can significantly delay healing and increase scar formation. In addition, burn wounds create an ideal environment for bacterial growth due to the loss of the protective skin barrier.[3,4]

TOPICAL AGENTS AND WOUND DRESSING

The epidermis is the largest organ of the body. It is essential in regulating fluid flow and body temperature, enabling various sensations such as cold, heat, pain, and touch. The skin comprises three main layers: the epidermis, dermis, and subcutaneous tissue. These layers work together to protect against pathogens while also allowing certain substances to pass through in a semipermeable manner. Although the skin possesses a natural self-regeneration ability, this ability can be hindered in various physiopathological conditions such as burns. In the case of burns, the vasculature is partially or fully damaged, limiting the factors and cells necessary for regeneration to reach the wound site. This vascular damage can result in delayed wound closure and an increased risk of complications such as pain, infection, and scarring.[25]

Various wound dressings are available, each with specific characteristics and indications. The selection of an appropriate dressing depends on the type and condition of the wound, as well as the individual patient's needs. Burn wound dressings possess several characteristics and functions contributing to effective wound healing. Moist wound healing is generally preferred over dry wound healing as it promotes faster and more effective healing. In addition, the dressing should help retain moisture in the wound bed, preventing desiccation (excessive drying) of the wound while avoiding maceration (overhydration and softening of the surrounding healthy skin). Burn wound dressings should have the capacity to absorb excess wound exudate to maintain an optimal moisture balance in the wound. Excessive exudate

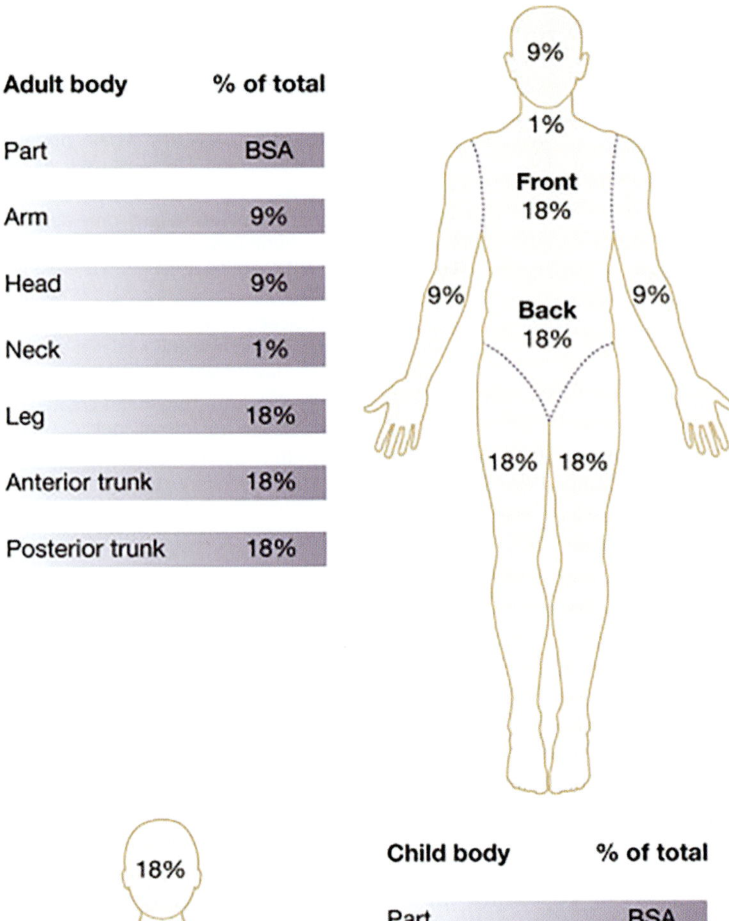

Child body	% of total
Part	BSA
Arm	9%
Head and neck	18%
Leg	14%
Anterior trunk	18%
Posterior trunk	18%

18%
Front 18%
9% 9%
Back 18%
14% 14%

Fig. 15.12 Estimation of burn size using the rule of nines. *BSA*, Body surface area. (Reprinted (in part) with permission from American Burn Association. *Advanced Burn Life Support™ Manual*; 2023. Available from: https://ameriburn.org/abls. Copyright© 2023 American Burn Association.)

can impede healing and increase the risk of infection. A primary function of burn wound dressings is to provide a barrier against bacteria and other pathogens. They should have antimicrobial properties or act as a physical barrier to prevent contamination and infection. Burn dressings may have properties that promote the formation of new blood vessels (angiogenesis) and facilitate the growth of connective tissue. The dressing should not impede blood circulation to the wound site, as adequate blood flow is essential for delivering oxygen, nutrients, and immune cells. The dressing should not adhere to the wound bed, as this can disrupt the healing process and cause pain on removal. Easy detachment and quick debridement of the dressing are desirable qualities. The dressing should be hypoallergenic and nontoxic to avoid adverse reactions or sensitivities in the patient. The dressing should be sterile when applied to prevent infection and ensure aseptic wound care.[3,5,25]

Topical agents are applied to open wounds after each cleansing and debridement to prevent or manage infections and relieve pain. In addition, topical antibiotics are vital for ischemic wounds where the delivery of antibiotics systemically may be compromised due to reduced blood flow.

In the case of maturing healed burns, mild lotions can be used to relieve dryness and itching. Moisturizers are essential to prevent healed wounds from cracking or splitting. It is important to avoid lotions containing alcohol as alcohol can further dry out the skin. Fragrance-free moisturizers are recommended to minimize the risk of hypersensitivity

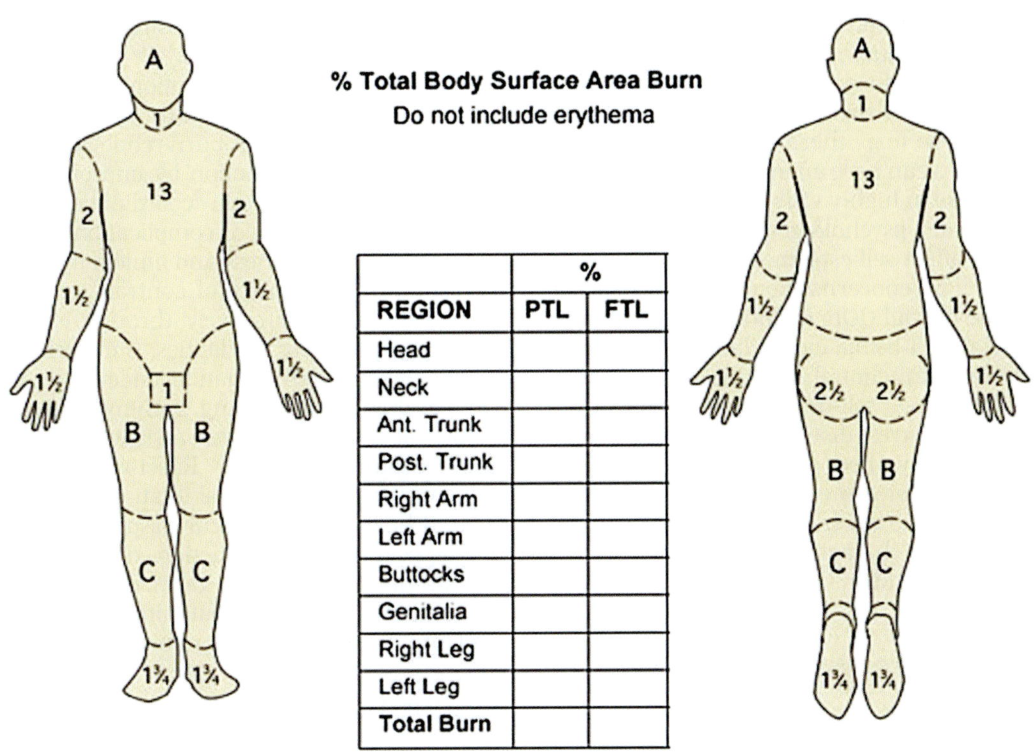

REGION	% PTL	% FTL
Head		
Neck		
Ant. Trunk		
Post. Trunk		
Right Arm		
Left Arm		
Buttocks		
Genitalia		
Right Leg		
Left Leg		
Total Burn		

AREA	Age 0	1	5	10	15	Adult
A = ½ of head	9½	8½	6½	5½	4½	3½
B = ½ of one thigh	2¾	3¼	4	4½	4½	4¾
C = ½ of one lower leg	2½	2½	2¾	3	3¼	3½

Fig. 15.13 The Lund and Browder method of determining total body surface area. *FTL*, Full thickness loss; *PTL*, partial thickness loss. (From *Thermal Burns*. Elsevier Point of Care; 2018.)

reactions triggered by perfumes. Moisturizers can also be beneficial when applying splints, orthotics, or prosthetic devices to patients with healed burns or scars. They help protect the skin from desiccation and shear forces that can lead to further skin damage or discomfort.[3–5,25]

Psychology of Burn Injury

Recovery from a burn injury involves physical healing and addressing various psychological issues that burn survivors may face. These issues can significantly impact their overall well-being and QOL. Burn injuries often result in physical disabilities, scarring, and functional limitations.[4] Coping with these changes and adjusting to a new normal can be challenging for survivors.[5,26] Burn survivors may grieve the loss of their preinjury physical appearance, abilities, independence, or lifestyle. They may also experience grief related to the loss of relationships, employment, or other life aspects.[19,27] The experience of a major burn injury can be traumatic, leading to posttraumatic stress symptoms such as intrusive thoughts, nightmares, hypervigilance, and avoidance.[28] Anxiety and depression are also common psychological reactions to trauma. In addition, burn survivors may experience chronic pain, difficulty sleeping, and body image concerns due to scarring and changes in physical appearance. Survivors may struggle with adapting to the emotional and psychological aftermath of the burn injury, such as changes in self-esteem, self-confidence, and self-identity.[26,28–32]

Among the most common manifestations of psychosocial distress for burn survivors following an injury are sleep disturbance, depression, body image dissatisfaction, and acute and posttraumatic stress. Burn survivors and their families must know that these psychosocial issues are common and a normal part of recovery. Recognizing and understanding these challenges can help individuals and their support systems anticipate and cope with them effectively.[26,32] It is also crucial to seek professional help from mental health professionals experienced in trauma and burn care to provide appropriate support and interventions throughout the recovery journey.[5,27,28,30]

Various factors can influence self-esteem in burn patients. Gender can affect self-esteem, as societal and cultural factors may affect how individuals perceive themselves based on their sex identity. In addition, the type of occupation or employment can impact self-esteem, as burn injuries may affect one's ability to work or engage in their desired profession.[19] The location, type (e.g., thermal, chemical, electrical), and site of the burn can have an impact on self-esteem, as visible burns or those in highly visible areas (such as the face) may have a greater psychological impact.[28] In addition, burn scars can affect self-esteem, as individuals may feel self-conscious or have concerns about their appearance and body image. The overall QOL, including physical, psychological, and social well-being, can influence self-esteem in burn patients. Pain, functional limitations, and social interactions can impact their self-perception.[30,32] The development of posttraumatic stress disorder (PTSD) following a burn injury can negatively affect self-esteem, as individuals may experience intrusive memories, avoidance, and emotional distress related to the traumatic event.[27,28,31,33,34] Box 15.2 shows preburn characteristics that place burn patients at higher risk of PTSD.

Rehabilitation Intervention

While significant advancements have been made in improving the survival rates of severe burn patients, the focus has now shifted towards comprehensive rehabilitation to address the functional and social aspects of recovery. Healthcare professionals strive to improve burn survivors' long-term outcomes and QOL by effectively managing burn scar contractures and optimizing rehabilitation protocols. Early and aggressive physical and occupational therapy are key components of burn care. These therapies focus on preserving and improving joint mobility, muscle strength, and functional abilities. Rehabilitation plays a crucial role in minimizing the impact of burn scar contractures.[22] The duration of rehabilitation treatment is also an important factor. Prolonged and consistent therapy sessions are necessary to achieve optimal outcomes. Rehabilitation programs for burn patients typically involve a combination of exercises, stretching, splinting, scar management techniques, and assistive devices.[36–38]

The goals of burn rehabilitation can vary depending on the individual patient's needs and the severity of their burn injury. The primary objective of burn rehabilitation is to restore and maximize physical function by improving range of motion (ROM), muscle strength, coordination, and balance.[38–41] Contractures are a major complication in burn patients that can lead to joint stiffness and limited mobility. The goal is to prevent the development of contractures and, if they occur, to manage them effectively through exercises, stretching, splinting, and other modalities. Burn rehabilitation aims to enable patients to regain independence in performing ADLs, such as dressing, grooming, bathing, and eating, which may involve adaptive techniques, assistive devices, and training in compensatory strategies.[36] Effective scar management is an integral part of burn rehabilitation. The goal is to optimize wound healing, reduce scar tissue formation, and improve the appearance and function of scars. Techniques may include massage, pressure garments, silicone sheets, and topical treatments.[36] These goals aim to improve the overall QOL and functional outcomes for burn survivors.[22,37,42–46]

Box 15.2 Risk Factors for Posttraumatic Stress Disorder Following Burn Injury

Preburn characteristics

- Personality
- History of alcohol and substance abuse disorders
- History of depression and other affective disorders

Acute stress symptoms

Anxiety related to pain

Type and severity of baseline symptoms of posttraumatic stress disorder

Injury characteristics

Female sex

Visibility of burn injury

Social support

Coping strategies

Modified from Herndon DN. *Total Burn Care*. Elsevier Health Sciences; 2007.[35]

WOUND HEALING AND SCAR FORMATION

Burn wound healing typically occurs in distinct phases, each characterized by specific cellular and molecular events (Fig. 15.14). The initial phase, hemostasis, involves the formation of a blood clot to stop bleeding. Platelets aggregate at the site of injury, releasing factors that initiate clotting. The clot helps to stabilize the wound and creates a temporary barrier against pathogens. The inflammatory phase is a critical phase that promotes the recruitment of immune cells to the wound site. Neutrophils are the first responders, followed by macrophages. These cells clear debris, release growth factors, and regulate the inflammatory response to facilitate the subsequent phases. The inflammatory phase also involves the formation of new blood vessels and the migration of fibroblast and epithelial cells into the injured area. Treatment focuses on wound care, facilitating vascular growth, and preventing wound contamination. The proliferative phase involves the generation of new tissue to replace the damaged area. Fibroblasts synthesize collagen, which provides structural support to the wound. Blood vessels form (angiogenesis) to supply oxygen and nutrients to the healing tissue. Epithelial cells at the wound edges migrate and proliferate to cover the wound surface. Treatment focuses on promoting epithelialization and encouraging proper alignment of newly deposited collagen fibers. Lastly, the remodeling phase is when the newly formed tissue is strengthened and reorganized. Collagen fibers realign along the lines of mechanical stress, improving the wound's tensile strength. Excess collagen is broken down, and scar tissue gradually matures and remodels. It is important to note that wound healing is a dynamic process, and the phases can overlap and interact. The duration and progression of each phase can vary depending on factors such as the size and depth of the wound, the presence of underlying health conditions, and the effectiveness of wound management.[20,25,47]

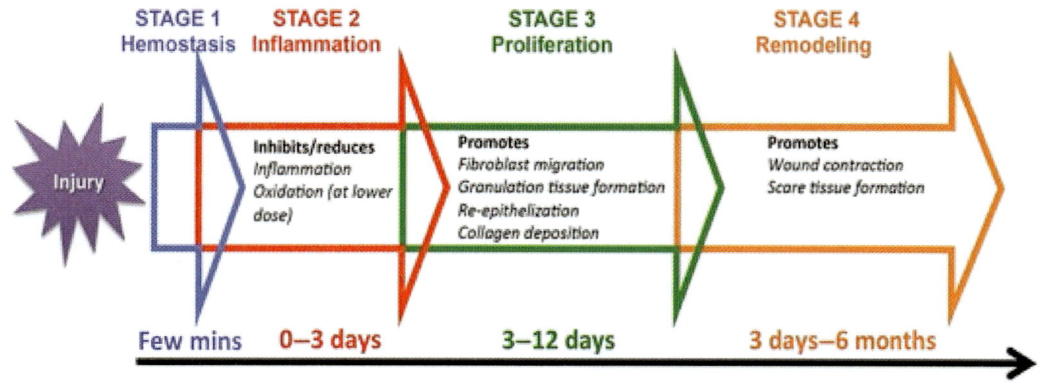

Fig. 15.14 Phases of burn wound healing. (From Akbik D, Ghadiri M, Chrzanowski W, Rohanizadeh R. Curcumin as a wound healing agent. *Life Sci.* 2014;116(1):1–7. doi:10.1016/j.lfs.2014.08.016.)

Burn scar formation is a complex process that occurs during burn healing. The severity and depth of the burn injury influence the extent and characteristics of scar formation. Inflammatory cells, such as neutrophils and macrophages, infiltrate the injured area and release cytokines, growth factors, and enzymes that regulate wound healing, including scar formation. During the proliferative phase, granulation tissue develops at the burn site. Granulation tissue consists of new blood vessels, collagen, and fibroblasts. Fibroblasts produce collagen, which provides structural support to the healing wound.[48] During the wound-healing process, macrophages and specific fibroblast subtypes release enzymes called matrix metalloproteinases that help break and remodel collagen. This collagen degradation is necessary for the normal healing process and tissue remodeling. Initially, the newly synthesized collagen fibers are disorganized and immature. As the wound healing progresses, specialized cells called myofibroblasts align the collagen fibers along the lines of mechanical stress, increasing the wound's tensile strength.[47,49] Burn scars are comprised of dense collagen bundles that replace the normal skin structure. Compared to normal skin, burn scars often lack hair follicles, sweat glands, and sebaceous glands. The scar tissue may appear thick, raised, and red.[1,48,50–52]

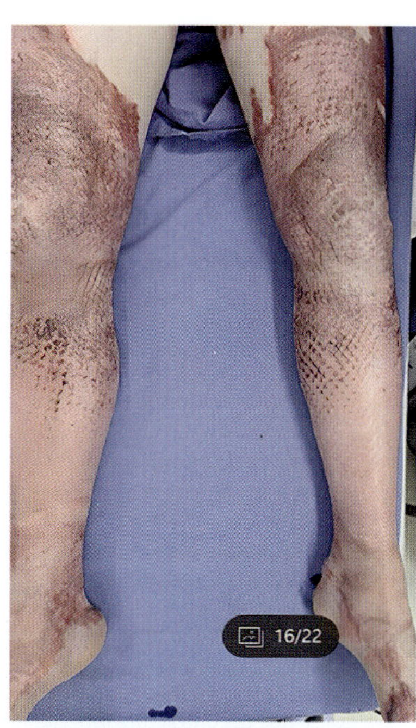

Fig. 15.15 Hypertrophic burn scars to both lower extremities. (From Joo SY, Cho YS, Lee SY, Seo CH. Regenerative effect of combined laser and human stem cell-conditioned medium therapy on hypertrophic burn scar. *Burns.* 2023;49(4):870-876.[115])

In cases where collagen synthesis exceeds its breakdown, hypertrophic scars can develop. These scars are raised above the normal skin surface and may appear red, thick, and fibrous. Hypertrophic scars remain within the boundaries of the initial wound (Fig. 15.15). Keloid scars extend beyond the boundaries of the original wound (Fig. 15.16).[48–50,53–55] Several factors can influence the formation and characteristics of burn scars and are shown in Box 15.3.

The management of burn scars involves a multidisciplinary approach of surgical and nonsurgical interventions. Early intervention and a comprehensive rehabilitation program can help optimize functional outcomes and improve the appearance and quality of burn scars. Burn scars can have significant impacts beyond their appearance and can be associated with various symptoms.[48,50] Burn scars can be painful, and up to 47% of patients may experience pain associated with their scars.[56] The pain can be constant or intermittent and may vary in intensity. It can interfere with daily activities and QOL. Itching is a common symptom associated with burn scars. It can be persistent and bothersome, affecting up to 67% of burn patients 2 years after the burn injury. Pruritus can be distressing, disrupt sleep, cause frustration, and impact psychological well-being. Some individuals may experience heightened sensitivity or hypersensitivity in and around the burn scar. The scar tissue may be more sensitive to touch, temperature changes, or even clothing rubbing against it, which can cause discomfort and affect daily activities. Burn scars can cause tightness or stiffness in the surrounding tissues. This can limit the ROM and flexibility, particularly if the scar is located near joints or areas that require movement. It can affect functional abilities and mobility.[23,48,53,54,57–59]

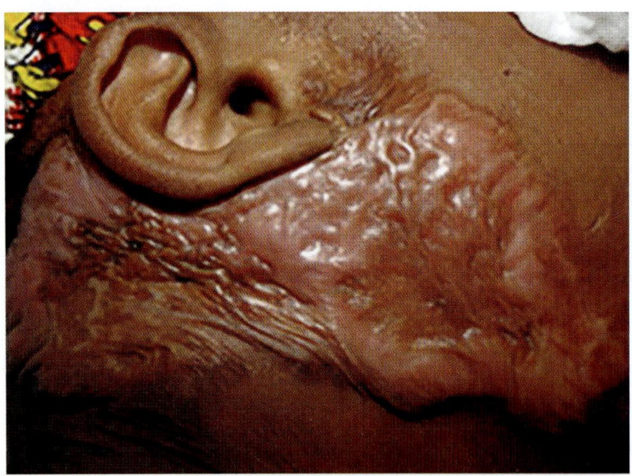

Fig. 15.16 **Keloid scars are benign dermal fibroproliferative raised and extend beyond the margins of the original wound.** (From Patel PA, Bailey JK, Yakuboff KP. Treatment outcomes for keloid scar management in the pediatric burn population. *Burns.* 2012;38(5):767–771.[116])

Box 15.3 **Factors That Influence Burn Scar Formation**

Factor	Result
Burn depth and severity	Deeper and more severe burns are more likely to result in extensive scar formation.
Infection	Burn wounds that become infected are at a higher risk of developing more pronounced scars.
Timing and effectiveness of wound care	Proper wound care, including early debridement and appropriate dressings, can help minimize scar formation.
Genetic predisposition	Individual genetic factors may influence the tendency to develop hypertrophic scars or keloids.
Patient age	Younger patients tend to have more robust wound-healing responses, which can contribute to increased scar formation.
Location and function of the burn site	Scars on joints or areas subject to frequent movement may be more problematic due to contracture formation and functional limitations.

OPERATIVE SCAR MANAGEMENT

Surgery is commonly used to correct scar contractures that cause functional deficits or deformities. Various surgical techniques are available for releasing scar contractures.[60] Split-thickness or full-thickness skin grafts are where healthy skin is taken from another part of the body (donor site) and transplanted onto the scarred area. Skin grafts can help replace scar tissue and improve functionality and appearance. Skin flaps involve moving nearby healthy tissue and blood supply to cover a scarred area. Skin flaps can provide better blood circulation and support for healing. Z-plasty is a surgical technique used to reposition and lengthen scars. It involves creating small triangular skin flaps on either side of the scar and rearranging them in a zigzag pattern. Z-plasties can help release tension and improve the flexibility and appearance of scars.[61] Tissue expansion involves inserting a balloon-like device called a tissue expander under the nearby healthy skin. Over time, the expander is gradually filled with saline solution, which stretches the skin and creates new, healthy tissue. The expanded tissue can then be used to cover the scarred area. It is recommended to defer surgery until at least 6 months after the burn injury or until the scar has matured sufficiently. This allows for a better assessment of the scar's characteristics and ensures the surgical intervention is performed appropriately. While surgery can alleviate scar-related problems, it is important to note that it also creates a new wound, which undergoes its own scar maturation process.[61] Rehabilitation is necessary after reconstructive surgeries to prevent the effects of contracture from recurring. Rehabilitation includes interventions to improve ROM, function, and overall recovery.[60]

NONOPERATIVE SCAR MANAGEMENT

Scar assessment tools have been developed to standardize the evaluation of scars. While there is no universally accepted gold standard, two commonly used tools are the Vancouver Scar Scale and the Patient and Observer Scar Assessment Scale.[56,62–64]

The Vancouver Scar Scale incorporates clinician ratings of pigmentation, pliability, vascularity, and height to assess scars. It provides a standardized framework for evaluating scar characteristics (Box 15.4).[65]

The Patient and Observer Scar Assessment Scale is another widely used tool. It includes a clinician assessment and incorporates the patient's perspective. In addition to the clinician's evaluation of pigmentation, pliability, vascularity, and height, the Patient and Observer Scar Assessment Scale includes patient assessment of pain, pruritus, color, stiffness, thickness, and irregularity. This scale recognizes the importance of considering the patient's scar experience, including subjective factors such as pain and itchiness.[56,63,67,68]

Efforts have been made to supplement these subjective assessment scales with objective measures. Objective measurement devices, such as spectrophotometers, are used to measure scar erythema (redness). Elastomers can assess scar pliability, while calipers can measure scar height and thickness. Histopathologic examination of scar biopsies is often performed to describe the cellular changes associated with a specific intervention. By utilizing both subjective and objective measures, scar assessment tools provide a comprehensive evaluation of scars and assist in monitoring changes over time or in response to different treatments.[54,62,67]

Compression therapy is a widely accepted and commonly used treatment for scars, regardless of their type and severity. It has been used in burn treatment since the 1970s due to its noninvasive nature and minimal associated complications. Compression therapy involves using compression garments (Fig. 15.17), which are often prescribed prophylactically for patients who have undergone surgical management or whose burn injuries have taken more than 14 days to heal. Burn scar supports can be fabricated to fit almost any body part, including the face, torso, upper extremity, hand, and lower extremity.[23]

The mechanism of compression therapy is twofold. First, it restricts blood supply to the scar area, which is thought

Box 15.4 Vancouver Scar Scale Ratings for Assessing Burn Scar

Pigmentation

0 = Normal (scar color closely resembles that of the rest of the body)
1 = Hypopigmentation
2 = Hyperpigmentation

Pliability

0 = Normal
1 = Supple (flexible with minimum resistance)
2 = Yielding (gives way to pressure)
3 = Firm (inflexible, not easily moved, resistant to manual pressure)
4 = Banding (ropelike tissue that blanches with extension on the scar)
5 = Contracture (permanent shortening of scar, producing deformity or distortion)

Vascularity

0 = Normal (scar color closely resembles that of the rest of the body)
1 = Pink
2 = Red
3 = Purple

Height

0 = Normal (flat)
1 = Raised less than 2 mm
2 = Raised less than 5 mm
3 = Raised more than 5 mm

Modified from Sullivan T, Smith J, Kernoda J, et al. Rating the burn scar. *J Burn Care Rehabil.* 1990;11(3):256–260.[66]

to regulate collagen synthesis by reducing the oxygen and nutrients delivered to the site. This restriction of collagen production helps maintain levels similar to those in normal scar tissue. Second, the mechanical loading exerted by compression aids in flattening and realigning the collagen bundles present in the scar tissue. It is shown that compression should exceed capillary pressure without compromising arterial flow, with pressure between 20 and 30 mm Hg being the conventional standard. Overall, the evidence suggests that compression therapy can lead to flatter, less vascular, more pliable, more functional, and esthetically pleasing scars. It is an effective treatment option that has stood the test of time in managing scars resulting from burns.[52,69–73]

Silicone has been found to be effective in treating established hypertrophic scars. Studies comparing silicone sheets with placebo in treating hypertrophic burn scars found that silicone sheets significantly improved scar pigmentation, vascularity, pliability, and pruritus.

The mechanism of action of silicone in scar treatment is not entirely understood. It has been hypothesized that silicone inhibits fibroblast activity through hydration and occlusion, activates collagenase through warming, and polarizes scar tissue due to the static negative charge of silicone. However, evidence also suggests hydration and occlusion are the main mechanisms explaining silicone's efficacy.[52] Overall, silicone has shown effectiveness in improving the appearance and symptoms associated with hypertrophic scars. Its ability to hydrate and create an occlusive environment plays a significant role in its efficacy, as demonstrated by various studies comparing silicone with other occlusive dressings.[23,70,72]

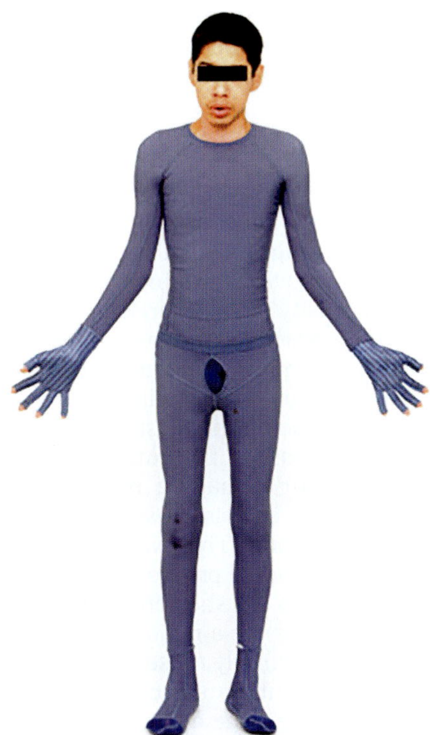

Fig. 15.17 **Custom-made pressure garments may be fabricated for the entire body.** (From Serghiou MA, Ott S, Cowan A, Kemp-Offenberg J. Burn rehabilitation along the continuum of care. In: *Total Burn Care.* Vol. 47. Elsevier; 2018:476–508 e4.)

Scar massage techniques are often employed in the treatment of hypertrophic scars. Various manual massage techniques minimize scar tissue fibrosis and alleviate adhesions. The specific method applied may vary depending on factors such as scar age and the inflammatory status of the scar tissue.[23] Gentle pressure applied to the epidermis may be used for scars in the early stages or with ongoing inflammation. This technique involves applying mild pressure while moving the skin in a specific direction. For mature scars, a moderate pressure technique can be used, which includes creating a skinfold and performing small rotations in different directions. These manual massage techniques improve scar flexibility, reduce tightness, and enhance tissue mobility. Trained therapists typically perform these interventions, which can be tailored to the specific needs and characteristics of the scar.[52,70]

Burn Rehabilitation Interventions

The rehabilitation of patients with burns involves a wide range of interventions that are used to optimize functional outcomes. While various interventions are available, the focus here will be on the use of splints, orthoses, and prosthetic devices. A comprehensive rehabilitation program aims to optimize physical function, enhance independence, promote psychological well-being, and facilitate the individual's reintegration into daily activities and society.

THERAPEUTIC EXERCISE

The primary goal of exercise in burn rehabilitation is to preserve and maintain the functional integrity of joint structures and muscle strength, which is typically achieved by actively or passively moving the joints and muscles.[24,46] The frequency and intensity of the exercise regimen may vary depending on the severity of the injury and the extent of joint involvement. As important and effective as exercise is in burn rehabilitation, some individuals may be reluctant to exercise (and some therapists may be reluctant to encourage them) because of the anticipation of increased pain or anxiety about damaging newly healing tissue. Frequent and regular exercise sessions are essential to achieve optimal outcomes. The exercise program should be adjusted as the individual progresses in their rehabilitation journey.[37,74] Due to the shortening and tightening of scar tissue, contractures are a major clinical complication for burn patients, particularly those with deep dermal and full-thickness burns. Contractures can significantly impact joint mobility and impair the ability to perform activities such as walking, transferring, fine motor tasks, and ADLs.[43] These limitations can have a profound effect on the overall functional abilities and QOL of burn survivors.[36,38,39,44,45,74]

ROM limitation of joints is a common complication following burn injuries, and it can persist from the initial admission to the hospital for years after the accident.[38] Several factors contribute to ROM limitation at different stages of the healing process. In the acute phase, edema, pain, fear, postsurgical effects, wound contraction, and general mental and physical weakness can all contribute to restricted ROM. Edema and pain in the surrounding tissues can make it challenging to move the affected joint. Fear and psychological distress may lead to guarded movements and avoidance of certain motions. Postsurgical effects, such as immobilization or the presence of dressings, can restrict joint movement.[22] The overall weakness and decreased muscle strength during the acute phase can also affect joint mobility. As the healing progresses and the acute phase resolves, ROM limitation becomes increasingly influenced by scar tissue.[53,74] Scar contraction is a natural part of the healing process, and as scars form, they can cause tissue tightness and restrict joint mobility. Scar contracture is the progressive tightening and shortening of scar tissue, leading to significant ROM limitation. Scar contractures can occur due to excessive scar tissue formation, inadequate scar management, or the natural healing process itself.[43] To address ROM limitation, early and aggressive rehabilitation interventions are crucial.[45,46,75]

Active Exercises

After a burn injury, there are several challenges that may make exercise difficult, including edema, pain, loss of skin elasticity, and wound contraction. However, exercise plays a crucial role in burn rehabilitation and can help address these challenges.[45] Edema is a common issue in the early stages of burn recovery and can contribute to joint stiffness. Active exercise is valuable in reducing edema by promoting circulation and lymphatic drainage. Therapists may use positioning techniques, compressive wraps, or devices to control edema in conjunction with exercise. Pain tolerance varies among individuals and can be a barrier to exercise. Therapists must help patients understand the importance of activity despite the pain involved. It is important to note that many individuals experience pain and stiffness relief after exercise, which can motivate them to continue with therapy sessions. Patients who understand the benefits of exercise may be encouraged to support and motivate others who are newly injured or struggling with their exercises. Loss of skin elasticity and wound contracture can lead to general stiffness, which may persist during the scar maturation process, particularly for those who develop hypertrophic scars. Exercise targeting the areas most vulnerable to scar formation should begin as early as possible after admission.[36,75] Early introduction of an exercise routine helps control edema, relieve stiffness, and prevent loss of strength and ROM. Active exercises are preferred for ROM exercises in burn patients due to their wide range of benefits.[46]

Early exercise activity has been shown to shorten the hospitalization stay for burn patients.[45] Ongoing research focuses on further investigating the effects of early exercise in burn rehabilitation.[46] Strengthening exercises play a critical role throughout the entire continuum of burn rehabilitation to prevent muscle atrophy. These exercises can begin during the acute rehabilitation phase. Resistive exercises are utilized to maintain or increase muscle strength, ROM, proprioception, and coordination. However, during the acute rehabilitation phase, implementing strengthening exercises may be challenging due to the patient's level of consciousness and comprehension. Therefore starting with simple exercises and gradually progressing as the patient's status improves is recommended.[40]

Isometric exercises are particularly beneficial when a patient is on bed rest, as they help maintain muscle strength with minimal energy expenditure. Isometric exercises involve contracting muscles without joint movement. One advantage of isometric exercises is that they help prevent the loss of muscle contraction, which can occur during prolonged immobilization.[37] Additionally, isometric exercises assist in maintaining muscle strength.[22,74]

The therapist can also apply manual resistance during exercises, which involves providing gentle resistance as the patient contracts their muscles or attempts motion against the resistance. Another approach is having the patient maintain a specific position while applying resistance. Incorporating strengthening exercises, including isometric exercises and manual resistance, is important in burn rehabilitation to prevent muscle atrophy, improve muscle strength, and enhance functional outcomes. The exercises should be tailored to the individual's capabilities and gradually progress as the patient's condition improves.[22,40,75]

Passive Exercise and Stretching

Passive ROM exercises are essential in preventing contractures, maintaining joint mobility, and elongating tissues when a patient is unable or unwilling to actively move through their available ROM. These exercises involve the therapist or caregiver moving the patient's limbs without any active effort from the patient. While passive ROM exercises require less energy expenditure from the patient, they do not provide the same benefits as active exercises.[22] When a patient is unable to actively move a joint through its full range, passive exercises are used to prevent joint stiffness and improve ROM. Passive exercises allow the assessment of the quality and quantity of joint motion.[37,75] By manually moving the patient's joints, they can evaluate any limitations, restrictions, or abnormalities in joint movement. This information is essential for monitoring progress and planning further interventions.[19,43]

Passive exercise and stretching are integral components of burn care to maintain ROM, assess joint motion, and elongate tissues. Burn injuries can cause scar formation, restricting joint mobility and leading to contractures. Passive exercises can help elongate and stretch soft tissues like muscles, tendons, and ligaments. By applying controlled and sustained stretches, passive exercises can help improve tissue flexibility and promote optimal alignment and function after a treatment session of ROM, and stretching, positioning, or splints are utilized to maintain the achieved ROM in burn care. These techniques help to ensure that the joints remain in the desired position, promoting the preservation of ROM and preventing the development of contractures.[37,43,75]

Exercise equipment commonly found in rehabilitation settings can be appropriate for patients with burns and their benefits in the rehabilitation process. Therapists play a crucial role in determining when and how to incorporate specific equipment into the patient's plan of care based on their individual needs and goals.[22] One example is using reciprocal overhead pulleys to increase the ROM in the upper extremities. The pulleys provide a controlled and guided movement pattern, allowing patients to perform exercises that stretch and mobilize their shoulders, elbows, and wrists to help improve joint flexibility and function. Bicycle ergometers can be utilized for both upper and lower extremity exercises in burn rehabilitation. They assist with promoting joint motion, providing resistance to strengthen muscles, and can contribute to cardiovascular conditioning. Patients can perform exercises while seated on a stationary bike, adjusting the resistance and intensity as needed.[19,22]

Gait Training

Gait training is an essential exercise for individuals with burned lower extremities. It serves multiple purposes in the recovery process and is significant in restoring functionality and promoting healing. Ambulation involves movement of the lower extremities, which helps maintain and improve joint mobility. Regular ambulation exercises can prevent joint stiffness and contractures that can occur as a result of prolonged immobilization. Gait training requires the activation of lower extremity muscles, including those that may have been affected or weakened due to the burn injury. Ambulation stimulates blood flow, which is crucial for delivering oxygen and nutrients to the burned tissues, promoting healing, and preventing complications like deep vein thrombosis. Walking also assists in reducing swelling in the lower extremities by activating the muscles and the pumping action of the calf muscles. Burn injuries can affect balance and coordination, making it challenging for individuals to walk safely. Gait training exercises, performed under supervision, if necessary, help improve balance and coordination, reducing the risk of falls and promoting a safer gait pattern.[23] Lastly, ambulation not only has physical benefits but also provides psychological benefits. It allows individuals to regain their independence, boost their confidence, and improve their overall well-being. It can also help reduce the psychological impact of being immobilized for an extended period.[76,77]

Early ambulation is often encouraged when the patient's medical condition allows it, and they are considered stable. However, several factors can make ambulation challenging for some patients. Patients with significant muscle weakness may struggle to support their weight and maintain balance while walking. Individuals experiencing significant pain may find engaging in ambulation uncomfortable or even intolerable. In cases where patients have undergone skin grafting, there is a risk of graft shearing or damage during ambulation, which requires careful monitoring and precautions.[1,23] Individuals with lower extremity burns often experience gait deviations due to compromised joint function and other factors related to their injury. The hip and knee may not fully flex during the initial swing phase of walking, leading to a shortened step length and decreased foot clearance. The knee may not fully extend during the terminal swing phase, resulting in a lack of forward propulsion and reduced step length. Instead of the heel making initial contact with the ground, the entire foot may contact the ground simultaneously during the initial contact phase of gait, which can be due to decreased ankle dorsiflexion and/or pain. Lack of ROM in ankle plantar flexion or hesitation in performing controlled knee flexion can impact the loading response phase essential for weight transfer. The knee may excessively flex during midstance, affecting stability and weight distribution during walking. Insufficient heel-off and weight shift onto the forefoot during terminal stance can impact push-off and forward progression. The knee may not flex sufficiently during preswing, affecting swing phase initiation and stride length. These gait deviations can vary depending on the location, size, and depth of the burn injury, as well as individual pain levels. Gait training is crucial for individuals with burns to address these deviations and optimize their walking pattern.[76,77]

PHYSICAL AGENTS

Modalities can be used in burn rehabilitation to address different treatment goals. These modalities include functional electrical stimulation, transcutaneous electrical nerve stimulation (TENS), ultrasound, paraffin, and hydrotherapy. It is essential to exercise caution when applying any modality in burn care, as healing and recently healed skin can be very sensitive. Scar tissue may have varying levels of sensory deficit. Heat, cold, coupling agents, and electrode adhesives can lead to skin breakdown. Thorough pretreatment and posttreatment inspection of the treatment site are crucial to minimize the risk of adverse effects.[1] The use of specific modalities in burn rehabilitation should be based on individual patient needs, therapeutic goals, and professional judgment. Close monitoring and assessment of the patient's response to these modalities are important to ensure safety and optimize outcomes.[4,5]

Functional electrical stimulation (FES) involves using electrical currents to stimulate specific muscles to help restore function and improve muscle strength disuse and immobility. By delivering electrical impulses to the muscles, FES can help maintain muscle mass, prevent muscle atrophy, and facilitate functional movements. FES can increase joint flexibility and improve ROM by facilitating controlled muscle contractions. FES interventions in burn care are tailored to the individual patient's needs and rehabilitation goals. Electrical stimulation parameters, such as intensity, frequency, and duration, can be adjusted based on the patient's condition and response. FES can be incorporated into a comprehensive rehabilitation program, progressing as the patient's condition improves.[78,79]

TENS uses low-intensity electrical currents applied to the skin to help alleviate pain. The effectiveness of TENS in burn pain management has been evaluated in various studies. Results have been mixed, with some studies reporting positive outcomes in terms of pain reduction, while others have shown no significant differences compared to control interventions or sham TENS. The variability in study designs, treatment parameters, and patient populations contributes to the conflicting findings. The location and severity of the burn injury, the stage of wound healing, and individual patient characteristics should be considered when determining the appropriateness and effectiveness of TENS therapy. TENS is often used as part of a multimodal approach to pain management in burn care.[78,79]

Ultrasound therapy utilizes high-frequency sound waves to provide deep heating to tissues, reducing pain and improving ROM. The effectiveness of ultrasound in decreasing pain or improving movement in burn patients is still debated in the literature. While ultrasound therapy has been used in burn care for its potential benefits, the available evidence regarding its effectiveness in this population is limited and inconclusive. The use of ultrasound therapy for pain reduction in burn patients has been investigated in several studies. Some studies suggest that ultrasound may be beneficial in reducing burn-related pain, while others have found no significant difference compared to control treatments or sham ultrasound. The heterogeneity of the studies, variations in treatment parameters, and small sample sizes contribute to the ongoing debate regarding the effectiveness of ultrasound for pain management in burns. Similarly, the effects of ultrasound therapy on improving ROM in burn patients are still debated. Some studies have reported a positive impact on joint flexibility and ROM, while others have found no significant differences compared to control treatments. The variability in treatment protocols, differences in outcome measures, and limitations in study designs contribute to the conflicting results.[7,79]

Paraffin therapy involves immersing the affected body part in a mixture of paraffin wax and mineral oil. The gentle heat from the paraffin and the skin-softening properties of the mineral oil can provide relief and promote tissue flexibility. Paraffin therapy has been used as a part of scar management in burn care. The wax's heat and moisturizing effects can help soften and flatten scars, improve their appearance, and enhance the overall flexibility and mobility of the affected areas.[1,7,79]

The use of hydrotherapy in burn care has evolved, and some aspects have changed over time. Hydrotherapy, specifically water immersion, was commonly used for wound cleansing in burn care. It was believed to assist in removing necrotic tissue and debris from the burn wounds. The literature has reported hydrotherapy for dressing removal and exercise in burn care. However, it is important to note that hydrotherapy is no longer indicated for wound cleansing due to the risk of cross-contamination. If hydrotherapy is used, precautions similar to those employed in open wound care are necessary to minimize the chances of infection. Hydrotherapy has been utilized to provide a supportive and low-impact environment for exercise and mobility training in burn patients. Water buoyancy reduces the body's weight-bearing load, allowing patients to perform exercises and movements with less stress on their joints and muscles. The use of hydrotherapy in burn care has been associated with pain relief due to the analgesic effects of warm water. Immersion in warm water can promote relaxation, decrease muscle tension, and alleviate pain.[1,4,79]

POSITIONING

Proper positioning is crucial in minimizing burn scar contracture development and promoting optimal healing in burn patients. Appropriate positioning aims to prevent contractures and maintain functional alignment of the affected body part during healing. Proper positioning is fundamental for patients who are unable to move or exercise. Using manufactured positioning devices or simple techniques, such as positioning the limbs, head, and neck in neutral alignment, can help maintain proper positioning and prevent complications. Suggestions of positions for a patient with burns are shown in Box 15.5. It helps to counteract the forces of gravity, edema, and muscle imbalances that can contribute to the development of scar contractures. Burn injuries can affect various anatomical sites, and each patient's specific needs for positioning and splinting may vary. Therefore various devices and splints may be required to address the unique requirements of each affected body part. Burn centers increasingly utilize appropriate positioning and

Box 15.5 Preferred Positions for Patients With Burns

Neck	Extension, no rotation
Shoulder	Abduction (90–110 degrees)
	External rotation
	Horizontal flexion (10–15 degrees)
Elbow and forearm	Extension with supination
Wrist	Neutral or slight extension
Hand	Functional position (dorsal burn)
	Finger and thumb extension (palmar burn)
Trunk	Straight postural alignment
Hip	Neutral extension/flexion
	Neutral rotation
	Slight abduction
Knee	Extension
Ankle	Neutral or slight dorsiflexion
	No inversion
	Neutral toe extension/flexion

splinting techniques in the acute care phase. Splints can be applied to the affected area while the patient is sedated or asleep to minimize edema and maintain proper alignment. Once the patient's mental status improves, splints can be used to maintain the burned regions in positions of function during sleep or sedation, which helps to optimize functional outcomes and prevent contractures. The splints can be temporarily removed for wound checks and active motion exercises.[1,19,22,75,80,81]

Proper positioning is crucial in managing acute burn and postsurgical edema. By appropriately positioning the affected body parts, edema can be controlled, reducing the risk of complications and promoting healing. Positioning plays a vital role in preventing and treating scar contractures. Identifying sites at risk for contracture formation during the initial evaluation allows therapists to implement counteractive positions as part of the therapy plan. To prevent potential burn scar contractures, the body area affected by the burn should be positioned opposite to the direction of contractile forces, which means positioning the body in a way that counteracts the tendency of contractile forces to draw the body into a fetal position—initiating a positioning program and activity early after the burn injury increases the success of contracture prevention (Fig. 15.18). Postexercise positioning helps to prolong the benefits gained from therapeutic activities. By positioning the body in a specific way after exercise, the effects of the exercise can be maximized.[1,22,23,43,75,80,81]

Positioning does not necessarily require expensive or intricate equipment. Simple items such as pillows, blankets, towels, or gauze rolls can effectively support and elevate body parts in desired positions. Positioning requires close monitoring and collaboration among the clinical team members and family to maintain the desired positions consistently. By incorporating appropriate positioning techniques into the burn rehabilitation program, the risk of complications, such as scar contractures, can be reduced, and optimal functional outcomes can be achieved. Positioning should begin immediately on admission to the burn center and continue throughout the rehabilitation process. Consistency and continuity in positioning are important for achieving optimal functional outcomes.[1,19,23,44]

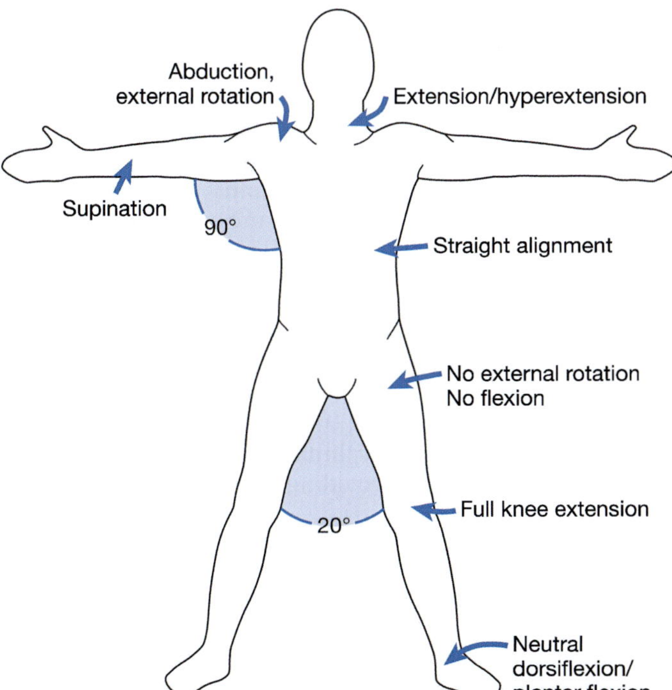

Fig. 15.18 Suggested positioning guidelines to prevent contracture. (From Cifu DX. *Braddom's Physical Medicine and Rehabilitation (e-book)*. Elsevier Health Sciences; 2020.)

The quote "the position of comfort is the position of deformity" is relevant to burned patients with serious injuries. This means that if a patient consistently maintains a position of comfort, such as a flexed or contracted position, it can lead to the development of fixed deformities or contractures over time.[80] The fetal position is often described as the position of comfort for individuals with burn injuries. This position provides temporary relief and reduces pain. However, maintaining it throughout the healing process can lead to fixed deformities and impair functional outcomes. Improper positioning can lead to deformities and impair functional outcomes. Therefore the positioning program aims to counteract contractile forces while maintaining optimal function. By implementing a comprehensive and patient-centered positioning program, burn rehabilitation therapists can significantly reduce complications, promote optimal healing, and improve functional outcomes for burn patients.[22,43,75]

Splinting and Orthotics

Hippocrates described burn scars as "tetanus," and Wilhelm Fabry illustrated a splint to treat a hand for hyperextension scar contractures.[82] In the early to mid-1900s, patients with burns were placed in splints immediately on admission to the hospital to prevent contraction; splints were removed for brief periods to permit wound care. Most burns were not covered by skin graft until at least 5 weeks after injury. The advent of surgical excision and grafting in the mid-1900s decreased the time required for a burn to heal. As a result, prophylactic splinting became a less standard procedure, and in the late 1970s and early 1980s, active exercise became the primary treatment method used by PTs working with burn patients.[83] The term "splint" is commonly used to refer to devices that assist with positioning and support of the affected body areas. Although the terms "splint" and "orthotic" have slightly different connotations, they are often used interchangeably in burn care.

Splints or orthotics are valuable in burn rehabilitation as they help maintain proper positioning, prevent contractures, and support functional movement. Splints can protect vulnerable structures, such as healing wounds, grafts, or exposed tendons/joints, by immobilizing and supporting them. These devices are typically custom made or adapted to the individual's specific needs and can support and protect healing tissues, promote proper alignment, and facilitate functional activities. The specific design and features of splints may vary depending on the individual's needs, the location and extent of the burn, and the stage of healing. Burn rehabilitation therapists work closely with patients to determine the most appropriate splinting strategies and ensure that they effectively support optimal functional outcomes.[1,19,21,23,44,84]

Splints are used to preserve and maintain the available ROM in joints affected by burns. They help prevent contractures and stiffness by holding the joints in positions that promote optimal alignment and functional movement. Splints also correct or prevent soft-tissue contractures, which occur when muscles, tendons, or other soft tissues become shortened or tightened. Splints help elongate the contracted tissues and restore or improve ROM by applying a continuous or intermittent stretch to the affected tissues. Splints can help suppress scar formation by applying gentle, controlled pressure to the healing tissues. This pressure can help reduce excessive scar tissue formation and promote more favorable scar remodeling. The specific goals at each phase may include edema control, pressure relief, tissue elongation, and graft protection.[1,19,23,25,43,75,84,85]

A thorough understanding of mechanical force systems and their application is crucial for achieving optimal outcomes. By spreading the pressure over a larger surface area, the therapist can minimize the risk of pressure sores or skin breakdown that may result from concentrated pressure. Manipulating the positioning and alignment of the splint and its components can increase the mechanical advantage, optimizing the forces applied to the tissues to help achieve desired outcomes more effectively. Proper placement and adjustment of straps are essential for achieving the desired mechanical effects. Straps should be positioned strategically to control and distribute forces while maintaining comfort and minimizing pressure points. The therapist should consider the rotational and translational forces acting on the joints and tissues and design the splint accordingly to minimize detrimental effects and promote proper alignment and movement. The concept of reciprocal parallel forces or three-point fixation involves applying forces in opposite directions or using multiple points of contact to stabilize and align the affected joint or tissue. This approach can help counteract contractile forces and promote proper positioning. The therapist should be aware of the torque effect, which refers to the rotational force applied around an axis. Understanding and utilizing the principles of torque can help optimize the mechanical effects of the splint on the affected area.[19,21–23,25,75,80] The advantages and disadvantages and indications and contraindications of therapist-fabricated splinting and burn care are summarized in Box 15.6.

Various materials can be used for burn splinting, depending on the patient's specific needs and the rehabilitation program's goals. Thermoplastic materials, such as low-temperature thermoplastics (e.g., Aquaplast, Orfit), are widely used in burn splinting. These materials become pliable when heated and can be molded to the desired shape to provide customized support and immobilization. They offer excellent conformability, durability, and the ability to be easily adjusted or remolded. Prefabricated orthotic components, such as outriggers, hinges, and joint stabilizers, can be incorporated into burn splints to provide additional support and control. These components are often made of lightweight materials like aluminum or plastic and can be attached to thermoplastic splints or other supportive structures. Soft foam padding, such as foam rolls or foam pads, enhances patient comfort and distributes pressure more evenly when wearing a splint. Foam padding can be applied underneath the splinting material to provide cushioning and prevent pressure points or skin irritation. Velcro straps are used for securing and adjusting the splint. They offer a convenient and adjustable method of securing the splint while allowing for easy removal and reapplication. Velcro straps are available in various lengths, widths, and strengths to accommodate different splinting needs. Elastic or neoprene materials can be used in splints that require flexibility or gentle compression. These materials provide a degree of stretch and can be beneficial for certain applications such as splinting joints that require controlled mobility or for providing compression to manage edema.[19,23]

Although evidence-based research on specific splint designs in burn care is limited, the field benefits from the collective experience and knowledge of providers specializing in burn rehabilitation. These professionals continually refine and adapt their approaches based on clinical outcomes and patient feedback, leading to a variety of commonly used splint designs that have demonstrated effectiveness in managing burn-related complications and promoting optimal functional outcomes.[22,23,80,85,86]

Box 15.6 Advantages, Disadvantages, Indications, and Contraindications of Therapist-Fabricated Splints in Burn Care

Advantages

Maintains or increases (serial or dynamic) joint position
Can be used during any phase of healing
Custom formed for each individual
Adjustable
May protect tissue (e.g., exposed tissues such as tendon or joint capsule, or skin from pressure)

Disadvantages

Potential for skin breakdown
Shearing may occur if not properly fit or fixed over a joint
May be difficult for nontherapist to apply

Indications

Need for positioning specific joints
Wound or scar contraction
Decreased joint range of motion
Need for safeguarding anatomic structures
Need for conforming scar tissue
Uncommunicative or nonresponsive patient

Contraindications

Direct application onto fragile tissue
Constrictive fixation strapping or wraps

Devices should

Not cause pain
Be designed with function in mind
Be cosmetically appealing
Be easy to apply and remove
Be lightweight and low profile
Be constructed out of appropriate materials
Allow for ventilation to prevent skin/wound maceration[7]

NECK

The neck should be positioned in a neutral or slightly extended position, approximately 15 degrees, without any rotation. This positioning helps maintain proper alignment and prevents excessive traction on the chin that could lead to mouth opening. Various strategies can be used to achieve the desired neck position. Placing the individual on a short mattress in the supine position helps maintain the desired position. Placing a rolled towel or foam cushion behind the upper back, along the scapular line, provides support and helps keep the desired neck extension.

Pillows should be avoided in cases of anterior neck burns. Using pillows may lead to flexion contractures, which can restrict neck mobility. Anterior neck burns can lead to several complications. Burns on the anterior neck can cause scar tissue formation, leading to a tightening of the skin and muscles. Skin tightening can limit mobility, making it difficult to extend the neck fully. Burns may damage the natural contours of the neck, leading to an altered appearance. Burns in the anterior neck region can affect the muscles involved in chewing, resulting in difficulties with mastication.[21,23]

In the case of anterior neck burns, a conforming custom thermoplastic collar can be fabricated. This collar is designed to provide support and maintain the desired neck position. It is custom made to fit the individual's neck and can help prevent flexion contractures (Fig. 15.19). A molded conformer splint addresses flexion contracture and promotes scar healing. It is made from a rectangular piece of low-temperature thermoplastic splinting material. After heating, the splint is molded directly on the patient's neck. The splint helps prevent neck flexion contracture by supporting and maintaining the neck in an extended position. It also exerts compression on the forming scar, aiding in scar management. Padding is added to protect vulnerable areas, and a velcro strap is attached to the back of the neck to secure the splint. Due to the splint's occlusive nature and its bony prominence coverage, it must be removed frequently to inspect the skin for any signs of irritation or breakdown.[21,23]

In cases where the wounds do not involve the chin extensively, soft cervical collars can effectively provide positioning, pressure, and contour for individuals with anterior neck burns. These collars can help maintain proper alignment, provide support, and assist in preventing contractures and promoting healing. The collar may not offer as much support or resistance to movements that could contribute to contractures. Philadelphia collars are rigid cervical collars that provide more comprehensive support and coverage, including over the chin. They are designed to restrict movement and provide greater stability to the neck. A Watusi-type collar can be used to provide isolated and direct pressure to a thicker scar band. This type of collar is designed to target and address scar tissue specifically. Patients with anterior neck burns may exhibit neck rotation or lateral flexion on one side, leading to a lateral neck contracture or torticollis. To prevent torticollis, a lateral neck splint can be fabricated. This splint conforms to the patient's head, lateral neck, and anterior/posterior shoulder, providing support and promoting proper alignment.[23] Other creative neck splints include the neck ring orthosis (Fig. 15.20), which uses plastic tubing (similar to the Watusi-type splint) to maintain cervical alignment and pressure over burn scars.[87]

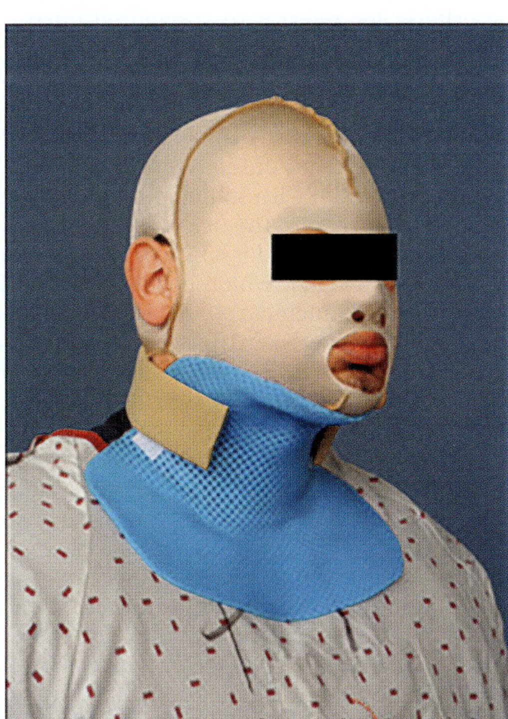

Fig. 15.19 An anterior neck conformer helps prevent neck flexion contractures. (From Serghiou MA, Ott S, Cowan A, Kemp-Offenberg J. Burn rehabilitation along the continuum of care. In: *Total Burn Care.* Vol. 47. Elsevier; 2018:476–508 e4.)

AXILLA AND SHOULDER

Burns involving the axilla and shoulder can lead to adduction contracture and webbing of the axillary folds. This deformity can have functional implications, making it difficult for individuals to reach and use their arms overhead, which are essential components of many functional activities. Webbing of the axillary folds refers to the formation of scar tissue that connects the skin and soft tissues of the

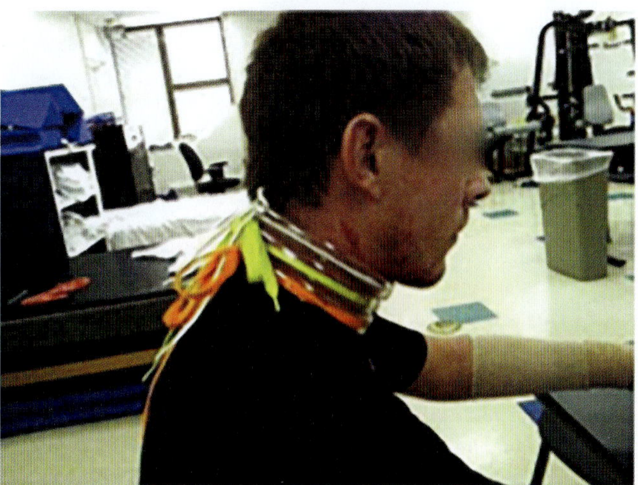

Fig. 15.20 Neck ring orthosis. (From Fletchall S. Neck ring orthosis. *Burns Open.* 2021;5(4):103–105.)

axillary region, creating a web-like appearance. This can further restrict shoulder movement and contribute to functional limitations.[21,23,88] A shoulder abduction splint (airplane splint) is often used to prevent adduction contractures and maintain proper shoulder joint alignment. This splint (Fig. 15.21) keeps the arm abducted and externally rotated to counteract the inward pull of the scar tissue. It can be custom made or commercially available. The figure-of-eight axillary strap (Fig. 15.22) provides compression, support, and contouring for the axillary region in burns or postburn healing cases. It is often used in conjunction with an airplane splint to enhance its effectiveness. By combining the figure-of-eight axillary wrap with an airplane splint, the aim is to achieve multiple benefits. The airplane splint helps maintain proper positioning and support for the shoulder and axilla, while the figure-of-eight wrap provides compression for contouring and elongation of the skin surface. This combination can help prevent contractures, promote healing, and improve the overall appearance of the axillary area.[23,89]

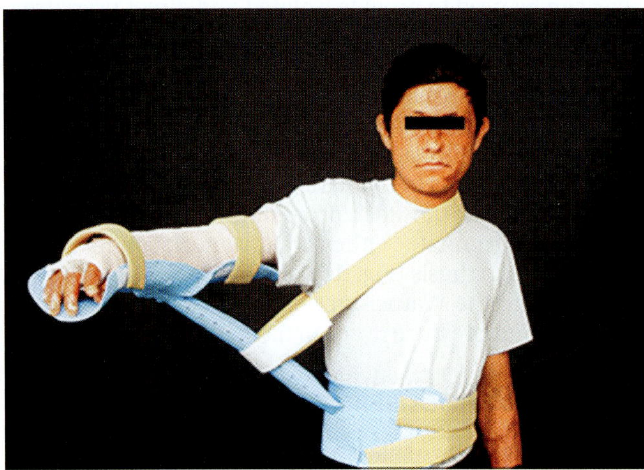

Fig. 15.21 A shoulder abduction splint (airplane splint) may be fabricated to accommodate wound dressings and promote healing while maintaining the shoulder abducted. (From Serghiou MA, Ott S, Cowan A, Kemp-Offenberg J. Burn rehabilitation along the continuum of care. In: *Total Burn Care.* Vol. 47. Elsevier; 2018:476–508 e4.)

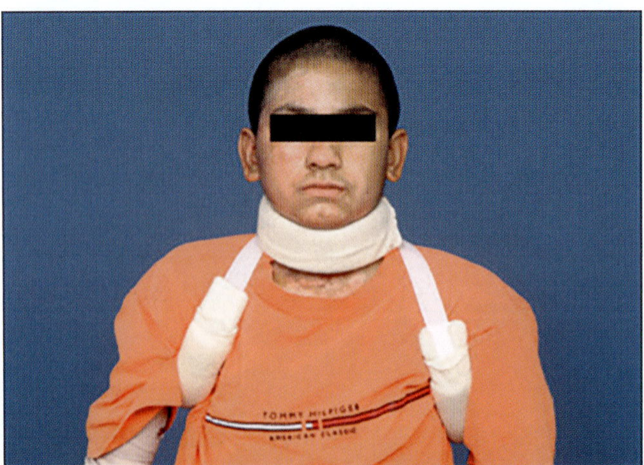

Fig. 15.22 A figure-of-eight axillary strap provides a constant stretch of the axillary skin surfaces. (From Serghiou MA, Ott S, Cowan A, Kemp-Offenberg J. Burn rehabilitation along the continuum of care. In: *Total Burn Care.* Vol. 47. Elsevier; 2018:476–508 e4.)

ELBOW AND FOREARM

Burns involving the elbow and forearm can lead to deformities such as elbow flexion contractures and pronation contractures. A conformer splint is commonly used to support and position the elbow joint to prevent these contractures. The conformer splint can be designed as either an anterior or posterior gutter or trough, depending on the patient's specific needs. The splint is fitted to the arm, extending from the proximal third of the upper arm (brachium) to the distal third of the forearm. In addition to static splints, dynamic elbow splints can be used to address contractures. These splints are designed to provide prolonged, gentle, and sustained stretch to the elbow joint, either in extension or flexion. The purpose of dynamic splinting is to gradually correct contractures by applying controlled tension and promoting ROM. Dynamic splints can also be custom-fabricated or purchased commercially for forearm contractures involving pronation and supination.[23,90–93] It is important to note that the elbow plays a significant role in the overall function of the hand. Achieving a full or near-full ROM in elbow flexion is more important for overall function than achieving full or near-full extension. The flexion range allows for activities that involve reaching, grasping, and manipulating objects, which are crucial for daily functioning.[21]

WRIST AND HAND

Hands are involved in over 80% of all severe burns.[55] While hand burns may not contribute significantly to overall mortality rates, they are still crucial for successful reintegration into society and professional life after hospital discharge. Although hand burns make up less than 5% of the TBSA affected by burns, they are considered severe injuries that meet the criteria for referral to specialized burn centers. These centers provide individualized care for hand burns, recognizing the importance of preserving hand function and optimizing the outcome of hand injury rehabilitation. By providing specialized care for hand burns, burn centers aim to improve functional outcomes and help individuals reintegrate into their daily lives, including professional and social activities that require the use of hands.[92,94] The most common deformity after a dorsal burn is the claw hand deformity (see Fig. 15.24), which positions the digits into hyperextension of the metacarpophalangeal (MCP) joints, flexion of the interphalangeal (IP) joints, loss of transverse metacarpal arch, adduction contracture of the thumb, flexion contracture of the wrist, and shortening of the dorsal skin. Box 15.7 shows a list of the most common postburn hand deformities.[55,90,95]

Orthotic intervention plays a vital role in managing burn injuries to the hand. Without appropriate early splinting and positioning, a typical intrinsic minus posture develops in a severely burned hand that is initially mainly due to swelling of the hand. The injured hand takes the characteristic position of wrist flexion, hyperextension of the MCP joints, and flexion of the IP joints (Fig. 15.23). Orthoses are used to protect healing wounds and grafts, guide forces, and align collagen during the rehabilitation process. They serve to prevent and correct burn scar contractures and deformities, ultimately aiming for optimal functional outcomes. When severe burns occur to the hand, not only the

Box 15.7 Postburn Hand Deformities

- First web adduction contractures
- Web space contractures
- Dorsal skin contractures
- Digital flexion contractures
- Boutonnière deformity
- Dorsal skin deficiency
- Digital loss secondary to ischemia
- Median and ulnar nerve compression syndrome

Modified from Wolfe SW, Pederson WC, Kozin SH, Cohen MS. *Green's Operative Hand Surgery (e-book)*. Elsevier Health Sciences; 2021.

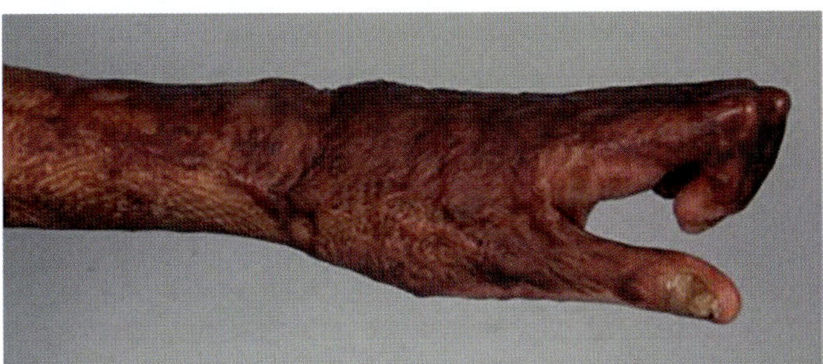

Fig. 15.23 **The most common deformity after a dorsal burn is the claw hand deformity.** (From Kelly BM, Berenz T, Williams T. Orthoses for the burned hand. In: *Atlas of Orthoses and Assistive Devices*. Elsevier; 2019:170–175.)

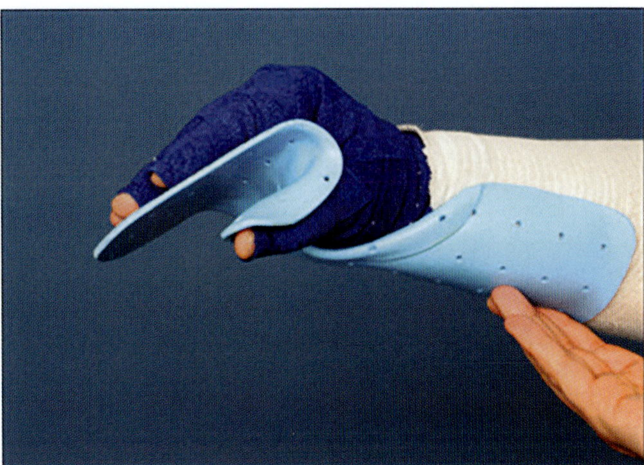

Fig. 15.24 **The intrinsic plus position hand splint (burn hand splint) positions the hand appropriately to prevent contractures and preserve function.** (From Serghiou MA, Ott S, Cowan A, Kemp-Offenberg J. Burn rehabilitation along the continuum of care. In: *Total Burn Care*. Vol. 47. Elsevier; 2018:476–508 e4.)

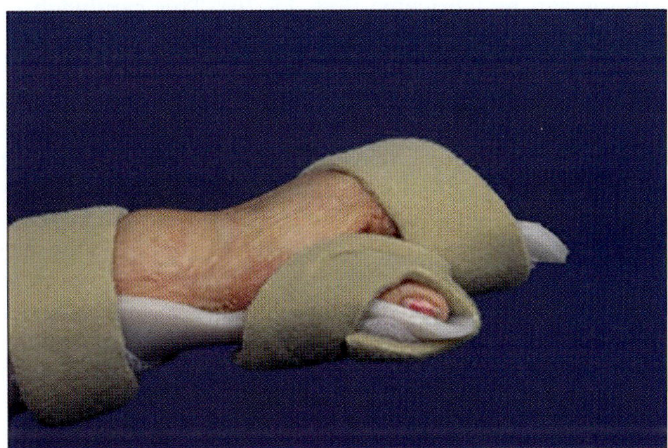

Fig. 15.25 **A palmar extension splint to stretch a palmar contracture.** (From Serghiou MA, Ott S, Cowan A, Kemp-Offenberg J. Burn rehabilitation along the continuum of care. In: *Total Burn Care*. Vol. 47. Elsevier; 2018:476–508 e4.)

skin but also deep structures such as tendons, muscles, joints, nerves, and vessels can be affected. Therefore therapists involved in burn rehabilitation must have a comprehensive understanding of the anatomy and kinesiology of the entire upper extremity. Preventing flexion or extension contractures of the hand and fingers and maintaining the web space of the thumb are crucial in managing burn injuries. The selection of the most suitable splint for an individual depends on the specific joint or joint complex involved and the desired anticontracture position. Overall, a well-designed splint should be comfortable to wear, provide the desired joint position and support, and allow for proper hand and finger function. By following the prescribed precautions, wearing schedule, and instructions, the individual can maximize the benefits of the splint and facilitate the healing and recovery process.[55,90,96]

The antideformity splint is the most common splint used at the wrist and the hand. This splint is designed to position the wrist and hand in a functional position (Fig. 15.24). A modification of this splint, the pan splint, positions all finger joints in extension. In cases of severe circumferential burn injuries to the hand, the fabrication of an orthosis that positions the hand in extension is necessary. One such orthosis is the resting pan extension orthosis (Fig. 15.25). This orthosis provides specific positions and alignments to support optimal healing and prevent complications. The orthosis promotes extension of the wrist joint, positioning the hand in a more extended position rather than a flexed posture, which helps counteract the tendency for contractures and promotes the stretching of tissues for optimal healing. The orthosis includes a component that extends the thumb in a radial and palmar direction.[97] This positioning helps maintain the web space between the thumb and fingers and prevents contractures. The orthosis is designed to extend the MCP and IP joints of the fingers, which prevents flexion contractures and helps maintain tissue extensibility.[55,90,96]

Fingers can sustain very severe injuries that require special attention and custom orthoses. Custom finger orthoses can be utilized for scar contractures on the dorsal or volar surface of the digits. These orthoses are individually fabricated to provide targeted support, alignment, and pressure to the affected areas. Finger gutter or trough splints are used to treat individual fingers based on the same principles used in elbow conformer splints.[55,90,96]

In cases where compliance with orthotic wear is challenging, particularly in pediatric patients, the IP joints of the fingers can assume a flexed position, which may result in pressure points on the fingertips or flexion contractures of the IP joints. To address this issue, a "sandwich" or bivalved

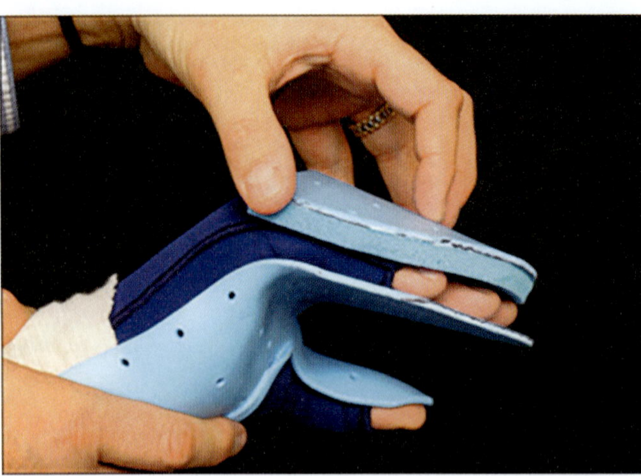

Fig. 15.26 The "sandwich" hand splint prevents proximal interphalangeal flexion contractures. (From Serghiou MA, Ott S, Cowan A, Kemp-Offenberg J. Burn rehabilitation along the continuum of care. In: *Total Burn Care*. Vol. 47. Elsevier; 2018:476–508 e4.)

orthosis can be fabricated (Fig. 15.26). This sandwich or bivalved orthosis provides comprehensive support and protection to the fingers. The volar component extends the fingers, preventing flexion contractures and pressure points on the fingertips. The dorsal shell adds stability and distributes pressure evenly across the fingers. The volar component extends from the proximal phalanges (clearing the MCP joints) to the distal phalanges of digits 2 to 5. The purpose of this component is to maintain the fingers in extension and prevent flexion contractures. The dorsal component consists of a thermoplastic shell that is fabricated to fit over the dorsum of digits 2 to 5. It extends from the proximal phalanges to the fingertips. The shell is padded with foam for comfort and to distribute pressure evenly.[55,90,96]

TRUNK AND PELVIS

Patients with burns involving the anterior trunk are susceptible to developing kyphosis, a forward curvature of the upper spine. Clavicular straps in a figure-of-eight design can be employed to counteract the flexion forces and promote proper posture. These straps help position the shoulders in retraction, preventing excessive flexion in healing upper trunk burns.

Individuals with burns affecting the mid and lower trunk can use commercial corsets or thoracolumbar spinal orthotics. These orthotic devices assist in maintaining posture and preventing postural abnormalities caused by scar contracture.[21,23]

In the case of burns affecting the pelvis, groin, and hip, the primary concern is the potential development of hip flexion and adduction contractures. To address this issue, hip abduction splints can be used. These splints are reinforced with a spreader bar or an anterior hip spica splint to keep the hip abducted, which helps prevent contractures and maintains proper hip joint alignment. Unilateral or asymmetric burns affecting the neck, axilla, trunk, and groin can lead to contractures that cause lateral curvature of the spine and scoliosis. The extent and severity of the contracture will determine the level and amplitude of the spinal curvature. The site and severity of the contracture will vary, resulting in different degrees of scoliosis. A hip or knee flexion contracture can lead to pelvic obliquity, which imposes a lateral lumbar curve, which means that when there is a contracture causing one hip or knee to be flexed more than the other, a tilted or oblique pelvis can result, leading to an additional lateral curve in the lower back or lumbar region of the spine. Commercially available corsets or thoracolumbar spinal orthotics can be prescribed to individuals with mid and lower trunk burns if their posture is compromised by scar contracture. These orthotic devices provide external support and help maintain proper spine alignment, promoting better posture and reducing the impact of contractures on the trunk. Hip abduction splints are designed to hold the hip joint in an abducted position, preventing the formation of contractures and maintaining proper alignment. Hip abduction splints are often reinforced with a spreader bar or an anterior hip spica splint to ensure optimal positioning and stability.[21,23,80]

LOWER EXTREMITY

Burn injuries to the anterior or posterior surface of the lower extremity that extend over the knee joint can lead to knee flexion contractures. In cases of deep anterior burns, the joint may be exposed, potentially causing damage to the patellar tendon. Deep posterior burns can result in the formation of bridging scars. It is essential to position the knee in full extension to address these issues, which can be achieved and maintained using a splint or, in severe cases, skeletal traction. Skeletal traction is applied until efficient quadriceps function is restored, and the patient can ambulate. Night splints should be worn to prevent scar contracture from developing. Knee splints for burn injuries may involve using a custom-made thermoplastic knee conformer on the posterior aspect of the knee or a soft knee immobilizer. These orthotic devices help maintain the knee in extension and provide support and protection during the healing process.[23,80,98,99]

Burn injuries affecting the ankles and feet can pose challenges for splinting due to these areas' complex structure and arthrokinematics. The specific location of the burn will determine the risk of contracture, either in the plantar flexion or dorsiflexion direction or potentially both.

Posterior foot drop splints or anterior/posterior ankle conformers are commonly fabricated as ankle splints to address these concerns. The choice of splint will depend on the specific needs of the individual and the nature of the burn injury. Posterior foot drop splints are designed to prevent or correct contractures that cause the foot to drop in a plantar flexed position. These splints support the ankle and hold it in a neutral or slightly dorsiflexed position to maintain proper alignment and prevent the development of contractures. The Multi Podus System (Fig. 15.27) is a specialized orthotic device that provides support and immobilization while relieving pressure on specific areas, such as the heel. By offloading pressure on vulnerable regions, these splints help prevent the development of pressure ulcers, which can be a concern in patients with limited mobility or compromised skin integrity due to burns. Anterior or posterior ankle conformers are orthotic devices that are molded to fit the shape of the ankle and foot and can be customized based on the location and extent of the burn.[100] These

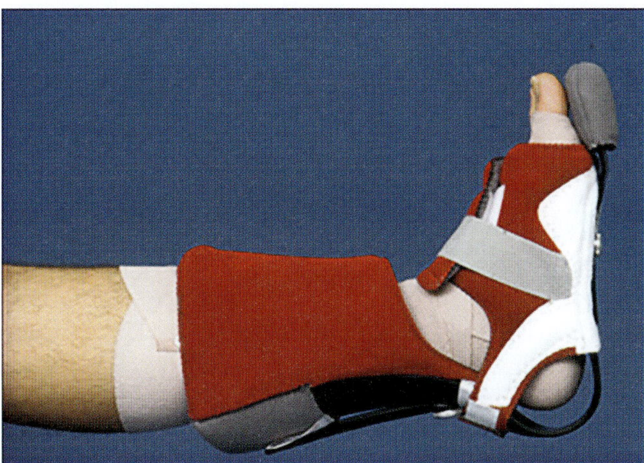

Fig. 15.27 The Multi Podus splint is utilized to position the burned foot appropriately and prevent heel and malleoli skin breakdown. (From Serghiou MA, Ott S, Cowan A, Kemp-Offenberg J. Burn rehabilitation along the continuum of care. In: *Total Burn Care*. Vol. 47. Elsevier; 2018:476–508 e4.)

conformers provide support, protection, and compression to the affected area, helping to prevent contractures and promote healing.[21,23]

Contracture deformities of the feet after burn injuries present a complex problem that requires a multidisciplinary approach in burn rehabilitation. Various options for managing these deformities are available, including orthopedic shoes with or without modifications, orthotic inserts, ankle-foot orthoses (AFOs), and heel lifts. Orthopedic shoes play a crucial role in lower extremity orthotics and can be used to correct deformities of the burned foot. The shoes can be modified to accommodate specific needs. Common modifications may include arch pads, molded foot thermoplastics, tongue pads, and metatarsal bars. These modifications help distribute forces appropriately, reduce pressure on sensitive or deformed structures, and promote even weight bearing along the plantar aspect of the foot. In addition to orthopedic shoes, orthotic inserts can be used to provide additional support, cushioning, and alignment correction. These inserts are designed to fit inside the shoe and can help improve foot function, reduce pain, and address specific foot deformities or imbalances. Heel lifts are another option that can be used to address leg-length discrepancies or to modify the biomechanics of the foot and ankle. They are placed inside the shoe to elevate the heel and provide additional support or correction. For more severe deformities or cases where additional support and control are needed, AFOs may be prescribed. AFOs are custom-made or prefabricated devices encompassing the ankle and foot, providing stability, alignment correction, and improved gait mechanics.[80] These devices can be designed to address specific contracture deformities and facilitate proper foot positioning and function.[21,100]

It is essential for individuals with foot contracture deformities after burn injuries to work closely with a healthcare team experienced in burn rehabilitation. They can assess the specific needs and goals of the individual and determine the most appropriate orthotic interventions, including selecting proper footwear, modifications, and additional orthotic devices to optimize function and promote healing. Regular evaluation and adjustment of the orthotic interventions may be necessary to achieve the desired outcomes.[21,23]

FACE AND MOUTH

Burns to the ears may require various strategies to protect and manage the affected areas as they heal. Strapping ear cups made of thermoplastic or foam can provide protection and cushioning for burned ears. An ear conformer can be custom made to prevent the rim of the ear from contracting toward the head and help maintain its shape. Internal ear canal splints can also be fabricated and adjusted as needed to prevent ear canal narrowing. Pressure on the ears can be prevented by using a soft circular foam that can be positioned posteriorly to the head to elevate the ears off the bed's surface.[101] Nasal obturators may be required to keep the nostrils open, and they can be adjusted as the circumference of the nostrils changes.[23,102]

Burns to the head and neck can lead to impairment of facial nerve function, resulting in weakness or paralysis of facial muscles, affecting facial expressions, eye closure, and overall facial symmetry. Sensory loss may also occur, decreasing sensation in the affected areas. Injuries to the eyelids resulting from burns can be challenging and may give rise to various complications.[23] One common complication is burn contracture, which can cause the eyelids to tighten and pull away from the eyeball, resulting in ectropion. Ectropion is characterized by the eyelid turning outward and can lead to problems with tear drainage, dryness, and cornea exposure. Eyelid injuries can also lead to corneal exposure, where the eyelids do not adequately protect the cornea. Corneal exposure can result in dryness, irritation, and potential damage to the cornea, which is the transparent front part of the eye. Furthermore, contracture of the canthi (the outer or inner corners of the eye) can occur due to eyelid injury.[21] Canthal contracture can cause the eyelids to become tightly pulled together, resulting in functional and cosmetic issues. Initiating a comprehensive rehabilitation program in a timely manner is crucial for managing facial burns. Such a program aims to address the functional and esthetic aspects of the burn injury, reduce potential complications, and optimize overall outcomes for the patient. In the postacute phase, facial scar hypertrophy may occur.[21] To manage this, high thermoplastic transparent masks, such as the Uvex and W-clear masks or silicone elastomer facemasks (Fig. 15.28), can be fabricated. These masks provide pressure therapy and help with scar maturation. Additionally, semirigid low thermoplastic opaque masks may be fabricated based on the state of scar maturation.[103,104]

Microstomia is a condition where the mouth opening becomes restricted due to scar tissue formation and can lead to difficulties in oral hygiene, speech articulation, and proper containment of food and saliva within the mouth. Oral incompetence refers to the inability to maintain an adequate lip seal, leading to drooling and an increased risk of aspiration. Burns can cause scarring and contracture of the lips, resulting in eversion (rolling outwards) of the lip tissues, and can contribute to functional and esthetic concerns, such as difficulty with oral hygiene, impaired speech, and compromised lip seal. Burns affecting the tongue, lips, and oral cavity can impact speech production and articulation. Scarring and limited mobility of the affected structures can lead to difficulty forming sounds and clear speech. Microstomia and oral incompetence can make proper oral

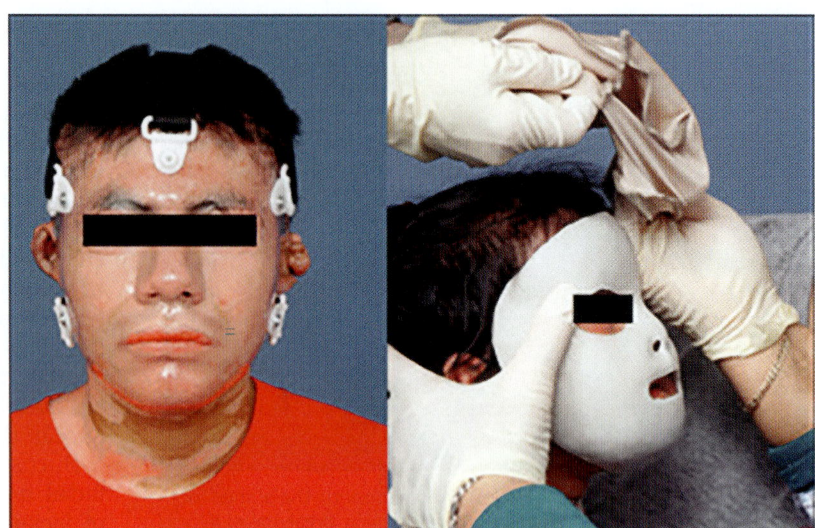

Fig. 15.28 A Uvex clear face mask or a silicon elastomer face mask provides pressure to the face to prevent scar hypertrophy and preserve facial features. (From Serghiou MA, Ott S, Cowan A, Kemp-Offenberg J. Burn rehabilitation along the continuum of care. In: *Total Burn Care.* Vol. 47. Elsevier; 2018:476–508 e4.)

hygiene practices difficult, increasing the risk of oral infections, dental decay, and periodontal diseases.[103] To prevent oral microstomia, mouth splints can be custom made by a therapist or obtained commercially (see Fig. 15.28). They can be static or dynamic, designed to provide a horizontal or vertical mouth opening. In cases of severe microstomia, compliance can be an issue and an orthodontic commissure appliance that attaches to the teeth may be fabricated by an orthodontist. Stacked tongue depressors are also used to help reverse oral microstomia (Fig. 15.29).[23,102,103,105,106]

ADDITIONAL CONSIDERATIONS

Materials such as tongue depressors or elastic wraps can be used as temporary splints to provide initial support and increase ROM in certain situations. These makeshift splints can serve as a temporary solution until more stable and durable splinting materials can be obtained or custom made. Tongue depressors, when secured with gauze wrapping, can provide a rigid structure to immobilize or support a joint temporarily and can be used to stabilize a joint and prevent undesired movement during the early stages of injury or rehabilitation. Stacked tongue depressors can also be used to help reverse oral microstomia.[107] However, they are not as versatile or durable as specialized splinting materials. Elastic wraps can be used to create dynamic splints by applying controlled tension to promote joint movement and increase ROM. They can provide gentle support and assistance during active exercises or functional activities. While elastic wraps can be helpful in some instances, they may not offer the same level of stability and control as custom made or commercially available splinting materials.[23,96]

Serial casts can also be used to provide end-range positioning for contracted scar tissue. Serial casting involves applying a series of casts over time to gradually stretch and lengthen the scar tissue (Fig. 15.30). The process begins with applying a cast that positions the affected joint or tissue at its current ROM. After this time, the cast is removed, and the joint or tissue is assessed for any improvements in ROM. If there is progress, a new cast is applied, incrementally increasing the stretch or ROM compared to the previous cast. This process is repeated with each cast application, gradually working towards the desired end-range position. Serial casting allows for controlled and progressive scar tissue stretching over time. It is often combined with other therapeutic interventions, such as manual therapy, stretching exercises, and functional activities to maximize the benefits.[21,23,96]

For patients with special rehabilitative complications after burn injury, such as exposed tendons or peripheral neuropathy, splints can be valuable in protecting and supporting these areas. For patients with exposed tendons, it is essential to keep the tendons moist with ointment-based gauze or biological dressings to promote healing. The limb is then splinted in a position that keeps the tendon slack, reducing tension and allowing for proper healing. Aggressive exercise should be avoided to prevent further damage or complications.[21,23,96]

Peripheral neuropathy, both idiopathic and secondary, can occur due to burn injury. Splints can be used to support and protect affected limbs, and careful monitoring of the patient's position, tightness of dressings, and fit of splints is necessary to avoid over-elongation or compression of peripheral nerves, which can worsen the neuropathy. In cases where there is a temporary or long-term neurologic deficit, such as drop foot, splints can be custom-fit to help overcome these deficits and improve functional mobility.[21,23,96]

When using splints to manage burn wounds, it is important to consider the risk of contamination and infection. Splints worn over open wounds can potentially serve as a source of microorganisms and may contribute to the risk of infection. Effective cleaning strategies for burn splints are crucial to minimizing contamination risk. Simply washing and drying the splint may not eliminate all microorganisms. One recommended method for cleaning burn splints is using a quaternary ammonia solution. This solution, typically prepared by adding 1 ounce of quaternary ammonia to a gallon of water, is 100% effective as a cleaning agent for splints.[108]

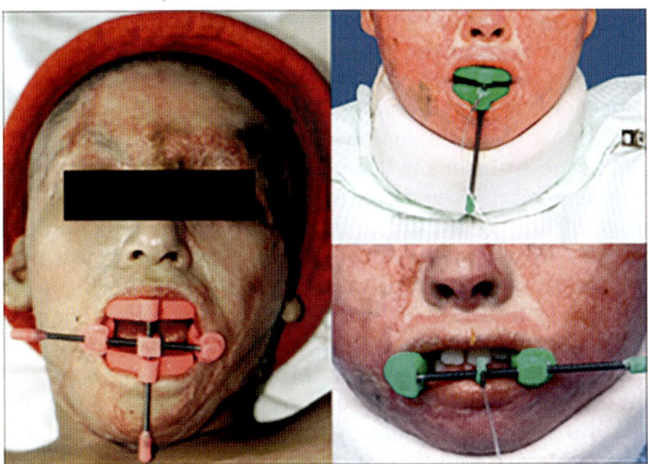

Fig. 15.29 Horizontal, vertical, and circumferential mouth-opening devices are utilized to correct oral microstomia. (From Serghiou MA, Ott S, Cowan A, Kemp-Offenberg J. Burn rehabilitation along the continuum of care. In: *Total Burn Care.* Vol. 47. Elsevier; 2018:476–508 e4.)

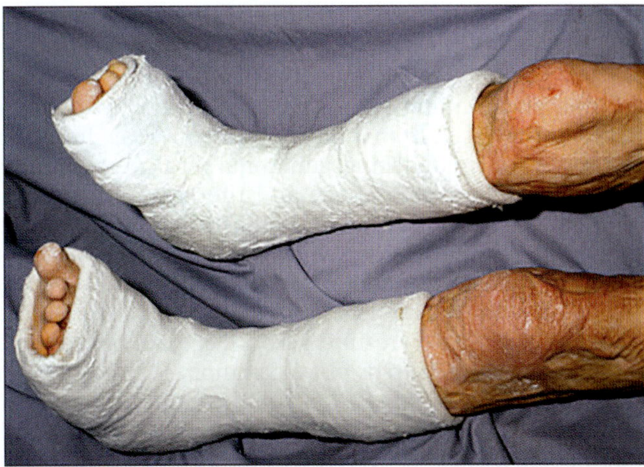

Fig. 15.30 Serial casting provides prolonged, gentle, sustained stretch and aids in tissue elongation and correction of contractures without pain. (From Serghiou MA, Ott S, Cowan A, Kemp-Offenberg J. Burn rehabilitation along the continuum of care. In: *Total Burn Care.* Vol. 47. Elsevier; 2018:476–508 e4.)

Case Example 15.1 **A Patient With Burns of Both Upper Extremities**

M.J. is a 17-year-old girl who was injured in a house fire 3 weeks ago and sustained 11% total body surface area burns to her face and both upper extremities. Facial burns were partial thickness in depth and spontaneously healed within 2 weeks. The burn injuries affecting both arms from midbrachium down each forearm and the dorsum of each hand were full thickness and required skin grafting for wound closure. Skin-grafting procedures were completed during the first 2 weeks of hospitalization in a series of three surgeries.

QUESTIONS TO CONSIDER

- What tests and measures would be most appropriate to document and track changes in M.J.'s ROM, strength, endurance, and functional status? How might they need to be modified or adapted because of the severity of her burns?

How will the medical care for her healing partial-thickness facial burns and her full-thickness, grafted upper extremity burns differ in terms of:

- Pain control
- Likelihood of scarring
- Wound care

- What factors might influence the maturation of burn scars in this young female?
- At this point in time, what are the primary rehabilitation goals for this young female? How do rehabilitation goals change over the stages of wound healing (inflammatory, proliferative, and maturation)?
- What joints are most at risk for developing contracture in the early phases of healing? What positions would be optimal to reduce risk of contracture development? What type of orthosis might you recommend at this time? What other interventions would be important to consider as she progresses through the stages of wound healing?
- What passive and active exercise strategies might you recommend to enhance range of motion (ROM), flexibility of healing tissues, strength, and endurance?
- What education and supportive strategies might be necessary?
- How long would you expect M.J. to be involved in rehabilitation activities? How will you assess whether your interventions are accomplishing the rehabilitation goals?

INTERVENTIONS AND OUTCOMES

When M.J. is not immobilized after surgery, she is involved in a treatment program that includes upper extremity mobility exercises and strengthening exercises and an aerobic conditioning exercise program. Early ROM is generally mildly limited because of edema and wound contraction. After the skin-grafting procedures, ROM at all affected joints is improving, with the exception of declines in left elbow extension and left hand metacarpophalangeal flexion (digits 2 through 5). An anterior elbow-conforming splint is fabricated for the left arm, and a functional position splint with approximately 40 degrees of metacarpophalangeal flexion is made for the left hand. Both splints are made of thermoplastic material and secured with hook-and-loop material strapping. These splints are applied during rest periods, naps, and the night to prevent further loss of ROM. When awake, M.J. participates in therapy sessions and a home program of passive stretching and active exercise of all the affected joints, with emphasis on the troublesome left elbow and hand. Use of the splints is discontinued after 2 weeks because the ROM has improved to normal.

Amputation and Prosthetics in Burn Rehabilitation

Amputations can occur among burn patients, often as a result of electrical insults but also from severe thermal injuries. These amputations have physical and psychological consequences that can significantly impact the patient's QOL.[23] People with epilepsy are also vulnerable because they often have prolonged exposure to the burn source during a seizure.[109] Burn injuries and frostbite injuries can sometimes lead to the necessity of amputation, especially when the wounds are deep or associated with severe tissue trauma. In some cases, amputations may also be performed due to uncontrolled infection that cannot be effectively treated. Patients with burns who require limb amputation may experience complications that can delay the process of fitting and training with a prosthetic limb. These complications may arise from multiple wound or scar sites, skin grafting on the residual limb, additional surgical procedures unrelated to the amputation, and the catabolic atrophy resulting from the burn injury. Postoperative complications following amputation, such as edema, phantom pain, and the formation of neuromas or bone spurs, can also affect individuals with burns who have undergone amputation. In cases of amputation resulting from electrical injuries, the formation of bone spurs is more common. When the burn injury affects more than 20% of the TBSA, there is a higher risk of developing HO, which is the abnormal formation of bone in soft tissues. However, it is important to note that clinically challenging cases of HO are relatively rare, occurring in only a small percentage of patients.[23,109–112]

Prosthetics play a crucial role in rehabilitating amputees and are designed, fabricated, and fitted by certified prosthetists. Each prosthetic device is individualized to meet the specific needs of the patient. The amputation's location and level dictate the prosthetic device's type and design. Different amputation levels require different prostheses, such as below-knee prostheses, above-knee prostheses, or upper-limb prostheses. The shape and contour of the remaining limb stump, also known as the residual limb, are essential in ensuring the prosthesis's proper fit and comfort. The prosthetist will take careful measurements and assess the unique characteristics of the residual limb. The functional needs and goals of the patient must be considered when designing the prosthesis and include assessing the patient's mobility requirements, such as walking, running, or engaging in specific activities or sports.

The patient's cognitive abilities and understanding of prosthetic use and care are considered. The design of the prosthesis should be user-friendly and easy for the patient to operate. The prosthetist considers the patient's vocational needs and any specific requirements related to their occupation. The prosthesis should facilitate the patient's ability to perform their job effectively. The patient's hobbies, recreational activities, and leisure pursuits are considered to ensure that the prosthesis accommodates and enhances their participation in these activities. The cost and affordability of the prosthesis are considered, along with the available financial resources of the patient. In addition to these factors, the prosthetic device should be comfortable to wear, easy to don and doff, lightweight, and constructed with durable materials. Its appearance should also be cosmetically appealing to the patient. Despite these concerns, patients with burn-related amputations are successfully rehabilitated with standard protocols.[23,109–112]

SKIN CONDITION

For individuals with skin graft sites on the residual limb following amputation, the fragility of the skin becomes a significant concern. The skin graft or fragile scar tissue may not tolerate pressure and shear forces well, developing blisters or small open wounds when exposed to the forces exerted during walking or prosthetic use. In such cases, wearing the prosthesis is often discontinued until the new wound has adequately healed. Areas associated with prosthesis use, such as the shoulder or scapula under an upper extremity prosthesis harness, may also experience similar issues with wound breakdown if they have undergone skin grafting or have fragile scars. In some patients, however, a free tissue transfer must be substituted for the split-thickness skin graft. Free tissue transfers provide excellent coverage of amputated limbs, but these transfers take time to develop protective sensation and may break down if weight bearing is started before this occurs. Soft-tissue involvement of the legs and arms is often extensive, and multiple soft-tissue debridements and skin grafts are usually necessary for patients who survive the initial onset of meningococcal disease. Meticulous care to maximize limb length and joint function can significantly enhance patient outcomes. Neuromas are frequent due to extensive loss of overlying skin and subcutaneous tissue. Although the presence of a skin graft or fragile scar may initially delay or prolong prosthetic training, most patients with burn-related amputations eventually succeed in using their prostheses on skin-grafted limbs. It is important to note that advances in prosthetic socket suspension and lining materials, such as "antishear" technologies, can benefit individuals with burn-related amputations. These advancements aim to minimize shear forces and provide better support and comfort for the residual limb, reducing the risk of skin breakdown and improving overall prosthetic fit and function.[23,110–112]

DELAYED FITTING

For patients with extensive burns affecting a large percentage of their TBSA, multiple surgical skin-grafting procedures are often required to cover the burn wounds adequately. These repeated surgeries can lead to delays in prosthetic fitting and training. After each surgical procedure, patients may be placed on postoperative bed rest for 2 to 7 days to facilitate initial healing of the grafted area. During this time, the limb may be positioned in a way that is less than optimal for prosthetic use to protect the new graft site and promote healing. This temporary positioning is necessary to ensure the graft's success and reduce the risk of complications. Conscientious wrapping of the residual limb can help manage swelling, provide support, and protect the graft site. Close monitoring of the healing process and implementing appropriate wound care techniques can help mitigate the difficulties associated with repeated surgical procedures and promote successful prosthetic fitting.[23,110–112]

STABILIZATION OF BODY WEIGHT

Patients with burns commonly experience weight loss due to hypermetabolism. The body's metabolic requirements can increase significantly, almost doubling, in response to a large burn. Despite receiving nutritional supplementation, individuals with significant burns often experience catabolic weight loss at a slower pace. In recovery, most individuals gradually regain the weight lost during the catabolic phase. However, this weight stabilization may take some time, and it can be challenging to fit a permanent prosthesis until the patient's weight has sufficiently stabilized. During the period of weight fluctuation, temporary sockets may need to be revised or refabricated to accommodate the

Case Example 15.2 A Patient With Amputation After Electrical Burns

C.T. is a 32-year-old male who was injured when a metal ladder he was using to trim tree branches made contact with overhead electrical wires. He sustained 35% total body surface area burns to his face, trunk, both upper extremities (including the right axilla), and his right lower leg. A right transhumeral amputation and a right transtibial amputation were required because of significant tissue damage from the electrical current. The amputations were performed on the third day after the burn; both residual limbs required several revisions of the amputation sites. Both residual limbs were successfully covered with a skin graft by the sixth day after the initial amputation.

QUESTIONS TO CONSIDER

- What tests and measures would be most appropriate to document and track changes in C.T.'s ROM, strength, endurance, and functional status? How might they need to be modified or adapted because of the severity of his burns?
- Given the cause of his burns, what are the possible issues related to wound healing, contracture formation, and preprosthetic care that will influence your clinical decision-making? What are the most pressing rehabilitation goals considering both his burns and his amputations in this early period of rehabilitation? In the months ahead?
- What will pain management and wound healing be like for someone like C.T., who has undergone amputation after electrocution, compared with someone with thermal burns who has had skin grafting?
- What factors will influence C.T.'s readiness for prosthetic fitting for this transtibial limb? For his transhumeral limb? What is C.T.'s prognosis for prosthetic use at both transtibial and transhumeral levels? How might the presence of skin grafts influence the prosthetist's recommendation for socket type and suspension of the prostheses? How will maturation of the residual limb and likely changes in body weight over time influence prosthetic fit and function?
- What are the key components in your preprosthetic plan of care for C.T.'s residual limbs? How might tissue healing influence his progression through prosthetic training? What passive and active exercise strategies might you recommend to enhance ROM, flexibility of healing tissues, strength, and endurance?
- What education and supportive strategies might be necessary for this young male with serious burns and amputation?
- How long would you expect C.T. to be involved in rehabilitation activities? How will you assess whether your interventions are accomplishing the rehabilitation goals?

INTERVENTIONS AND OUTCOMES

Although C.T. was fitted with a transtibial prosthesis within 3 weeks of skin grafting, the fitting of C.T.'s initial upper extremity prosthesis must be postponed because of the time required to obtain closure of the remaining burn wounds on the right upper extremity (6 weeks). Given the extent of his burns, signal sites for a myoelectric (externally powered) prosthesis are difficult to identify. Thus C.T. is fit with a conventional body-powered transhumeral prosthesis with a hook as a terminal device. Deep burns on both shoulders and the left trunk further delay (10 weeks) this fitting because of intolerance of the newly healed skin to the prosthetic harness.

C.T. quickly becomes functional with his transtibial prosthesis, although susceptibility to pressure requires a special antishear, pressure-distributing liner. During the fitting and training delays for his transhumeral prosthesis, an aggressive treatment program, including mobility and strengthening exercises, is directed at the right upper extremity. The residual limb is also shaped with compression wraps and stockinet. C.T. also participates in similar mobility and strengthening exercises for other affected areas, as well as an aerobic exercise program to improve his endurance.

Twelve weeks after injury, C.T. is fit for and begins formal training with his prosthesis (dual-control cable system). There is one incident of skin breakdown under the harness over the left scapula. This area is dressed and padded with dense foam. There are no further incidences of skin breakdown. C.T. is discharged from physical therapy associated with the amputation 15 weeks after injury.

During his episode of care for rehabilitation and prosthetic training, C.T. endured several delays in management of his amputations as a result of the care related to other burn injuries, particularly those in strategic anatomic regions. It was important to maintain focus on preparation of the transtibial residual limb for containment within and functional use of the prosthesis and to prepare his transhumeral residual limb and opposite arms for the figure-of-eight harness and control system. Much of C.T.'s rehabilitation care concentrated on mobility ROM and strength (especially of his upper extremities and the shoulder girdle) and endurance training.

changing shape and size of the residual limb. This process allows for adjustments to be made as the patient's weight gradually stabilizes. The goal is to ensure the permanent prosthesis's proper and comfortable fit once the weight has reached a more stable state, which helps optimize the fitting and function of the prosthesis and promotes the patient's overall recovery and mobility.[23,110–112]

Education

Burn patients play a vital role in their rehabilitation and recovery process. Involving the patient early on and including their family members or caregivers as part of the burn care team is essential for successful outcomes. Education is a crucial component of burn rehabilitation, and it should cover various aspects of care and self-management. Topics such as proper skin care, exercise programs, using pressure supports (such as cushions or garments), positioning techniques, and adherence to splint protocols are important areas to focus on during the educational process. The effectiveness of education can be assessed by the patient's and caregiver's ability to demonstrate knowledge and understanding of the rehabilitation program. This may involve practical demonstrations, discussions, and active participation in learning activities. Reinforcement, reasoning, and reassurance should be incorporated into the educational process to enhance understanding and engagement. By providing education and empowering the patient and their caregivers with knowledge and skills, they can actively participate in their care and recovery, promoting a sense of control, fostering independence, and enhancing their ability to manage their condition outside the hospital setting. Continuous communication, follow-up sessions, and periodic assessments can further reinforce education and ensure that the patient and their caregivers are equipped with the necessary knowledge and skills to optimize their recovery and long-term well-being.[23,30,45,90,113]

Summary

Individuals recovering from burn injuries require a multidisciplinary approach involving the expertise of various healthcare providers. Rehabilitation professionals play a crucial role in many aspects of postburn care, working collaboratively with other healthcare team members. A critical aspect of rehabilitation professionals' involvement is in wound care and surgical grafting procedures. They contribute their expertise in assessing and managing the healing process, monitoring wound progress, and providing interventions to promote optimal healing and minimize complications. Education about the burn rehabilitation process is another key responsibility of rehabilitation professionals. They help patients and their caregivers understand the recovery journey, manage expectations, and provide guidance on self-care techniques, such as proper skin care, scar management, and prevention of contractures and deformities. Preventive care is also a significant focus for rehabilitation professionals who work to minimize the risk of hypertrophic scarring, contractures, deformities, and subsequent disabilities through early and proactive interventions, including the use of splints or orthotic devices to maintain proper alignment and prevent contractures, as well as exercise prescription tailored to the individual's needs. Rehabilitation professionals are knowledgeable in designing and fabricating splints to support and protect healing tissues, promote optimal positioning, and prevent complications. They also prescribe and guide patients through exercise programs encompassing stretching, flexibility, strengthening, and endurance training, addressing specific functional goals. In cases where individuals require prosthetic limbs, rehabilitation professionals collaborate with prosthetists to prescribe and provide training for using adaptive and assistive devices, such as prostheses, to enhance gait and activities of daily living. They work closely with patients to ensure a proper fit, functionality, and training for optimal prosthetic utilization.

References

The complete listing of the References are available in the accompanying enhanced eBook version included with the print purchase of this textbook. Visit Elsevier eBooks+ (eBooks.Health.Elsevier.com) to access this content.

16 Prescription Wheelchairs: Seating and Mobility Systems

SUSAN HALLENBORG VENTURA AND KATHERINE BENDIX

LEARNING OBJECTIVES

On completion of this chapter, the reader will be able to do the following:

1. Describe the three components of prescription wheelchairs.
2. Develop recommendations to meet minimal-to-moderate seating and mobility needs.
3. Identify clients in need of referral to specialized wheelchair clinics.
4. Apply biomechanical principles to establish customized solutions for common seating and mobility problems.
5. Apply basic principles of wheelchair prescription to generate the least costly and least complex prescriptions.
6. Generate documentation to detail medical justification for prescribed seating and mobility solutions.
7. Educate clients and others about the importance of proper fit and function of wheelchair components.

There are approximately 3.3 million people in the United States who rely on wheelchairs for functional mobility.[1] They range from very young children who are unable to attain the ability to ambulate, to very old adults who have lost the ability because of various disabling conditions. Some clients need temporary assistance with mobility for illnesses or injuries that cause impairments that are expected to resolve over time. Others will need them for the remainder of their lives.

Contrary to common understanding, wheelchairs are a complex form of assistive technology. Well-prescribed wheelchairs can optimize environmental access and participation,[2] whereas poorly considered prescriptions can cause problems ranging from discomfort to very serious injury.[3] Careful measurements and the provision of supports needed to optimize postural alignment and access to mobility features are important, even for clients who will use the most basic wheelchairs.

A wheelchair is composed of a seating system (the postural support structure), a frame (the supporting structure), and a mobility system (the propelling structure) (Fig. 16.1).[4] All three components provide different functions but must form an integrated unit for efficient and safe wheeled mobility and optimization of the client's functional potential.

No single strategy works for every client. Each person is unique, with his or her own set of problems and goals, so each requires an individualized approach to problem solving.[5] The use of some basic principles to guide the wheelchair prescription process will help ensure comprehensive coverage of concerns as well as avoid overprescription and costly errors.

Principles of Seating and Mobility

PRINCIPLE 1: ADDRESS SEATING BEFORE MOBILITY

The degree to which the client can maintain a balanced, upright posture with dynamic stability while seated in the wheelchair will determine the outcomes of many functional activities, including the method used to propel the wheelchair. For example, if "propping" with the upper extremities is needed to maintain postural alignment, the client will be unable to simultaneously use his or her upper extremities to propel the wheelchair. Seating solutions should be identified before making a final decision about mobility options.[6]

PRINCIPLE 2: STRIVE FOR OPTIMAL POSTURAL ALIGNMENT

It is helpful to envision an anatomically advantageous seated posture when designing seating solutions, even though variations from this position are common. Truly optimal solutions are those that meet the medical, functional, and personal goals of each client. The seated posture illustrated in Fig. 16.2 can be considered optimal for wheelchair positioning in the same way the anatomical position is considered optimal when standing. It provides a reference point from which to describe deviations and provides a goal for the provision of seating supports. The optimal seated position for wheelchair use is characterized by a neutral pelvic position in which there is no rotation, no obliquity, and a slight anterior tilt. The hips are flexed to a minimum of 90 degrees with neutral to slight abduction and neutral to slight external rotation. The knees are flexed to a minimum of 90 degrees, and the ankles and feet are supported on footplates. The trunk is positioned in midline with preservation of the natural curves of the spine. The head is supported over level shoulders to allow the eyes to be forward facing and horizontal. When voluntary motor control is present in the upper extremities, they should be relaxed and supported at rest to minimize shoulder and neck strain and be unencumbered by contact with the seating or mobility systems during functional activities. Clients who have limited motor control may need external support to maintain the upper extremities in neutral alignment. The optimal wheelchair seated position described here provides a stable base of support, minimizes postural discomfort and stress, and optimizes functional potential from the seated position.

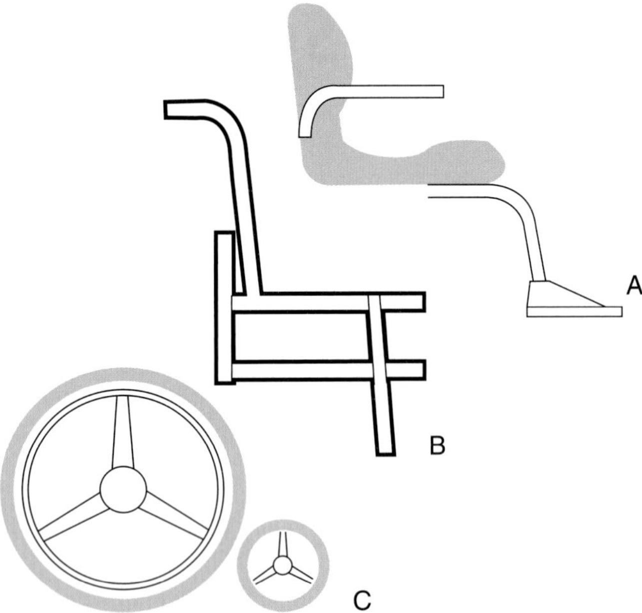

Fig. 16.1 The three components of the wheelchair include the postural support (A), the supporting structure (B), and the propelling structure (C).

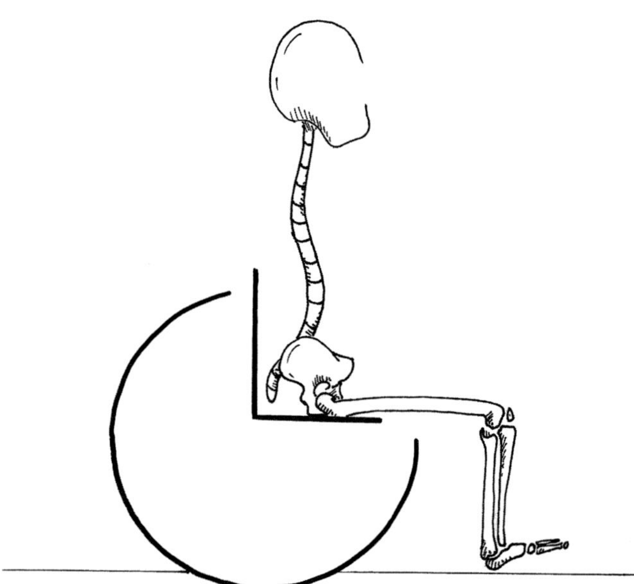

Fig. 16.2 Optimal postural alignment in wheelchair sitting. (Courtesy Annmarie Sherrick.)

PRINCIPLE 3: APPLY SEATING SOLUTIONS IN A PROXIMAL TO DISTAL DIRECTION

Postural support must be introduced thoughtfully, beginning with the base of support, which is composed of the pelvis and the lower extremities. Capturing the best possible pelvic alignment often corrects postural problems in more distal areas of the body. This approach will help ensure that only the essential amount of external support is provided, which will result in the least costly and least restrictive solution.[7] Best outcomes are those that allow the client to move freely to take advantage of available motor control to participate to the greatest possible degree in all mobility-related activities of daily living (MR-ADLs).[8] For example, the presence of a flexible scoliosis in the thoracic spine does not necessarily call for the addition of lateral trunk supports. As discussed later, this common postural deviation may be easily eliminated with adjustments made within the seat cushion to correct a flexible pelvic obliquity.

PRINCIPLE 4: PROVIDE CORRECTION BEFORE ACCOMMODATION

The evaluation process will reveal whether postural problems are fixed or flexible. The goal is always to provide the greatest amount of correction possible without causing discomfort or risk of injury. It is common to discover semi-flexible postural problems when working with clients who have long-standing impairments. In those cases, the goal is to find the balance between correction and accommodation while aiming to achieve midline orientation of the trunk and upper body and the best possible dynamic stability. Fixed postural deformities require custom-contoured solutions to prevent the progression of deformity when possible; distribute weight-bearing forces over the largest possible surface area; and upright, balanced sitting for functional activities.

PRINCIPLE 5: MEASURE ACCURATELY

It is of vital importance to identify the client's optimal postural alignment before taking measurements. This will ensure proper sizing of the wheelchair and its component parts. Measurements of the client should be checked against simulated solutions. In some cases, the client's existing equipment can be used to form the basis of determining the best size and configuration of the new equipment. Clients who are being assessed for the first time will need to be provided with simulation by using a close approximation or mockup of what will be prescribed. Waugh and Crane provide an excellent online resource to guide therapists through the process of measuring the client and support surfaces.[9]

The Seating System

The seating system can be considered an orthosis. It is a device that applies external forces to achieve dynamic stability, correction, or compensation for loss or absence of function.[8,10] A seating system provides the support needed to achieve optimal postural alignment for safe, comfortable, and functional wheelchair positioning.

Table 16.1 provides an overview of considerations for the evaluation process used to establish seating interventions. The table is arranged by body segment, beginning with the pelvis, which is central to the base of support in sitting. The need for seating interventions should be considered first at the pelvis and then progress in a more distal direction as outlined. Each body segment described includes the desired posture (relative to the optimal seated position described previously), common deviations seen at that body segment, possible causes for the deviations, common presenting symptoms, and examination

Table 16.1 Postural Evaluation by Body Segment: Possible Causes and Examination Procedures

Body Segment	Desired Posture	Common Deviations	Possible Causes	Common Symptoms	Examination Procedures
Pelvis	■ Slight anterior tilt ■ Neutral lateral tilt ■ Neutral rotation ↓ ■ Shifts center of gravity anterior to spine → ■ Assists with upright posture	Posterior tilt (sacral sitting)	Physical: ■ Proximal hypotonia ■ Extensor hypertonia ■ Limited hip flexion ■ Tight hamstrings Equipment: ■ Seat belt on or above ASIS ■ Seat depth too long ■ Hammock effect of sling seat and back	Skin/soft tissue: ■ Breakdown of the skin over the sacrum Pain: ■ Back and neck Posture: ■ Compensatory kyphosis ■ Hips and knees extended, adducted and internally rotated	Posture: ■ Compare pelvic position sitting in wheelchair to sitting on a firm mat Flexibility: ■ Assess active and passive range of motion of pelvis and hip joints ■ Measure thigh length on both sides Wheelchair: ■ Assess condition and appropriateness of wheel-chair components
		Obliquity	Physical: ■ Asymmetrical strength or muscle tone ■ Fixed (structural) scoliosis Equipment: ■ Hammock effect of sling seat ■ Solid seat insert or cushion tilted on one seat rail	Skin/soft tissue: ■ Breakdown of the skin over the lower ischial tuberosity Pain: ■ Hip, back, neck Posture: ■ Scoliosis ■ Asymmetrical height of pelvic crests	
		Forward rotation of the pelvis on one side	Physical: ■ Lumbar scoliosis with rotational component Equipment: ■ Thigh length discrepancy with seat depth fitted to the longer side ■ Seat too high for person who propels with one LE (rotates pelvis forward to functionally lengthen the stronger LE for propulsion)	Skin/soft tissue: ■ Ischial or trochanteric breakdown Pain: ■ Low back Posture: ■ Pelvis drifts to one side of w/c ■ Functional or actual leg length discrepancy	
Hips	■ Flexion at or >90 degrees ■ Neutral to slight abduction Neutral to slight exter-nal rotation ↓ ■ Discourages flexor or extensor synergies ■ Wide base of support increases stability	Extension, adduc-tion, internal rotation	Physical: ■ Posterior pelvic tilt ■ Extensor tone ■ Limited hip flexion ■ Hip dislocation ■ Windswept deformity (high side of pelvis) Equipment: Seat depth too short	Skin/soft tissue: ■ Sacral breakdown Pain: ■ Hips, back and/or neck Posture: ■ Compensatory kyphosis ■ Posterior pelvic tilt ■ Knee extension, ankle plantarflexion	■ ROM assessment of both hips ■ Isolated motor control ■ Tonal assessment ■ Reflex assessment ■ Tonic labyrinthine supine ■ Tonic labyrinthine prone ■ Symmetrical tonic neck reflex ■ Asymmetrical tonic neck reflex
		Excessive flexion, abduc-tion, external rotation	Physical: ■ Anterior pelvic tilt ■ Proximal hypotonia or weakness ■ Windswept deformity (low side of pelvis) Equipment: ■ Abductor pommel too wide or too far proximal	Skin/soft tissue: ■ Pressure on distal, lateral thigh(s) as they press against the w/c sides Pain: ■ Low back Posture: ■ "Frog leg" position	■ ROM assessment of both hips ■ Isolated motor control ■ Tonal assessment ■ Reflex assessment ■ Tonic labyrinthine supine ■ Tonic labyrinthine prone ■ Symmetrical tonic neck reflex ■ Asymmetrical tonic neck reflex

(Continued)

Table 16.1 Postural Evaluation by Body Segment: Possible Causes and Examination Procedures—Cont'd

Body Segment	Desired Posture	Common Deviations	Possible Causes	Common Symptoms	Examination Procedures
Knees	Flexion near 90 degrees ↓ ■ Discourages extensor tone ■ Minimizes stress on two joint muscles	Excessive knee flexion	Physical: ■ Short hamstrings ■ Hypertonic hamstrings Equipment: ■ Footrests too far back on w/c	Skin/soft tissue: ■ Pressure on popliteal fossa Pain: ■ Paresthesias legs and feet Posture: ■ Feet slip off footrest posteriorly	■ ROM assessment both knees ■ Isolated motor control ■ Muscle tone, reflexes ■ Equipment—footrest hangers and footplates
		Excessive knee extension	Physical: ■ Dominant extensor tone Equipment: ■ Footrests too far forward on w/c ■ Seat depth too long	Skin/soft tissue: ■ Sacral pressure Pain: ■ (See posterior pelvic tilt) Posture: ■ Feet are too far forward on footplates ■ (See posterior pelvic tilt)	
Feet	■ Neutral dorsiflexion/plantarflexion Plantigrade foot, supported on footplate ↓ ■ Avoids stimulation of reflex activity ■ Helps to maintain functional ankle ROM	Excessive dorsiflexion with eversion	Physical: ■ Component of LE flexor synergy ■ Stimulation of plantar-grasp reflex Excessive knee flexion ■ Limited ankle plantarflexion Equipment: ■ Excessive pressure on metatarsal heads from poorly placed footplates	Skin/soft tissue: ■ DF contractures ■ Pronated foot Pain: ■ Fatigue and discomfort in the ankles Posture: ■ Heel(s) the only part of the foot in contact with footplates	■ ROM assessment both feet and ankles ■ Isolated motor control ■ Muscle tone, reflexes ■ Equipment—footrest hangers and footplate adjustability
		Excessive plantarflexion with inversion	Physical: ■ Component of LE extensor synergy ■ Stimulation of positive supporting reaction or other primitive reflex pattern ■ Limited ankle dorsiflexion ■ Equipment:Footrests too low ■ Feet not fully supported on footplates	Skin/soft tissue: ■ Plantarflexion contractures ■ Supinated foot Postural: ■ "Drop foot"	
Spine	"Plumb line" posture with slight lumbar and cervical lordosis, slight thoracic kyphosis ↓ ■ Minimize stress on trunk musculature ■ Provides mechanically stable alignment, minimizing available lateral flexion and rotation of spine	Scoliosis	Physical: ■ Compensatory righting for a pelvic obliquity ■ (See pelvic obliquity) Equipment: ■ (See pelvic obliquity)	Skin/soft tissue: ■ Breakdown in skin fold created by concavity ■ Unilateral ischial breakdown Pain: ■ Hip, back, neck Posture: ■ Pelvic obliquity ■ Windswept hips ■ "Habitual" leaning to one side	■ Assess symmetry of shoulders, pelvic crests ■ Assess alignment of spinous processes ■ Assess flexibility of spine ■ Assess equipment ■ Seat, back, belt ■ Footrest hangers and footplates
		Excessive kyphosis thoracic and lumbar spine and excessive lordosis of the cervical spine	Physical: ■ Compensatory righting for a posterior pelvic tilt ■ (See posterior pelvic tilt) Equipment: ■ (See posterior pelvic tilt)	Skin/soft tissue: ■ Breakdown thoracic spinous processes Pain: ■ Neck and back Posture: ■ Posterior pelvic tilt ■ Hip extension, adduction, internal rotation	

Table 16.1 Postural Evaluation by Body Segment: Possible Causes and Examination Procedures—Cont'd

Body Segment	Desired Posture	Common Deviations	Possible Causes	Common Symptoms	Examination Procedures
Shoulder Girdle	Neutral with regard to scapulae protraction or retraction	Scapular protraction	Physical: ■ Increased flexor tone in upper extremities ■ Hypotonia Equipment: ■ Sling back support ■ Concave back support	Skin/soft tissue: ■ Breakdown inferior border of scapulae Pain: ■ Rhomboids area Posture: ■ "Winging" of scapulae	■ Assess alignment, symmetry and position of scapulae relative to spinous processes ■ Assess active scapulae muscle control ■ Assess passive scapulae motion ■ Assess equipment—back support
		Scapular retraction	Physical: ■ Increased extensor tone in upper extremities ■ Hypotonia with proximal "fixing" Equipment: ■ Inadequate block against strong extensor pattern	Skin/soft tissue: ■ Breakdown, spine of scapulae Pain: ■ Upper back Posture: ■ Shoulders externally rotated, adducted and retracted	
Head	Midline vertical, eyes horizontal	Laterally flexed	Physical: ■ Scoliosis with compensatory righting ■ Less than fair head control ■ Asymmetrical muscle tone Equipment: ■ Inadequate proximal support (pelvis, trunk, or head)	Skin/soft tissue: ■ Irritation from backrest or headrest causing skin breakdown or hair loss Pain: ■ Neck Posture: ■ Uneven shoulder height (scoliosis) ■ Even shoulder height (lack of head control)	■ ROM of the neck ■ Head control ■ Functional assessment ■ Muscle tone ■ Equipment ■ Proximal support structures ■ Back support ■ Head support
		Increased cervical lordosis	Physical: ■ Increased flexion of trunk with compensatory righting to bring the eyes to midline, horizontal Equipment: ■ Inadequate proximal support	Skin/soft tissue: ■ Irritation of skin near the occipital protuberance Pain: ■ Neck Posture: ■ Kyphotic spine Or ■ Increase lumbar lordosis	
Upper Extremities	Relaxed, free for propulsion or other functional activities	Required for postural support on tray or armrests	Physical: ■ Paralysis of upper extremities Equipment: ■ Inadequate proximal support	Skins/soft tissue: ■ Breakdown near elbows Pain: ■ Shoulders Posture: ■ Leaning on one or both UEs	■ Observation ■ Functional assessment ■ Isolated motor control ■ Tonal assessment ■ Reflex assessment ■ Tonic labyrinthine supine ■ Tonic labyrinthine prone ■ Symmetrical tonic neck reflex ■ Asymmetrical tonic neck reflex

ASIS, Anterior superior iliac spine; *DF*, dorsiflexion; *LE*, lower extremity; *ROM*, range of motion; *UEs*, upper extremities; *w/c*, wheelchair. Always begin postural evaluation with assessment of the pelvis and move in a proximal to distal direction from the base of support. These are general guidelines only—optimal position varies according to medical and functional needs.

procedures that may be helpful in identifying the underlying causes for the deviations observed.

Care must be taken to provide the least possible external support to facilitate the use of any available voluntary motor control to avoid interference with functional activities. It is also important to distribute the forces associated with corrective components of the seating system over the greatest possible surface area to ensure comfort and soft-tissue protection.[8] This is especially true for clients who have both motor and sensory impairments, because they are at increased risk for pressure-related damage to the skin and underlying soft tissues.[11,12]

Pressure ulcers occur when unprotected weight bearing results in ischemia of the skin and soft tissues, especially those surrounding bony prominences. The propensity for developing pressure ulcers is exacerbated by many factors, including cumulative pressure and shear forces caused by sitting for extended periods of time, the experience of high pressures for short periods of time, impaired sensory and motor function, and poor sitting posture.[13] Other mediating factors include the presence of heat and moisture buildup between the skin and the seating system, illness, and inadequate nutrition and hydration.[14–16] Chronic problems with pressure ulcers can have a devastating effect on quality and extent of life,[17,18] so prevention is of paramount importance in developing seating interventions. Proper size and set up of the wheelchair are essential to pressure management.[19] Equally important are the strategic use of external postural supports that offer pressure-relieving properties, client education/training in weight-shifting and monitoring strategies, and, if needed, the addition of active seating options such as tilt or recline.[12]

As already mentioned, all seating interventions begin by addressing seating concerns at the pelvis and lower extremities, as these regions of the body form the base of support in sitting. Key to success is identifying appropriate seat and back supports to assist with positioning the pelvis, distribution of weight-bearing forces over the largest possible pressure-tolerant areas, and/or offloading any areas that have a history of soft-tissue breakdown.[20]

Both passive and active pressure-relieving technologies are available. Passive technologies are the most commonly prescribed and consist of wheelchair cushions and related seating components that increase the surface area for weight bearing through the processes of envelopment and/or redistribution of weight-bearing forces. Areas at high risk for breakdown include the ischial tuberosities, the sacrum, and greater trochanters, while more pressure-tolerant areas include the distal femurs and fleshy areas of the buttocks. Many pressure-relieving cushions, such as the one shown in Fig. 16.3, accomplish both goals by combining a shape that redistributes weight-bearing forces with air- or fluid-filled inserts to achieve envelopment.

Active technologies include dynamic seat cushions and/or the use of wheelchair frames that permit tilt, recline, or standing. Dynamic seat cushions typically consist of a series of alternating chambers. A motor pumps air or fluid through chambers to change the configuration of the support surface gently and continuously, much like an alternating-pressure mattress used in hospital beds for clients who are unable to change position. Power or manual tilt (Fig. 16.4), recline (Fig. 16.5), or standing systems (Fig. 16.6) alternate weight-bearing surfaces by changing the client's position in space to periodically off-weight areas of concern.

Comfort and functional outcomes are as important as postural alignment and soft-tissue protection.[21] Clients need to feel secure in their seating systems to function optimally. Individuals who experience discomfort or feelings of insecurity when seated report dissatisfaction with their equipment, which may lead to equipment abandonment.[22]

The process of identifying priorities for seating systems can be quite challenging. It may be necessary to make compromises to achieve the overall best outcome for the client. For example, consider a client who has been using an air-filled cushion with excellent pressure management, but this cushion does not provide the necessary corrective forces to achieve optimal postural alignment. The team may recommend an alternative intervention that meets all identified needs, but the client may resist that option. The obligation of the team is to educate the client about the risks and benefits of recommended and preferred equipment so he or she can make an informed choice. Health professionals should remember that the client is the only one who can decide what is best for his or her circumstances. Forcing choices on an individual is likely to have negative consequences. The

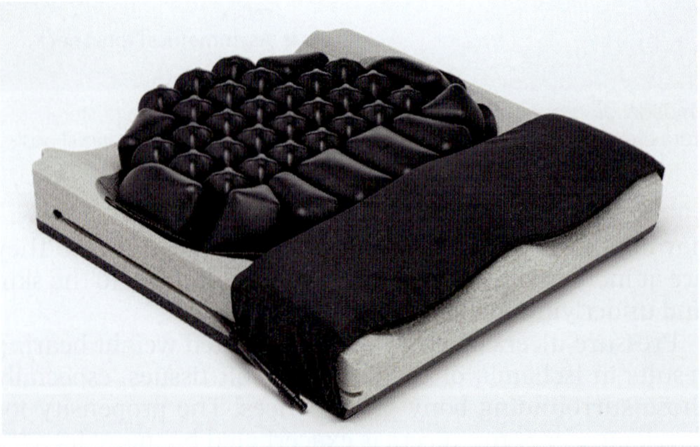

Fig. 16.3 Hybrid cushion includes a contoured base for redistribution of pressures and air-filled bladder to achieve envelopment. (Courtesy Permobil Inc.)

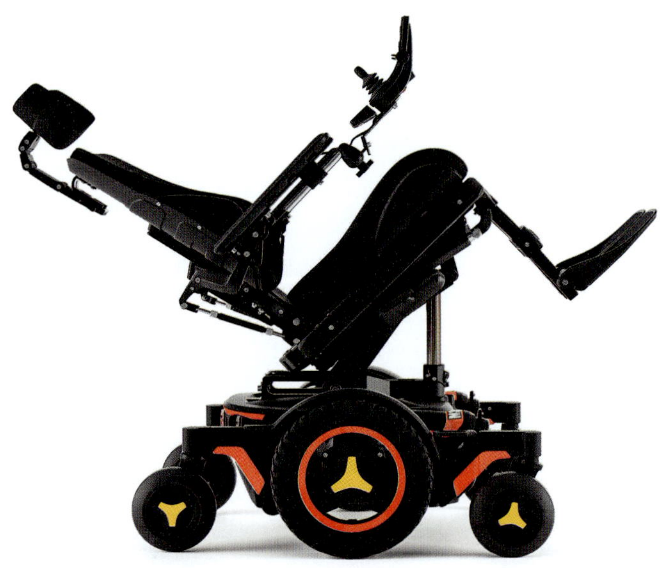

Fig. 16.4 Power wheelchair with power tilt. (Courtesy Permobil Inc.)

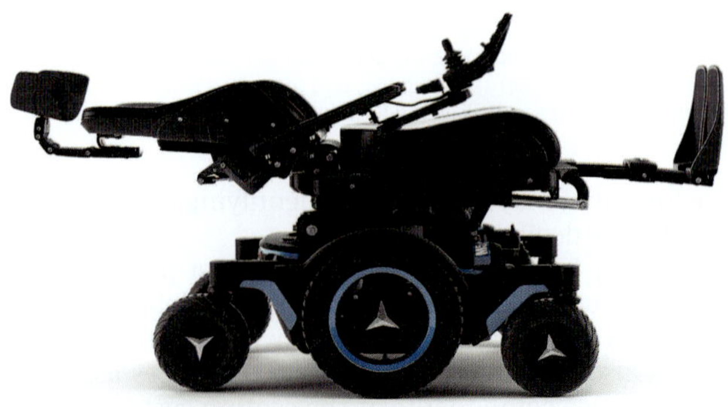

Fig. 16.5 Power wheelchair with power reclining back and elevating leg rests. (Courtesy Permobil Inc.)

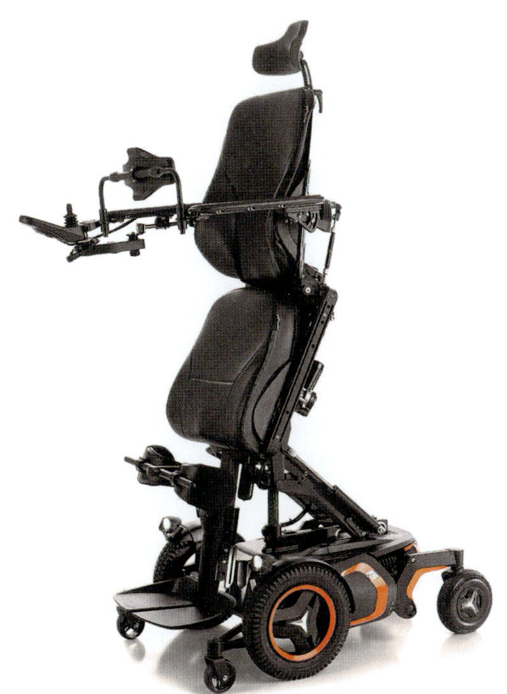

Fig. 16.6 Power wheelchair with power standing feature. (Courtesy Permobil Inc.)

best solution is one that meets all the needs identified to the greatest extent possible but yields optimal client satisfaction.

Clinicians need to be familiar with the types of commercially available seating options so they can educate their clients and make appropriate recommendations. While familiarity with specific brands and models is beneficial, it is more crucial to understand the key properties and features offered by different seating solutions. The rehabilitation technology supplier, a member of the healthcare team, is available for consultation to ensure that the selected seating options align with the desired outcomes and meet the clients' specific needs.

What is of utmost importance is for clinicians to be able to identify seating problems and whether they are flexible or fixed. Flexible deformities can be corrected within the seating system, whereas fixed deformities cannot be corrected so will need accommodation. Table 16.2 provides an overview of common fixed and flexible problems that occur at each segment of the body, beginning with the pelvis. Generic solutions are proposed, and these can be matched to commercially available products with the help of the rehabilitation technology supplier. Categories of available seating components and their properties are discussed here.

SEATING COMPONENTS

Seating components vary according to shape, size, and component materials. Prescribed components must work together to provide optimal positioning, comfort, function, and soft-tissue protection.[23] The two main components of the seating system are the seat and back supports. These work together to support the pelvis in a neutral position in all three planes of available movement: anterior/posterior tilt in the sagittal plane, rotation in the horizontal plane, or obliquity in the frontal plane. Most clients, even those who use wheelchairs on a temporary basis, will benefit from some form of support beyond the upholstery offered on standard wheelchairs.[24] The seat and back material that is standard on most wheelchairs offers little resistance to forces that impact pelvic positioning, which may include gravity, tonic reflex activity, and hypertonicity.

The three most common postural deviations of the pelvis include the posterior pelvic tilt, pelvic obliquity, and pelvic rotation.[25] Each of these deviations impact posture in other regions of the body. The most common is the posterior pelvic tilt, which occurs in response to the gravitational pull on the pelvis in unsupported sitting. A posterior pelvic tilt is accompanied by flexion of the lumbar and thoracic regions and hyperextension of the cervical spine, because automatic righting reactions work to center the upper body over the base of support and right the eyes to a forward facing, horizontal orientation.[26] The posterior pelvic tilt and associated postural deformities are illustrated in Fig. 16.7. This posture is associated with abnormally high spinal disk pressures and impaired respiratory function which contribute to fatigue and discomfort after prolonged sitting.[27]

Another common postural deviation stems from the pelvic obliquity, which is shown in Fig. 16.8. This posture is often associated with clients who have asymmetrical muscle tone. For example, clients who have increased muscle tone on the right side of the body may present with a right pelvic obliquity—that is, the pelvic crest on the right side of the body sits higher compared to the left side. This position of the pelvis results in asymmetrical positioning of the hips and thighs, as well as a scoliosis of the spine, with the convexity of the curve occurring on the opposite side. Correction of the pelvic obliquity with well-prescribed seat and back supports may resolve the other asymmetries without additional seating interventions, depending on the degree to which the asymmetries are flexible. Pelvic obliquity caused by abnormal muscle tone may be accompanied by pelvic rotation, depending on the distribution of hypertonicity that is acting on the pelvis and lower extremities.

Table 16.1 outlines possible causes of the posterior pelvic tilt, pelvic obliquity, and pelvic rotation. It is important to look beyond the presenting symptoms to identify the cause of pelvic deviations, because the information obtained will help determine whether the seating system will need to provide correction or accommodation. Further, the extent to which external postural support is needed in other areas of the seating system will depend on the amount of correction that can be achieved at the pelvis.

When postural deviations are flexible, correction can generally be accomplished through the action of three counteractive forces: an inferior force from the seat cushion to capture the ischial tuberosities, a posterior force from a back support to capture the posterior superior iliac spines of the pelvis, and an anterior corrective force that can be established either with an anterior positioning strap or the introduction of hip flexion into the seating system (so the knees sit higher than the hip joints). These three counteracting forces will work together to achieve neutral pelvic alignment if adequate flexibility is present.

Accommodation of pelvic deviations is needed when deformities are fixed, because application of external forces to an immovable pelvis will likely result in excessive pressure buildup, pain, and ultimately soft-tissue injury such as a pressure ulcer. Care must be taken to provide a supportive

Table 16.2 Common Problems and Possible Solutions for Wheelchair Seating

Body Segment	Common Problems	Possible Solution(s)
Pelvis	Flexible posterior tilt	■ Supportive seat and back with belt placed between 60 and 90 degrees to seat rails (distal to ASIS) ■ "Squeeze" frame (inclinable seat) to increase hip flexion and capture the pelvis in good alignment
	Fixed (structural) posterior pelvic tilt	■ Accommodate the pelvis by opening up the seat to back angle >90 degrees
	Flexible obliquity	■ Supportive seat and back with belt placed between 60 and 90 degrees to seat rails (distal to ASIS)
	Fixed obliquity	■ Accommodate by building up under the high side of the obliquity
Hips	Hip adduction	■ Proper pelvic position ■ Removable abductor pommel placed at most distal point on seat at midline
	Hip extension—flexible	■ Proper pelvic position ■ Increase flexion past 90 degrees with inclinable seat
	Hip extension—fixed	■ Accommodate by opening up to seat to back angle
Thigh	Thigh length discrepancy	■ Proper pelvic position ■ Asymmetrical seat or cushion depth
Knees	Flexion contracture	■ Accommodate with shorter seat depth and footplates that extend posteriorly
	Extension contracture	■ Accommodate with elevating leg rests (preferably fixed vs. adjustable to prevent asymmetries) and unnecessary addition of weight
Feet	Fixed deformities	■ Support with foot cradle, adjustable angle footplate, heel loops, toe straps, as needed
Spine	Poor trunk control, no asymmetries	■ Proper pelvic alignment ■ Lateral supports mounted on high back ■ Tilt-in space wheelchair
	Fair trunk control, no asymmetries	■ Lateral supports mounted to a high back
	Flexible scoliosis	■ Proper pelvic position ■ Three- (to four-) point pressure system
	Fixed scoliosis	■ Proper pelvic position, three-point pressure system for support ■ Total contact system may be needed to ensure skin protection
	Flexible kyphosis	■ Proper pelvic position ■ Lumbar support on tilt-in space system ■ Clavicular pads if needed
	Fixed kyphosis	■ Accommodate with concave backrest and soft, supportive materials
Shoulder girdle	Excessive protraction	■ Firm back ■ Clavicular pads ■ Lap tray
	Excessive retraction	■ Concave back support, lap tray, humeral wings on tray
Head and neck	Poor head control	■ Proper pelvic alignment ■ Tilt-in space wheelchair frame ■ Posterior headrest ■ Increase support with lateral and anterior support as needed and tolerated
	Fair head control	■ Removable headrest, used especially for travel
	Cervical hyperextension	■ Proper alignment of pelvis and spine

Always begin at the pelvis when attempting to solve postural problems.

seat and back, but the goal shifts from achieving correction to achieving comfort and support. These goals are achieved with the use of soft, accommodative materials that are capable of enveloping bony prominences, distributing weight-bearing pressures to the largest possible pressure-tolerant surface area, and creating an upright, balanced posture that maximizes the functional capacity of the client.

Commercially available seating components vary in their ability to provide the correction or accommodation needed, and clients will respond differently to available options, depending on body shape and composition, perceptions of comfort, esthetic preferences, and other factors. Successive trials with different options may be needed to identify the best solutions for individual clients.

The lowest cost seating components are solid, padded seats and backs. They are the easiest to manufacture and may provide some benefits over standard fabric upholstery. However, their planar (noncontoured) shape is not effective in accommodating contoured body surfaces, which creates the potential for high pressure buildup in the areas of bony prominences. Fortunately, many manufacturers offer contoured seating components, which distribute weight-bearing forces more effectively.[28]

Two types of contoured surfaces exist: (1) precontoured (generically contoured) and (2) custom contoured. The design of precontoured seats and backs is based on average anthropometric measurements,[29] and they come in a variety of sizes to fit most wheelchairs and clients.

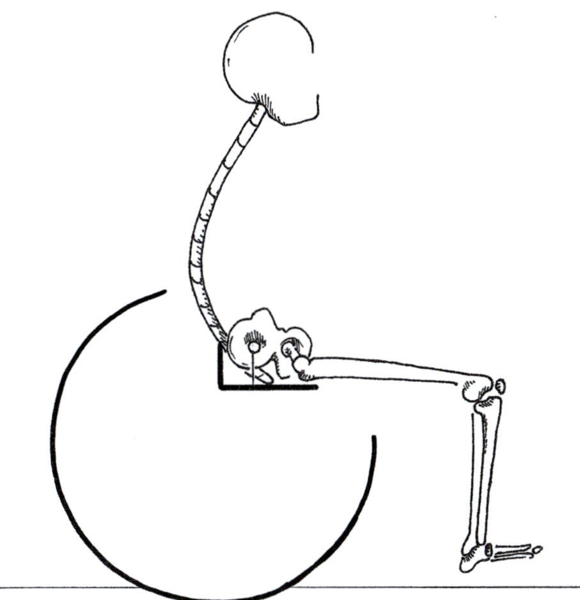

Fig. 16.7 Posterior pelvic tilt and associated postural deformities, including flexion of lumbar and thoracic spines and hyperextension of the cervical spine. (Courtesy Annmarie Sherrick.)

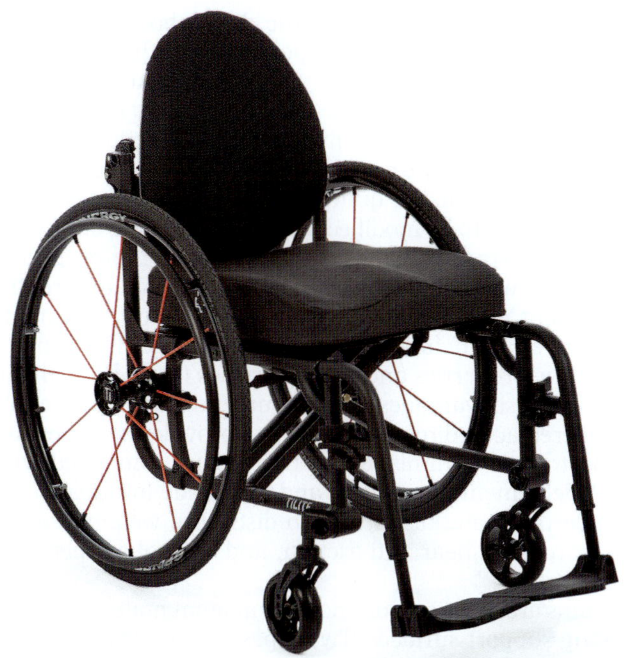

Fig. 16.9 Precontoured seat and back. (Courtesy Permobil Inc.)

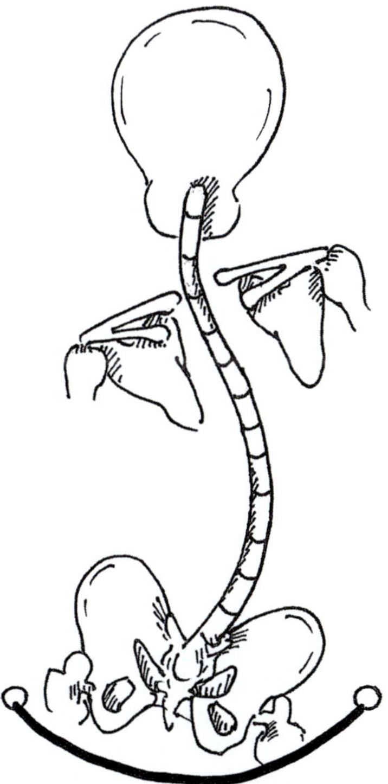

Fig. 16.8 Left pelvic obliquity with compensatory right C-curve scoliosis. (Courtesy Annmarie Sherrick.)

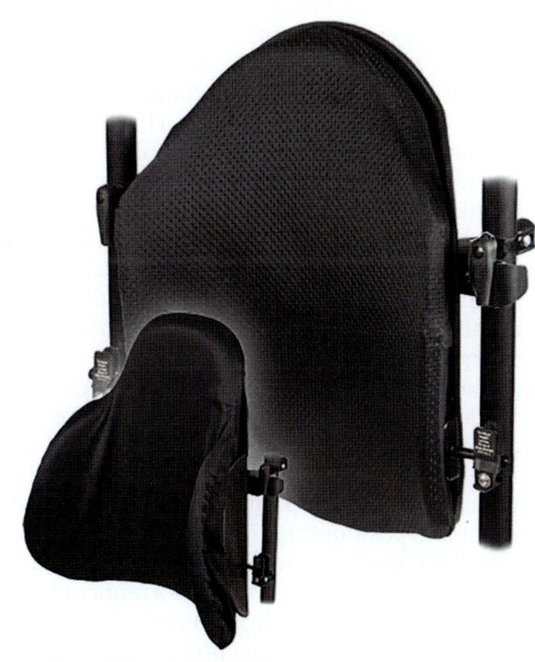

Fig. 16.10 Back rest with lateral supports. (Courtesy Sunrise Medical, Fresno, California.)

See Fig. 16.9 for an example of precontoured seat and back cushions. These seat/back options are designed to support neutral alignment of the pelvis and the natural curves of the spine. Some back supports also provide lateral supports to assist with side-to-side balance, as shown in Fig. 16.10. The effectiveness of these surfaces for either postural support or pressure management depends not only on the properties of their component materials but also on the precision of fit, so careful measurement and matching the client to available options is key to successful outcomes.

Custom-contoured surfaces are constructed directly from the shape of the client. Many technologies are available to assist with the development of custom-contoured cushions, including hand-shaping foam, computer-assisted design/computer-assisted manufacturing systems, and "foam-in-place" technologies, among others.[30] These systems are designed to record the shape of the client's body as precisely as possible to manufacture support surfaces that match the contours of that individual. Custom-contoured systems are generally reserved for use with clients who have severe, fixed musculoskeletal deformities and little ability to move actively. They offer the best option for distribution of weight-bearing forces but are quite costly, restrictive, heavy, and offer no ability to be modified if the client's needs change.

It is important to gain knowledge about the properties associated with the materials used to manufacture the component parts of seating systems. The most commonly used materials include foams, air, gel, or a combination of these. The properties and characteristics (including advantages and disadvantages) of each material must be carefully considered according to its ability to provide the necessary support while minimizing the risk factors associated with the development of pressure and soft-tissue injuries. These include the materials' ability to distribute weight-bearing forces, reduce shear and friction, and control temperature and moisture.[16,20,31]

Foams are the most common component material used in making support surfaces. Two types of foam are available: elastic (available as either a closed-cell or open-cell material) and viscoelastic. Both types have advantages that make them well suited for use in postural supports as well as disadvantages that must be considered. Elastic foams deform in proportion to the applied load, which helps them reduce peak pressure over bony prominences.[31] They do not, however, provide good envelopment, and they tend to insulate heat and keep it near the body. Viscoelastic foams are temperature sensitive, meaning they become softer and more compliant at higher temperatures.[31] This characteristic helps them provide even better pressure distribution than elastic foams, but clinicians must carefully assess individual clients' reactions to the warming effect in areas of concern.

Fluid-filled cushions are often composed of materials such as air, gel, or viscous fluids that are enclosed in one or more compartments.[31] Most of these products provide greater immersion into the cushion, thus distributing pressure over larger areas of the body and reducing pressures at bony prominences (see Fig. 16.3). The type of material used in the cushion influences both skin temperature and the moisture buildup where the support surface contacts the body.[32] Understanding the different kinds of materials helps the clinician select an appropriate seat cushion for pressure management and positioning.

Covers used for seating components are also important to consider, because they can alter the performance characteristics of the underlying supportive materials.[32] An inflexible cover will prevent a cushion from providing optimal envelopment, and those that have high friction coefficients will override the benefits of cushion materials that were selected for their low friction coefficients. Cover materials also need to be resilient, easy to clean, in some cases moisture resistant, and esthetically pleasing to the client.

Once the team has identified the best seat and back supports to achieve optimal proximal alignment, consideration can be given to more distal body segments, beginning with the lower extremities. Table 16.1 provides evaluation guidelines for all remaining regions of the body. Table 16.2 presents common problems and possible solutions, and Table 16.3 describes different seating components and accessories with their relative advantages and disadvantages.

It is generally desirable to minimize stress or stretch on the hamstring muscles when positioning the lower extremities, so the knees should be flexed to 90 degrees or more with the footrests positioned as close to the wheelchair frame as possible without interfering with the caster wheels. This also accomplishes a related goal of achieving the smallest possible overall turning radius of the wheelchair. Footrest options will generally depend on the selection of the frame of the wheelchair. Some are integral components of the frame (Fig. 16.11), whereas others are designed to be removable for ease of transfers and other functional activities as shown in Fig. 16.12.

It is important to account for the thickness of the seat cushion when determining the length of the footrest to be ordered. Manufacturers consider "minimal footrest extension" to be the distance between the standard upholstery and the top of the footplate, but this does not account for the thickness of an added seat cushion. For example, if the client's measurement between the popliteal fossa and the foot is 17″ and he or she will be sitting on a 3″ cushion, the minimum footrest extension needed on the chair as delivered will be 14″.

Trunk positioning can be considered once the base of support is optimized (pelvis and lower extremities). The seat and back supports chosen to achieve optimal pelvic positioning will likely have a positive impact on resultant posture of the trunk, but it may be necessary to provide additional postural support if motor control of the upper body is limited. For example, lateral trunk supports may be needed to support the client in midline. These may be provided as integral components to the backrest or attached to the frame to enable some adjustability (see Fig. 16.10).

Back height is an important consideration. The minimum recommended height of a back support is one that captures the posterior superior iliac spines of the pelvis to provide pelvic stability. Clients who have functional use of the upper extremities for manual propulsion or other activities will need a back support that is no higher than the inferior angle of the scapulae to permit freedom of movement of the shoulder girdles. Back supports that reach the top of the shoulders are generally reserved for clients who have poor trunk control and no functional movement of the upper extremities.

The specific height chosen will depend on how much trunk support is needed and whether other accessories, such as lateral trunk supports or a headrest, will be used because they will need a point of attachment. "Back height" specified by wheelchair manufacturers is the distance between the top of the standard seat upholstery and the top of the standard back upholstery. The measurement needed for the wheelchair prescription must account for the seat cushion thickness, just as it had to be considered for the footrest measurement. Here, the prescribed height of the back support will be the patient's measurement from the bottom of the buttocks in sitting to the height of the desired back support on the client, *plus* the thickness of the cushion. For example, if the patient needs a back support that reaches a height that is just below the inferior angle of the scapulae and their body measurement from buttocks to inferior angle is 14″, the total prescribed back height will be 17″.

Table 16.3 Advantages and Disadvantages of Various Wheelchair Components

Wheelchair Component	Options	Advantages	Disadvantages
Leg and foot supports	■ Swing-away footrests	■ Lightweight support for lower extremities ■ Removable for transfers	■ Add to weight of wheelchair (vs. platform) ■ Require maintenance ■ Require management by wheelchair user
	■ Flip-up foot platform	■ Lightweight ■ Few moving parts ■ Very stable ■ Often allows increased knee flexion angle; more comfortable and compact for user	■ Very little adjustability ■ Both lower extremities supported at same angle ■ Unable to accommodate moderate or severe ankle contractures ■ Not removable; may interfere with transfers for some users
	■ Manual elevating leg rests	■ Allows multiple leg positions ■ May prevent some dependent edema (true edema management also requires recline or tilt to elevate the legs above the heart level) ■ May increase lower extremity comfort	■ Heavier than standard leg supports ■ Many moving and adjustable parts; higher maintenance needs ■ More strength and dexterity needed to manage
Arm supports	■ Flip-back armrests	■ Stable arm support ■ Typically lightweight ■ Easy to manage	■ Multiple moving parts ■ Require maintenance to work properly ■ May not be adjustable enough for all individuals
	■ Tubular swing-away armrest	■ Extremely lightweight ■ Easy for wheelchair user to manage ■ Requires very little hand dexterity and strength	■ May not feel stable to user ■ May not tolerate extreme or repeated stresses ■ Attachment hardware requires maintenance
	■ Detachable, adjustable-height armrest	■ Support upper extremities in multiple positions ■ Removable for transfers	■ Heavier ■ More moving parts; higher maintenance requirement ■ May be difficult for users to manager, especially to replace parts on the wheelchair
	■ Desk-length armrest	■ Allow wheelchair user to approach tables, sinks, desks for improved function ■ Lighter in weight than full-length arm supports	■ May not provide adequate support during transfers ■ Do not provide full arm support
	■ Full-length armrest	■ Provide full arm support ■ Provide improved support during transfers	■ Heavier than desk-length arm ■ Do not allow close approach to tables, sinks, or desks
Wheel locks	■ Pull-to lock	■ Allow closer access for transfers to surfaces ■ Move away from wheels so hands do not hit with propulsion	■ May be more difficult to lock
	■ Push-to lock	■ Lock easily and securely	■ May interfere with propulsion ■ May interfere with transfers
	■ Under-seat or scissor locks	■ Complete clearance for hands during propulsion ■ No interference in transfers	■ Significantly better balance and coordination required for locking and unlocking ■ More difficult to adjust

Head or neck supports are needed for clients who have poor head control or if the wheelchair will be equipped with the ability to tilt or recline. Head and neck rest pads come in a variety of shapes and styles. There are also many hardware attachment options. The type that is prescribed will depend on related functional needs of the client.

Upper extremity support will vary from none to those that provide full support of the forearms and hands of clients who have no active motor control of the upper extremities. Some considerations include the need to have removable armrests to facilitate independent and obstacle-free transfers, adjustable height to assist with different functional activities, and those that can move with the backrest as the wheelchair is reclining. Options, advantages, and disadvantages are presented in Table 16.3.

The Frame

The wheelchair frame is closely integrated with both the seating and mobility systems of the wheelchair. It provides a solid base for the attachment of seating components and facilitates the client's access to the mobility structures. Table 16.4 provides an overview of wheelchair configurations for clients needing long-term, permanent solutions for seating and mobility.

Manual wheelchair frames can be folding or rigid in structure. Folding frame wheelchairs have two side frames attached by a center cross brace to permit folding the chair from side to side. Rigid frame chairs consist of side frames that are welded together to act as a single unit. Rigid frame chairs can be reduced in size for transportation purposes by folding the back onto the seat and removing the rear wheels if the chair is equipped with quick-release axles. Rigid frame wheelchairs are more efficient to propel because they are lighter in weight and none of the propulsion force applied by the user is absorbed by moving parts.

Standard weight manual wheelchairs (such as those used in hospitals) typically have steel frames. They are very durable but also heavy to propel and lift. Lightweight wheelchairs are usually made of aluminum, and ultralight wheelchairs are typically composed of aluminum, titanium, or carbon

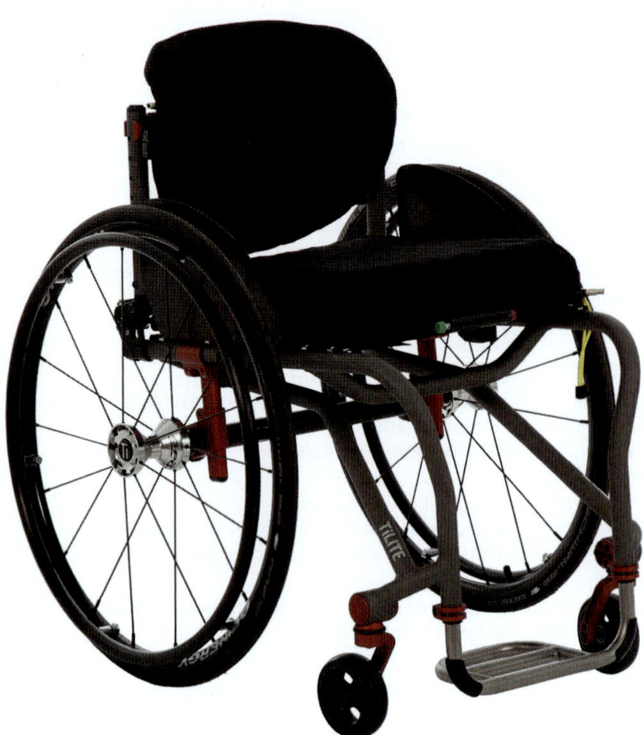

Fig. 16.11 Rigid frame ultralight wheelchair with integrated foot support. (Courtesy Permobil Inc.)

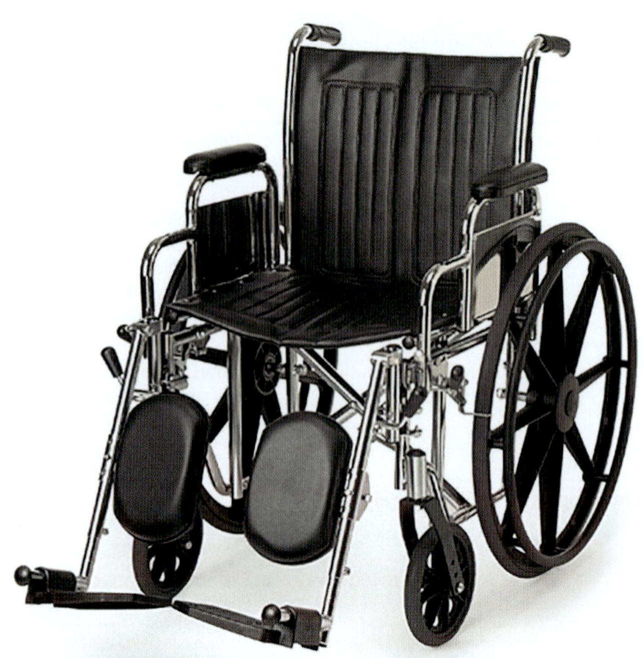

Fig. 16.12 Manual wheelchair with cross-brace folding mechanism. (Courtesy Sunrise Medical, Fresno, California.)

fiber. Aluminum is widely available, easy to weld, and typically less costly, but it can rust and corrode when exposed to the elements. Aluminum provides a stiffer ride, and this can offer some advantage on smooth terrain. Titanium has a very high strength-to-weight ratio, and therefore less material is needed to build a frame. The result is an overall lighter frame that does not corrode and has inherent vibration dampening. Titanium costs more than aluminum, so justification of the medical need to third-party payers can be challenging. Carbon fiber offers many functional advantages to other options because it is extremely light and durable, but it remains cost prohibitive in most cases.

Some manual wheelchair frames offer options, such as adjustable rear axle plates and front caster housings, to move the seating system forward, back, up, or down on the wheel base to increase propulsion efficiency, enhance maneuverability, and reduce the risk of overuse injuries.[33] Some clients will be unable to achieve functional independence with manual wheelchairs regardless of how lightweight or optimally configured, so power wheelchairs must then be considered.

A power wheelchair is composed of a power base over which the seating system is placed. The power base houses the motors, batteries, and software options. Both manual and power wheelchairs can be equipped with special function frames, such as tilt, recline, standing, or elevation. These features require additional medical justification and assist with pressure redistribution, positioning, pain management, physiological functions, comfort, and functional independence.[34,35]

Recliner frames, such as the one shown in Fig. 16.5, permit an increase in the seat-to-back angle. They are typically paired with elevating leg rests to allow the client to assume a full supine position. This can be advantageous for pressure redistribution, self-catheterization, change in hip angle for pain management, and to allow for gravity to assist with positioning. Caution should be used when prescribing recliner frames for clients who have spasticity, as the change in the hip angle can trigger spasms and disrupt overall positioning. Movement to and from sitting can also increase shear forces, which contribute to the development of pressure ulcers.

A tilt frame allows the client to remain in one position because the seat-to-back angle is fixed. Pressure redistribution is accomplished by tilting the upper portion of the frame over the lower portion, as shown in Fig. 16.4. Tilt is often a better option for clients with hypertonicity for the reasons mentioned previously.

Seat elevators are only available on power chairs. They allow the client to raise or lower the seat height relative to the ground, which can increase functional independence in activities such as transfers.

Standing frames, such as the one shown in Fig. 16.6, are available on both manual and power wheelchairs. They are integrated into the base and allow the client to achieve a standing position while being supported by the seat and back of the wheelchair. Standing is associated with many physiological benefits, including tone management, an increase in bone density, facilitation of bowel and bladder regulation, and pressure redistribution. It also provides advantages for environmental access and social participation.

The Mobility System

The mobility structure provides the means of propelling the wheelchair. It is composed of the drive wheels, caster wheels, tires, and client interface component, such as the hand rims on a manual wheelchair or joystick on many

Table 16.4 Wheelchair Configurations for Clients Needing Long-Term, Permanent Solutions

Wheeled Mobility Device	Advantages	Disadvantages	Possible Application
Semiadjustable manual wheelchair (lightweight)	■ Simple to use ■ Folds for transportation ■ Lighter weight than standard wheelchair ■ Partial adjustability ■ Easier to propel ■ Durable ■ Will accommodate custom seating	■ Not custom fit ■ Lack of axle adjustability may limit manual propulsion by user ■ Still may be too heavy for many users	■ Intermittent or temporary use ■ Possible use for in-home applications if environment tolerates
Fully adjustable manual wheelchair with a folding frame (ultra-lightweight)	■ Very light frame ■ Maximal adjustability, especially of rear axle position ■ Custom fit to user ■ Accommodates custom seating ■ Accommodates to uneven ground by flexing ■ Folds side-to side for easy transportation	■ Many adjustable or removable parts ■ More complex design, requires more maintenance ■ Some propulsion energy lost in flex of frame	■ Full-time wheelchair user with permanent disability ■ User wants to transport in trunk of vehicle ■ Environment includes travel over uneven surfaces
Fully adjustable manual wheelchair with a rigid frame (ultra-lightweight)	■ Very light frame ■ Maximal adjustability, especially of rear axle position ■ Custom fit to user ■ Fewer removable or adjustable parts than folding frame ■ Accommodates custom seating	■ Does not accommodate to uneven terrain as easily as folding frame ■ May be more difficult to transport in trunk of car (less compact when folded)	■ Full-time wheelchair user with permanent disability ■ User wants most efficient system for propulsion ■ Used mainly indoors or on even terrains
Power assist manual wheelchair	■ Light frame ■ Maneuvers such as manual wheelchair ■ Minimizes stress on shoulders	■ Heavier than nonpower assist ■ More difficult to disassemble for transport	■ Lightweight manual wheelchair user with limited endurance or shoulder limitations ■ Manual wheelchair user with long-distance ambulation needs or difficulty managing outdoor terrain independently
Tilt-in-space frame wheelchair	■ Allows rotation in space for pressure management or other benefits ■ Available for both manual and powered wheelchairs	■ Frame often heavier and bulkier ■ Usually does not fold for transportation ■ If on manual wheelchair, typically has small rear wheels, requiring an attendant to propel	■ Wheelchair user requires rotation in space for pressure management or other medical reason, such as respiratory disease
Reclining frame wheelchair	■ Allows for change in seat-to-back angle, often to full supine position ■ Available for both manual and powered wheelchairs	■ Frame often heavier and bulkier ■ Rear wheels set further back to provide larger base of support when in recline position ■ Difficult to propel if used with manual wheelchair	■ Used when a need for change in seat to back angle is required ■ Used for pressure management ■ May be used for self-care in wheelchair ■ May be used when supine bed transfers are required ■ Often used when building sitting tolerance during initial rehabilitation
Powered scooter	■ Allows simple-to-learn powered mobility ■ Good outdoor access ■ Swivel seat for ease of transfers ■ Baskets and other accessories for function, such as shopping	■ Only one access method ■ Large turning radius; difficult to use in many homes ■ Does not accommodate custom seating; few seating support options	■ Used with individuals who have limited endurance ■ Often used for primarily outdoor mobility purposes
Powered wheelchair	■ Full access to powered mobility for both indoor and outdoor use ■ Multiple access methods possible ■ Accommodates custom seating supports ■ Accommodates power seating options, such as tilt or recline	■ Heavy ■ Requires van for transportation ■ Less maneuverable than manual wheelchair ■ Requires more initial training for optimal safety and function	■ Individuals who cannot propel manual wheelchair effectively ■ Used for indoor and outdoor mobility for long distances ■ May be used in work or school applications for part-time manual wheelchair users

power wheelchairs. Goals of the mobility system focus on the facilitation of movement within the client's environment and commonly:

1. Provide independent mobility in all environments of interest to the client.
2. Provide speed and agility that equals or exceeds gross motor abilities of "typically functioning" age-related peers.
3. Maximize participation in all MR-ADLs.
4. Minimize energy expenditure and prevent injury through ergonomically sound design.

Selection of the client's most reliable source of motor control is key to prescribing the most appropriate mobility system.[4] The access method can be entirely manual, entirely power, or manual with power assistance. Table 16.5 summarizes the indications, advantages, and disadvantages of the various wheeled technologies.

MANUAL WHEELCHAIRS

Manual wheelchairs typically have two sets of wheels. The two large wheels range in size from 20″ to 26″ and are located in the rear. Two smaller caster wheels can range from 3″ to 8″. They are connected to the front of the

Table 16.5 Mobility Options: Considerations, Common Problems, and Possible Solutions

Propulsion Type	Indications	Considerations	Common Problems	Possible Solution(s)
Manual wheelchair: bilateral upper extremity (UE)	Clients who have adequate UE strength to achieve functional mobility (speed, distance, endurance)	■ Weight of chair ■ Adjustability to optimize positioning and UE alignment for propulsion ■ Availability of accessories needed, including appropriate wheel/caster sizes, tires, footrests, etc. to fit environmental and lifestyle needs	Physical: ■ Shoulder and wrist pain ■ Excessive shoulder abduction ■ Short propulsion stroke Equipment: ■ Inadequate seating system ■ Seat too wide ■ Seat too high ■ Rear axle position too far back ■ Wheelchair tipping backward on inclines	■ Lightweight frame and accessories to decrease strain ■ Narrower wheelchair to optimize UE to push rim alignment ■ Upright postural alignment with appropriate seating system ■ Align seating system to achieve elbow flexion of 100–120 degrees when hands are at the top of the push rims ■ Rear axle in line with or anterior to center of shoulder joint ■ Education for proper propulsion ■ technique to decreased coefficient of drag on push rim ■ Consider use of antitippers during training phase
Manual wheelchair: unilateral upper and lower extremity	Hemiplegia	■ Rear wheel alignment for UE propulsion ■ Low seat to allow LE propulsion	Physical: ■ Posterior pelvic tilt ■ Short propulsion strokes on rear wheel ■ Inadequate heel → toe progression during propulsion Equipment: ■ Casters interfering with feet ■ Nonfunctional thigh not fully supported due to height of footrest to allow for ground clearance ■ Footrest supporting nonfunctional LE bottoms out on ramps	■ Pelvic belt and/or shorter seat depth to prevent posterior pelvic tilt during foot propulsion ■ Top of cushion to floor measurement less than or equal to patient measurement of popliteal fossa to bottom of foot ■ Optimize seat width and axle position for UE propulsion ■ Split seat to allow for hip flexion, increased thigh support, and more clearance for footrest on side of impairment ■ 6″ or smaller caster to increase clearance for foot propulsion
Manual wheelchair: unilateral UE (one arm drive)	Impaired motor control in all but one UE	■ Requires larger hand to grasp and propel two rims on stronger side ■ Added weight to frame and additional step for folding ■ High risk for overuse syndrome	Physical: ■ Shoulder and wrist pain ■ Difficulty maneuvering chair on all surfaces and tight spaces	■ Consider power options
Power assist wheels	Manual wheelchair user with shoulder painImpaired shoulder or hand function	■ Increased weight of each wheel increases difficulty when folding or propelling in fully manual mode ■ Allows for mobility over a variety of terrain with less strain to shoulder/wrist joints ■ Requires additional maintenance ■ Increased overall width of chair to accommodate power components in axles	Physical: Increased shoulder pain experienced when loading wheelchair into vehicle	■ Consider wheelchair van ■ Second set of lightweight rear wheels to use as a backup
Power wheelchair: joystick controller	Unable to propel manual wheelchair but has consistent and reliable volitional control capable of activating a joystick	■ Environmental access—requires ramps and elevators ■ Increased maintenance requirements over manual ■ Permits independence for clients who cannot propel manual wheelchairs ■ Limited options for community transportation ■ Proportional control of the wheelchair is possible	Equipment: ■ Joystick in the way of transfers and pulling up to tables Physical: ■ Difficulty with control when ataxia is present	■ Consider swing-away hardware for obstacle-free transfers ■ Adjust wheelchair programming to decrease responsiveness to involuntary movements ■ Consider manual wheelchair as a backup

Table 16.5 Mobility Options: Considerations, Common Problems, and Possible Solutions—Cont'd

Propulsion Type	Indications	Considerations	Common Problems	Possible Solution(s)
Power wheelchair: sip and puff	No reliable motor control of upper or lower extremities	■ Requires increased training/ maintenance ■ Oral motor control is needed ■ Nonproportional control so minimal option to vary speed "on the fly" ■ Difficulty conversing when driving the chair ■ Additional steps in activation needed to access power seat functions	Equipment: Difficulty tracking on uneven ground Physical: ■ Disruption of seated position can cause client to lose access to controller ■ Client fatigue	■ Consider specialized path correction system ■ Provide secondary emergency shutoff system ("kill switch") to avoid accidents ■ Modify drive parameters to fine tune driving ■ Train client and caregivers in the use of positional markers to increase reliable access to controller ■ Chest strap and pelvic belt to ensure proper alignment ■ Attendant control as a backup ■ Manual wheelchair as backup
Power wheelchair: head array system	Availability of reliable head/ neck control	■ Requires increased training, set up and maintenance ■ Nonproportional control so cannot vary speed "on the fly" ■ Additional steps in activation needed to access power seat functions	Equipment: ■ Difficulty tracking on uneven ground ■ Equipment malfunction with greater number of more intricate parts Physical: ■ Hairstyle and head wear can impact proximity switches ■ Neck pain and fatigue	■ Consider specialized path correction system ■ Modify drive parameters to fine tune driving ■ Chest strap and pelvic belt to maintain proximity to switches ■ Optional attendant control ■ Shorter hairstyle/low ponytail/no hats ■ Manual wheelchair as a backup

wheelchair frame by caster housings. Casters swivel to permit steering and maneuverability of the chair. Rear wheels are composed of tires mounted on rims that are connected to their hubs by metal spokes (called *spoked wheels*) or synthetic spokes (called *mag wheels*). Push rims (sometimes called *hand rims*) are attached to the outside of the wheels. They are slightly smaller in diameter than the wheels and are the access point for propulsion and maneuverability.

Factors to consider when selecting the most appropriate wheels include weight and the environment in which they will most often be used. Spoked wheels are lighter but require more maintenance and are not well suited for moist environments. Mag wheels require little maintenance but add weight to the wheelchair, and performance may be affected by extreme temperatures.

Standard wheelchairs offer few options in the selection of wheel size or configuration. Most are equipped with 24″ rear wheels and 8″ front casters. Higher cost models, including lightweight and ultra-lightweight wheelchairs, can be equipped with different sized wheels and casters, as well as adjustable rear axle and caster housings. These features permit the adjustment of the client's orientation in space to improve alignment for positioning or propulsion efficiency. The degree to which these features can be adjusted depends on the wheelchair frame. Figs. 16.12 and 16.13 illustrate the differences between the standard and ultralight options for adjustability.

Adjustable rear axle and caster housings are important for clients who use wheelchairs on a full-time basis, because they are at a higher risk of developing overuse injuries with associated pain and loss of function from repetitive movements.[21,36,37] The two main areas of focus are the shoulders (e.g., rotator cuff tears) and wrists (e.g., carpal tunnel syndrome).[38]

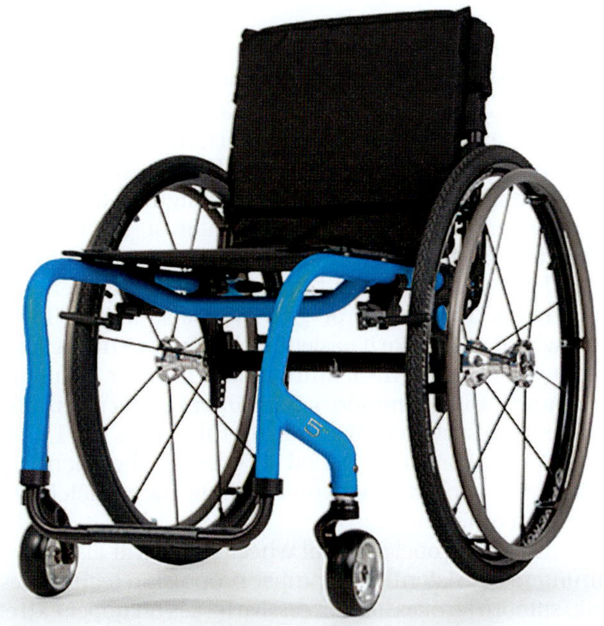

Fig. 16.13 Ultralight wheelchair with rigid frame. (Courtesy Sunrise Medical, Fresno, California.)

Ease of bilateral upper extremity manual wheelchair propulsion is maximized when the wheelchair is as light and as small as possible and the client's weight is distributed rearward (with the seat moved back in relation to the rear wheels) to decrease rolling resistance.[39] Research has determined that the optimal upper extremity to push rim position allows for 100 to 120 degrees of elbow flexion when the client's hand is resting on the top of the push rim (Fig. 16.14).

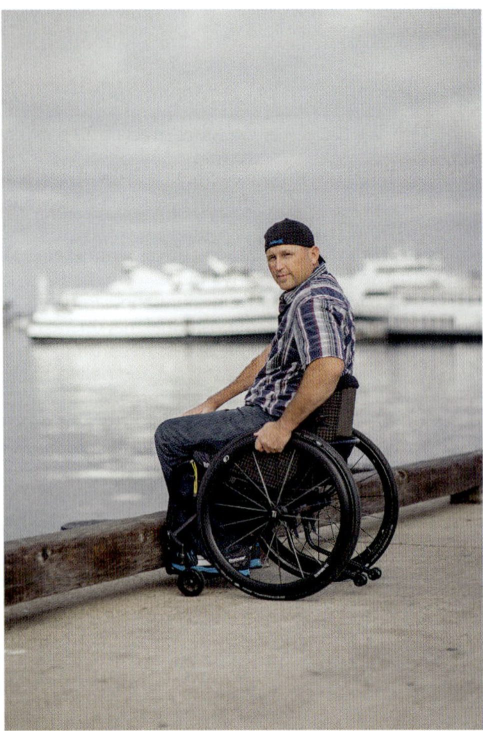

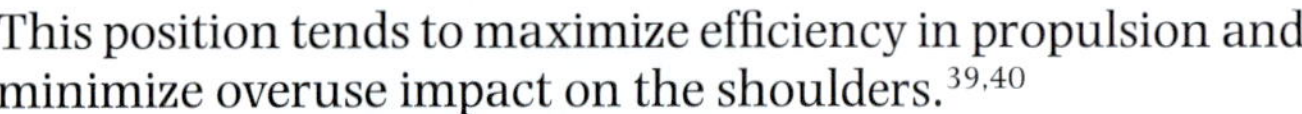

Fig. 16.14 Optimal upper extremity to push rim position for manual wheelchair propulsion. (Courtesy Permobil Inc.)

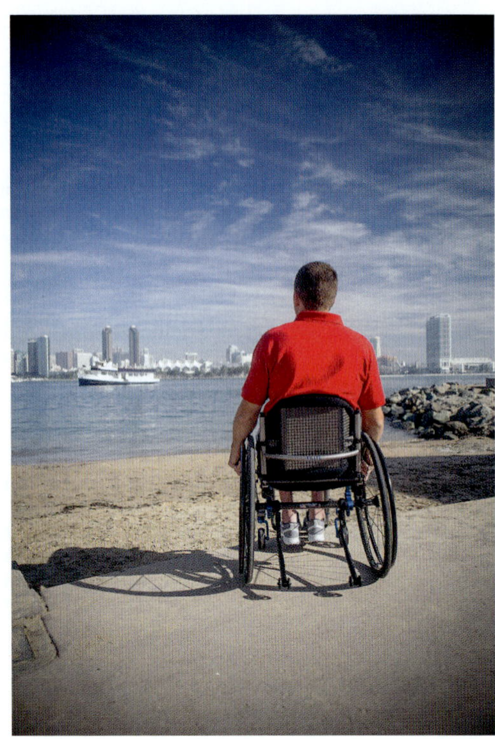

Fig. 16.15 Anti-tip tubes with wheels. (Courtesy Permobil Inc.)

This position tends to maximize efficiency in propulsion and minimize overuse impact on the shoulders.[39,40]

Wheelchair propulsion biomechanics, wheelchair configuration, and training are all important considerations in the prevention of injuries. Clients will need training to effectively manage wheelchairs that are configured to maximize propulsion efficiency. The client's center of gravity will be shifted to a position that is lower than what it would be in a standard wheelchair, and this may make transfers more challenging. The center of gravity is also shifted further back, which will make it easier for the chair to tip backward (into a "wheelie"). This feature makes it easier to navigate curbs and other common environmental barriers, but it may be necessary to utilize anti-tip tubes (Fig. 16.15) during the initial training period to prevent the client from tipping over backward when propelling the wheelchair up ramps and other inclines.

Clients who propel manual wheelchairs will also require training to consistently use proper propulsion techniques.[41] Long, smooth strokes limit excessive forces on upper extremity joints and decrease the rate of loading on the push rims. In contrast, short, choppy pushes are associated with higher energy expenditure and the development of repetitive use syndromes. Allowing the hands to drop below the rims during the "recovery" (nonpropulsion) phase of the stroke aids in smooth motion and protects the shoulders from injury.[39]

Clients who do not have functional use of both upper extremities can use other propulsion techniques.[42] Those with hemiplegia typically use one upper and lower extremity to achieve functional manual wheelchair propulsion. The stronger upper extremity manages the push rim on the rear wheel for propulsion in tandem with the lower extremity, which also manages directional control and variations in speed and acceleration. Clients who lack reliable motor control in both upper extremities may propel their wheelchairs with their feet, bypassing the use of the push rims altogether. Lower extremity propulsion mandates careful prescription of the seat height to achieve optimal heel-toe progression, and this typically requires smaller rear wheels and casters, as well as adjustable axle plates and caster housings.

Clients who have functional use of only one upper extremity *may* be able to propel manual wheelchairs with one arm drive or lever drive systems.[43] These options connect the axles of both drive wheels (either with a dual push rim or a lever system) so that the client can control both wheels and have effective directional control from one side of the chair. This method is very taxing, however, and can only be used for short distances. A power wheelchair option is typically a better solution.

Power assist wheels may be an alternative for some clients who are at high risk for overuse injuries but are not quite ready to consider the accessibility challenges associated with power wheelchairs.[44] Power assist wheels are interchangeable with the rear wheels on manual wheelchairs, and this is easily accomplished on chairs equipped with quick-release axles. The difference between a manual rear wheel and a power assist rear wheel is the presence of batteries and motors within the hubs of the wheels. The client propels power assist wheels with the push rims in the same way, but the physical effort is boosted by the power assist motors, making it possible to travel longer distances and/or travel over more challenging terrains with less risk of repetitive strain injuries. Power assist wheels are heavier than standard wheels, so it is more difficult to remove them if folding the wheelchair for car transport. It is also challenging to propel or have a caregiver push the wheelchair if the power assist wheels are broken. However, clients may easily interchange them with nonmotorized wheels when power assist wheels need maintenance or repair.

POWER WHEELCHAIRS

One of the most important decisions for any client is that of manual versus power mobility. Both mobility systems have advantages and disadvantages, and overall function is greatly affected by this decision. Conditions and impairments that often indicate the need for power mobility include the following:

1. Severe upper extremity or upper trunk weakness leading to an inability to propel any type of manual wheelchair
2. Ataxic or uncoordinated movement of the upper extremities
3. Endurance limitations, whether from neuromuscular or cardiopulmonary impairment
4. Progressive conditions that will likely lead to loss of upper extremity strength or poor endurance (e.g., amyotrophic lateral sclerosis or multiple sclerosis)
5. Orthopedic problems in the upper extremity joints (e.g., arthritis or preexisting rotator cuff or carpal tunnel impairments)
6. Environments that require long-distance travel on a regular basis or travel over rough terrain

Once a determination has been made that power mobility is necessary, one of the next decisions is the access method for control of the device.[45]

Scooters are the least complicated versions of power mobility devices. Propulsion is activated by the client through a tiller that is directly connected to the front wheel of the device. Scooters are typically only appropriate for clients who require minimal assistance with positioning and travel on very limited terrains, including indoor surfaces and smoother outdoor surfaces.

Power wheelchairs can be equipped with mid-wheel drive (Fig. 16.16), front wheel drive (Fig. 16.17), or rear wheel drive (Fig. 16.18). The drive wheels are connected to the motors that control the speed and acceleration of the wheelchair in response to a joystick or other client access method, including switch arrays, sip and puff, and head-controlled devices, among others. These options make it likely that even clients with significant impairments and functional limitations can achieve independent mobility. For example, clients who have Duchene muscular dystrophy tend to lose gross motor control while retaining fine motor control of the fingers. A joystick can be programmed to respond to the smallest joystick excursions to achieve full speed of the wheelchair. Other motor impairments can be accommodated, such as the need to ignore extraneous movements caused by tremors or muscle spasms.[46,47]

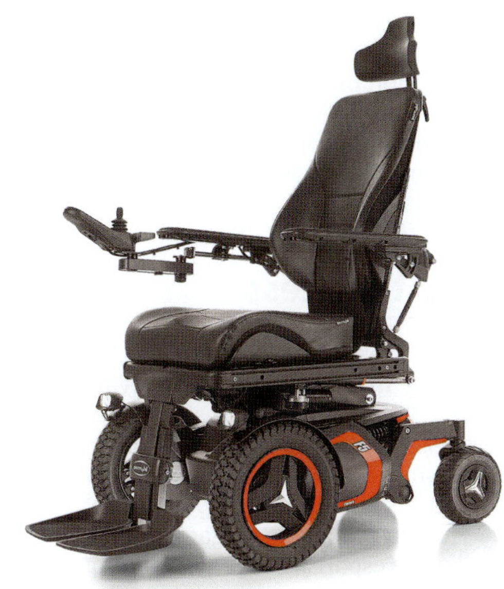

Fig. 16.17 **Front wheel drive power wheelchair.** (Courtesy Permobil Inc.)

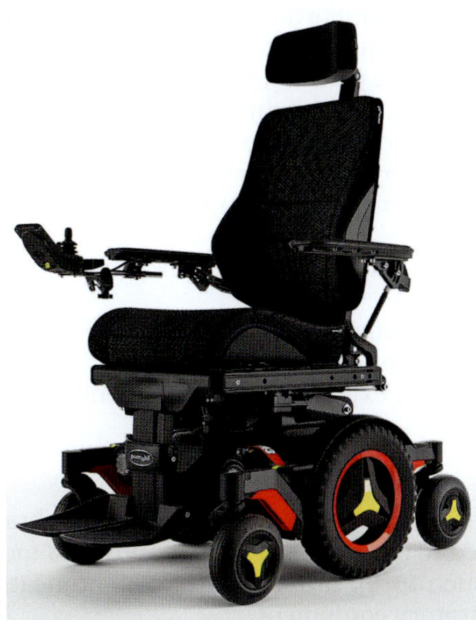

Fig. 16.16 **Mid-wheel drive power wheelchair.** (Courtesy Permobil Inc.)

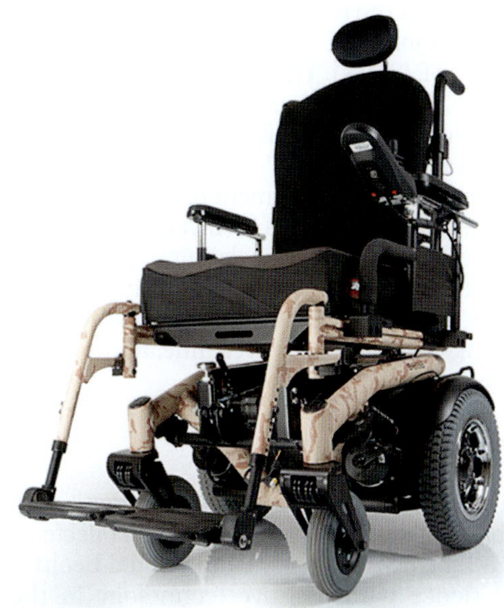

Fig. 16.18 **Rear wheel drive power wheelchair.** (Courtesy Sunrise Medical, Fresno, California.)

Assessment for the appropriate method of access depends first on achieving the best seating solutions to optimize any available source of reliable motor control. Some input methods, such as sip and puff and head control systems, require longer training periods. A thorough evaluation with multiple episodes of training may be required before the best access method is selected.

Special care is needed for the prescription of power wheelchairs. Clinicians must be able to provide adjustments in many of the drive parameters, including but not limited to speed, acceleration, starting and stopping, turning and changing directions, locking, unlocking, and free-wheeling.

Regardless of the type of wheelchair that is being recommended, a detailed client assessment is needed to identify which options are appropriate for each client. Clients with significant impairments and functional limitations will benefit from the experience of specially trained clinicians who work with complex rehabilitation technology on a regular basis. Errors in prescription or ordering will come at great costs to the client, not only in dollars but in overall functional potential. Less experienced clinicians are encouraged to refer clients to wheelchair clinics for recommendations and prescriptions.

The Seating and Mobility Assessment Process

The seating and mobility assessment is a highly complex process involving multiple component evaluations, tests, and measures.[21] The client's needs should be considered in the broadest possible context. This will ensure appropriate recommendations, provide meaningful outcome measures, and justify requests for third-party payment.[48–50]

Specially trained clinicians, organized in a team structure, are usually responsible for performing seating and mobility assessments. The team may include a physical therapist, occupational therapist, speech-language pathologist, a physician, a rehabilitation technology supplier, and other professionals identified as important by the client. It is particularly helpful if one or more of the rehabilitation professionals and the rehabilitation technology supplier are Assistive Technology Professionals/Seating and Mobility Specialists (ATP/SMSs). These two credentials are provided by the Rehabilitation Engineering and Assistive Technology Society of North America (RESNA) to recognize expertise in wheelchair prescription.[51] Some third-party payers will not consider requests for payment of certain types of wheelchairs unless an ATP/SMS is involved in the recommendation and delivery of the wheelchair.[52] The team engages in assessment, prescription, and training. All aspects of the process must be carefully documented to ensure funding, tracking of client needs over time, and accuracy of the medical record.

SUBJECTIVE/HISTORY

A detailed history is an essential component of a seating and mobility assessment. Information collected typically includes all medical diagnoses and related health information, experience with assistive technology in the past, a description of the client's usual daily activities, the home and other environments in which the equipment will be used, transportation needs of the client, and details about potential funding sources. The information collected will help the team establish goals and interventions and often translates into the best justification for any recommendations.

DIAGNOSES AND RELATED HEALTH INFORMATION

All diagnoses and related impairments and limitations are relevant to the assessment process. First, determine if the client relies solely on a wheelchair for mobility or if some ambulation potential exists (with or without assistive devices). Third-party payment may be in jeopardy if the team fails to establish a clear justification of need for the seating and mobility systems. It is important to know the dates of onset of the client's diagnoses and whether impairments are static or progressive in nature.

Information about associated health concerns is also important. Note the presence of difficulties with breathing, cardiovascular or circulatory problems, seizure disorders, bowel and bladder incontinence, nutrition and digestion, medications and side effects, previous or planned surgeries, orthopedic concerns such as subluxation or dislocation of the hip or shoulder, osteoporosis, other orthotic interventions (including leg, foot, or trunk orthoses), history of pressure ulcers or other skin conditions, sensation, pain, visual deficits, hearing deficits, and cognitive and behavioral problems.[53] Diagnostic information and related health concerns have a direct impact on the selection of seating and mobility components, as well as approval of insurance coverage of prescribed equipment.

PRIOR EXPERIENCE WITH ASSISTIVE TECHNOLOGY

It is helpful to fully understand the client's experiences with assistive technology. Some clients will be referred for assessment of need for a first wheelchair, but others will have important experiences that need specific exploration. The age, make, and model of any devices currently in use should be recorded, along with the sizes of all items and their present condition. It is important to note the client's posture and function while using this equipment and to determine and document why the person has been referred for assessment. Helpful considerations might include the following:

1. Did the client outgrow the equipment?
2. Did the equipment meet or exceed its expected life span?
3. Has there been a change in medical condition or functional status?
4. What does the client like/dislike about the current equipment?
5. How is the current equipment used, and is that use appropriate and effective?
6. What, if any, experience has the client had with other equipment?
7. What are the client's goals for any modifications or new seating or mobility devices?
8. Does the client use any other assistive technology that will need to interface with the seating and mobility systems, such as an augmentative communication device or respiratory equipment?

MOBILITY-RELATED ACTIVITIES OF DAILY LIVING

The client's home environment or other environments in which the equipment will be used must be understood, including those accessed for school, work, or recreation.[21] Ask the client to describe typical activities of daily living that will involve the use of the wheelchair, including methods of transfer, optimal height of the wheelchair seat for transfers to other surfaces, and techniques used to accomplish self-care, vocational, and avocational activities.

Information about the mode of community transportation (e.g., car, adapted van, public transportation, school-provided transportation) is important to ensure that the new seating and mobility systems will be compatible with what is still in use. Even small differences in the size and configuration of new devices can create problems. Consider van tie-down systems and the clearance available if the client enters a van using an automatic lift. It is better to anticipate these needs than to discover them once a new wheelchair is delivered.

FUNDING SOURCES

Most clients will seek third-party payment for seating and mobility systems. Prescribers will need to be familiar with the rules and regulations of potential payers from the start of the prescription process to ensure that any necessary documentation is targeted to the requirements of the funding agency. The most common payers are Medicare (federal insurance), Medicaid (state insurance), and private health insurance companies. Some clients may be eligible for benefits from the Veteran's Administration if the need for a wheelchair is related to illnesses or injuries that resulted from service in the armed forces. Medicare and Medicaid are government agencies that are regulated by the Centers for Medicare and Medicaid (CMS). Federal regulations that affect Medicare change periodically in response to policy changes, and states have some flexibility to alter Medicaid rules beyond those established by CMS. Clinicians can rely on their rehabilitation technology suppliers to keep them up-to-date about coverage trends.

PHYSICAL EXAMINATION AND ASSOCIATED CONSIDERATIONS

The physical examination begins with observation of the client as he or she enters the clinic. Make note of any postural deviations, difficulties with wheelchair propulsion, overall movement quality, and evidence of discomfort. Information gleaned from the subjective assessment helps the team to hone in on potential areas of concern, even those that go beyond the scope of the seating and mobility assessment team. For example, the history of pressure ulcers will need to be addressed with the prescription of an appropriate seating system and a means to achieve intermittent pressure relief, but it also may be appropriate to refer the client to other health professionals for counseling on nutrition, bowel and bladder management, or other medical issues.

A gross assessment can be made by conducting a review of major systems, including a quick screen of the functions associated with cardiovascular, pulmonary, integumentary, musculoskeletal, neuromuscular systems, as well as the communication and cognitive abilities of the individual.[54]

Components of the cardiovascular and pulmonary assessments include determination of blood pressure, heart rate, pulse oximetry, respiratory rate, and edema. Skin condition must be assessed, particularly those areas of the body that are prone to pressure buildup within the seating system. Direct observation of any affected areas is essential.

Gross assessment of musculoskeletal and neuromuscular status includes a quick screen of available range of motion in all major joints and recording of the client's height and weight. The client's ability to propel and other aspects of wheelchair management provides general information about the neuromuscular system. Cognitive function and the client's ability to communicate can be observed while collecting information throughout the assessment process.

TESTS AND MEASURES USED IN SEATING AND MOBILITY ASSESSMENTS

The gross review of systems helps determine anything that requires more comprehensive assessment with specific tests and measures. The examination should take place with the client in different positions, including assessment of postural alignment in the current wheelchair, sitting and supine on a mat, and simulation of any proposed interventions.

Many tests and measures are used during the seating and wheeled mobility examination process. Some are necessary for all clients, and others are used only in particular instances and are determined based on the client's presenting symptoms. See Table 16.1 for common symptoms encountered during seating assessments. The table is arranged according to body segments (beginning with the pelvis) and presents possible physical and equipment causes for presenting symptoms, as well as examination procedures that can be used to identify underlying causes.

Many of the tests and measures used are incorporated into the mat evaluation, with observation of the client in seated and supine positions. The team assesses the following with the client seated on the edge of the mat: postural asymmetries, sitting balance, available range of motion in the spine and pelvis, functional abilities (e.g., transfers and reaching), and the influence of abnormal muscle tone and reflex activity on posture and function.

Results obtained in sitting are compared with those discovered in the supine mat evaluation. This position is often used for measuring specific joint range of motion, strength, coordination, and the influence of abnormal muscle tone and reflexes (and how this differs in supine compared with sitting). Attention must be paid to isolated hip joint mobility; orthopedic deformities such as pelvic asymmetries, hip joint subluxations or dislocations; and flexibility of the spine and pelvic regions.[21]

Examination in both supine and sitting positions offers an important means to assess the flexibility of postural deformities. Gravitational pull on the body influences postural reactions differently in each position. Postural deformities that are present during the sitting assessment but disappear in the supine mat evaluation can be considered flexible and may be correctible in the seating system. In contrast, postural asymmetries that are present in sitting and remain unchanged in supine should be considered fixed. Attempts to correct them in the seating system will result in pain and/or soft-tissue injury.

Simulation techniques are helpful.[53] Hand simulation is often performed with the client seated on the mat. The therapist uses his or her hands to mimic forces that can be applied by components of the seating system. This technique helps the therapist determine if external supports will provide the desired effect on the client's posture, how much force is required, and the optimal location and direction of the force that needs to be applied.[21]

A seating simulator offers a means to verify the results of the hand simulation. This device is a highly adjustable wheelchair frame with many interchangeable components.[55] It is first preset to provide the desired supports; then the client sits in it so the therapist can determine if the settings produce the desired postural and functional outcomes.

The third simulation method involves the use of commercially available seating and mobility products that offer a close approximation of those that are being considered by the team. This approach provides the advantage of testing the actual components that may be prescribed to determine their effectiveness in meeting the established goals and helpful evidence to support funding requests made to third-party payers.

A variety of more specialized tests and measures may be indicated for some clients. These include pressure mapping (Fig. 16.19),[56] custom-contour seat simulation, pulse oximetry and other circulatory assessments during simulation, and functional wheelchair propulsion testing.[57] These specific measures are generally not appropriate for all seating and mobility assessments but can be mixed and matched according to the needs of the client. All these tests and measures provide the therapist with the necessary information required for the evaluation and determination of final equipment selections.

Examination findings should be organized according to body segment for easy translation into necessary interventions. Table 16.1 details the desired seated posture for each body segment, common deviations and associated symptoms, possible physical and equipment causes, and the examination procedures that should be used to determine the underlying cause of deviations. Specific information about neuromuscular, musculoskeletal, cardiopulmonary, and integumentary status is collected using standardized tests and measures as the client progresses through the examination process. It is helpful to decide which tests and measures can be performed in each position (sitting in the existing equipment, sitting on the edge of the mat, and laying supine) to minimize the need to have the client change positions.

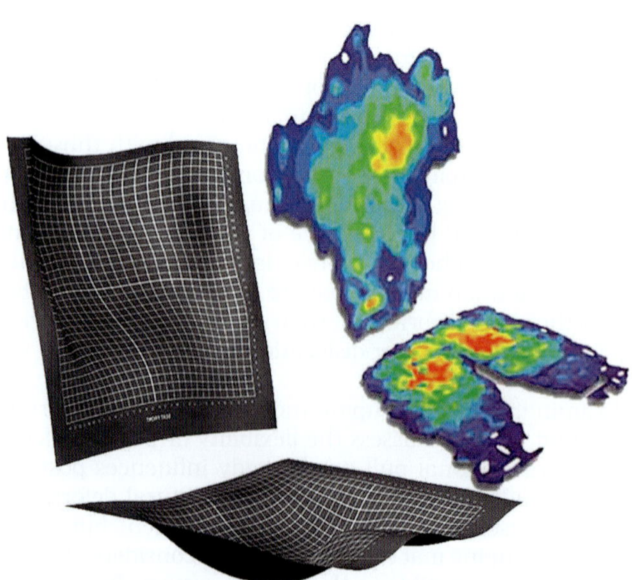

Fig. 16.19 Image of CONFORMat. (Courtesy Tekscan, Inc., South Boston, Massachusetts.)

Neuromuscular

Evaluators should make note of any weakness, incoordination, influence of abnormal muscle tone causing asymmetries, and/or hyperflexed or hyperextended posturing causing variations from the optimal postural alignment in sitting. It is important to compare seated postures in current equipment to seated postures on the mat, because inappropriate equipment may be a contributing cause to presenting problems. The results of the neuromuscular assessment are an important factor in identifying an appropriate intervention. For example, asymmetrical muscle tone in the trunk can cause lateral trunk flexion and ultimately scoliosis if left unchecked. The use of carefully placed lateral trunk supports in combination with a tilt-in space frame may inhibit the reflex activity responsible and help to keep the client aligned after intermittent spasms. It is important to note whether neuromuscular conditions are static or progressive, because seating and mobility systems designed for individuals with progressive disorders will need to be easily modified to meet the client's needs over the expected life of the wheelchair, which is typically 3 to 5 years.

Musculoskeletal

The musculoskeletal assessment will reveal the need to correct or accommodate postural deformities. Every attempt should be made to correct flexible postural problems to prevent them from becoming fixed problems. For example, the common postural deviations caused by a flexible posterior pelvic tilt can often be corrected by providing three carefully placed external forces to maintain the pelvis in neutral alignment. Clients who present with fixed postural deformities will need accommodation to envelope and protect any rigid bony prominences and distribute weight-bearing forces to prevent discomfort and soft-tissue injury.

Cardiopulmonary

Some clients will present with impairments and limitations in the cardiovascular system, which may translate into the need to provide extra soft-tissue protection if the client has vascular problems that limit the ability to heal. More commonly, cardiopulmonary impairments limit endurance and may indicate the need for a power wheelchair for functional mobility, even when upper extremity function may be adequate to propel a manual wheelchair.

Integumentary

Any existing problems with the integumentary system should be addressed by making accommodations to protect areas of existing skin or soft-tissue injury to minimize the risk of future damage. This is accomplished by prescription of a cushion that is capable of offloading any areas of the body that have a history of skin breakdown and distributing all seating pressures across the largest possible surface area of more pressure-tolerant body parts.[20,21]

Comorbidities

Many clients who rely on the permanent use of a wheelchair for seating and mobility will present with impairments and limitations of more than one system. Interventions then may require a careful risk/benefit analysis about how much correction, accommodation, and compensation is needed. For example, a client with significant musculoskeletal deformities, paralysis, and abnormal muscle tone will present with many challenges that must be addressed. It will be important to balance multiple needs to optimize outcomes of function, comfort, skin protection, and other factors identified as important by the client.

The data collected during the examination process is matched to commercially available seating and mobility components to develop a seating system that corrects or accommodates postural problems identified, a wheelchair frame that can provide the desired body-in-space positioning, and a mobility system capable of providing the client with a safe and efficient means of locomotion in all environments of interest.

Ordering the Wheelchair

Inadequate support or improper fit of the wheelchair can lead to a variety of problems for both seating and mobility, so even those clients who require a wheelchair on a temporary or part-time basis should be prescribed a wheelchair that fits properly and provides a minimally supportive seat and back to avoid injury or secondary impairments. Manufacturers of standard wheelchairs provide guidelines for measuring clients and their environments of intended use to ensure the best fit possible. See Table 16.6 for standard wheelchair dimensions and Table 16.3 for accessories that can be used to personalize the wheelchair to help meet the client's individual and environmental needs.

Clients who require full-time, permanent use of a wheelchair will require more than basic fit and support to address impairments and limitations and should be referred to a team of specialists at a wheelchair clinic as previously discussed.[50] All members of the team help to generate the plan of care, specific interventions, and a comprehensive wheelchair prescription that will meet all needs identified through the evaluation process. Each team member plays a vital role in helping ensure the best outcome through service coordination, ongoing communication with all parties involved, and clear documentation of the process.

The physical or occupational therapist typically assumes the role of lead coordinator of the process. He or she helps to ensure that the prescription moves through all required steps so the client can receive the equipment in a timely manner. The therapist works closely with the rehabilitation technology supplier to identify specific manufacturers' products to meet the client's goals and needs identified in the assessment process. The therapist incorporates those details into a letter of medical necessity. This document is the key to obtaining approval of third-party payment.

The letter of medical necessity must be clear, concise, and comprehensive, as well as consistent with the guidelines for coverage specified by the funding source. The purpose of this letter is to provide a clear picture of the client and the equipment being recommended. This letter must contain several elements.

The introductory paragraph should describe the client in detail, including the diagnoses and associated limitations and impairments, onset dates, prognosis, a summary of the history and the systems review, as well as the reason for any unusual requests. For example, most wheelchairs are expected to last a minimum of 3 to 5 years. Requests to pay for new equipment within that timeframe must be accompanied by a convincing argument as to why the replacement is needed.

Next, detailed information is provided about the specific tests and measures used during the examination and outcomes of the evaluation. These include, but are not limited to, the individual's functional status, strength, range of motion, musculoskeletal deformities, neuromuscular status, abnormal muscle tone or reflex findings, and the results of the simulation processes. This information can be organized and reported on a standardized form or in a narrative style.

The seating and mobility assessment will have revealed problems associated with the musculoskeletal, neuromuscular, integumentary, and cardiopulmonary systems. It is important for the therapist to document the relationship between the impairments and limitations identified and the seating and mobility interventions that are being recommended to justify the medical need for each component of the seating and mobility system. Each part of the system must be specified and accompanied by medical and/or functional justification to support the selection. Third-party payers may also require an explanation about why lower cost options were not effective for the client.

Finally, a summary of the client information and contact information for the primary therapist and the prescribing physician should be provided so that the funding source may contact these individuals if any questions arise during

Table 16.6 Standard Wheelchair Configurations for Clients Needing Short-Term, Temporary Solutions

Frame	Seat Size	Seat to Floor	Back Height	Seat and Back	Armrests Styles	Footrest
Adult sizes	16–22″ wide (in 2″ increments) by 16 or 18″ deep	19 ¾″	16 ½″	Sling-style upholstery	■ Fixed full or desk length ■ Removable full or desk length	■ Fixed with flip-up footplates ■ Swing-away/removable footrests ■ Swing-away/removable elevating leg rests with calf pads
Hemi height	18 × 16 or 16 × 16	17 ½″	16 ½″			

the review process. Meticulous preparation of the letter of medical necessity may mean the difference between efficient funding of the seating and mobility system and a long, drawn-out review process that could delay the delivery of equipment by several months.

The rehabilitation technology supplier assumes primary responsibility for all aspects of the intervention once the letter of medical necessity has been provided. He or she is responsible for submitting the medical documentation to the third-party payer, along with a detailed cost invoice of all parts of the wheelchair being requested. The rehabilitation technology supplier also acts as the conduit for any questions that arise during the review process. Once funding is approved, the rehabilitation technology supplier orders the prescribed equipment (often from several different manufacturers), assembles the equipment according to the specifications prescribed, and notifies the therapist that the seating and mobility system is ready for delivery. The client then returns to the seating clinic for fitting, adjustment, and training. Delivery is a critical element in the intervention process and directly affects the outcomes related to the use of the equipment.

Delivering the Wheelchair

Delivery of equipment may occur several months after the examination and prescription process for all but very basic wheelchair prescriptions. It is important for the therapist to ensure that the status and needs of the client have not changed since the initial seating and mobility assessment. The delivery process includes making necessary adjustments as well as training the client and any caregivers in the use, maintenance, and care of the equipment.[50] Instructions should be provided in multiple formats (i.e., verbal, demonstration, and in writing) and must include review of the owner's manuals provided by the equipment manufacturers. The client should have the opportunity to function in and use the equipment during the delivery process to ensure that the goals established during the examination process have been effectively attained.

Regardless of the type of wheelchair selected or the access method chosen, intensive training of the person using the wheelchair is necessary.[50] Training takes place across settings and over time. Wheelchair skills are typically introduced during inpatient rehabilitation, but training usually continues after discharge until the new client gains independence with advanced skills. Initial training may begin with loaner or temporary equipment used to assess options and designs that will allow optimal mobility before a wheelchair prescription is finalized. Additional training is typically necessary once the permanent wheelchair and associated equipment have been delivered.

Clients who use manual wheelchairs need training in the safe use of equipment, which includes effective management of obstacles in all environments typically accessed (home, community, work, and leisure settings). They need to learn how to perform or direct basic maintenance of the equipment (including cleaning procedures and maintaining moving parts) and know when and whom to contact if something out of the ordinary occurs with the wheelchair.

Clients who use power wheelchairs often require more extensive periods of training to achieve optimal safety, mobility, and function.[45] This training must include management of indoor terrain and obstacles, such as turning in tight spaces, managing door frames and transitions between flooring surfaces, and negotiating other indoor obstacles, such as elevators. Training should also include outdoor terrain, such as ramps, curbs, side slopes, grassy surfaces, gravel surfaces, and safe operation on crowded sidewalks or when crossing streets. If a power seating system is prescribed (e.g., tilt or recline), the client must be educated regarding the proper and safe use of this system, including how often to use it and under what conditions it should (and should not) be used.

Although the assessment and prescription for a wheelchair usually takes place in a specialty clinic, functional training after delivery of the equipment is typically provided by outpatient or home care therapy services. Therapists who are unfamiliar with any aspects of the new equipment or training protocol can obtain assistance from the prescribing clinicians and/or rehabilitation technology supplier.

Follow-Up

The final component of an adaptive seating evaluation is reexamination, also known as follow-up.[50] Periodic reexamination of equipment and client needs is essential to maintain optimal function. Most seating and mobility equipment has a usable life span of 3 to 5 years, but shorter life spans can be expected if the client is particularly active or if the equipment is used in harsh or demanding environments. It is important to establish appointments for reexamination to evaluate whether the client's needs continue to be met by the equipment. It is also important for the client to be prepared to independently assess the need for follow-up with clinicians or the rehabilitation technology supplier. The client is the most knowledgeable person regarding the adequacy of the equipment over time, so it is important to provide the information needed to recognize the need for adjustments, modifications, repairs, and eventual replacement.

State of the Art

The science and art associated with wheelchair prescription is still in its infancy. There is a great deal of interest among clinicians to increase the availability of evidence to support clinical decision-making in the practice of wheelchair seating and mobility.[58,59] Some work has been done to develop and validate outcome measures to facilitate evidence-based practice in this field,[57,60,61] but few randomized controlled clinical trials have been conducted.[58,62,63]

More effort has been focused on the development of national seating and wheelchair standards. RESNA has been actively working toward the development of wheelchair position papers, as cited throughout this chapter. These guides are intended to provide objective information to consumers and clinicians about the safety and performance of wheelchairs. The standards established have provided a platform for research into characteristics of wheelchairs that are most beneficial to consumers and assist with justification for third-party payment of higher-quality products based on ultimate cost-effectiveness.[64,65]

Summary

Wheelchairs are essential aids for daily living for people with mobility impairments. They have the capacity to impact virtually every aspect of life in a positive or negative way, including health, happiness, vocational potential, avocational pursuit, and environmental access. Recommendations must be considered carefully and be as unique as the individual for whom the wheelchair is being prescribed. Even clients who require the most basic wheelchairs deserve careful assessment to ensure proper fit and function over the expected life of the wheelchair. Insurance companies typically cover the cost of a wheelchair every 3 to 5 years, so it is of critical importance to make sound recommendations to ensure client safety, comfort, and function.

References

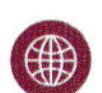

The complete listing of the References are available in the accompanying enhanced eBook version included with the print purchase of this textbook. Visit Elsevier eBooks+ (eBooks.Health.Elsevier.com) to access this content.

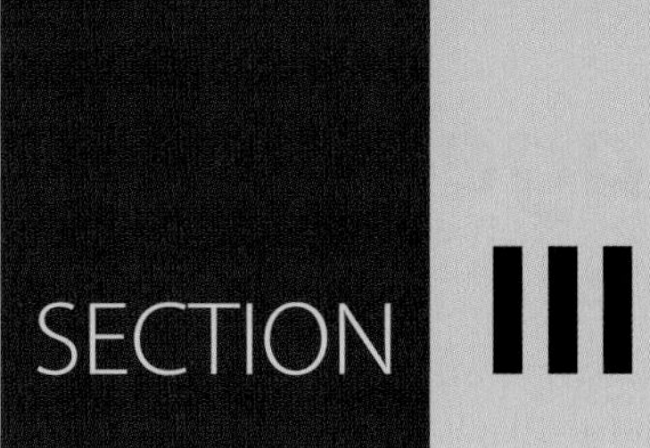

Prostheses in Rehabilitation

17

Etiology and Management of Amputation*

SHENG-CHE YEN, MARIE B. CORKERY, AND KEVIN K. CHUI

LEARNING OBJECTIVES

On completion of this chapter, the reader will be able to do the following:

1. Identify the major causes and epidemiology of limb loss.
2. Discuss major risk factors for dysvascular/neuropathic-related amputation.
3. Discuss major risk factors for trauma-related amputation.
4. Discuss major causes for trauma-related amputation.
5. Discuss major causes for congenital amputation.
6. Describe racial disparities in amputation.
7. Identify key issues considered by the rehabilitation team when they are caring for people with limb loss.

Throughout the history of medicine, amputation has been a relatively frequently performed medical procedure and has often been the only available alternative for complex fractures or infections of the extremities. The earliest amputations were generally undertaken to save lives; however, their outcomes were often unsuccessful—many resulted in death from shock caused by blood loss or the onset of infection and septicemia in those who survived the operation. In these early amputations, removal of the compromised limb segment as quickly as possible was essential. With the advent of antisepsis, asepsis, and anesthesia in the mid-19th century, physicians focused increasingly on the surgical procedure and conservation of tissue.[1] Today, when amputation is necessary, surgery is undertaken with consideration for the functional aspects of the residual limb. This chapter reports on the etiology of amputation or limb loss in the United States. The important factors contributing to the incidence and prevalence of limb loss are presented. An overview of key concerns regarding the rehabilitative process and expected outcomes for persons with limb pathology resulting in limb loss are discussed.

Surveillance data on persons living with limb loss are limited because there is no national database in the United States for compiling data specific to persons with amputation. Information on persons with amputation is derived from a variety of sources including information on hospital discharge diagnoses. The key statistics on limb loss in the United States was summarized by National Limb Loss Resource Center and was presented in an infographic.[2] In brief, there are approximately 2.1 million people living with limb loss, and 185,000 people undergo amputation annually.[3] More amputations occur among males than among females, and amputation rates increase steeply with age.[4] It is estimated that the number of people living with limb loss will increase to 3.6 million by the year 2050, which is more than double that from 2005 (Fig. 17.1).[3]

The majority of amputations are performed in the lower extremity,[3] and more than 150,000 people undergo lower extremity amputations in the United States annually.[5] Jessica Lo et al.[6] reviewed the direct costs related to lower extremity amputation reported in the literature[7-10] and presented these costs in 2019 values. In summary, the total projected lifetime healthcare costs after lower extremity amputation was approximately $878,927; the mean cost of a lower extremity amputation procedure due to peripheral vascular disease was approximately $20,207; the total inpatient cost for adults older than 66 was approximately $32,136; the mean cost per inpatient stay for diabetes-related lower extremity amputation was approximately $24,010. The high costs create a burden on the healthcare system.

Lower extremity amputation is a major cause of functional limitations. In a retrospective study, the 1-year ambulatory rate following a major lower extremity amputation was 46.1%.[11] The limitations in ambulation can have significant impact on patients' ability to return to work. A review article found that the rate of return to work after a lower extremity amputation was approximately 66%.[4] Mackanzie et al. reported that more than 50% of patients were not able to return to work in 84 months after lower extremity amputation.[12] In military service, 42.2% of service members were determined to be fully disabled and not able to return to duty following a transfemoral amputation.[13]

Causes of Amputation

Limb loss occurs for a variety of reasons, and the majority result from a disease process (Fig. 17.2).[4] Most amputations result from vascular conditions and neuropathy, and they are often associated with diabetes. Traumatic loss of a limb is the second most common cause of amputation, followed by cancer and congenital limb deficiencies. This section discusses each of these causes of amputation.

*The author extends appreciation to Dr. Milagros Jorge, whose work in prior editions provided the foundation for this chapter.

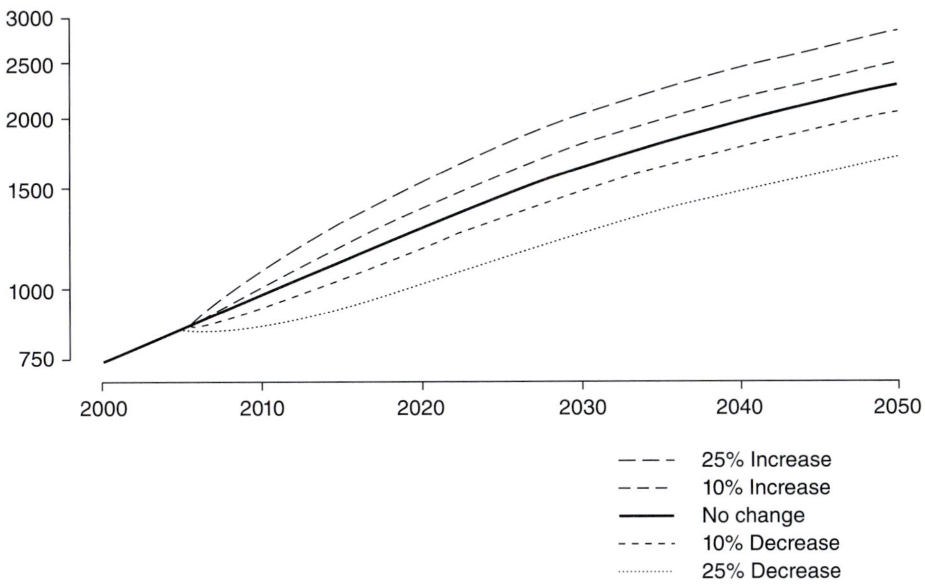

Fig. 17.1 Projected number of Americans living with limb amputation from years 2000 to 2050.[3]

VASCULAR CONDITIONS AND NEUROPATHY

Peripheral Artery Disease and Diabetes

The health condition most frequently related to amputation is peripheral artery disease (PAD) complicated by neuropathy.[14,15] PAD has variable clinical presentations ranging from asymptomatic to intermittent claudication and ischemia. Intermittent claudication is a significant cramping pain, usually in the calf, that is induced by walking or other prolonged muscle contraction and relieved by a short period of rest. Loss of one or more lower extremity pulses is an indication of ischemia. In arteriosclerosis obliterans, at least one major arterial pulse (the dorsalis pedis artery at the ankle, popliteal artery at the knee, or femoral artery in the groin) is often absent or markedly impaired. The prevalence and incidence of PAD are both sharply age related, rising more than 10% among patients in their 60s and 70s. The prevalence of more severe or symptomatic disease seems to be higher among males than among females.[16]

The risk factors of developing PAD include smoking, advanced age, hypertension, hyperlipidemia, and most importantly, diabetes.[16] The "2016 American Heart Association/American College of Cardiology Guideline on the Management of Patients With Lower Extremity Peripheral Artery Disease" states that diabetes is an important risk factor for the development of PAD.[17] The presence of diabetes increases the risk of adverse outcomes among patients with PAD, including progression to chronic limb ischemia and amputation.[18] The number of persons with diabetes in the US population continues to rise. According to the National Diabetes Statistics for 2022, 37.3 million people have diabetes, which accounts for 11.3% of the US population.[19]

Diabetic foot ulceration is a common complication of diabetes mellitus that often results in lower extremity amputation.[20] Elevated blood sugars associated with diabetes damage blood vessels and nerve fibers and impair

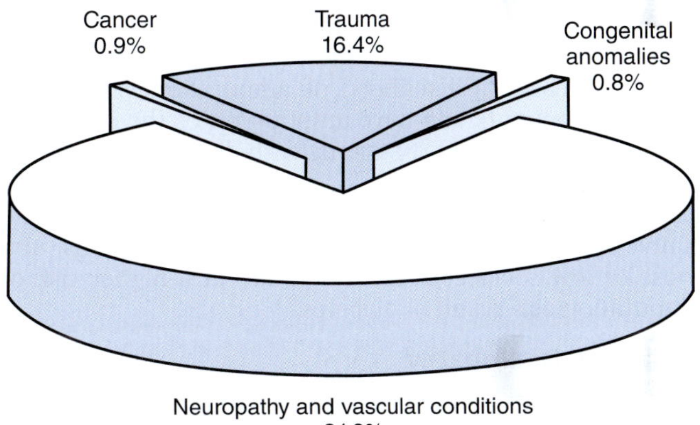

Fig. 17.2 Causes of amputation in percent. The majority of amputations result from a disease process.[4]

circulation. Nerve damage causes peripheral neuropathy, a condition of loss of sensation to the feet. The loss of protective sensation in the feet would not alert an individual to foreign substances in their shoes, such as pebbles or gravel. This lack of awareness can lead to blisters or other minor injuries. Once the skin is broken, sores on the feet may not heal because of poor circulation. The damaged tissues are eventually required to be removed through amputation. In addition to foot ulceration, other clinical factors that contribute to lower limb amputation in persons with diabetes include lower extremity infection due to nonhealing neuropathic foot ulcers, severe ischemic pain, absent or decreased pulses, local necrosis, osteomyelitis, systemic toxicity, acute embolic disease, and severe venous thrombosis.

Diabetes is a leading cause of nontraumatic lower extremity amputation in the United States.[21] Incidence of lower extremity amputations in the diabetic population compared to the nondiabetic is higher, with relative risks varied between 7.4 and 41.3.[22] Between 2% and 5% of individuals with PAD and without diabetes and between 6% and 25% of those with diabetes eventually undergo an amputation.[4,23] While there were declining rates of diabetes-related nontraumatic lower extremity amputations between 1990 and 2010,[24,25] this progress may have been reversed recently.[26] A recent study found that the amputation rates per 1000 adults with diabetes decreased by 43% between 2000 and 2009, but it rebounded by 50% between 2009 and 2015.[26] The reversal was more prominent in young and middle-aged adults and was driven more by males than females.[26] The cost of health care for persons with chronic diseases such as diabetes and PAD is estimated by the American Diabetes Association (ADA) at $330 billion per year, and a major cost associated with diabetic medical care is attributed to lower limb amputation.[27]

In individuals with diabetes, the prevalence and severity of dysvascularity increases significantly with age and the duration of diabetes, particularly in males. The incidence of lower extremity amputation among persons with diabetes is almost 50% higher for males than for females.[16] Initial amputation may involve a toe or foot; subsequent revision to transtibial or transfemoral levels is likely to occur with progression of the underlying disease. In individuals with diabetes, dysvascular disease increases the risk of a nonhealing neuropathic ulcer, infection, or gangrene, all of which increase the likelihood of amputation. Some 20% to 50% of patients will have amputation of the contralateral leg in 1 to 3 years.[28] Patients with diabetes who are 65 years of age or older account for most diabetes-related lower extremity amputations. In addition, African-American and Native American patients, residents of rural regions, and those of low socioeconomic status are at a higher risk of amputation as a result of diabetes.[14]

Peripheral Neuropathy

Peripheral neuropathy is the most common risk factor for foot ulcers in people with diabetes.[29]

The ADA defines diabetic peripheral neuropathy as "the presence of symptoms and/or signs of peripheral nerve dysfunction in people with diabetes after the exclusion of other causes."[30] There is no gold standard for diagnosing diabetic peripheral neuropathy.[30] Its symptoms are similar to those of peripheral neuropathy of other sources: numbness or reduced ability to feel pain, muscle weakness, difficulty walking, and serious foot problems.

Neuropathy is as important and powerful as dysvascular disease as a predisposing factor for lower extremity amputation. More than 80% of all nontraumatic amputations in diabetic patients are the result of foot ulcers.[31] Peripheral neuropathy is suspected when one or more of the following clinical signs are present: (1) deficits of sensation (loss of Achilles and patellar reflexes, decreased vibratory sensation, and loss of protective sensation); (2) motor impairments (weakness and atrophy of the intrinsic muscles of the foot); and/or (3) autonomic dysfunction (inadequate or abnormal hemodynamic mechanism, tropic changes of the skin, and distal loss of hair).[32] The resulting loss of thermal, pain, and protective sensation increases the vulnerability of the foot to acute high-pressure and repetitive low-pressure trauma.

Patients may also experience significant numbness or painful paresthesia of the foot and lower leg. Individuals with peripheral neuropathy may not be aware of minor trauma, pressure from poorly fitting shoes along the sides and tops of their feet, or pressure from thickening plantar callus, all of which contribute to the risk of ulceration, infection, and gangrene. Motor neuropathy and associated weakness and atrophy contribute to the development of bony deformity of the foot. The bony prominences and malalignments associated with foot deformity change weight-bearing pressure dynamics during walking, further increasing the risk of ulceration. Peripheral neuropathy is one of the most crucial precursors of foot ulceration, especially in the presence of dysvascular disease. Nonhealing or

Case Example 17.1 A Patient With Dysvascular Disease–Related Amputation

T.S. is a 67-year-old African-American male with a 10-year history of type 2 diabetes mellitus. Until 2 years ago, he smoked one pack of cigarettes daily, but he quit after coronary artery bypass grafting following an acute myocardial infarction. He became insulin dependent at the time of his myocardial infarction and cardiac surgery. His comorbid medical problems include hypertension, managed pharmaceutically with a beta blocker, and moderate vision loss secondary to diabetic retinopathy.

T.S. underwent complete transmetatarsal amputation of the left foot 6 months earlier because of a nonhealing plantar ulcer under the second and third metatarsal heads that had progressed to osteomyelitis. Three weeks earlier, intermittent claudication of the right calf became severe enough to warrant medical attention. On evaluation, T.S. was noted to have a neuropathic ulcer under his first metatarsal head, probing to bone. Doppler studies were monophasic, suggesting that the vascular supply required for healing was inadequate. Arteriography indicated a markedly diminished distal arterial flow to the foot but an adequate arterial supply to the mid-tibial level. T.S. had failed a revascularization attempt with stent placement.

After an interdisciplinary meeting involving his internist (who helps him manage his diabetes), cardiologist (who helps him manage his hypertension and heart disease), vascular surgeon (who oversaw this evaluation), physical therapist and prosthetist (who explained the process of rehabilitation), social worker (who explained services and support available to those with amputation), and family, T.S. concurred with the recommendation for an "elective" transtibial amputation. Two weeks after his surgery, he was impatiently waiting for his wound to heal to the point where he could begin prosthetic training.

QUESTIONS TO CONSIDER

- What possible medical and physiologic factors contributed to this patient's loss of limb?
- What impact will his current health status and comorbid conditions have on his prognosis for rehabilitation, both in terms of eventual outcome and in the duration of this episode of care?
- What plan of care for the preprosthetic phase of his rehabilitation would you propose?
- How would the International Classification of Functioning disablement framework apply to T.S.?

infected neuropathic ulcers precede approximately 80% of nontraumatic lower extremity amputations in individuals with diabetes.[31]

Outcomes of Amputation Secondary to Vascular Conditions and Neuropathy

The morbidity and mortality risks associated with diabetes and vascular disease continue after amputation. Death in the years immediately after amputation is not uncommon. One-third of elderly people receiving lower limb amputation die within a year of surgery.[33,34] A systematic review reported that the 5-year mortality rate was very high, ranging from 53% to 100%.[35] Because PAD and neuropathy occur in a symmetric distribution, the risk of subsequent reamputation of the ipsilateral site or amputation of the contralateral lower extremity is high. Dillingham and colleagues report that 26% of patients required another amputation procedure within a 12-month period.[34] The most common causes of death in persons with amputation include complications of diabetes, cardiovascular disease, and renal disease.

TRAUMATIC AMPUTATION

The second leading cause of amputation is trauma. Traumatic amputation is defined as an injury to an extremity that results in immediate separation of the limb or will result in loss of the limb as a result of accident or injury.[36] Trauma-related amputation occurs most commonly among young adult males but can happen at any age to individuals of either sex. Common causes of trauma-related amputation include motor vehicle traffic injuries, fall injuries, firearm injuries, and machinery injuries.[37,38] In 2002, a study found a decreasing trend in the incidence of trauma-related major amputation.[4] This reduction may be attributable to the implementation of new safety regulations, the development of safer farm and industrial machinery, improved safety in work conditions, and medical advancement in techniques for salvaging traumatized limbs.

Using the National Trauma Databank, a study analyzed the epidemiology of trauma-related amputation between 2002 and 2004.[39] Approximately 1% of the patients with trauma in this database received amputation. Amputations were most often performed in the age group 31 to 45 years and the majority was male (76.8%). Approximately 76.9% had digit amputation while 23.1% had limb amputation. Among patients with a single-limb amputation, approximately 59% had a lower extremity amputation while approximately 41% had an upper extremity amputation. Below-knee amputation was the most performed amputation in the patients who received a lower limb amputation.

Military service members are a major population having trauma-related amputation. US engagement in military operations in Afghanistan, Iraq, and Syria, including Operation Freedom's Sentinel (Afghanistan), Operation Inherent Resolve (Iraq and Syria), Operation New Dawn (Iraq), Operation Iraqi Freedom (Iraq), and Operation Enduring Freedom (Afghanistan), has caused more than 1600 service men and women to sustain traumatic amputations or limb loss.[40] In these individuals, approximately 69% had a single-limb loss and approximately 31% had multiple-limb losses.[41]

Because the mechanism of injury in traumatic amputation is variable, this type of amputation is usually classified according to the severity of tissue damage. The extent of injury to the musculoskeletal system depends on three interacting factors: (1) movement of the object that caused the injury; (2) the direction, magnitude, and speed of the energy vector; and (3) the particular body tissue involved. Traumatic amputation can be categorized as partial or complete. In partial traumatic amputations, at least half the diameter of the injured extremity is severed or damaged significantly. This kind of injury can incur extensive bleeding because all of the blood vessels involved may not be vasoconstrictive. A second type of traumatic amputation occurs when the limb becomes completely detached from the body. As much as 1 L of blood may be lost before the arteries spasm and become vasoconstrictive.

For optimal outcome, surgical intervention for revascularization or treatment of the amputated site is usually necessary within 6 to 8 hours after the accident.[42] One of the primary efforts of the surgical team for a person with lower extremity amputation is to preserve limb length to the extent that healing is possible.[43] Replantation is the surgical procedure to reattach the part of the body that has been amputated.[44] When replantation is considered, the window of opportunity is much narrower. The decision to replant is a difficult one and is influenced by the patient's age and overall health status, the level of the extremity injury, and the condition of the amputated part (Table 17.1). Replantation has been most successful in the distal upper extremity. The goal of upper extremity replantation is to provide a mechanism for functional grasp rather than solely for cosmetic restoration of the limb. The period of recovery and rehabilitation after replantation is often significantly longer than that after amputation.

Persons with trauma-related amputation undergo extreme physiologic changes as well as psychologic trauma.

Table 17.1 Indications and Contraindications for Replantation of Amputations

INDICATIONS FOR REPLANTATION
■ Amputations in children
■ Multiple finger and hand amputations
■ Thumb
■ Single-finger injuries
■ Ring avulsion injuries
CONTRAINDICATIONS TO REPLANTATION
■ Severe crush injury
■ Prolonged warm ischemia, especially of muscle
■ Severe contamination
■ Medical comorbidities that can affect anesthesia, healing, therapy, or ability to cooperate with care
■ Life-threatening injuries
■ Refusal to accept blood transfusions or blood products in cases of major amputations

The indications and contraindications are not absolute, and the decision for replantation is best made by the patient and physician after a discussion of the potential outcome, benefits, risks, possible complications, and available alternatives to the replantation. This discussion is very dependent on the surgeon's judgment of the potential outcome for a given patient.
From https://www.microsurgeon.org/replantation.php.

Case Example 17.2 **A Patient With Traumatic Amputation**

C.J., a 20-year-old female, was on active duty with the National Guard in Afghanistan when a rocket-propelled grenade hit her convoy and she sustained significant shrapnel injuries to both lower extremities. After emergency care on the ground, C.J.'s condition was considered critical enough to warrant immediate transport to a military hospital in Germany. Trauma surgeons at the center determined that her wounds were severe enough to require midlength transtibial amputation on the right and a long transfemoral amputation on the left. Because of wound contamination from shrapnel and debris and a resulting high risk of infection, C.J.'s surgical wounds were initially left open (unsutured) while local and intravenous antimicrobials were administered. After several days of care, C.J. was returned to the operating room for revision and closure of her wounds. She now has significant edema and serosanguineous drainage on the right limb with a small area of wound dehiscence in the middle of the suture line. Although the left residual limb is not as edematous, the suture line is inflamed and ecchymotic, with more than a dozen healing puncture wounds from shrapnel fragments over the anterior and lateral thigh. Once she is medically stable, C.J. will be moved to a military rehabilitation hospital in the United States for preprosthetic care and rehabilitation.

QUESTIONS TO CONSIDER

- Given the circumstances of these traumatic amputations, how does this patient's prognosis differ from that of the previous patient (Case Example 17.1) with a dysvascular/neuropathic amputation?
- How might the rehabilitation of this patient be similar to or different from that of the patient in Case Example 17.1 in terms of eventual outcome and duration of care?
- What plan of care would you implement to promote wound healing?

With the sudden loss of a body part, the patient may experience an extended period of grieving. Addressing the patient's psychologic as well as physical needs is important for optimal outcome. An interdisciplinary team approach to rehabilitation is the most effective means of addressing the comprehensive needs of a patient who has unexpectedly lost a limb to trauma.[44]

CANCER

The third cause of limb loss is cancer related—primary cancer or secondary cancer due to metastatic disease. There are a number of cancers that can affect the limbs and may present the need for amputation.[45] Primary bone cancers are extremely rare; they account for less than 1% of all cancers.[46] The three most common forms of bone cancer are (1) osteosarcoma, (2) chrondosarcoma, and (3) Ewing sarcoma. These cancers arise from the growing end of long bones (osteosarcoma), and cartilage (chondrosarcoma). Ewing tumors occur primarily in the bone (Ewing sarcoma of bone) or soft tissue (extraosseous Ewing tumor). Ewing sarcoma can develop in any bone, but it is most often found in the pelvis, femurs, ribs, or scapula. The American Cancer Society's estimates for primary cancers of the bones and joints in 2022 was reported as 3910 total new cases.[46] The estimated number of deaths from bone and joint cancers was reported as 2100.[46]

The tumor most commonly associated with amputation is osteosarcoma, which primarily affects children and adolescents in the 10- to 24-year-old age group.[47] A second peak in incidence occurs in adults, primarily males aged 80 to 84 years.[47] Osteosarcoma Surveillance, Epidemiology and End Results (SEER) data from the US National Cancer Institute from 1975 to 2018 reported 5016 (86%) cases of primary osteoscaroma and 680 cases (14%) of subsequent osteosarcoma.[47] Osteosarcoma incidence by age group was as follows: 382 osteosarcoma cases in the youngest age group (0–9 years old) with an age-adjusted incidence rate of 1.9 per million; 2312 osteosarcoma cases in the 10- to 24-year-old age group, which represented nearly 50% of all osteosarcoma cases in the SEER 18 database; 1411 cases in the 25- to 59-year-old age group with an osteosarcoma incidence rate of 1.9 per million. There were 908 cases among individuals older than 60. The incidence of osteosarcoma in this oldest age group was 2 per million in the most recent decade.[47] Multiple factors have been shown to contribute to developing osteosarcoma, most commonly race, sex, and age. A higher incidence rate of the diagnosis is registered among young males of African origin.[47,48] The American Cancer Society reports a 5-year relative survival rate of 77% for patients with localized nonmetastatic osteosarcoma.[49] When the cancer has metastasized, the 5-year survival rate is 26%.[49]

Clinically, osteosarcoma can be divided into two stages: localized and metastatic. Localized osteosarcoma refers to the cancer, affecting only the bone and the tissues in which it developed. It can then further be categorized into resectable and nonresectable stages, based on the viability of surgically removing the tumor. The metastatic stage of osteosarcoma shows that the cancer has spread from the original site to other organs, most commonly the lungs, making it more difficult to treat.[46,48] Osteosarcoma typically occurs at or near the epiphyses of long bones—especially the distal femur, proximal tibia, or proximal humerus—during times of rapid growth. Most patients have a history of worsening, increasingly deep-seated pain, sometimes accompanied by localized swelling. Children with osteosarcoma are vulnerable to pathologic fracture, an event that often prompts diagnosis. Currently amputation is no longer the primary intervention for osteosarcoma. Since the early 1990s, the need for amputation in osteosarcoma has been greatly reduced by advances in early detection, imaging techniques, chemotherapy regimens, and limb resectioning and salvage procedures. With the development of new surgical techniques for limb salvage, including bone graft and joint replacement, and advancements in chemotherapy and radiation, the incidence of amputation as a consequence of osteosarcoma has decreased significantly. Up to 90% of patients can be treated with limb salvage surgery.[49-52]

Tumor resection followed by limb reconstruction frequently provides a functional extremity. Weight bearing is limited, and the limb is protected by an orthosis early in rehabilitation. Once satisfactory healing has occurred, full weight-bearing and near-normal activities can be

Case Example 17.3 A Patient With Osteosarcoma

R.K. is a 16-year-old male high-school student who sustained an unexpected fracture of the distal femur in a collision during playoffs for the state soccer title. He had experienced increasing lateral knee pain during the previous 4 weeks but had not complained to his coaches or parents for fear he would have to "sit out." Examination in the emergency department revealed a swollen and tender distal femur and knee. A radiograph showed a fracture just proximal to a radiodense lesion of the medial femoral condyle, including the articular surfaces of the knee. Magnetic resonance imaging indicated that the tumor extended posteriorly, close to the neurovascular bundle in the popliteal fossa. Biopsy confirmed osteosarcoma. The orthopedic surgeon and oncologist reviewed the options for limb salvage and amputation with R.K. and his parents, recommending amputation because the location of the tumor precluded the wide clear margins at the knee required for endoprosthetic knee replacement or cadaver allograft salvage strategies. R.K.'s fractured limb was stabilized in a knee orthosis while a preoperative course of chemotherapy was undertaken and the possibility of metastasis to the lungs was evaluated by further testing. Resection of the tumor to a midlength transfemoral level of amputation was planned once the initial course of chemotherapy had been completed, to be followed by a second course of chemotherapy. R.K. and his family were encouraged by visits from a survivor of osteosarcoma who had had a transfemoral amputation 7 years earlier and was now a competitive runner at the national and paralympic level.

QUESTIONS TO CONSIDER

- How does the diagnosis of a serious cancer affect the rehabilitation of young people with medically necessary amputations?
- What psychologic factors must be considered?
- What physiologic factors must be considered?
- What are the similarities and differences in the prognosis and plan of care for this patient with cancer-related amputation as compared with the previous patients with dysvascular/neuropathic and trauma-related etiologies in terms of eventual outcome and duration of this episode of care?

resumed. Amputation is typically reserved for nonresectable tumors.[52] Amputation for osteosarcoma is associated with advanced age, advanced stage, larger tumors, greater comorbidities, and lower income.[51]

CONGENITAL LIMB DEFICIENCY

Congenital limb deficiencies, also known as limb reduction deficits or congenital amputation, are relatively rare. They refer to the absence of a limb or part of a limb at birth. Congenital limb deficiency rates of 5.15 per 10,000 live births in the United States from 2010 to 2014 have been reported.[53] There are 2026 estimated cases of congenital limb deficiency annually in the United States, occurring in approximately 1 in 1943 births.[53] Most are due to primary intrauterine growth inhibition or disruptions secondary to intrauterine destruction of normal embryonic tissues. The upper extremities are more commonly affected and radial deficiencies are more common than ulnar.[54] Upper limb deficiencies in children vary from minor abnormalities of the fingers to major limb absences. Embryologic differentiation of the upper limbs occurs most rapidly at 5 to 8 weeks' gestation, often before pregnancy has been recognized or confirmed. During this period the upper limbs are particularly vulnerable to malformation. The etiology of limb malformation is unclear. Potential contributing factors cited in the research literature include (1) exposure to chemical agents or drugs, (2) fetal position or constriction, (3) endocrine disorders, (4) exposure to radiation, (5) immune reactions, (6) occult infections and other diseases, (7) single-gene disorders, (8) chromosomal disorders, and (9) other syndromes of unknown cause.[54,55]

An infant with a congenital limb deficiency may be missing an entire limb or just a portion of one. Commonly, if the entire limb is absent, it is termed "amelia." The International Standards Organization/International Society of Prosthetists and Orthotists (ISO/ISPO) system is the standard for classifying congenital limb deficiency.[56] In this system deficiencies are categorized into two basic types: transverse and longitudinal. Transverse deficiencies occur across (or transverse to) the long axis of the limb. Transverse deficiencies are described by the level at which the limb terminates. See Table 17.2 for descriptions of levels of transverse deficiencies.

In transverse deficiency, the limb develops to a point and then ceases to develop; it resembles an amputation residual limb in which the limb has developed normally to a particular level beyond which no skeletal elements are present. Terminal transverse defects, when the terminal part of the limb is completely missing, are more common than intercalary deficit, when some part of the limb is missing but the terminal part is present, even if malformed.[55] In longitudinal deficiencies, a reduction or absence occurs within the long axis of the limb, but normal skeletal components are present distal to the affected bones. Longitudinal deficiencies are named for the bones partially or totally affected and the fraction missing. [56] See Table 17.3 for descriptions of longitudinal deficiencies. Longitudinal deficiencies are differentiated into further subgroups: preaxial (radial and tibial side), postaxial (ulnar and fibular side), and axial (central). See Table 17.4 from the Centers for Disease Control and Prevention[55] for the types of limb deficiencies by axis and segment involved.

Table 17.2 International Standards Organization (ISO) Descriptions of Levels of Transverse Deficiencies of Upper and Lower Limbs

Body Part	Transverse Deficiency
Shoulder and pelvis	Total
Upper arm and thigh	Total, upper third, middle third, lower third
Forearm and leg	Total, upper third, middle third, lower third
Carpal and tarsal	Total or partial
Metacarpal and metatarsal	Total or partial
Phalangeal (finger or thumb or toe)	Total or partial

Adapted from Nelson et al.[56]

Table 17.3 International Standards Organization (ISO) Descriptions of Levels of Longitudinal Deficiencies of Upper and Lower Limbs

Body Part	Deficiency Classification
Scapula	Total or partial
Clavicle	Total or partial
Humerus	Total or partial
Radius	Total or partial
Ulna	Total or partial
Carpus	Total or partial
Metacarpals	Total or partial
Phalanges	Total or partial. 1, thumb; 2, index; 3, middle; 4, ring; 5, little
Ilium	Total or partial
Ischium	Total or partial
Pubis	Total or partial
Femur	Total or partial
Tibia	Total or partial
Fibula	Total or partial
Tarsus	Total or partial
Phalanges	Total or partial. 1, great toe; 2,3,4,5

Adapted from Nelson et al.[56]

Table 17.4 Types of Limb Deficiencies by Axis and Segment Involved[55]

Complete Absence	All segments	Amelia
	Intercalary	Absence or severe hypoplasia of part of limb with normal or nearly normal terminal segment, including: ■ typical and atypical intercalary defects ■ femoral hypoplasia
Longitudinal	Preaxial	Radial, tibial, first digit/toe (with or without involvement of second digit/toe).
	Axial	Hand/foot only: Third ray involved (with or without second and fourth ray) Includes typical split-hand/foot and split-hand/foot monodactyly type
	Postaxial	Fifth digits/toes (with or without fourth digit/toe involved)
Mixed		Any other combination of two or more subtypes; for example, femoral-fibula-ulnar complex

Adapted from CDC. *Limb Reduction Defects/Limb Deficiencies*. Centers for Disease Control and Prevention. Published March 17, 2021. https://www.cdc.gov/ncbddd/birthdefects/surveillancemanual/quick-reference-handbook/limb-reduction-defects-limb-deficiencies.html; 2021.

The use of prosthetics is a common intervention for children with congenital limb deficiencies. Sometimes surgery is necessary to prepare the existing limb for the most effective use of a prosthesis, especially after periods of rapid growth. The goals of prosthetic training for the child should be to enhance the function of the limb and provide a cosmetic replacement for a missing limb. Rehabilitation efforts are designed with the child's cognitive, motor, and psychological development in mind. Children with congenital limb deficiencies are a special population and may require surgical revision during or after periods of significant growth or after conversion to a more functional level for prosthetic fitting.

Levels of Amputation

Amputation can be performed as a disarticulation of a joint or as a transection through a long bone. The level of amputation is usually named by the joint or major bone through which the amputation has been made (Table 17.4).[4] See Fig. 17.3 for amputation levels above the knee, Fig. 17.4 for transtibial amputation levels, and Fig. 17.5 for foot amputation levels. An amputation that involves the lower extremity can affect an individual's ability to stand and walk, requiring the use of prosthetics and, often, an assistive device for mobility. Amputation involving the upper extremity can affect other activities of daily living, such as feeding, grooming, dressing, and a host of activities that require manipulative skills. Because of the complex nature of skilled hand function, prosthetic substitution for upper limb amputation does not typically restore function to the same degree as that of lower extremity prosthetics. The amputation surgeries that are most commonly performed due to dysvascular conditions involve the lower extremity. They include toe (33.2%), transtibial (28.2%), transfemoral (26.1%), and foot amputations (10.6%).[57] Ankle disarticulation (Syme), through-knee, hip disarticulation, and hemipelvectomy amputations constitute an additional 1.5% of all amputations.[57] Of the approximately 150,000 nontraumatic leg amputations every year in the United States most cases occur in patients with diabetes.[58] One study found that diabetes-related amputations accounted

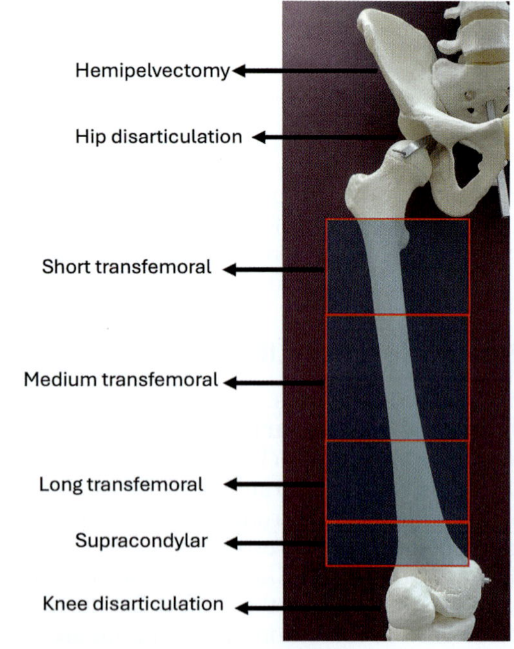

Fig. 17.3 Amputation levels above the knee.

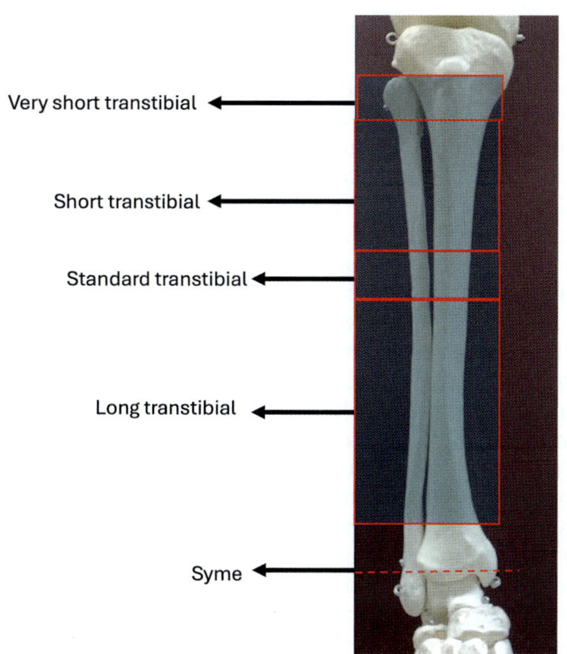

Fig. 17.4 Transtibial amputation levels.

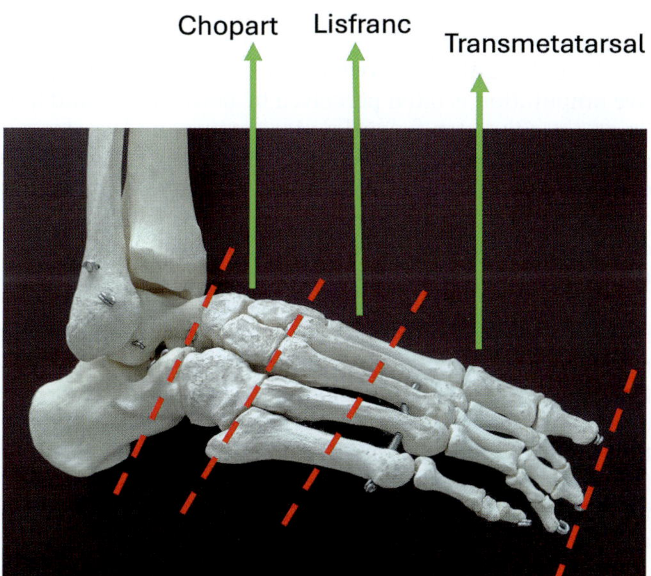

Fig. 17.5 Foot amputation levels.

for 75% of all adult hospitalizations for nontraumatic lower extremity amputation in 2015.[26] National US data have shown that diabetes-related nontraumatic lower extremity amputations have recently increased following a period of decline, particularly among young and middle-aged adults.[21] Amputation rates per 1,000 people with diabetes decreased by half from 8.5 in 2000 to 4.4 in 2009; however, from 2009 onward rates increased to 4.8. Overall increases were in rates of toe and foot amputations, while rates of transtibial and transfemoral continued to decline

Table 17.5 Terminology Used to Describe the Site of Lower Extremity Amputation

Site	Terminology
Toe	Phalangeal
Forefoot	Ray resection (one or more complete metatarsal)
	Transmetatarsal (across the metatarsal shaft)
Midfoot	Partial foot (e.g., Chopart, Boyd, Pirogoff)
At the ankle	Syme
Below the knee	Transtibial (long, standard, short)
At the knee	Knee disarticulation
Above the knee	Transfemoral (long, standard, short)
At the hip	Hip disarticulation
At the pelvis	Hemipelvectomy

over time.[21] Similar trends have been reported in Medicare beneficiaries without diabetes, but the overall amputation rates in this population are substantially lower.[26] Geiss et al. examined 2000–15 data from the Nationwide Inpatient Sample (NIS) of the Agency for Healthcare Research and Quality data from the NIS and the National Health Interview Survey from 2000 to 2015. They found increases in diabetes-related amputation among young and middle-aged adults, driven largely by minor amputations, increases in younger and middle-aged adults and men, and by increases in minor amputations, mostly of the toe.[26] Individuals with diabetes tend to have more minor amputations such as toe or first ray, compared with individuals who have peripheral vascular disease, who have more major limb amputations. However, the frequency of subsequent amputation is also higher in individuals with diabetes.[57] One study found that one out of every five patients undergoing any version of a partial first ray amputation eventually required a more proximal reamputation.[59] Trauma accounts for approximately 5.8% of lower limb amputations and is the most common cause of amputation in the second and third decade of life.[57] Cancer accounts for approximately 0.8% of total amputations and is the most common cause of amputation between the ages of 10 and 20 years.[57]

Today the majority of transtibial and transfemoral amputations are performed with an understanding of wound healing and the functional needs and constraints of prosthetic fitting so that rehabilitation outcomes are usually positive. Other levels of amputation, although less commonly performed, continue to pose challenges for the surgeon, prosthetist, physical therapist, and patient during prosthetic fitting and rehabilitation.

Racial Disparities in Amputation

Evidence indicates that certain racial and ethnic groups are at increased risk for lower extremity amputation. This increased risk appears to be linked to a higher prevalence of diabetes complicated by PAD. The ADA reports that "African Americans and Hispanics are over 50% more likely to have diabetes as non-Hispanic whites."[27] African Americans are two to four times more likely to lose a limb as a result of diabetes complications.[4] Compared to non-Hispanic White people, non-Hispanic Black people were more than twice as likely to be hospitalized for lower limb amputations in 2017.[60] Metropolitan areas with greater numbers of African-American residents are associated with higher amputation rates.[61] Compared to White Americans, Black Americans are less likely to receive procedures that can prevent amputation.[62]

Based on the available 2012 data, hospital admissions for lower extremity amputations in Hispanic people 18 years of age and older with diabetes were 50% higher than those for non-Hispanic White people.[63] Research into the epidemiology of race and ethnicity is advancing to further elucidate the essential contributing factors. The Hispanic Community Health Study/Study of Latinos, sponsored by the National Heart, Lung, and Blood Institute and six other centers as well as the National Institutes of Health, indicates that the prevalence of diabetes in the Hispanic community has variability based on country of origin, length of stay in the United States, as well as access to health care.[63]

Compared to non-Hispanic White adults, American Indian and Alaska Native adults have rates of diabetes that are three times higher,[64] and lower extremity amputation has become a common complication in these populations.[65] Why these populations have a significantly higher rate of lower extremity amputation is unclear. Potential contributors include a genetic or familial predisposition to diabetes, a higher prevalence of hypertension and smoking, or both. Health promotion and education efforts that target this high-risk population (including programs aimed at the effective management of diabetes, minimization of other risk factors, and special foot care programs for early detection of neuropathic and traumatic lesions) are effective strategies to reduce the likelihood of amputation. Further research is necessary to better understand the causes of racial differences in amputation rates and to identify and promote health initiatives that will alleviate this excess risk among minority populations.

Rehabilitation Issues for the Person With an Amputation

Several factors influence the success of rehabilitation after amputation. These include age, health status, cognitive status, sequence of onset of disability, concurrent disease and comorbidity, and the level of amputation.[66] With anticipated growth in the aging segments of the population and the presence of chronic dysvascular conditions, amputation in the US geriatric population will probably double from 28,000 to 58,000 per year by 2030.[67] The number of persons living with limb loss will more than double from 1.6 million in 2005 to 3.6 million in 2050. Prosthetic, physical therapy, and healthcare needs will increase to ensure continued independence, quality of life, and participation in activities of daily living among these individuals. Persons with limb loss will require considerable rehabilitation resources.[5,10]

Evidence-based efforts to reduce the incidence of lower extremity amputation in persons with diabetes through improved public awareness and evidence-based management of PAD are recommended.[58,68] The American Heart Association has proposed several policy and legislative changes directed at improving public awareness and management of individuals with PAD with a goal of reducing nontraumatic amputations by 20% by 2030.[58] These include measures to improve prevention, diagnosis, and management of individuals with PAD; regulation of tobacco products; affordable, accessible, and equitable medical care for all patients with PAD; professional education; and funding to support PAD research.[58] Large clinical centers have demonstrated the effect of early intervention for the diabetic population by using an interdisciplinary team approach to preventive care.[69] Interventions to prevent PAD and neuropathy should target smoking cessation programs as well as exercise, dietary, and pharmaceutical interventions to obtain better control of hypertension, hyperlipidemia, and hyperglycemia.[70] These efforts are likely to further reduce the incidence of amputation and other complications among people with diabetes. For those with existing PAD or diabetic neuropathy, intensive foot care programs should focus on the prevention of ulceration and early intervention to prevent the expansion of small lesions as well as their infection and the development of gangrene.[17] Foot care programs are most effective if they develop in a team setting and focus on patient education. Surgical revascularization procedures are performed to avoid amputation in persons with chronic foot ulceration. The revascularization procedures include vascular bypass, angioplasty, stent placement, and end-stage limb-salvage procedures.[23]

The decision to undergo amputation often follows a long struggle to care for an increasingly frail foot by the patient, family, and healthcare providers. In this circumstance, elective amputation is often perceived by both patient and family as a positive step toward a more active and less stressful life. The interdisciplinary team approach best addresses the complex needs of the individual with diabetes, including clinical evaluation, determination of risk status, patient education, footwear selection, decision making about amputation, and rehabilitation after surgery.

The physical rehabilitation[71] process for persons with amputation occurs in different stages, beginning with a postoperative acute phase, where positioning, skin protection, sensory and proprioceptive training, joint range of motion, and muscle strengthening occur in conjunction with general conditioning activities. This leads to functional training for independence in mobility including transfer skills, balance exercises, wheelchair mobility, and ambulation with assistive devices that extends to the subacute phase of rehabilitation. The preprosthetic phase includes management of the residual limb including wound care, edema control, shaping, desensitization, and increasing joint and muscle flexibility. Strengthening of the trunk as well as the extremities is essential for prosthetic use. Traditionally, physical therapists have focused on the ability to perform functional activities such as walking, turning, and managing ramps and other uneven or unpredictable surfaces safely, independently, and efficiently with and without a prosthesis. Physical therapists assist physicians and prosthetists in determining an individual's readiness for prosthetic fitting and are often involved in decisions about prosthetic components. After initial fitting, physical therapists coordinate prosthetic training, consulting with prosthetists if problems with prosthetic alignment arise. Once these basic mobility activities are mastered, the therapist can serve as a consultant to assist the person with amputation in returning to preamputation employment and leisure activities. The rehabilitation process for persons with lower limb amputation is aimed at maximizing functional mobility outcomes. In order to achieve functional ambulation, prosthetists and physical therapists must address issues of residual limb or phantom pain management,[72] muscle strengthening,[73] balance, and ambulation training.[74,75]

The Clinical Practice Guidelines for rehabilitation of lower limb amputation, developed by the US Department of Veterans Affairs and the US Department of Defense, recommend the use of reliable and validated objective outcome measures throughout rehabilitation.[76] These should include self-report and performance-based measures.[77] Functional outcome measures such as the Amputee Mobility Predictor to assess functional mobility and The Timed-Up-and-Go test to assess balance are recommended in individuals with lower limb loss.[76,78] Quality-of-life indicators and outcome measures ultimately evaluate the success of the rehabilitation process.[79-81]

As many as 70% of persons with a lower extremity amputation report using their prosthesis on a full-time basis: putting it on in the early morning, wearing it all day, and taking it off in the evening.[79] Two major reasons for limited use or nonuse are generally cited: physical discomfort when walking with the prosthesis and psychologic discomfort. The wide variation reported in the success of functional ambulation with a prosthesis after below-knee amputation appears to be related to age and concurrent disease.[80] Healing time, indicated by time between surgery and fitting for the first prosthesis, correlates with age but not with the cause of amputation. Age is also more important than the etiology of amputation in predicting the total length of time in rehabilitation and achievement of functional ambulation: older adults with amputation are likely to require a longer rehabilitation period to accomplish an ambulatory status equal to that of the younger group.[82] Although most people recovering from amputation achieve some level of upright mobility, a smaller percentage of older persons with concurrent chronic disease become functional ambulators as compared with younger persons who had amputations because of trauma or osteomyelitis. Today, US veterans with traumatic amputations have greater options for returning to active duty than were available in the recent past due to the prosthetic and rehabilitation training provided in Veterans Administration medical centers. US military service

Table 17.6 Members and Roles of the Multidisciplinary Team for Rehabilitation After Amputation

Team Member	Role
Physician	Often serves as coordinator of the team
	Assesses need for amputation, performs surgery, monitors healing of suture line
	Monitors and manages patient's overall medical care and health status
	Monitors condition of remaining extremity for patients with peripheral vascular disease (PVD), neuropathy, or diabetes
Physical therapist	Provides preoperative education about the rehabilitation process and instruction in single-limb mobility
	Designs and manages a preprosthetic rehabilitation program that focuses on mobility and preparation for prosthetic training
	Evaluates patient's readiness for prosthetic fitting; can make recommendations for prosthetic fitting
	Designs and manages a prosthetic training program that focuses on functional ambulation and prosthetic management
	Monitors condition of the remaining extremity for patients with PVD, neuropathy, or diabetes
Prosthetist	Designs, fabricates, and fits the prosthesis
	Adapts the prosthesis to individuals, adjusts alignment, repairs/replaces components when necessary
	Monitors fit, function, and comfort of the prosthesis
	Monitors condition of the remaining extremity for patients with PVD, neuropathy, or diabetes
Occupational therapist	Assesses and treats patients with upper extremity amputation, monitors readiness for prosthetic fitting, recommends components
	Assists with problem solving in activities of daily living for patients with upper or lower limb amputations
	Makes recommendations for environmental modification and assistive/adaptive equipment to facilitate functional independence
Social worker	Provides financial counseling and coordination of support services
	Acts as liaison with third-party payers and community agencies
	Assists with patient's and family's social, psychological, and financial issues
Dietitian	Evaluates nutritional status and provides nutritional counseling, especially for patients with diabetes or heart disease or those who are on chemotherapy or are recovering from trauma
Nurse/nurse practitioner	Monitors patient's health and functional status during rehabilitation
	Provides ongoing patient education on comorbid and chronic health issues
	Monitors condition of remaining extremity for patients with PVD, neuropathy, or diabetes
Vocational counselor	Assesses patient's employment status and potential
	Assists with education, training, and placement

Modified from May B. Assessment and treatment of individuals following lower extremity amputation. In: O'Sullivan SB, Schmitz TJ, eds. *Physical Rehabilitation: Assessment and Treatment*. Davis; 1994:379.

members injured in Afghanistan and Iraq who sustained limb loss—including transfemoral and transradial levels of amputation—have remained on active duty and continue to serve successfully. The typical age at the time of initial lower limb dysvascular amputation is between 51 and 69 years; therefore consideration must be given to the special rehabilitation needs of the older patient. The complexity of issues during rehabilitation of the older adult who is undergoing an amputation is often compounded by comorbidity, fragile social supports, and limited resources.[80] In patients with dysvascular conditions, concomitant cerebrovascular disease can have a more complicated rehabilitation process. A preamputation history of stroke or occurrence of stroke during the course of rehabilitation is not uncommon. Similarly, cardiovascular disease can limit endurance and exercise tolerance; endurance training becomes a critical component of the postamputation preprosthetic rehabilitation program.

Optimal rehabilitation care begins with consultation and patient and family education efforts before surgery. A specialized interdisciplinary team most effectively provides this presurgical and perisurgical care (Table 17.6). Team members often include a surgeon, physical therapist, certified prosthetist, occupational therapist, nurse or nurse practitioner, recreational therapist, psychologist, and social worker. The patient and family members are active and essential members of the team as well. Effective communication provides the team with the necessary information to develop a tentative treatment plan from the time of amputation to discharge home.

Persons with trauma-related amputation undergo extreme physiologic changes as well as psychological trauma. With the sudden loss of a body part, the patient may experience an extended period of grieving. Addressing the patient's psychological as well as physical needs is important for an optimal outcome. An interdisciplinary team approach to rehabilitation is the most effective means of addressing the comprehensive needs of a patient who has unexpectedly lost a limb to trauma.[76]

With a specialized treatment team and the use of new lightweight, dynamic prosthetic designs, the potential for rehabilitation of the older patient has increased significantly in the past decade. At the time of surgery, special consideration is given to the optimal level of amputation. This is a particularly important concern for the older patient. The selection of the surgical level of amputation is probably one of the most important decisions to be made for the patient undergoing an amputation. A lower limb prosthesis ideally becomes a full-body weight-bearing device. However, bony prominences, adhesions of the suture line scar, fragile skin and open areas, shearing forces at the skin/socket interface, and perspiration can complicate this function. The energy cost of ambulation[83] must be considered, especially for older patients with significant deconditioning or comorbid conditions. The higher the level of amputation and loss of joints, long bone length, and muscle insertion, the greater the impairment of normal locomotor mechanisms. This leads to increased energy costs in prosthetic control and functional ambulation and a greater likelihood of functional limitation and disability.

Preservation of the knee joint seems to be a key determinant in determining the potential for functional ambulation and successful rehabilitation outcome. Persons with transtibial amputation who have an intact anatomic knee joint demonstrate a more energy-efficient prosthetic gait pattern and postural responses; they are more likely to ambulate without additional assistive devices (e.g., walkers, crutches, canes). They are also more likely to be full-time prosthetic wearers than are persons with transfemoral amputation. The benefits of preserving the knee, particularly among older adults, are so crucial that a transtibial amputation may be attempted even with the risk of inadequate healing; this may necessitate later revision to a higher level.[84]

The patient with a bilateral transfemoral amputation faces additional rehabilitation challenges. The significant increase in energy consumption that is required can prevent long distance ambulation. Many older patients, as well as younger persons with bilateral transfemoral amputation, may choose wheelchair mobility as a more energy efficient and effective means of locomotion. Ambulation potential depends on cardiac function, strength, balance, and endurance.[84] Options for prosthetic components for the older person with an amputation have increased dramatically in the past 20 years. Selecting the most appropriate components for the individual requires input from the entire rehabilitation team in close communication with the patient and family members.

Rehabilitation Environment

Traditionally, preprosthetic and early prosthetic programs have occurred in rehabilitation departments of acute care hospitals. However, in today's healthcare arena, where length of stay in acute or tertiary care facilities is very limited, early prosthetic rehabilitation is more than likely to begin in the home through home care physical therapy services, in the community through ambulatory preprosthetic rehabilitation, or in a skilled nursing facility. Patients who qualify for a subacute rehabilitation or skilled nursing home stay would also receive the preprosthetic rehabilitation programs necessary to prepare for prosthetic use after limb loss. In this environment, the care is specialized for the older person with an amputation. A quality subacute rehabilitation or skilled nursing facility should have the complement of professional services and essential postamputation rehabilitation treatment team necessary to address the complex needs of this group of patients., Today's healthcare environment does not offer older persons with an amputation an acute inpatient rehabilitation stay until they are ready for prosthetic fitting or after they have received the prosthesis and are ready for intensive rehabilitation with the device. For patients with multiple medical complications, rehabilitation may be continued in a subacute setting or skilled nursing facility. For patients without complications and with a strong social support network, an outpatient rehabilitation program may be preferable. This plan allows them to reintegrate into the home and community while maintaining support of the rehabilitation team. The most effective care and rehabilitation for individuals undergoing an amputation requires the skills and ongoing support of an integrated rehabilitation team.

Summary

Amputation and limb loss can occur as a result of trauma or health conditions (nontraumatic). Amputation can affect persons of all ages. Most nontraumatic amputation surgeries are performed in older citizens who have dysvascular disease with or with diabetes mellitus. Traumatic amputation occurs in US military service men and women engaged in military operations in Afghanistan, Iraq, and Syria, where explosive devices often cause limb loss to soldiers. Traumatic amputations are also the result of motor vehicle accidents, the use of power tool and firearms, and recreational activities. Congenital amputations occur rarely, and amputation due to cancer persists as a medical concern but is diminishing with the new surgical approaches and limb-salvage techniques. Medical advances in the treatment of persons with dysvascular disease and diabetes mellitus offer encouragement that the rise in amputations in the elderly population will decrease in the coming years. The improved education initiatives directed at preventing diabetic foot ulcers or early management of persons with diabetic foot ulcers also provide encouragement that the rate of amputation in persons with diabetes mellitus and dysvascular disease will decrease. Advances in the field of prosthetics enable young, athletic persons with limb loss to return to active lifestyles including return to active military service for injured service men and women. The rehabilitation process after amputation is essential for making sure that patients have the opportunity to maximize their functional abilities and quality of life. Although the rehabilitation phases after amputation may present many challenges for patients, their families, and the professionals involved in their care, they also provide many opportunities for success and reward. An optimal outcome after amputation is best achieved through interaction with a patient-centered, interdisciplinary healthcare team. With effective physical rehabilitation and prosthetic care, most individuals with amputations can return to a level of activity and lifestyle similar to that of their preamputation status.

References

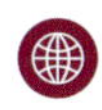

The complete listing of the References are available in the accompanying enhanced eBook version included with the print purchase of this textbook. Visit Elsevier eBooks+ (eBooks.Health.Elsevier.com) to access this content.

18 High-Risk Foot and Wound Healing

HEIDI CHEERMAN, EDWARD MAHONEY, AND MILAGROS JORGE

LEARNING OBJECTIVES

On completion of this chapter, the reader will be able to do the following:

1. Explain the relationship between diabetes and the risk of developing foot disorders and delayed wound healing.
2. Identify the interactive factors that contribute to pressure ulceration injury in persons with vulnerable feet.
3. Describe the components of a thorough foot examination for persons with vulnerable feet at risk for pressure injury.
4. Explain the importance of each component in a thorough wound examination.
5. Compare and contrast the efficacy and drawbacks of the most commonly used options for reducing pressure to promote healing and prevention in the vulnerable foot.
6. Determine which wounds would benefit from the addition of therapeutic modalities.
7. Develop a comprehensive treatment plan to manage vulnerable feet, including those with delayed healing of open wounds.
8. Describe the revised National Pressure Injury Advisory Panel pressure injury staging system.

The thought of losing a limb has to be one of the most frightening things a person will ever face. For the majority of the population, the idea likely conjures up some sort of catastrophic event that can be pushed to the back of the mind as something that is unlikely to occur. Unfortunately, individuals with vulnerable feet, or feet with a high risk for injury, face the very real possibility of losing a limb in the foreseeable future. A high-risk foot is one that has an underlying disease process that puts the tissues at a greater risk of tissue breakdown. In many cases the foot wound is the result of an underlying disease such as diabetes, a condition that will negatively affect wound healing. Diabetes is the leading cause of nontraumatic lower extremity amputation.[1] The number of persons with diabetes and prediabetes in the US population continues to rise. According to the National Diabetes Statistics 2022, an estimated 37.3 million people of all ages, or nearly 11.3% of the US population, has diabetes.[2] Nighty-six million US adults have prediabetes, and 48.8% of Americans age 65+ have prediabetes.[2]

Persons with diabetes often develop peripheral neuropathy and lose sensation to the feet, which can predispose them to injury due to insensate feet. Insensate feet fail to respond to prolonged pressure or mechanical stress, which can lead to skin irritation and pressure sores such as heel ulceration or plantar surface ulceration. Often there is delayed wound healing due to neuropathic changes, impaired circulation, and edema. Delayed wound healing can result in wound site infection, tissue necrosis, and amputation. Early intervention in the instruction of proper foot care for persons with diabetes and in the management of skin abrasions, pressure sores, and open wounds is a preventive measure for avoiding foot ulceration and lower extremity amputation.[3]

This chapter addresses the clinical management of persons with vulnerable feet at high risk for skin breakdown due to pressure injuries that result in foot ulceration and place the individual at risk for foot amputation or limb loss. The importance of conducting a comprehensive physical examination that includes assessment of the vascular, sensory, motor, and autonomic systems, as well as a mobility assessment and footwear inspection, will be introduced. Current interventions and evidence-based treatment strategies aimed at preventing wounds to vulnerable feet or seeking to minimize delayed wound healing will be discussed. Wound management through proper wound assessment, the use of electrotherapeutic and other modalities for infection control and healthy tissue proliferation, the importance of offloading pressure techniques such as using total contact casts (TCCs) and other pressure-relieving strategies, and the use of clinical approaches that seek to prevent recurrence of injury to vulnerable feet will be highlighted in the chapter.

Normal Wound Healing

To fully appreciate the impact of different disease states on wound healing, it is necessary to begin with an understanding of normal wound healing. Wound healing involves a coordinated interaction of three phases: inflammation, proliferation, and remodeling.[4] Although these stages do overlap to some degree, they are discussed individually for purposes of clarity. The body's first response to injury during the inflammatory phase is to stop the bleeding at the site of injury through a process known as hemostasis. In response to an injury, platelets, which are formed in bone marrow and are free floating in the vascular system, are attracted to the injury site. The platelets also undergo activation promoting a coagulation cascade, which causes them to change from a round shape into a sticky form that enables them to adhere to the injured area.[5] The platelet plug may be enough to stop the bleeding in minor injuries, or it may be augmented by the coagulation cascade to form a larger clot. An in-depth discussion on the coagulation cascade is beyond the scope of this chapter. In terms of wound healing, coagulation is only one part of the role of the platelet. The second role, which is critical to wound healing, is the secretion of numerous growth factors and cytokines that set the stage for later phases of wound healing.

The first cells to arrive at the wound site in response to the coagulation cascade are granulocytes, which are a form of white blood cells. Neutrophils are the most abundant of the granulocytes and are found in the wound within 24 hours after injury. These cells are nonspecific and phagocytic, which is crucial for disposing of damaged cells in the area. Other granulocytes include phagocytic eosinophils and basophils, which release histamine. The next leukocytic cells to respond are monocytes, which become macrophages in the wounded area. Macrophages are phagocytic but can also be thought of as growth factor factories because they play such a critical role in producing the growth factors that guide the remainder of the healing process.

Toward the latter stages of the inflammatory response, the wound is well into the proliferative phase of healing. The goal of this phase is to resurface the wound with a layer of viable epithelium. For this to occur, a well-vascularized dermal matrix is laid down in the wound bed. To accomplish this, new blood vessels are formed (neovascularization), and collagen is created by fibroblasts (fibroplasia). At the same time, new skin is being produced through the process of reepithelialization, and wound contraction is occurring, which helps to approximate the wound margins and make the resultant scar smaller. The duration of this phase is greatly influenced by the size of the wound but is generally considered to last up to several weeks. Despite wound closure, the healing process is not yet complete as tissues continue to remodel. In fact, the remodeling phase is by far the longest and can last for more than a year from wound closure until the tissues have reached their maximum strength. Even after the wound has completely remodeled, it will not regain the same strength that uninjured tissue has and will continue to require close monitoring and protection to prevent reulceration.

Assessment of the High-Risk Foot

According to the most recent data from the Centers for Disease Control and Prevention, diabetes is the leading cause of nontraumatic lower extremity amputation.[6] With that in mind, it is of particular importance to assess the patient's diabetes status (Fig. 18.1).

Following a thorough review of systems, a quick but thorough objective examination of the foot should occur. This examination should include assessments of the vascular, sensory, motor, and autonomic systems, as well as a mobility assessment and footwear inspection.

VASCULAR ASSESSMENT

It could be argued that a thorough vascular assessment is the most crucial aspect of the evaluation of vulnerable feet. Not only can impaired blood flow be a causative agent for the development of ulceration, it will also impact healing of ulcers regardless of the etiology. A clinical vascular examination can be performed quickly and help the clinician decide if circulation is adequate or if further, more advanced testing is required. The examination should begin with an assessment of the pedal pulses (dorsalis pedis and posterior tibial). Pulses can be recorded as present or absent or can be graded on a more qualitative basis (Fig. 18.2):

0 = Unable to palpate
1+ = Barely perceptible
2+ = Weak
3+ = Normal
4+ = Bounding pulse; possible Charcot joint or aneurysm

A study by Mohammedi and colleagues found that the absence of peripheral pulses was a strong independent predictor for risk of outcomes, such as peripheral artery disease (PAD), for individuals with type 2 diabetes.[7] These findings support the examination of peripheral pulses that may ameliorate early detection and medical management of vascular complications, especially for individuals who may have limited healthcare access to technical resources. The assessment of pulses should not be used alone to determine the extent of arterial compromise but should be correlated with other findings from the clinical examination.

The ankle-brachial index (ABI) is a simple, noninvasive clinical test that should be applied to diagnose PAD. ABI assessment is the "gold standard" for screening and diagnosing PAD.[8] In an effort to standardize the measurement technique when obtaining an ABI value, in 2012 the American Heart Association (AHA) developed a scientific position statement entitled "Measurement and Interpretation of the ABI."[9] The ABI is the ratio of the systolic blood pressure at the ankle (pedal arteries) to the blood pressure in the upper arm (brachial artery). The ABI should be performed by a clinician who has received specific education and training in the measurement technique using proper equipment. The AHA recommends using Doppler. The Wound Osteotomy and Continence Nursing society reports the ABI obtained using a pocket Doppler is interchangeable with vascular laboratory tests to detect PAD.[10] The systolic pressure is recorded in both arms, unless contraindicated (lymphedema, dialysis port), and the higher of the two values should be used. In the foot the dorsalis pedis and posterior tibial artery are both assessed and the highest value is used (Fig. 18.3).

Normal: 1 to 1.29

- Borderline: 0.91 to 0.99
- Mild PAD: 0.71 to 0.90
- Medium severe PAD: 0.41 to 0.7
- Severe PAD: <0.4

$$\text{ABI} = \frac{\text{Highest ankle systolic pressure}}{\text{Highest brachial systolic pressure}}$$

A normal ABI is 1.0, which indicates normal arterial blood flow to the foot. An ABI value of less than 0.9 should

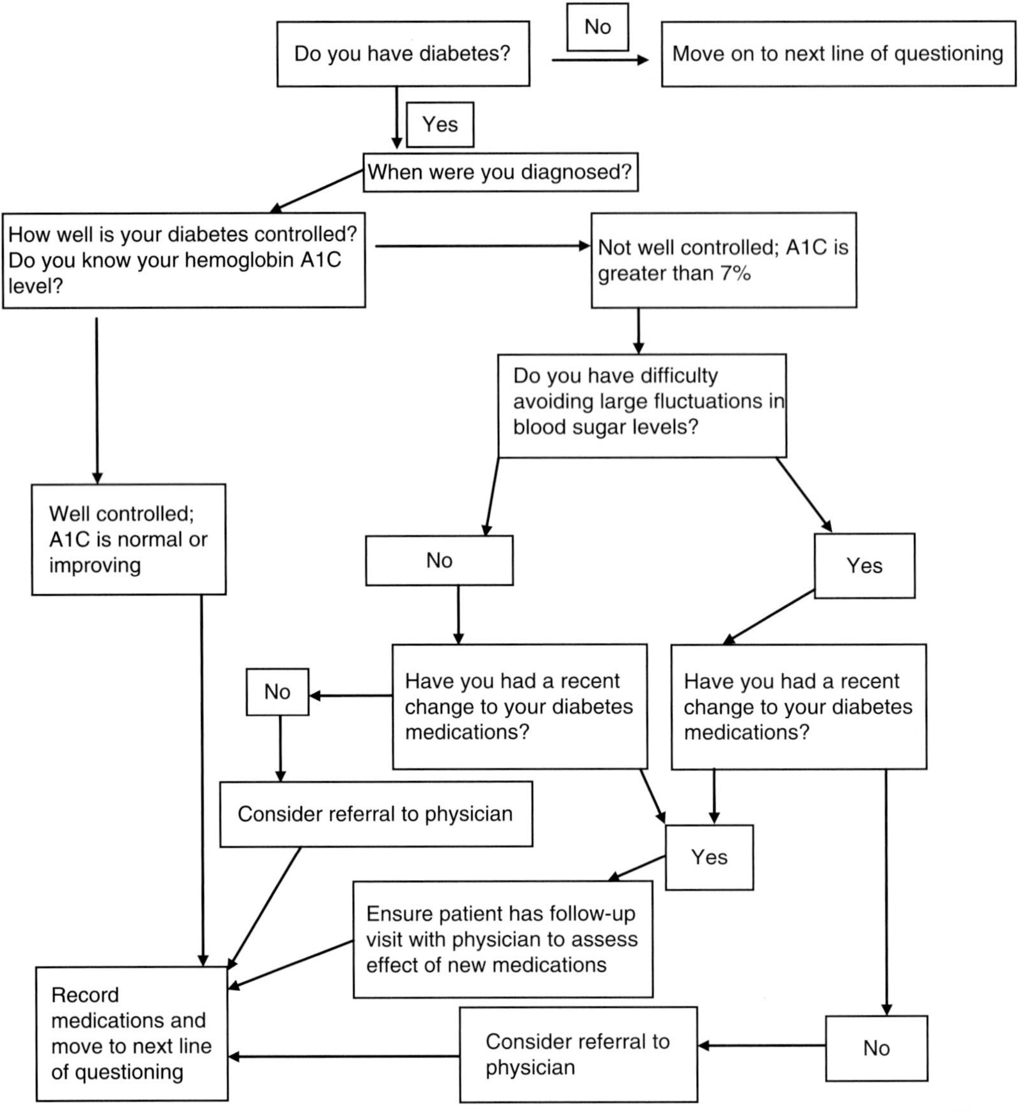

Fig. 18.1 Flow sheet for diabetes assessment.

be referred to the referring physician, who may in turn make a referral to a vascular specialist for further testing. In the case of individuals with long-standing diabetes, an ABI greater than 1.2 may be obtained because of calcified vessels in the lower extremity. If this is the case, the ABI value is of no significance as it pertains to arterial flow and further testing is required.

One test that can be performed is the toe pressure test. By using a specially designed cuff that fits over the digit and a Doppler flowmeter, the pressure in the digital arteries, which are less affected by calcification, can be assessed (Fig. 18.4). A systolic toe pressure greater than 50 mm Hg is generally considered normal; an increased risk of amputation and failure to heal is associated with pressures less than 30 mm Hg.[10]

Another noninvasive vascular assessment technique is transcutaneous oxygen pressure ($TcPO_2$). Low $TcPO_2$ measurement, a measurement of skin perfusion, is a predictor of ulceration[4] and healing.[11] Studies have found that the use of abnormal toe systolic pressures and $TcPO_2$ measurements[12,13] can predict poor outcomes.[14] In general, no single noninvasive test provides enough information to make decisions about vascular intervention. Analysis is usually done by a vascular specialist who interprets the results of a combination of tests.

If signs of arterial insufficiency are present and the patient has a foot wound, or if the patient has none of the typical symptoms of ischemia but has a nonhealing wound despite adequate control of infection and external pressure, referral for further vascular evaluation is warranted. Many patients have significant arterial disease but few clinical signs, such as pain or open wounds, that warrant the risks involved with an invasive vascular procedure. They should still be educated in foot care and proper shoe fit. Because better circulation may be necessary to heal an open wound than to keep unbroken skin intact, the goal for patients with arterial insufficiency is to prevent foot wounds from occurring.

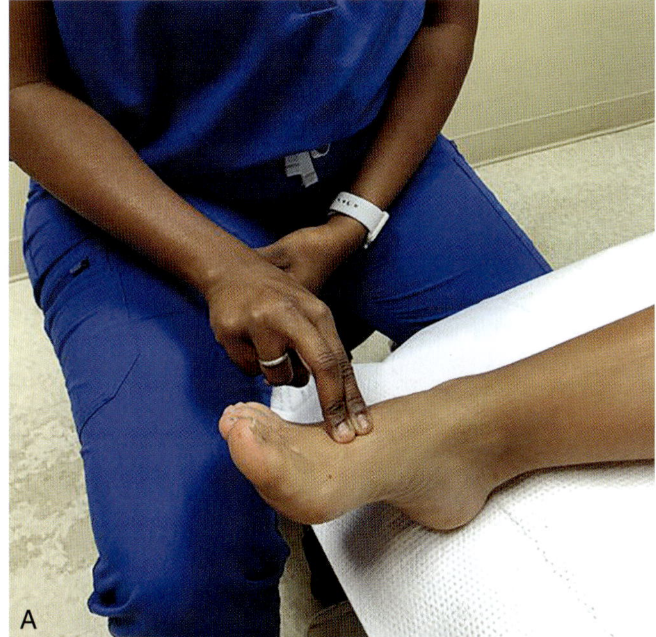

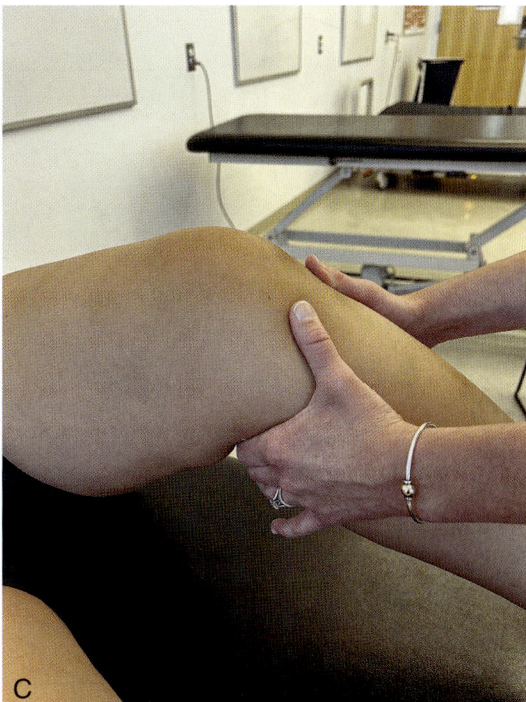

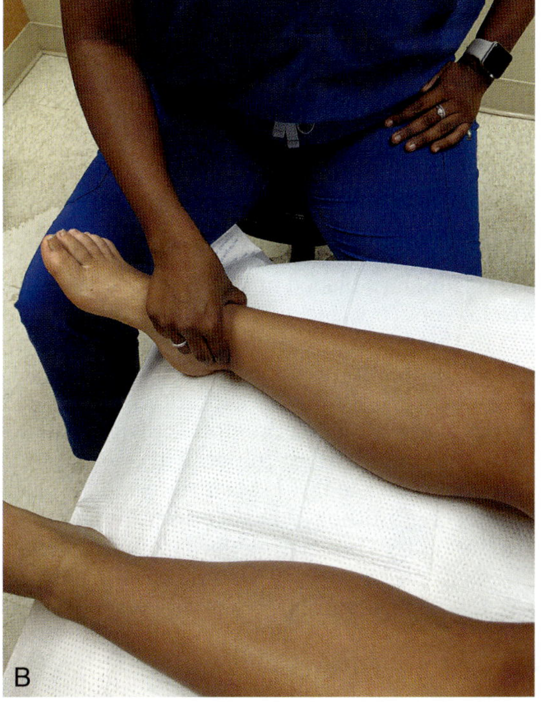

Fig. 18.2 Palpation of pedal pulses. (A) Dorsalis pedis pulse. (B) Posterior tibial pulse. (C) Popliteal pulse.

SENSORY ASSESSMENT

Patients in all settings, with many different diagnoses, may have impaired sensation. Diabetes is the most common reason for impaired sensation, but it is also associated with chronic alcoholism, syphilis, Hansen disease (formerly leprosy), spinal cord injury, and peripheral nerve injuries. Regardless of the cause, when the ability to perceive an external stimulus is diminished, it increases the risk for ulceration. In patients with diabetes, a loss of protective sensation is the leading cause of foot ulceration.[15,16] Simply put, if a patient cannot feel discomfort, there is no stimulus to change anything. In the case of a foot rubbing on a shoe or brace, an individual with intact sensation will stop to address the problem because of discomfort, whereas the person with impaired sensation may be unaware of the problem until the shoes are removed and blood is seen on the sock.

Protective sensation can be assessed in several different ways in the clinic, with very little special equipment needed. The two simplest methods are Semmes-Weinstein monofilaments and tuning forks. A 5.07 monofilament, which takes 10 g of perpendicular force to bend, is the most widely used clinical tool for the assessment of protective sensation (Fig. 18.5).

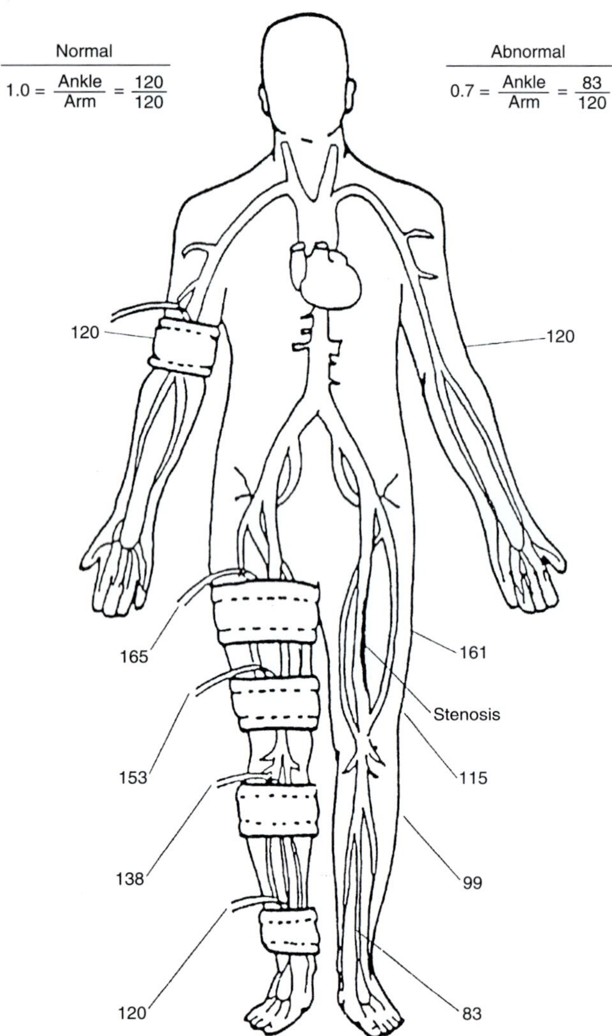

Fig. 18.3 Ankle-brachial index ratio of pedal systolic pressure and brachial systolic pressure.

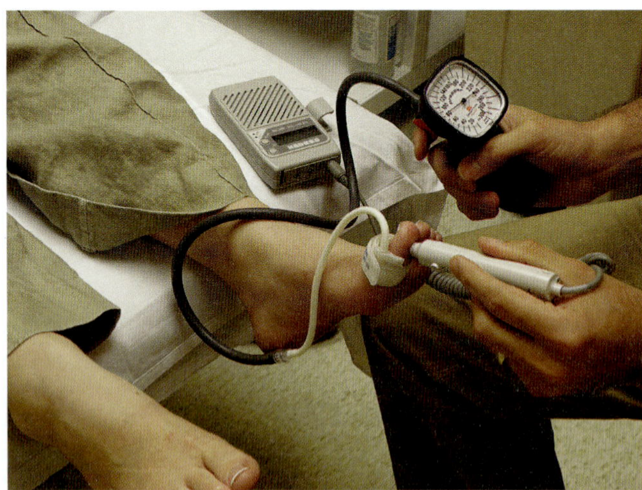

Fig. 18.4 Toe cuff for the assessment of digital blood flow.

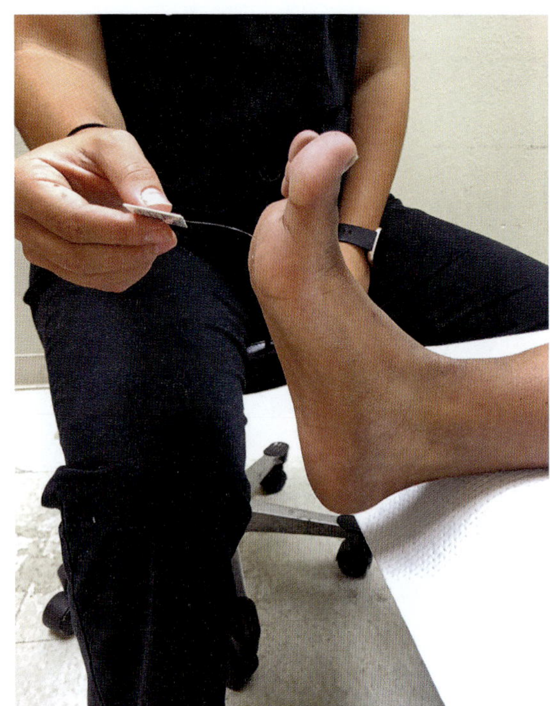

Fig. 18.5 Semmes-Weinstein monofilament.

The patient is instructed to close his or her eyes, and the monofilament is applied perpendicular to the skin surface with enough pressure to cause it to bend. Inability to sense the monofilament is considered to be a positive test for the loss of protective sensation. Care must be taken to avoid areas with thick callus, because the test results will not be valid. Alternatively, a tuning fork can be used for vibratory testing. A study by Oyer and associates found a vibrating 128-Hz tuning fork placed on the toe was more sensitive to the onset of neuropathic changes than monofilament testing.[17,18] In this testing procedure a clanging tuning fork is placed on the area to be tested and remains there until the subject can no longer feel the vibration. The tuning fork is then quickly moved to an area of known intact sensation on either the subject or examiner. If the vibration can still be felt in that site, the test is positive for a loss of vibratory sensation. Other authors[19] have found similar results using similar methods with tuning forks of different frequencies, for example, 512 Hz, which may be more convenient because the 512-Hz tuning fork is smaller (Fig. 18.6).[19]

MOTOR ASSESSMENT

A thorough musculoskeletal evaluation is necessary to determine a given patient's likelihood for ulceration. Deformities and abnormal biomechanics often change pressure distribution in the foot and can lead to discomfort, callus, and, ultimately, ulceration. The clinician can begin to assess for motor impairments while the patient is seated. The wear pattern on shoes, as well as the presence of calluses on the foot, can identify potential pathologies that ultimately may lead to ulcer formation. Following a visual inspection of the feet and footwear, a musculoskeletal examination that includes reflexes, strength, and range of motion should be performed. Particular attention should be paid to toe extension and dorsiflexion range of motion because limitations in either one greatly increases weight-bearing forces through the forefoot in the latter stance phases of gait. This becomes

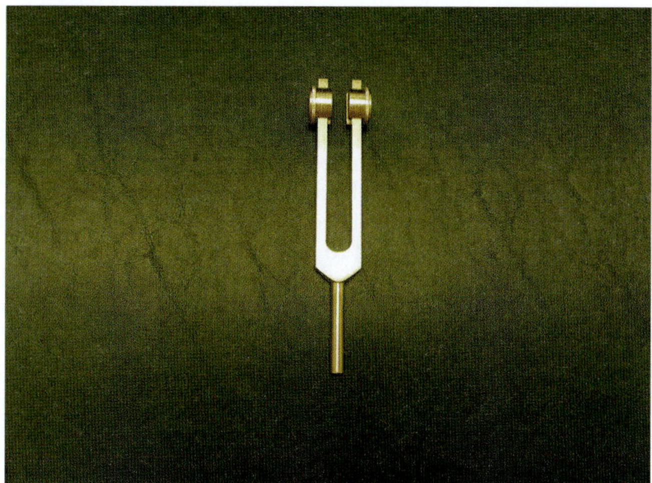

Fig. 18.6 Tuning fork for the assessment of neuropathy.

increasingly important to assess if the patient has diabetes, because a loss of dorsiflexion has been widely documented in that population. If a patient is ambulatory, a gait assessment should be a standard part of the high-risk foot assessment.[20] Major deviations from the normal gait pattern can be assessed with a quick visual inspection. For example, patients with peroneal nerve injuries have difficulty with foot clearance and have a shorter loading response, which increases pressure at the forefoot. Alternatively, a patient could have increased forefoot pressure in terminal stance as a result of limited dorsiflexion range of motion. A mild limitation in motion may present as an early heel rise, whereas a more severe restriction can lead to excessive knee flexion for clearance during the swing phase of gait. With a static foot assessment, it may be apparent that both individuals have increased forefoot pressure, but the cause would not be known, with the result that the optimal intervention could not be selected. With careful gait analysis, the clinician can determine the cause of the pressure and choose appropriate interventions, such as a rocker bottom shoe to substitute for the midfoot rocker in the first case or an orthosis to aid in dorsiflexion in the second case. Chapter 5 provides an in-depth review of the gait assessment.

Many of the deformities that occur as a result of motor neuropathy are more subtle than the previous examples. As neuropathy advances, the intrinsic muscles atrophy and become weaker, leading to muscle imbalances and changes in joint alignment.[19,21] When tissues over these joints are then loaded, they are unable to withstand the same amount of pressure and begin to break down. As extensor muscles on the dorsum of the foot overpower flexor muscles of the plantar aspect, the net result is extension at the metatarsophalangeal joint, which increases pressure at the plantar aspect of the metatarsal head (MTH). This occurs with both claw and hammer toe deformities, the difference being that claw toes are characterized by flexion of both interphalangeal (IP) joints, whereas hammer toes have flexion at the proximal IP and extension at the distal IP joint. Care must also be taken to protect the distal tips of the toes, as well as the dorsum of the IP joints, because these areas are easily injured from rubbing on shoes. Persons with diabetes who have motor neuropathy may develop a high-risk foot, commonly referred to as an "intrinsic minus" foot because of the impairment in function of the small muscles of the foot. The intrinsic minus foot presents as a pes cavus (high arch) deformity with prominent MTHs. Compounding matters is the distal migration of the metatarsal fat pad into the toe sulcus as a result of muscle imbalance. Now the metatarsal region has increased pressure because of the foot shape, as well as the loss of fat pad over the MTH that would normally increase the total surface area being loaded.[22]

Partial foot amputation is another deformity that alters plantar pressure distribution. Because the surface area to carry the force of body weight is smaller, pressure on the remaining structures increases. Studies that have looked at great toe amputation in patients with diabetes have found an increase in plantar pressure and the development of new deformities and ulcerations after amputation.[23,24] As loss of parts of the foot occurs, the mechanics of the foot change, transferring stresses to new areas with the potential for ulceration.

Plantar ulceration has been associated with lower extremity peripheral neuropathy and excessive plantar pressures.[25] Pressure on the soft tissues of the foot is related to three variables: the magnitude of the force applied to the foot, the amount of surface over which the force is applied, and the length of time over which the force is sustained. Because much of the focus in treating and preventing foot ulcers is on reducing pressure, one must understand the relationship of pressure to these three variables. The following formula should be considered:

$$\text{Pressure} = \text{Force}/\text{Area}$$

As indicated, anything that increases the magnitude of the force applied to the foot or decreases the area over which the force is applied increases pressure and makes tissue damage more likely. Immediate injury can occur from extremely high force applied over a small area, as when a patient steps on a tack or piece of glass. Injury occurs because tremendously high pressure exceeds the tensile strength of the skin. Pressure on the foot can also become excessive when a moderate amount of force is repeatedly applied over a small surface area—when bony deformities cause small localized areas of weight bearing or when partial foot amputations decrease the patient's weight-bearing surface. The force applied to the foot (body weight) remains essentially the same, but the actual pressure on the tissues is greater because of reduction of the surface area. In patients with diabetes, factors such as limited joint mobility, structural abnormalities, and previous amputation[26] can lead to increased force or decreased surface area. All of these are associated with increased plantar pressures and ulceration.

Further complicating this picture is the time factor. In looking at tissue ischemia and resultant ulceration, Kosiak found an inverse relationship between the amount of pressure applied to tissues and length of time that the pressure was sustained.[27] Low pressures sustained over long periods of time caused tissue necrosis. This is the mechanism of tissue injury when decubitus ulceration occurs in bedridden, poorly mobile patients. Tissue necrosis also occurs along the medial or lateral borders of the feet or tops of hammer toes when patients wear shoes that are too tight. Kosiak found that as the magnitude of pressure increased, fewer hours were necessary to induce injury.

The most common cause of skin breakdown in the neuropathic foot is repeated bouts of moderate pressure during everyday walking.[28] For health professionals who care for patients with diabetic foot problems, two facts from this research hold particular significance. First, when the inflammatory changes (heat and swelling) began to persist from 1 day to the next, breakdown of the tissue was prevented by discontinuing the repeated stress. Second, breakdown was prevented by either decreasing the amount of pressure per repetition or by reducing the number of repetitions.

AUTONOMIC ASSESSMENT

Autonomic changes represent the third category of changes associated with polyneuropathy.[29,30] With roles including the regulation of moisture and blood flow, as well as controlling hair and nail growth and overall skin integrity, the autonomic system is crucial to healthy feet. Cracks and fissures in the foot, as well as nail pathologies, can predispose people to ulceration or infection. Because these are all end products of autonomic dysfunction, patients need to be educated on how to prevent them from occurring. Patients with autonomic dysfunction, most commonly from diabetes, should be educated to moisturize their feet often so as to avoid drying and cracking of the skin. Creams or non–alcohol-based lotions should be applied liberally to the feet and legs, but the areas between the toes should be avoided because the excess moisture can lead to fungal infections. Not only is moisturized skin more comfortable, it is also stronger and less likely to develop cracks and fissures, which are easy entries for infections. If nails are too thick to be trimmed safely at home with regular nail clippers, the patient should be encouraged to seek professional help for nail care.

One of the most damaging outcomes related to dysfunction of the autonomic system is diabetic neuropathic osteoarthropathy, also known as Charcot foot. This destructive process can significantly alter the bony architecture of the foot and can lead to excessive plantar pressures[31] and subsequent ulceration if left unchecked (Fig. 18.7). This process was first recognized in patients with syphilis during the 19th century by Jean-Martin Charcot. Although several neuropathic diseases, including syphilis and Hansen disease, can cause a Charcot arthropathy, it is most commonly seen in persons with diabetes.[31] Charcot foot is a progressive disorder that leads to joint dislocation, fractures, and deformity of the foot.[32]

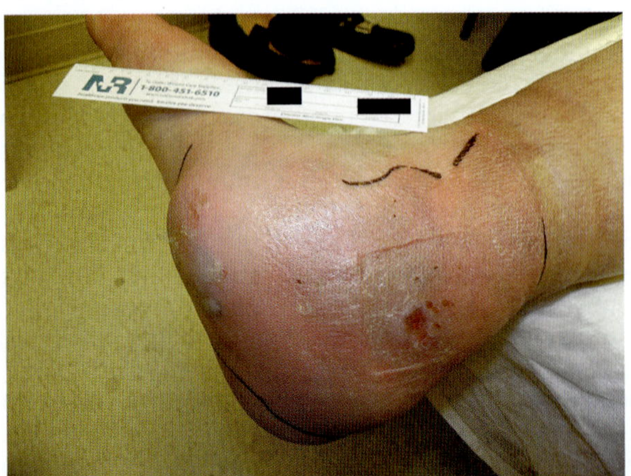

Fig. 18.7 Charcot foot with ulceration, infection, and deformity.

Charcot surmised that when the proper functioning of the autonomic system was impaired by disease, it led to an increase in blood flow to the bones, which then led to bone resorption. Over time, this became known as the neurovascular theory.[33] A second theory states that development of a Charcot foot is related to trauma in an insensate foot. Because of the lack of sensation, there is no perception of the trauma, and thus no adjustments to compensate for it. If the joint continues to be loaded, it will stay inflamed and eventually break down. This became the neurotraumatic theory.[34] Charcot foot is thought to be an inflammatory process.[35] The underlying cause is persistent hyperglycemia and microvascular disease, leading to nerve injury via osmotic changes and ischemia.[35] There is sensory neuropathy, loss of pain sensation, and the incidence of trauma including recurrent microtrauma. On clinical examination, the foot is erythematous and edematous, has an elevated skin temperature, and has reduced sensation to nociceptive pain and pressure.[36]

Charcot foot can become debilitating if not recognized early enough to arrest the development of the rocker bottom deformity that is characteristic of the disease. It is often misdiagnosed because no single diagnostic test can confirm its presence. Medical history, clinical manifestations, and radiographic findings all must be considered. Unfortunately, the clinical presentation of a red, hot, swollen foot often leads to the diagnosis of cellulitis, which is treated with antibiotics. During the time the patient is being treated with antibiotics for an infection that does not exist, they are continuing to damage the foot by walking on it. Radiographs taken in the acute phase are not sensitive to the development of neuropathic fractures, and bone scans do not differentiate Charcot foot from osteomyelitis.[37] Magnetic resonance imaging, although a costly imaging technique, is extremely useful for evaluating the foot and ankle in suspected Charcot neuropathy and is capable of identifying bone injury prior to complete fracture.[37]

Charcot foot should be suspected if a patient with neuropathy presents with sudden onset of localized swelling, warmth, and erythema in the absence of an open wound. Appropriate treatment for Charcot foot should be initiated until this condition is ruled out on further testing. During acute Charcot arthropathy, joint destruction can be minimized by immobilization in a TCC and avoidance of weight bearing until signs of healing become apparent (decreased temperature, decreased swelling, and improved radiographic findings). Both lack of compliance with non–weight bearing and use of orthotic devices in place of cast immobilization have shown prolonged healing times.[38] When cast immobilization is discontinued, the use of an orthotic device for continued protection of the joints during the initial return to weight bearing should be considered.[39]

The architectural changes that occur in the foot secondary to neuropathic osteoarthropathy result in high-pressure areas. Because of this, following the period of immobilization and limited weight bearing, patients with a history of Charcot foot must be provided with appropriate footwear to stabilize the foot and reduce plantar pressure. Surgical intervention may be indicated for unstable or severely malaligned fractures or dislocations, which create problems with recurrent ulceration, fitting of shoes, ability to ambulate, and recalcitrant ulcers.[40] Some of these procedures require months of immobilization and avoidance of weight bearing, which can be difficult for many patients with diabetes and neuropathy. Such surgery is usually advocated only if nonsurgical management fails.

FOOTWEAR ASSESSMENT

The analysis of the high-risk foot truly begins before the patient sits on the examination table. The type and appearance of the footwear they are wearing can give insight as to the cause of their pathology. Shoes that either do not fit properly or are excessively worn can cause problems, including blisters, calluses, and wounds. On the other hand, shoes that someone refuses to wear are not useful as they will just sit in the closet.

Characteristics of the proper shoe for the high-risk foot include:

- Snug fit at the heel to prevent pistoning (moving up and down) of the heel
- Wide toe box to accommodate for deformities such as bunions and hallux valgus
- Deep toe box to accommodate claw/hammer toes and molded inserts
- Fashionable enough that the patient will wear the shoes

It is recommended that people shop for new shoes in the mid-to-late afternoon to ensure the best fit. Because foot size changes throughout the day, a shoe purchased to fit the foot early in the morning may be too small by late evening, and conversely a shoe bought at night may be too large for the foot in the morning.

GAIT AND BALANCE

Motor neuropathy causes weakness of foot and ankle musculature that may result in gait deviations that change plantar pressure patterns or contribute to instability. Gait and balance are also affected by damage to sensory nerves, which leads to an inability to sense where the foot is in space. The use of ankle-foot orthoses or shoe modifications may help restore a more normal gait, stabilize joints, or improve balance.[39] Studies have found that patients with peripheral neuropathy secondary to diabetes have problems with gait and postural stability.[41,42] In examining a patient with a high-risk foot, physical therapists must include not only the patients' foot problems but also their overall functional status. To reduce the morbidity associated with falls, recommendations that address safety and function should be included in the treatment plan.[43]

Wound Assessment

Although it is clear that the most effective way to prevent amputations is to avoid getting wounds in the first place, that is not always possible. When a wound does develop, regardless of the etiology, a thorough wound assessment becomes a necessity. The comprehensive wound assessment begins with a thorough patient history, which helps the clinician not only gain a better understanding of the cause of the wound, but also forecast healing rates of the wound more accurately. It is often helpful to take the entire patient history prior to undressing the wound, because there is a tendency to focus solely on the wound once it is visible and forget about other factors that may be important.

Once the patient history is reviewed, the wound can be carefully undressed. In addition to the components already discussed for the evaluation of the high-risk foot, the assessment also includes an examination of the immediate wound and periwound area. The wound should be assessed for location, color, odor, size/depth, and drainage type and amount, and the periwound tissues should be assessed for any abnormalities (Fig. 18.8).

LOCATION

After a thorough medical history has been taken, the examiner may have a good hypothesis as to the cause of a wound before even seeing it. The objective examination can either confirm or refute this hypothesis. One of the first objective findings that should be documented is wound location. Although traumatic wounds can occur in any anatomic location, many of the common wound etiologies tend to occur most frequently in certain areas. Diabetic foot (neuropathic) ulcers are most common on the plantar aspect of the digits and MTHs, more specifically, the great toe and first MTH, but they can occur in any area of high stress.[25] Ulceration secondary to neuropathy is also common on the dorsum of the toes, as well as bony prominences, such as the lateral aspect of the first and fifth MTHs and the base of the fifth metatarsal, and anywhere a shoe or brace may be rubbing. Wounds secondary to vascular insufficiency can occur in any location that has impaired blood flow but are most frequently found on the toes, dorsum, and lateral aspects of the foot, as well as the lateral leg. In contrast, wounds of venous origin tend to be in what is often referred to as the "gaiter" area, just proximal to the medial malleolus. It should be noted that these are general guidelines, and an accurate diagnosis cannot be made based solely on location. When describing wound location, the clinician should be as precise as possible, often using bony landmarks as descriptors. This becomes increasingly important when multiple wounds are present.

WOUND COLOR

A simple designation for wound color is to use the red-yellow-black staging system, which was first published in the United States in 1988 and had been used in Europe prior to that.[44] Red wounds are generally healthy, well vascularized, and progressing through the normal stages of healing. The red appearance is attributed to the deposition of highly vascularized collagen, known as granulation tissue. This tissue is fragile and may bleed with excessive force or friction. Granulation tissue that bleeds with minimal pressure or has a dusky appearance is called *friable* and should be investigated further as it is typically a sign of increased bacteria present in the wound. Yellow wounds indicate fibrinous slough or infection is present. Slough has a stringy, adherent characteristic and can be removed by a variety of methods, which are discussed later in this chapter (see section "Preparing the Wound Bed by Eliminating the Source of Inflammation or Infection"). Wounds also may have a black appearance, which signifies the presence of eschar. Eschar is often hard to the touch but can be soft or boggy if there is a lot of fluid present. In most cases, it is beneficial to remove the eschar because the necrotic tissue promotes the proliferation of bacteria. Several instances when this is not advised are intact eschar on heels and vascular wounds that would not be able to heal following débridement. In addition to the red-yellow-black system that is focused on the dermis, the clinician must also be aware of deeper structures that may be apparent in the wound bed. The first tissue encountered beneath the dermis is known as subcutaneous tissue, fat, or adipose. This should have a pale yellow, moist appearance when healthy but dries out and darkens when it is nonviable. Healthy muscle has a bright red color, and the striations are often visible in the tissue. Damaged muscle takes on a dusky gray appearance with a much-less-pliable texture. The remaining structures that will be encountered in a deep wound bed—ligaments, tendons, bone—all should be white if well vascularized. If these tissues are compromised, they will take on a dusky yellow appearance and continue to darken as damage proceeds.

Subjective exam:

Pain: Last dressing change:

Comments:

Objective exam:

Mode of arrival:

Assistive device:

Wearing prescribed dressings/footwear?

Wound location:

If other, enter location:

Wound stage:

Wound color:

Color	Pre-débridement	Post-débridement
	%	%
	%	%
	%	%

Odor:

Size: cm²

L: W: D:

Drainage amount:

Drainage type:

Periwound:

Nails:

Edema:

Sensation:

Pulses: (L) (R)

DP		
PT		
Popliteal		
ABI		

Range of motion:

Special Tests: Results:

Fig. 18.8 Wound assessment flow sheet. *ABI*, Ankle-brachial index *DP*, dorsalis pedis; *PT*, posterior tibial.

Comments:

Treatment:

Wound cleansed with

Débridement performed today? Débridement type:

Modalities:

Dressings: Offloading:

Comments:

Assessment:

Tolerance to treatment:

Comments:

Plan:

Comments:

Follow up:

Nails:

Edema:

Sensation:

Pulses: (L) (R)

DP		
PT		
Popliteal		
ABI		

Range of motion:

Special Tests: Results:

Fig. 18.8 Cont'd

For documentation purposes, the use of percentages is helpful in describing the wound color. For example, a wound could be 80% red, with 20% firmly adhered yellow fibrin. It is also suggested that the percentage should be documented before and after treatment if there is any significant change in the wound appearance. The use of clinical pathways and other intervention strategies such as dedicated foot clinics in the diagnosis and treatment of patients with diabetes at risk for foot ulceration can improve patient outcomes by reducing the need for lower extremity amputation.[45]

ODOR

One of the most troubling aspects of a wound from a patient's perspective is odor. Most significant wounds will have some odor when dressings are removed. As a clinician, it is important to know whether or not the odor is caused by infection or simply from the dressing having been in place for an extended period. Before making this determination, dressings should be removed and the wound should be rinsed with sterile water or saline. Odors that are eradicated are likely caused by drainage on the dressings. This is especially true of occlusive dressings, such as hydrocolloids. If cleansing the wound does not eliminate the odor, it is more likely caused by necrotic or infected tissue. Wounds with a strong odor often contain anaerobic and aerobic bacteria and are referred to as *polymicrobial*; anaerobic bacteria create odor by releasing compounds including putrescine and cadaverine. These odors can be extremely strong and are often described as acrid smelling. Aerobic bacteria also are capable of producing foul odors. Because the strength of an odor is subjective, it is recommended that descriptions such as sweet, fishy, necrotic, putrid, and the like also be included in the assessment of the odor. Infection should be considered when previously odor-free wounds develop an odor, but it should also be pointed out that some infections do not produce any odor at all.

SIZE

Wound size should be documented on a routine basis because it is an easy way to monitor progress in wound healing. For most wounds, unless they are perfectly symmetric, a diameter or even length and width may not give an accurate representation as to the true size of the wound. When length and width are used, the largest length is recorded, and the width is recorded perpendicular to the length. Although improvements can be seen as these numbers decrease, it is difficult to accurately calculate a total surface area for the wound or a percent area reduction because wounds are irregularly shaped. Alternative methods include photography with a transparent film over the wound, wound tracings with transparent film, and digital cameras that can calculate the surface area of the wound. Newer technologies using smartphone applications for wound imaging and measurement are being developed. All of these options enable the clinician to calculate surface area and percent reduction in size.

Regardless of the method used to calculate wound size, the orientation of the wound should be standardized to ensure that subsequent measurements are assessing the same dimension. Bony landmarks can be used for this purpose, but it is most common to describe length in a cephalocaudal (head-to-toe) fashion and width perpendicular to that. Unfortunately, the largest dimensions of most wounds will not line up perfectly with axes along the cephalocaudal and perpendicular plane. For this reason, many clinicians describe wound orientation using a clock face, with 12 o'clock being at the head and 6 o'clock at the feet. Using this system, a wound could be described as 6 cm in length from 10 o'clock to 4 o'clock and 3 cm in width from 1 o'clock to 7 o'clock. Undermining, tunneling, or any other abnormality in the wound can also be described using the clock face, which will help with consistency in measurement, especially if another clinician is measuring the wound.

DEPTH

A thorough understanding of anatomy is necessary for accurate staging of wounds. In turn, accurate staging of wounds relies on being able to assess wound depth properly. Before depth can be measured, the wound must be free of nonviable tissue so the wound base can be visualized or probed. The wound can then be probed with a sterile probe held perpendicular to the skin surface. Because wounds do not all have a uniform depth throughout, the deepest point should be measured and the location where the measurement was taken should be documented. After the depth measurement is obtained, wounds can be classified in several ways, depending on the etiology. Table 18.1 reviews different wound classification systems that rely on wound depth as a part of the staging criteria.[46–49] The revised pressure injury classification system by the National Pressure Injury Advisory Panel includes illustrations that clarify proper staging of pressure injuries.

DRAINAGE

The ideal wound will have enough moisture to prevent desiccation of the wound bed, but not so much that it causes breakdown of periwound tissues. The characteristics of wound drainage will vary depending on multiple factors, including wound location, vascular status, and presence of infection. Drainage should be classified by amount and type to accurately describe what is occurring in the wound. Assessing the amount of drainage is somewhat subjective in that it is not practical, or even possible in many cases, to weigh the amount of exudate from the wound. Instead, the clinician describes the amount of exudate along a continuum, such as the following one:

None→Scant→Minimal→Moderate→Heavy→Copious

This can be difficult to quantify, especially for the inexperienced clinician, because different dressings will absorb vastly different amounts of fluid and thus could make a heavily draining wound appear drier, or vice versa. Wounds with underlying arterial insufficiency tend to be drier because less circulation is getting to the wound bed, whereas patients with wounds that are venous in nature often experience heavy drainage because of the edema present. When the amount of exudate increases and a reason is not clearly stated that relates to the change, such as changes in treatment approach (i.e., surgical intervention to increase blood flow, discontinuation of compression therapy, or resting in dependent positions), then infection should be considered as a likely cause. The presence of infection causes the wound to remain in the inflammatory phase of wound healing, which results in increased drainage. Infected wounds often exhibit purulent drainage, which can be yellow, green, tan, or even creamy or cloudy. These wounds often require a combination of local and systemic agents to treat the infection. In addition to purulent drainage, drainage can also be serous (watery), sanguineous (bloody), or serosanguineous (pink or reddish, watery).

PERIWOUND SKIN

The area immediately surrounding a wound, known as the *periwound skin*, should be assessed carefully because

Table 18.1 Wound Classification Systems

Classification System	Intended Wound Etiologies	Grades	Comments
Wagner[46]	Diabetic foot	0 = Intact skin 1 = Superficial ulcer 2 = Deep ulcer (through dermis) 3 = Infection 4 = Partial foot gangrene 5 = Full foot gangrene	
University of Texas[47]	Diabetic foot	A0 = Preulcerative or postulcerative lesion AI = Superficial wound AII = Involves tendon or capsule AIII = Involves bone or joint	Letter stage changes as follows: B = Infection C = Ischemia D = Infection and ischemia
Partial/full	All wounds	Partial = Involves epidermis and up to part of the dermis Full = Involves structures deep to the dermis	
Burns[48]	Burns	Superficial = Epidermis only Superficial partial = Superficial dermis involved Deep partial = Deep dermis involved Full thickness = Subcutaneous tissue involved Subdermal = Muscle, tendon, bone involved	Some experts do not make a distinction between full-thickness and subdermal burns, because both require surgery to heal[129]
National Pressure Injury Advisory Panel[49]	Pressure injury stages	1 = Nonblanchable erythema; skin is intact 2 = Partial-thickness skin loss with exposed dermis 3 = Full-thickness skin loss; fascia or any structure deep to fascia are not visible 4 = Full-thickness skin and tissue loss with exposed or palpable fascia or subfascial tissues (muscle, tendon, ligament, capsule, bone) Unstageable = Full-thickness pressure injury: Obscured full-thickness skin and tissue loss and slough. Deep tissue injury = Nonblanchable with deep red, maroon or purple discoloration	When teaching about the unstageable pressure injury, explain it is termed "unstageable" because the wound base cannot be visualized, not because the clinician cannot determine the stage of injury. Important to explain the difference between a nonblanchable stage 1 that should resolve with proper offloading and nonblanchable with deep tissue injury, which is likely to open to a larger wound.

it can give clues as to the state of the wound. Evidence of excessive pressure, excess moisture, decreased vascularity, and the presence of infection can all be found in the periwound skin with a quick visual inspection and palpation. Table 18.2 lists periwound findings and their significance.

In addition to the factors listed in Table 18.2, the amount of soft tissue over prominent areas also can be assessed. Decreased amounts of soft-tissue bulk have been identified in persons with diabetic neuropathy in comparison with persons without diabetes used as controls.[50] With less soft tissue present, peak pressures at the prominent areas are increased, which increases the likelihood of ulceration.

Wound Management

The larger concept of wound bed preparation and wound healing involves understanding the source of the wound and addressing the patient in a holistic manner.[51,52] The acronym "TIME"[53] is used to highlight key factors that must be addressed:

T = Tissue management
I = Inflammation and infection control
M = Moisture balance
E = Epithelial (edge) advancement

Successful wound-healing interventions can be categorized into a few essential steps, which are discussed in detail. These overlapping steps include:

1. Preparing the wound bed by eliminating the source of inflammation or infection.
2. Providing an optimal wound-healing environment.
3. Reducing further trauma to the wound.
4. Keeping the wound healed once it has closed and preventing new ulcers from forming.

PREPARING THE WOUND BED BY ELIMINATING THE SOURCE OF INFLAMMATION OR INFECTION

The current model of infections that is most widely used involves the interaction between the host response and the amount of bacteria present in the wound. As outlined by this model, a patient with a healthy immune response is able to tolerate a higher bacterial load without developing signs of infection than a patient with an impaired immune response. The amount of bacteria in a wound is usually described on a continuum from sterile to a systemic infection. Sterile wounds have no bacteria, whereas systemic infections have overwhelmed the wound with bacteria and cause systemic immune responses. Intermediate stages include contaminated wounds, characterized by bacteria that is present but not invading the tissue; colonized wounds that are still capable of healing despite invading bacteria; and critical

Table 18.2 Periwound Skin Assessment

Appearance	Description	Significance
Callus	Area of hyperkeratosis, typically in response to high pressures[53,127,128]	Frequently associated with neuropathy and/or bony deformity. Indicates area susceptible to breakdown[127]
Blister	Fluid-filled area causing separation of epidermis from dermis	Shearing forces from rubbing on shoes, brace, bed, etc.; may also be caused by adhesive dressings on skin
Erythema	Redness	Indicates inflammation caused by local stress or infection; redness in immediate periwound area is normal in acute wounds, but excessive redness or redness that persists for 30 to 60 min after the stress is removed requires intervention; erythema associated with infection is often well demarcated; if red streaks are noted (lymphangitis), consult physician because it is a sign of spreading infection
Maceration	Changes in tissue caused by excessive moisture	Can lead to skin breakdown; may be a result of excessive sweating, heavy wound drainage, incontinence, or inappropriate dressings
Induration	Hardening of the tissue because of edema	Chronic edema impairs wound healing; induration is often associated with infection or venous disease
Hemosiderin	Brownish discoloration of the skin around a wound. Associated with deposition of hemoglobin in extravascular tissues	Often associated with venous disease
Excoriation	Wearing away of the skin	Indicates an area of trauma; often preceded by maceration and/or blistering
Presence of scars	A scar is the final result of a previous injury	May give clues to the chronicity of the problem as well as the extent of damage in the area
Temperature	Can be palpated or assessed with infrared thermometer; is typically compared with adjacent areas or to contralateral side	Nonspecific indicator of inflammation; helpful to monitor "hot spots" that may be at risk of breakdown, or for resolution of a Charcot fracture
Edema	Swelling in the tissues	Bilateral edema suggests a systemic problem; unilateral edema indicates a localized problem; can occur with infection, inflammation, venous dysfunction, and lymphedema; consider Charcot foot if insensate
Other changes	Taut, shiny, hairless, cracked skin	Taut, shiny skin with a loss of hair indicates impaired blood flow; cracked skin is associated with aging, diabetes, or vascular disease. Important to moisturize skin frequently

colonization in which the bacteria are overwhelming the immune system and are creating a localized response.[53–55] It is in the colonized and critically colonized wounds, and in infected wounds in conjunction with systemic medications, that selective débridement, modalities, and topical dressings are most helpful in optimizing the wound environment.

An effective means of reducing inflammation and infection risk is removal of the tissue that may harbor bacteria, through a process known as *débridement*. There are many ways débridement can be performed,[56] and all of them are within the scope of practice of the physical therapist except for surgical débridement. Because surgical débridement may involve the excision of viable and nonviable tissue to ensure that all of the necrotic or infected tissue is removed from the area, it is called *nonselective débridement*. Slightly less aggressive is sharp débridement. Sharp and surgical débridement both use sterile sharp instruments to remove tissue, but the tissue that is being débrided is limited to nonviable tissue in sharp débridement. For this reason, sharp débridement is referred to as *selective débridement*. Despite being widely accepted, or perhaps because it is so widely accepted as a standard of care, there is limited evidence on the effectiveness of sharp or surgical débridement. Débridement with sharp instruments is the quickest way to remove undesirable tissue, but is also the riskiest method and is best used by the experienced clinician. Risks can be minimized by using the appropriate equipment and assessing the patient thoroughly to ensure that they do not have any of the contraindications/precautions listed in Box 18.1.

In addition to sharp and surgical débridement, mechanical, acoustic, enzymatic, larval, and autolytic forms of débridement are also viable options. Of these, all are classified as selective with the exception of mechanical débridement. Mechanical débridement can be performed using a variety of methods, including abrasion, wet-to-dry dressings, and whirlpool. All of these methods may remove nonviable tissue but can be detrimental to healthy tissue and, if used at all, should be limited to cases in which the majority of the wound is nonviable.

Historically, whirlpools were frequently included in the treatment plan for an individual with a wound. Proposed benefits were increasing blood flow to the area because of the warm water, as well as the ability to remove dressings and necrotic tissue. The whirlpool also has many shortcomings as a wound care modality, including the risk of cross-contamination, unregulated pressures on the wound, exacerbation of dependent edema, and excessive maceration. As a result, pulsatile lavage with suction (PLWS) has largely replaced the whirlpool as the hydrotherapy of choice for wound management. There are no

Box 18.1 **Contraindications and Precautions to Sharp and Surgical Débridement**

- Medically unstable patient (surgical only)[129]
- Dry gangrene or lack of vascular supply to heal wound[129]
- Intact, dry eschar on heel[130]
- Impaired clotting mechanism or on anticoagulants[52]
- Pyoderma gangrenosum[130]
- Clinician without a thorough knowledge of anatomy of the area to be débrided

absolute contraindications to the use of PLWS, but care must be taken around exposed vessels, vital organs, and fistulas. Precautions must also be taken to reduce the risk of cross-contamination, including using personal protective equipment, treating in a private room, using a shield to prevent backsplash, and disposing of single-use components properly.

PLWS delivers a stream of irrigating solution (irrigant) such as saline or saline with antibiotic. The irrigant solution that can be directed at the area of interest to débride slough and reduce bacterial counts on the wound.[57] It appears that the effectiveness of lavage improves as the amount of irrigant used to flush out bacteria is increased.[58] With PLWS, the water pressure can be controlled and can be delivered within the safe range of 4 to 15 psi, which is effective at removing nonviable tissue and bacteria without traumatizing healthy tissue.[58] For the purposes of reducing bacterial levels, the higher end of that range is recommended, because nearly 85% of bacteria can be removed from a wound with 15 psi. Acoustic, or ultrasonic, energy is the newest form of débridement to enter the wound care arena.[59] Currently, there are several ultrasonic débridement devices on the market that are capable of performing selective débridement. These devices are classified as low-frequency (kilohertz range, as opposed to megahertz with conventional ultrasound) and high-intensity ultrasound devices. Early studies demonstrated effectiveness of these devices at increasing fibrinolysis, improving blood flow to the wound, and reducing bacterial counts, and may be faster than sharp débridement in many cases.[60–62] Recent studies support the evidence that ultrasonic debridement is a safe and efficient method of debridement,[63] and that it is a therapeutic intervention that may contributed to reduced costs for nonhealing wounds.[64] One systemic review in the past 5 years compared healing outcomes for nonsurgical sharp debridement and low-frequency ultrasonic debridement in diabetic patients and identified no significant differences.[65] However, this review was only based on two studies that met the inclusion criteria. Although capable of producing extremely rapid débridement and a reduction in bacteria, the use of ultrasonic débridement remains cost-prohibitive for clinics that do not specialize in wound healing. For that reason an in-depth discussion of ultrasonic débridement is not included in this chapter.

The remaining forms of débridement tend to be slower but are less harmful to healthy tissue. Larval therapy, aka maggot therapy, biosurgical debridement, or biologic debridement involves the use of sterile maggots, which secrete enzymes to liquefy necrotic tissue but have no negative effect on granulation tissue.[66] A hindrance to this type of debridement is the "ick" factor associated with maggots; however, a review of the recent international literature may lead to more acceptance. A qualitative study from Brazil in 2020 identified proper education about the treatment as an important factor related to increased acceptance among patients. Those patients also expressed positive outcomes related to pain and odor reduction, overall wound improvement, and increased levels of hope.[67] A Turkish study compared negative-pressure wound therapy to larval therapy following revascularization in patients with peripheral arterial disease and ischemic wounds. Results of that prospective randomized trial showed a higher percentage of patients in the negative-pressure therapy group required subsequent amputation and only 18.2% of the wounds healed compared to 92.3% in the larval therapy group.[68] Unlike larval therapy where enzymes are excreted, enzymatic débridement involves the application of a topical agent to the wound surface. The enzyme works to denature the protein in the necrotic tissue on the wound bed.[69] Autolytic débridement uses the body's own self-produced enzymes to rid a wound slowly of necrotic tissue.[69] In a moist wound, phagocytic cells and proteolytic enzymes can soften and liquefy the necrotic tissue, which is then digested by macrophages. These débridement strategies should not necessarily be thought of as independent of each other. For example, sharp débridement is often done in conjunction with enzymatic or autolytic débridement. All of the forms of débridement serve to reduce the risk of infection by removing the energy source for the bacteria. There also are interventions that specifically target the bacteria rather than the necrotic tissue.

Over the past several decades, the number of dressings that have been developed to reduce bacteria in the wound has increased dramatically. These include a variety of dressings that contain silver, methylene blue, gentian violet, polyhexamethylene biguanide (PHMB), iodine, or honey. It is important to consider antimicrobial dressings as one component of a comprehensive treatment, and not a cure. As an example of how these dressings can be a beneficial addition to a wound care plan, a randomized control trial comparing ultrasonic debridement with ultrasonic debridement in combination with a PHMB dressing revealed that the addition of the antimicrobial dressing led to significantly lower bacterial counts, reduced pain, fewer wounds that deteriorated, and more wounds that reduced in size.[70] Antimicrobial dressings have been shown to be superior to nonantimicrobial dressings in the reduction of bacteria, but there is insufficient evidence to state one antimicrobial dressing is superior to another in terms of promoting wound healing.[71,72] These dressings are available in so many varieties, ranging in absorptive capacity, adhesive versus nonadhesive, amorphous versus sheet form, and the like, that there is likely a good option for nearly any wound type. What is most important to remember is that none of these dressings should be used as a replacement for systemic antibiotics.

It is common to use topical antimicrobial dressings along with systemic medications, especially in the case of arterial insufficiency. For example, a patient with a diabetic foot ulcer may have an infected toe with poor vascularity. In this case the amount of the systemic antibiotic getting to the infected area may be limited and could benefit from a topical agent to reduce the degree of surface bacteria. There are several problems with the continued use of antimicrobial dressings, namely cost and the concern over developing resistance. Because they are impregnated with antimicrobial agents, these dressings are more expensive than a comparable nonantimicrobial dressing and are not intended to be used for the duration of wound healing. Likewise, there is some concern in the wound care community that overuse of silver dressings may lead to the development of resistant strains of bacteria in the future, similar to what happened with the widespread use of antibiotics.

In addition to antimicrobial dressings and the interventions already discussed, several biophysical agents including electrical stimulation[73] and ultraviolet light, also referred to as phototherapy,[74] have strong evidence supporting their use in the management of infections. Phototherapy includes the use of ultraviolet light, as well as laser light. Electrical stimulation units and ultraviolet light equipment are likely to be found in most physical therapy clinics because these modalities have been standard equipment in their practice for decades, although the use of ultraviolet light is much less common than it once was. An in-depth discussion of stimulation parameters is beyond the scope of this chapter, but a brief description will be provided. Electrical stimulation for wound healing is typically delivered using high-voltage pulsed current. This has short intervals of time where a high amount of voltage causes current to flow in one direction, followed by a much longer time where no current is flowing. The unidirectional flow of current is important because charged particles will be drawn toward the oppositely charged electrode and repelled from the like-charge electrode, just as a positive pole and negative pole on a magnet will stick together and two positives will push each other apart. This concept is known as *galvanotaxis* and is the basis for the use of electrical stimulation in tissue healing. When the goal is to treat an infection, the current recommendation is to place an ionic silver (Ag^+) dressing or gel on the wound surface and cover that with the positive pole (anode).[75] In this setup, the silver will be repelled from the electrode into the tissue where it can interact with bacteria and the bacteria can be attracted to the anode because both gram-negative and gram-positive bacteria carry a net negative charge. The negative pole (cathode) can be placed approximately 15 to 30 cm away. The treatment electrode may be placed on the immediate periwound skin or directly in the wound. If stimulation is applied directly to the wound, the wound must be filled with hydrogel- or saline-moistened gauze. Treatment is usually continued until signs of infection are no longer present or until progress halts, at which time polarity is reversed to jumpstart healing.

Ultraviolet C light is another modality used for the treatment of infected wounds. Ultraviolet therapy is effective in reducing microorganisms in colonized wounds and promoting granular tissue formation, reepithelialization, and sloughing off necrotic tissue. Studies show the use of ultraviolet phototherapy has a shorter mean time to complete wound healing when compared with a control group.[76,77]

PROVIDING AN OPTIMAL WOUND-HEALING ENVIRONMENT

As mentioned previously, it is somewhat of an artificial delineation to break wound healing down into different steps because there is so much overlap. Early in the wound-healing process the primary goal may be removal of nonviable tissue, as mentioned in the previous section, but selective débridement would be of no use if concurrent steps were not taken to optimize the wound-healing environment. Once bacteria in the wound are controlled and an adequate arterial supply is ensured, the focus of therapy can shift to moist wound healing. Moist wound healing includes the use of dressings and, in some cases, compression therapy to create a wound bed that is neither too wet (macerated) or too dry (desiccated) to be suitable to wound healing. An analogy to a beach is commonly used to help explain this concept, in which the optimal wound environment is the wet sand and suboptimal environments are underwater or on dry land.

To create a moist wound bed, the clinician must have a good understanding of the wound etiology and a familiarity with the available wound-care dressings. Certain wounds, such as those associated with infection, venous insufficiency, and lymphedema, tend to drain heavily and require absorbent dressings, whereas wounds without an adequate blood supply tend to be dry and often require the addition of moisture. With the appropriate use of cleansing agents, protection of the periwound skin, and selection of suitable dressings, wound healing can be positively influenced. Educating a patient about appropriate cleansing agents is particularly important if a patient will be cleansing the wound at home. The patient should be educated not to scrub the wound and to avoid the use of harsh chemicals such as bleach, iodine, hydrogen peroxide, alcohol, or surgical scrub brushes for daily cleansing, unless specifically prescribed for the management of a heavily colonized wound. Although some of these chemicals can be extremely effective at controlling bacteria, they are all cytotoxic and can impede wound healing. The general rule of thumb "if you wouldn't put it in your eye, don't put it on your wound" works well. For healthy granulating wounds, normal saline or sterile water are effective for mild cleansing and the removal of small particles of adhered dressing that may be present. Some wounds have bacteria that are adhered to the surface forming a matrix known as a biofilm. In these cases a noncytotoxic wound surfactant is a better option.

Once the wound is clean, consideration can shift to the periwound area. This skin is vulnerable to injury from adhesive dressings or excess wound drainage, but damage can be limited or prevented with the use of a skin protectant. There are literally hundreds of dressings on the market, making it impractical, if not impossible, to keep up with all of them. By having a general understanding of each class of dressings, the clinician should be able to choose a dressing that is not only safe but effective in the management of the wound at hand. Table 18.3 outlines the characteristics of some of the most commonly used classifications of dressings.

No single dressing is intended to treat a wound through all phases of wound healing, nor is every patient with the same diagnosis going to respond the same. It is important to reassess the characteristics of the wound at each patient visit to ensure that the optimal dressing is being used. Factors such as ease of use, the patient's ability to change the dressing independently, how often it will need changing, the degree of discomfort associated with dressing changes, and cost need to be considered. For example, a hydrocolloid is easy to apply but would not be cost-effective for a wound that needs to be changed twice per day, and a transparent film may be inexpensive and easy to use but inappropriate for an individual with poor periwound skin integrity. When wounds cannot be closed immediately, dressings may be used until wound closure or until it is suitable for a surgical procedure such as a flap, graft, or application of a cultured tissue product (CTP). Lower extremity diabetic foot ulcers treated with CTPs were less likely to result in amputation,

Table 18.3 Common Wound Care Dressings

Indication	Dressing Type	Contraindications	Comments
Absorption	Alginate	Excessively dry wounds	Secondary dressing required
		Full-thickness burns	
	Hydrofiber	None	Secondary dressing required
	Foam	Excessively dry wounds	Adhesive and nonadhesive varieties
			Absorptive capacity varies between brands
Active bleeding	Alginate	Excessively dry wounds	Secondary dressing required
		Full-thickness burns	
	Silver nitrate	Skin hypersensitivity	Effective on hypergranulation
Add moisture	Hydrogels	Moderate to heavy exudate	Gel or sheet forms
Maintain moisture	Hydrocolloids	Local or systemic infection	May increase wound odor at dressing removal
		Caution with fragile periwound skin	
	Transparent films	Cavity wounds	May decrease need for unnecessary dressing changes because wound can be visualized
		Tracts, tunnels, undermining	
		Infection	
		Excessive exudates	
Fragile skin	Silicone	None	Reduces scarring
			May be used to prevent an absorbent secondary dressing from adhering
Antimicrobial	Silver	Avoid use with enzymatic débriders	Most dressing classifications have a silver version
	Honey	None	Requires secondary dressing
	Polyhexamethylene biguanide	Avoid gauze-based dressing overexposed nerves, vessels, and tendons	Important to keep gauze moist to avoid adhering to wound bed
	Methylene blue/gentian violet	Full-thickness burns	Requires premoistening with sterile water or saline
			Requires secondary dressing
	Cadexomer iodine	Iodine sensitivity	Sheet and gel forms available
		Hashimoto thyroiditis	Requires secondary dressing
		Nontoxic nodular goiter	
		Graves disease	
		Pregnant or lactating females	
Débridement	Hydrocolloid	Local or systemic infection	May increase wound odor at dressing removal
		Caution with fragile periwound skin	
	Transparent film	Cavity wounds	No absorptive capacity
		Tracts, tunnels, undermining	
		Infection	
		Excessive exudates	
	Collagenase	Hypersensitivity to collagenase	Requires daily application
		Do not use with silvers	Requires secondary dressing
	Gauze	Directly on healthy granulation tissue	Wet-to-dry dressing is not recommended; if used, it should be restricted to necrotic wounds
		Exposed nerves, vessels, tendons	Effective as a secondary dressing

emergency department visits, and hospitalization compared to wounds not treated with those advanced products.[78] Other emerging technologies that have been shown to be beneficial in the healing of diabetic wounds include platelet-rich plasma,[79,80] and autologous fat grafts.[81] It is outside the scope of practice for rehabilitation professionals to perform these procedures; however, as support for these interventions grows, awareness that they exist is becoming more important.

Acute wounds in an otherwise healthy individual may heal without difficulty if appropriate dressings are used. In chronic wounds or patients with impaired wound-healing potential, the use of certain biophysical agents can stimulate wound healing. Electrical stimulation, pneumatic compression, negative-pressure wound therapy, ultrasound, and laser have all been shown to be effective in the management of wounds. The reader may refer to any biophysical agents textbook for an in-depth discussion of each of these agents and correct procedures for use. The majority of evidence supporting electrical stimulation for wound management is at least 20, and in some cases more than 50 years old. Very little recent data exists to support or refute the claims of electrical stimulation as an intervention for wound healing, but a 2022 systemic review suggests that it appears beneficial for diabetic foot ulcers, but further investigations are needed.[82]

Low laser light therapy is also used for the treatment of wounds.[83,84] The results of the use of low laser light therapy to promote wound healing have been variable with low or no efficacy in the past.[84] Recent investigations show promising results of various forms of laser therapy in comparison to other modalities. Improved diabetic foot ulcer healing rates were seen when wounds were treated with CO_2 laser versus those treated with a surgical approach,[85] and when low level laser therapy was compared to hyperbaric oxygen therapy during the first 4 weeks.[86] Treatment with gallium aluminum arsenide lasers resulted in faster rates of wound closure compared to light-emitting diode therapy and both modalities improved neuropathic symptoms, which has the potential to impact healing of diabetic foot ulcers if the patient is more aware of weight bearing.[87]

REDUCING FURTHER TRAUMA TO THE WOUND

Regardless of the advanced wound care dressing used, wounds will not heal unless the wound can be protected from further trauma. In most cases, trauma comes in the form of weight-bearing forces. In a bed-bound individual, dynamic air mattresses and air-fluidized beds are used to disperse forces, which in turn, reduce the amount of pressure at the wound site and allow it to heal. For persons who are more active, offloading can be even more of a challenge because there is a balance that needs to be met between maintaining function and providing pressure relief to the wound. This is the dilemma faced by a person with drop foot who needs an ankle-foot orthosis to walk effectively, but the orthosis is causing a wound on the plantar aspect of the fifth MTH. The challenge for the clinician is to offload the foot so that the wound can heal as quickly as possible, enabling the patient to return a previous level of function.

Many of the advances in pressure reduction strategies for the foot have come about because of diabetes. As a result of the neuropathic and arterial changes discussed previously, many of these individuals will develop foot ulcers that require offloading. Many of these wounds would respond well to several weeks of complete bed rest because all weight-bearing forces would be eliminated from the bottom of the foot. This is not practical for most patients, and even if it were a possibility, it is not without risk (e.g., blood clots, deconditioning, pressure injuries). Maintaining non–weight bearing at home is also a major challenge for most patients. When a patient sustains an orthopedic fracture to the foot, pain serves as negative feedback and prevents the person from weight bearing. In the presence of neuropathy, the sensation of pain is diminished so the deterrent from putting the foot on the floor is absent. Although non–weight bearing or partial weight bearing is encouraged through the use of an assistive device, it is prudent to assume the device will not be used all the time and to protect the foot as if you intend weight bearing to occur.

Total Contact Casting

The gold standard for offloading the neuropathic foot has traditionally been total contact casting (TCC) (Fig. 18.9). Initially used in the management of Hansen disease (formerly leprosy), TCC was first brought to the United States by Dr. Paul Brand.[88] Using the simple equation, pressure = force/area, it is evident that pressure can be reduced by reducing the amount of weight (force) going through the wound and by increasing the total area that the patient's weight is spread over. TCC has intimate contact with the entire plantar aspect of the foot, with the exception of the wound location. This serves to increase the weight-bearing surface area and reduce the force through the wound. In addition, immobilization of the ankle in neutral prevents dorsiflexion and weight transfer toward the front of the foot during the late stance phases of gait. TCC reduces vertical and shear forces acting on the foot.

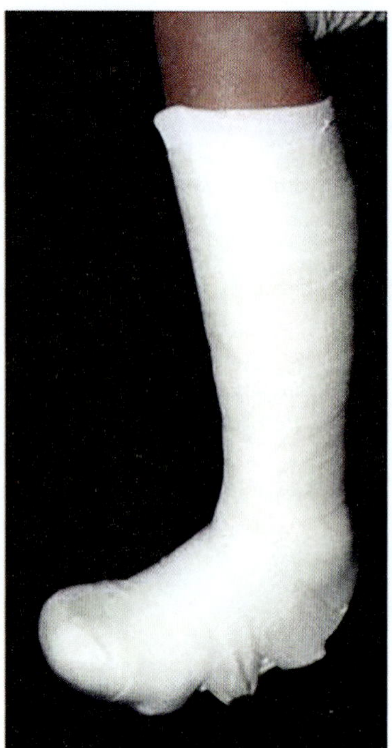

Fig. 18.9 Total contact cast.

Numerous studies report favorable results in healing diabetic foot ulcers with the use of TCC.[88–92] Three randomized control studies found that TCC for patients with neuropathic foot ulcers had 90% healing and healed in a shorter time span compared with patients who did not have total contact casting but had other offloading strategies such as non–weight-bearing status, use of walker aid, and/or use of removable air cast.[93–95] Traditional TCC was made of plaster material, which required the patient to be non–weight bearing for at least 24 hours. Many clinics currently do a combination of plaster and fiberglass or all fiberglass casts to allow patients to return to weight bearing more quickly. The initial TCC also had contact with the entire foot, including the wound. Since that time, a modified approach in which the wound site is isolated has been shown to reduce pressure significantly more than the true "total contact" method.[96]

Proper application of TCC requires additional training, and although the experienced clinician may see the benefit, the complexity may deter others from utilizing this offloading method. Prefabricated TCC kits exist as an alternative to tradtional TCC. These kits may be easier to apply and have demonstrated similar outcomes to traditional TCC.[97] Although it has demonstrated superiority in offloading,

TCC is not appropriate for all cases. It should not be used in cases of excessive drainage, vascular insufficiency, infection, or fluctuating edema and for wounds that are deeper than they are wide. Because the condition of the foot cannot be monitored while it is enclosed in a cast, the patient must be able to recognize the warning signs indicating the need to have the cast changed. These signs include excessive swelling of the leg that causes the cast to become too tight, loosening of the cast that allows the foot and leg to move within the cast, a sudden increase in body temperature or of blood glucose level that might indicate infection, staining and drainage through the cast, excessive odor from the cast, new complaints of pain, and damage to the cast.

Removable Cast Walkers

Despite being the gold standard for offloading the neuropathic foot, TCC is not widely used because of concerns over iatrogenic complications, as well as a lack of experience among clinicians. In its place, removable cast walkers have become the most widely used method to offload the foot. The removable cast walker is an orthotic device with double uprights fixed at a 90-degree angle to a rocker-soled walking platform. As with TCC and the walking splint, the fixed position of the ankle prevents propulsion at the forefoot, where the greatest pressures tend to occur. Removable cast walkers are available from various manufacturers. Because they are not custom made for each patient, care must be taken when fitting the device to ensure that it accommodates the contours of the patient's foot and ankle, particularly in the area of the uprights. A custom-molded insert can be added to most manufactured walkers.

Instant Total Contact Cast

A major advantage of TCC over the removable walker is the forced compliance because of the inability of the patient to remove the cast. Because the cast cannot be removed, it is ensured that the wound is being offloaded 24 hours per day. Several studies show the removable cast walkers to be comparable with TCC for pressure reduction.[98,99] However, other investigators report faster healing times with TCC as opposed to removable cast walkers.[93–95] Under the assumption that the seemingly conflicting data was a function of the cast walker being removed, researchers designed studies that compared TCC and removable cast walkers to cast walkers that were made nonremovable by wrapping them with a layer of fiberglass (Fig. 18.10). These nonremovable cast walkers were named instant total contact casts (iTCCs). Results of one study found the iTCC to be equivalent to TCC in the proportion of wounds that healed in 12 weeks,[100] whereas the second study found healing rates with the iTCC to be comparable with healing rates of conventional TCC in previous studies and superior to the removable cast walker.[101] Based on the available evidence, the iTCC is a viable option for a neuropathic wound, especially for the clinician that has not been trained in the application of, or does not have the time to apply, TCC.

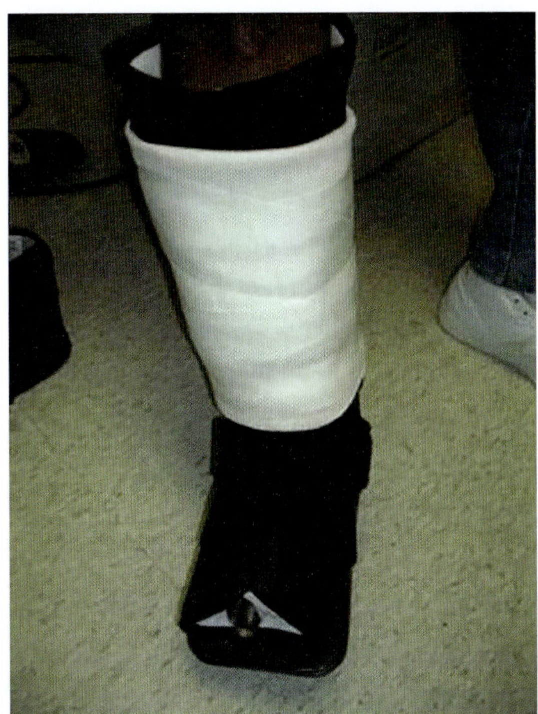

Fig. 18.10 Instant total contact cast fabricated by applying fiberglass to a removable cast walker. (Miller J, Armstrong DG. Offloading the diabetic and ischemic foot: solutions for the vascular specialist. *Semin Vasc Surg*. 2014;27(1):68–74.)

Wound-Healing Shoes

The cast, splint, and cast walker should all be considered as therapies of choice to offload neuropathic ulcerations. It is tempting to use less-restrictive devices because those that cover the leg seem like such an inconvenience to the patient. For most patients, putting them in devices that will be less than optimally effective is doing them a disservice. In some cases where a cast is contraindicated or the leg will not fit in a cast walker, devices that go only as high as the ankle may be useful. One of these devices is the wedge shoe, which has an elevated toe portion in relation to the heel so as to offload the forefoot (Fig. 18.11). The wedge shoe causes the body weight to shift back toward the heel, decreasing forces at the forefoot, albeit not to the same extent as the devices that transfer weight up the leg.[102] For pressure to be reduced, the area to be offloaded must be distal to the fulcrum of the shoe. To maximize pressure reduction, patients should be instructed to take short steps with the contralateral leg. This ensures that they do not propel over the wedge, causing contact between the distal end of the shoe and the ground. In clinical experience, this is often difficult for patients to do, and the telltale "clicking" of a patient in a wedge shoe can usually be heard as soon as the patient walks into the clinic. When a patient takes a large enough step to allow the front of the shoe to hit the ground, pressure at the forefoot is increased but may still be less than if the patient were ambulating in a regular shoe because of the rigidity of the wedge shoe's sole. This rigidity serves to reduce the transfer of weight toward the forefoot that typically happens in terminal stance, but it does not isolate the at-risk area in relation to the rest of the forefoot. The addition of a custom-molded insert with a relief area has been shown to be effective at addressing this problem.[90]

The issue of compliance with the wedge shoe, and all shoe offloading devices, remains a question. On the one hand, it could be argued that wedge shoes are less cumbersome, so are more likely to be worn; and on the other hand that they

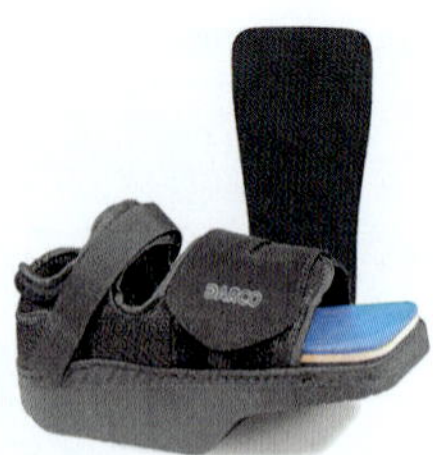

Fig. 18.11 **OrthoWedge shoe.** (Courtesy Darco International, Huntington, West Virginia).

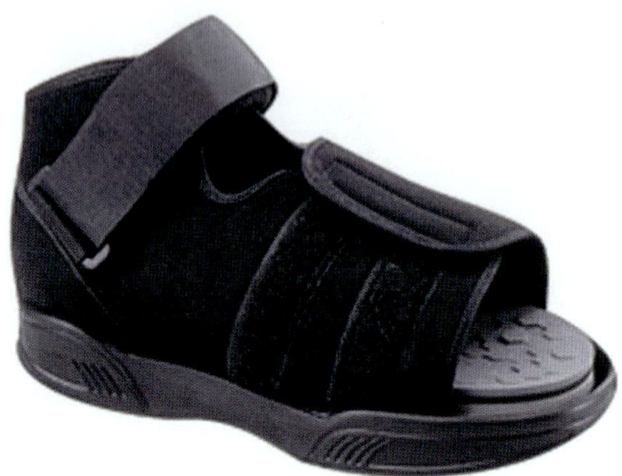

Fig. 18.12 DH wound-healing shoe, which has pegs that can be removed. (© Össur.)

are easier to remove, making it more likely that the foot will be left unprotected. Another issue is that wedge shoes are difficult for patients with limited dorsiflexion and could actually increase forefoot pressure if a patient has a limited range of motion. Walking in a wedge shoe feels very unnatural because of the functional leg-length discrepancy created. This can be difficult to manage for patients with balance issues and can also lead to back discomfort. Finally, one last drawback to the wedge shoe is that it cannot be used to offload bilaterally because it shifts the patient's weight too far posteriorly.

An alternative shoe-type device to the wedge shoe is a shoe with modifiable insoles.[103] An example of this device, the DH shoe by Royce Medical Co. (Ossur North America, Aliso Vejo, California), has an insole with pegs that can quickly be removed to relieve pressure to the at-risk area (Fig. 18.12). Advantages of this shoe type versus the wedge shoe include the ability to offload any part of the foot, not just the forefoot, a flat sole that is safer for those with balance issues, and the ability to offload bilateral feet simultaneously. A disadvantage to this type of shoe is that the flexible sole allows for a toe break during the gait cycle, which allows weight to transfer anteriorly.

Other Pressure-Relieving Options

There are several temporary offloading options[104,105] that can be applied directly to the foot in cases in which the previous described options either are unavailable or undesirable. The first option is adhesive felted foam (Fig. 18.13).[104] A custom-fit piece of ¼-inch felt-backed foam is adhered to the plantar surface of the foot. A U-shaped aperture is cut in the foam to reduce pressure around the ulcer. The margins

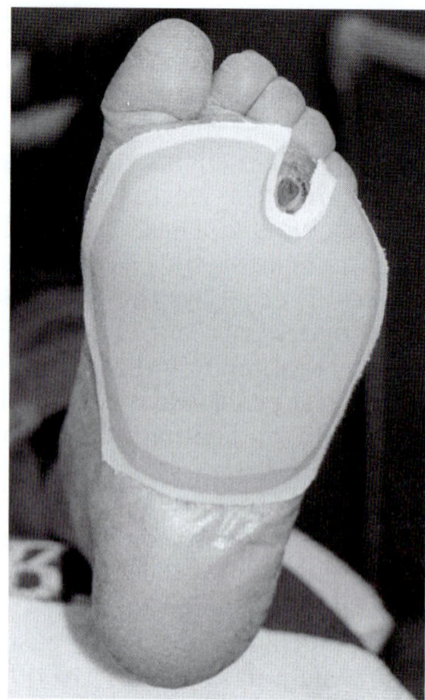

Fig. 18.13 Felted foam pressure relief. Edges of the foam have been beveled.

of the aperture are positioned close to but not overlapping the wound edge, extending distally beyond the wound. The entire plantar surface of the foot must be examined to identify all vulnerable spots that need accommodation before the pad is applied. For forefoot ulcers, the pad extends proximally along the midfoot to increase the weight carriage in this area. All edges of the foam pad should be beveled to minimize chances of skin breakdown from edge pressure. When a bony deformity is particularly prominent, an additional layer of foam can be used to relieve pressure adequately from the ulcer site. A thin dressing is placed flatly over the ulcer. A healing sandal is used for ambulation. If the area is preulcerative or postulcerative, an extra-depth shoe can be worn. The felted foam should be thought of as temporary because the pressure relief provided by the foam pad decreases significantly by the fourth day.[106] Consequently, changing the pad every 3 or 4 days might be beneficial.

Felted foam is generally well accepted by the patient. Because this method allows for easier mobility than TCC or walking splint, patients tend to walk more. This may not be desirable considering the possible effect of cumulative pressure. Despite walking more, patients using felted foam as an offloading method seem to respond well to the therapy as measured by the percentage of wounds that heal and the amount of time they take to heal.[107-109] The major benefit of the felted foam appears to be constant wear time, without the excess bulk and seems to be a good option for patients that tend to walk barefoot, even though they are instructed not to.

Another temporary form of offloading is the football dressing. The football dressing was first proposed by Rader and Barry as a simple alternative to TCC for neuropathic ulcers.[110] The football dressing involves three layers of cast padding: the first is fan-folded over the toes, the second is wrapped circumferentially around the foot, and the third covers up to the lower one-third of the leg. A layer of gauze is then applied and covered with an elastic wrap. Although there are limited data that support the use of the football dressing, a retrospective analysis of its use found it to have comparable effectiveness compared with the published data for TCC and iTCC for the management of wounds across the spectrum on the University of Texas Diabetic Foot Classification System.[110] Some clinicians have had success using the football dressing in conjunction with a removable cast walker to ensure that the foot has some degree of protection even if the cast walker is removed.[111]

Prevention of ulceration or reulceration

The simplest and most cost-effective way to treat a wound is to avoid getting one in the first place. This is best accomplished through risk identification, patient education, fitting with appropriate footwear, and follow up for routine care. Being able to classify patients based on their risk for developing ulceration is critical for the proper management of each individual. One of the most widely used risk classifications was developed by the International Working Group on the Diabetic Foot (IWGDF). This classification system has been shown to predict foot complications (Table 18.4).[112–114]

In 2008 Lavery and associates published a revision of the IWGDF classification system.[115] In their new model, risk category 2 was divided into two groups, labeled 2 A and 2B. Group 2 A included patients with sensory neuropathy and deformity, and group 2B consisted of patients with peripheral arterial occlusive disease. Group 3 was divided into those with a history of an ulcer (3 A) and those with a history of amputation (3B). When they applied this new classification system to 1666 patients with diabetes, they found that there were significantly more foot complications in the "B" groups than in the "A" groups. In addition, they found that there was little clinical difference between groups 1 and 2 A and suggested those two groups could be combined. These changes led to the development of the Texas Foot Risk Classification (Table 18.5). Unlike this classification that looks at the risk for ulceration, a retrospective study published by Sayiner et al. in 2019 identified the characteristics of diabetics who underwent amputation.[116] Of the 400 diabetic patients with foot wounds they investigated, 143 (35.75%) had to have a foot amputation. Proteinuria, longer history of smoking, previous ulcerations and amputations, ulcers with gangrene, coronary and peripheral artery disease, hypertension, and male sex were all identified as effective predictors for the need to have an amputation.

Once a patient's risk factors have been identified, patient education can be tailored to the individual patient's needs. It is often helpful to have a small pamphlet or flier available for patients to take home that outlines what is safe and unsafe for them to do. A comprehensive educational pamphlet should include skin care, skin inspection, and footwear guidelines as shown in Box 18.2. Recommendations should be adjusted based on the patient's individual needs; for example, performing nail care at home would not be advisable for a patient with vascular compromise or who has difficulty reaching or seeing his or her feet.

Risk stratification is also important in determining the most appropriate footwear for a patient. Patients in the Texas Foot Risk Classification category 0 do not typically require special footwear but should be educated on proper shoe fit. The proper shoe should match the contours of the foot and should be comfortable at the time of purchase (no break-in period). High-risk patients should have the width and length of their feet measured every time they buy a new pair of shoes. It is also a wise investment for each clinic that deals with high-risk feet to obtain a shoe-measuring device (Fig. 18.14), because many problems can be avoided with proper fitting shoes. Width is measured across the widest part of the forefoot, typically across the MTHs, with the patient standing. Two measurements need to be taken for shoe length; one is the heel-to-toe length and the other is the heel-to-arch length. This extra measurement helps to ensure that the toe break in the shoe is in line with the MTHs. If the heel-to-toe and heel-to-arch lengths are the same, then that is the correct shoe size. If they are different, the patient should be fit with the larger of the two sizes. Patients should be instructed to try on new shoes in the mid-to-late afternoon, after they have been on their feet for most of the day to account for fluctuating edema. If they shop in the morning, they risk having shoes that are too tight by evening, and if they wait until evening to shop, shoes may be too large in the morning. A well-fitting shoe should have approximately one thumb's width between the longest toe and the end of the shoe, and the material on the dorsum of the shoe should be pinchable if the shoe is not too narrow or shallow. Patients who have a loss of sensation and no other risk factors (category 1 of original IWGDF) also do not require protective footwear but may benefit from a soft nonmolded insert in the shoe. It is important that they are educated on what to look for in a shoe. High heels increase forefoot pressure, shoes with narrow toes squeeze the foot, thongs can irritate between the toes, and slip on shoes do not stay in place very well. A supportive shoe allows the foot to stay in proper biomechanical alignment while remaining relaxed. Athletic shoes and shoes made with more flexible materials are excellent options for this low-risk group because they reduce pressure in comparison with leather shoes.[117,118]

Table 18.4 International Working Group on the Diabetic Foot Risk Classification

Risk Category	Definition
0	No neuropathy
1	With neuropathy, no deformity or peripheral vascular disease
2	With neuropathy and deformity or peripheral vascular disease
3	History of ulceration or amputation

Table 18.5 Texas Foot Risk Classification

Risk Group	Characteristics
0	No neuropathy or arterial disease
1	Neuropathy present
2	Arterial disease present
3	History of ulceration
4	History of amputation

From Lavery LA, Peters EJ, Williams JR, et al. Reevaluating the way we classify the diabetic foot: restructuring the diabetic foot risk classification system of the International Working Group on the Diabetic Foot. *Diabetes Care.* 2008;31(1):154–156.

Box 18.2 Guidelines for Preventative Foot Care

Skin care

DO:
- Wash feet daily. Dry them well, especially between the toes.
- Apply a thin coat of moisturizer to feet daily, avoiding between the toes.
- Trim toenails after washing and drying feet.
- Cut toenails straight across; smooth any sharp edges with an emery board.
- Have a podiatrist handle any thickened or ingrown toenails.
- Thin thick corns or calluses by gently using a pumice stone or by professional care.
- Check water temperature with a thermometer or elbow before bathing.
- Wear socks at night if feet are cold.
- Use sunscreen on the tops of feet during the summer.
- Ask healthcare provider to check feet at each visit.

DO NOT:
- Soak feet. This can dry them out and cause cracking.
- Use moisturizer between toes. Moisture between the toes allows germs to grow.
- Cut corns and calluses.
- Use chemical agents, corn plasters, strong antiseptics, or adhesive tape on feet, because they can damage skin.
- Use hot water bottles or heating pads, because they can burn feet.

Foot Self-Inspection

DO:
- Inspect all surfaces of the feet daily (including between the toes) for signs of injury: reddened areas, blisters, cuts, cracks, or sores.
- Report any injuries to a healthcare provider immediately.
- Feel for areas of increased temperature.
- Check for tender areas on the bottom of feet.
- Use a mirror if necessary to see the bottom of feet.
- Have a family member, friend, or healthcare professional check feet if necessary.

DO NOT:
- Wait to report problems to a healthcare provider. Early attention can often prevent small problems from becoming big ones.

Footwear

DO:
- Wear shoes that fit the size and shape of feet and leave room for any necessary insoles.
- Ask a healthcare provider to recommend the correct type of shoe.
- Break in new shoes slowly, checking feet frequently for signs of irritation. Report signs of irritation to a healthcare provider.
- Keep shoes and insoles in good repair.
- Always wear socks or stockings with shoes, wearing a clean pair daily.
- Before putting on shoes, check for rough areas, torn linings, or loose objects that can injure a foot.

DO NOT:
- Walk barefoot (use slippers at night, special shoes or sandals for the beach).
- Wear socks that are too baggy or have holes or prominent seams.
- Wear socks or stockings that are constricting at the top.
- Wear sandals with thongs between the toes.

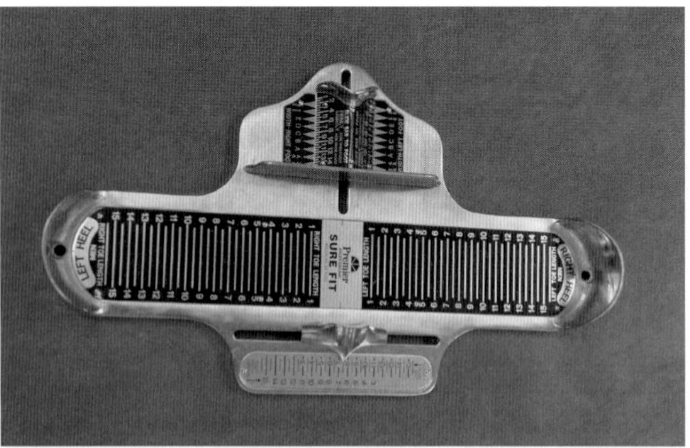

Fig. 18.14 Brannock foot measuring device. (Courtesy The Brannock Device Co., Liverpool, New York).

For higher-risk groups, specialty footwear, including custom insoles and extra-depth or molded shoes, is indicated. Custom inserts are molded to the foot and reduce pressure at the heel and forefoot compared with flat insoles by spreading weight-bearing forces over a larger area.[119] The ideal insert strikes the perfect balance between durability and cushioning. No single material has been identified that accomplishes both tasks effectively, so most orthotics are fabricated with several different materials.[120] Although these multidensity insoles seem to strike a balance between support and pressure relief, they are thicker than a flat insole and require the use of an extra-depth shoe. Custom-molded insoles in combination with extra-depth shoes are effective at preventing recurrent ulceration in diabetics (Fig. 18.15).[119,121]

One of the most difficult times in the wound-healing process is the transition from "treatment" footwear to everyday footwear. These patients comprise group 3 in the Texas Foot Risk Classification. Because most people with a diabetic foot ulcer see the return to normal footwear as a goal, it is often tempting for both the patient and clinician to rush this process once the wound has completely epithelialized. At this point in the healing process, the wound may not be mature enough to handle the pressure increase from the treatment shoe to a regular shoe. As an intermediary, some of the shoe-type offloading devices mentioned earlier in this chapter can serve as a bridge between treatment devices that

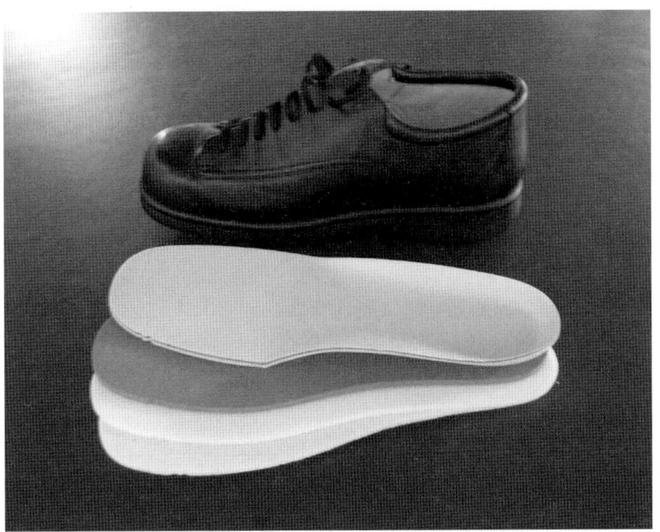

Fig. 18.15 Extra-depth shoe with removable insoles.

immobilize the ankle and permanent footwear. Depending on the degree of deformity, individuals in these risk groups will need to be fit with custom insoles and either extra-depth or custom-molded shoes.[122] For added pressure relief, areas surrounding the postulcerative site can be built up with firmer materials to transfer weight away from the maturing tissue. To reduce the risk of blisters caused by shear forces, any adjustments should be made to the underside of the insole so the foot remains in contact with a smooth surface. Rather than relying on white socks to make it easier for the patient to see if they are bleeding somewhere, a more appropriate strategy, particularly in this transition phase, is to monitor for signs of increased warmth as that indicates an at risk area for ulceration or reulceration.[123] When elevated temperatures are detected, the patient can reduce strain on the tissues by reducing activity, returning to previous offloading footwear, or both.

More aggressive shoe modifications can be used for those who require pressure reduction beyond what in-shoe modifications can achieve. The most effective of these modifications is adding a rocker bottom to the outer sole of the shoe (Fig. 18.16). Diabetic shoes with molded inserts and rocker bottom soles decrease pressure at the heel and forefoot and simultaneously increase midfoot pressures, which is typically a less vulnerable area.[122] A review by Cavanagh reported mixed results pertaining to the effectiveness of rocker bottom soles but notes several major flaws in the studies that found them to be ineffective.[124] The reduced pressure associated with the rocker sole has been shown to be clinically significant because it reduced the recurrence rate compared with patients wearing their own shoes.[125]

Many of the strategies used for patients transitioning back to permanent footwear following an ulceration can be applied to the Texas Foot Risk Classification group 4, or more simply, those whose status is postamputation. Pressure relief remains critical, and rocker bottom shoes are effective in limiting the transfer of weight anteriorly, but there are some unique complications associated with transmetatarsal amputations. Depending on the amputation site, the long extensors of the foot may be damaged or be put at a mechanical disadvantage relative to the intact plantar flexors which attach to the posterior heel. The result of this imbalance is an equinus deformity which increases pressure at the distal end of the foot. A second problem is proper shoe fit. A short shoe that is fit to the amputation can reduce pressure on the distal foot but also increases pressure on the contralateral foot; however, short shoes were not well received by patients because of cosmesis. Appearance may seem trivial in relation to preventing the recurrence of an ulcer, but it is naïve to overlook appearance. If shoes are disliked so much that they are not worn, they serve no purpose at all. Along the same line of reasoning, patients need to be educated about the importance of not only wearing their shoes while outside but also in the house, where shoes are frequently removed. If this is not feasible, some other form of offloading, such as a customized sandal, may be helpful to increase compliance with offloading. Conversely, a full-length shoe is more cosmetically pleasing but may increase shear forces as a result of the foot sliding forward in the shoe. When a full-length shoe is combined with a rigid rocker bottom and a custom-molded insert, pressures at the forefoot of both the involved and contralateral foot were reduced compared with a regular shoe with a toe filler.[126] Persons wearing this combination also had faster walking speeds and physical performance test scores compared with patients in regular footwear with a toe filler. Based on these findings, the best option for those in risk category 4 is a full-length, rigid rocker bottom shoe, with a custom-molded insole.

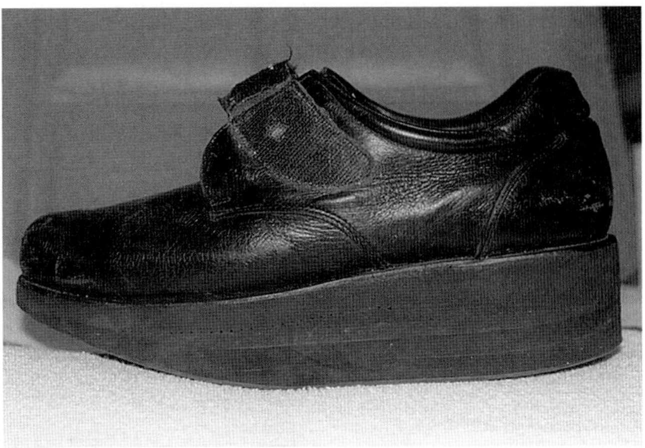

Fig. 18.16 Rocker bottom shoe.

Summary

The largest group of people with vulnerable feet at risk for vascular, sensory, motor, and autonomic changes that can result in wounds that fail to heal and are the source of loss of toes, foot, or limb is the population of individuals with diabetes. With an ever-increasing number of individuals diagnosed with diabetes, it is important that the clinician be able to identify risk factors so as to reduce future complications. This chapter reviewed the assessment of the vulnerable foot, as well as a comprehensive wound evaluation.

Applicable interventions were provided and organized according to the treatment goal to assist with the development of a successful treatment plan. Finally, footwear recommendations based on risk stratification were discussed to ensure that clients are given the best chance to return to their activities without ulcer formation or recurrence.

References

The complete listing of the References are available in the accompanying enhanced eBook version included with the print purchase of this textbook. Visit Elsevier eBooks+ (eBooks.Health.Elsevier.com) to access this content.

19 Amputation Surgeries for the Lower Limb

PATRICK D. GRIMM AND BENJAMIN K. POTTER

LEARNING OBJECTIVES

On completion of this chapter, the reader will be able to do the following:

1. Understand the most common indications for lower extremity amputation and compare and contrast the key methods of assessment used to decide when amputation is necessary.
2. Determine the most appropriate level of amputation based on resultant biomechanics and the need for adequate soft tissue coverage as well as appreciate the surgical techniques used to manage bone, soft tissue, nerves, and blood vessels during lower extremity amputations.
3. Anticipate postoperative care requirements, common complications, and expected outcomes following lower extremity amputation.
4. Provide an overview of the most commonly used surgical approaches as well as special considerations for each level of amputation.
5. Describe current areas of active research in the field of lower extremity amputation in regards to prosthesis anchorage, methods of active prosthesis control, and strategies for treatment and prevention of amputation-related neuromas.

Introduction

Approximately 180,000 lower extremity amputations are performed in the United States each year.[1] The most common reasons to perform an amputation include vascular insufficiency, trauma, or neoplasm. Overall, more than 90% of lower extremity amputations are performed as a result of vascular disease, with a significant portion of those patients carrying a diagnosis of diabetes mellitus.[2] The amputation of a limb is a truly life-altering event, affecting the physical, functional, and psychological dimensions of a person's world[3]; however, when done for the right reasons and with the appropriate technique, an amputation can be an important step towards recovery—amputation surgery therefore should be approached as a reconstructive procedure, not merely an ablation or afterthought of treatment failure.

The primary aim in performing an amputation is removal of the diseased, ischemic, mangled, or otherwise nonfunctional portion of the extremity. Once accomplished, the surgeon can then focus on reconstruction with the goal of creating the best possible conditions for the rapid return of maximal function and improved quality of life.

Although surgical technique is a key determinant in the success of an amputation,[4] other important factors include adequate preoperative counseling,[5] close postoperative follow-up with appropriate management of comorbidities and complications during the perioperative period,[6,7] and a properly implemented rehabilitation plan.

This chapter provides an overview of the indications for lower extremity amputations, surgical principles and techniques, postoperative care, commonly encountered complications, and future directions in the field of lower extremity amputations. Rehabilitation professionals play a vital role in the care of lower extremity amputees. Indeed, the surgical procedure and immediate perioperative care represent but a small fraction of the long path towards recovery. The goal of this chapter is to help rehabilitation professionals care for amputees by cultivating a better understanding of the rationale behind the surgical procedures performed and the expected postoperative course.

Indications for Lower Extremity Amputation

DYSVASCULAR AND NEUROPATHIC DISEASE

Prevalence and Risk Factors

Peripheral artery disease (PAD) is a term that includes a variety of disease processes that affect noncardiac, nonintracranial arteries, the most common of which is atherosclerosis.[8] A basic understanding of this disease is important given that up to 90% of lower extremity amputations in the United States are due to dysvascular disease.[2] One of the strongest risk factors for developing peripheral artery disease is diabetes mellitus (DM), reflected by the fact that 70% of patients who have amputations for dysvascular limb also have DM.[9]

The overall prevalence of PAD in the United States, across all ethnicities, is estimated to range from approximately 2% in persons 40 to 49 years of age to 20% or higher in persons older than age 80 years.[10] Risk factors for PAD include history of smoking, DM, untreated or poorly managed hypercholesteremia, untreated or poorly managed hypertension, kidney dysfunction, and chronic inflammation.[11] Significant morbidity and mortality is associated with PAD. It is estimated that one in four individuals with PAD undergoes some form of amputation, one in three will likely die within 5 years of diagnosis, and only one in four will survive more than 10 years after diagnosis.[12–14] Comorbid conditions that amplify risk of death in the year following PAD-related amputation include congestive heart failure, renal failure, and liver disease, as well as postoperative systemic sepsis.[15]

Patient Assessment

The assessment of an individual with compromised peripheral circulation begins with a careful and detailed health history and review of risk factors, continues with physical examination and routine blood work, and is followed by additional imaging or invasive tests as needed.[8,16]

A common symptom of chronic arterial vascular insufficiency is claudication. This vascular-related pain has been described as a deep aching, cramping, muscle fatigue, or tightness that develops during physical activity and dissipates with rest. Although most common in the superficial posterior compartment (gastrocnemius and soleus) of the lower leg, claudication can occur in any muscle with compromised blood supply, including the muscles of the thigh and hip. Claudication is the result of accumulation of lactic acid as a byproduct of anaerobic metabolism during muscle contraction. When an individual has persistent pain while at rest (i.e., "rest pain"), nocturnal recumbent pain, or ischemic skin lesions, the individual is classified as having critical limb ischemia, and is at high risk of amputation if revascularization fails or cannot be undertaken.[17]

Acute or sudden occlusion of an arterial vessel is marked by constant and unrelenting pain and may be accompanied by feelings of tingling, numbness, or coldness as peripheral nerves of the lower limb are affected by ischemia.[18,19] The signs of acute limb ischemia can be remembered as the 5 Ps: pain, paresthesia, pallor, poikilothermia (cold skin), and pulselessness. Although a limb with chronic arterial insufficiency demonstrates dependent rubor, the skin of an acutely compromised limb may be quite pale or blanched distal to the site of occlusion. Acute occlusion is often an emergent situation, requiring pharmacological or surgical intervention to restore blood flow to the limb.

The physical exam is an essential component of any patient assessment and provides key information for decision-making. The examination begins with visual inspection of the lower extremity and feet, concentrating on skin condition, presence or absence of hair, and nail condition.[8] Open wounds, callus, ecchymosis, dry necrosis, erythema, mottling, and altered pigmentation are documented. Wounds that lie under or are surrounded by callus on the plantar or weight-bearing surfaces of the foot are most likely neuropathic ulcers. Dry, blackened, or moist gangrenous wounds in the nail beds and between toes are likely signs of vascular insufficiency. Although "healthy" traumatic wounds often display clear serosanguineous drainage, any thickened, yellowish, or foul-smelling discharge from a wound suggests soft tissue or bone infection. When evaluating diabetic foot ulcers, the depth of ulceration and vascular supply to the region significantly guide treatment decisions (Table 19.1). Motor neuropathy may cause atrophy of the intrinsic muscles of the foot, allowing stronger flexor muscles to pull the toes into a claw deformity.[20] These newly created pressure points are at risk for ulceration. Protective sensation (as measured by perception of Semmes-Weinstein 5.07 filament), as well as touch, pressure, vibration, and position sense, are likely to be impaired or inconsistent.[21] Additionally, impairment of the autonomic system often causes dry, tight, shining, easily cracked skin, as well as altered blood flow to the bones of the foot, increasing risk of Charcot arthopathy in addition to ulceration.[22,23]

Table 19.1 Wagner Classification of Diabetic Ulcers and Common Treatment Recommendations

Grade	Description	Treatment
0	Skin intact but foot at risk	Accommodative footwear or total contact casting
1	Localized superficial ulcer	Total contact casting, ± irrigation and débridement
2	Ulcer deep to tendon, bone, ligament, or joint	Surgical débridement, irrigation, antibiotics, total contact casting, correction of deforming forces
3	Deep abscess or osteomyelitis	Surgical débridement, irrigation, antibiotics, total contact casting, correction of deforming forces, may require partial foot amputation or ray resection
4	Gangrene of toes or forefoot	Local amputation—partial foot or ray resection
5	Gangrene of entire foot	Amputation

Adapted from Anakwenze OA, Milby AH, Gans I, et al. Foot and ankle infections: diagnosis and management. *J Am Acad Orthop Surg*. 2012;20:684–693.

Vascular Examination

The least invasive and simplest strategy used to assess adequacy of vascular supply to the distal limb is palpation of distal lower extremity pulses at the dorsalis pedis and posterior tibial arteries, popliteal pulse at the knee, and femoral pulse at the groin. If all pulses are palpable, it is highly likely that there is adequate circulation to heal a neuropathic ulcer. Absent distal pedal pulses do not, however, confirm vascular insufficiency; pedal pulses are nonpalpable in up to 10% of the general population.[24] Further exam should proceed in a stepwise, systematic fashion, beginning first with measurement of the ankle-brachial index (ABI).[8,25] This noninvasive method measures the systolic blood pressure at the level of the ankle and compares it with the systolic blood pressure of the brachial artery above the elbow. Values less than 0.9 indicate PAD, while values above 1.4 are suggestive of poorly compressible arteries due to calcification. A word of caution—it has been estimated that 30% of patients with critical limb ischemia have a normal or near normal ABI due to this phenomenon—thus physical examination remains critical and additional, more sensitive testing may be indicated.[26] Further noninvasive tests (Table 19.2) include measurement of the toe brachial index (normal ≥0.7) and transcutaneous oximetry (>30 mm Hg suggests adequate perfusion for wound healing).[27] Segmental leg pressures, pulse volume recording, and duplex ultrasound may also be considered. (Refer to Chapter 18 for a detailed description of noninvasive assessment strategies.) Imaging modalities that outline the specific arterial anatomy are magnetic resonance angiography (MRA) and computed tomography angiography (CTA) (Fig. 19.1).[28,29] In addition to the workup of chronic vascular disease, CTA is a valuable tool in the evaluation of suspected vascular injury in the setting of an acute trauma[30] (Fig. 19.2A and B).

Finally, conventional arteriography is indicated in symptomatic patients being considered for revascularization procedures. This invasive strategy involves local surgical placement of a catheter into the femoral artery in the groin

Table 19.2 These noninvasive methods of vascular assessment help determine the severity of peripheral vascular disease and may predict the likelihood of wound healing following surgical intervention

Test/Measure	Normal Values	Abnormal Findings
Capillary refill time	Elevation of limb 20 s	Delayed refill or persistent blanching
	Return to dependent position	Rubor of dependency
	Pressure on toe or nail	
	Blanch, then refill in 1–2 s	
Refill after occlusion	Inflation of blood pressure cuff at thigh for 5 min	>10 s: impaired arterial perfusion
	On release, flush to normal skin color at toes within 10 s	
Venous refill time	Elevation of the limb 2 min	>10 s: impaired arterial perfusion
	Return to dependent position	<10 s: valvular incompetence of veins
	Veins on dorsum of foot refill in 10 s	
Doppler ultrasound	Triphasic on auscultation	Biphasic: mild vascular impairment
		Monophasic: significant impairment
		Absent: complete occlusion
Ankle-brachial index	0.9–1	<0.9 impaired arterial flow
		<0.5 unlikely to heal distal wound
Segmental blood pressure	<15 mm Hg drop in systolic pressure between adjacent sites (groin, thigh, just below knee, and at ankle)	>20 mm Hg decrease: possible occlusion
		>10 mm Hg: possible vessel calcification
Pulse volume recordings	Sharp peaks at each recorded site	Flattening on recording: occlusive disease
	Similar across left and right extremities	
Transcutaneous oxygen pressures	>40 mm Hg suggest healing of ulcer or surgical incision is likely	<20 mm Hg predict nonhealing of ulcer or surgical incision
Duplex scanning	Low velocity ratio; constant hue and intensity of image	Velocity ratio >4 or peak velocity >400 cm/s indicates >75% stenosis

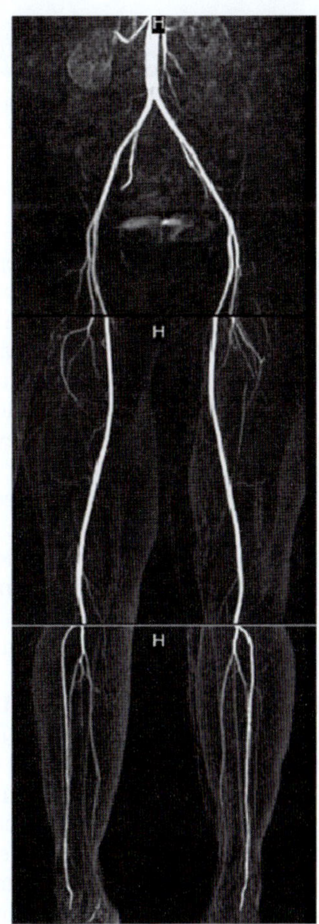

Fig. 19.1 Results of a computed tomography angiography in an individual with intact circulation.

(or alternatively, the axillary, radial, or subclavian arteries), followed by introduction of radiopaque dye into the arterial tree and exposure to radiation.[31] While this method generally provides excellent visualization of vascular anatomy, drawbacks include difficult delineation in distal or heavily calcified vessels and the risk of kidney injury with nephrotoxic contrast agents.[25]

Indications for Amputation Versus Revascularization

Peripheral arterial disease or DM may result in a nonviable or threatened limb due to occlusive vascular disease, neuropathic-related reasons, or frequently, a combination of both.[18,32] The management and prognosis for each of these groups are somewhat different. Vascular bypass surgery,[33] percutaneous endovascular stents,[34] or the use of thrombolytic intervention[35] may preserve the limbs of those with large-vessel vascular disease without significant microvascular dysfunction or neuropathy. Persons with a combination of diabetes and vascular disease are the most likely to require amputation; advanced age and multiple comorbidities (e.g., cardiovascular and cerebrovascular disease, kidney disease, and visual impairment) provide additional challenges for healing, early mobility after amputation, and the prosthetic rehabilitation process. Furthermore, chronic wounds resulting from either vascular insufficiency or neuropathy further jeopardize the viability of the extremity by providing an avenue for infection. When infected neuropathic or vascular wounds fail nonoperative management, amputation may be indicated, sometimes on an urgent or emergent basis.[36–38]

The management of peripheral artery disease is a complex undertaking and consultation with a vascular surgeon

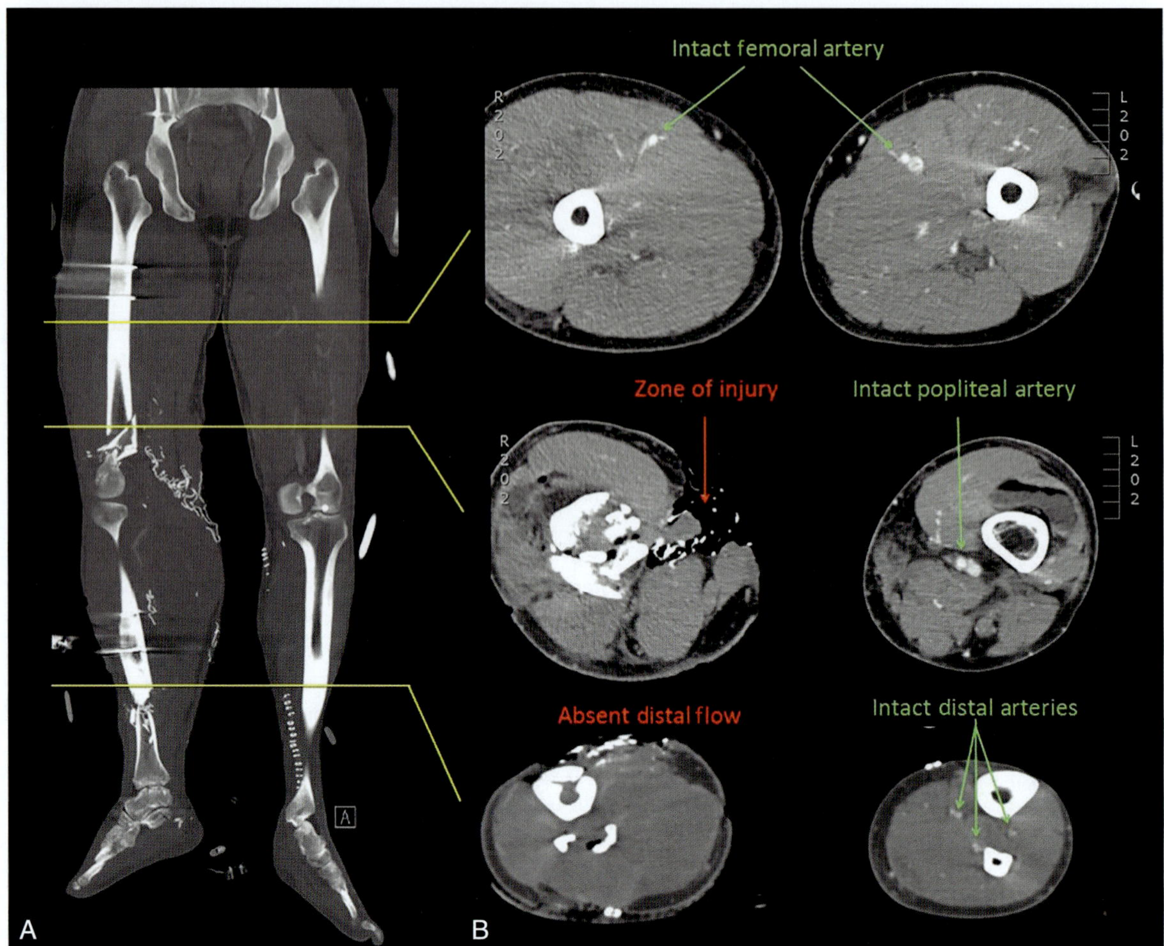

Fig. 19.2 (A) Coronal computed tomography of lower extremity in a patient who sustained a blast injury; (B) axial cross-section of computed tomography angiography proximal to the zone of injury, at the zone of injury, and distal to the zone of injury. Note the absence of flow to the distal vasculature in the limb. Vascular repair in this patient was not successful, resulting in a transtibial amputation.

is advised to determine revascularization options as well as determination of which amputation level is most likely to heal. This complexity is reflected the by numerous classification systems that have been designed to describe the disease process, and in limited cases, direct therapy.[39] Without timely revascularization, amputation rates approach 40% and population-based studies have shown amputation rates for critical limb ischemia to be highest in regions of the country with the least intensive vascular care.[40–42] The optimal approach to critical limb ischemia (endovascular vs. open surgical techniques) has yet to be defined; however national trends have recently reported an increase in the proportion of endovascular procedures as compared to open procedures, as well as a decrease in major amputations performed.[43] The results of a multicenter randomized controlled trial Best Endovascular versus Best Surgical Therapy in Patients with Critical Limb Ischemia (BEST-CLI) found a reduced risk of major adverse limb events with open surgical intervention (42.6%) versus endovascular therapy (57.4%) in patients with a viable segment of saphenous vein. For those requiring an alternative bypass conduit there was no statistical difference in major adverse limb events between the open surgery cohort (42.8%) and the endovascular cohort (47.7%).[44]

Amputation is often the best option when arterial anatomy precludes bypass or if severity of disease is such that bypass cannot salvage irreversibly ischemic and gangrenous tissue. Patients with complex medical conditions at high risk for intraoperative and postoperative complications may also be considered for amputation to minimize the risk of serial vascular procedures.[45] Revascularization can also be considered as an adjunct to amputation in an attempt to improve healing and preserve amputation level.[46] However, given the systemic nature of the disease process and associated comorbidities, revision to a more proximal amputation level commonly occurs. Reamputation rates vary by amputation level—approximately 34% of foot and ankle amputations and 15% of transtibial ampuations progress to more proximal level of limb loss.[2] Since vascular and neuropathic disease are systemic illnesses, these patients are at risk for compromise of both lower limbs.[47] After amputation of one limb, careful monitoring of vascular status and skin condition and appropriate conservative care of the intact limb and foot are essential. This is particularly true in the postoperative-preprosthetic period when there is single-limb ambulation with assistive devices, as well as in the months and years following initial amputation.[48,49]

TRAUMA

Incidence and Patient Population

In the United States, trauma accounts for up to 6% of all lower extremity amputations with the most common causes being motor vehicle accidents, falls, firearms, or machinery; however, due to the greater life expectancy of trauma-related amputees, around 20% of persons living with lower limb loss experience amputations due to trauma.[9,50] In areas of the world where there is current or recent armed conflict, traumatic amputations are more likely to be the result of improvised explosive devices, land mines, grenades, shrapnel, or direct gunfire.[51] Many of the injuries sustained by coalition personnel during the recent conflicts in Iraq and Afghanistan involved limb-threatening trauma.[52–54] Since 2001, more than 1700 service members have lost over 2300 limbs during the course of these conflicts.[55]

In contrast to amputations performed in the setting of vasculopathy, amputations following trauma are more likely to be performed on young, otherwise healthy individuals.[9] As a result, these patients often have the potential to return to a high level of function following amputation and are likely to be reliant on their residual limb and prosthesis for many years following their injuries.

Evaluation of the Threatened Limb

Depending on the mechanism of injury, trauma may result in an acute amputation or (more commonly) in open fractures with limb-threatening soft tissue damage (Fig. 19.3). Open fractures result in a high likelihood of infection as a consequence of introduced environmental microorganisms, ischemia caused by vascular compromise, and tissue necrosis due to direct damage.[56] The most commonly used classification scheme for open fractures, the Gustilo-Anderson classification, uses both wound size and vascular status to stratify the severity of the injury (Table 19.3). Although originally developed for open tibia fractures only, it is commonly applied to all extremity fractures and provides a common language to describe open injuries. The threatened limb must undergo a thorough assessment of both limb-specific and patient factors prior to proceeding with amputation or limb salvage. Considerations include severity of bone and soft tissue loss, adequacy of arterial blood supply, neuromotor and sensory function of the extremity, potential for prosthetic use, recovery time, and anticipated long-term functional status and quality of life.

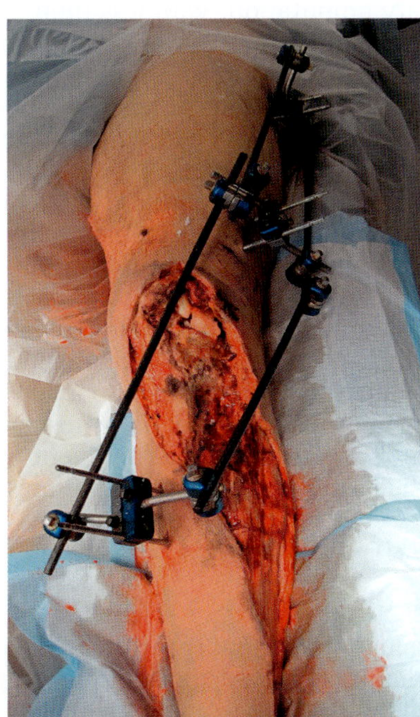

Fig. 19.3 Clinical photograph of a Gustilo-Anderson Type 3B distal femur fracture with external fixation in place. This patient ultimately required transfemoral amputation.

Limb Salvage Versus Reconstruction

Advances in trauma care and surgical techniques, including microsurgery and bone transport, have increased the likelihood that a traumatized limb can be preserved. However, not all limbs can or should be saved, which presents the surgeon and patient with an often difficult decision to make. Although there are a number of decision-making models available that attempt to quantify the factors involved when such a difficult decision is necessary (e.g., Predictive Salvage Index, Mangled Extremity Severity Score, Limb Salvage Index, Hanover Fracture Scale) few accurately predict the fate of an injured extremity, although specificity in predicting successful limb salvage is fair to good.[57–60] Suggested absolute indications for amputation include blunt or contaminated traumatic amputations, a mangled extremity in a critically injured patient in shock, or a limb with a warm ischemia time of greater than 6 hours.[61,62]

The best available evidence to guide decision-making comes from the Lower Extremity Assessment Project (LEAP), a multicenter, prospective observational study that tracked outcomes for 601 patients with limb-threatening injuries that underwent either limb salvage or amputation.[63] In light of important limitations, such as the lack of randomization, the study remains controversial and has been cited by advocates of both limb salvage and amputation. What the LEAP data have shown is that long-term outcomes (e.g., return to work, perceived health status) are generally poor for both primary amputation and successful limb salvage and reconstruction patients. Furthermore, outcomes are often driven more by economic, social, and personal resource factors rather than the initial treatment selected.[63,64]

Table 19.3 Gustilo-Anderson Classification of Open Fractures

Type	Description
1	Open clean wound <1 cm in length
2	Open wound >1 cm and <10 cm without extensive soft tissue damage
3A	Open wound >10 cm with extensive soft tissue damage but able to be closed
3B	Open wound that requires rotational or free tissue transfer for bony coverage
3C	Associated vascular injury that requires repair for viability of the limb

Adapted from Gustilo RB, Anderson JT. Prevention of Infection in the treatment of one thousand and twenty-five open fractures of long bone, retrospective and prospective analyses. *J Bone Joint Surg Am.* 1976;58(4):453–458.

A multivariate analysis of factors influencing surgeons' decision to perform a primary amputation in the LEAP study found a clear hierarchy with degree of soft tissue injury by far the most important component, followed by nerve function, vascular status, and extent of bony injury.[65] However, the mere absence of plantar sensation, once thought to be an important indicator of the need for amputation, has been found not to impact outcomes as the majority of patients regain sensation by 2 years after injury, and some of those with allegedly normal sensation on presentation lose this function.[65,66] Overall complication rates for both limb salvage and amputation groups are significant—however, the complication profiles (and the expected surgical course) differ between the two.[67] Given the need for multiple reconstructive procedures, patients undergoing limb salvage generally have much higher rates of rehospitalization and can expect for complications to occur for up to a year following initial injury.[67] In contrast, complications in patients undergoing amputation generally resolve within 6 months. Individuals and their families must be informed of the pros and cons of limb salvage versus amputation, including risk of infection and failure, as well as intensity and timeframe for rehabilitation and likelihood of returning to premorbid functional levels.[68]

In terms of the cost of care, early expenditures for both limb salvage and reconstruction were found to be similar. As might be expected due to the frequent need for multiple surgical procedures associated with limb salvage, rehospitalization costs were much higher in the reconstruction group. However, the substantial cost of prosthetic devices resulted in overall higher costs at 2 years for the amputation group. The lifetime cost of amputate care is estimated to be three times higher, again primarily due to prosthesis-related expenses.[69]

Considerations Unique to Traumatic Amputations

Initial management of trauma patients with a limb-threatening injury should focus on patient stabilization, resuscitation, and control of hemorrhage followed by thorough debridement of all contaminated wounds. An aggressive initial debridement should be performed, with removal of all devitalized muscle, skin, and bone that is devoid of soft tissue attachments. Wounds are then irrigated with normal saline, using gravity or low flow irrigation.[70] In the vast majority of cases, definitive closure should not be attempted at the time of initial debridement. Serial debridement allows for nonviable tissue to declare itself, thus allowing for judicious removal and preservation of soft tissue that can help preserve the length of the residual limb.[56] Accordingly, guillotine style amputations should be avoided in most instances, as this unnecessarily sacrifices soft tissue coverage. Diligent preservation of viable soft tissue may result in flaps of viable muscle and skin that do not fit classically described flaps for amputation closure and thus are considered atypical flaps or "flaps of opportunity." Generally, irrigation and debridement is performed every 48 to 72 hours until the wound is considered clean and devoid of nonviable tissue, and the patient medically stable and suitable for attempted closure. Negative pressure wound therapy is a useful tool in managing open wounds during frequent trips to the operating room (Fig. 19.4), and local antibiotic delivery via antibiotic impregnated polymethylmethacrylate (i.e., bone cement) beads is a common tactic utilized in the hope of mitigating infection.[56,71] The timing of wound closure is a matter of clinical judgment and, in certain cases, definitive closure may include the use of split thickness skin grafts, local flaps, or free tissue transfers in an effort to preserve amputation length.[72] Although associated with high complication rates, fixation of fractures proximal to a traumatic amputation can performed to preserve functional joint level or salvage residual limb length.[73]

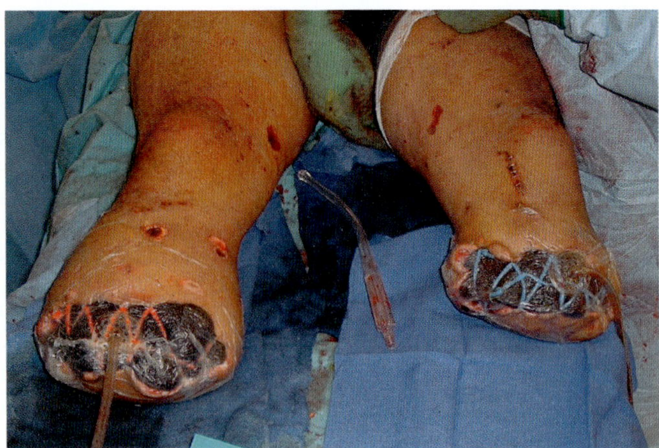

Fig. 19.4 Patient with bilateral traumatic transtibial amputations with negative pressure wound therapy in place. This technique allows for efficient management of open wounds in between multiple surgical debridements. Note also the elastic vessel loops in place on each wound, allowing for continuous tension to prevent retraction of the skin edges and preserve maximal soft tissue coverage.

NEOPLASM

Incidence and Patient Population

Neoplasm represents the least common indication for lower extremity amputation, with less than 1% of amputations performed for malignant or locally aggressive bone or soft tissue tumors.[2] The term sarcoma refers to malignant tumors that arise primarily from embryonic mesoderm and can be broadly categorized into tumors of bone or soft tissue. Seventy five percent of all extremity sarcomas are observed in the lower extremities.[74,75] The incidence of tumors of bone and soft tissue demonstrate two age peaks: the first occurs in adolescents and young adults (e.g., osteosarcoma, Ewing sarcoma), with a second peak in mid- and late-life adults (especially metastatic).[76] Advances in diagnostic imaging, chemotherapy, radiation therapy, and reconstructive surgical techniques have made limb salvage a viable option in the treatment of many tumors. Currently, consideration of amputation as a treatment option is limited to only the most aggressive tumors. Rates of amputation at tertiary centers for extremity sarcoma are reported to be less than 10%.[77]

Evaluation of the Patient

The initial evaluation of a patient with a suspected bone or soft tissue tumor includes a detailed history, physical exam, and plain radiographs of the anatomic region of concern. Further cross-sectional imaging with magnetic resonance imaging (ideally) and/or computed tomography helps to characterize the lesion location, size, extent, and relationship

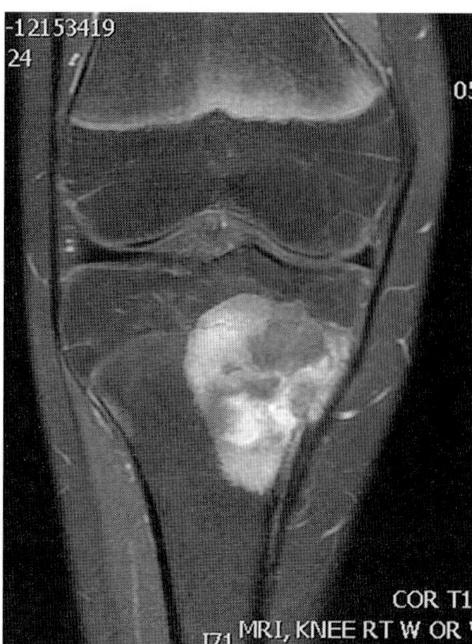

Fig. 19.5 Coronal T1 postcontrast sequence of the knee demonstrating a malignant neoplasm (osteogenic sarcoma) of the proximal tibia.

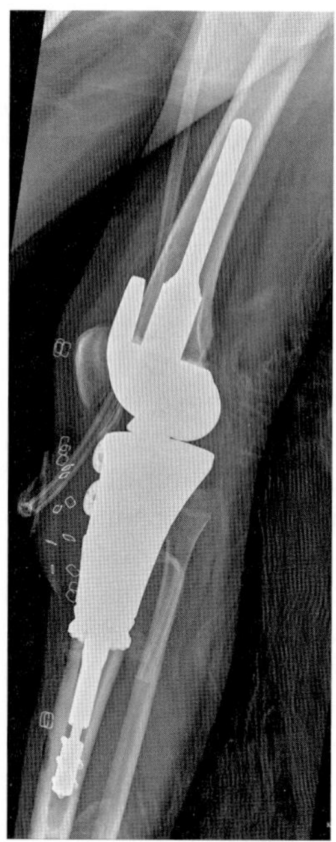

Fig. 19.6 Postoperative lateral radiograph of the same patient's knee shown in Fig. 19.4, now with a custom megaprosthesis utilized for limb-sparing surgery.

to vital neurovascular structures (Fig. 19.5). Other studies such as bone scan or positron emission tomography may be indicated in certain cases. While a select few types of lesions can be diagnosed by imaging alone, many will require biopsy to obtain a tissue diagnosis.[78] Patients requiring biopsy should be referred to an orthopedic oncologist. Prior studies have demonstrated significantly higher rates of diagnostic error for biopsies performed at referring institutions. Moreover, biopsies not performed by the treating surgeon frequently result in alterations to treatment and an ultimate change in the patient's clinical course.[79] The optimal care of patients with a musculoskeletal tumor requires a team of professionals, including an orthopedic oncologist, radiologist, pathologist, radiation oncologist, and medical oncologist.

Therapists must also be aware of the impact of chemotherapy and radiation treatments on healing soft tissue and bone, on peripheral sensation, and on physiological response to exercise and activity, as well as the individual's overall health status, immune response, prognosis, and level of energy.[80,81] The most successful rehabilitation programs are individualized and adapt to any adverse effects of concurrent therapeutic interventions. Individuals with recent diagnosis of bone cancer often find significant support in interacting with others who have previously rehabilitated from limb-sparing or amputation surgery.[82]

Limb-Sparing Surgery Versus Amputation

Historically, most tumors of bone were managed by amputation with adjunctive chemotherapy or radiation.[83] In the modern era, current reconstruction techniques using allograft bone, endoprostheses, and arthroplasty, along with a combination of multiagent chemotherapy, radiation, or isolated limb perfusion with tumor necrosis factors may be used in an effort to preserve the limb[84–87] (Fig. 19.6). These strategies have significantly reduced the number of tumor-related amputations performed each year. Amputation may be necessary when there is large, multifocal, high-grade, sarcoma, pathological fracture, significant involvement of neurovascular structures, or if the tumor is chemoresistant.[88–91] Amputation may also be indicated in the case of local recurrence following previous limb salvage.[91] The decision to perform limb salvage or amputation is multifactorial but centers around four important considerations: impact of treatment choice on patient survival, short- and long-term morbidities, the function of a salvaged limb versus a prosthesis, and psychosocial impact on the patient.[92] The potential for recurrent disease and subsequent metastases or death have been the primary concerns over attempts at limb salvage surgery in the setting of malignant disease. However, a landmark study published in 1982 found no difference in overall or disease specific survival in patients with soft tissue sarcoma that were randomized to major amputation or limb-sparing surgery with adjuvant radiotherapy.[93] Subsequent studies for other types of sarcoma have confirmed that limb salvage surgery does not jeopardize survival. Indeed, multiple recent meta-analyses of amputation versus limb salvage for osteosarcoma found a higher 50-year survival rate for limb salvage procedures without an increased risk of local recurrence.[94–96] In the modern era, patients that undergo primary amputation for an extremity sarcoma are more likely to have had loss of function of the limb due to tumor involvement or lacked a feasible salvage option due to the need to remove critical limb structures or to achieve appropriate tumor margins.[77]

Patients should be counseled with regards to morbidity associated with limb-sparing surgery as well as with amputation. Although limb-sparing surgeries can vary drastically, these procedures generally are associated with a higher rate of perioperative morbidity than amputation. Many complications are related to large endoprosthetic implants used to reconstruct resected bone. Frequently encountered complications include aseptic loosening, deep infection, instability, and implant or periprosthetic fracture.[85] Infection rates following endoprosthetic reconstruction of lower extremity tumors are approximately 10% and has been reported as high as 25% in some series, far higher than for conventional arthroplasty.[97] Nearly 10% of patients who undergo limb salvage initially may ultimately require an amputation, most commonly due to local recurrence or infection.[98] A long-term study of pediatric patients with lower extremity sarcoma treated initially with limb salvage surgery found a nearly 18% risk of late amputation at 25 years after diagnosis. Male gender and prosthetic joint reconstruction were independently associated with an increased likelihood of late amputation.[99]

Objective measures such as survival or local recurrence are relatively straightforward to collect. In contrast, the effect of treatment choice on an individual's function or quality of life is far harder to measure. In general, no studies have demonstrated a difference in functional outcomes for limb salvage or amputation for oncologic indications.[100] However, more proximal levels of amputation (i.e., proximal to the knee) are generally associated with greater functional limitations. Limb salvage, rather than amputation, at these levels has been shown to result in better measures of gait efficiency, but the impact on a patient's perception of quality of life is less clear.[101,102]

LIMB DEFICIENCY DISORDERS

Limb deficiency disorders encompass a wide range of congenital anomalies that involve hypoplasia or aplasia of one or more of the bones of the appendicular skeleton. Lower limb deficiency disorders are estimated to occur in approximately 2 per 10,000 live births.[103] Nearly half of patients with lower limb deficiency are born with major anomalies of the internal organs, axial skeleton, or central nervous system.[103,104] Deficiencies are broadly categorized as transverse or longitudinal.[105] Transverse deficiencies are perpendicular to the long axis of the limb thus resulting in the amputation of the limb at the level of the deficiency, such as the congenital absence of a foot. In contrast, longitudinal deficiency affects the long axis of the limb, as in the absence of a fibula. Transverse deficiencies are the most common type, often due to amniotic bands.[103] The rehabilitation, prosthetic, and eventual elective surgical management of children with limb deficiency is linked to age-appropriate developmental status, with the goal of enhancing function while minimizing deformity.[106] The reader is referred to Chapter 29 for in-depth information on developmentally appropriate preprosthetic and prosthetic activities for mobility and skill, as well as discussion of the therapist's and prosthetist's role in counseling and educating the family and child about rehabilitation and prosthetic alternatives.

Orthopedic management of children with congenital limb deficiency focuses on enhancing appropriate growth of the residual limb, maintaining relatively equal limb length or proximal joint levels, enhancing joint function, and ensuring appropriate prosthetic fit. Surgical treatment options include a wide variety of interventions, ranging from relatively simple such as minor revisions to optimize the shape of the limb to more complex such as surgical distraction procedures to lengthen bone, conversion to a conventional level of amputation or disarticulation or, in select instances, reconstruction involving a combination of surgical reorientation and arthrodesis.[107–110]

By way of example, children with severe partial longitudinal deficiency of the femur (proximal focal femoral deficiency) may be managed with a Van Nes procedure, known as a rotationplasty, in which the tibia is repositioned 180 degrees and fused to the residual femur (if present) or pelvis so that the reversed ankle can function as a knee joint[111] (Figs. 19.7 and 19.8). Alternatively, isolated arthrodesis of the knee and ankle disarticulation can achieve a weight-tolerant residual limb that closely resembles a traditional transfemoral residual limb.[108] Deficiencies of the fibula or tibia

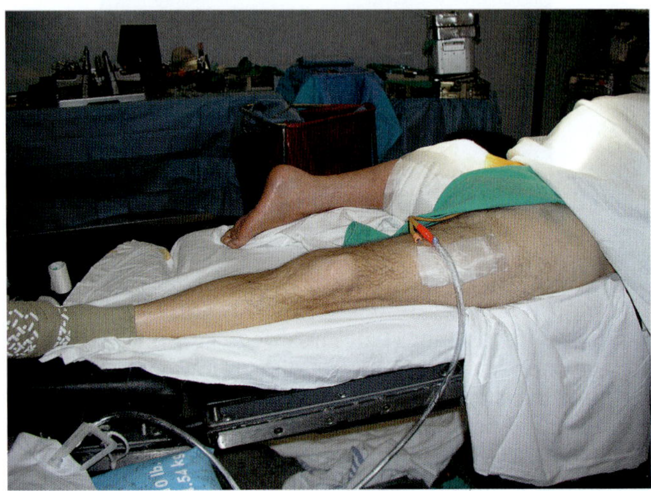

Fig. 19.7 Clinical photograph of patient who underwent right lower extremity rotationplasty for a malignant neoplasm in the right thigh. Note the right ankle has been rotated 180 degrees from its native orientation to function as a knee joint.

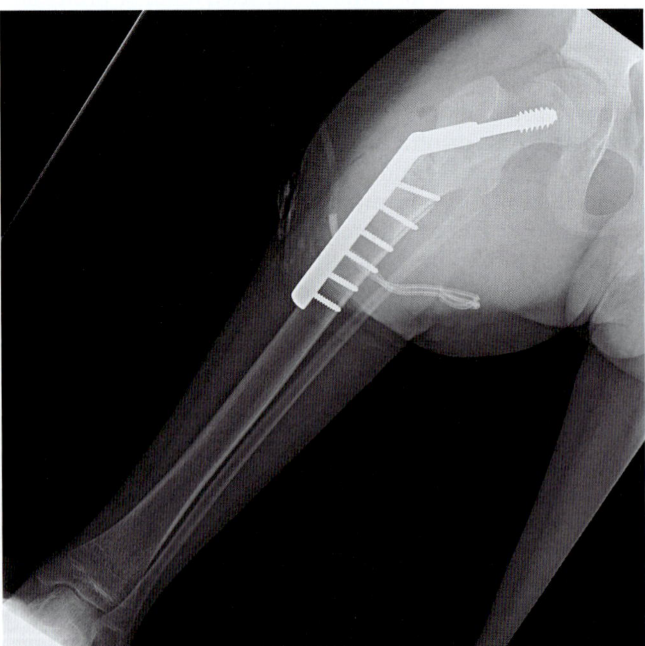

Fig. 19.8 Radiograph of same patient in Fig. 19.6 demonstrating fixation of tibia to the proximal residual femur. The ankle has been positioned at the same level as the contralateral knee.

may be managed, depending on the severity of the defect and resulting deformity, by custom footwear and shoe lift, epiphysiodesis, corrective osteotomy, limb lengthening, ankle disarticulation, or conversion to traditional transtibial amputation. [112,113] Regardless of the treatment option selected, the goal is to maximize ambulatory capability by creating a functional limb that is equal to the contralateral side.

Surgical Principles of Amputation

DETERMINING THE LEVEL OF AMPUTATION

Determination of the appropriate level of amputation is guided by two principles: soft tissue coverage and preservation of residual limb length. An adequately vascularized soft tissue envelope must be present to ensure successful healing.[114] Preoperative physical examination and other previously mentioned measures such as the ankle-brachial index, transcutaneous oximetry, and angiography provide key information about the adequacy of blood flow to the threatened portion of the extremity. In the setting of traumatic amputations, repeat examination of remaining soft tissue during serial irrigation and debridement prior to definitive closure aids in the determination of viable tissue.[56] Residual limb length plays an important role in the mechanical work able to be performed as well as with prosthesis options and fit. Furthermore, as many functional anatomic joints as reasonably possible should be preserved. The energy required for ambulation increases significantly with more proximal amputations.[115,116] Remaining muscles and joints must compensate for the absence of muscle function distal to the level of amputation. For example, patients with transfemoral amputation adapt to limb loss with trunk and pelvic movement asymmetries to facilitate weight transfer during walking. In contrast, patients with transtibial amputations do not demonstrate the need for such adaptations.[117]

At times, tension occurs between the goals of length preservation and adequate soft tissue coverage. For individuals with plantar neuropathic ulcers and osteomyelitis, for example, a transmetatarsal amputation has the potential to preserve the ankle joint and permit functional gait without prosthesis and is often less difficult for individuals to accept psychologically.[118] If there is delayed or failed healing, however, the risks of complications associated with limited activity and bedrest (e.g., further deconditioning, pneumonia, deep venous thrombosis, decubitus ulcer) and repeated anesthesia if surgical revisions to more proximal levels become necessary can be significant.[119] In these instances an initial surgery at the transtibial level might improve the chances for optimal rehabilitation outcome.[120] In individuals with traumatic crush injury to the proximal tibia but intact knee joint, an extremely short transtibial residual limb may actually be more difficult to manage prosthetically than a long transfemoral residual limb: the reduced surface area around a short residual tibia and fibula for weight bearing within the socket increases pressure on the skin and soft tissue of the residual limb, reducing functional wearing time of the prosthesis despite the advantage of preservation of the anatomical knee joint. Put succinctly, limb length should be preserved so long as it does not result in a nonhealing, painful, or dysfunctional residual limb. This includes atypical, novel, or extralong amputations such as a transtibial amputation below the level of the mid-tibia. Due to both poor soft tissue coverage as well as limited space available for prostheses, these levels risk leaving the patient with the limitations of both the more proximal and more distal amputation levels, without the full benefits of either.

TECHNICAL CONSIDERATIONS

Bone

Following amputation, the residual bone of the limb will be required to transmit force between the body and the prosthetic device. This transmission of force may occur either through the end of a resected bone as in a transfemoral amputation or through a disarticulated joint as in a Syme amputation. To accommodate this function, residual bone should be surgically contoured to allow for a smooth weight-bearing surface. Bony prominences not covered by adequate soft tissue should be resected.

Soft Tissue and Muscle

Careful management of skin and muscle at the site of amputation allows for the creation of a durable soft tissue envelope that can withstand the stress of weight bearing and prosthetic fit. Furthermore, appropriate muscle coverage can allow for improved control and alignment of the residual limb.[121,122] In general, there are two ways of securing muscle about the end of a residual limb: myoplasty or myodesis. Myoplasty involves suturing of a residual muscle to its antagonist over the end of the residual limb to create physiologic tension between the two muscle groups. However, this is generally not recommended in isolation as tension may not be achieved and deep bursa formation may occur as a result of the unstable muscle mass.[56,121] Myodesis involves suturing residual muscle and fascia directly to bone through drill holes or to the periosteum. This technique results in the most structurally stable construct and allows for secure soft tissue padding, preserved muscle bulk, and functional muscle use during ambulation.[123,124] In the absence of myodesis, residual muscles are likely to experience greater atrophy and contractures may result from unbalanced muscle units. Skin flaps should be kept as thick as possible, particularly in the setting of dysvascular amputations as the underlying subcutaneous tissue provides blood flow to the skin. In certain patients without compromised circulation, split thickness skin grafts, local rotational flaps, or free tissue transfer can be utilized in "heroic" efforts to preserve length and amputation level, particularly just distal to the knee or elbow.[72,125] Patients should be counseled that although these techniques result in successful preservation, they are associated with frequent complications. While it is important to achieve adequate soft tissue coverage, this effort should not be taken to the extreme. Excessive, often hypermobile skin and soft tissue at the end of the limb should be avoided as it interferes with both prosthesis wear and control.

Nerve

Following transection of a peripheral nerve, regenerating axons from the proximal portion form a disorganized mass of abnormal nerve as they attempt to reconnect with the distal stump. While presumably all transected nerves form a neuroma, not all are symptomatic. Ebrahimazed et al. found a 13% rate of symptomatic neuromata in transtibial amputations, and a 32% rate in transfemoral amputations.[126,127] Surgical management is frequently required—symptomatic neuromata were the indication for 11% of revision procedures in a retrospective review of 300 consecutive combat-related lower extremity amputations.[128] A neuroma is most likely to be symptomatic when it forms in an anatomic region where it is exposed to pressure, stretch, or vascular pulsations. A multitude of both prophylactic and therapeutic techniques have been described to address symptomatic neuromata; however, there is no clear gold standard treatment or prevention option.[129–131] At present, the most commonly performed and simplest procedure is a traction neurectomy in which the nerve is pulled distally and then transected.[132] On transection, the nerve retracts into the limb, ideally in an area of robust soft tissue coverage. This does not prevent neuroma formation but rather is intended to place the transected nerve end in an area with robust soft tissue padding well away from ligated vessels and the end of the residual limb. Recently, there have been a number of promising techniques for nerve management in the setting of amputation as discussed later.

Vessels

Special attention should be paid to hemostasis and management of blood vessels. The use of tourniquet during the procedure allows for improved visualization and hemostasis intraoperatively and has not been shown to result in increased healing complications, even in the case of severe peripheral arterial disease.[133,134] Major vessels should be identified and ligated with nonabsorbable suture. Larger blood vessels, such as the popliteal artery, should be double ligated, particularly in patients with normal blood flow. The tourniquet should be deflated prior to closure and meticulous hemostasis obtained. Suction drains are routinely used to prevent accumulation of a hematoma postoperatively.

Postoperative Care

DRESSINGS

The completion of the surgical procedure is but the first stage of the intervention. A multidisciplinary team of physical medicine specialists, physical therapists, occupational therapists, and prosthetists is required to achieve the ultimate goal of restoring function via fitting of an appropriate prosthetic limb. The average time to prosthetic fitting varies widely, depending on the level of amputation as well as patient- and healthcare system–related factors. For transtibial amputations, the time to prosthetic fitting following amputation has been reported to range between 19 and 76 days.[135] Our preference is to fit most traumatic, oncologic, and congenital amputations between 4 and 6 weeks postoperatively. This period is substantially longer for dysvascular patients to ensure that adequate superficial and deep wound healing, which is slower in such patients, has occurred.

The primary concerns in the transition from amputation to functional residual limb are adequate wound healing, edema control, prevention of joint contractures, and rapid return to activity. Toward those ends, a number of philosophies exist with regards to postoperative dressings and wound care. For the most part, patients are kept non-weight bearing on the involved extremity until the wounds are healed. Commonly used dressing techniques include soft dressing, rigid dressings, and immediate postoperative prosthesis (IPOP). When a soft dressing is used, a sterile dressing is applied to the surgical incision and the limb is wrapped in a compressive bandage. The limb is kept elevated and, depending on the amputation level, elastic shrinkers are applied as soon as postoperative drains are removed. Alternatively, rigid dressings consist of a well-padded plaster of Paris splint or cast that is applied to the limb at the conclusion of surgery (Fig. 19.9). Potential advantages of rigid dressings include edema control, prevention of joint contractures, and a shorter time to prosthetic fitting.[135] On the other hand, soft dressing may be better suited for amputations with tenuous skin closure as it allows for greater ease of wound inspection and decreased risk of pressure ulceration. Removable rigid dressings (RRDs) may provide the best of both techniques by providing the benefits of a rigid dressing with regard to contracture prevention and protection from external trauma, while at the same time providing ease of access for regular wound inspection.[136] Regardless of the selected technique, the goals remain the same: reduced edema, controlled pain, contracture prevention, and a stable limb volume that is healed and amenable to prosthetic fitting.

As suggested by the name, a patient with an IPOP is fitted with a temporary prosthesis immediately following surgery. Reported advantages include early ambulation and rehabilitation, which may reduce the sequelae of prolonged immobilization as well as providing a psychologic benefit.[137–139]

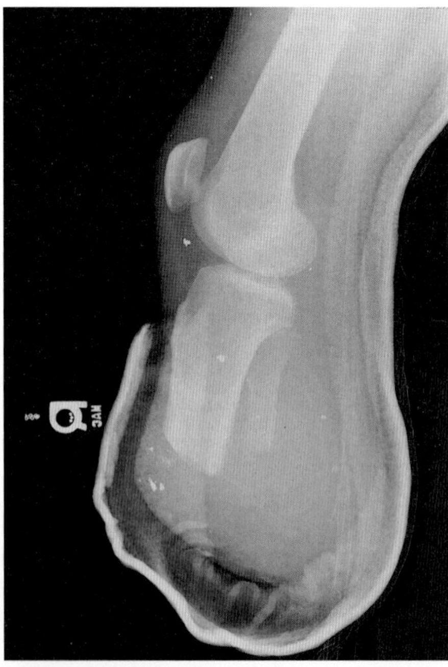

Fig. 19.9 Postoperative lateral radiograph of transtibial amputation demonstrating rigid plaster of Paris splint, molded to keep knee in an extended position. Note that the splint material stops short of the patella, an area with prominent subcutaneous bone that is prone to ulceration with rigid dressings.

However, the success of this technique has been demonstrated in primarily nontraumatic-related amputations and concerns persist regarding wound healing and early detection of infection that may preclude early mobilization.[56]

PAIN MANAGEMENT

Patients undergoing lower extremity amputation commonly experience significant acute postoperative pain, with studies reporting moderate-to-severe residual limb pain in 30% to 53% of patients.[140,141] Patients with acute postoperative pain are thought to be at higher risk for developing chronic residual limb pain; thus, much effort has been devoted to optimizing postoperative pain management following amputation.[141] Current recommended strategies include a multimodal approach using interventional methods with perineural regional or epidural analgesia and pharmacologic agents including acetaminophen, nonsteroidal antiinflammatories, gabapentin, ketamine, and opioid therapy as well as so-called alternative measures (e.g., acupuncture, biofeedback) as needed.[142] Given the complexity of analgesic techniques and the multiple classes of medication involved, consultation with a pain medicine specialist should be strongly considered, both for optimization of perioperative pain control and for management of potential chronic pain issues.

Complications

Unfortunately, complications frequently occur following lower extremity amputations. Complications can range from minor, such as superficial wound necrosis, to major, such as need for reamputation at a more proximal level or death. A study of 2879 patients who underwent a major amputation following trauma found a 27.5% rate of major postoperative complications.[50] Data from the LEAP study further lend insight into complication profiles after trauma-related amputations. Over the course of 24 months following surgery, a total of 128 complications were reported in 149 patients who underwent amputation during the initial hospitalization. Wound infection (34.2%), wound necrosis (13.4%), phantom limb pain (13.4%), and "stump" complications (10.7%) were most frequently reported.[67] Complications following amputations for vascular insufficiency are also regrettably common, with one multicenter prospective clinical database study finding an overall complication rate of 43%, with nearly 20% of patients being readmitted to the hospital within 30 days of the index procedure.[143] Minor amputations are also subject to complicated postoperative courses. One retrospective study of 717 patients undergoing toe and transmetatarsal amputations found a readmission rate of 13.9% with infection, ischemia, and nonhealing wounds as the leading causes. Nearly all (95%) of those readmitted underwent reamputation, with almost two-thirds (64%) requiring a transtibial or more proximal amputation.[144] Risk factors for readmission were largely nonmodifiable, including hypertension, peripheral artery disease, and renal insufficiency.

WOUND HEALING

If wound healing problems are encountered, the initial step in evaluation should be reevaluation of the amputation level. This is of particular relevance for dysvascular amputations. Previously mentioned objective measures including ABI and transcutaneous oxygen levels should be utilized to determine healing potential.[145] Two other key and potentially modifiable risk factors include nutrition and smoking status. Multiple authors have cited a cutoff of less than 3.5 g/dL albumin and total lymphocyte count less than 1500 cells per cubic millimeter as markers of malnutrition and a potential risk factor for wound healing following amputation.[146–149] At a minimum, nutritional intake should be optimized in the postoperative period and if possible, preoperatively. Smoking compromises cutaneous blood flow velocity, increases the risk of microthrombi, and has been shown to be associated with a 2.5 times higher risk of infection and reamputation in smokers as compared to nonsmokers.[150] Similarly, being a current smoker predicted more complications (odds ratio = 1.8) in transfemoral amputations performed due to critical limb ischemia.[151] In the trauma patient population, current smokers with limb-threatening open tibia fractures were found to be twice as likely to develop an infection compared to nonsmokers.[152] Though often difficult, the topic of smoking cessation should be discussed with patients undergoing amputation. Patients may benefit from counseling, nicotine replacement therapy (itself a vasoconstrictor), and pharmacologic agents such as antidepressants.[153]

FLUID COLLECTIONS

The risk of developing a postoperative hematoma can be mitigated by meticulous hemostasis during the procedure, the use of drain, and adequate compression via either soft or rigid dressings. Surgical dogma suggests that a hematoma can compromise wound healing by serving as a culture medium for bacterial infection and may require evacuation in the operating room. However, the presence of an acute postoperative fluid collection is not indicative of an infection in and of itself. In a study of patients with combat-related amputations, over half demonstrated fluid collection within the early (<3 months) postoperative period[154] (Fig. 19.10). The only factors associated with return to the operating room and a diagnosis of infection were clinical findings of erythema, warmth, and wound drainage. Nonetheless, given the incidence of postoperative infection following both trauma and vascular-related amputations, wounds should be monitored closely.[67,155]

During the perioperative period, standard guidelines for the prevention of surgical site infection should be followed, including timely administration of antibiotics preoperatively, careful antiseptic technique, and thorough irrigation with normal saline in the setting of traumatic injuries. Topical, intrawound antibiotic application has been shown to decrease residual limb infection in combat-related amputations.[156]

HETEROTOPIC OSSIFICATION

Following amputation, particularly high-energy traumatic amputations, bone may form in the soft tissues surrounding a residual limb. This process, known as heterotopic ossification (HO), has been noted to occur in nearly 65% of high-energy, combat-related amputations[157] (Fig. 19.11). While

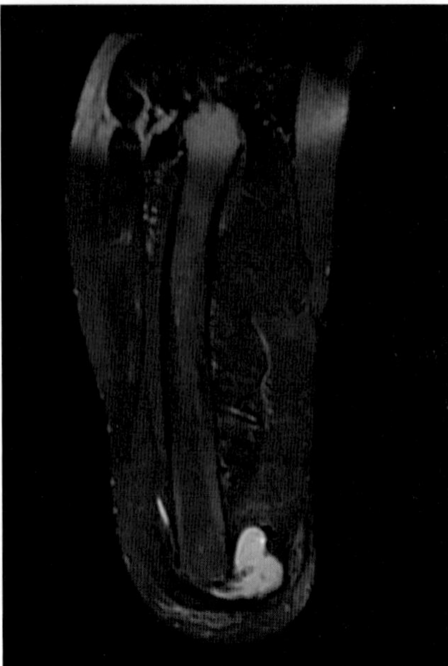

Fig. 19.10 Sagittal T2 sequence magnetic resonance imaging of transfemoral amputation demonstrating fluid collection at the distal end of the residual femur.

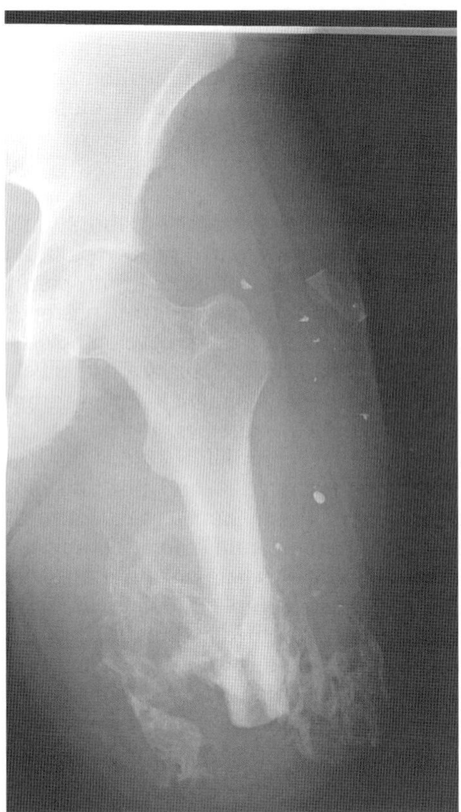

Fig. 19.11 Radiograph of transfemoral amputation with severe heterotopic ossification surrounding the distal portion of the residual femur.

asymptomatic HO can simply be observed, surgical excision is the only available treatment option for prominent subcutaneous bone that interferes with prosthetic fit and wear. In a study of reoperation following combat-related lower extremity amputations, HO excision was found to be the second most common indication (24%) for return to the operating room.[128] The etiology of posttraumatic HO is thought to be due to a combination of both local wound conditions and a systemic inflammatory response to injury.[158] Nonsteroidal antiinflammatory therapy and low-dose irradiation are effective measures for prevention of HO following total hip arthroplasty and surgical treatment of acetabular fractures, but concerns over both safety and feasibility in trauma-related amputations have led to a search for alternate prophylactic agents.[159–162] Bear in mind that HO does not occur exclusively in combat-related amputations—a retrospective review of 158 civilian patients with lower limb amputations found a 23% rate of HO, although the severity of HO formation and need for surgical excision was less than reported in military cohorts.[163] These differences are attributed to the lower incidence of blast mechanism and generally less severe systemic injury patterns found in civilian trauma.[157]

PAIN

While the true prevalence of chronic amputation-related pain is unknown, several cross-sectional survey studies of patients with amputation suggest that more than 70% of individuals experience some degree of amputation-related pain, regardless of time since amputation.[164,165] Pain can be broadly categorized into phantom limb pain (PLP), residual limb pain (RLP), or pain due to distant causes, such as a herniated disc. Phantom limb pain is defined as painful sensations perceived in the missing portion of the amputated limb while residual limb pain is perceived to originate from the residuum itself. The exact pathophysiology of phantom limb pain remains unclear, but is thought to be the result of a complex interaction between the central nervous system, peripheral nervous system, and psychological factors.[166] Current methods of treatment include three broad categories: pharmacologic (nonsteroidal antiinflammatory drugs, acetaminophen, opioids, antidepressants, anticonvulsants, N-methyl-D-aspartate (NMDA) receptor agonists), invasive (neurectomy, cordotomy, sympathectomy, spinal cord stimulation), and nonpharmacologic/noninvasive (mirror therapy, biofeedback, hypnosis, acupuncture). Regrettably, to date there are no treatments that provide for complete relief of PLP. A recent review of phantom limb pain highlights the substantial prevalence of this complication (up to 80%) as well as the lack of evidence based interventions to treat this vexing problem.[167] The authors emphasize the importance of a multimodal approach within an interdisciplinary team, and recent surgical advances such as targeted muscle reinnervation (TMR) and regenerative peripheral nerve interfaces (RPNIs), discussed below, may provide an enduring solution to PLP.

RLP can most frequently be attributed to issues with prosthetic fit. Most sockets require an intimate fit to maximize function and avoid focal pressure points. If pain is increased with prosthetic wear, an evaluation for fit and alignment should be considered. Other reasons for residual limb pain include infection, edema, or dermatologic problems. Point tenderness within the residual limb may result from bursa, muscle, bone spurs, or neuroma formation. Several promising techniques are being investigated in regards to neuroma management and will be discussed in greater detail at the end of the chapter.

Outcomes

As previously discussed, functional outcomes are intimately related to both level of amputation and the disease state leading to amputation. Distal amputations with more preserved anatomic joints result in greater patient mobility with more efficient energy expenditure.[115,168] In general, patients with trauma-related amputations are younger and have fewer medical comorbidities, resulting in superior functional outcomes. Patients undergoing dysvascular amputations, on the other hand, have generally dismal overall survival, much less functional outcomes. One large retrospective study found an overall survival rate of 69.7% at 1 year and 34.7% at 5 years.[169] Notably, survival for patients with transfemoral amputations was significantly worse (50.6% and 22.5%) than for transtibial amputations (74.5% and 37.8%). A separate study of major dysvascular amputations found that of those patients surviving 2 years after amputation, only half remained functionally ambulatory.[170]

Once again, the data from the LEAP study provide considerable insight into functional outcomes following trauma-related amputations. In the cohort of 161 patients who underwent amputation, functional outcomes at 2 years were generally poor, with similar Sickness Impact Profile scores amongst patients with transtibial, through knee, and transfemoral amputations.[171] However, self-selected walking speeds were higher in the transtibial cohort as compared to the transfemoral cohort and a higher percentage of patients with transtibial amputations were able to walk independently on uneven ground. Of note, patients with through knee amputations fared worse than patients with either transtibial or transfemoral amputations, a finding that contrasted with the principles of length preservation in amputation surgery. Patients with through knee amputations had lower self-selected walking speeds, less independence in transfer, walking, or stair climbing, and also needed more help with physically demanding tasks, thus calling in to question the wisdom of a through knee amputation. The authors of the study surmised that worse functional outcomes were seen in this cohort as a result of limited soft tissue coverage at this level (i.e., long posterior flaps containing the gastrocnemius muscles generally used to cover this region are frequently absent in trauma-related amputations, and were not present in 12 of the 17 through knee amputations in that study).

A meta-analysis including 3105 patients with trauma-related lower extremity amputations lends further understanding of expected functional outcomes.[172] The author found that patients with transtibial amputations consistently demonstrates better outcomes than more proximal amputations across all outcome measures, including 36-Item Short Form Survey (SF-36) physical components score. A significantly higher proportion of patients with transtibial amputations (72%) and through knee amputations (78%) were able to walk a distance greater than 500m as compared to transfemoral amputations (55%) or bilateral amputations (50%). However, a significantly higher percentage of patients with through knee amputation (85%) reported painful symptoms associated with the residual limb and wore their prosthesis considerably less. Overall, 70% of patients with a lower extremity amputation were able to return to work, with no statistical difference between amputation levels. However, the subgroup analysis of military patients found that only 16% of patients with a transtibial amputation were able to return to duty while 11% of patients with a transfemoral amputation returned to duty. While not as profound, decreased rates of return to duty were also demonstrated in a retrospective review of US military service members with lower extremity amputation; overall less than 50% were able to return to active duty.[173] Of particular note, this study also reported a nearly 40% rate of depressive symptoms and almost one-fifth of patients screened positive for posttraumatic stress disorder. Although these statistics include both amputation and limb salvage patients, the point remains the same: the loss of a limb is a major life event and can have significant psychosocial impact. Findings were similar in a study of the civilian trauma population. Of 569 patients enrolled in the LEAP study, 48% screened positive for a likely psychologic disorders at 3 months and, at 2 years following injury, one-fifth reported severe phobic anxiety or depression.[174] Despite the prevalence of these mental health concerns, only 22% of patients had received mental health services at 2 years after injury. Individuals caring for persons with limb loss must be aware of the prevalence of mental health concerns in this patient population, and should facilitate access to appropriate mental health resources whenever possible.[175]

Patients with lower extremity amputations are also subject to a number of secondary health effects, mostly related to reduced mobility and biomechanical changes to ambulation patterns.

Rates of both hip and knee osteoarthritis in the intact limbs of unilateral amputees have been found to exceed that of the general population, potentially due to the increased demand placed on these joints.[176] Similarly, over half of amputees report bothersome levels of back pain at a rate roughly twice that of general population.[164,165] Delayed ambulation and proximal levels of amputation have also been associated with the development of low bone mineral density in patients sustaining trauma-related amputations.[177] Finally, amputation affects more than just the musculoskeletal system—there has been a long-studied association between amputation and subsequent cardiovascular risk—including the development atherosclerosis and abdominal aortic aneurysms.[178–181] Further concerns include obesity and secondary diabetes at increased rates.[182]

Amputations of the Foot and Ankle

Amputations of one or more toes (digit, phalanx) or part of the foot are the most frequently performed surgeries in older individuals, often secondary to a nonhealing, often infected, neuropathic plantar ulcers. Individuals most vulnerable to development of plantar ulcers usually present with a combination of sensory impairment (loss of protective sensation); autonomic dysfunction (dry and brittle skin); foot deformity resulting from weakness of the intrinsic muscles of the foot; and impaired circulation that, although adequate to sustain an intact limb, is insufficient to allow healing to occur.[183] In these situations, it is especially important to determine (before amputation) the point at which limb circulation is sufficient for successful healing of the residual foot. Bear in mind that physical deconditioning due to prolonged bedrest and systemic complications associated with repeat surgical revisions of a poorly healing amputation can substantially compromise the rehabilitation process and jeopardize the potential for a positive outcome. Amputations of the foot may also be the result of severe crush injury, land mine explosion, shrapnel wounds, or similar acute trauma to the foot. Those with partial foot amputation may require adaptive footwear, shoe filler, a passive prosthesis, or accommodative foot orthoses, and may be referred to physical therapy for gait training with an appropriate assistive device.

AMPUTATIONS OF THE TOES

Phalangeal (digit) amputations are performed most often due to vascular insufficiency, failed conservative management of a neuropathic ulcer on the plantar toe surface, or when there is infection or osteomyelitis of the phalanges.[184] Digit amputation can be performed at the distal, middle, or proximal interphalangeal joints or with removal of the metatarsal head.[185] Adequate circulation for healing of the surgical wound is a prerequisite to amputation surgery at this distal level.

For removal of digits, sagittal flaps are typically used (Fig. 19.12). If there will also be resection of metatarsal head, the surgeon may opt to use a "racquet" incision. The digits are removed, either by disarticulation through the joint or transection through the shaft of the digit, using an oscillating saw. Amputation of the base of the great toe should preserve at least 1 cm of the proximal phalanx so as to allow for some retained plantar flexion at the metatarsophalangeal joint.[186] Complete loss of the hallux results in dysfunction in toe off, particularly noticeable during rapid walking or running.[187] If the base of the proximal phalanx is preserved, at least one sesamoid bone should also be saved to maintain weight-bearing function of the first metatarsal. In the case of disarticulation at the metatarsophalangeal articulation, sesamoids should be removed to prevent undue plantar pressure, particularly in the neuropathic patient.[186]

Amputation of the lesser toes causes relatively little gait disturbance; however, leaving only one or two toes in a diabetic patient may lead to concentrated pressure and subsequent ulceration and thus it is advisable to remove all of the toes in this setting.

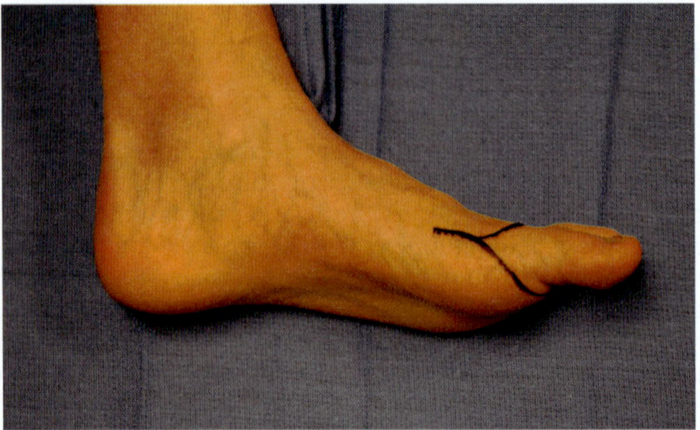

Fig. 19.12 Incision for disarticulation at the metatarsophalangeal joint. When skin conditions allow, a long plantar flap should be fashioned.

Surgical wounds are closed in a standard fashion, with the goal of a tension free primary closure.

Toe separators may be included in the postoperative dressing to prevent drift of the remaining toes into the defect made by the amputated digit.[186]

Patients may be kept non–weight bearing, or alternatively, hindfoot weight bearing only until the incisions are well healed. The individual is encouraged to keep the limb elevated as much as possible: education about avoiding prolonged dependency of the limb (i.e., elevating the limb while sitting) is essential. A stiff sole postoperative shoe may be used to protect the forefoot for several weeks or months following surgery, before returning to normal footwear. Individuals with dysvascular and neuropathic disease benefit from custom-fabricated accommodative orthosis to distribute plantar pressures and minimize the risk of developing additional neuropathic ulcers on plantar surfaces of the remaining digits and metatarsal heads.

Ray Resection

A ray resection involves removal of the toe and all or part of its corresponding metatarsal. This procedure is performed most commonly in the setting of vascular disease, neuropathic ulcer or osteomyelitis. Regrettably, many patients undergoing partial ray resection will require reamputation at a more proximal level.[188] Border-ray resections (the first and fifth rays) are easier to perform and generally have better functional outcomes than central ray resections.[189] The gap left by central ray resection may cause difficulty with skin closure, necessitating more proximal resection of the central ray to allow the adjacent rays to drift centrally.[186]

The residual metatarsal (if any) is beveled at a 30- to 45-degree angle so that there will be no sharp edge to damage tissue during the late stance phase, as body weight rolls over the distal plantar surface of the healed residual limb. If multiple rays are resected, skin graft may be required for wound closure.[190] Given the high rates of failure of this type of amputation at baseline, however, our preference is to recommend and proceed to a more proximal level of amputation if advanced skin or soft tissue coverage is required.

Ray resection may be the surgery of choice for problems of the fourth and fifth rays: as long as the first through third rays are intact, there is minimum compromise to forward progression in gait on the healed residual limb. When the first and second rays must be removed, however, there is significant disruption of weight bearing forces during walking and high risk of ulceration; a complete transmetatarsal amputation managed with custom footwear with a rocker bottom often has better functional outcome than leaving the third through fifth rays intact.[191,192]

The deformity that results when multiple rays have been amputated may require an accommodative orthosis or a prosthetic filler in the shoe, along with adaptive or custom footwear to protect the residual limb from high pressures resulting from altered biomechanics during forward progression and propulsion when walking.

Transmetatarsal Amputation

A complete transmetatarsal amputation (TMA) is resection of all five metatarsals proximal to the metatarsal head. In this surgery, the goal is to preserve as much length of the shaft of the metatarsals and healthy plantar skin as possible so that the resulting residual limb will be long enough for an effective biomechanical lever for forward progression over the foot during gait and will have enough plantar surface such that higher shear forces and pressures exerted on the shortened forefoot during the late stance phase of gait will not compromise skin condition.[193] It is difficult to predict whether primary healing is possible after TMA in persons with diabetes and critical limb ischemia. A systematic review of reoperation and reamputation after transmetatarsal amputation reported a 33.2% rate of major amputation following the index procedure.[119]

To perform a transmetatarsal amputation a fish mouth style incisions is made on the dorsal foot just proximal to the metatarsal heads, and continues in a curvilinear arc along the plantar surface almost to the base of the toes (Fig. 19.13A and B) This type of incision creates a long plantar flap that will be sutured closed after bony and soft tissue elements have been excised. An oscillating saw is used to transect each of the metatarsals, and then the toes are plantar flexed to allow careful dissection of the soft tissue that will be used as the posterior flap from the bony structures being removed. The tendons and sheaths of extrinsic muscles of the foot, as well as distal attachments of intrinsic muscles, are transected; the plantar surface of residual metatarsals are beveled or rounded; and any distal nerves are resected under slight tension and allowed to retract into the residual limb. The normal cascade of the metatarsals should be recreated, progressing from distal medial to proximal lateral (Fig. 19.14A). When possible, all five metatarsal bases should be preserved for better midfoot balance and to reduce the risk of Charcot breakdown in neuropathic patients.[186] The plantar flap can be secured to the residual metatarsals via drill holes and then trimmed and debulked to fit appropriately to the dorsal incisions for a smooth wound closure.[194]

Although only tendon insertions involving toes are lost with this amputation level, muscle imbalance between dorsiflexors and plantar flexors increases as the length of a transmetatarsal residual limb decreases. This leaves individuals with short residual metatarsals at risk of developing equinovarus deformity in an already vulnerable foot. Tendon transfers are commonly performed to restore balance to the transmetatarsal residual limb.[195,196] Achilles lengthening is performed to provide greater ankle dorsiflexion, ultimately reducing distal plantar pressures on the residual forefoot.[197] A retrospective study of 85 patients undergoing TMA found a 35% rate of recurrent ulceration in patients undergoing TMA alone as compared to 3% in the cohort that underwent TMA with concomitant achilles tendon lengthening.[198]

A standard dressing and compressive wrap is applied following the procedure. Limited mobility and non–weight-bearing ambulation is usually recommended in the immediate postoperative period however, some authors have reported success with application of total contact cast and immediate weight bearing following the procedure.[194] Gradual progression to full weight bearing with an assistive device (walker, crutches, single cane) and independent ambulation without an assistive device is determined by skin condition of the residual limb and the individual's previous ambulatory status, postural control, and functional

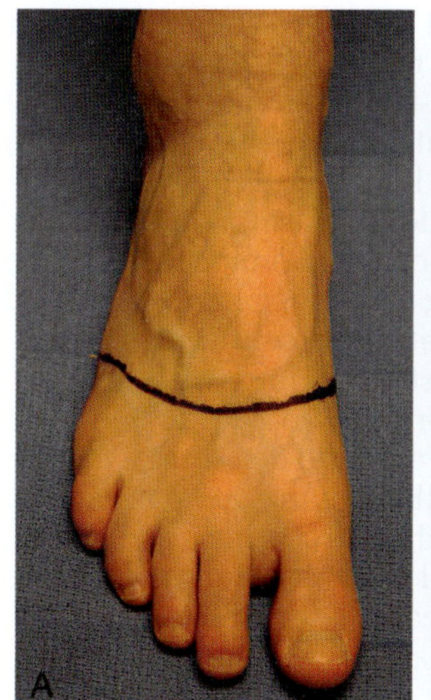

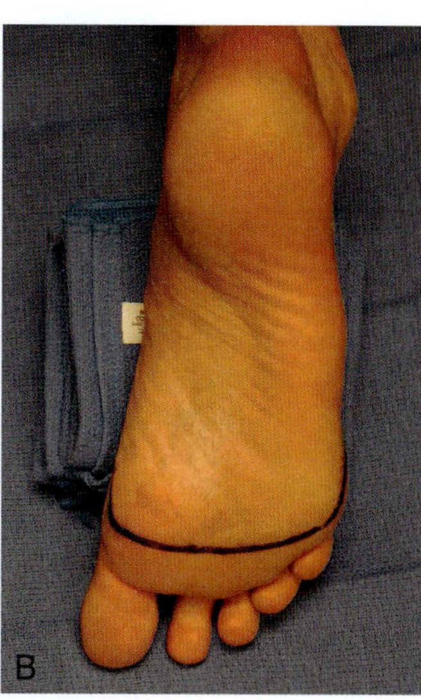

Fig. 19.13 Dorsal (A) and plantar (B) incisions for transmetatarsal amputation, note that plantar flap is longer than dorsal flap to allow coverage over the end of the transected metatarsals.

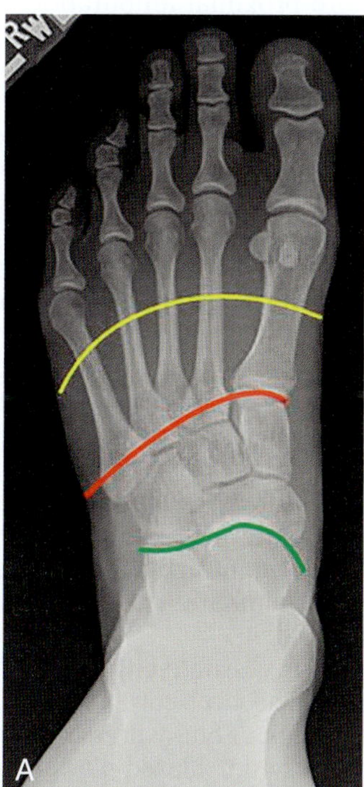

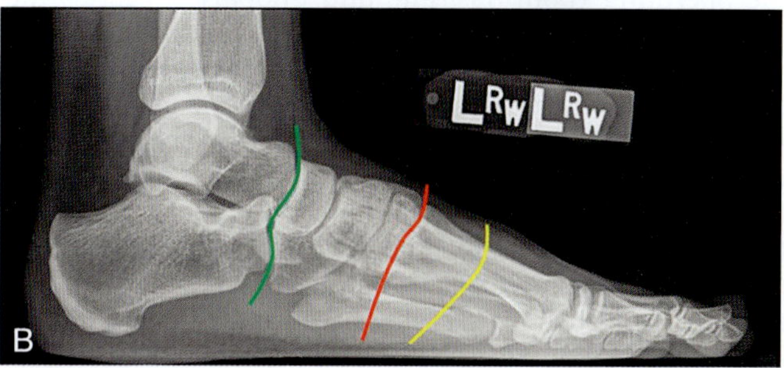

Fig. 19.14 Anterior-posterior (A) and lateral (B) radiographs of the foot with the transection levels for transmetatarsal (*yellow*), Lisfranc or tarsometatarsal (*red*), and Chopart or midtarsal (*green*) amputations.

level. Many individuals benefit from wearing a sneaker or oxford with forefoot filler and a rocker bottom applied to the sole to dissipate higher weight-bearing forces on the distal plantar residual limb in the late stance phase; those with short residual transmetatarsal limbs may require a custom shoe that encompasses the ankle or a custom thermoplastic ankle-foot orthosis to counteract muscle imbalance leading to equinovarus position during the swing phase of gait and to ensure efficient heel strike at initial contact and appropriate forward progression in stance. Those with polyneuropathy should be cautioned not to go barefoot, even in their home environment: their ability to detect injury to the plantar (or dorsal) surface of the foot may be significantly compromised. An open wound (neuropathic or traumatic in origin) on a transmetatarsal residual limb that becomes infected or fails to heal often leads to revision to the transtibial amputation level.

AMPUTATIONS OF THE MIDFOOT

Within the midfoot, amputations can be performed via disarticulation of the tarsometarsal joints (Lisfranc procedure) or midtarsal joints (Chopart procedure) (Fig. 19.14A and B) Both Lisfranc and Chopart amputations are often preferable to more proximal amputations as both procedures maintain the calcaneus and its tough, weight bearing skin. The operative approach and postoperative care for both surgeries is similar to that of a transmetatarsal amputations. The surgical incision is made more proximally across the dorsum of the foot, and a long posterior/plantar flap is created to wrap upward toward the dorsal incision when the surgical wound is closed. In a Lisfranc procedure, the forefoot is excised from the midfoot through the tarsometatarsal joint, usually leaving the "keystone" base of the second metatarsal in place to maintain a transverse arch of the midfoot. The distal attachments of the peroneus brevis, peroneus longus, extensor hallucis longus, and anterior tibialis may be repositioned during surgery in an attempt to restore balance between muscle groups controlling dorsiflexion/plantar flexion and inversion/eversion positioning of the foot at rest and during walking.[199] In a Chopart procedure, the disarticulation takes place in the joints between the talus and navicular and between the calcaneus and cuboid.

Both procedures necessitate either lengthening or complete sectioning of the heel cord in an effort to prevent equinovarus deformity. A bulky dressing with an compressive wrap or a slightly dorsiflexed plaster cast is applied in the operating room. Lisfranc and Chopart surgeries may be used for individuals with significant traumatic injury or bone or soft tissue tumor in the forefoot; they are rarely used for individuals with dysvascular or neuropathic limbs.[193] Although both approaches preserve the ability to bear weight through the calcaneus, there is even greater likelihood of development of the equinovarus deformity and prosthetic fitting can be challenging. A retrospective study of 18 patients undergoing Chopart amputation for a diabetic foot infection reported a 94% rate of wound complications and low rate (44%) of successful ambulation with a prosthesis, leading the authors to recommend judicious patient selection when performing amputation at this level.[200] Persons with a midfoot-level residual limbs typically require custom footwear and orthoses that control the residual limb above the ankle for protection during activity and to ensure biomechanically sound, safe ambulation.[201]

SYME AMPUTATION

The most commonly performed amputation involving the hindfoot is the Syme procedure, a surgical technique that disarticulates the tibiotalar joint (i.e., ankle), trims the malleoli to create a flat weight-bearing surface, and repositions the fat pad and soft tissue of the heel under the distal tibia and fibula (Figs. 19.15 and 19.16). Although the Syme procedure reduces leg length with removal of the calcaneus and talus, a well healed distal residual limb is pressure tolerant for ambulation with a prosthesis and, if necessary, for short distances (e.g., emergencies, getting to the bathroom at night) without a prosthesis.[186] As such, energy expenditure in patients with Syme amputations is nearly equivalent to age-matched controls.[168] A variation of the Syme procedure, known as a Pirogoff amputation, retains the weight-bearing portion of the calcaneus and fuses it to the distal tibia. A recent systematic review of Syme amputations found a vascular etiology as the indication for amputation in 65% of patients.[202] The most common complications in adults included residual limb pain (25%), ulceration or infection (23%), need for reamputation (20%), and skin problems (18%).

The surgical incision for Syme amputations extends along the anterior ankle from medial to lateral malleoli and then curves downward around the plantar (posterior calcaneus) surface to outline what will be the distal pad of the residual limb. After sharp incision through skin and subcutaneous tissue, toe extensor and dorsiflexor tendons are cut and the anterior capsule of the ankle is exposed. The foot is passively plantar flexed so as to access and open the joint capsule medially to laterally (with care to preserve the posterior tibialis artery going to tissue that will be the pad of the residual limb) and to disarticulate the talus. The posterior joint capsule, posterior tibialis tendon, and flexor hallucis longus tendon are transected. The periosteum of the calcaneus is carefully stripped and preserved for use in

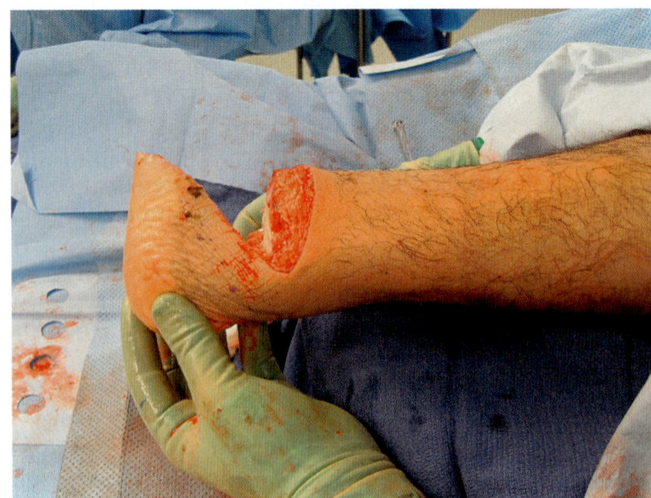

Fig. 19.15 Intraoperative photograph of a Syme amputation prior to securing heel pad to the distal end of the tibia.

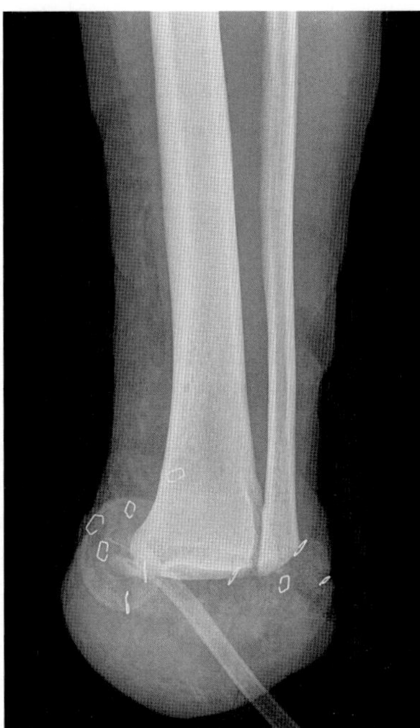

Fig. 19.16 Postoperative anterior-posterior AP radiograph of a Syme amputation showing disarticulation through the tibiotalar joint and resection of the medial and lateral malleoli.

attaching the posterior flap/fat pad to the tibia later in the procedure. The Achilles tendon and plantar soft tissue are then dissected from the calcaneus, and the amputated foot completely removed. Plantar tendons and any remaining intrinsic muscle tissue are excised from the posterior flap/fat pad. The distal tips of the medial and lateral malleoli are removed using an oscillating saw, level with the articulating surface of the tibia. Oblique drill holes in the medial, lateral, and anterior edges of the tibia and fibula are used to secure preserved periosteum and posterior heel pad in place. The continued viability of the heel pad is a key component to a successful outcome. A prolonged period of non–weight bearing (usually at least 6 weeks) is essential to ensure that the heel pad is not disrupted until it is firmly healed in place. Depending on the condition of the residual limb, the individual may be ready for initial prosthetic fitting by 6 to 8 weeks following amputation. Initial prosthetic training must be with careful partial weight bearing and an appropriate assistive device, with frequent inspection of the integrity and positioning of the distal pad.

Transtibial Amputation

Transtibial amputation represents the "work horse" and by far most common amputation level in the lower extremity. This level typically has positive surgical and rehabilitative outcomes, as long as there is sufficient circulation for healing of the residual limb.[127,203] Standard surgical teaching suggests an ideal length of 2.5 cm of residual limb for every 30 cm of patient height, typically resulting in a bone length of 12.5 to 17.5 cm[204]; our preference is to add 1 to 2 cm of length to this calculation, although ensuring adequate soft tissue padding and patient height (26–29 cm of space from the residual limb to the ground or contralateral heel pad is recommended for prosthetic fitting options) remains critical. As residual tibial length decreases toward the tibial tubercle, mechanical advantage of knee flexors exceeds that of knee extensors, making it difficult to extend the knee enough to advance a prosthesis during swing and for controlled (eccentric) knee extension for stability in the early stance phase. Because the surface area for weight bearing within the socket decreases as the length of the residual limb decreases, limb length, the likelihood of discomfort, skin irritation, and limited use of a transtibial prosthesis increases. Conversely, in long residual limbs, the larger total surface area to distribute pressures within the socket and long lever arm potentially enhance prosthetic control, although there is a risk of chronic skin irritation and discomfort along the sharp edge of the distal-anterior tibial crest. Recent advances in prosthetic materials and design can accommodate, to some degree, for the biomechanical and prosthetic fitting challenges of a long residual limb (i.e., with more than 66% of original tibial length) or of a short residual limb (i.e., preserving 33% or less of original tibial length). Comfort in the prosthesis, quality of gait, and energy cost of ambulation seem to be best balanced when the level of amputation maintains tibial length between 12 and 15 cm.[205]

Depending on the condition of the skin and soft tissue, as well as the circumstances that have led to the decision to amputate, the surgeon selects from a number of surgical approaches. The most commonly used approach is the long posterior (myofasciocutaneous) flap described by Burgess in the 1960s. This technique preserves the highly vascular gastrocnemius as well as all anterior compartment muscles beyond the residual tibia, brings the flap up and forward, and positions the suture line across the distal-anterior residual limb below the cut surface of the tibia (Fig. 19.17).[206]

In dysvascular patients, muscles of the anterior compartment can be susceptible to necrosis which may cause delayed healing and potential revision to a higher level. A modification of the posterior flap procedure described by Bruckner removes all of the tibialis anterior as well as the bulk of the soleus to the level of the residual tibia. The modified Bruckner method also removes the fibula.[207] Despite the theoretical advantages, no clear benefit of these techniques has been demonstrated in the literature.[208] A third modification, first described by Ertl in 1949 as an osteomyoplastic amputation with tibiofibular synostosis, incorporates a bone bridge between the distal tibia and fibula for added stability.[209]

When a posterior flap cannot be achieved, the surgeon may create equal anterior-posterior skin flaps in which the incision runs in a U shape medially to laterally across the bottom of the residual limb, or equal medial-lateral flaps, in which the incision runs in a U from anterior to posterior across the bottom of the residual limb (Fig. 19.18). The surgeon may even use a long medial or long lateral flap that positions the incision on the distal opposite side of the limb.[210] To date, there is no evidence to show a benefit of one type of incision over another.[211] In the setting of trauma, atypical flaps may be required to achieve optimal soft tissue coverage while maintaining residual limb length.[56] In all approaches the surgeon seeks to retain enough soft tissue so that there is little or no tension across the closed incision, but not so much that there will be redundant skin and tissue that might challenge prosthetic fitting.

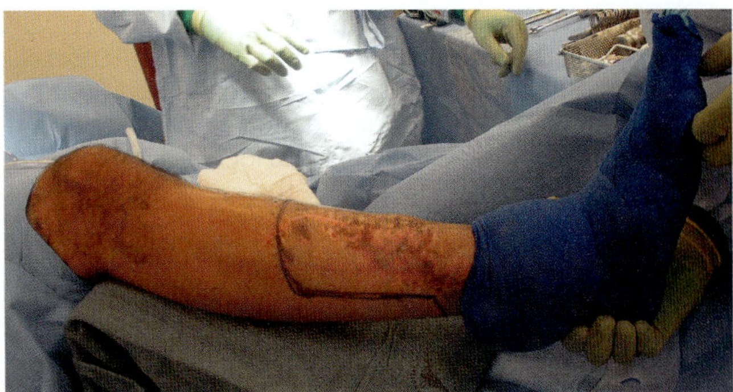

Fig. 19.17 Preoperative photograph of the skin incision for a transtibial amputation. As is commonly the case, a long posterior skin flap was used to cover the end of the residual limb.

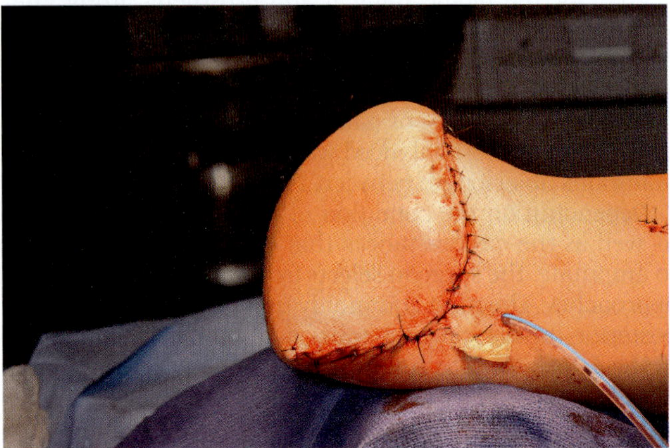

Fig. 19.18 Postoperative photograph of an atypical flap used to cover a transtibial amputation. In this case, only the saphenous nerve was intact to skin at the level of the amputation, thus a medially based, saphenous neurocutaneous flap was used to provide the patient with a sensate residual limb end.

MODIFIED BURGESS PROCEDURE

The intended tibial length is marked and a line for the anterior incision is drawn, sweeping into a distally curved posterior flap. The anterior incision is made through skin and then soft tissue to the periosteum of the tibia, and subcutaneous blood vessels are clamped. Next, muscles in the anterior compartment are incised so that the anterior tibial artery, vein, and deep peroneal nerve can be identified, clamped, transected, and ligated.[208] Soft tissue is carefully removed from around the fibula approximately 2 cm shorter than the residual tibia. An oscillating saw is used to transect the fibula. The surgeon then cuts the tibia, taking care to bevel the anterior edge to minimize risks of potential irritation and ulceration and/or bursa formation. The skin and subcutaneous incision are now continued along what will become the posterior flap. Once the amputated limb has been removed, the posterior tibial and peroneal arteries and veins are clamped. Major nerves are grasped with gentle traction, resected at the most accessible proximal point, and allowed to retract into the residual limb.[56] The soleus muscle is then dissected from the medial and lateral heads of the gastrocnemius and removed to debulk the posterior flap for optimal wound closure. The blood vessels of the posterior and lateral compartments are clamped, transected, and ligated. high-energy injuries may lead to the disruption of the interosseous membrane between the residual tibia and fibula. The surgeon may opt to perform a bone bridge synostosis as previously discussed, or a more proximal suture bridge construct alone in an effort to achieve tibiofibular stability.[212] This, theoretically, minimizes the likelihood symptomatic distal fibular instability during subsequent activity and prosthetic use. The tourniquet is deflated, any bleeding small vessels are electrocauterized or sutured, and hemostasis is restored. The beveled anterior tibia is smoothed with a rasp and a myodesis is performed by securing the posterior compartment musculature to the tibia, usually via drill holes.[206] The incision is closed over drains in a tension free manner.

As previously discussed, a soft or rigid dressing may be applied. The patient is encouraged to keep the knee of the residual limb in full extension; elevation over a pillow leads to hip and knee flexion contracture that will be problematic later in rehabilitation.

Physical therapy usually begins in the first days after surgery, with transfers, and single-limb ambulation with a walker or crutches. Bedside commodes and wheelchairs with removable armrests assist self-care and mobility and reduce the risk of falls.

Staples or sutures typically remain in place for 3 weeks; if there are indications of delayed healing, the surgeon may opt to leave every second or third suture in place longer, reinforcing the incision with adhesive wound closure strips when staples have been removed. Gentle mobilization of soft tissue begins to prevent adherence of the incision scar to underlying fascia and bone. Casting for initial prosthesis occurs only when there has been adequate closure of the surgical wound and the circumference of the distal and proximal portions of the residual limb below the knee is nearly equal. For some individuals this may occur within 3 weeks; for others it may require several months.

MODIFIED BRUCKNER PROCEDURE

The modified Bruckner procedure is based on the premise that, for individuals with significant PAD, risk of postoperative muscle necrosis will be less likely if the muscles most susceptible to ischemia are removed during surgery.[208] For that reason, anterior and lateral compartment muscles, as well as the lateral gastrocnemius, are excised. In addition, the soleus and its large venous plexus are removed to reduce the risk of postoperative thrombosis.[208] The fibula is also removed, especially if the residuum is short, to create a limb that will be more tolerant of pressure within the prosthetic socket. The operation otherwise proceeds as described for the modified Burgess procedure.

MODIFIED ERTL PROCEDURE

In theory, the creation of a distal synostosis allows for a more stable weight bearing interface and less painful residual limb; however, these theories have not been substantiated in the literature in terms of functional outcomes. Retrospective reviews comparing the modified Burgess technique and the modified Ertl technique found similar functional outcomes between the groups but noted a higher rate

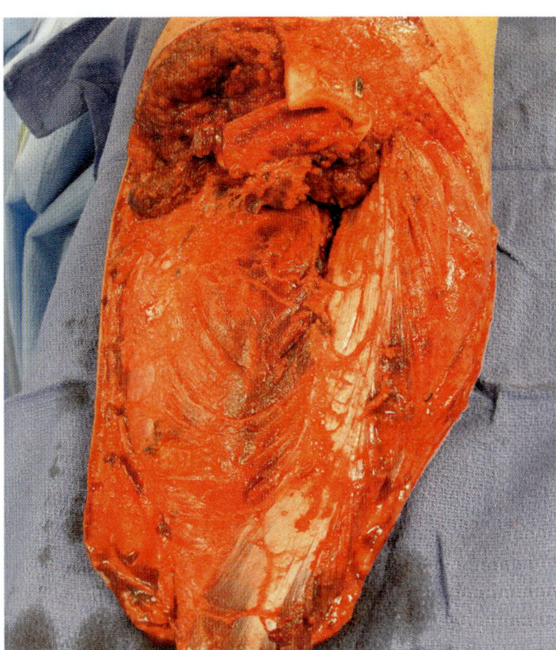

Fig. 19.19 Intraoperative photograph of a modified Ertl transtibial amputation. A cut segment of fibula is secured with a TightRope device between the tibia and and fibula. Note also, the long posterior flap of posterior compartment musculature preserved to close over the end of the residual bone.

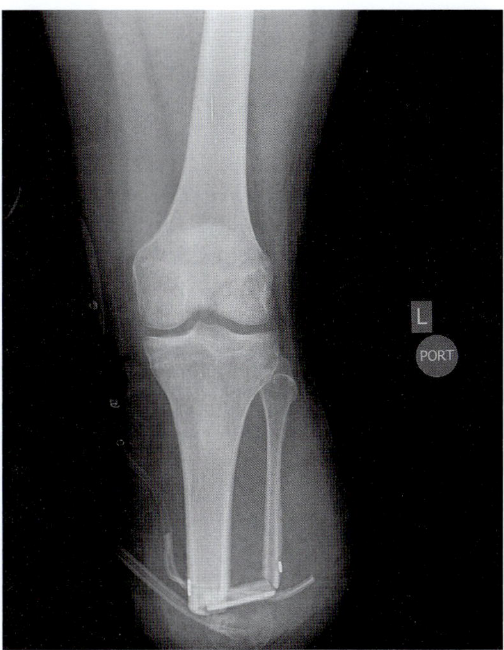

Fig. 19.20 Postoperative radiograph of modified Ertl transtibial amputation with bone bridge secured in place by a TightRope. The metallic buttons are visible on the medial cortex of the tibia and the lateral cortex of the fibula.

of reoperations in the Ertl group, many of which were bone bridge related.[213,214] The preliminary results of a prospective multicenter randomized trial comparing the Burgess and Ertl techniques found no difference in functional outcomes between the groups and a higher rate of complications in the Ertl technique group.[215,216]

The distal bone bridge can be constructed from a variety of sources, however a segment of the amputated fibula is most commonly used.[209] In many instances, more bony length can be preserved, resulting in a cylindrical residual limb with some end-bearing capacity for prosthetic use. This procedure is most typically used in young, healthy individuals expected to be very active using their prosthesis, especially for those in the military.[217] Initial preparation of the limb is similar to that of a posterior flap procedure. A segment of bone is harvested from the amputated fibular shaft, sized to bridge the space between tibia and fibula of the residual limb, but other sources of bone may also be used, such as a portion of residual tibia in the setting of a revision amputation[218] (Fig. 19.19). The inner edges of the tibia and fibula may be notched to allow the bone bridge to fit securely between them. The bone bridge may be secured in place in a number of ways; for example, use of compression screws, or running a "TightRope" (Arthrex Inc, Naples, Florida) suture through a hole drilled in the fibula, then through the shaft of the bone bridge, then through a hole drilled in the tibia[209] (Fig. 19.20). Because of the extensive dissection required, this technique uses more operative time (and more time under anesthesia and with tourniquet in place) than the modified Burgess and Bruckner surgeries.[219] Consequently, it is generally contraindicated for patients with multiple comorbidities or those who are medically frail.

Knee Disarticulation

In previous centuries, before development of surgical anesthesia and antibiotics, simple knee

disarticulation surgery often had a much more favorable outcome than transtibial amputation.[220] Because this surgery does not transect major muscle mass, it can be done in less time and with significantly less blood loss than transtibial or transfemoral amputation. Additionally, simple disarticulation through the knee joint disrupts only the tissue compartment of the joint itself, making postoperative infection in fascia, muscle, or bone much less likely. The femoral condyles, with their cartilaginous covering, are designed to tolerate weight bearing, and preservation of the entire femur provides mechanical advantage to the prosthetic wearer.

The residual limb heals without much atrophy, requiring less socket replacement or revision early on, allowing fitting with a definitive prosthesis in less time than the typical transtibial or transfemoral residual limb. Additionally, this surgery preserves the growth plate of the distal epiphysis, an important consideration in children.[106] For individuals with severe bilateral vascular disease who are nonambulatory before surgery, the extra length of the femurs provides a larger base of support in sitting, enhancing postural control.[221]

The length of an intact femur, along with the anatomy of the condyles, creates several important challenges to prosthetic fit and function in terms of choice and placement of the prosthetic knee unit, which affects energy cost, as well as efficiency of prosthetic gait. The bony, bulbous residual limb of those who undergo a simple knee disarticulation also creates a challenge regarding donning and doffing the prosthesis (Fig. 19.21). Surgical techniques developed by

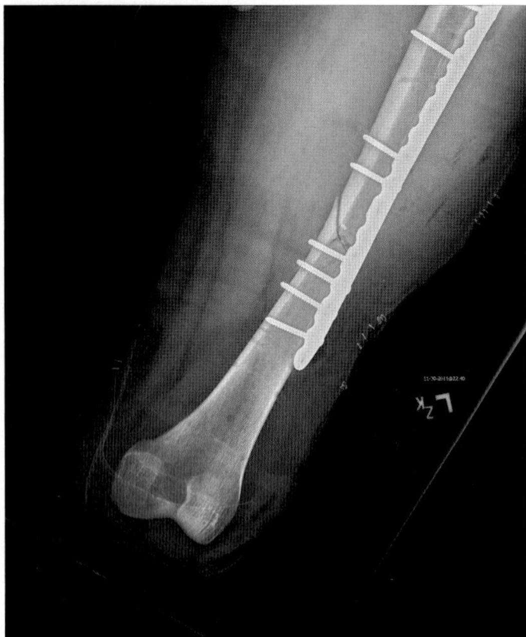

Fig.f 19.21 Anterior-posterior radiograph of a knee disarticulation. The bulbous medial and lateral condyles of the femur can cause difficulty with prosthetic fit. The proximal femur fracture was fixed using a plate and screws. Although associated with frequent complications, fixation of proximal fractures preserves overall amputation length.

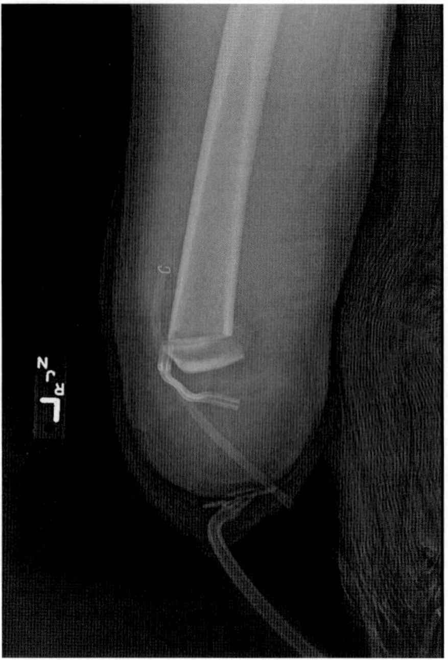

Fig. 19.22 Lateral radiograph of Gritti-Stokes knee disarticulation in which the femoral condyles are transecting just proximal to the joint and the patella is attached to the metaphyseal bone.

Mazet and Hennessy in the 1960s removed the patella and trimmed the medial and lateral condylar surfaces to address the problems associated with bulbous distal anatomy.[222]

In 1977 Burgess recommended removal of 1.5 to 2 cm of the distal condyles to permit placement of a newly developed four-bar prosthetic knee unit closer to what had been the anatomical axis of the knee.[223,224] Some surgeons advocate modifying the patella and then fusing it to the intercondylar notch of the femur to maintain quadriceps tension, or sectioning the femoral condyles and fusing the patella to the transected femur while leaving the adductor magnus insertion intact. The latter is known as a Gritti-Stokes amputation[225–227] (Fig. 19.22). Typically either equal sagittal flaps or a long posterior flap are used to provide additional “cushion” for weight bearing through the distal residual limb.[116] Proponents of simple knee disarticulation, without modification of the distal femur, suggest that the combination of reduced rates of infection, better primary healing, larger surface areas for weight bearing, and advances in prosthetic design and technology lead to better functional outcome and higher rates of prosthetic use. However, these theoretical benefits, particularly in the setting of traumatic amputations, have been called in to question by recent studies, as previously discussed.[171,172] After detailed patient counseling, we still prefer knee disarticulations to long transfemoral amputations in most cases when viable gastrocnemius muscle remains for distal soft tissue coverage.

The skin incision is planned to create either equal medial and lateral flaps approximately half of the anteroposterior diameter of knee in length or a long posterior flap. The patellar tendon is transected at the tibial tubercle, as well as the medial and lateral collateral ligaments just above the menisci. Next, the knee is slightly flexed and the infrapatellar fold is cut. This provides access to the cruciate ligaments, allowing the surgeon to free them from their attachment to the tibia. The posterior joint capsule is carefully cut, with attention to keeping neurovascular structures in the popliteal fossa intact, while exposing the femoral attachment of the gastrocnemius muscle. The popliteal artery and vein and saphenous vein are clamped and ligated, and the tibial, common peroneal and saphenous nerves are transected under traction and allowed to retract into the residual limb. The surgeon then cuts through the gastrocnemius at the distal musculotendinous junction, and the lower leg is removed.

When transcondylar modification is desired, an oscillating saw is used to trim the edges of the condyles before irrigation. In preparation for closure the patellar tendon is sutured to the anterior and posterior cruciate ligaments (Fig. 19.23), and the cut edge of the gastrocnemius muscle is sutured to the anterior joint capsule (myoplasty). If no patellofemoral fusion is to be attempted, the patella may either be retained or excised. Advantages of retention include creating improved prosthetic suspension and rotational control. Advantages of excision include no risk of breakdown over the subcutaneous patella and no theoretical risk of symptomatic patellofemoral arthrosis or motion at the expense of deadspace creation. Either way, we recommend performing a suprapatellar synovectomy in an effort to minimize postoperative fluid collection risk and accelerate the scarring in of the residual extensor mechanism. The hamstring tendons are transected distally and allowed to retract or, preferably, secured to the posterior joint capsule. The lateral and medial flaps are positioned with approximated edges, and subcutaneous tissues are sutured closed. Finally, the outer layer of skin is closed using staples or sutures.

A soft or rigid dressing may be applied. Some or all of the staples or external sutures are removed at 2 to 3 weeks,

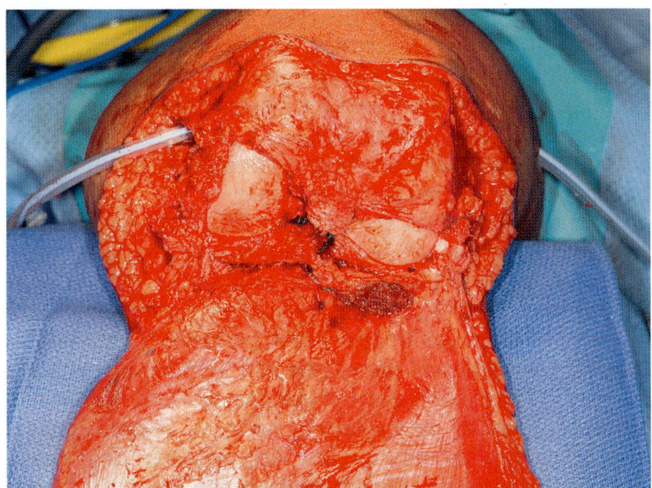

Fig. 19.23 Intraoperative photograph of knee disarticulation. In this case, the patella has been removed and the residual extensor mechanism sutured to the cruciate ligaments. Note again, a long posterior muscle flap consisting of the medial and lateral gastrocnemius muscles is preserved for closure.

depending on the condition of the incision. Readiness for a training prosthesis is determined by full healing of the surgical incision, typically between 3 and 8 weeks after surgery.

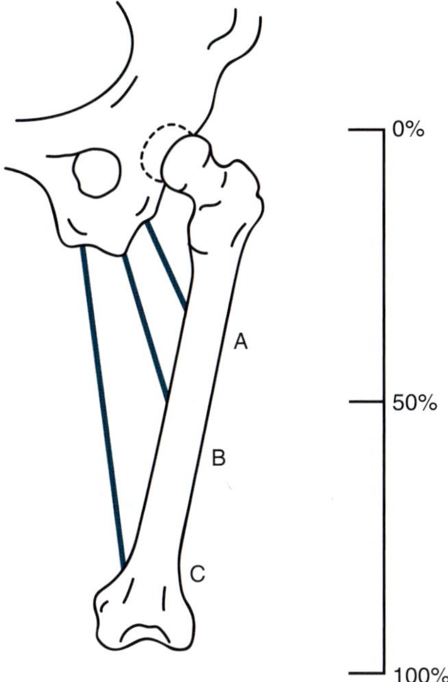

Fig. 19.24 Diagram of point of attachment and line of pull for the (*A*) adductor brevis, (*B*) adductor longus, and (*C*) adductor magnus, as they relate to femoral length. As the length of the residual femur decreases, power and efficiency of adductor muscles groups are increasingly compromised.

Transfemoral Amputation

When deciding on where to transect the femur, it is important to consider vascular status, muscle insertions, and residual limb biomechanics. For those patients requiring transfemoral amputation, function and prosthetic control improves as length of residual femur increases. Preservation or reattachment of the adductor brevis, adductor longus, and especially adductor magnus provides sufficient power for stabilization of the residual limb in adduction during stance so that the abductors can work to keep the pelvis level during prosthetic gait[123,228,229] (Fig. 19.24). Preservation of femoral length and of muscle mass via myodesis, rather than resection through muscle belly, results in a stronger residual limb that is more easily fit and has better prosthetic control.[124,230] It also reduces the risk of developing hip abduction and flexion contracture during rehabilitation and over the individual's lifetime (Fig. 19.25). The surgeon must work with the viable thigh tissue to create a residual limb that is balanced in muscular power, provides a long enough lever to allow hip extensors to control prosthetic knee stability in stance, and has as smooth and sensate a skin surface as possible.

Equal anteroposterior flaps, equal mediolateral flaps, or a long flap from any one limb surface that will be approximated to the opposite limb surface at closure may be used. The fascia and muscle of the quadriceps and adductors are transected as far distally as possible, and the femur is scored at the desired level of amputation. The femur is cut with an oscillating saw, and the distal bone is retracted anteriorly so that the surgeon can access posterior structures. The hamstrings and tensor fascia lata are incised and transected as distally as possible. Major vessels are ligated. The sciatic nerve is ligated, cut while under traction, and allowed to

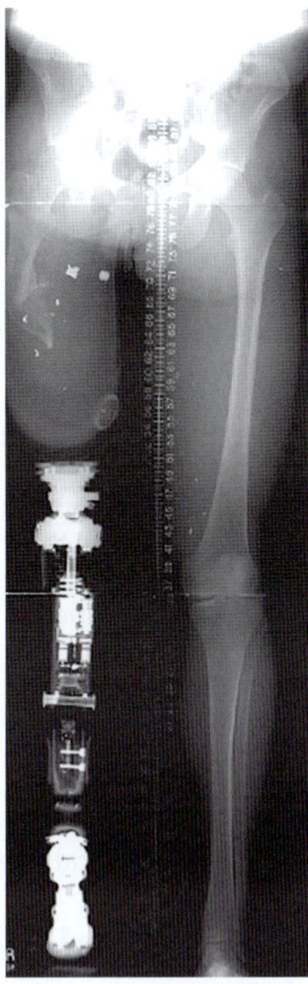

Fig. 19.25 Standing radiograph of a patient with a short transfemoral amputation. In the absence of native adductor musculature insertions or adductor myodesis, the residual limb assumes an abduction deformity, particularly noticeable on this standing radiograph.

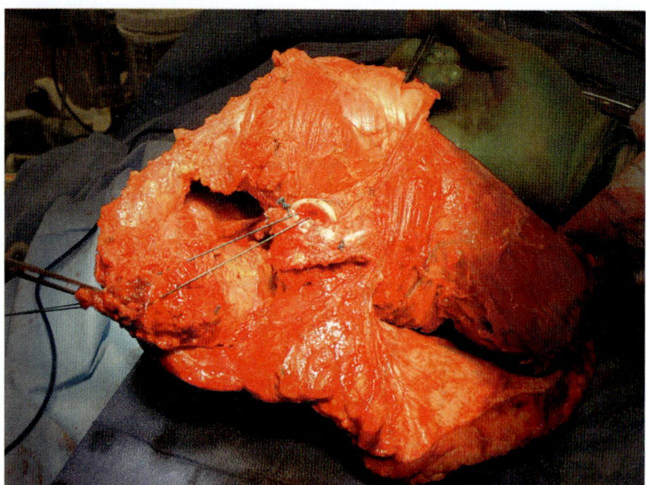

Fig. 19.26 Intraoperative photograph of an adductor and medial hamstring myodesis during a transfemoral amputation. Notice that the sutures pass through drill holes in the residual femur to provide stable anchor point.

retract into hamstring muscle tissue. The sharp edges of the residual distal femur may be shaped and smoothed with a rasp or file. Muscle can be secured via either myoplasty or myodesis, however myodesis results in the most stable construct.[121] The adductor muscles are pulled under the distal femur medially to laterally and sutured to the lateral femur by drill holes; this may be reinforced with additional drill holes medially to prevent subluxation and loss of tension in the adductor myodesis (Fig. 19.26). The hamstrings are sutured to the distal femur or the quadriceps, which is pulled under the distal femur in an anterior-to-posterior direction over the repositioned adductor, attaching it to the posterior surface of the femur. The fascia, subcutaneous tissue, and skin are then closed in a layered fashion. The goal is to create a tapered, cylindrical residual limb with few "dimples" or redundant tissues. A soft or rigid dressing is applied. If a soft dressing is used, it may be helpful to use a long compressive wrap that includes the waist in a hip spica configuration.

Mobility training and early preprosthetic positioning exercises (to encourage positioning of the residual limb in hip extension and adduction) are optimally initiated the day after surgery, and single-limb gait training with an appropriate assistive device follows as soon as the individual can tolerate increasing activity. Strategies for consistent gentle soft tissue compression are initiated as soon as possible using an compressive wrap, elasticized stockinette, and eventually a commercially available "shrinker." Staples or sutures remain in place for 3 weeks or more, perhaps being removed in successive stages to ensure a solid wound closure. Fitting for initial prosthesis is, as in all other levels of amputation, determined by the condition of the suture line; for some patients this may occur as early as 3 or 4 weeks postoperatively, and for others several months after surgery.

Hip Disarticulation and Hemipelvectomy

Amputation at the level of the hip or pelvis is an amputation of last resort and represents high-risk surgery that may be indicated for patients with severe trauma, uncontrollable sepsis, failed revascularization, widespread metastases, or malignant bone or soft tissue tumors.[231–233] The complex anatomy of this region and relative rarity of these procedures present a significant surgical and rehabilitative challenge. These surgeries are best performed in facilities with an experienced interdisciplinary team.

Hip disarticulations account for only 0.5% of all lower extremity amputations and perioperative mortality rates have been reported between 0% and 44%.[2,231,234] In contrast to hemipelvectomy, this procedure preserves the pelvis thereby allowing weight bearing through the ischium in an appropriately fit prosthesis and improved sitting balance. Even the preservation of the iliac wing, however, may improve potential for prosthesis wear. A racquet shaped skin incision allows creation of a large posterior flap of skin, subcutaneous tissue, and gluteal muscle mass for wound closure. The incision begins at the medial edge of the anterior superior iliac spine, continues along the inguinal ligament to just below the ischial tuberosity and gluteal crease, and then arches upward over the greater trochanter and anterior thigh back to the anterior superior iliac spine. The surgeon must carefully free neurovascular structures in the inguinal region, as well as detach each of the many surface and deeper muscles that cross the hip joint, starting with the anterior and medial groups, then moving laterally and posteriorly. The gluteal muscles are detached from the greater trochanter but kept in place on the pelvis to be part of the posterior flap. The head of the femur is dislocated from the acetabulum. The residual gluteal muscles are then sutured to the inguinal ligament and anterior pelvic periosteum, although adductor and quadriceps-based flaps have been described for cases in which the gluteal muscles are absent or compromised. Incisions are closed in standard layered fashion over deep drains. Compression is provided by soft elastic spica wrap. Limited periods of sitting, mobility, and transfer training, as well as ambulation on the contralateral limb using a walker or crutches, begins as soon as the patient is medically stable and able to tolerate increasing levels of activity, optimally within 2 to 3 days after surgery. Special attention must be paid to the sitting posture, with minimal time spent in a posteriorly tilted "sacral sitting" position, to ensure skin integrity. Patient and family education must include efforts to carefully protect the surgical site during movement and activities of daily living. An early referral to the prosthetist for fabrication of a custom thermoplastic RRD may occur in the week immediately following surgery. Fitting for initial prosthesis, as in amputation at all other levels, is determined by rate and adequacy of healing of the surgical site.

Hemipelvectomy, as classically described, amputates the pelvic ring via disarticulation of the pubic symphysis anteriorly and the sacroiliac joint posteriorly. Variations of this procedure include the extended or modified hemipelvectomy. An extended hemipelvectomy includes portions of the sacrum, lumbar spine, and/or contralateral pelvis. A modified, or partial, hemipelvectomy resects less than the entire innominate bone[235] (Fig. 19.27). A functional limb requires an intact lumbosacral plexus, femoral neurovascular bundle, and hip joint. When two out of these structures are nonfunctional, amputation is usually the best option.[114] The procedure itself is one of the most technically

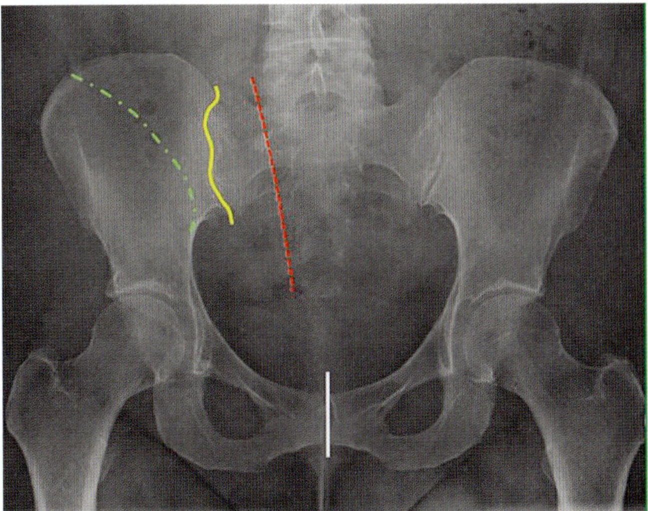

Fig. 19.27 AP pelvis radiograph with levels of resection for a modified (*green dashed line*), standard (*yellow line*), and extended (*red dashed line*) hemipelvectomy. Anteriorly, the pelvis is transected at the pubic symphysis (*white line*).

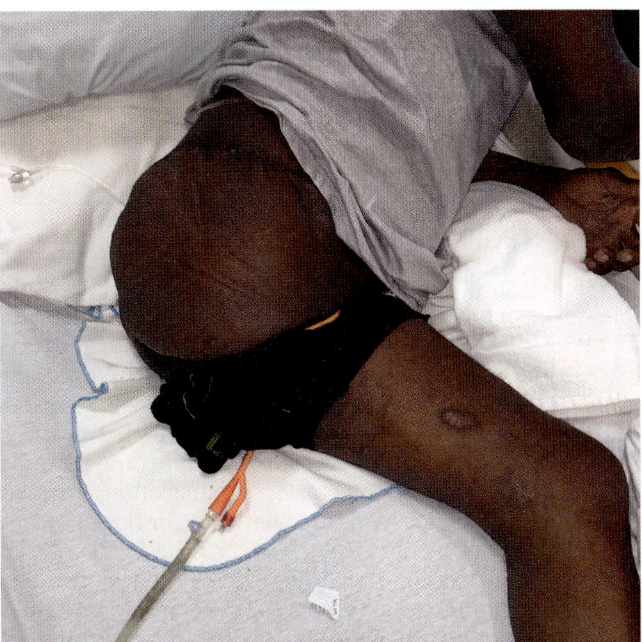

Fig. 19.28 Clinical photograph of patient who underwent hemipelvectomy with an anterior based quadriceps flap for closure.

demanding and invasive surgeries performed in orthopedics; the median blood loss for hemipelvectomy in a series preformed for resection of musculoskeletal tumors was found to be over 3 L.[236] Given the proximity of vital neurovascular structures and intraabdominal contents, a thorough understanding of the anatomy and meticulous surgical technique is required to safely perform this procedure.

The surgical technique for a hemipelvectomy varies based on planned soft tissue coverage as well as the degree of bony resection indicated. Beginning anteriorly, superficial abdominal musculature is incised to expose the iliacus and the iliac fossa is cleared by blunt dissection. Major blood vessels from the iliac artery are sequentially ligated. Posteriorly, a flap including the gluteal fascia and the medial portion of the gluteus maximus is elevated off of the iliac crest. The paraspinal musculature of the lumbosacral spine is divided from iliac crest and the gluteus maximus elevated from the sacrotuberous ligament, coccyx, and sacrum. The remaining muscles crossing the hip joint are divided and the femoral nerve and lumbosacral nerve trunk are transected. The hip is then abducted and the pubic symphysis is divided followed by transection of the sacral nerve roots. Disarticulation is then performed through the sacroiliac joint with a scalpel and osteotome. The pelvic floor muscles are divided under tension and the process of closure may begin. Soft tissue coverage options include posterior based flaps (most common), anterior based flaps, or free tissue transfer from viable distal portions of the amputated limb, known as fillet flaps[237,238] (Fig. 19.28). In the absence of viable distal limb tissue, a combination of random pattern flaps and split thickness skin graft may be required.[239] With advances in surgical and anesthetic techniques, mortality rates for hemipelvectomy have improved from historical rates of nearly 50% mortality to less than 10% in more recent series.[240,241] Nonetheless, overall complication rates remain high, with one large series of 160 patients finding a morbidity rate of 54%, most commonly due to infection and flap necrosis.[242] Mobilization and transfer training may need to be deferred until the individual is well enough and nutritionally supported enough to tolerate increased levels of activity. Furthermore, given the high rates of soft tissue complications, infection, and flap necrosis, prolonged sitting and pressure on the flaps utilized for closure and coverage are best deferred until at least early wound healing has been achieved.

In the absence of bony support, custom fit prostheses allow weight bearing through compression of the residual tissue and musculature of the amputated side.[235] At this amputation level, energy expenditure for ambulation with a prosthesis is increased by approximately 125% as compared to able bodied controls.[243] No significant difference in energy expenditure for ambulation was demonstrated between hip disarticulation and hemipelvectomy. A recent retrospective review of 43 patients who underwent hip disarticulation or hemipelvectomy found that 43% were able to successfully use a prosthetic limb.[244] In a long-term follow-up of 76 patients with war-related pelvic level resections, 70% wore a prosthesis routinely.[245] Notably however, 60% required a double crutch for ambulation and 80% reported upper extremity pain, likely a reflection of the increased demands placed on the upper extremity for use of ambulatory aids. Given both the cumbersome nature of prosthesis fitting, wear and use at this level, as well as the increased energy expenditure of ambulation, many patients with a sound contralateral lower extremity prefer single leg ambulation with crutches. As with more distal amputation levels, functional outcomes are tied to the disease state leading to amputation. Of 63 patients who underwent hip disarticulations, only 2 of 37 patients with vascular disease were fitted with a prosthesis and could ambulate. In contrast, all 24 patients who had a hip disarticulation for oncologic reasons were able to ambulate in a prosthesis.[246]

In summary, pelvic level resections are technically challenging procedures associated with a high rate of complications and variable postsurgical outcomes. When possible (i.e., the surgery is not emergent) patients and their families should be counseled extensively regarding the potential surgical and rehabilitative course. A multidisciplinary team capable of managing all phases of care remains critical.

Future Directions

OSSEOINTEGRATION

Over 150 years have passed since the first patent for a suction socket for lower extremity amputees was filed during the Civil War.[247] Despite many surgical and prosthetic advances in this time period, the traditional suction-based patient-prosthesis interface continues to be both most commonly utilized and a source of difficulty, mostly related to ulceration, folliculitis, sweating, loss of suspension, and pain. An alternative approach, known as osseointegration, bypasses many of the problems associated with conventional socket-based interfaces by attaching the prosthesis directly to the bone of the residual limb (Fig. 19.29). The concept of bony healing to metal fixtures was first demonstrated successfully in dental implants by Dr. Per Invar Brånemark and is now a commonplace procedure in the world of oral reconstructive surgery.[248] In the 1990s, Per Invar's son, Dr. Rickard Brånemark, led a team of surgeons and prosthetists in efforts to develop a transcutaneous osseointegrated implants for patients with limb loss.[249] Since that time, the initial implant system and treatment protocols have been refined and the concept of osseointegration has expanded to treatment centers around the world including Germany,[250] the Netherlands[251] the United Kingdom,[252] Australia,[253] and in the United States[254] where a clinical trial is under way with a US Food and Drug Administration Humanitarian Use Device designation.

To date, clinical outcomes have been published on four separate implant systems—the Osseointegrated Prosthesis for the Rehabilitation of Amputees developed by Dr. Branemark in Sweden, the Integrated Leg Prosthesis developed by Dr. Aschoff in Germany, and Osseointegrated Prosthetic Limb developed in Australia by Dr. Al Muderis and the Percutaneous Osseointegrated Prosthesis developed at the University of Utah. An in-depth review of the different types of implants currently in use is beyond the scope of this chapter, however the principle benefits and challenges associated with each remain similar and warrant further discussion. Interested readers are directed to recent review articles summarizing advancements in the field of osseointegration.[255–257]

Indications

As a developing technique, indications for lower extremity osseointegration are not yet clearly, nor uniformly, defined. In most instances, this procedure has only been offered to patients who have demonstrated considerable difficulty with their conventional socket-based prosthesis. The prosthesis-residual limb interface at the transfemoral level has long been problematic—a large soft tissue envelope around the residual femur reduces load transfer to the skeleton and compromises control and stability. As a result, for lower extremity amputations, this technique has been implemented primarily for those with transfemoral limb loss, but has been reported at the transtibial level as well.[258–260] The procedure is generally, although not absolutely, contraindicated in patients with peripheral vascular disease and/or diabetes due to presumably higher risk of infection and likely shorter anticipated survival.

Implant Fixation

Depending on the protocol utilized, the osseointegration procedure may be performed in one or two stages.[249,261] In the staged procedure, only the intramedullary portion of the implant is placed in the first stage and the incision is closed (Fig. 19.30). After a predetermined period of time (between

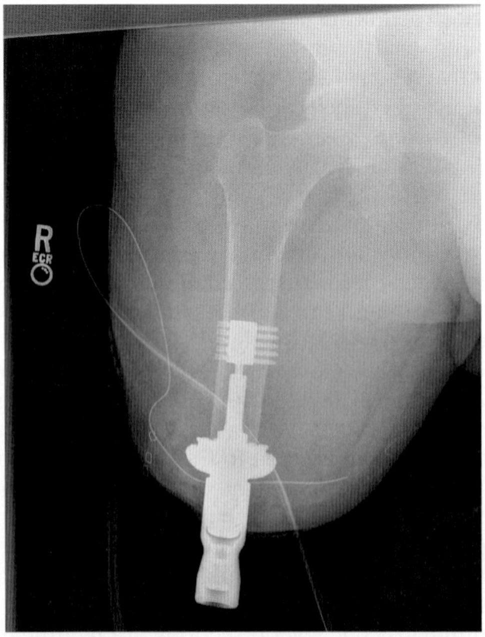

Fig. 19.29 AP radiograph of transfemoral osseointegration. The transcutaneous portion penetrates the soft tissue envelope and provides a point of direct attachment for a prosthetic limb.

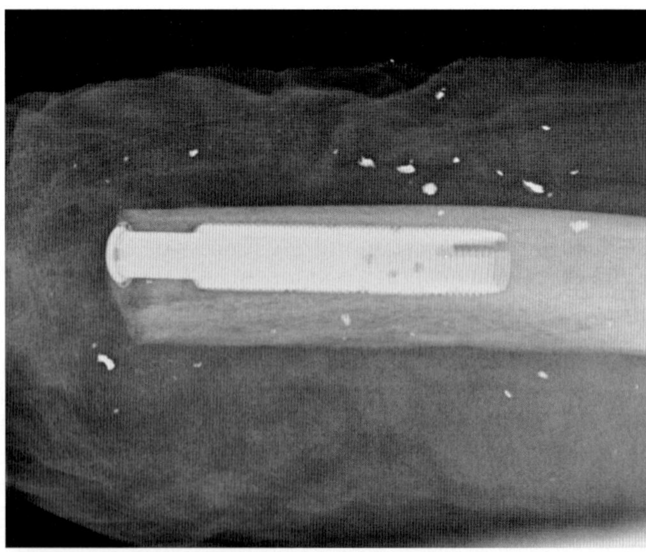

Fig. 19.30 Lateral radiograph following stage one of the osseointegration procedure using the OPRA (Osseointegrated Prosthesis for the Rehabilitation of Amputees) device. Only the fixture is placed and the incision is closed. With time, bony ingrowth occurs at the threaded titanium surface of the implant.

6 weeks and 6 months, depending on the protocol) the transcutaneous portion of the device is implanted in stage 2. Stable fixation can be achieved by bony ingrowth into the implant—either a threaded titanium implant or a press-fit porous metal surface.[249,253,262] Additional strategies for fixation included interlocking screws or the use of an axially loaded device anchored by transfixion pins.[253,254] While all devices achieve some degree of primary stability at the time of implantation, bony ingrowth is required for durable results.[262]

Skin-Implant Interface

The skin-implant interface presents a primary challenge in the successful application of osseointegration in patients with limb loss. The transcutaneous portion of the device allows continuous exposure of underlying subcutaneous tissue to the outside environment (Fig. 19.31). Although soft tissue management strategies at the time of implantation vary, regardless of technique the patient is left with a permanent stoma around the implant, a site that, unsurprisingly, is colonized with bacteria.[263] Recent literature has documented an overall lower rate of soft tissue infections utilizing a shallow soft tissue envelope at the skin penetration site, rather than bulky flaps.[264] The skin-implant interface requires daily care and remains at risk of infection, which is greatest in the early postoperative period but lasts throughout the life of the implant.

Rehabilitation Protocol

Although time points vary between practitioners, rehabilitation follows a similar trajectory for all implant systems. Following implantation, a period of restricted weight bearing is enforced with gradual progression to full weight bearing as the implant achieves bony ingrowth and the muscles controlling the residual limb adapt to direct skeletal weight bearing once more. Not infrequently, muscular and myodesis-related pain persist up to 1 year following implantation, but function frequently improves to better than baseline, socket-based outcomes much sooner.[251]

Complications

The most commonly reported complication associated with osseointegration is infection. Superficial infection has been reported as high as 55% in some series, although the majority of these can be treated with antibiotics alone.[265] The long-term risk of osteomyelitis in transfemoral osseointegrated implants has been estimated at 20% at 10 years, with an associated 9% risk of implant removal due to infection.[266] Although more recent results suggest improvements over these rates as implant designs and implantation technique have evolved, these findings nonetheless represent an important baseline both for patient counseling purposes and to improve on moving forward. Deep infections requiring implant removal are particularly problematic as this may result in further shortening of the residual limb. Longer term (5 years or longer) follow-up studies of transfemoral implants have commonly reported mechanical complications, most frequently involving transcutaneous adapters or abutments.[267–269] Other potential complications such as aseptic loosening (2%–6%) and periprosthetic fracture (0%–4%) occur at a lower rate.[250,263,265,270]

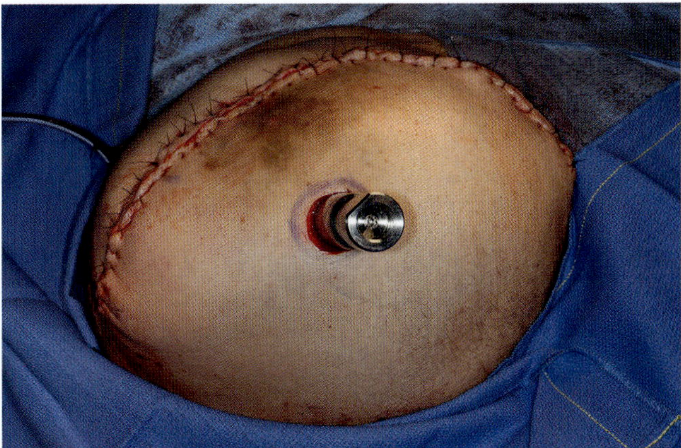

Fig. 19.31 Postoperative photograph of transfemoral amputation with transcutaneous portion of the osseointegrated device in place. The opening, or stoma, around the implant is at risk of infection and must be monitored carefully.

Outcomes

In addition to avoiding problems related to the limb implant interface, osseointegrated implants allow for physiologic weight bearing, improved range of motion at the proximal joint, and osseoperceptive (i.e., osseoproprioception) sensory feedback[249] (Fig. 19.32). These factors ultimately result in more frequent prosthetic wear and use and, as has been shown in multiple studies, improved quality of life.[253,261,265,271] Additionally, transfemoral osseointegration appears to allow for more efficient movement, with one study finding decreased walking energy costs at the 2-year follow-up and 30% increase in the number of patients able to ambulate 500 m without stopping.[272] At the 1-year follow-up, a prospective, case control study of 22 patients found significantly increased prosthetic use, improved 6-Minute Walk Test, decreased oxygen consumption during treadmill walking at self-selected velocity, and overall improved prosthesis-related quality of life.[270] A comparative study of quality of life in patients with transfemoral amputations using either socket prostheses or osseointegrated prostheses found fewer prosthesis associated problems and higher prosthesis associated quality of life in patients with osseointegration.[273]

In short, osseointegration has the potential to tremendously improve the quality of life for select lower extremity amputees. However, it is not without risk. Continued long-term follow-up is required, in addition to further research to optimize the skin-implant interface, mitigate infection, and improve bony fixation.

ACTIVE LOWER LIMB PROSTHESES AND THE HUMAN-MACHINE INTERFACE

Unlike passive or semiactive prostheses, an active prosthesis is capable of providing net positive work—an essential capability of any device that seeks to recreate the functionality of the missing portion of a limb. More than 20 active or powered prostheses have been described in the literature, including solutions for both transfemoral and transtibial amputations.[274] However, to harness the full benefit of a powered prosthesis, the user must be able to control its movement. Control strategies vary but may require the press of button or exaggerated body movements to switch

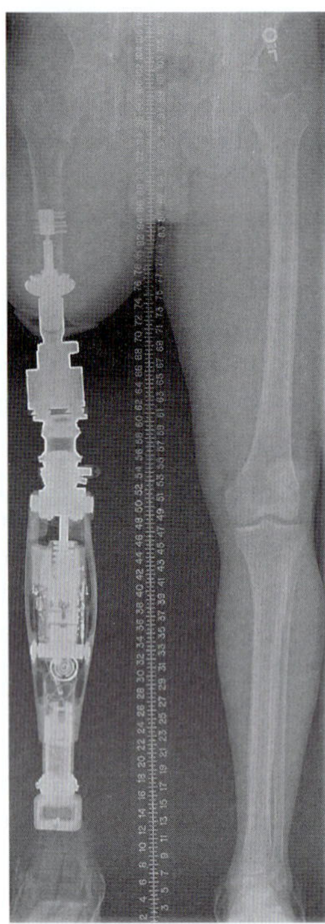

Fig. 19.32 Standing radiograph of a patient with a transfemoral osseointegrated device attached to lower extremity prosthesis. In addition to other advantages, skeletal attachment of the prosthesis allows for direct weight bearing through the residual femur resulting in improved sensory feedback known as osseoproprioception.

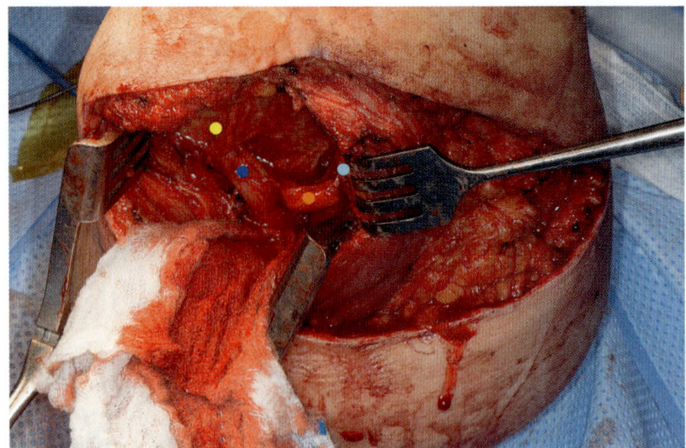

Fig. 19.33 Intraoperative photograph of targeted muscle reinnervation. The sciatic nerve has been separated into tibial and peroneal divisions. On the left, the tibial division (*blue dot*) has been coapted to motor nerve of the semimembranosus (*yellow dot*). On the right, the peroneal division (*orange dot*) has been coapted to a motor nerve to the biceps femoris (*light green dot*).

between modes of locomotion.[275,276] These solutions fall short of the ultimate goal—intuitive, volitional control of the powered prosthesis.

However, there are promising developments within this field. Muscle contractions in the residual limb generate electromyographic (EMG) signals that can be detected by surface electrodes. Neural information obtained from these electrodes is then used to control prosthetic movements, essentially identical to what upper extremity amputees have utilized for the last several decades with myoelectric prostheses. When combined with pattern recognition algorithms, this approach has been demonstrated to improve control of powered leg prostheses by reducing classification error across ambulation modes and during transitions between ambulation modes.[277] Technical challenges to this approach include signal noise, latency, and the lack of proprioceptive or haptic (i.e., sensory) feedback.

A technique known as TMR was developed initially in an effort to improve the capability of upper extremity myoprostheses to match the demands of functional tasks such as reaching or grasping.[278] This procedure surgically connects transected residual peripheral nerves to motor nerves that control muscles which are otherwise nonfunctional as a result of the amputation (Fig. 19.33). The muscle, once reinnervated by the donor nerve, acts as a biologic amplifier—volitional contraction produces EMG signal that can be interpreted by surface electrodes and used for prosthetic control. Impressive improvements, namely reduced error rates, seamless transitions between modes of ambulation, and the ability to reposition the limb in space while nonambulatory have been demonstrated in a patient who underwent TMR following a trauma-related knee disarticulation.[279] As promising as these developments are a persistent challenge remains in obtaining a reliable, high-quality EMG signal, particularly in the setting of a traditional socket fit prosthesis.

Since the 1960s, researchers have investigated intramuscular EMG signal recording in hopes of bypassing the problems associated with surface recordings.[280,281] Recent work has shown these intramuscular devices to be equivalent to or better than surface EMG in real time testing of patients with upper extremity amputations.[282] Future possibilities include permanently implanted devices that wirelessly transmit signal to the prosthesis.[283]

The agonist-antagonist myoneural interface (AMI) is yet another emerging approach to improve neural control of advanced limb prostheses. In this technique, agonist and antonist muscle groups (typically discarded or myodesed as part of traditional amputations) are maintained in the residual limb and coapted in series so that the contraction of the agonist muscle results in stretch of the antagonist group, and vice versa. The efferent signals from contracting muscles that controlled now absent distal joints can be relayed via surface EMG to myoelectric prostheses, resulting in intuitive control of prosthetic joints (i.e., efferent signal from the ankle AMI, consisting of tibialis anterior coapted to the lateral gastrocnemius, allows for dorsiflexion and plantar flexion of a prosthetic ankle joint). Furthermore, mechanoreceptors within the muscles of the AMI allow for natural proprioreceptive feedback, allowing for sensation of prosthetic joint position, speed, and torque. First investigated in a large animal model, AMI has been implemented in pilot studies in human subjects at both the transtibial and transfemoral amputation levels with promising early results.[284–286]

Investigators are also working towards providing sensory feedback from the amputated limb. Targeted sensory innervation follows the similar principles to TMR, except that a sensory nerve rather than a motor nerve is coapted to target motor nerve branch. Subsequent ingrowth of the nerve through the muscle and overlying skin results in regained sensation to touch, temperature, and proprioception.[287,288] Finally, a technique known as RPNI has been developed in an effort to create a long-term, stable interface with transected peripheral nerves. In this technique, a free muscle graft is wrapped around the end of the transected nerve along with an implantable electrode on the muscle's surface. Once reinnervated the muscle serves a bioamplifier of both afferent and efferent signals—stimulation of the implanted electrode may allow for somatosensory feedback in addition to bioprosthetic control.[289–291] To date, the concept has been demonstrated in animal studies only.

In truth, it may be the combination of these techniques—osseointegration, peripheral nerve interfaces, implanted electrodes, pattern recognition algorithms and powered prostheses—that provides the ideal replacement for an amputated limb. In 2014 Ortiz-Catalan et al. reported 1-year follow-up of a patient with a transhumeral amputation who had received an osseointegrated implant with imbedded, transosseous leads to muscle for EMG signal detection and to a peripheral nerve for sensory feedback.[292] These complementary techniques allowed for a bidirectional interface in which the patient has been able to intuitively control the movement of the limb and naturally perceive sensory feedback. Although such a combination of procedures is far from the standard care for upper extremity amputations, much less lower extremity amputations, these are exciting developments for patients with limb loss and those who care for them.[293,294]

Neuroma Prevention and Treatment

Amputation through an extremity necessarily requires transection of peripheral nerves. Invariably, this results in the formation of disorganized regenerating nerve tissue, known as a neuroma, which may or may not become symptomatic. Symptomatic neuromata are most frequently discussed in the context of transtibial and transfemoral amputations, in part because of the larger cross-sectional diameter of nerves at these levels and also because partial foot amputations are most frequently performed due to vasculopathy and/ or neuropathy in which peripheral nerve function is often severely compromised. It has been estimated that neuroma-related pain affects 13% of transtibial amputees and 32% of transfemoral amputees.[126,127] These symptoms often require surgical intervention—approximately 10% of revision procedures in combat-related amputations are due to symptomatic neuromata.[126–128]

A multitude of prophylactic and therapeutic techniques have been described for symptomatic neuroma prevention, with none being clearly superior or optimal; however, several recently developed techniques shows promising results and deserve specific mention.

As discussed previously, TMR was initially developed as a method of improving myoelectric prosthesis control in upper extremity amputations. Subsequently, many patients reported complete resolution of their neuroma-related pain following TMR procedures.[295] The rationale to explain this finding is as follows: coaptation of the residual nerve to recipient motor nerve branches encourages organized regeneration into the denervated muscle. The recreation of physiologic continuity prevents disorganized axonal regeneration by giving the nerve "somewhere to go, and something to do".[296] The technique has been utilized in lower extremity amputations with promising results, although long-term follow-up data have not been published.[275,297] The highest level of evidence study published to date, a randomized controlled trial comparing TMR to neuroma excision and burial for postamputation pain, found that TMR improved phantom limb pain and trended towards improved residual limb pain.[298] Additional prospective and retrospective case series have likewise demonstrated a reduction in RLP and and PLP, with investigators utilizing this technique for both prophylaxis and treatment.[299,300] Durable results with TMR have been reported at intermediate follow-up and complications rates are not increased relative to patients undergoing amputation alone.[301,302] Early work suggests that TMR performed at the time of the index amputation may result in improved pain scores as compared to patients undergoing TMR in a delayed fashion for postamputation pain.[303]

RPNIs have also been proposed as a treatment for symptomatic neuromata.[304] In this technique, the neuroma is excised and a free muscle graft is wrapped around the residual nerve end. A recent study of RPNI performed at the time of major extremity amputation found that compared to a control group, patients treated with RPNI had a lower incidence of symptomatic neuroma formation (0% vs. 13%) and reduced phantom limb pain (51% vs. 91%).[305]

To date, no studies have directly compared outcomes of TMR relative to RPNI.[306] However, these strategies may best work in a complementary fashion, with TMR utilized for more frequently symptomatic nerves (sciatic, peroneal, tibial) and RPNI reserved for less problematic nerves (sural, saphenous) or for instances of insufficient nerve length or quality or the absence of a suitable target.[307,308]

These techniques for neuroma prevention and treatment represent promising solutions to a vexing problem following amputation. Further prospective, comparative studies are required to better determine the superiority of any one strategy.

Summary

Understanding the epidemiology of limb loss is key to meeting the perioperative and rehabilitative needs of this patient population. No matter the indication for amputation, the decision to remove some or all of a limb is frequently challenging and always life altering. However, amputation should be viewed not as a treatment failure—when done with appropriate technique and with a multidisciplinary team approach, a positive functional outcome can result. In selecting the appropriate level of amputation, several factors must be carefully considered: the likelihood of successful healing of the surgical wound; the preservation of the ankle and knee (if possible) to minimize the impact on energy cost of gait and postural control; and the creation of a residual limb with adequate skin surface and soft tissue robustness, length, and dimensions for prosthetic fitting and function. Appropriate management of bone, muscle, nerves, and skin remain essential to a successful outcome. Even with flawless technique, complications are frequent and patients require consistent follow-up in the perioperative period for appropriate management. Although many principles can be applied to all amputations, each individual amputation level has its own key technical points. In the future, amputation surgery may routinely involve a number of novel techniques, all of which have been developed with goal of creating a painless residual limb that provides maximum functional benefit to the patient.

References

The complete listing of the References are available in the accompanying enhanced eBook version included with the print purchase of this textbook. Visit Elsevier eBooks+ (eBooks.Health.Elsevier.com) to access this content.

20 Postoperative and Preprosthetic Care

TAMARA N. GRAVANO AND KELLY ALLEGRO

LEARNING OBJECTIVES

On completion of this chapter, the reader will be able to do the following:

1. Plan a comprehensive examination for an individual with recent lower extremity amputation, selecting appropriate tests and measures and documentation strategies.
2. Use information gathered in the examination, evidence from the clinical research literature, and knowledge of postoperative care to evaluate individuals with recent lower extremity amputation.
3. Formulate an appropriate physical therapy (PT) movement system diagnosis and prognosis for rehabilitation for individuals with recent lower extremity amputation.
4. Develop appropriate short- and long-term goals and estimate duration, frequency, and intensity of care in the postoperative, preprosthetic care of an individual with recent lower extremity amputation.
5. Develop an appropriate PT plan of care for single-limb mobility, residual limb care and wound healing, and preprosthetic rehabilitation.
6. Describe strategies to monitor progress and to adapt and advance the plan of care during the preprosthetic period of rehabilitation.
7. Describe strategies to evaluate outcomes of postoperative, preprosthetic rehabilitation.

Patient-Client Management After Amputation

INDIVIDUALS WITH A NEW AMPUTATION

In the early days following surgery, the person with a new amputation will likely experience acute surgical pain and will likely be grieving the loss of their limb. The immediacy of pain combined with a sense of loss may make it difficult for those with recent amputation to recognize their potential for a positive rehabilitation outcome.[1] Older persons with dysvascular or neuropathic limb loss may have had time to physically and psychologically prepare for an elective amputation after a prolonged period of managing a poorly vascularized foot or nonhealing neuropathic ulcer. Therefore they may be less distressed about losing their limb than younger persons who suddenly lost a limb in a traumatic accident or other medical emergency. However, whatever the circumstances leading to amputation, losing one's limb requires significant psychological adjustment.[1] Early education and discussion about rehabilitation and the person's ultimate goals are extremely important.

PATIENT-CENTERED CARE AND MULTIDISCIPLINARY TEAMS

In response to the number of military personnel with traumatic amputations and older veterans with dysvascular amputation, the Departments of Defense and of Veterans Affairs have adopted interdisciplinary, patient-centered care as the ideal model for rehabilitating persons with amputation.[2–4] There is a growing number of female veterans with amputations. In a recent qualitative study, female veterans with lower extremity amputation expressed similar concerns as their male counterparts, such as the importance of available, well-fitting prostheses and the central role of the provider-patient relationship. However, they also noted unique needs such as formal opportunities for social support and peer interaction for female veterans with lower extremity amputation and ensuring clinical interactions are sex-sensitive and free of bias.[2] The physical therapist and prosthetist, as members of the rehabilitation team, will interact with surgeons, patients, and family members as decisions about surgical levels, plans for postoperative care, potential for prosthetic use, and prosthetic rehabilitation plans are made. For persons facing elective amputation because of dysvascular disease, a period of physical therapy (PT) intervention before surgery can positively impact postoperative outcomes.[4]

In the days immediately after amputation, this initial stage of acute care and early rehabilitation sets the stage for the eventual return to functional mobility, the ability to return to valued activities, and participation in key family and social roles.[4] Although the immediate goals of each interdisciplinary team member vary, all ultimately lead toward independence and return to the preferred lifestyle of the person with a newly amputated limb. To accomplish this, the team must use a holistic and comprehensive approach to address the person's comorbid burden of illness, psychological and developmental needs, and long-term functional, vocational, and leisure goals. Surgical and medical team members are most concerned about the healing suture line and overall health status, especially for individuals with vascular insufficiency and those at risk of infection after traumatic amputation.[5] Nursing professionals provide general medical and wound care as the suture line heals and administer medications for pain management.[5–7] Registered dieticians assess the patient's nutritional needs related to wound healing and exercise demands.[8] Physical and occupational therapists focus on enhancing the patient's early mobility, self-care, assessment of the potential for prosthetic use, control of edema and pain management, donning and doffing dressings and shrinkers for optimal shaping of the residual limb, and prevention of secondary complications.[8]

The prosthetist may fabricate an immediate postoperative prosthesis (IPOP) or an early postoperative prosthesis (EPOP), or a semirigid dressing (SRD) and begins to consider which prosthetic components and suspension systems will ultimately be most appropriate, given the individual's characteristics, abilities, and functional needs.[8,9] The person with a new amputation and their family are often most concerned about pain management and what life will be like with limb loss.[10] A psychologist, social worker, vocational counselor, or school counselor is involved as needed to help with psychological adjustment and to organize long-term rehabilitation care or community resources in preparation for discharge.[4] A spiritual leader, such as a priest or rabbi, can also be a valuable resource for the person with a new amputation, the family, and the team.

Although the multidisciplinary team can vary in size, depending on patient needs and practice settings, the member at the team's center is the individual with a new amputation and their caregiver(s).[4,11] Coordinated communication among all team members, including the opportunity for the amputee and their family members to ask questions and voice concerns, is more important in this early postoperative and preprosthetic period than during the prosthetic prescription process and training later in the rehabilitation process. This early period sets the stage for the individual's expectations and, ultimately, success as an individual with limb loss.[3,9] The unique training, clinical expertise, and individual roles of each team member contribute, in a collaborative process, to developing a rehabilitation plan that best meets the needs and optimizes the potential of the individual who has lost a limb.[6] The team must agree on the timing and prioritization of specific rehabilitative interventions to meet the goals defined for each patient. Effective communication and strong relationships among the surgeons, orthopedists, or trauma teams who perform the majority of amputations and the rehabilitation team substantially improve the quality of patient care and assist the rehabilitation process.

This chapter focuses on the roles of rehabilitation professionals who work with persons with a new amputation in the days and weeks immediately after surgery. It explores how surgical pain and phantom sensation are managed, strategies for controlling postoperative edema, and methods for assessing a patient's prosthetic fitting readiness. Interventions are identified that help a person with a new amputation gain competence with single-limb mobility tasks. Evidence-based exercises that provide the foundation for successful prosthetic use are provided. The strategies for patient management are organized around the model outlined in the American Physical Therapy Association's Guide to Physical Therapist Practice (Fig. 20.1).[12]

Examination

Ideally, for those undergoing an "elective" amputation, the rehabilitation team will meet with the individual and caregivers before surgery to begin collecting information that will be used to guide intervention and provide information about the rehabilitation process. The rehabilitation team should provide patients and their families with information regarding surgical interventions, rehabilitation programs, prosthetic options, and potential outcomes while establishing realistic goals.[3] Preoperative interaction may not always be possible, primarily when an amputation occurs after failed revascularization, acute and severe limb ischemia, severe infection, or civilian or combat-related traumatic injury. If a preoperative assessment is not

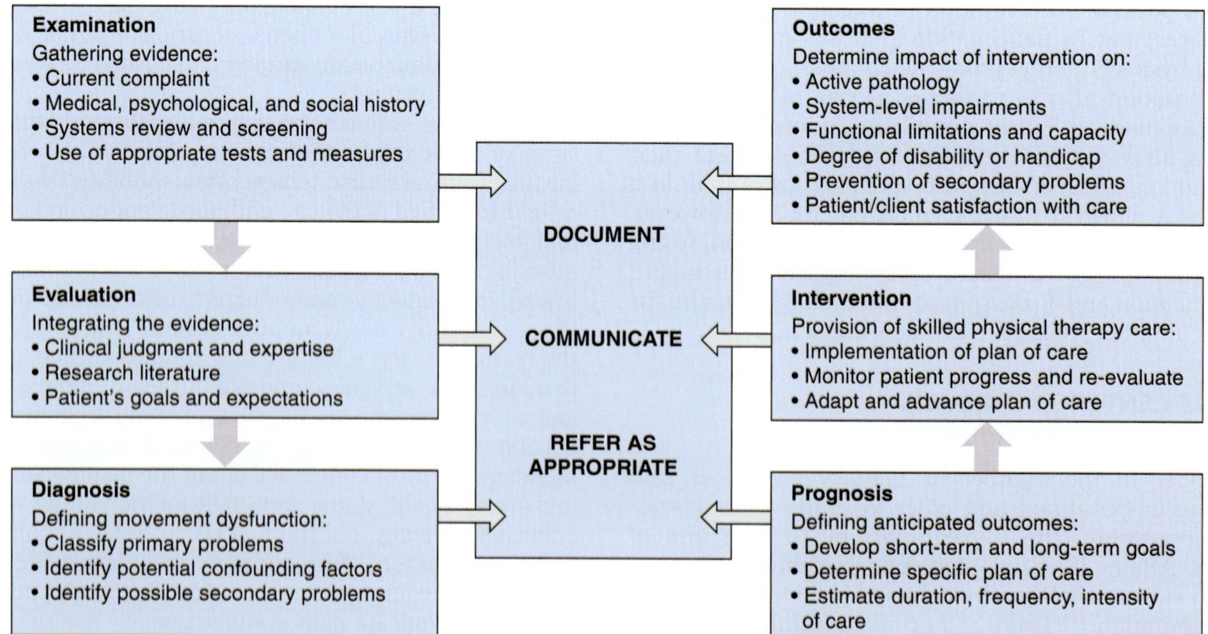

Fig. 20.1 The components of a systematic and effective patient-client management process. (Adapted from http://guidetoptpractice.apta.org/, with permission of the American Physical Therapy Association. Who are Physical Therapists? Guide to Physical Therapist Practice. © American Physical Therapy Association. All rights reserved.)

possible, referral to rehabilitation should be made as soon after surgery as possible; delaying referrals often leads to contracture formation, further cardiovascular and musculoskeletal deconditioning, delayed prosthetic fitting and training, a greater risk of dependency, and a higher risk of reamputation, institutionalization, and mortality.[13,14] Box 20.1 summarizes the components of a comprehensive assessment for persons with lower extremity amputation.

Whenever the first contact with the individual and family occurs, the rehabilitation team begins by gathering baseline information to guide the rehabilitation process's planning and implementation. This initial information is collected in three ways: developing a complete patient-client history, reviewing physiologic systems to identify important comorbidities that will affect the rehabilitation process, and using appropriate tests and measures to identify impairments and functional limitations to be addressed in the rehabilitation plan of care.[12] Prioritize the following: initial healing of the surgical site, pain management, volume control of the residual limb, bed mobility, and transfers. Examination in the preprosthetic period (in an outpatient, home care, or subacute setting) will add more detail to determine the potential for a prosthetic prescription.

PATIENT-CLIENT HISTORY AND INTERVIEW

Rehabilitation professionals use several strategies to gather information about an individual's medical history. In the acute care setting, the process usually begins with a review of the individual's current medical record or chart, as well as previous medical records (if available). The chart

Box 20.1 Comprehensive Assessment for Patients With Lower Extremity Amputation

History (Data Collected From Chart Review and Interview)

Demographics	Age, sex, primary language, race/ethnicity
Social history	Family and caregiver resources, other social support systems
Occupational history	Employment or retirement status, typical work and leisure activities
Developmental status	Physical/motor, perceptual, cognitive, and emotional dimensions
Living environment	Characteristics and accessibility of "home" environment, projected discharge destination
Current condition	Reason for referral, current concerns/needs, previous medical/surgical interventions for current condition
Past medical history	Prior hospitalizations and surgeries; smoking, alcohol, or drug use (past and present)
Family history	Health risk factors for vascular and cardiac disease
Medications	Prescription medication for current and other medical conditions
	Over-the-counter medications typically used
Functional status	Current and prior abilities and functional limitations (ADLs/IADLs)

Systems review (concurrent/comorbid disease and impairment related to prognosis for and participation in rehabilitation)

1. Cardiopulmonary and cardiovascular systems
2. Endocrine and metabolic systems
3. Musculoskeletal system
4. Neuromuscular system
5. Gastrointestinal and genitourinary systems

Tests and measures (areas for specific assessment)

Pain	Presence of phantom limb sensation or pain
	Postoperative pain and pain management strategies
	Muscle soreness related to altered movement patterns
	Joint pain related to motion or comorbid arthritis, etc.
Anthropomorphic characteristics	Residual limb length (bone length, soft tissue length)
	Residual limb girth, redundant tissue ("dog ears," adductor roll)
	Residual limb shape (bulbous, cylindrical, conical)
	Assessment of type and severity of edema
	Effectiveness of edema control strategy being used
	Overall height, weight, body composition
Skin/integument	Assessment of surgical wound healing
	Assessment/management of adhesions and existing scar tissue
	Other skin problems (other incisions, grafts, psoriasis, cysts, etc.)
	Integrity of remaining foot/limb, especially if neuropathic or dysvascular etiology of amputation
Circulation	Palpation/auscultation of lower extremity pulses, residual and intact limbs
	Skin temperature and presence of trophic changes, residual and intact limbs
	Skin color and response to elevation or dependent position, residual and intact limbs
	Claudication time and distance, impact on function

(Continued)

Box 20.1 Comprehensive Assessment for Patients With Lower Extremity Amputation—cont'd

Range of motion/muscle length	Range of motion, soft tissue length, and joint contracture
Joint integrity	Ligamentous integrity or joint instability
	Structural alignment or joint deformity
	Integrity or inflammation of synovium, bursae, cartilage
Muscle performance	Current muscle strength of upper extremity, trunk, lower extremity
	Muscular power for functional activity
	Muscular endurance for functional activity
	Potential for improvement
Motor function	Motor control, including dexterity, coordination, agility, tone
	Motor learning, including previous use of ambulatory aids, prostheses
Upper extremity function	Power and strength of upper extremity and of trunk
	Ability to use upper extremity in functional activities
Aerobic capacity	Blood pressure, heart rate, respiratory rate (at rest, as well as during and following activity)
	Perceived exertion, dyspnea, angina, during functional activity
	Overall level of physical fitness and functional capacity
Attention/cognition/emotion	Level of consciousness, sleep patterns
	Ability to learn and preferred learning style
	Cognitive dysfunction screening (delirium, depression, dementia)
	Motivation, attention/distractibility, learning styles
Sensory integrity	Protective sensation of residual and remaining limb
	Superficial sensation: light touch, sharp/dull, pressure, temperature
	Proprioception: kinesthesia, position sense
Mobility	Changing position in bed (rolling, scooting, coming to sitting)
Postural control	Static, anticipatory, reactionary balance, in sitting, standing, during functional activities
Transfers	Ability to transfer to/from bed, toilet, wheelchair, mat, tub/shower
Assistive/adaptive equipment	Assistive devices/adaptive equipment currently being used
Ambulation and locomotion	Ability to use ambulatory aid safely for single-limb gait
	Ability to use wheelchair safely
	Adaptations/equipment necessary for patient's living environment
Gait and balance	Assessment of postural control in quiet standing, reaching, ability to stop/start, change direction, and alter velocity while walking
	Reaction to unexpected perturbation, at rest and during activity
	Observational gait assessment, identification of gait deviations
	Kinematic gait assessment (e.g., speed, stride length, cadence)
	Energy cost or efficiency of locomotion/gait, perceived exertion and dyspnea
	Ability/safety to manage uneven terrain, stairs, ramps, etc.
Posture	Resting posture in sitting, standing, other positions
	Alteration in posture due to loss of limb segment
Self-care	Ability to perform basic ADLs
	Ability to perform IADLs
	Availability of assistance and preparation of caregivers
Community/work reintegration	Analysis of roles/activities/tasks
	Functional capacity analysis, determination of essential functions
	Analysis of environment, safety assessment
	Assessment of need for adaptation
Prosthetic requirements	Potential for functional prosthetic use
	Readiness for prosthetic fitting/prescription
	Appropriate prosthetic design, components, suspension

ADLs, Activities of daily living; *IADLs*, instrumental activities of daily living.

Adapted from American Physical Therapy Association. *The Guide to Physical Therapy Practice; Pattern K: Impaired Gait, Locomotion, and Balance, and Impaired Motor Function Secondary to Lower Extremity Amputation. Guide to Physical Therapist Practice 4.0.* American Physical Therapy Association; 2014. http://guidetoptpractice.apta.org/content/1/SEC2.body.

review provides a broad overview of the individual's health, comorbidities, medications, prior and current functional status, and details about the surgical procedure. Data that other healthcare team members have generated in their examination and evaluative processes are quite relevant to PT care to avoid redundancy in the examination and in planning what additional information will be necessary to collect during subsequent interviews and discussions with the individual and family caregivers.

The interview process provides vital information about the individual's priorities and concerns so that they can be appropriately integrated into the care plan. The physical therapist may also gather supplementary information from the clinical research literature to assist in the subsequent development of prognosis and plan or care, especially if the individual's situation is unusual or complex.[15]

Demographic and Sociocultural Information

The information gathered when reviewing history often begins with basic demographics such as age, sex, race/ethnicity, primary language, and level of education. The data helps us to appropriately target communication during our interaction with an individual with recent limb loss. It is also important to build an understanding of the individual's sociocultural history, including beliefs, expectations and goals, preferred behaviors, and family and caregiver resources, as well as access to and quality of informal and formal support systems.[16–18] There is some evidence regarding the benefits of a formal peer support system for individuals with recent limb loss.[19] Peer visits are found to be most beneficial when individuals are matched according to age, sex, and amputation level. A comprehensive examination includes an assessment of both physical and psychological components regarding the amputation and use of a new prosthetic.[17] Each factor is a potentially significant influence on the individual's engagement in the rehabilitation process. Rehabilitation professionals also gather information about the individual's employment status and task demands, roles and responsibilities within the family system, leisure interests and hobbies, and previous and preferred involvement in the community (access, transportation, and key activities). In addition, information about smoking, alcohol intake, and other previous substance use/abuse, as well as the individual's coping style and preferred coping strategies, help the team to understand better how the individual may behave in the postoperative period. This information is essential in developing a prognosis and plan of care; it helps rehabilitation professionals to better define the long-term goals and anticipated outcomes of rehabilitation.

Developmental Status

Another piece of information that informs an appropriate rehabilitation plan of care is the physical, cognitive, perceptual, and emotional developmental status of the individual and their caregivers, as well as an understanding of the family system as an organization.[20,21] Although the relevance of developmental status is most apparent when the individual being examined is a child, the perspective afforded by understanding of life span development is valuable for individuals with recent amputation of any age. Examples of factors that evolve over the life span that affect an individual's participation in rehabilitation include postural control, motor abilities, perceptual abilities, willingness to take risks, problem-solving, coping styles and strategies, and limb dominance. Observation and interchange during the interview process help the therapist to determine if further clinical examination of developmental status will be necessary.[21]

Living Environment

Rehabilitation professionals gather information about the characteristics of an individual's physical living environment.

- They ask about getting into and out of the house (e.g., how far is it from the car to the house?
- What surfaces will be encountered moving from the car to the house?
- Are there steps and railings at the entry?
- What are the distances between the primary living areas that the person will have to navigate?
- How accessible and functional are each of the primary living areas in the home for those using ambulatory aids or a wheelchair for mobility?
- Is it possible to adapt the home if necessary?
- What adaptive equipment is already available?
- What type of assistance is likely to be routinely available?
- What type of equipment is expected to be acceptable for the individual and family?).

Asking about the individual's ability to drive, access to public transportation, or plans for alternatives for transport once discharged from the acute care setting is important. This may determine the necessary services and where they will be provided.

- Will the individual return to their home environment on discharge from acute care?
- If so, will they require home care, or is transportation available for follow-up appointments with physicians and outpatient rehabilitation?
- Alternatively, will the individual have an interim stay in another healthcare facility for further rehabilitation?

This information will help set rehabilitation priorities and begin the discharge planning process.[21]

Health, Emotional, and Cognitive Status

During the interview, the rehabilitation professional's impression of the individual's general health status that initially developed during chart review broadens. The rehabilitation professional asks questions to discern how the person perceives their health and ability to function in self-care, family, or social roles. They assess the individual's understanding of the current situation, prognosis, and expectations about the rehabilitation process. They may explore the person's coping style, response to stress, and preferred coping skills and strategies.[22,23] This conversation also reveals the individual's current emotional status, ability to learn, cognitive ability, and memory function. A person who undergoes an amputation may struggle with body image and struggle to maintain satisfaction with their quality of life.[24] Because increased levels of depression, anxiety, and body image issues are associated with sexual dysfunction in individuals with lower-limb amputation, the therapist should screen for depression and be prepared to select appropriate referral sources.[3,23]

Because rehabilitation involves physical effort, it is essential to understand the person with a recent amputation's usual level of activity and fitness and their readiness to exercise. Is physical activity a regular part of the preamputation lifestyle? Has there been a period of prolonged inactivity before surgery?[24] Will any other health habits, such as smoking and the use of alcohol or other substances, affect the individual's ability to do physical work and ability to learn or adapt?[24–26]

Medical, Surgical, and Family History

Potentially critical medical conditions that may influence postoperative/preprosthetic rehabilitation include diabetes, cardiovascular disease, cerebrovascular disease, obesity, neuropathy, renal disease, congestive heart failure (CHF), uncontrolled hypertension, and preexisting neuromuscular or musculoskeletal pathologic conditions or impairments, such as stroke or osteoporosis.[27,28] Each of these has a potential impact on wound healing, functional mobility, and exercise tolerance during rehabilitation. Healing and risk of infection are also concerns for those with compromised immune system function, whether from diseases such as human immunodeficiency virus (HIV)/acquired immunodeficiency syndrome (AIDS), those on transplantation medications, those involved in chemotherapy or recent stem cell transplantation, or those using medical steroids.[29] Wound healing, skin condition, and endurance may be issues for persons currently undergoing chemotherapy or radiation treatments for cancer.[30,31]

A review of the individual's surgical history provides additional information that helps rehabilitation professionals anticipate the individual's response to physical activity. Has the individual had a cardiac pacemaker or defibrillator implanted? Has there been previous amputation of toes or part of the foot of either the newly amputated or "intact" limb? Are there recent surgical scars to be aware of (e.g., following revascularization before amputation)? Has there been a total joint replacement or lower extremity fracture that might affect rehabilitation activities and prosthetic component selection?

The "laundry list" of comorbidities and previous surgeries identified in the chart review does not necessarily mean the individual is in poor health. Many individuals manage chronic illnesses and conditions quite effectively. Although they may have less functional reserve than those without a pathologic condition, they have the potential for positive rehabilitation outcomes.[32]

Physical therapists must also be aware of the results of tests and diagnostic procedures other team members have undertaken as part of their examination and evaluation. These might include preoperative cardiac or peripheral vascular studies, electrocardiogram, stress tests, pulmonary function tests, radiographs, CT, MRI, urinalysis, and laboratory tests for various components of blood (e.g., hemoglobin [Hb], cell counts, cultures). Physical therapists must recognize potential physiologic signs and symptoms that may occur when a laboratory value is out of range.[33] Comparison of the individual's test results to established norms provides an index of overall health status and tolerance of activity levels. Monitoring laboratory test values (e.g., white blood cell [WBC], hematocrit, Hb, platelet, the international normalized ratio, partial prothrombin time, glycosylated Hb, and blood glucose levels) and oxygen saturation levels provide ongoing information about general health status and exercise/activity tolerance, allowing the therapist to adapt the intervention to the individual's potentially changing condition.[33]

Because many medications used to manage postoperative pain affect thinking and learning, it is crucial to understand what pain management strategies are in place and when medication is typically administered.[7,34,35] Given the likelihood of cardiovascular comorbidity in older adults with vascular disease and diabetes, it is also essential to understand what cardiac medications are being administered and how these medications affect response to physical activity and position change. It is not unusual for persons who have been immobile or on bed rest to be at risk of postural (orthostatic) hypotension, especially if they are taking medications to manage hypertension.[33] In addition, given the stress of the surgery and hospital environment, especially if the amputation was performed under general anesthesia, there is the possibility of temporary postoperative delirium or difficulty with learning and memory.[36] If confusion is observed, clarifying typical preoperative cognitive status is important by speaking with family and caregivers.

Current Condition

A review of the operating room report in the medical record provides information about surgical procedure, drain placement, method of closure, and planned postoperative wound and limb-volume strategies being used. When combined with knowledge of pain management strategies and demographic information, this information guides early postoperative/preprosthetic care. Physical therapists use this information to identify potential issues with healing, determine educational needs for the person with a new amputation, develop strategies for early positioning of the residual limb, identify potential issues affecting prosthetic fit, and prepare the residual limb for wearing a prosthesis. Determining how comorbidities and injuries are being actively managed is also important because these affect readiness for early mobility, learning, and memory. Impressions of the individual's psychological state, fears, and expectations round out the baseline with which the person will begin early rehabilitation.

SYSTEMS REVIEW

In the acute care setting, there has likely been a fairly comprehensive review of physiologic systems as a component of preoperative work-up (or emergency care in the case of traumatic injury). Rehabilitation professionals find the results of such review in the medical record's physician notes and intake forms. The therapist may choose to screen or evaluate in more detail if the information in the record is insufficient or lacks detail related to functional status and response to increasing activity and exercise. The review of systems must include the anatomic and physiologic status of the cardiovascular, cardiopulmonary, integumentary, musculoskeletal, and neuromuscular systems, as well as communication, affect, cognition, language, and learning style.[37]

Ongoing screening as rehabilitation progresses will help identify the onset of secondary problems and postoperative complications that require medical intervention or referral to other team members. Deterioration in cognitive status or onset of new confusion over a relatively short period of time is especially important to watch for because it is often the first indication of dehydration, adverse drug reaction, or infection (e.g., pneumonia, urinary tract infection, infection of the surgical construct) in older adults.[37]

TEST AND MEASURES

In the postoperative/preprosthetic period, physical therapists use a variety of objective tests and measures to determine the severity of impairment and functional limitation. These measures establish a baseline that will be used to determine PT movement-related diagnosis, prognosis, and assess outcomes of the rehabilitation process.[12] Table 20.1 lists

Table 20.1 Examples of Tests and Measures Important in the Postoperative, Preprosthetic Period

Category	Examples of Test or Measurement Strategy
Aerobic capacity, endurance	Heart rate at rest, % maximal attainable in activity Arm ergometry, single-limb bicycle ergometry, combined upper extremity/lower extremity ergometry Respiratory rate at rest, during activity Ratings of perceived exertion or dyspnea
Anthropometric characteristics	Residual limb length Residual limb circumference Description of edema type and location
Arousal, attention, cognition	Mini-Mental State Examination, Mini-Cog Delirium scales Depression scales (e.g., Geriatric Depression Scale, Centers for Epidemiologic Studies Depression scale) Saint Louis University Mental Status (SLUMS) Montreal Cognitive Assessment (MOCA)
Balance	Static postural control (various functional positions) Anticipatory postural control in functional activity Reaction to perturbation Specific balance tests (e.g., Berg, Functional Reach)
Circulation	Palpation of peripheral pulse Skin temperature
Gait and locomotion	Use of assistive devices Level of independence, cueing, or assistance required Time and distance parameters (velocity, cadence, stride) Pattern and symmetry Perceived exertion and dyspnea
Integumentary integrity	Condition of the incision Nature and extent of drainage Condition of "intact" limb Skin color, turgor, temperature
Joint integrity and mobility	Manual examination of ligamentous integrity Documentation of bony deformity
Mobility	Observation of bed mobility (e.g., rolling) Observation of transitions (e.g., supine-sit) Observation of description of level of assistance, cueing required transfers (various surfaces, heights)
Muscle performance	Strength: manual muscle test, handheld dynamometer Power: isokinetic dynamometer, manual resistance through range at various speeds of contraction Endurance: 10 repetitions maximum, or maximum number contractions, time to fatigue
Neuromotor function	Observation of quality of motor control in activity Observation of efficiency of motor planning Determination of stage of motor learning with new or adapted tasks Muscle tone Reflex integrity
Pain	Description of nature or type of pain Visual analog scale for intensity of pain Body chart for location of painful areas Description of factors to increase/decrease discomfort
Range of motion/muscle length	Goniometry Functional tests (e.g., Thomas test, straight-leg raise)
Self-care and home management	Observation of BADLs and IADLs BADL and IADL rating scales
Sensory integrity	Protective sensation (Semmes-Weinstein filament) Proprioception and kinesthesia Visual acuity, figure-ground, light/dark accommodation Vestibulo-ocular function during position change Hearing impairment (acuity, sensitivity to background noise)

BADLs, Basic activities of daily living; *IADLs*, instrumental activities of daily living.

examples of tests and measures appropriate for the postoperative/preprosthetic period. Although most strategies are similar to those used in general PT practice, some may need to be adapted to accommodate the condition or length of the residual limb (e.g., the point of application of resistive force during manual muscle testing of knee extension strength after transtibial amputation). However, whenever the measurement technique is altered, the reliability and validity of the data collected may be questionable, and the data generated may be less precise. Therapists often begin with an examination at the level of impairment and then move on to functional assessment.

Assessing Acute Postoperative Pain

The individual with a new amputation will likely be coping with significant acute postoperative pain and may be distressed by the sense that the limb is still in place (phantom sensation) after amputation. Pain is a subjective individual experience and should be assessed in a standardized manner. Physical therapists use assessments that document the nature of pain, the location of pain, and the intensity of discomfort the individual is experiencing. These include descriptors generated by the individual with recent amputation or circled on a pain checklist, body maps, visual analog scales, provocation tests, or specific pain indices or questionnaires developed for postsurgical patients (Fig. 20.2).[38,39]

McGill Pain Questionnaire

Part 1: Where is Your Pain?

Please mark, on the drawings below, the areas where you feel pain.
Put "E" if the pain is external
Put "I" if the pain is internal
Put "EI" if the pain is both internal and external

Part 2: What Does Your Pain Feel Like?

Some of the words below describe your PRESENT pain. Circle ONLY those words that best describe your pain right now. Leave out any category that is not suitable. Use only a single word in the appropriate category—the one that applies the best.

1	2	3	4
Flickering Quivering Pulsing Throbbing Beating Pounding	Jumping Flashing Shooting	Pricking Boring Drilling Stabbing Lancinating	Sharp Cutting Lacerating
5	**6**	**7**	**8**
Pinching Pressing Gnawing Cramping Crushing	Tugging Pulling Wrenching	Hot Burning Scalding Searing	Tingling Itchy Smarting
9	**10**	**11**	**12**
Dull Sore Hurting Aching Heavy	Tender Taut Rasping	Tiring Exhausting	Sickening Suffocating
13	**14**	**15**	**16**
Fearful Frightful Terrifying	Punishing Grueling Cruel Vicious Killing	Wretched Blinding	Annoying Troublesome Miserable Intense Unbearable
17	**18**	**19**	**20**
Spreading Radiating Penetrating Piercing	Tight Numb Drawing Squeezing Tearing	Cool Cold Freezing	Nagging Nauseating Agonizing Dreadful Torturing

Part 3: How Does Your Pain Change With Time?

1. Which word or words would you use to describe the *pattern* of your pain?

1	2	3
Continuous Steady Constant	Rhythmic Periodic Intermittent	Brief Momentary Transient

2. What kind of things *relieve* your pain?

3. What kind of things *increase* your pain?

Part 4: How Strong is Your Pain?

People agree that the following five words represent pain of increasing intensity. They are:

1	2	3	4	5
Mild	Discomforting	Distressing	Horrible	Excruciating

To answer each question below, write the number of the most appropriate word in the space beside the question.

1. Which word describes your pain right now? ________
2. Which word describes your pain at its worst? ________
3. Which word describes it when it is least? ________
4. Which word describes the worst toothache you ever had? ________
5. Which word describes the worst headache you ever had? ________
6. Which word describes the worst stomach-ache you ever had? ________

A

No pain at all |———————— 100 mm ————————| Worst possible pain

B

Fig. 20.2 Examples of tools used to document pain and discomfort. (A) McGill Pain Questionnaire. Descriptor groups: sensory (1–10), affective (11–15), evaluative (16), and miscellaneous (17–20). (B) The visual analog scale. (A, Modified from Melzack R. The McGill pain questionnaire; major properties and scoring methods. *Pain.* 1975;1(3):277–299. B, From Bijur PE, Silver W, Gallagher EJ. Reliability of the visual analog scale for measurement of acute pain. *Acad Emerg Med.* 2001;8(12):1153–1157.)

It is also important to assess how severely pain interferes with functions, what activities or conditions increase the pain, and what positions or strategies have helped manage the postoperative pain. Documentation of pain management strategies is also important: narcotic and opioid medications potentially impact attention, learning ability, and response time during movement and balance activities.[40,41]

Phantom Sensation and Phantom Pain

It is estimated that ~95% of individuals with limb loss experience residual limb pain, phantom limb pain, or both. *Residual limb pain* is commonly described as pain that occurs at the surgical site.[34] *Phantom limb pain* is a type of neuropathic pain described as shooting pain, severe cramping, or a distressing burning sensation that may be localized near or distal to the surgical site.[1,34,42] Phantom limb pain is typically episodic, lasting days, weeks, months, or even years in some cases.[35] Phantom limb pain can migrate into more proximal regions of the amputated limb, known as *telescoping pain*. Fortunately, fewer than 15% of those experiencing phantom pain rate it as severe or constant; most experience transient mild-to-moderate discomfort that does not interfere with usual activity. Phantom pain is more likely in those with longstanding and severe preoperative dysvascular pain and those requiring amputation after severe traumatic injury.[43,44]

Female sex, limb loss of the upper extremities, and presence of chronic pain are all reported risk factors for phantom limb pain.[34,43]

In contrast to residual pain and phantom limb pain, *phantom limb sensations* are typically described as nonpainful numbness, tingling, tickling, or pressure distal to the surgical incision of the residual limb.[7,34] In most cases, if the individual reports significant phantom sensation or pain, careful inspection of the residual limb helps to rule out other potential sources of pain, such as a neuroma or an inflamed or infected surgical wound. A neuroma may form any time a nerve is cut. Despite multiple surgical techniques to prevent neuromas, such as electrocautery, perineural closure, and silastic capping, most surgeons will cut the nerve proximal to the bone stump and allow it to retract into the stump, hoping to avoid a painful neuroma.[45] Phantom limb sensation and pain tend to decrease over time, whether the amputation resulted from a dysvascular/neuropathic extremity or a traumatic injury.[43,44]

Assessing Residual Limb Length and Volume

The length and volume of the residual limb are important determinants of readiness for prosthetic use, as well as socket design and components chosen for the training prosthesis.[46,47] Initial measurements can be made at the first dressing change. Changes in limb volume are tracked by frequent remeasurement during the preprosthetic period of rehabilitation. This is important because discomfort from the poorly fitting socket is the most common reason for clinical visits for individuals with recent limb loss.[46,47]

The two components of *residual limb length* are the actual length of the residual tibia or residual femur and the total length of the limb, including soft tissue. Measurements are taken from an easily identified bony landmark to the palpated end of the long bone, the incision line, or the end of soft tissue. In the transtibial limb, the starting place for measurement is most often the medial joint line of the knee; an alternative is to begin measurement at the tibial tubercle (Fig. 20.3A). The starting place for measurement in the transfemoral limb can be the ischial tuberosity or the greater trochanter (see Fig. 20.3B). Precise notation must be made about the proximal and distal landmarks used for the initial measurement to ensure consistency in the subsequent measurement process. Table 20.2 presents a descriptive classification schema for residual limb lengths.

Residual limb volume is typically assessed by serial circumferential girth measurements with a tape measure.[48,49] For persons with transtibial amputation, circumferential measurement begins at either the medial tibial plateau or the tibial tubercle and is repeated at equally spaced points to the end of the limb (Fig. 20.4). For those with a transfemoral amputation, measurement begins at either the ischial tuberosity or the greater trochanter. It is also repeated at equally spaced points to the end of the residual limb. The interval between measurements should be documented (i.e., every 5 cm or every inch) for consistency and reliability in future measurements. Prosthetists use a variety of

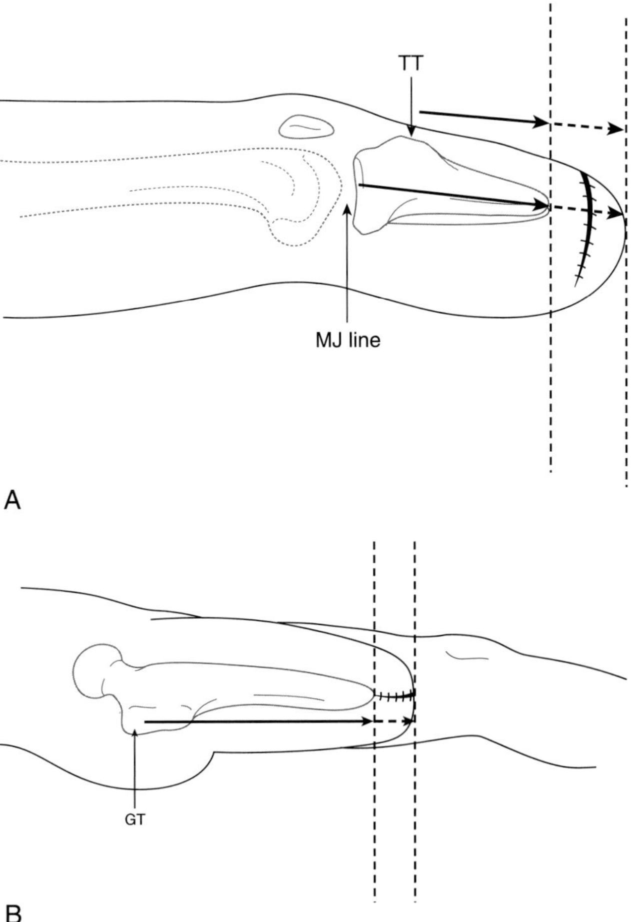

Fig. 20.3 (A) Medial view of a left transtibial residual limb. Limb length is measured to the end of the tibia *(solid arrow)* and to the end of soft tissue *(dotted arrow)* from a bony landmark such as the medial joint *(MJ)* line or tubercle of the tibia *(TT)*. (B) Lateral view of a right transfemoral residual limb. Limb length is measured from the greater trochanter *(GT)* or ischial tuberosity to the end of bone *(solid arrow)* and to the end of soft tissue *(dotted arrow)*.

Table 20.2 Residual Limb Lengths and Associated Prosthetic Consequences[46–49]

Segment	Level	Preserved	Inches	Centimeters	Functional Outcome
Adult tibia	Intact	100%	14.5 ± 1.2	36.9 ± 3.0	Effective walking ability
Transtibial residual limb	Short	< 35%	<5 especially if < 3	<12.7 especially if <7.6	Insufficient knee extension strength and power for prosthetic control; intolerance of weight-bearing pressures applied to skin and soft tissue by a prosthetic socket
	Standard	35%–50%	5–7	12.7–17.8	Effective prosthetic control for safe and energy-efficient gait; relatively comfortable prosthetic fit
	Long	>50%	> 7	> 18	Distal anterior discomfort and skin irritation in sitting and during swing limb advancement related to high socket pressure at limb-socket interface.
Adult femur	Intact	100%	17.1 ± 1.1	43.5 ± 2.8	Effective walking ability
Transfemoral residual limb	Short	<35%	<5	<15.2	Insufficient hip extension and abduction strength and power for stance control when using prosthesis
	Standard	35%–50%	5–8.5	15.2–21.8	Effective prosthetic control for safe and energy-efficient gait; relatively comfortable prosthetic fit
	Long	>50%	>8.5	>21.8	Long lever arm enhances prosthetic control in stance but may limit choice of prosthetic knee units (if residual limb length and knee unit length exceeds femur length of intact limb)

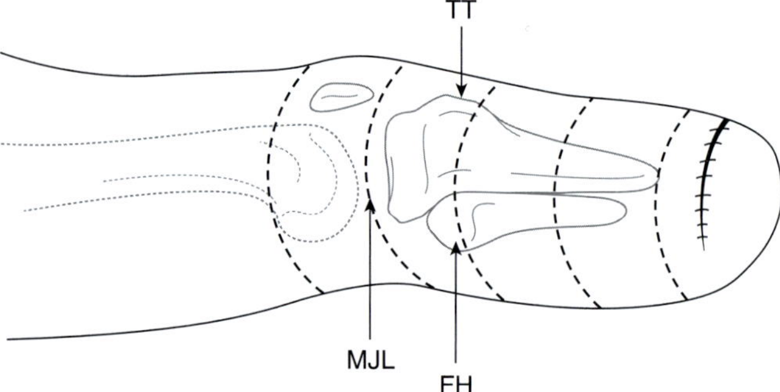

Fig. 20.4 Limb volume and shape of a transtibial residual limb is assessed by taking successive circumferential measures *(dotted lines)* from a bony landmark such as the medial joint line *(MJL)* to the suture line. *FH*, Fibular head; *TT*, tibial tubercle.

technology-based volumetric measurement strategies to capture residual limb anthropomorphic characteristics to guide socket fabrication digitally.[48,49]

One determinant of readiness for prosthetic fitting is a comparison of the proximal and distal circumference of the limb. Often, referral for prosthetic fit is made when the distal limb circumference measurement is equal to or no more than ¼-inch greater than the proximal limb circumference. Ideally, with adequate control of edema and compression, the transtibial residual limb will mature into a tapered cylindrical shape with a distal circumference slightly less than the proximal circumference. The transfemoral limb typically develops into a more conical shape, with a distal circumference significantly less than the proximal circumference. A smaller distal circumference is desirable so that shear forces on soft tissue will be minimal when the prosthesis is donned and used.

Assessing Integumentary Integrity and Wound Healing

Assessment of skin condition and both of the patient's limbs' vascular, sensory, and motor status is imperative. There are many risk factors for skin problems postamputation. Comorbidities such as peripheral vascular disease and diabetic neuropathy can increase the risk of skin breakdown and infection after amputation.[50] During the assessment, there is an opportunity to introduce the individual with a new amputation and their family to strategies that are likely to be used for compression and edema control after surgery. Instructing the individual and family about the proper positioning of the residual limb is also important, as well as the need to maintain knee extension and neutral hip alignment to minimize soft tissue tightness and joint contracture.

The physical therapist should inspect the limb at every visit because changes in dermatologic integrity can occur at any time and result from many causes, including direct physical trauma, edema, irritation, and infection. If the limb has excessive tissue or loose skin beyond the end of the bone, skin or tissue folds, or adherences at the terminal end, prosthetic fitting and use may be complicated by skin problems.[50] Skin inspection should begin immediately and continue daily.

In most settings, the surgeon who performed the amputation assesses the condition of the surgical site at the initial dressing change. This can occur as early as the first postoperative day when soft dressings and elastic wraps have been used or if the residual limb has been casted in a rigid dressing on the third postoperative day.[50,51] After this initial appraisal, the status of the surgical wound is assessed by the nurse or physician at each dressing change. In some settings, the physical therapist is charged with inspecting the residual limb to monitor the stage of healing of the incision and the limb's shape, length, sensory integrity, and volume; the therapist works closely with the surgeon in postoperative wound management and timing of prosthetic replacement.

The wound is carefully examined with each dressing change, and the quantity and quality of drainage from the wound are documented. Initially, drainage will be sanguineous (primarily bloody); typically, as the surgical wound begins to heal over the next few days, drainage transitions to serosanguineous and eventually to serous exudate. Much of this early drainage is absorbed by the wound dressing. Significant amounts of bright red arterial blood (hemorrhage) or darker venous blood (draining hematoma) should be reported to the surgeon for further assessment. As preoperative, perioperative, and postoperative antibiotic administration is the standard of care,[52–56] the incidence of postoperative infection of the incision is decreasing. A study of over 21,000 diabetic patients with lower extremity amputation between 2005 and 2017 determined a 6.8% postoperative infection rate, down from nearly 25%.[55] The authors found that the factors of below-knee amputation, smoking, preoperative sepsis, and obesity were associated with a higher risk of postop infection.[50] Increasing amounts of drainage, as well as thickening, discolored exudate, foul odor, or enlarged lymph nodes proximal to the limb, may signal an infection of the wound; this must be immediately reported to the physician, especially if it occurs in persons who are immunocompromised or whose limbs may have been environmentally contaminated during a traumatic injury.[50] Infection can significantly delay healing, increase the length of acute care stay, require revision of the surgical construct or reamputation to a proximal level, increase the risk of deconditioning and contracture development associated with bed rest, and compromise rehabilitation outcomes.[57,58]

In the first several postoperative days, signs of inflammation (e.g., erythema, edema, elevated tissue temperature surrounding the incision) are likely present along the incision line secondary to tissue trauma sustained during surgery.[57] The wound's edges should be closely approximated for effective primary healing; any areas of wound separation (dehiscence), scab or eschar formation, ecchymosis, or other signs of tissue fragility or decreased viability must be carefully documented and monitored. Clinicians watch for signs of epithelial resurfacing across the incision and the development of a healing ridge along the incision. Prolonged edema delays wound healing because the associated pressure compromises angiogenesis, which, in turn, increases the risk of wound ischemia, tissue necrosis, infection, and the need for revision to a higher level.[59–61] Risk of residual limb osteomyelitis should be suspected when delayed healing and residual limb pain persist in the weeks and months following amputation.[58,62] Persons with a recent or current smoking history are more likely to experience significantly delayed healing following amputation.[60,63,64]

Negative Pressure Wound Therapy (NPWT) has been shown to have a positive effect on wound healing.[65,66] Recent evidence shows the effectiveness of NPWT for surgical wounds healing by primary closure and suggests it can reduce the risk of infection.[65] Similarly, another study focused on using NPWT combined with other treatments for chronic tibia osteomyelitis and demonstrated infection control and improved wound healing time.[62]

Many persons with traumatic, elective, or other nondysvascular amputation have achieved sufficient healing and limb volume control within 2 weeks to use a prefabricated adjustable prosthesis or to be casted for their initial (preparatory, training) prosthesis (Fig. 20.5).[64] Those with amputation secondary to vascular disease often require 4 to 8 weeks or more to achieve adequate healing and limb shaping to allow for prosthetic casting; this is greatly influenced by the strategy used to manage edema in the immediate postoperative period.[67] The surgeon may begin to remove sutures or staples from the incision as early as 10 to 14 days after surgery. Initially, every other or every third suture/staple can be left in place to guard against wound dehiscence; remaining sutures or staples are removed over successive days. The surgical wound is often reinforced with Steri-Strips when sutures or staples are removed to protect the incision from shearing forces during preprosthetic activity and early prosthetic training. The Steri-Strips can remain on the limb for 2 or more weeks after removing the sutures/staples. Gait training with a prosthesis can cautiously begin, with the surgeon's approval, when clear evidence of primary healing is found, even if several sutures have been left in place to protect an area along the incision line that has been slow to fully close.[67]

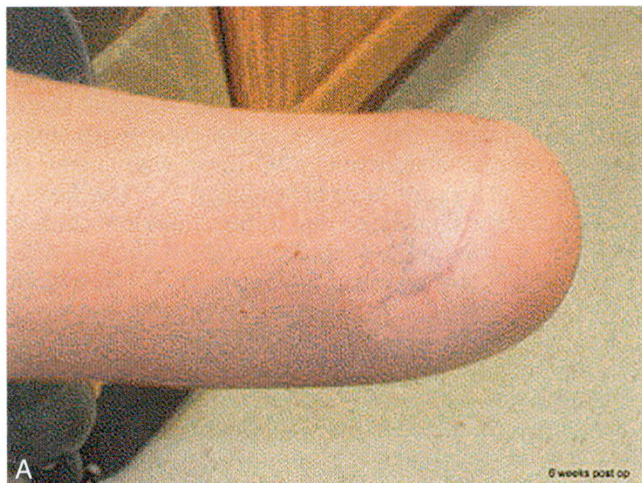

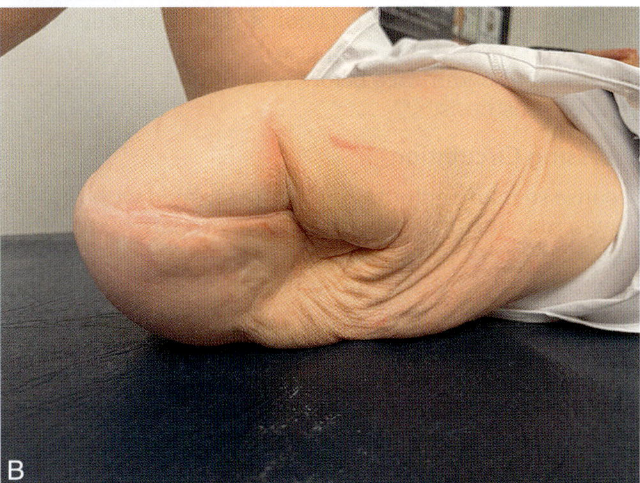

Fig. 20.5 (A) A well-healed, transtibial residual limb with posterior flaps after successful shaping. This residual limb could be described as cylindrical, with little redundant tissue present. (B) Healed, elective, dysvascular transfemoral amputation, with several invaginated scars. (From Stewart JD, Anderson CD, Unger DV. The Portsmouth modification of the Ertl bone-bridge transtibial amputation: the challenge of returning amputees back to active duty. *Oper Tech Sports Med.* 2005;13(4):222–226.)

Age alone should not be a limiting factor when assessing the potential for prosthetic use. Evidence supports a return to independent ambulation for older adults rehabilitating in a skilled nursing facility despite other comorbidities.[68]

Successful independent prosthetic use was associated with their prior level of function and having a below-knee amputation (vs. a higher level of amputation) without phantom pain.[69] However, delayed healing of the surgical wound may postpone prosthetic use. Older persons with diabetes and vascular insufficiency and those who smoke are particularly at risk for delayed healing.[60,61,69] The healing process can also be delayed due to infection, immunosuppression, or traumatic damage sustained during activity or in a fall days or weeks after surgery.[69,70] Nutritional status is a significant determinant of wound healing in the early postoperative and preprosthetic period; individuals with compromised nutritional status are more likely to experience delayed wound healing and are at greater risk of postoperative infection and cardiopulmonary and septic complications.[71] When transcutaneous oxygen and carbon dioxide are carefully monitored, persons with minor nonhealing incisional wounds (1 cm × 1 cm) can safely use a pneumatic prosthesis temporarily to preserve/improve mobility and endurance before being fitted with their customized prosthesis.[67,69]

Assessing Circulation

Because so many amputations are associated with the dyad of vascular insufficiency and polyneuropathy, examining and monitoring the vascular status and skin integrity of the remaining (intact) limb and the residual limb is critical. One criterion for determining the level of amputation is the likelihood of healing of the surgical construct.[8,14] Surgeons caring for persons with dysvascular limbs typically determine the status of peripheral circulation using both noninvasive and invasive tests before amputation; however, delayed healing or failure of the suture line to close sometimes occurs even with careful preoperative evaluation. In the days and weeks after amputation surgery, team members watch for signs of vascular compromise that might threaten adequate surgical wound closure. There is an increased risk of mortality in older adults when a secondary, higher-level amputation is warranted, whether due to failed revascularization or disease progression.[61,62,68] In a study of amputees aged 70 and older, the mortality rate after reamputation increased by 4% per year of age.[68]

The remaining limb becomes much more vulnerable to skin and soft tissue damage because of increased biomechanical stress associated with single-limb mobility following amputation surgery.[50,72] Surgeons should attempt to leave a thick muscle flap with ample vascular supply at the end of the stump, as much as 5 cm distal to the bone, to allow sufficient padding.[45] Physical therapists must examine the residual limb using noninvasive strategies to assess the adequacy of blood flow, including skin temperature and turgor, skin color at rest and after a position change, palpation, or auscultation of pedal and popliteal, and/or femoral pulses, segmental blood pressures, and calculation of an ankle-brachial index. A thorough baseline assessment enables the team to identify and respond to any circulatory problems that might develop as rehabilitation continues.

Assessing Range of Motion and Muscle Length

A near-normal range of motion (ROM) in the proximal joints of the residual limb is paramount for effective prosthetic use.[73] Persons with recent limb loss are at risk of developing soft-tissue contracture at the proximal joint to amputation during the preprosthetic period. The risk of hip and knee flexion contracture formation is associated with spending long periods of time sitting in a wheelchair or resting in bed before and after amputation. Other factors that contribute to the risk of flexion contracture formation include the protective flexion withdrawal pattern associated with lower extremity pain, muscle imbalances that result from loss of distal attachments, and the loss of tonic sensory input generated by weight bearing on the sole of the foot.[74,75] Because limitation in the lower extremity ROM can have a significant impact on the quality and energy efficiency of prosthetic gait, it is essential to assess and monitor ROM.[75] Equally important is implementing strategies to prevent or minimize contracture development as early in the postoperative, preprosthetic period as possible.[73,75]

For persons with transtibial amputation, definitive measurement of hip ROM is possible with standard goniometric techniques. With the loss of the malleolus as a distal reference point, accurate measurement of knee extension ROM can be challenging, especially when there is a short residual limb (Fig. 20.6). Familiarity with the normal anatomy of the tibia improves the therapist's positioning of the mobile arm of the goniometer and the accuracy of measurement. For individuals with transtibial and transfemoral amputation, the Thomas test may be an effective tool for determining the severity of hip flexion (Fig. 20.7A–C). Full hip extension is critical for prosthetic knee stability when walking with a transfemoral prosthesis.[73] The accuracy of standard goniometric measurement of hip adduction and abduction decreases as residual limb length decreases. There is no practical way to assess the rotation of the transfemoral residual limb.

Hip flexion ROM limitations will likely result in increased lumbar lordosis when standing and walking with a prosthesis later in rehabilitation. Attempts to achieve an upright posture over the prosthesis in the presence of hip flexion contracture can lead, over time, to excessive mobility of the lumbosacral spine and the development of low back pain when walking with a prosthesis.[76] Individuals with bilateral transtibial amputation and those who wear a transfemoral prosthesis are much at risk for this problem: Secondary spinal dysfunction and low back pain can be more disabling than the original amputation.[73,76] Attention to the importance of achieving near-normal joint ROM and soft-tissue excursion early in the preprosthetic period has a powerful impact on effective prosthetic use long term.

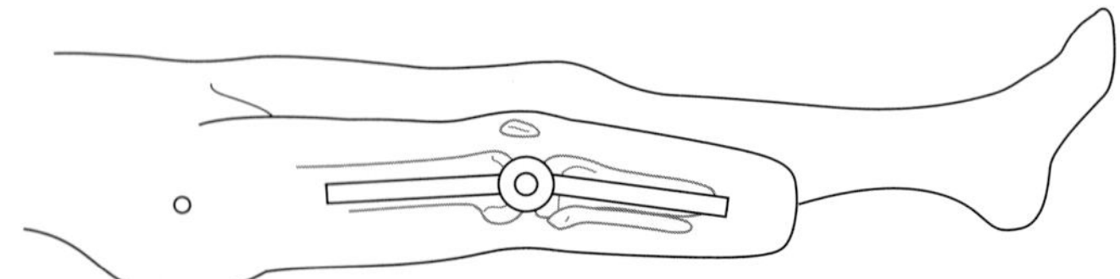

Fig. 20.6 Measurement of knee extension for persons with transtibial amputation requires an understanding of the normal anatomy of the tibia to compensate for loss of the distal malleolus as a point of reference for the mobile arm of the goniometer.

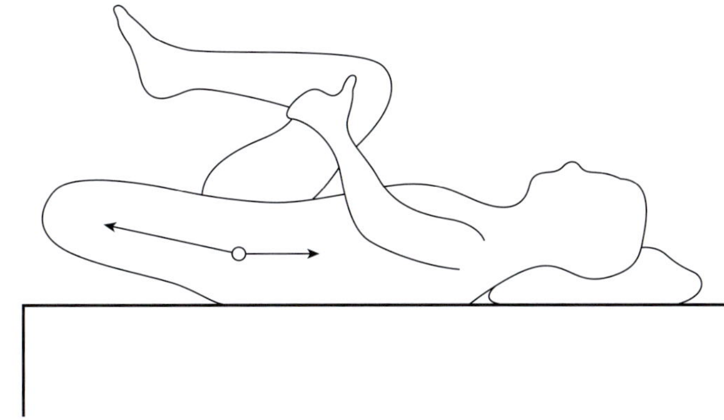

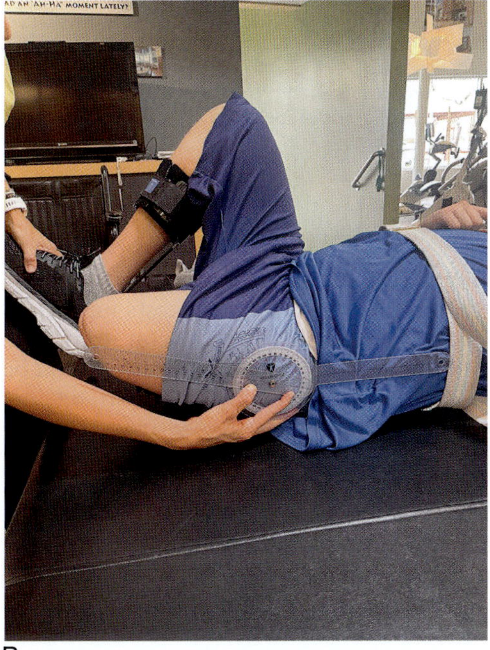

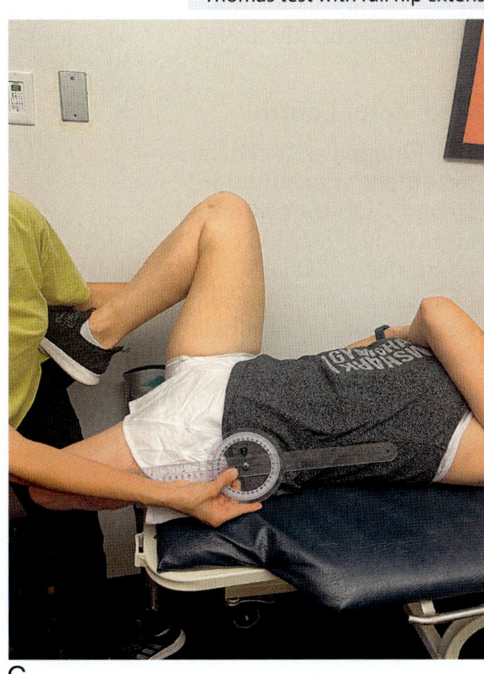

A B C

Fig. 20.7 (A) The Thomas test can be used to assess the tightness or contracture of hip flexors for patients with transtibial and transfemoral residual limbs. The patient is positioned in supine with both limbs flexed toward the chest and the pelvis in slight posterior tilt. While the opposite limb is supported in place, the residual limb is gently lowered toward the support surface. Tightness or contracture of hip flexors causes the pelvis to move into an anterior tilt before the limb is fully lowered. (B) Measuring hip extension of the residual limb using the Thomas test. The patient is unable to achieve full hip extension. (C) Thomas test with full hip extension achieved.

When sitting or lying in bed, the natural tendency is for the lower limb to roll outward into a slightly flexed, abducted, and externally rotated position. Excursion of the hip is important to assess; tightness of external rotators may be masked by apparent tightness of hip flexors or abductors. The functional length of two-joint muscles is also important to consider. Adequate hamstring length is essential if the person with recent transtibial amputation is to maintain a fully extended knee when seated. If the knee is held in extension by a rigid dressing or thermoplastic splint, hamstring tightness will pull the pelvis into a marked posterior tilt. Instead of sitting squarely on the ischial tuberosities, the person with hamstring tightness sits in a kyphotic position with weight shifted onto the sacrum.[73,76] This compromised postural alignment increases the risk of spinal dysfunction, skin irritation, and pressure injury formation. Tightness in the rectus femoris, sartorius, and tensor fascia latae can interfere with advanced mobility skills, such as kneeling while transferring to and from the floor. Even simple mobility skills, such as the ability to transition from sitting to standing to prepare for a transfer, transtibial amputees have demonstrated an asymmetric weight distribution pattern with a tendency to prefer to weight bear over the intact limb.[77,78] The therapist should be aware of the need to incorporate symmetric weight acceptance to both limbs in preparation for higher-level activities such as ambulation.

Assessing Joint Integrity and Mobility

For individuals with transtibial limb loss, the alignment and ligamentous integrity of the knee will be an important determinant of socket design, suspension strategy, and, eventually, the dynamic alignment of the prosthesis. Specific assessment of the joint function of the residual limb is often deferred to later in the preprosthetic period when there has been primary healing of the surgical site; however, history of previous ligament injury or tear of the meniscus and concurrent degenerative joint disease or existing bony deformity (e.g., genu recurvatum, genu valgus, or genu varum) should be noted during the initial assessment.

The special tests used to assess knee function in those with limb loss are the same as those used to evaluate joint integrity in individuals with musculoskeletal dysfunction in intact limbs. They include joint play, medial and lateral gap tests to assess the integrity of the collateral ligaments, anterior and posterior drawer tests to assess cruciate integrity, and various tests for a meniscus tear.[79,80] However, the techniques must be adapted to the length of the residual limb; the loss of the foot means the examiner's distal point of stability is moved upward on the limb, compromising the biomechanical advantage, as well as the accuracy of the examiner. It may be helpful to first examine the knee of the intact limb using traditional hand placement to get a sense of the individual's baseline, then move the distal hand upward on the intact limb and repeat the examination using hand placement appropriate for the residual limb. Comparison of distal and proximal test results of the intact limb provides a frame of reference for subsequently testing the knee of the residual limb.[79,80]

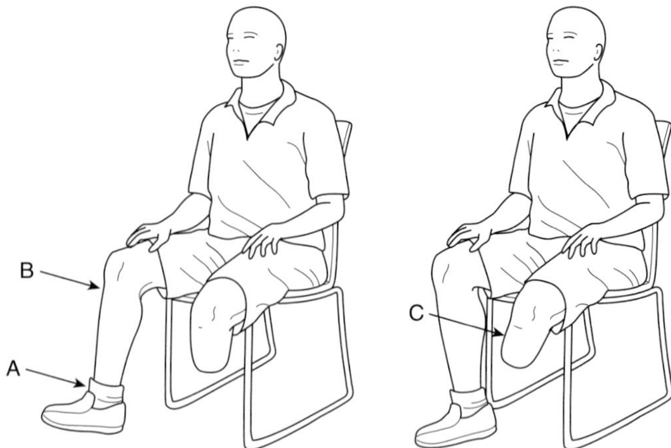

Fig. 20.8 Suggested points of force application to improve accuracy of manual muscle test (MMT) for knee extension strength in a transtibial residual limb. *A*, Standard MMT position on the remaining limb. *B*, Moving the point of force application proximally on the intact limb provides a frame of reference for subsequent testing (*C*) of the residual limb.

Assessing Muscle Performance and Motor Control

Assessment of strength and muscle function is a crucial component of preprosthetic and prosthetic rehabilitation, although definitive strength assessment is postponed until there is adequate healing of the surgical site to protect the new incision from sheer forces. The strength of key muscle groups at the next most proximal joints can be specifically assessed with standard manual muscle testing or handheld dynamometry techniques.[81,82] Given time constraints during the initial assessment, the therapist may opt to use functional antigravity activities to screen for impairments of strength and power of the remaining limb and trunk, specifically testing the strength of particular muscles if functional problems are identified.

For those with transtibial amputation, observation of active knee flexion and extension strength is used to determine if at least a grade of fair (a rating of three out of five) is present until the physician determines sufficient wound healing has been accomplished.[81,82] For those with a transfemoral amputation, assessment of hip muscle strength beyond active antigravity fair muscle grade must also be postponed pending incisional healing.

Definitive strength testing can be implemented once the surgeon and rehabilitation team confirms proper healing of the incision site cannot be compromised by externally applied resistance. Because of the length of the residual limb, the examiner must apply the resistive force at a more proximal position on the extremity than is defined by the standard manual muscle test technique. With an altered manual contact, the mechanical advantage of the examiner is reduced, and the subjective sense of strength grade may be inflated. This modified point of force application affects the validity of test results. Many therapists attempt to maximize validity by first testing the intact or remaining limb (assuming similarity of strength between the patient's limbs), using a standard technique to assign a muscle grade (Fig. 20.8*A*). The intact limb is then retested with a more proximal hand placement, simulating the position for testing of the residual limb (see Fig. 20.8*B*). This grade serves as a point of reference when the residual limb is tested (see Fig. 20.8*C*). For persons with transtibial amputation, the functional strength of hip extensors can be assessed with the individual lying supine, a small bolster or towel roll positioned under the lower thigh of the residual limb, and the intact limb held flexed against the trunk (Fig. 20.9A). The ability to lift the pelvis (bridge) from the supporting surface by pushing downward into the bolster suggests functional hip extensor strength. Functional hip extension strength is tested similarly on the opposite limb. Hip abduction can be tested in a side-lying position (residual limb down) against a bolster, asking the individual to push downward to raise the pelvis off of the supporting surface (see Fig. 20.9A–C). These positions can also be used as strengthening exercises to repeatedly lift body weight in concentric, holding (at the top), and eccentric (controlled lowering) contraction.

Observation of functional activities can identify if there are impairments in these types of muscle functions. More specific testing of power can be accomplished using an isokinetic apparatus set at varying speeds or by asking the person to move at varying speeds against manual resistance.

Assessment of the ability to switch between types of muscle contraction can be accomplished by providing manual resistance while asking the individual to "contract," "hold," and "let go slowly" for key muscle groups. An example of a key functional activity in which this type of control is important is rising from sitting to standing and returning to a seated position. Many persons can generate adequate force in the intact lower extremity to stand up but have difficulty controlling their descent back to sitting—"plopping" back into their seat. This is especially true for individuals who have been inactive or on prolonged bed rest.[83]

If there is any indication of previous or current neuromuscular dysfunction, examination of tone and motor control is also important. Assessment of muscle tone includes deep tendon reflexes (DTRs), response to passive movement of limbs and trunk (hypotonicity or hypertonicity, rigidity), placement and drop tests, coordination and fine motor tests (e.g., rapid alternating movement; fine, quick tapping or clapping), as well as observation of any abnormal synergy pattern, tremors, or involuntary movement.[79,82] Qualitative assessment of the individual's ability to initiate, sustain,

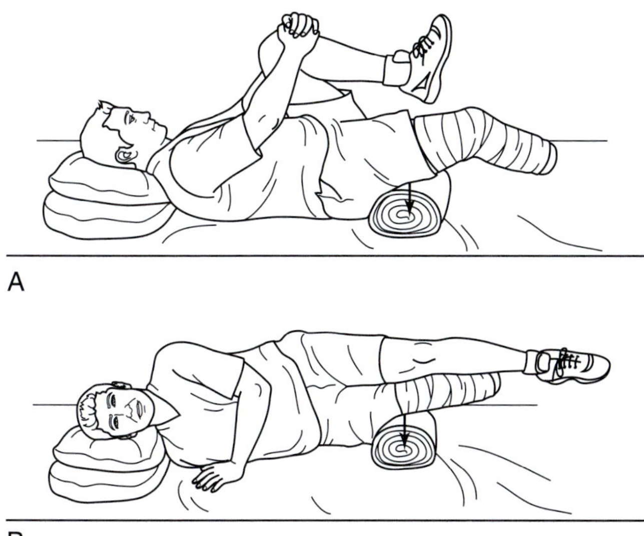

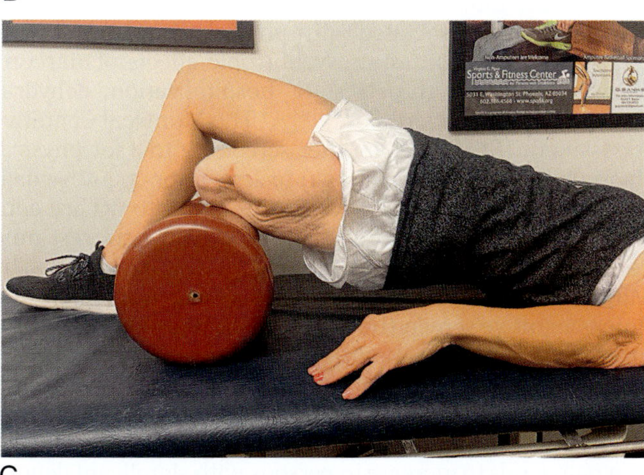

Fig. 20.9 Strategies for functional testing of hip extensor (A) and hip abductor (B) muscle strength following transtibial amputation. A small bolster or firm towel roll is positioned at the distal thigh, and the individual attempts to lift the pelvis from the supporting surface. In persons with transfemoral amputation, these positions can be used once sufficient healing of the surgical construct has occurred. These positions can later be used, with body weight as resistance, for concentric (lifting), isometric (holding), and eccentric (controlled lowering) strengthening exercises. (C) Functional strength testing of the hip extensors for an individual with transfemoral limb loss.

and terminate movement during functional activities will help the therapist identify motor control issues that may need to be addressed as part of the care plan.

Assessing Upper Extremity Function

Following lower-limb amputation, individuals rely heavily on their upper extremities to complete functional mobility tasks such bed mobility, transfers, and wheelchair mobility. It is important to screen for deformity or other musculoskeletal or neuromuscular impairments involving the upper extremity due to the increase in demand of the upper body. Many of those with dysvascular- and neuropathic-related lower extremity amputation have age-related degenerative joint disease that might make use of a wheelchair or an assistive device challenging.[79,82] Screening for functional strength and muscle endurance of muscles that stabilize the shoulder and elbow identifies individuals who would benefit from a progressive resistive exercise program targeting the upper extremity to enhance their ability to transfer and ambulate.[84]

Polyneuropathy, in a "stocking-glove" distribution, is the most common neuromuscular impairment encountered in those with diabetes who have undergone lower extremity amputation. Diabetic polyneuropathy affects all extremities—not only the sensory system, but also the voluntary motor and autonomic systems.[85,86] For this reason, it is important to at least screen for distal upper extremity sensory loss, weakness of intrinsic muscles of the hand, and autonomic impairment (e.g., postural hypotension) during the preprosthetic period. Compromised upper extremity sensation and functional strength may affect the type of assistive device used for mobility, compression strategy for the residual limb, and, eventually, selection of a suspension strategy for the prosthesis.[87,88]

Assessing Aerobic Capacity and Endurance

Determining baseline (resting) vital signs (e.g., pulse, blood pressure, respiratory rate, blood oxygen levels via pulse oximetry) is the first step in assessment of aerobic capacity and endurance. Screening for orthostatic (postural) hypotension is important for any individual who has sustained a period of inactivity and bed rest, especially if the individual is older, is on medications that blunt blood pressure response, or has a history of autonomic dysfunction from a peripheral or systemic pathologic condition.[87,89] Change in vital signs during transfers or early mobility training and the time to return to resting baseline values provide information about responsiveness to exercise. Soon after surgery, anxiety about pain or risk of injury during activities may contribute to a physiologic "fight-or-flight" response, influencing vital signs.[90] A calm and focused demeanor on the part of the therapist, as well as explanation and education about what will happen and the reason for the assessment, can help an individual with recent amputation to better manage fears and concerns.

Ratings of perceived exertion and dyspnea are useful assessment strategies in the postoperative/preprosthetic period, both to assess how the person with new amputation is tolerating increasing activity and to help the individual target an appropriate level of activity.[91,92]

Upper extremity ergometry, single-leg cycling tests, or combined upper- and lower-limb ergometry tests have been used as indexes of aerobic capacity for those who have recently lost a limb if definitive testing is indicated.[92–96]

Given the similarities in etiology and impact of peripheral vascular, cardiovascular, and cerebrovascular disease, many persons with dysvascular amputation are likely to be at risk for, or have even had, heart attack (myocardial infarction [MI]) or brain attack (stroke).[97–99] The rehabilitation team must be alert for early signs and symptoms of cardiac compromise as the person with new amputation begins transfer and single-limb mobility training. Individuals who have had previous cardiac rehabilitation following MI, angioplasty, or coronary artery bypass may better understand the importance of conditioning exercise as part of their preprosthetic program. Assessment of the quality of motor control and tone is imperative if there is a history of stroke.[90]

Assessing Attention and Cognition

Assessing cognitive function in individuals who have undergone limb loss is crucial for several reasons:

1. Rehabilitation Planning: Cognitive function assessment helps in developing an individualized rehabilitation plan for people with limb loss. Understanding the person's cognitive abilities allows healthcare professionals to tailor rehabilitation strategies to their specific needs, ensuring better outcomes and optimizing the use of prosthetic limbs or assistive devices.[82,100–102]
2. Prosthetic Device Use: Using a prosthetic limb effectively requires cognitive skills such as attention, memory, problem-solving, and coordination. Assessing cognitive function helps identify potential challenges and limitations individuals may face when learning to use a prosthetic device. This information enables healthcare providers to provide appropriate support and training to enhance the person's ability to control and adapt to the prosthetic limb.[100–102]
3. Safety Considerations: Cognitive impairments can affect safety during daily activities and mobility for individuals with limb loss. Assessing cognitive function helps identify any deficits that may increase the risk of accidents, falls, or other safety concerns.[100–102] By recognizing these risks, healthcare providers can implement strategies to mitigate them, such as recommending modifications to the environment or providing additional supervision or support.

Dysvascular limb loss refers to limb loss resulting from vascular conditions, such as peripheral arterial disease or diabetes-related complications. Nondysvascular limb loss includes traumatic amputations or those caused by cancer or congenital conditions.

Individuals with dysvascular limb loss, particularly those with diabetes, may be at a higher risk of cognitive impairments. Diabetes-related factors like high blood sugar levels, vascular damage, and the risk of stroke can affect cognitive function. Conditions like diabetic neuropathy and peripheral vascular disease may lead to reduced blood flow to the brain, potentially causing cognitive deficits. While individuals with nondysvascular limb loss may also experience cognitive changes, the risks are generally lower compared to dysvascular limb loss.[103–105] Traumatic limb loss or congenital conditions do not inherently carry the same risk factors for cognitive impairment as vascular diseases.[105] However, traumatic injuries that resulted in limb loss can occasionally be associated with traumatic brain injury (TBI), which can lead to cognitive deficits. It is important to note that the risks and impact on cognitive function can vary widely among individuals, and each case should be assessed individually. Additionally, the presence of other factors, such as age, overall health, and comorbidities, can influence cognitive function in both dysvascular and nondysvascular limb loss cases.[101,103] Therefore a comprehensive assessment by healthcare professionals is essential to determine the specific cognitive function risks and develop appropriate interventions for individuals with limb loss. Because cognitive status is not always linear, several examination measures exist to quantify difficulties with recall, attention, memory, registration, and orientation. They should be administered periodically to identify and monitor cognitive problems. The following examination tools are suggested, though not an exhaustive list.

The Saint Louis University Mental Status (SLUMS) examination is a 30-item screening questionnaire that tests for orientation, memory, attention, and executive functions. The SLUMS is used to detect mild neurocognitive disorder, a condition that often precludes dementia (Fig. 20.10A).[106–109] The norms are dependent on education level. For those with a high school education, scores of 27 to 30 indicate normal cognitive function (25–30 for less than high school education). Dementia is suspected for scores 20 and below for high school graduates and scores 19 and below for less than high school.[106] Other measures of cognitive function include the Mini-Mental State Examination (MMSE), and the SLUMS is comparable to the MMSE and possibly better at detecting mild neurocognitive disorder.[106,107] In older adults, the most common form of cognitive impairment is delirium.[100,101] This temporary and typically reversible problem is associated with physiologic stressors (e.g., clearing from anesthesia, psychotropic effects of narcotic pain medications, the stress of hospitalization, dehydration, onset of infection).[102,104,108,109] The Montreal Cognitive Assessment (MOCA) is another screening tool for physical therapists that has been shown to screen for cognitive deficits better than the MMSE.[107] Scores of 26 to 30 are considered normal, and scores of 25 and below suggest mild cognitive impairment to dementia (see Fig. 20.10B). The Mini-Cog (see Fig. 20.10C1 and C2) is another example of a quick cognitive screen that is useful for identifying the progression of cognitive impairment.

Cognition and the ability to learn may also be compromised by depression associated with mourning the loss of one's limb.[110–112] Perception of acute surgical pain and phantom pain tends to increase in persons with significant depression following amputation and those who view amputation as a catastrophic event.[112,113] Persons whose amputation was traumatic (accident-related, combat-related, or work-related) often must also contend with significant anxiety, anger, or posttraumatic stress disorder and may require psychiatric referral for posttraumatic stress disorder symptoms that hamper rehabilitation.[112,113] Measures commonly used to evaluate depression in the preprosthetic period include the Geriatric Depression Scale, the Beck Depression Inventory, and the Center for Epidemiological Studies Depression Scale.[114,115] Anxiety following amputation can be assessed using the Hospital Anxiety and Depression Scale and the Geriatric Anxiety Inventory.[116–118] Scores indicating moderate-to-high levels of delirium, depression, or anxiety should prompt referral to mental health services for further evaluation and intervention. Participation in rehabilitation often reduces levels of depression and anxiety[115,117]; it can be more informative to track how scores change over a period of time than to interpret a single value. An observational cohort study of 49 adults with nontraumatic lower extremity amputations used the Hospital Anxiety and Depression scale to examine anxiety levels and found higher rates of preoperative anxiety in patients undergoing transtibial amputation compared with transfemoral amputees. When the authors compared below knee amputation (BKA) with above knee amputation groups, a higher level of anxiety was noted in the BKA group, which significantly decreased postoperatively.[104]

VAMC

SLUMS Examination

Questions about this assessment tool? E-mail aging@slu.edu.

Name__________ Age __________

Is patient alert? __________ Level of education __________

Department of Veterans Affairs

Score	Points	Item
__/1	(1)	**1. What day of the week is it?**
__/1	(1)	**2. What is the year?**
__/1	(1)	**3. What state are we in?**
		4. Please remember these five objects. I will ask you what they are later. Apple Pen Tie House Car
		5. You have $100 and you go to the store and buy a dozen apples for $3 and a tricycle for $20.
	(1)	**How much did you spend?**
__/3	(2)	**How much do you have left?**
		6. Please name as many animals as you can in one minute.
__/3		(0) 0-4 animals (1) 5-9 animals (2) 10-14 animals (3) 15+ animals
__/5		**7. What were the five objects I asked you to remember?** 1 point for each one correct.
		8. I am going to give you a series of numbers and I would like you to give them to me backwards. For example, if I say 42, you would say 24.
__/2		(0) 87 (1) 649 (1) 8537
		9. This is a clock face. Please put in the hour markers and the time at ten minutes to eleven o'clock.
	(2)	Hour markers okay
__/4	(2)	Time correct
__/2	(1)	**10. Please place an X in the triangle.**
	(1)	**Which of the above figures is largest?**
		11. I am going to tell you a story. Please listen carefully because afterwards, I'm going to ask you some questions about it. Jill was a very successful stockbroker. She made a lot of money on the stock market. She then met Jack, a devastatingly handsome man. She married him and had three children. They lived in Chicago. She then stopped work and stayed at home to bring up her children. When they were teenagers, she went back to work. She and Jack lived happily ever after.
	(2)	**What was the female's name?**
__/8	(2)	**When did she go back to work?**
	(2)	**What work did she do?**
	(2)	**What state did she live in?**
______		**TOTAL SCORE**

AD MAJOREM DEI GLORIAM · IHS

Department of Veterans Affairs

SAINT LOUIS UNIVERSITY

AGING SUCCESSFULLY

SCORING

HIGH SCHOOL EDUCATION		LESS THAN HIGH SCHOOL EDUCATION
27-30	Normal	25-30
21-26	MNCD*	20-24
1-20	Dementia	1-19

* Mild Neurocognitive Disorder

A

Fig. 20.10 (A) The Saint Louis University Mental Status Examination. (B) The Montreal Cognitive Assessment. (C1 and C2) The Mini Cog. (A, From http://aging.slu.edu/pdfsurveys/mentalstatus.pdf; Tariq SH, Tumosa N, Chibnall JT, Peri III HM, Morley JE. Mild cognitive impairment and dementia is more sensitive than the Mini-mental Status Examination (MMSE)—a pilot study. *J Am Geriatr Psych*. 2006;14:900–910. B, Copyright Nasreddine Z, MD. Copies are available at http://www.mocatest.org/; C1 and C2, Available from https://mini-cog.com/.)

For those with amputation as a result of dysvascular problems, the underlying mechanism for peripheral arterial disease (PAD), cardiovascular disease, and cerebral vascular disease is the same; in population studies, persons with severe PAD tend to have more cognitive impairment than those without PAD.[119–121] There is a positive relationship between level of cognitive resources (e.g., memory, executive function, problem-solving ability), the ability to walk with a prosthesis, and postamputation adjustment and quality of life.[119–121] Cognitive impairment should not preclude postoperative rehabilitation and prosthetic prescription: supervised use of ambulatory assistive devices and, eventually, prostheses may improve safety during self-care and reduce overall caregiver burden.[120]

Assessing Sensory Integrity

Early in the postoperative period, screening of sensory function (vision, hearing, and somatosensation) is aimed at determining if strategies for enhancing communication may be necessary and if the individual has sufficient

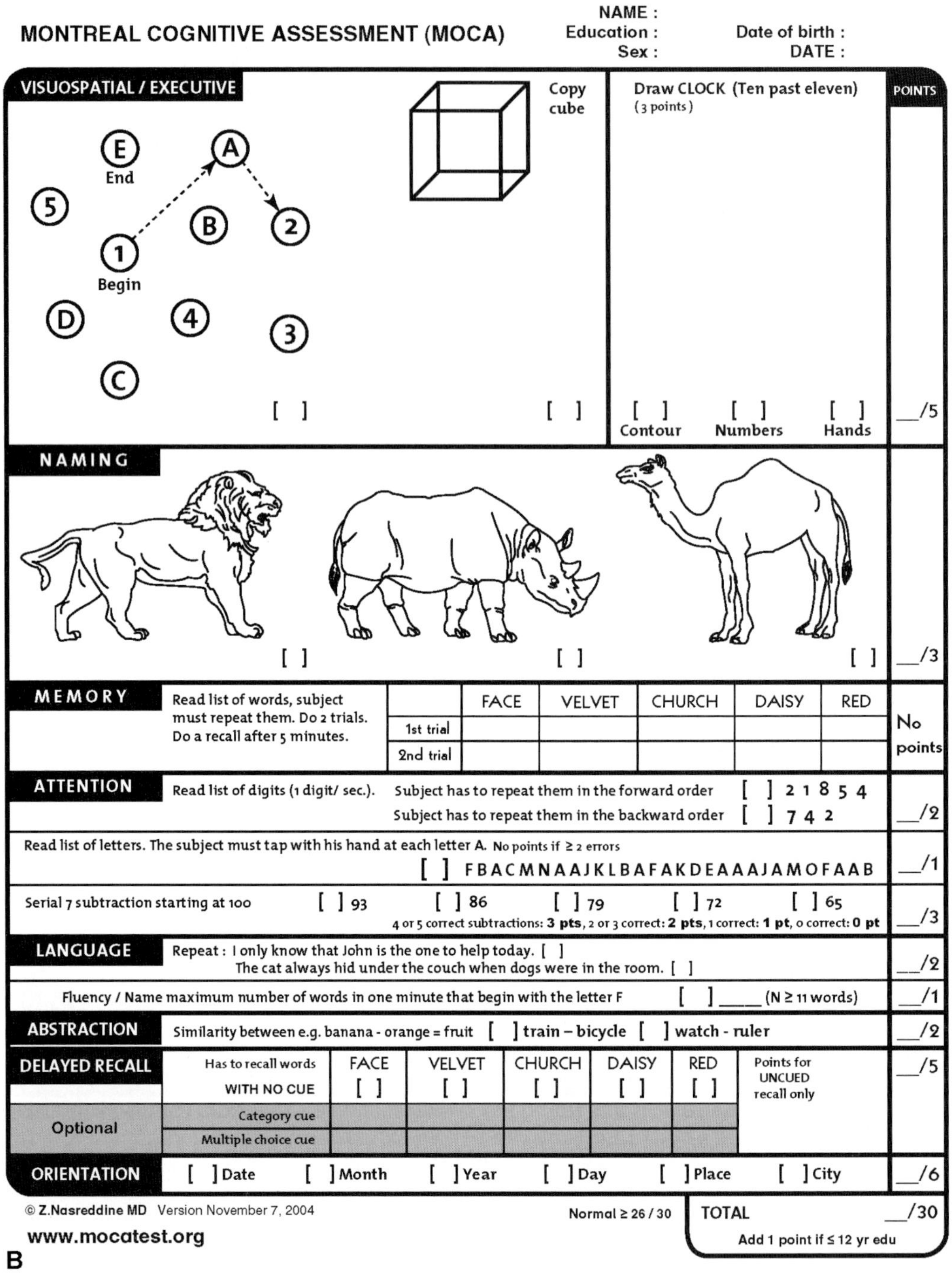

MONTREAL COGNITIVE ASSESSMENT (MOCA)

NAME :
Education :
Sex :
Date of birth :
DATE :

		POINTS
VISUOSPATIAL / EXECUTIVE	E End, A, 5, B, 2, 1 Begin, D, 4, 3, C [ ] — Copy cube [ ] — Draw CLOCK (Ten past eleven) (3 points) [ ] Contour [ ] Numbers [ ] Hands	__/5
NAMING	[ ] [ ] [ ]	__/3

MEMORY	Read list of words, subject must repeat them. Do 2 trials. Do a recall after 5 minutes.		FACE	VELVET	CHURCH	DAISY	RED	No points
		1st trial						
		2nd trial						

		POINTS
ATTENTION	Read list of digits (1 digit/ sec.). Subject has to repeat them in the forward order [ ] 2 1 8 5 4 Subject has to repeat them in the backward order [ ] 7 4 2	__/2
	Read list of letters. The subject must tap with his hand at each letter A. No points if ≥ 2 errors [ ] F B A C M N A A J K L B A F A K D E A A A J A M O F A A B	__/1
	Serial 7 subtraction starting at 100 [ ] 93 [ ] 86 [ ] 79 [ ] 72 [ ] 65 4 or 5 correct subtractions: **3 pts**, 2 or 3 correct: **2 pts**, 1 correct: **1 pt**, 0 correct: **0 pt**	__/3
LANGUAGE	Repeat : I only know that John is the one to help today. [ ] The cat always hid under the couch when dogs were in the room. [ ]	__/2
	Fluency / Name maximum number of words in one minute that begin with the letter F [ ] ____ (N ≥ 11 words)	__/1
ABSTRACTION	Similarity between e.g. banana - orange = fruit [ ] train – bicycle [ ] watch - ruler	__/2

DELAYED RECALL	Has to recall words WITH NO CUE	FACE [ ]	VELVET [ ]	CHURCH [ ]	DAISY [ ]	RED [ ]	Points for UNCUED recall only	__/5
Optional	Category cue							
	Multiple choice cue							

		POINTS
ORIENTATION	[ ] Date [ ] Month [ ] Year [ ] Day [ ] Place [ ] City	__/6

© Z.Nasreddine MD Version November 7, 2004
www.mocatest.org

Normal ≥ 26 / 30 TOTAL __/30
Add 1 point if ≤ 12 yr edu

B

Fig. 20.10, cont'd

"data-collection" mechanisms in place to monitor the surgical wound condition, to inspect the condition of the remaining foot and limb, and to scan the environment in preparation for and during functional activities.[122–125] Sensory integrity is also a factor influencing the selection of prosthetic components and suspension method.

Given the age and common morbidities of those with vascular and neuropathic etiology of amputation, it is quite likely that some degree of visual impairment will be present in this group.[126] If the individual typically wears glasses for daily function, glasses should be worn during the examination and subsequent intervention. Simple strategies to reduce glare, increase contrast (e.g., handgrips on walkers), and enhance acuity (e.g., large, simple, bold type on written instructions) can help those with common age-related visual changes be more functional during the post-operative/preprosthetic period.[126]

Similarly, there are cumulative age-related changes in structure, physiology, and function of the auditory system to be aware of when interacting with older persons with a recent amputation.[127] Attention to the ability to hear and interpret sound is vital when examining persons with

Mini-Cog©

Instructions for Administration & Scoring

ID:__________ Date:______________

Step 1: Three Word Registration

Look directly at person and say, "Please listen carefully. I am going to say three words that I want you to repeat back to me now and try to remember. The words are [select a list of words from the versions below]. Please say them for me now." If the person is unable to repeat the words after three attempts, move on to Step 2 (clock drawing).

The following and other word lists have been used in one or more clinical studies.[1-3] For repeated administrations, use of an alternative word list is recommended.

Version 1	Version 2	Version 3	Version 4	Version 5	Version 6
Banana	Leader	Village	River	Captain	Daughter
Sunrise	Season	Kitchen	Nation	Garden	Heaven
Chair	Table	Baby	Finger	Picture	Mountain

Step 2: Clock Drawing

Say: "Next, I want you to draw a clock for me. First, put in all of the numbers where they go." When that is completed, say: "Now, set the hands to 10 past 11."

Use preprinted circle (see next page) for this exercise. Repeat instructions as needed as this is not a memory test. Move to Step 3 if the clock is not complete within three minutes.

Step 3: Three Word Recall

Ask the person to recall the three words you stated in Step 1. Say: "What were the three words I asked you to remember?" Record the word list version number and the person's answers below.

Word List Version: _______ Person's Answers: ______________ ______________ ______________

Scoring

Word Recall: ______ (0-3 points)	1 point for each word spontaneously recalled without cueing.
Clock Draw: ______ (0 or 2 points)	Normal clock = 2 points. A normal clock has all numbers placed in the correct sequence and approximately correct position (e.g., 12, 3, 6 and 9 are in anchor positions) with no missing or duplicate numbers. Hands are pointing to the 11 and 2 (11:10). Hand length is not scored. Inability or refusal to draw a clock (abnormal) = 0 points.
Total Score: ______ (0-5 points)	Total score = Word Recall score + Clock Draw score. A cut point of <3 on the Mini-Cog™ has been validated for dementia screening, but many individuals with clinically meaningful cognitive impairment will score higher. When greater sensitivity is desired, a cut point of <4 is recommended as it may indicate a need for further evaluation of cognitive status.

C1

Fig. 20.10, cont'd

concurrent confusion caused by postoperative delirium or acquired brain injury after trauma who may also have impaired attention. Simple strategies to enhance the ability to listen and hear include dropping the pitch of the speaking voice; speaking more slowly and projecting the voice without shouting; maintaining direct eye contact; interacting in as quiet an environment as possible; and augmenting what is said with directive gestures, simple diagrams, or brief written instruction in large print.[127] Ensuring that hearing aids are in place and functional is crucial during interviews and for patient/family education. Importantly, hearing aids typically amplify all sound; attention to volume and complexity of background noise must always be considered.

In examining somatosensation, the therapist is screening for areas of diminished sensation and areas of hypersensitivity or dysesthesias on the surface of the residual limb and the remaining limb.[127] For those with a neuropathic-dysvascular disease, it is imperative to ascertain if there is adequate protective sensation (ability to perceive the 5.07 Semmes-Weinstein filament consistently) on weight-bearing surfaces of the intact limb, which will be

Clock Drawing

ID:__________ Date:______________

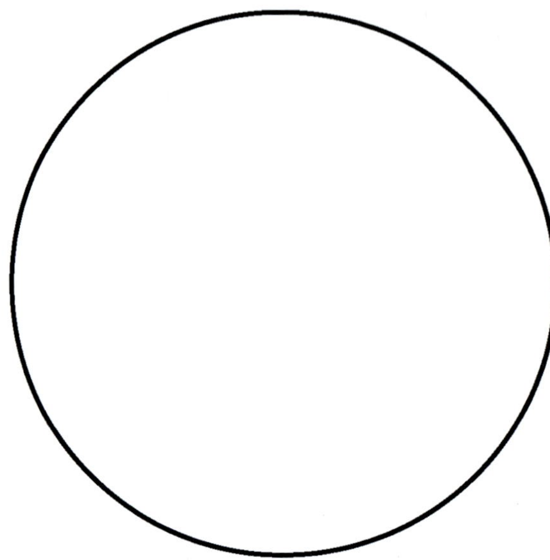

References

1. Borson S, Scanlan JM, Chen PJ et al. The Mini-Cog as a screen for dementia: Validation in a population based sample. J Am Geriatr Soc 2003;51:1451–1454.
2. Borson S, Scanlan JM, Watanabe J et al. Improving identification of cognitive impairment in primary care. Int J Geriatr Psychiatry 2006;21: 349–355.
3. Lessig M, Scanlan J et al. Time that tells: Critical clock-drawing errors for dementia screening. Int Psychogeriatr. 2008 June; 20(3): 459–470.
4. Tsoi K, Chan J et al. Cognitive tests to detect dementia: A systematic review and meta-analysis. JAMA Intern Med. 2015; E1-E9.
5. McCarten J, Anderson P et al. Screening for cognitive impairment in an elderly veteran population: Acceptability and results using different versions of the Mini-Cog. J Am Geriatr Soc 2011; 59: 309-213.
6. McCarten J, Anderson P et al. Finding dementia in primary care: The results of a clinical demonstration project. J Am Geriatr Soc 2012; 60: 210-217.
7. Scanlan J & Borson S. The Mini-Cog: Receiver operating characteristics with the expert and naive raters. Int J Geriatr Psychiatry 2001; 16: 216-222.

v. 01.19.16

C2

Fig. 20.10, cont'd

subject to repeated loading during single-limb ambulation.[127] Standard sensory testing protocols for light touch, point, and generalized pressure (am I touching you? yes/no), the ability to localize (where am I touching you?), and temperature discrimination (hot/cold) are used and often documented on a body chart.[127,128] This information is used to guide patient-family education about skin inspection and wound care, as well as decisions about appropriate socket-limb interface for a prosthetic prescription. Screening for proprioceptive and kinesthetic awareness at intact joints provides information that will be useful when designing interventions for postural control and, eventually, prosthetic gait training.[127–130]

Sensory testing requires that the individual be able to concentrate and focus so as to respond when a stimulus is presented. The reliability of sensory testing is diminished in individuals with confusion or delirium or if the examiner uses a consistent (predictable) pattern or rhythm during testing.[127,130] To minimize the likelihood of "lucky guesses" in those with suspected sensory impairment, it may be helpful to test specific sites multiple times, in random order and variable timing, documenting the number of accurate responses versus the number of times stimulated (e.g., 0/3, 1/3, 2/3, or 3/3) at each testing site.

Noting how the individual with a new amputation perceives the residual limb is also important; is the individual willing to look at the limb, watch it during dressing changes, touch it, or freely move it? One challenge in the preprosthetic period is to assist the incorporation of this "different" limb in the person's body image and self-perception.[16–19,23,130] Some individuals with dysvascular-neuropathic disease continue to perceive their limb as fragile and needing protection. Those with traumatic amputation may become emotionally distressed when confronted with objective evidence of their loss. These situations may interfere with the readiness to wear and use a prosthesis effectively. Awareness of the person's emotional response to their altered body guides the therapist in patient education and intervention activities aimed to accomplish adaptation of body image necessary for effective prosthetic use.

Assessing Mobility, Locomotion, and Balance

An individual with recent amputation may find that simple mobility tasks (rolling over, coming to sitting/returning to supine, transitioning from sitting to standing) are more difficult than anticipated following surgery. With the reduction of body mass that results from lower extremity amputation, for example, the individual's functional center of mass (COM) shifts slightly upward and to the opposite side of the body; the degree of the shift is directly related to the amount of body mass removed during amputation surgery.[131] When this alteration in body mass is paired with deconditioning associated with bed rest, performance of mobility tasks degrades. It is important to document baseline functional status and to discern how much that altered body mass, altered muscle performance, and even fear of pain or of falling may be contributing to difficulty in moving. These alterations in COM may require adaptation of strategies used before surgery for postural control; most persons with recent amputation can effectively adapt their postural control mechanisms by practicing activities that require them to anticipate or respond to postural demands.

One of the most worthwhile aspects of preoperative assessment is determination of the usual (previous) and current (postoperative) ambulatory status of the person with new amputation. The therapist is interested in the individual's familiarity with the use of assistive devices (e.g., walker, crutches, canes); need for assistance to assume standing and while walking; typical distances walked before surgery; the overall effort (energy cost) of walking; the frequency of walking; any other factors or comorbidities that limit walking; and the type of walking environment the person is most likely to encounter after discharge from acute care (e.g., level inside, uneven outside, stairs, and ramps). Self-reports and direct observation of walking provide this information. Preamputation ambulatory status is a very strong predictor of functional postoperative prosthetic use.[132,133]

At this early point in rehabilitation, the priority is safety and the functionality of walking rather than quality and preciseness of the gait pattern. Detailed observational gait analysis is typically deferred until training with the prosthesis begins. Quantitative kinematics (e.g., cadence, gait speed, step, or stride length) and ratings of perceived exertion can be used to establish a baseline early in the postoperative period as a benchmark for progression and readiness for discharge. Individuals with new amputation must be able to use a step-to or swing-through gait pattern with the type of walker or crutches that provides adequate stability and energy efficiency with the least activity restriction.[134,135] Once gait training with the prosthesis begins, the strategies of resisted gait and functional training have been found to be more effective than supervised walking in improving gait performance.[136]

In acute care settings, initial examination and gait training are likely to focus on level, predictable surfaces in a relatively closed environment. The ability to manage on various surfaces in active and open environments is examined as care progresses; discharge from acute care approaches; and preprosthetic rehabilitation continues at home, in subacute settings, or on an outpatient basis. The individual with a recent amputation using an assistive device in single-limb ambulation must be able to walk forward, sideways, and backward, change direction, turn, and manage stairs and inclines to be safe and functional in the home environment. Familiarity with and effectiveness of propulsion and maneuverability of a wheelchair are likely to be important in the preprosthetic period for the individual and family caregivers.

Determining the effectiveness of the individual's postural control is also key. This includes stability in quiet sitting and standing; anticipatory postural adjustments in reaching, in transitions from sitting to standing, and during locomotion; and reactionary postural adjustments when there is unexpected perturbation or unpredictable environmental conditions (e.g., a wet area on the floor, an area rug that may shift when stepped on). Although objective mobility measures such as the Tinetti Performance Oriented Mobility Assessment and Berg Balance Scale are used clinically for persons with a recent amputation, the reliability, validity, and norms for safe or impaired performance are not well documented in the research literature.[137–141] The Functional Reach test is a valid and specific measure of balance for individuals at the final prosthetic phase after lower-limb amputation, and it correlates with the Timed Up and Go (TUG) test.[140] There is evidence of differences in limits of stability between patients with vascular and nonvascular unilateral transtibial amputation (UTA) and patients without amputation. When center of gravity excursion end points were measured across all three groups, the patients with vascular UTA had substantially reduced stability limits compared with patients without amputation and those with nonvascular UTA.[142]

The Amputee Mobility Predictor (AMP) (Fig. 20.11) is a 21-item performance-based outcome measure that can determine preprosthetic and prosthetic balance and mobility capabilities, as well as change over time for preprosthetic and prosthetic rehabilitation.[133,143-145] Minimal detectable change (MDC) for the AMP is reported to be 3.5 points.[146] Providing an opportunity for the individual to assess their capabilities during sitting, standing, and ambulation with or without an assistive device allows the physical therapist to identify physical limitations with balance, postural control, and mobility skills. This also helps the individual to anticipate what mobility will be like while the residual limb heals and while awaiting the prosthesis. There are two

AMPUTEE MOBILITY PREDICTOR ASSESSMENT TOOL – AMPnoPRO

Initial instructions: Testee is seated in a hard chair 40-50cm height with arms. The following maneuvers are tested without the prosthesis. Advise the person of each task or group of tasks prior to performance. Please avoid unnecessary chatter throughout the test and no task should be performed if either the tester or testee is uncertain of a safe outcome. One attempt only per item Maximum of 2 days allowed to complete assessment

The right limb is: □ PF □ TT □ KD □ TF □ HD □ intact The left limb is: □ PF □ TT □ KD □ TF □ HD □ intact

NAME: **ASSESSOR:** **DATE:** **TIME:**

Item			COMMENTS
1.Sitting Balance Sit forward without backrest, with arms folded across chest for 60s.	Cannot sit upright independently for 60s Can sit upright independently for 60s	=0 =1	
2.Sitting reach Reach forwards and grasp the ruler using preferred arm (Tester holds ruler 26cm beyond extended arm midline to the sternum, or against the wall, intact foot midline)	Does not attempt Cannot grasp or required arm support Reaches forward and successfully grasps item	=0 =1 =2	
3.Chair to chair transfer 90° Chair height between 40-50cm , allowed to use aid but no armrests	Cannot do or requires physical assistance Performs task but unsteady or needs contact guarding Performs independently	=0 =1 =2	
4.Arises from chair–single effort Chair height between 40-50cm, tester asks patient to cross arms over chest. If unable, uses arms or assistive device	Unable without physical assistance Able, uses arms/assistive device to help Able without arms	=0 =1 =2	
5.Arises from chair-multiple effort Chair height between 40-50cm, multiple efforts allowed without penalty	Unable without physical assistance Able but requires >1attempts Able to rise in one attempt	=0 =1 =2	
6. Immediate standing Balance(1st 5 secs) Standing on one leg, timing commences at initial hip extension	Unable Able, but requires use of arms for support Able without arm support	=0 =1 =2	
7. Standing balance :30seconds 1st attempt do not use arm support, if unable, may use arm support on 2nd attempt	Unable Able, but requires use of arms for support Able without arm support	=0 =1 =2	
8. (Amypro only)			
9. Standing balance: standing reach Reach forward and grasp the ruler 26cm beyond preferred arm midline to the sternum or against a wall	Unable Able, but requires use of arms for support Able without arm support	=0 =1 =2	
10. Standing balance: nudge test Standing on one leg, tester gently pushes on subjects sternum with palm of hand 3 times (ONLY if safe to do so)	Begins to fall, needs catching catches self using arms for support Steady, toes come up for equilibrium reaction	=0 =1 =2	
11. Standing balance: eyes closed 30sec.	Unsteady or uses arm support Steady without arm support	=0 =1	
12. Standing balance: picking object off the floor Object is placed 30cm in front of patient, midline	Unable Able, but requires use of arms for support Able without arm support	=0 =1 =2	
13. Stand to sit Patient is asked to sit in chair with arms crossed over chest. If unable, allow use of hands	Unable, or falls into chair Able, but uses arms for support Able, without use of arms	=0 =1 =2	
14. Initiation of gait Patient is asked to hop with an aid and observed for hesitancy	Any hesitancy or multiple attempts to start No hesitancy	=0 =1	
15. Hopping 8 meters a) Step length b) Foot clearance (discourage deviations incl. Circumduction, foot sliding or shuffling	a) Does not advances 30cm on each hop Advances minimum of 30cm each hop b) Unable to clear foot without deviations Clears foot on every step	=0 =1 =0 =1	
16. Step continuity	Stopping or discontinuity between hops Hops appear continuous	=0 =1	
17. Turning 180° turn to sit in chair	Unable to turn without physical assistance No assistance, 4 or more hops to turn No assistance, 3 or less hops to turn	=0 =1 =2	
18. Variable cadence Patient is asked to hop 4 meters, and repeat a total of 4 times. Speeds are to vary from slow, fast, fast and then slow (ONLY if safe to do so)	Unable to vary cadence Able to vary cadence, but asymmetrical step lengths used or balance compromised Able without asymmetry or balance compromise	=0 =1 =2	

Fig. 20.11 Items of the Amputee Mobility Predictor scale. (With permission from Amputee Mobility Predictor (AMP, AMPPro or AMPnoPro). Copyright©1999 Advanced Rehabilitation Therapy, Inc. Miami, Florida.)

versions of the AMP: The Amputee Mobility Predictor with a prosthesis (AMPPro) is for people wearing a prosthesis and the Amputee Mobility Predictor without a prosthesis (AMPnoPRO) is used when a prosthesis is not worn. The total AMPPro score ranges from 0 to 47 and on the AMPnoPro from 0 to 43 and can determine a person's appropriate K-Level mobility according to the Medicare Functional Classification Level scale. Only the 21-item AMP and aforementioned scoring range can differentiate K-Level mobility or should be considered an AMP instrument. Higher scores indicate better mobility.[143,144,147] Because the AMP is used for persons with unilateral or bilateral transtibial limb loss, the AMP-Bilateral (AMP-B) was developed for people with bilateral transfemoral or transfemoral-transtibial amputations. The AMP-B has been shown to determine the mobility and functional capabilities of service members with bilateral lower-limb loss. Similar to the AMP, the AMP-B is strongly correlated with the 6-Minute Walk Test.[148] AMP-B scores range from 0 to 47, based on modifications to the original AMP scoring.[148,149]

A self-reported mobility scale, the Prosthetic Limb Users Survey of Mobility (PLUS-M), has been shown to have moderate correlation with AMP scores and TUG test times among people with lower-limb loss.[150] For those individuals with high levels of mobility, the Comprehensive High-Level Activity Mobility Predictor (CHAMP) has been shown to correlate with the 6-Minute Walk Test for service members with lower-limb loss.[151–153]

Assessing Posture, Ergonomics, and Body Mechanics

In assessing symmetry of alignment in sitting and standing, the physical therapist must differentiate between habitual or preferred postures from fixed postures, malalignments, and deformities. This might be accomplished by noting whether a particular postural orientation is maintained during different functional activities and whether the individual with new amputation can change position or alignment when so directed. Quantitative measures to document abnormalities in posture and alignment include comparison with vertical and horizontal using plumb line and grids, goniometry and angle assessment, and passive movement.

Given the typical age group of persons with dysvascular-neuropathic etiology of amputation, there may be kyphosis associated with osteoporosis, especially if there is a history of pathologic compression fractures of the spine.[134,141,142] Assessing the health and function of the lumbar spine in standing and during reaching and lifting activity (including excursion of hamstrings and flexibility of hip flexors and adductors) is important because of the likelihood of developing low back pain with the use of a prosthesis if there is contracture. This is especially true for individuals with a transfemoral or any bilateral amputation level.[154,155] Considering back health early in the preprosthetic program is a health promotion/wellness activity that is a worthwhile investment in time and effort. Over time, persons with amputation are likely to develop osteopenia or osteoporosis of the residual limb; those with transfemoral amputation may be at increased risk of pathologic hip fracture as they age.[155,156]

Assessing Self-Care and Environmental Barriers

In the acute care setting and in many acute rehabilitation centers, the Acute Care Index of Function is used to assess basic mobility, cognitive status and impairment, and activity limitations and can assist the healthcare team to determine discharge location. There are 20 items, scored as the level of assistance required to perform each from unable, dependent, or independent.[157]

In the postacute setting, one option to assess functional outcomes is the Activity Measure for Post-Acute Care (AM-PAC) and the related "6-Clicks" Inpatient Short Form. Based on the World Health Organization's International Classification of Disability and Function model (ICF), the AM-PAC measures the amount of difficulty and assistance required to perform basic mobility, daily activity, and applied cognitive functions. The "6-Clicks" short form is a quick measure to assist in predicting acute care hospital discharge destinations that is compatible with many electronic medical records and the Functional Independence Measure tool.[158]

An individual's ability to transfer to and from the toilet, in and out of the shower or bathtub, and in and out of a car, bus, or subway; to manage stairs, elevators and escalators; and to get up from the floor (in case of a fall) should be examined as the preprosthetic period advances. This is part of the assessment of readiness to return to the home environment or determine the need for continued rehabilitation. The rehabilitation team must also consider the individual's ability to dress, perform self-care and grooming activities, inspect their residual and remaining limbs, and function in typical food preparation roles and other instrumental activities of daily living (IADLs). A brief, preprosthetic instruction in activity of daily living (ADL) performance should be incorporated into the rehabilitation plan.[159]

The team assesses the family caregiver's ability to provide appropriate and adequate assistance at home if the individual needs help or guarding during functional activities. Discussion about what work and leisure activities are important for the individual to resume once home will guide the selection of appropriate adaptive equipment and adaptive movement strategies necessary to carry out important tasks and roles before receiving the prosthesis.

Finally, information about the accessibility of the person's living environment must be gathered to determine whether it is feasible to return home to function on a single limb during the preprosthetic period. The therapist may ask family members to measure doorway widths, determine whether there is adequate space for maneuvering a wheelchair, and consider the need for the installation of ramps to make entering/exiting the home both less effortful and safer.

Monitoring for Postoperative Complications

Many individuals undergoing amputation, whether related to an infected diabetic foot wound, peripheral vascular disease, or traumatic injury, carry a high comorbid burden of illness. Physical therapists must be aware of potentially life-threatening and rehabilitation-delaying complications in the postoperative, preprosthetic period. In-hospital mortality following amputation is estimated to be from 4% to 20%.[160,161] Predictors of mortality during this vulnerable time include significant renal disease, chronic obstructive pulmonary disease and CHF, previous MI or ischemic stroke, liver dysfunction, and age 75 years or older.[162,163] Transfemoral amputation and older age were found to have a higher proportion of early postoperative mortality.[163] Patients who require a blood transfusion during or following surgery tend to have both more postoperative complications and a greater risk of mortality.[164]

There is also a high risk of morbidity during the immediate postoperative period. The stress of surgery may contribute to problematic hyperglycemia and the need for insulin in persons with diabetes, even those who had not previously required insulin.[165] Cardiac complications for persons with diabetes, PAD, and coronary artery disease in the postoperative period include arrhythmia (with the associated risk of cerebral embolism), exacerbation of CHF, and new MI or stroke.[166–169] Bed rest and inactivity are associated with the risk of deep venous thrombosis and associated pulmonary embolism, risk of developing pneumonia, and risk of developing decubitus (pressure) ulcer on the heel of the intact limb or sacrum.[167,168,170] Placement of a catheter for urine collection increases the risk of urinary tract infection.[171] Infection of the surgical wound has been reported to be between 10% and 26% in dysvascular disease and 34% in those with amputation due to trauma.[163,166] Pneumonia, urinary tract infection, or infection of the wound may contribute to the development of sepsis and eventual multisystem organ failure.[166,170,171]

Correlations with higher pain levels and poor social support have been identified in a study of individuals with limb loss who experience complex regional pain syndrome. Careful screening of pain and psychosocial factors can help identify those most at risk.[172]

Case Example 20.1 An 89-Year-Old Female Facing "Elective" Transtibial Amputation for Severe Arterial Occlusive Disease of Her Right Foot

N.H. is a slight but energetic female referred to your interdisciplinary team for preoperative examination and education about the rehabilitation program she will be involved in after her planned transtibial amputation. She stands 5 feet 2 inches tall with slight kyphosis and weighs 101 lb. She rises to standing by scooting to the edge of her wheelchair (used for community mobility), then rocking back and forth several times to build momentum. She tells you that she spends her days reading the *New York Times*, writing to grandchildren and the few long-term friends still alive, cooking (with help to assemble ingredients and take things in and out of the oven), and talking to other "shut-ins" from her church on the phone. N.H. lives in the home of her youngest son, a 67-year-old who has recently undergone quadruple coronary artery bypass grafting and is recovering from an embolic stroke that left him with mild left hemiparesis. Grandchildren and great-grandchildren visit fairly often. According to her chart, N.H. has hypertension controlled by β-blockers, had a mild MI 15 years ago, has never smoked cigarettes, and enjoys a glass of wine with her evening meal. She had lens implants for cataracts bilaterally but still wears glasses to read. Over the past year, claudication has become an increasing problem, making it uncomfortable for her to walk from her bedroom at one end of the ranch-style home to the kitchen and family room at the other. When presented with the choice of revascularization versus amputation, she decided that, in the long run, she would rather take her chances with amputation surgery with spinal anesthesia than bypass graft with general anesthesia. She expresses concern that she is "very out of shape" because her walking has been so limited by ischemic pain. She has a good friend whose husband used a transtibial prosthesis for many years after losing his foot in a lawnmower accident; this has assured her that a prosthesis will allow her adequate mobility and function once she heals after surgery. She tells you she has come through many difficult times during her long life, and although sad at the prospect of losing her leg, she looks forward to being free of claudication pain and anticipates she will muster the determination necessary to get back on her feet.

QUESTIONS TO CONSIDER

- What additional data might you want to gather from the medical record to build your understanding of her current condition and medical prognosis?
- What are the most important questions to ask during your interview with N.H. and her son as you formulate her PT diagnosis and plan of care?
- Given her age and general health status, what additional review of physiologic systems would be important to carry out before surgery? Why have you chosen these systems? How might they affect her ability to participate in rehabilitation?
- What specific tests and measures, at an impairment level, will be important to do during your physical examination? How long do you think the assessment might take? How might you prioritize if your time with N.H. is limited? How reliable are the strategies that you have chosen? How precise does the information you are collecting at this preoperative visit need to be?
- What functional activities would you choose to assess before her surgery? What tests and measures will you use to document her functional status?
- What information would be important for you to share with N.H. and her son about the first few days after her surgery? Before discharge from acute care? During the preprosthetic period until she is ready to be casted for her initial prosthesis?
- Given the limited information currently available to you, what impression or expectations do you have about her postoperative care? How might this be different if she had a medical diagnosis of type 2 diabetes?

Case Example 20.2 A 25-Year-Old Male with Bilateral Traumatic Transtibial Amputations Sustained in a Construction Accident

P.G. is a construction worker that was pinned between the fenders of two vans when the driver of one van put the vehicle in reverse as P.G. was walking between them. He sustained severely comminuted and open midtibia and fibula fractures and significant damage to soft tissue and neurovascular structures. Tourniquets were placed on his limbs by emergency medical technicians responding to the 911 call. In the emergency department, trauma surgeons determined that neither of P.G.'s limbs met the criteria for limb salvage. Because the limbs were contaminated by dirt and debris from the job site, the surgeon performed bilateral open transtibial amputations to allow for frequent wound inspection. P.G. was placed on intravenous antibiotics. Three days after the operation, there is no sign of infection in either limb. Revision and closure of his residual limbs is scheduled for tomorrow, using an equal anterior and posterior flaps closure, leaving approximately 5 inches of residual tibia in length. Adjustable polypropylene, removable semirigid dressings (SRDs) are planned for compression and wound protection postoperatively.

A review of the medical record indicates that P.G. was in generally good health before his injury, although he has been a pack-per-day smoker since the beginning of high school. He was 6 feet 4 inches tall, weighing 210 lb before his injury. His only previous hospitalization was at age 17, for open-reduction, internal fixation of a midshaft right femoral fracture sustained in a motorcycle accident. P.G. has been married for 1 year, and his wife is 7 months pregnant. They live on the third floor of a three-family home in the ethnic city neighborhood where they grew up. Extended family members have kept vigil at the hospital since the accident to support P.G. and his wife. When not working, P.G. is an avid motorcycle rider, competing locally in both speed and distance events. He also participates in an intracity adult basketball league.

Pain management has been via a morphine pump; even with this, P.G. reports typical pain levels of 5 to 6 out of 10, increasing in severity during dressing changes. When you come to discuss his postoperative rehabilitation with him, he is in a semireclined position in bed, with both lower limbs

Case Example 20.2 **A 25-Year-Old Male with Bilateral Traumatic Transtibial Amputations Sustained in a Construction Accident—cont'd**

abducted and externally rotated at the hip, resting in apparent 20 degrees of knee flexion. He is anxious and quite angry over the situation, stating that he "can't believe this has happened" and "doesn't want to end up in a wheelchair" unable to work. The only experience he has with persons with amputation is an uncle with poorly controlled diabetes who had successive amputations of multiple toes as a consequence of vascular insufficiency, subsequently revised to transmetatarsal because of osteomyelitis of a neuropathic wound, and then to transtibial because of delayed healing. P.G.'s uncle's rehabilitation was complicated by a significant stroke a week after transtibial amputation, and although he wears a prosthesis, his mobility limitations keep him homebound.

QUESTIONS TO CONSIDER

- What additional data better understand P.G.'s current condition and medical prognosis?
- What are the most important questions to ask during your interview with P.G. and his family as you begin to formulate his PT diagnosis and plan of care?
- What additional review of physiologic systems would be important to carry out before surgery? Why have you chosen these systems? How might they affect his ability to participate in rehabilitation?
- What specific tests and measures, at an impairment level, will be important to do during your physical examination? How long do you think the assessment might take? How might you prioritize if your time with P.G. is limited? How reliable are the strategies you have chosen? How precise does the information you are collecting at this preoperative visit need to be?
- What functional activities would you choose to assess before his surgery? What tests and measures will you use to document his functional status?
- What information would be important for you to share with P.G. and his family about the first few days after the next surgery? Before discharge from acute care? During the preprosthetic period until he is ready to be casted for his initial prostheses?
- Given the limited information currently available to you, what impression or expectations do you have about his postoperative care? How might P.G.'s care be similar to or different from that of his uncle and the older female in the previous case?

Process of Evaluation, Diagnosis, and Prognosis

Understanding an individual's rehabilitation needs emerges as baseline data are collected and integrated with health professionals' clinical expertise and judgment and evidence from the clinical research literature. As part of the evaluative process, the team weighs factors likely to influence the rehabilitation program and begins to formulate a plan of care to address the individual's specific needs. The team identifies key problems that will need to be addressed, formulates a PT (rehabilitation) movement dysfunction diagnosis, estimates the level of function that will likely be reached and the time and intensity of intervention necessary to achieve it, specifies measurable goals that will be used to judge progression over time, and prioritizes interventions to be carried out as part of the rehabilitation program.

PHYSICAL THERAPY DIAGNOSIS

The PT diagnosis reflects the problems with body structure and function (impairments) and activity (functional limitations) the person with recent amputation encounters due to their surgery and current health status. The PT diagnosis differs from the medical diagnosis in that it focuses on the functional consequences of a condition at the level of the system and, more importantly, at the level of the whole person.[7]

The models used to frame the rehabilitation process have evolved from the process of disablement to a focus on enablement, based on the WHO International Classification of Functioning, Disability and Health (ICF).[173–175] The models provide a way of organizing the information collected in the patient-client interview and examination process to facilitate the development of a PT movement diagnosis, prognosis and goals, and plan of care. The statement of PT diagnosis for the particular individual begins with a prioritized list of activities to be addressed during the episode of care, followed by the contributing impairments of body systems and structures related to or resulting from the individual's constellation of active pathologic conditions and comorbidities. Formulating the PT diagnosis in this way clearly guides establishment of goals and appropriate interventions.

PLAN OF CARE: PROGNOSIS

Forecasting the length of the proposed episode of PT care and the potential for prosthetic replacement and rehabilitation can be challenging. Decisions must be informed by several factors:

1. The overall health, cognitive, and preamputation functional status of the individual;
2. The level of amputation as it affects prosthetic control and the energy cost of walking;
3. The likely contribution of prosthetic use to perform basic and IADLs for the individual or for the caregivers who will be assisting and managing daily function;
4. The resources (financial and instrumental) available to the individual during the entire rehabilitation process; and
5. Knowledge of the typical length of stay for patients with amputation in the setting where care is provided (i.e., acute care, inpatient rehabilitation, subacute care, home care, or outpatient care).

The premorbid factors that predict successful prosthetic use (i.e., rehabilitation potential) include the ability to walk functional distances in the months prior to surgery, the overall level of physical fitness, requiring little assistance in ADLs, and the ability to maintain single-limb stance without assistance.[176–178] Persons of advanced age often require a more extended rehabilitation but eventually become functional prosthetic users. Delayed wound healing (which delays prosthetic fitting), as well as knee and hip flexion contracture, reduce the likelihood of successful prosthetic use.[177,178] A long list of past or chronic illnesses does not predict poor rehabilitation potential: Approximately 75% of persons with amputation are able to return to independent living, managing multiple chronic conditions effectively to become highly functional prosthetic users.[179,180] Premorbid health conditions that make prosthetic use less likely (odds ratio > 2.0) include moderate-to-severe dementia, end-stage renal disease, and advanced coronary artery disease.[180,181] Persons with very low body mass (underweight) may have more difficulty with prosthetic ambulation and functional independence than those who are overweight and obese, given a similar comorbid burden of illness.[181] Hip extensor strength is a powerful contributor to overall function with a prosthesis for persons with both transtibial and transfemoral amputation.[182] Difficulty learning has more of an impact during the postoperative and preprosthetic period than does depression or anxiety.[183] The sooner an individual is fit for a prosthesis and begins rehabilitation following amputation, the more likely the individual will become a functional prosthetic user.[183]

Long-term outcome of function and survivorship following amputation is more difficult to forecast: The relatively high morbidity and mortality for patients with amputation secondary to vascular disease have been well documented.[184–186] Unless there is clear evidence that ambulation will not be possible and that provision of prosthesis will not improve the patient's mobility (e.g., reducing the amount of assistance that is necessary to transfer), prosthetic replacement should and must be considered.

A key component of prognosis is delineation of the frequency, intensity, and duration of the episode of care. In the acute care setting, hospitalization for an uncomplicated amputation may be 4 to 7 days and PT may occur for 30 to 45 minutes, once or twice daily. For frail or chronically ill older adults coping with multiple comorbidities, length of stay often increases to 21 or more days. For individuals with amputation as a result of trauma affecting multiple systems, the period of hospitalization depends on the severity of damage across all systems, so that duration of care may be longer. Postacute care occurs in inpatient rehabilitation settings (approximately 55%); subacute rehabilitation settings (approximately 21%); or by discharge to home with referral for in-home nursing and rehabilitation services (approximately 24%).[187] Discharge location is determined by overall health status and need for care, availability and capacity of family caregivers, the type of rehabilitation settings or care that is available in the area, and insurance and financial considerations. In subacute settings, for those on Medicare, the rehabilitation stay may be for a month or more, and care is much more intense, with PT typically occurring twice daily with an hour or more of PT and occupational therapy planned each day. Care provided at home and in outpatient settings may be somewhat less intense, occurring 3 times a week for an hour or more but is certainly supplemented by an active home program.

PLAN OF CARE: DETERMINING APPROPRIATE GOALS

Goals to be achieved during a particular episode of care are influenced by the setting in which care is provided. Although the overall goal of the preprosthetic period is to prepare the individual for prosthetic fitting and training, the specific goals of the acute care setting may be to achieve primary wound closure, initiate an effective strategy for compression, and achieve supervision or minimal assist in transfers and in locomotion using a wheelchair or ambulatory device on level surfaces during the days or week that the person is hospitalized. In subsequent subacute, home care, and outpatient settings, goals expand to include strengthening of core and key muscle groups; ensuring adequate ROM for prosthetic use; improving cardiovascular fitness; and achieving more advanced ADLs, IADLs, and mobility skills over a longer period of intervention.[188] An effective goal is directly linked to the impairments and functional limitation identified in the PT diagnosis and is stated in measurable terms so that progression can be assessed as postoperative and preprosthetic care continued (Box 20.2).

Box 20.2 Acute Care Goals for Case Example 20.1a

N.H. is an 89-year-old female with a recent transtibial amputation secondary to peripheral arterial disease. By the conclusion of this episode of care (projected 4–5 days), N.H. will be able to do the following:

- Actively participate in the inspection of her surgical wound during dressing changes and of her remaining limb.
- Describe and recognize signs of inflammation, dehiscence, ecchymosis, and infection along her incision site and of inflammation or developing neuropathic or vascular ulceration of her remaining extremity.
- Direct caregivers in properly applying her compressive dressing and removing her rigid dressing.
- Safely perform rolling and bridging activities, without assistance, for adequate bed mobility with perceived exertion of no more than 3 out of 10.
- Demonstrate active contraction into full-knee extension in supine and seated positions.
- Demonstrate understanding of proper stretching and flexibility for knee and hip extension in multiple functional positions.
- Safely rise and return from sitting to standing position from a standard armchair or wheelchair with minimal assistance and occasional verbal cues, with perceived exertion of 4 out of 10.
- Ambulate with contact guard and occasional cues, using a hop-to pattern with a standard walker for 25 feet, with a perceived exertion of 4 out of 10.
- Direct caregivers in assisting her with toilet transfers and clothing management during toileting and other self-care activities.

Case Example 20.2b **Determining a Physical Therapy Diagnosis for P.G. Following Revision of Bilateral Transtibial Amputations**

- You have collected the following information in your chart review, interview, and brief initial examination:
- *Surgery:* Underwent revision and closure of bilateral open amputation 2 days ago (under general anesthesia) with equal anterior and posterior flaps closures; 5.25-inch residual tibia on left, 4.75-inch residual tibia on right. Placed in bulky dressing and Ace wrap for compression, then into bilateral adjustable prefabricated semirigid dressings to hold knees in full extension and protect surgical construct. Moderate serosanguineous drainage noted at first dressing change. Wound edges slightly inflamed consistent with operative trauma. No dehiscence noted. Proximal circumference at joint line 10.25 inches bilaterally, distal circumference (4 inches below) of right residual limb 11.25 inches and of left residual limb 11 inches.
- *Postoperative health:* Elevated temperature postoperatively, with diminished breath sounds in posterior bases of lungs bilaterally. Radiograph suggests early pneumonia. Cough nonproductive.
- *Cognition/affect:* Signs of agitation and distress in recovery room, being mildly sedated for combination of pain relief and calming. Currently lethargic and somewhat distractible, requiring consistent cueing to stay on task during examination.
- *Pain/phantom sensation:* Reports postoperative pain at 7 out of 10 level. Complains of shooting pains in phantom right lower extremity and is distressed by "itchy" toes on phantom left lower extremity. Currently intravenous narcotics every 3 hours for pain management.
- *ROM/muscle length:* Reports "pulling" behind knees when head of bed elevated into long sitting position. Requests time out of semirigid dressing to allow knee flexion and to be more comfortable.
- *Muscle performance/motor control:* Able to actively extend both knees to approximately 10 degrees from full extension; stops because of "pulling" behind knee.
- *Upper extremity function and transfers:* Able to "push up" to lift body weight when assisted to bedside chair, requiring contact guard/minimal assist, using a sliding board to transfer.
- *Aerobic capacity/endurance:* Reports transfer effort 6 out of 10 on perceived exertion scale. Reports dyspnea 5 out of 10 immediately following transfer.
- *Rolls independently:* Able to come to sitting from side-lying with minimal assistance.
- *Postural control:* Maintained static sitting balance on edge of bed 2 minutes. Able to reach forward 7 inches, sideward more than 10 inches bilaterally, reluctant to turn and reach behind because of discomfort. Effective postural responses to mild perturbations forward and backward, moderate perturbations sideways.

QUESTIONS TO CONSIDER

- List all of the active pathologic conditions and comorbidities that will influence P.G.'s postoperative/preprosthetic care.
- List and prioritize the impairments, across physiologic systems and from a psychological perspective, that should be directly addressed or considered in his rehabilitation plan of care.
- List and prioritize the functional limitations that will be addressed during his acute care stay. Suggest additional functional limitations that will be addressed as his rehabilitation progresses at home or at a subacute or rehabilitation facility.
- List and prioritize disabilities that P.G. is likely to be concerned about and that the rehabilitation team will be attempting to minimize over the course of his care.
- Develop a definitive PT diagnosis for P.G. on the basis of the disablement model.
- Develop a rehabilitation prognosis for P.G. and explain or justify your expectations.
- Develop a list of prioritized goals for P.G. for the next 2 weeks in the acute care hospital. Expand these goals as if care would continue after discharge in a rehabilitation center, at home, or on an outpatient basis. What will the frequency, duration, and intensity of his rehabilitation sessions be? How will you judge if he is making progress toward achieving these goals?

Interventions for Persons With Recent Amputation

After limb loss surgery the focus shifts to preparation for prosthetic use.[189] Strategies for control of edema, pain management, and facilitation of wound healing are implemented. The ultimate goal postsurgical is to return the patient to their pre-surgical level of function. A recent study indicates that a majority of patients who undergo transtibial amputation due to diabetic complications report improved quality of life at least 1 year after the surgery.[190] This may be due to decreased pain and improved mobility compared with the previously nonfunctional lower extremity.[191] For persons with dysvascular or diabetes-related amputation, the condition of the remaining foot must be carefully monitored as single-limb mobility training begins.[189,190] Handling of the residual limb during dressing changes and skin inspection, as well as the consistent use of compression devices, helps to desensitize the residual limb, enhancing readiness for prosthetic use. Exercises to strengthen key muscle groups in the residual and remaining limb and to assist effective postural responses are implemented to assist function and prepare for prosthetic gait. Functional training in self-care and transfers begins in the acute care setting and is followed up in home care, subacute, or outpatient settings. The therapist may use a combination of manual therapy, therapeutic exercise, facilitation techniques, physical agents, and mechanical or electrotherapeutic modalities to help manage pain, assist healing, minimize risk of soft-tissue contracture, and enhance mobility. A rigid dressing or temporary socket may be fabricated or adapted to protect the residual limb while it heals.[189,190]

POSTOPERATIVE PAIN MANAGEMENT

Pain is a significant physiologic stressor that affects homeostasis and the patient's ability to concentrate and learn.[191,192]

Pain management after limb loss can be categorized as medical, nonmedical, or surgical treatments. Nonmedical and nonsurgical management is the preferred treatment amongst healthcare providers.[189,192] Patient characteristics and past medical history are typically what drive treatment decisions. In the early postoperative period, persons with recent amputation are faced with learning how to care for their new residual limb, including monitoring for signs of infection, using strategies to control edema, and appropriate positioning to minimize the risk of contracture formation. They must also learn a variety of new motor skills including exercises to preserve strength and ROM and how to protect their healing suture during functional mobility. If postoperative discomfort and pain are kept to a minimum, they can better learn and retain these new cognitive and motor skills. Similarly, preoperative anxiety and depression have been shown to influence pain intensity postoperatively, as well as chronic postamputation pain.[192] Healthcare professionals should be aware of these factors when designing a plan of care.

Pain can also be fatiguing and demoralizing; those with significant pain may be reluctant to participate fully in active rehabilitation programs because they fear that movement will only increase their pain. Individuals with significant pain may be erroneously labeled as unmotivated or uncooperative when their primary goal is to find a way to escape their discomfort. Importantly, although certain types of pain medications (opioid and narcotic analgesics) are effective in providing relief, they may compromise cognitive function or increase the risk of postural hypotension.[40] Therapists must be aware of the actions and side effects of the pain medication being used.

In the days immediately after amputation the goal is to minimize the intensity of acute postoperative pain. Prevention of pain is more effective than reduction of pain, thus those with recent limb loss are encouraged to request pain medication before pain becomes severe.[41] Effective management of postoperative edema is an important element in the control of postoperative pain as well.

MEDICAL TREATMENT FOR POSTOPERATIVE AND PHANTOM LIMB PAIN

A variety of pharmacologic and nonpharmacologic interventions have been used for individuals with significant phantom limb sensation or pain, although management of phantom pain is often challenging and frustrating.[193] Table 20.3 summarizes the results of a 2016 Cochrane Review focused on efficacy of pharmacologic management of phantom limb pain.[193] Current best evidence is, at best, limited as a result of differences in study methodology and design, insufficient control groups, and acuity/chronicity of the pain. Readers are encouraged to follow developing evidence from future randomized controlled trials of pharmacologic agents in the management of phantom limb pain. One strategy designed to impact development of phantom limb pain in the postoperative period is continuous analgesic infusion to control the severity of phantom limb pain in the immediate postoperative period; the success of this intervention varies with pharmacologic agents and the rate of their administration.[193–196] Pulse radiofrequency ablation[197] and botulinum toxin type A injection[198] show promise as possible interventions for severe longstanding phantom limb pain that has not been responsive to more conservative approaches. Sympathetic blocks appear to reduce pain intensity over the short term (up to 1 week) but not over the long term (up to 8 weeks).[199] Implantation of spinal cord stimulators has been explored for persons with severe, intractable phantom limb pain; however, results appear to be equivocal and complications of the implantation worrisome.[200] A variety of medications (e.g., amitriptyline, tramadol, carbamazepine, ketamine, morphine) can be used if phantom pain is disabling; however, efficacy appears to be low. Recent studies of ketamine for phantom pain indicate its effectiveness for acute and chronic postsurgical pain.[201,202] Use of epidural anesthesia during surgery and/or perineural infusion of local anesthetic for several days following surgery may help reduce phantom pain development.[203] Although many models or theories for phantom limb sensation and phantom pain have been proposed, the neurophysiologic mechanism underlying this phenomenon is not well understood.[204]

Physical Therapy for Postoperative and Phantom Pain (nonmedical, physical therapy treatment for postoperative and phantom pain)

The success of early rehabilitation is influenced by the effectiveness of postoperative pain management; for this reason, physical therapists must be aware of medications being used and be involved in assessing the effectiveness of the pain management strategy and its impact on patient learning and function. When epidural anesthesia has been used during surgery or in the immediate postoperative period, it is imperative that the patient's cognitive, autonomic, sensory, and motor function is carefully evaluated before transfer training and single-limb mobility activities are started. In whatever setting PT care is provided, it is important that administration of medications be timed so that pain control is optimal during PT activities. If the patient is experiencing phantom sensation or pain, the physical therapist plays an important role in educating the patient and family about these sensations. Due to the cortical component associated with phantom limb pain, psychological treatment alternatives such as relaxation techniques, guided imagery, hypnosis, biofeedback, or virtual reality activities may be effective adjuncts for pharmacologic interventions aimed at pain reduction.[34,205–208]

Transcutaneous electrical nerve stimulation (TENS) is speculated to be an effective adjunct for pain management by increasing blood flow, reducing muscle spasms, and blocking nociceptor neurons in the spinal cord. TENS may also play a role in the management of troubling phantom sensation in the immediate postoperative period; however, its efficacy in the prevention or management of phantom limb pain over time is not well supported in the clinical research literature.[34,208] There is limited evidence for the use of TENS to reduce phantom limb pain using low-frequency and high-intensity settings, although more studies are needed.[209]

Additional PT interventions that have been used to manage postoperative pain include mechanical stimulation (e.g., massage, vibration, percussion) and superficial heat (e.g., ultrasound, hot packs, cryotherapy) or cold; although

Table 20.3 Application of the WHO International Classification of Functioning, Disability and Health (ICF) Model, Completed Postoperatively, for Case Example 20.1a: N.H., an 89-Year-Old Female, Following Elective Transtibial Amputation Secondary to Severe Peripheral Arterial Disease

	Overall Health Status	Body Structure and Function (Physiological Systems)	Activity (Overall Functional Status)	Participation (Ability to Engage in Social Roles)	Buffers or Confounding Factors
Resources (preoperative)	Effective management of chronic conditions prior to surgery Intact cognitive status and effective executive function preoperatively Self-rated health "good" other than claudication	Effective vision and hearing Effective communication Highly motivated: determined to eventually return to own home	Previous use of walker and wheelchair Able to ambulate independently with assistive device functional (in home) distances Self-selected walking speed 0.85 m/s preoperatively Independent in self-care (toileting, bathing with tub seat and handheld shower, dressing) Independent in stair management, step up to step pattern, with rail	Active and engaged in community (church) Able to manage food preparation and cleanup with minimal assistance	Knowledge of successful prosthetic use by friend Understanding of the rehabilitation process: previous participation in cardiac rehabilitation Lives in one-story home, with ramp at entry Significant emotional and instrumental support available by a number of family caregivers
Active problems (examination findings)	Medical diagnosis: Peripheral arterial disease with critical limb ischemia Status post right transtibial amputation, posterior flap (2/15/12) Removable rigid dressing 2″ square ecchymosis suture line Moderate amount of serosanguineous drainage at mid suture line Postoperative pain (morphine pump) Comorbid conditions Hypertension (β-blockers) Status post MI (1997) Cataract (lens implants 6/12/07) Recent fall in hospital bathroom (2/17/12) Mild postoperative delirium with sundown syndrome Stress incontinence Possible osteoporosis Possible sarcopenia	Postoperative pain (4/10 VAS) Phantom sensation (cramping) Potential for delayed healing because of injury to surgical site sustained in fall Postoperative edema Limited excursion right knee flexion and hip extension ROM Less than 3/5 muscle strength right knee extension, hip abduction, hip extension Diminished functional core and upper extremity muscle strength Limited muscular endurance Limited cardiovascular endurance Limited short-term memory and distractibility (MMSE preoperation 28/30, postoperation 18/30) Hypersensitivity to touch and pressure bordering suture line Inadequate protective sensation left forefoot Impaired postural control in single-limb support (static and dynamic)	Difficulty with transitions Effortful but functional rolling side to side Minimal assistance to shift upward in bed (difficulty sustaining "bridge" position) Minimal assistance supine to/from sitting with directional cueing Moderate assistance sit to stand, with directional cueing Maximal assistance stand to sit with poor eccentric control upper extremity and left lower extremity Inability to ambulate functionally Moderate assist of 1, hop-to pattern in parallel bars, requires consistent cueing Step length 6 inches, perceived exertion 7/10, distance 10 ft Diminished exercise and activity tolerance Difficulty with toileting, dressing, and other self-care activities Quickly becomes frustrated and agitated when encounters difficulty with mobility and self-care tasks Possible difficulty with carryover of new learning from session to session until delirium clears Difficulty self-monitoring status of residual limb and remaining limb	Inability to function in typical premorbid roles in interactions with family at home Inability to function in premorbid roles in interactions with members of her communities (church, friends, extended family)	Left lower extremity claudication may limit activity

Physical Therapy Diagnosis: N.H. has difficulty with functional activity (mobility and transfers, ambulation, and self-care activities) secondary to postoperative dysfunction of body structure and systems (transient cognitive impairment, pain, impaired muscle strength and motor control, diminished endurance, limited range of motion of at key lower extremity joints, impaired postural control) related to recent transtibial amputation, postoperative delirium, and various comorbidities.

MI, Myocardial infarction; *MMSE*, Mini Mental Status Exam; *ROM*, range of motion; *VAS*, visual analog scale.

there are clinical reports of short-term pain relief, there are few studies that have carefully evaluated their efficacy.[210] For any PT intervention in the postoperative/preprosthetic period, it is imperative to pay careful attention to the healing status of the wound: wound closure must not be compromised by any intervention that is aimed at reducing discomfort or pain.

Energy-based medicine therapies (e.g., mind-body connection approaches, therapeutic touch, eye-movement reprocessing and desensitization, motor imagery) may be alternative approaches to the management of acute and chronic phantom limb pain, although there are few well-designed and well-controlled studies of their efficacy.[211,212] Mirror box therapy is being investigated as a strategy to minimize the development and severity of phantom pain after amputation.[205,213–215] This approach attempts to facilitate cortical reorganization by accessing the mirror motor and sensory neuron systems and prefrontal cortex in the brain.[216] In the most commonly used paradigm, persons with amputation attempted to move their "missing" limb while simultaneously moving and observing reflected image of the movement of the intact limb.[217] The degree of severity of phantom limb pain has been shown to positively correlate with the onset of relief, with the lowest levels of pain experiencing relief in the fewest number of sessions and the highest pain levels requiring the most amount of sessions before relief.[218] Although preliminary evidence suggests that mirror box therapy may be helpful, more carefully designed and controlled studies are necessary before it can be widely adopted for clinical use. Mirror therapy is not without adverse effects: Some individuals experience dizziness and disorientation, sense irritation in their residual limb, or do not tolerate the intervention, especially if mirror therapy is concurrent with traditional prosthetic training.[219] Still, despite all of the various forms of treatment for phantom limb pain, there appears to be no first-line treatment, indicating a need for further study.

LIMB VOLUME, SHAPING, AND POSTOPERATIVE EDEMA

The management of postoperative edema is important for four reasons: Edema control strategies are essential components of pain control, enhance wound healing, protect the incision during functional activity, and assist preparation for prosthetic replacement by shaping and desensitizing the residual limb.[7] A variety of postsurgical dressing and edema control strategies are available. These include soft dressings with or without Ace wrap compression, SRDs, various removable rigid dressings (RRDs) applied over soft dressings, or the application of a rigid cast dressing in the operating room.[220–222] An IPOP or EPOP is a rigid dressing with an attachment for a pylon and prosthetic foot.[223] Pneumatic IPOP/EPOP options are also available for early ambulation. Each option contributes to pain control, wound healing and protection, and preparation for prosthetic use in a significantly different way. The choice of strategy is determined by the etiology and level of amputation, the condition of the skin, the medical and functional status of the patient, access to prosthetic consultation and care, the preference and experience of the surgeon, and established institutional protocol. Table 20.4 compares characteristics of the most commonly used postoperative/preprosthetic options.

Soft Dressings and Compression

The traditional postoperative edema control and wound management strategy is a soft dressing with or without compression wrap. A nonadherent dressing is placed over

Table 20.4 Results of a Cochrane Review of Prescription Medications Used in the Management of Moderate-to-Severe Phantom Limb Pain and Their Side Effects

Medication	Class	Primary and Secondary Outcomes[a]	Adverse Effects Reported
Oral or IV morphine	Opioid	Short-term decrease in pain intensity Better sleep No impact on mood Satisfaction higher in oral versus IV	Sedation, fatigue, dizziness/vertigo, constipation, sweating, difficulty voiding, itching, respiratory depression
Ketamine or dextromethorphan	NMDA receptor antagonists	Short-term decrease in pain intensity Better sleep Better sense of well-being No impact on functional status	Sedation, hallucinations, loss of consciousness, hearing impairment, balance problems, insobriety
Gabapentin	Anticonvulsant	Trend toward short-term decrease in pain intensity No impact on mood No impact on functional status No impact on sleep	Somnolence, dizziness, headache, nausea
Amitriptyline	Tricyclic antidepressant	No impact on pain intensity No impact on mood No impact on functional status Negative impact on sleep	Dry mouth, drowsiness, blurred vision, dizziness, constipation, altered sleep, nausea/vomiting/diarrhea, tinnitus, urinary retention
Calcitonin infusion	Polypeptide hormone	Trend toward decreased intensity and frequency of phantom limb pain in persons with recent amputation	Facial flushing, nausea, sedation, dizziness
Lidocaine; bupivacaine	Anesthetics	No different than morphine	Stinging sensation at injection site

[a]Primary outcomes: change in phantom limb pain intensity; possible secondary outcomes: changes in mood (depression), functional status, quality of sleep, patient satisfaction with intervention, severity of adverse effects.
Adapted from Alviar MJ, Hale T, Dungca M. Pharmacologic interventions for treating phantom limb pain. *Cochrane Database Syst Rev*. 2016;10(10):CD006380.
NMDA, *N*-methyl-D-aspartate.

the suture line, sterile absorbent gauze fluff is then placed over this, and one or more rolls of gauze is loosely overwrapped in a figure-eight pattern around the residual limb. A compressive Ace bandage wrap may then be used in an effort to control some of the postsurgical edema and assist in shaping the residual limb. The use of Ace bandages is still the most frequently used immediate postsurgical option due to the cost effectiveness but limiting postsurgical edema is poor. Although this method continues to be the most frequently used immediate postsurgical option for patients with limb loss or when significant wound drainage and a high risk of infection are present, soft dressings with Ace wraps are ineffective for limiting postoperative edema.[221,222,224] Soft dressings cannot protect a healing incision from bumps, bruising, or shearing during activity or from fall-related injury. The other practical disadvantage of elastic Ace bandage compression of the residual limb is the need for frequent reapplication: Movement during daily activities quickly loosens the bandages, compromising the effectiveness of the compression. Most rehabilitation professionals suggest that Ace bandages should be removed and reapplied every 4 to 6 hours and should never be kept in place for more than 12 hours without rebandaging.[224]

Effective application of an Ace wrap requires practice, manual dexterity, and attention to details if the desired distal-to-proximal pressure gradient is to be achieved (Figs. 20.12 and 20.13).[74,224,225] It may be difficult for patients with limited vision, arthritis of the hands and wrist, limited trunk mobility, or compromised postural control to master this technique for independence in control of edema. Nurses, residents, surgeons, therapists, prosthetists, and family members (and anyone else who may be taking down the soft dressing to care for the wound) must be consistent and effective in reapplication of the Ace bandage if maximal control of edema is to be achieved. Ineffectively applied elastic wraps can lead to a bulbous, poorly shaped residual limb, which is likely to delay prosthetic fitting.[225] Tight circumferential wrapping can significantly compromise blood flow, compromising healing of the incision and even leading to skin breakdown.[225]

Some patients with bulbous or pressure-sensitive residual limbs do not tolerate Ace wrap for compressions. An alternative to these patients, as well as for those with limited dexterity, is application of an elasticized stockinet or Tubigrip sock (Seton Health Care Group TLC, Oldham, England). Both materials are available with various levels of elasticity; minimal to significant compression can be achieved, depending on the patient's tolerance of pressure. The double-layer method starts with careful application of a long piece of elastic stockinette or Tubigrip over the transtibial residual limb to midthigh level (Fig. 20.14). The remaining length of elastic stockinette or Tubigrip is turned or twisted 180 degrees (to minimize pressure over the new incision) and rolled over the residual limb as a second layer of compression. As residual limb volume decreases and the limb becomes more pressure tolerant, a stockinette or Tubigrip with progressively narrower diameters is used to increase compressive forces and assist limb shrinkage and maturation. These materials are relatively inexpensive, but they are not as durable as commercially available elastic shrinker socks.[221,224]

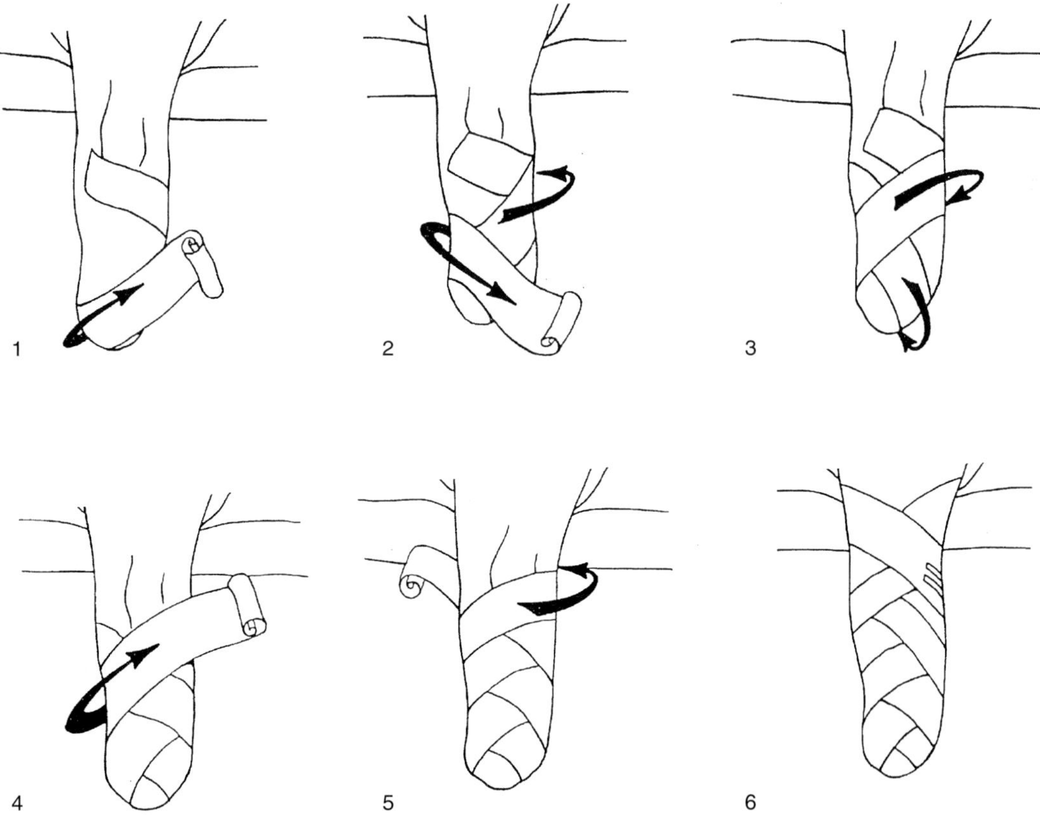

Fig. 20.12 The application of an effective Ace wrap to a transtibial residual limb uses successive diagonal figure-eight loops between the distal residual limb and thigh to create a distal-to-proximal pressure gradient. This creates a distal-to-proximal, tapering, cylindrical residual limb with minimal excess distal soft tissue. (Modified from Karacollof LA, Hammersley CS, Schneider FJ. *Lower Extremity Amputation*. Aspen; 1992:16–17.)

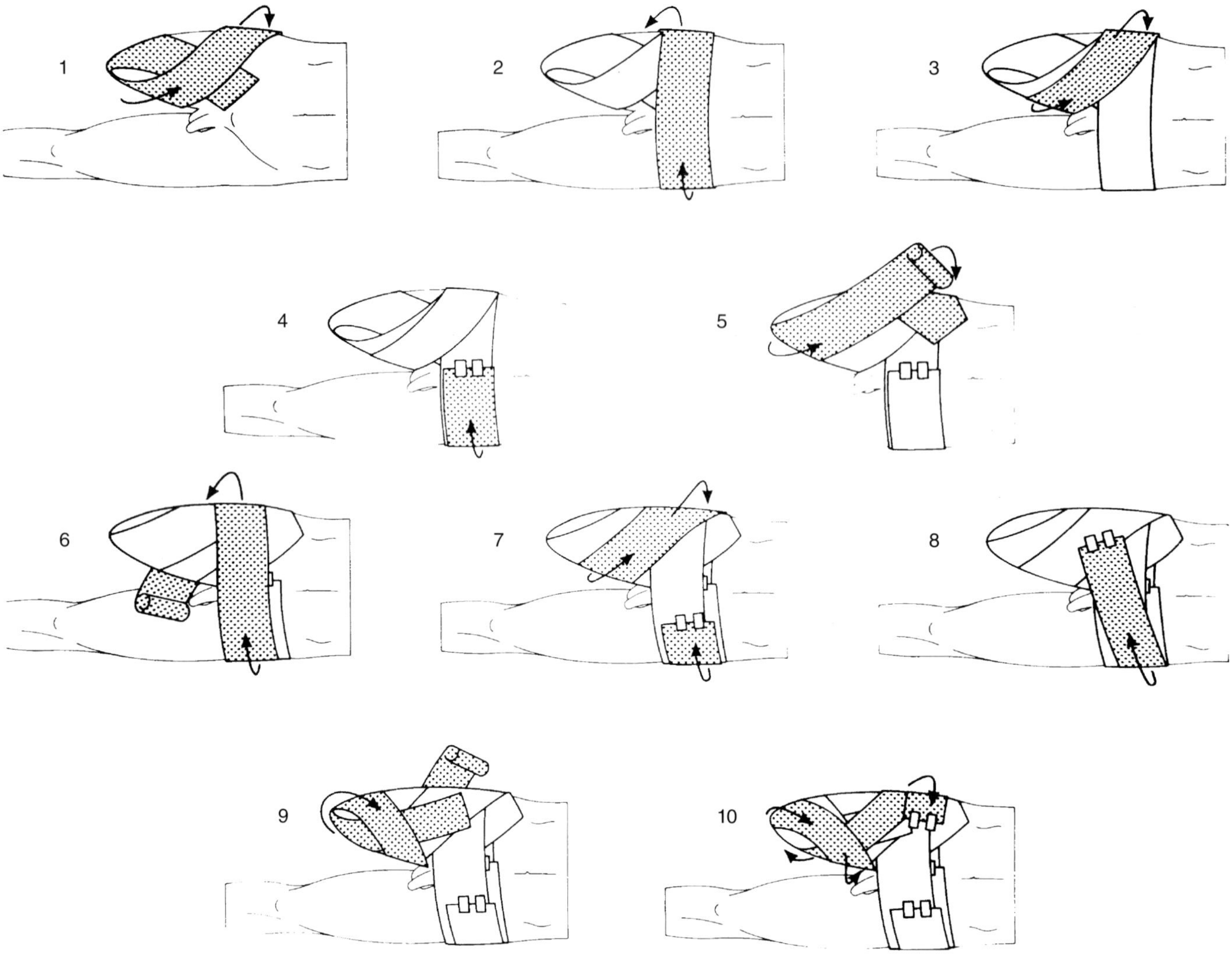

Fig. 20.13 The application of an effective Ace wrap to a transfemoral limb also strives to create a distal-to-proximal pressure gradient using a modified figure-eight pattern. For patients with transfemoral amputation, the wrap is anchored around the pelvis and applied to pull the hip toward hip extension and adduction. Note the importance of capturing soft tissue high in the groin within the Ace wrap to reduce the risk of developing an adductor roll of noncompressed soft tissue. (From May BJ. *Amputation and Prosthetics: A Case Study Approach*. F. A. Davis; 1996:84.)

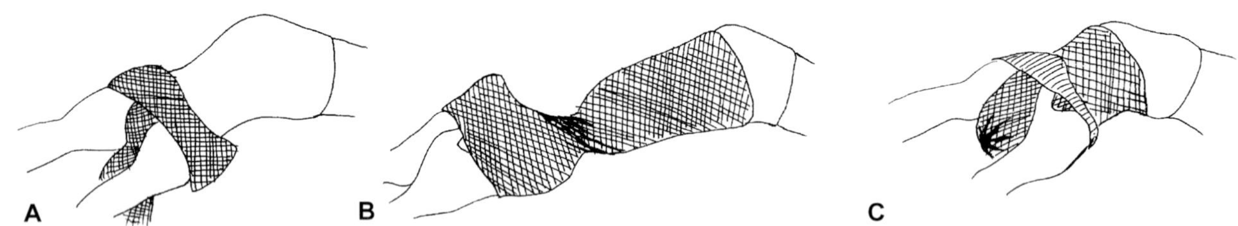

Fig. 20.14 One strategy to control edema and manage limb volume is to use a double layer of an elastic stockinet or Tubigrip to apply compressive forces to the limb. After the initial layer (A) has been smoothly applied, the stockinet is twisted closed (B) at the end of the limb, and the excess is applied (C) as a second layer of compression.

Pressure Garments: "Shrinkers"

Once the suture line has healed sufficiently, many prosthetists and therapists recommend the use of a commercially manufactured elasticized "shrinker" pressure garment whenever the prosthesis is not being worn (Fig. 20.15A and B).[3,225,226] These garments are designed to apply significant distal-to-proximal graded compressive force to the residual limb. Due to graded compressive forces, individuals with limited manual dexterity or upper extremity strength may have difficulty donning and doffing the shrinkers. Patients with recent amputation must be careful to minimize or avoid excessive shear forces over the incision as the shrinker is being applied. Although shrinkers are effective for control of edema and limb volume, it is not possible to create "relief" for bony prominences or pressure-vulnerable areas

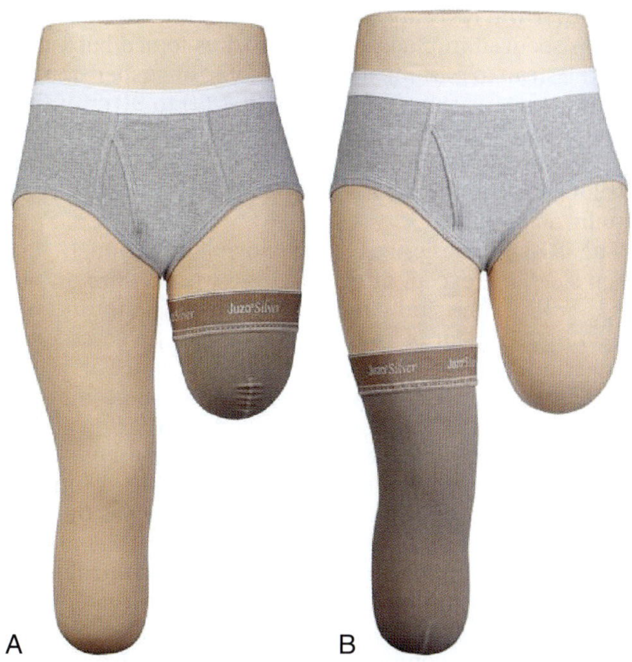

Fig. 20.15 Examples of commercially available transfemoral (A) and transtibial shrinkers (B) used for edema control and shaping of the residual limb. (From www.juzo.com.)

on the residual limb. As with other soft dressings, commercial shrinkers cannot protect the residual limb from trauma during daily activities or in the event of a fall. It is not unusual for patients to continue to use a shrinker for limb volume control, whenever they are not wearing their prosthesis, for 6 months to a year after amputation.[3]

Although a number of edema control options are available for persons with transtibial amputation, those with transfemoral residual limbs have fewer strategies from which to choose. Commercially manufactured shrinkers are more convenient to don and are more likely to remain in place than the more cumbersome Ace wraps, but those who choose this option must be just as careful to capture all the soft tissue high in the groin within the shrinker to avoid the development of an adductor roll, redundant tissue that may make prosthetic fitting more challenging. Another alternative for those with transfemoral amputation is a custom-fit Jobst pressure garment. Jobst garments can be fabricated either as a half-pant or full-pant garment; the full-pant garment achieves more consistent suspension and compression, especially for patients who are obese. A Jobst garment may be the only effective alternative for patients with short transfemoral amputation.

Because shrinkers, Tubigrip, and prosthetic socks worn over a healing residual limb are permeable, they absorb perspiration from the skin of the residual limb, as well as any drainage from the suture line. For this reason, they must be laundered daily in warm water and a mild soap. Cotton, wool, or elasticized materials do not tolerate the heat and turbulence of a clothes dryer; most prosthetists recommend that shrinkers and socks be smoothed out on a flat surface to dry. The person wearing the garment must have a sufficient number available to apply compression around the clock. In addition, sock changes are less frequent during the weekdays than on the weekends, and use of a daily "sock log" may help to facilitate proper sock use for volume management and comfort.[226]

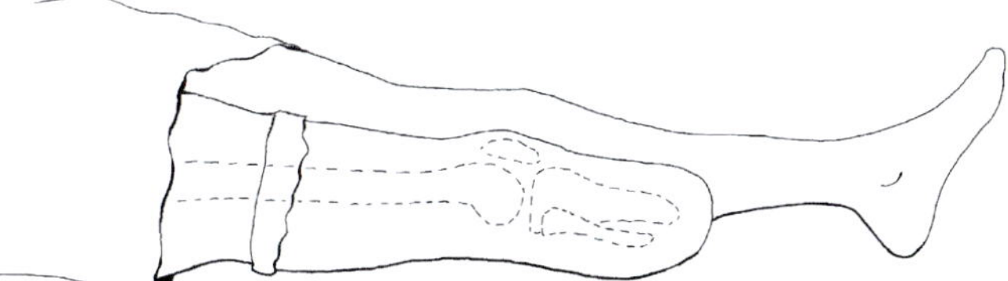

Fig. 20.16 A plaster or fiberglass cast, applied immediately after amputation in the operating room, is an effective method of edema control, protection of the residual limb, and prevention of knee flexion contracture.

Removable Rigid Dressings

The RRD is a "cap" cast worn over a soft or compressive dressing (Fig. 20.16).[227] This edema control strategy effectively protects the healing residual limb and helps to limit the development of edema. RRDs are used in three circumstances. For some individuals managed with a non-RRD applied in the operating room, the next step in postoperative edema control may be fabrication of an RRD. For others the RRD is applied instead of a cylindrical cast in the operating room. The RRD can also be fabricated after surgery for those initially managed with soft dressings and elastic bandages. The physical therapist may be responsible for fabrication of the RRD, working in collaboration with the surgeon, surgical nurse, or prosthetist.

The RRD has been shown to be more beneficial than soft dressings for reducing limb edema, increasing healing time, limb contouring, reduced external limb trauma, and prevention of knee contractures.[228,229]

One of its major advantages, when compared with a cylindrical cast, is the ability to doff (remove) and don (apply) the RRD quickly and easily to monitor wound healing and provide daily wound care. Use of an RRD also assists residual limb shaping and shrinkage; patients who wear RRDs are often ready for prosthetic fitting more quickly than those managed with soft dressings or Ace wraps alone.[230,231] Because the RRD limits the development of edema, it is an important adjunct in the management of postsurgical pain. The protective cap limits shearing across the incision site as the person recovering from amputation surgery moves around in bed or during therapy; this soft-tissue immobilization can assist wound healing.

The RRD is not as likely to become displaced or dislodged during activity when compared with Ace wrap compression. The ease of donning and doffing means that individuals with new amputation can quickly become responsible for this task component of caring for their residual limb. Because the RRD is removed and reapplied several times a day for wound care, the residual limb quickly becomes desensitized and tolerant of pressure, which assists transition to prosthetic wear. Fabrication and use of an RRD provide the opportunity to educate those new to prosthetic use about the fabrication of a preparatory prosthesis and the use of prosthetic socks to obtain and maintain socket fit.

The RRD is most appropriate for patients whose transtibial incision appears to be in the initial stages of healing.[230,231] Although the wound may be inflamed secondary to the trauma of surgery, no signs of infection, significant ecchymosis, or large areas of wound dehiscence should be present. Those with substantial drainage from their surgical wound requiring bulky soft dressings and frequent dressing changes are not good candidates for RRD; it is difficult to accommodate distally placed bulky dressings within the RRD shell. Those with fluctuating edema secondary to CHF or dialysis can be managed with an RRD if it is fabricated when limb volume is high: Layering prosthetic sock ply over the limb before putting on the RRD accommodates for volume loss. The RRD works best if distal residual limb circumference is no more than ½ inch larger than its proximal circumference. Compressive dressings may be more appropriate for patients with extremely bulbous residual limbs.

The residual limb is prepared for casting by first placing a protective layer of gauze fluff over the suture line.[3] The limb can be loosely wrapped in plastic wrap to assist removal of the completed RRD after casting. Next, a "sock" made from elasticized cotton stockinette or Tubigrip is applied over the limb, with particular care to avoid shearing across the suture line. Pieces of Webril or a similar filler material are layered around the limb to create reliefs within the RRD for bony prominences (i.e., tibial crest, fibular head, distal tibia) and the hamstring tendons. When the distal residual limb has a larger circumference, additional padding is added proximally to ensure the RRD will be cylindrical and easily donned. A long sock made from regular cotton stockinette is carefully donned over the padding; this will be the inner layer of the finished RRD. The outline of the patella marked on the stockinet will serve as a guide for trim lines after the cast has dried. Typically, two rolls of fast-setting plaster cast material are sufficient for an RRD. The residual limb is supported in full-knee extension, and successive layers of plaster are smoothed into place, building a cast with an anterior trim line at midpatella and a slightly lower posterior trim line to allow knee flexion without tissue impingement.

The cotton stockinette sock is then folded down over the cast at the knee, and several additional circumferential layers of plaster are used to finish and reinforce the proximal brim (to ensure the RRD can subsequently withstand repeated donning/doffing). An Ace wrap can be applied to provide additional compression while the plaster sets. Once the RRD has hardened sufficiently, the patient is asked to flex the knee slightly and the cast is carefully removed from the residual limb. The extra Webril or padding is pulled out of the RRD, and the inner surface is inspected for potentially problematic rough areas or ridges. Because the RRD is almost cylindrical, it is helpful to mark the front of the cast to ensure it is correctly donned.

Before the completed RRD is applied, one or two gauze pads are placed over the suture line for protection. A prosthetic sock, Tubigrip, elasticized stockinette sock, or commercially manufactured "shrinker" is carefully donned, with minimal shear stress across the suture line. Additional ply of prosthetic socks are used as needed to ensure a snug fit within the RRD. A small amount of Webril or other fluffy padding is placed in the distal anterior RRD to protect the distal tibia and suture line; then the RRD is carefully slipped onto the residual limb, aligning the markings on the front of the RRD with the patella for optimal fit. A small foam filler or cushion can be placed between the anterior brim and residual limb to minimize the risk of friction during activity. The outer Tubigrip or stockinet suspension sleeve is then rolled over the RRD and onto the thigh, the supracondylar strap is secured in place, and the sock is folded back down over the strap to minimize the risk of loss of suspension. The skin must be inspected within the first 60 to 90 minutes of initial fitting with an RRD to assess skin integrity and identify potential pressure-related problems. If no skin problems develop, routine wound inspection once per nursing shift is usually adequate.

The RRD is designed to be worn continuously, even when sleeping, except during routine wound care or bathing.[3,230,231] If the individual with recent amputation is expecting to be out of the RRD for more than several minutes, another form of compression such as a shrinker or several layers of Tubigrip must be available to minimize the development of edema. The individual wearing an RRD must be encouraged to report any localized pain or discomfort as signs of potential problems with RRD fit or function. Layers of prosthetic sock are added, over time, as the residual limb "shrinks." There is some evidence that polymer gel socks worn under an RRD may help to control edema and associated pain and reduce the time to prosthetic fitting.[3,230,231] Sometimes short distal socks are necessary to provide for distal compression without excessive proximal bulkiness that can prohibit donning. The consistent use of 12- to 15-ply socks to achieve appropriate fit usually indicates the need for fabrication of a smaller RRD. Significant change in the shape or configuration of the residual limb also requires fabrication of a new RRD.

The referral for fabrication of the initial (preparatory or training) prosthesis can occur within 12 to 17 days of surgery if the incision has healed sufficiently. Many individuals continue to use their RRD in conjunction with a shrinker for control of edema and limb protection whenever they are not wearing their prosthesis for as long as 6 months after surgery.

Removable Polyethylene Semirigid Dressings

An alternative to a plaster RRD is a removable polyethylene SRD.[3,230] Like the RRD, the SRD is an effective strategy for control of edema, protection of the healing incision, and shaping of the residual limb.[230] However, unlike the RRD, the SRD requires the skill of a prosthetist for fabrication. The prosthetist may take a negative mold of the patient's residual limb while in the operating room or when the rigid dressing is removed on the third or fourth postoperative day. A positive model is created using the negative mold and is modified to incorporate reliefs for pressure-intolerant areas of the residual limb. The polyethylene is heated and vacuum molded over the positive model in the same way a thermoplastic socket would be. The polyethylene SRD is often ready for delivery in 2 or 3 days after casting. When an individual is initially casted for a polyethylene SRD in the operating room before being placed in a plaster or fiberglass cast, the SRD may be delivered on the day the rigid plaster dressing is removed.

The polyethylene SRD has several advantages when compared with the plaster of Paris RRD. First, polyethylene is easier to clean; as a result, hygiene of the residual limb may be improved. The polyethylene SRD is lighter in weight and somewhat more durable than a plaster RRD; it does not melt if exposed to liquids. The flexibility of the material makes it easier to don and doff than the stiff plaster RRD. Because the polyethylene SRD closely resembles a transtibial socket, greater carryover about proper use of prosthetic socks for optimal fit in the socket of the initial (preparatory, temporary, or training) prosthesis is likely.

The major disadvantage of a polyethylene SRD is the cost associated with casting and fabrication. Because most residual limbs become progressively smaller with maturation in the weeks and months after amputation, several successfully smaller SRDs may need to be fabricated as the limb shrinks. In some settings, plaster RRDs are used until the initial prosthetic fitting. At that point the prosthetist makes a polyethylene SRD, in addition to the socket, for the training prosthesis. Some companies now offer a prefabricated adjustable SRD with Velcro closures as an alternative to the custom-molded polyethylene SRD.

Zinc Oxide–Impregnated Semirigid Dressing

Another postoperative strategy is the fabrication of an SRD using a zinc oxide–impregnated Unna bandage. Unna is most often used in the management of chronic venous stasis ulcers (Unna boot)[3]; because it appears to enhance healing, it has also been used as a strategy to control edema and facilitate healing following transtibial amputation.[3] As the Unna dressing dries, it provides nonelastic external support to the residual limb, preventing development of edema. The Unna dressing is basically a roll of gauze impregnated with zinc oxide, triglycerine, calamine, and gelatin. This pasty dressing easily adheres to the skin on application, drying to a semirigid leathery consistency within 24 hours. Typically, an Unna dressing would be applied to the residual limb immediately after wound closure in the operating room.[3] Although not as rigid and protective as an RRD or SRD, Unna paste dressings are more effective in limiting postoperative edema than are soft dressings and Ace wrapping.[3,230] An Unna SRD can be left on for as long as 5 to 7 days; if more frequent wound inspection is desired, it can be easily removed with bandage scissors. Because the Unna dressing remains in place for an extended period, fewer opportunities are available for limb desensitization and patient education about socket fit compared with those for the RRD and polyethylene SRD.

Nonremovable Rigid Dressings

Many surgeons opt to use a cylindrical plaster or fiberglass cast placed on the new transtibial residual limb in the operating room immediately after amputation (Fig. 20.17).[79,90] Rigid dressings accomplish three very important postoperative goals: (1) control of immediate postoperative edema (and subsequently, reduction of postoperative pain); (2) protection of the vulnerable newly sutured residual limb from inadvertent trauma during bed mobility, transfers, and single-limb ambulation; and (3) prevention of postoperative knee flexion contracture. All three of these goals help to reduce time to initial prosthetic fitting.[98,231]

A rigid dressing is a simple postoperative cast applied in the same way as a cast that is used to immobilize a fracture of the proximal tibia or distal femur. The newly sutured surgical construct is dressed with gauze, and a cottonette or Tubigrip "sock" is pulled over the residual limb. A layer of cast padding is applied smoothly over the stockinette, and extra cushioning is placed to protect the patella and femoral condyles. The knee is placed in as close to a fully extended position as possible, and fast-drying plaster of

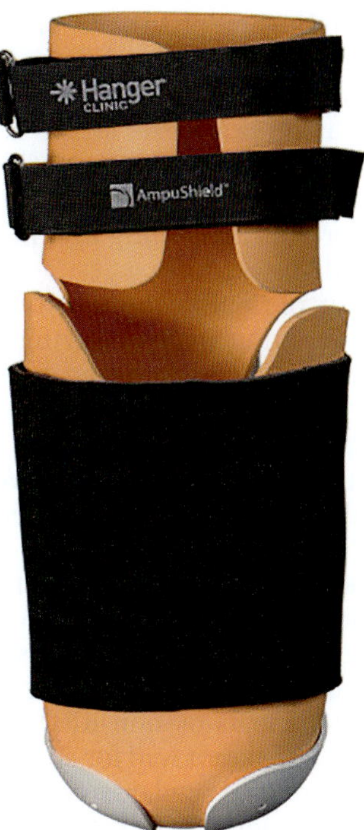

Fig. 20.17 **AmpuShield removable rigid dressing.** (From Reichmarnn JP, Stevens PM, Rheinstein J, Kreulen CD. Removable rigid dressings for postoperative management of transtibial amputations: a review of published evidence. *PM&R.* 2018;10(5):516–523.)

Paris or fiberglass casting material is wrapped around the limb, at least to the level of upper thigh (2–4 inches below the perineum). The stockinette is then folded over the proximal edge of the newly applied cast and is incorporated into one or two addition wraps of casting material to finish the proximal border of the cast.

Modifications of the cast as it is setting or drying, such as molding it to fit closely over the supracondylar thigh, are used to aide suspension. A strip of webbing may be incorporated on the anterior surface for attachment to a waist belt to further aid suspension. If the cast is to be used as the base for an IPOP (discussed in more detail later), the prosthetist modifies the cast as in a patellar tendon–bearing socket to ensure that weight-bearing forces are directed to pressure-tolerant areas of the limb and that bony prominences and the suture line are well protected.

The initial rigid dressing stays in place on the residual limb for 2 to 5 days postoperatively (or more), depending on the patient's condition and the surgeon's preference.[90,98,232,233] When the cast is removed, the status of the wound is carefully inspected. If the wound is healing well, the physician may opt for reapplication of the cast for an additional period, which varies by protocol used, of between 5 and 21 days. If the status of the wound is questionable or risk of infection high, an alternative method of edema control that allows more frequent wound inspection and care must be used. Some physicians opt to replace a thigh-encasing rigid dressing with an RRD after the first cast is taken off, regardless of wound status.

Application of a rigid cast, especially if it is the base of an IPOP (discussed later), requires careful attention to anatomy and alignment, well-developed manual skills, and a clear understanding of prosthetic principles. A poorly applied or inadequately suspended rigid dressing can lead to skin abrasions or pressure-related ulcerations over bony prominences, delaying prosthetic fitting until wound healing occurs.[234–238] Pistoning or rotation of the rigid dressing on the residual limb can apply distracting forces over the suture line, compromising healing and increasing the risk of ecchymosis or dehiscence.

A major criticism of thigh-level, non-RRDs is that the cast prevents visual inspection and monitoring of the new surgical wound and limits access for wound care.[239,240] Therefore a non-RRD may not be appropriate for those with significant risk of infection, especially if wounds were potentially contaminated during traumatic injury. Wound status can be monitored only indirectly, using body temperature, WBC count, size and color of drainage stains on the cast, and patient reports of increasing discomfort and pain as indicators of a developing infection.

There are several strategies physicians and prosthetists have to address to assess healing, while providing the protection and other benefits of non-RRD. One is to bivalve the cast so that it can be removed for short periods to allow wound care. Prefabricated rigid dressings, custom fit by the prosthetist to the individual with new amputation, are also available.[237–240]

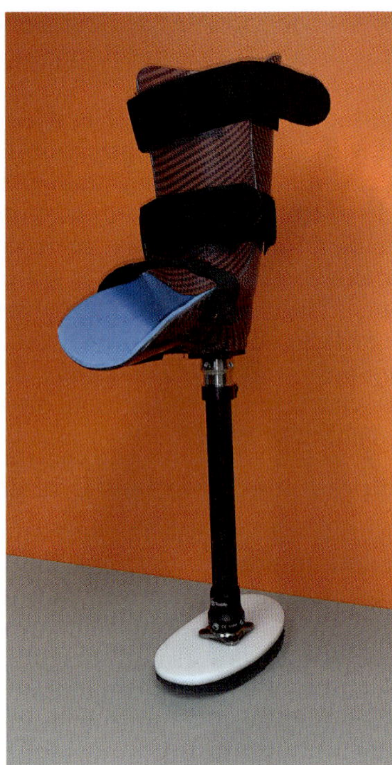

Fig. 20.18 Bent-knee prosthesis. (Courtesy Hanger Inc., Austin, Texas.)

Pneumatic Compression for Early Ambulation

The deconditioning associated with inactivity is a particular concern in the postoperative and preprosthetic periods. However, ambulation on a single limb can be quite challenging for persons with a high comorbid burden of illness. Although pneumatic compression (such as the air splints used for immobilization following acute fracture) is relatively inexpensive and can be quickly removed and reapplied for wound inspection, the compression tends to be uneven, so shaping of the residual limb is not as effective as other methods. The splint can be uncomfortably hot if worn for more than 20 to 30 minutes. However, its major benefit is that it allows early protected weight bearing on the residual limb; this is especially beneficial for individuals who are physically or functionally frail. The air splint provides limited mobility for patients who would not otherwise be ambulatory and may be a useful means of assessing the potential for prosthetic rehabilitation. Several air-filled early prosthetic options exist for compression in the postoperative and preprosthetic periods.[232] However, because regulation of the amount of weight bearing allowed within a pneumatic compression splint is difficult to control, the therapist must weigh the risks of placing too much pressure on the surgical wounds as compared with limited mobility. For this reason, many prosthetists prefer a non–weight-bearing rigid residual dressing.[232] Another option is the bent-knee prosthesis, which, when used with an RRD, removes weight bearing from the incision site yet does not prohibit ambulation[233] (Fig. 20.18).

When donning a pneumatic compression device for early ambulation, the suture line is covered with smooth gauze pads for protection. Prosthetic socks, stockinet, or Tubigrip is then applied over the residual limb before the air splint is inflated. Felt pads are strategically placed over the residual limb's soft dressing, or a shrinker loads pressure-tolerant areas (medial tibial flare and patellar tendon) while protecting pressure-sensitive areas (crest of the tibia and fibular head) after inflation of the air splint. The sleeve is zipped into place around the limb, and the limb is positioned in the frame before inflation. The sleeve is inflated with a hand or foot pump to an air pressure of 35 to 40 mm Hg. This low pressure sustains toe touch to partial weight without compromising capillary blood flow to the healing suture line. Recently a variety of prefabricated pneumatic immediate postoperative prostheses, with inflatable air bladders within an adjustable closure polyethylene "socket," have become available.[234–237]

Rigid Dressing as a Base for Immediate Postoperative Prostheses

When a non-RRD is to be used as an IPOP, a prosthetist joins the surgical team in the operating room during cast application to incorporate the features of a patellar tendon–bearing socket and an attachment for a pylon into the cast (Fig. 20.19).[238] Several felt or gel pads are positioned on the limb to direct and distribute weight-bearing forces more effectively onto pressure-tolerant areas (e.g., medial tibial flare, anterior muscle compartment, patellar tendon). The residual limb is then supported with the knee extended, and several layers of elastic or nonelastic plaster of Paris or fiberglass casting material are applied. The proximal edges of the cast are finished at the upper thigh (2–4 inches below perineum) level. Modifications of the cast (as it is setting) are used to aid suspension or, for an IPOP, to ensure weight-bearing forces are directed to pressure-tolerant areas. Pressure applied to the outside of the cast just above the femoral condyles captures normal femoral anatomy to create supracondylar suspension. For an IPOP, the prosthetist incorporates a patellar tendon bar, a broad "shelf" for the medial tibial flare, and a stabilizing popliteal bulge by applying manual pressure to these areas as the cast begins to set. The prosthetist also

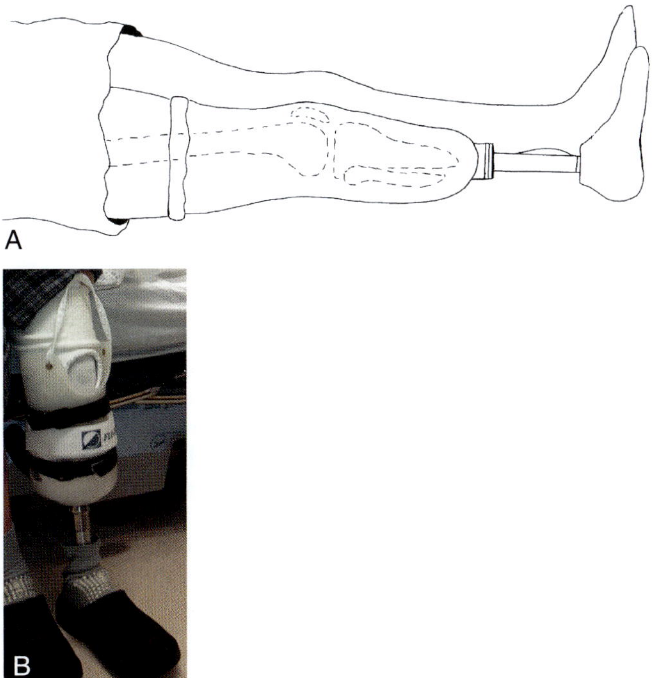

Fig. 20.19 (A and B) Incorporation of a pylon and features of a patellar tendon-bearing socket in an immediate postoperative prosthesis (IPOP) can facilitate early mobility in selected patients. (From Ali MM, Loretz L, Shea A, et al. A contemporary comparative analysis of immediate postoperative prosthesis placement following below-knee amputation. *Ann Vasc Surg*. 2013;27(8):1146–1153.)

incorporates a point of attachment and alignment into the distal cast for subsequent attachment of a pylon and prosthetic foot. Finally, the prosthetist or surgeon can incorporate a suspension attachment, which will connect to a waist belt, into the proximal anterior surface of the cast.

In a retrospective study of individuals who underwent a below-knee amputation, at 60 days postamputation 58% of those who received a rigid plaster or plastic IPOP were ready for prosthesis casting compared with 38% of those who received a soft dressing.[239] The early mobility afforded by application of an IPOP may be important physically and psychologically for individuals with new amputation who would otherwise be unable to achieve single-limb ambulation with a walker or crutches, especially those who are at significant risk of functional decline, physiologic deconditioning, or atelectasis and pneumonia secondary to inactivity and immobilization.[240,241] Although an IPOP replaces the amputated limb with a pylon and prosthetic foot, limited and protected weight bearing is essential in the early postoperative period: most physicians suggest toe touch or partial weight bearing. Shearing forces that result from excessive weight shift and repeated loading of the residual limb in an IPOP can compromise or delay wound healing.[238] Because of this risk, an IPOP is inappropriate for frail or confused individuals who are likely to be unreliable about limiting weight bearing. Many proponents of IPOP suggest that gradual controlled application of mechanical stress to healing connective tissues actually assists tissue modeling for better tolerance of the mechanical stresses of prosthetic wear and ambulation. Although the early application of mechanical stresses is apparently well tolerated by wounds with adequate blood supply, ischemic wounds tolerate only minimum stress in their healing phase.

Selecting the Appropriate Compression Strategy

In deciding which edema control and limb-shaping strategy is most appropriate, the rehabilitation team should consider the following questions:

1. Can the person don/doff the device independently? If not, is a family member available who can assist with this task?
2. Given the individual's physical characteristics and likely level of activity, will the device remain securely in place on the residual limb?
3. Will the device apply enough compression for effective progressive limb shrinkage?
4. Will the device apply enough compression for symmetric shaping of the residual limb?
5. Will the device protect the skin and healing suture line during daily activities, and does use of the device carry any risk of skin irritation or breakdown?
6. Is the device comfortable for the patient to use or wear over the long periods of time that are required for effective control of edema and limb shaping?
7. Is the device relatively cost effective in terms of fabrication, modification, and replacement?

Monitoring tissue tolerance and potential areas of pressure closely in whatever edema control method is chosen is very important, especially in the first few days and weeks after amputation. Although rigid dressings, IPOPs, and Unna dressing remain on the limb for extended periods, each other method of edema control and shaping should be removed and reapplied a minimum of three times each day to ensure appropriate fit and tissue tolerance in the acute phase of healing. When a rigid cast or IPOP is removed, it must be quickly replaced with an alternative compression device so that limb volume does not increase substantially. Individuals with recent amputation must wear the compression device at all times unless walking in a training prosthesis (even time out of compression during bathing should be as short as possible). Most people find that a compression device is necessary to maintain the desired limb volume for 6 months to a year after surgery. Some persons with mature residual limbs who have fluctuation in volume because of concurrent medical conditions continue to require compression well beyond the first postoperative year.[3,242–244]

Many people with amputation experience a transient increase in residual limb volume after showering or bathing; they often choose to bathe in the evening so that volume change does not interfere with prosthetic use. Those who prefer to bathe in the morning may need to use a compression device immediately after bathing to achieve optimal prosthetic fit and suspension, especially if suction suspension (which requires consistent limb volume) is used. Those who use prosthetic socks may require a few less ply of sock immediately after bathing but need to add a few more ply after a few hours as limb volume decreases.

SKIN CARE AND SCAR MANAGEMENT

It is important that the healing incision move without adherence to underlying deep tissue or bone as healing progresses. There must be sufficient gliding between skin and underlying layers of soft tissue after healing so that shear forces will be minimal while the prosthesis is donned and used for function. An adherent scar at the distal tibia can be quite problematic: If a point of adherence is present along an incisional scar, the mobility of tissues will be compromised. The resulting traction and shear forces are likely to lead to discomfort, skin irritation, and often recurrent breakdown of soft tissues with prosthetic use. Once primary healing has been established, the person with recent amputation learns to use gentle manual massage to enhance tissue mobility in preparation for prosthetic use. At first, this is performed above and below, but not across, the incision to minimize the risk of dehiscence.

When the wound is well closed and Steri-Strips are no longer necessary to support and protect the incision, gentle mobilization of the scar itself can begin. Handling of the limb during soft tissue mobilization and massage not only minimizes adhesion formation but also helps the individual to adapt his or her body image to include the postamputation residual limb and prepare for the sensory experience of prosthetic use.[241,242]

Persons with new amputation may have surgical scars from previous vascular bypass or from harvesting veins for coronary artery bypass surgery. These may require carefully applied soft tissue mobilization or friction massage to free adhesions and restore the mobility of the skin. Those with traumatic amputation may have healing skin grafts or abrasions from road burn, thermal injury, or electrical burn. In such cases, wound care and débridement are important components of preprosthetic rehabilitation. For individuals with healing burns or skin graft, the use of an appropriate compression garment or shrinker assists healing and maturation of skin, controls postoperative edema, and shapes the residual limb.

Once the sutures have been removed, normal bathing resumes and a routine for daily skin care is established. Most physicians, prosthetists, and therapists recommend daily cleansing of the residual limb with a mild, nondrying soap. Patting or gently rubbing the limb with a terry cloth towel until it is fully dry also helps to desensitize it in preparation for prosthetic use. A small amount of moisturizer or skin cream can be applied if the skin of the residual limb is dry or flaky. A limb with soft, healthy pliable skin is much more tolerant of prosthetic wear than a limb with tough, dry, easily irritated skin. Persons with new amputation and their caregivers are taught to inspect the skin of the entire residual limb carefully, using a mirror if necessary to visualize difficult-to-see areas. Areas over bony prominences that may be vulnerable to high pressure within the socket are especially important to assess.

Persons with amputation are as likely to have other dermatologic conditions such as eczema or psoriasis as the general population.[243–246] Those with hairy limbs or easily irritated skin may be more at risk of folliculitis and similar inflammatory skin conditions once the prosthesis is worn consistently. Effective early management of skin irritation or other skin problems is important: Serious skin irritation or infection precludes prosthetic use until adequate healing has occurred.

Some persons with new amputation mistakenly assume that something must be used to "toughen" the skin in preparation for prosthetic use. They may opt to rub the skin with alcohol, vinegar, salt water, or even gasoline, erroneously thinking that this will make the skin thicker and more pressure tolerant. In fact, these "treatments" can damage the skin, making it more susceptible to pressure-related problems. Patient and family education about effective cleansing and skin care strategies is essential in the early postoperative/preprosthetic period.

RANGE OF MOTION AND FLEXIBILITY

Persons with transtibial amputation are at significant risk of developing both knee and hip flexion contractures. Those with transfemoral amputation are very likely to develop hip flexion and external rotation contracture. Such contractures cause substantial problems for prosthetic fit and alignment, as well as on efficiency of walking with a prosthesis. Impairment of extensibility of two-joint muscles, such as the hamstrings and rectus femoris, may not be obvious when an individual is seated but may have profound impact on comfort when wearing a prosthesis during functional activities. For this reason, proper positioning is a key component of preprosthetic rehabilitation.

Prolonged dependence of the residual limb held in knee flexion when sitting also leads to development of distal edema, which can delay readiness for prosthetic fitting. Persons with transtibial amputation must maintain the knee in as much extension as possible, whether in bed, sitting in a wheelchair or lounge chair, or during exercise and activity. Although it may be comfortable to place a pillow under the knee when sitting or lying in bed, a more effective strategy is to position a small towel roll under the distal posterior residual limb to encourage knee extension (Fig. 20.20). Use of a wheelchair with elevating leg rests on the side of the amputation helps to keep the residual limb in an extended position, although a "bridge" between the seat and calf support may be necessary for those with short residual limbs. In some settings, the therapist fabricates a posterior trough splint from low-temperature thermoplastic materials; this splint supports the limb in knee extension when the individual with recent amputation is resting in bed or sitting in a wheelchair.

Manual stretching techniques will allow the PT to determine the end feel and tissue extensibility and should be employed periodically to assess progress. If the individual is able to assume prone position, the weight of the limb can be used to assist elongation of the hamstring muscles and soft tissue of the posterior knee (Fig. 20.21). A small towel roll positioned just above the patella effectively positions the limb for elongation. Although there is little conclusive evidence in the research literature about contracture management in persons with recent lower-limb amputation, evidence from studies of soft-tissue contracture following total knee arthroplasty suggest that prolonged stretching, dynamic splinting, and manual therapy may be effective following amputation as well.[247–249] Stretching programs also have a positive impact on the quality and efficiency of gait in older adults.[250] What is not well understood is the intensity necessary if stretching is to prevent or minimize degree of contracture formation, especially if there is also evidence of central nervous system dysfunction.[251–253] Intervention strategies currently used to target

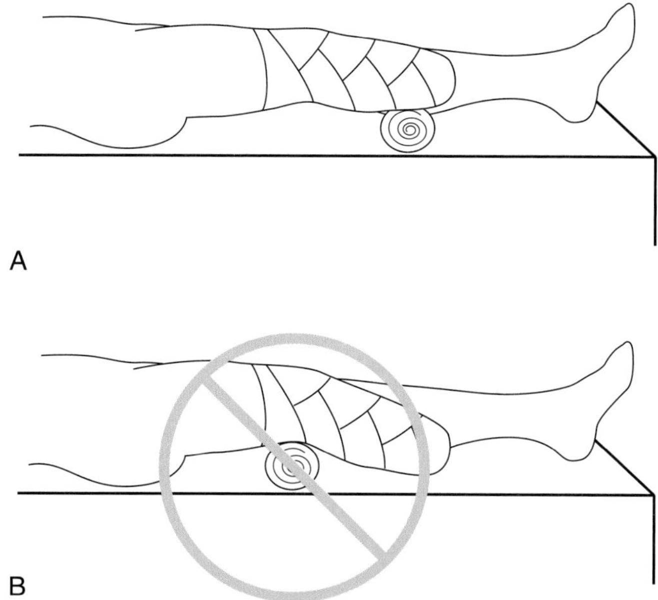

Fig. 20.20 The optimal position for individuals with recent transtibial amputation is in full extension. (A) A small rolled towel, bolster, or pillow placed under the distal posterior residual limb encourages knee extension, whereas (B) support under the knee makes the development of knee flexion contracture more likely.

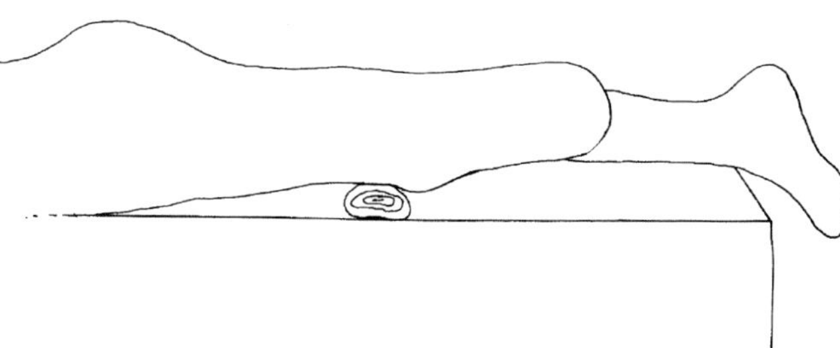

Fig. 20.21 Prone positioning for stretching of the posterior soft tissue and prevention of knee flexion contracture. A small towel roll placed just above the patella elevates the residual limb from the surface of the mat or bed. The therapist can use hold-relax or contract-relax techniques, or the patient can actively contract the quadriceps to elongate the hamstrings and posterior soft tissues.

joint ROM and flexibility include proprioceptive neuromuscular facilitation (PNF) hold-relax or contract-relax[254,255] and myofascial release.[256] Although the strength of the clinical research evidence on interventions for stretching and flexibility following lower-limb amputation is low, the consequences of not attending to risk of contracture development are substantially negative. Converging recommendations by experts strongly support that interventions aimed at contracture prevention or minimization are essential in the postoperative/preprosthetic period.[257–260] Persons with recent amputation are instructed on how to perform exercises (done at the bedside while an inpatient or at home while an outpatient) that are designed to elongate muscles and soft tissue to counteract the tendency to develop tightness, especially in two-joint muscles. Performed independently or with the assistance of a family member or caregiver several times a day, these stretching exercises are as important as individualized PT sessions during preprosthetic and prosthetic rehabilitation.

Significant hip flexion contracture can render a person with transfemoral amputation ineffective in controlling a prosthetic knee unit and walking with a prosthesis. Persons with recent transfemoral amputation tend to hold their residual limb diagonally outward when seated, unconsciously and automatically increasing their seated base of support to enhance postural stability. If they spend significant amounts of time in a seated position, development of hip flexor, abductor, and external rotator tightness is almost inevitable. PT interventions that elongate these soft tissues, including manual stretching, active exercise, and functional postural training, are used to counteract the tendency for tightness to develop.[255–261] Resting in a prone position with a towel roll under the distal anterior residual limb provides prolonged elongation for tight hip flexors. However, care must be taken to maintain a neutral pelvis or slight posterior tilt when lying prone. Excessive hip flexor tightness leads to lordosis of the lumbosacral spine.

MUSCLE PERFORMANCE

Most individuals do not achieve sufficient activity levels after lower-limb amputation. A recent study found that 61% of lower-limb amputees did not achieve the recommended 150 minutes of activity per week and that 33% were sedentary.[262] Rehabilitation professionals must promote physical activity participation beyond minimal functional levels but also encourage strength and aerobic conditioning to maximize health benefits. Strengthening programs have two goals: (1) remediation of specific weaknesses detected in the examination and (2) maximization of overall strength and muscular endurance for safe, energy-efficient prosthetic gait. Because functional activities require use of muscles at varying lengths and types of contraction, effective preprosthetic exercise programs include concentric, holding (isometric), eccentric, and cocontraction activities in a variety of positions and muscle lengths.[257–260] In the immediate postoperative period the specific strengthening program is often a combination of isometric and active isotonic exercise within a limited ROM of the joint just proximal to the amputation.[257–263] This strategy minimizes stress or tension across the incision while preserving and improving the strength of key muscle groups. It is as critical to include strengthening exercise for the intact (nonamputated limb) as for the residual limb. Core stability also needs to be addressed.

Incorporation of controlled exhalation during isometric contraction minimizes the risks to cardiac function and fluctuations of blood pressure that are associated with the Valsalva maneuver.[262] For persons with transtibial amputation, exercises to strengthen knee extension that are initiated within the first week of amputation might include "quad sets" in the supine position or "short arc quads" performed in the supine or sitting position. For those with transfemoral amputation, "glut sets" in the prone or supine position or "short arc" hip extension and abduction in a gravity-eliminated position would be initiated. Gailey and Gailey[260] recommend an exercise strategy of slow, steadily controlled, 10-second muscular contractions, followed by 5 to 10 seconds of rest, for 10 repetitions as one that is easily learned and physiologically sound. As wound healing is accomplished, exercises can be progressed to include active exercises through larger arcs of motion, active resistive exercise (using weights or manual resistance), or isokinetic training. Application of manual resistance during functional activities, as in PNF, allows the therapist to provide appropriate resistance as muscle strength varies throughout the active ROM while providing facilitation and augmented sensory feedback to the patient.[263] Progressive resistive exercise for strength development (low repetition–high load) and muscular endurance (high repetition–low load) are key and should also be included.[264–267] Isokinetic exercise, involving both concentric and eccentric contraction, allows the patient to develop muscle strength and control at a variety of movement velocities and has a marked positive impact on functional ability.[268–270] Isokinetic exercise, if prescribed properly, is well tolerated by older adults, even at speeds of 180 degrees per second angular velocity.[269]

For individuals with transtibial amputation, attachments of the quadriceps and hamstrings are typically intact and preprosthetic strengthening exercises emphasize control of the knee, as well as hip extensor and abductor strength for stability in stance. There is evidence that older males who are unable to develop knee extension force greater than 1.13 Nm/kg (measured by handheld isokinetic dynamometer, normalized by body weight) and older female who are unable to develop knee extension force greater than 1.01 Nm/kg have a high risk for functional decline, morbidity, and mortality.[268] These strength values may represent the minimum threshold for community function and could serve as evidence-based functional goals for persons recovering from transtibial amputation (both limbs) and transfemoral amputation (remaining limb). Those with transtibial amputation are also very likely to have deficits in muscle performance around the hip; strengthening programs must include hip abductors (for stance phase stability) and hip extensors,[260] much like those who are receiving rehabilitation following total knee arthroplasty.[271,272]

Persons with transfemoral amputation must develop strong hip extension capabilities to control the prosthetic knee unit. They must also have effective hip abduction power if the pelvis is to remain level during stance. It is vital to recognize that the distal attachments of the hamstrings, rectus femoris, sartorius, tensor fasciae latae/iliotibial band, adductor longus, and adductor magnus are relocated by myodesis or myoplasty or are lost entirely (for patients with short residual limbs) during transfemoral surgery. The combination of an altered line of pull and loss of muscle mass often creates an imbalance of muscle action around the hip.[273–275] The gluteus maximus, gluteus medius, and iliopsoas, with their intact distal attachments, are more powerful in determining resting hip position than the altered adductor group. If the tensor fasciae latae/iliotibial band and gluteus maximus become secondarily shortened, function of the adductor group is further compromised. Because of this imbalance, the physical therapist must consider activities that strengthen the remaining hip adductors, as well as hip extensors and hip abductors, to prepare the patient for effective postural control in sitting and standing and stance phase stability in prosthetic gait.[275]

General strengthening exercises for the trunk and upper extremities are also essential components of an effective preprosthetic exercise program. Back extensors and abdominal muscles play a principal role in postural alignment and postural control. Activities that involve trunk rotation or diagonal movements activate trunk and limb girdle muscles in functional patterns, addressing strength and flexibility for functional activities and enhancing reciprocal arm swing and pelvic control in gait. Upper extremity strengthening, targeting shoulder depressor and elbow extensors, enhances the patient's ability to use an assistive device for single-limb ambulation before prosthetic fitting.

ENDURANCE

Many older adults with dysvascular amputation begin rehabilitation with compromised cardiopulmonary endurance because of the effects of comorbid cardiac and pulmonary diseases and on deconditioning associated with inactivity and bed rest.[68] In persons with significant peripheral vascular disease without amputation, endurance training on treadmill improved endurance (6-Minute Walk distance) and physical function (Short-Form 36 physical functioning values).[276] In deconditioned individuals, a 2-Minute Walk Test may be a more appropriate test of aerobic conditioning than the 6-Minute Walk Test because it has been shown to be predictive of 6-Minute Walk Test distance for individuals with lower extremity amputations.[277] A distance of 113 m is necessary for patients to be likely to walk at least 300 m in the 6-Minute Walk Test to show potential as community ambulators.[277] There are significant differences in the 2-MWT performance between age, sex, cause of amputation, and level of amputation. A recent study of 100 individuals with lower-limb loss determined an average distance and gait speed of 143.8 m and 72.1 m/min, respectively. Males walked farther and faster than females, and younger individuals walked farther and faster than older individuals. Level of amputation also mattered, with longer residual limbs performing superiorly to those with short residual limbs.[278] Although treadmill training is not appropriate in the preprosthetic period, other strategies, such as cycle ergometer driven by the intact limb, upper extremity ergometer, or cycle/recumbent combined upper and lower extremity ergometers (e.g., NuStep Inc, Ann Arbor, Michigan) (Fig. 20.22), can be safely and successfully used for persons with lower-limb amputation.[279,280] Endurance and physical conditioning are predictors of prosthetic use: the ability to exercise at or greater than 50% of age-predicted maximum volume of oxygen consumption (VO_{2max}) differentiated between persons with amputation able to walk functional distances (100 m) with a prosthesis and those who were unable to do so.[281–283] Because energy cost of walking with a prosthesis increases as limb length decreases, endurance training is particularly important for persons with transfemoral amputation.[284–286] Energy expenditure increases with the level of amputation from transtibial to bilateral transfemoral, as much as 20% to 200%.[287,288] Persons with amputation can substantially improve level of fitness (VO_{2max}) and, with that, their potential for physical activity and prosthetic use.[287]

POSTURAL CONTROL

Loss of a limb shifts the position of the body's COM, moving it slightly upward, backward, and toward the remaining or intact extremity; the magnitude of this shift is determined by the extent of limb loss. The shift may have relatively little

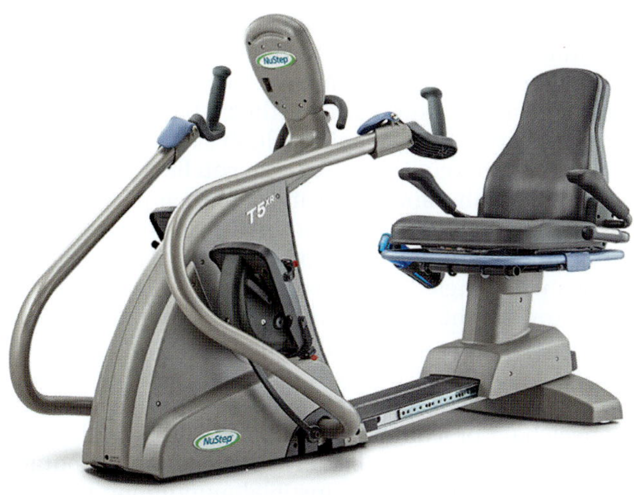

Fig. 20.22 Example of a combined upper and lower extremity recumbent ergometer appropriate for endurance exercise as part of the preprosthetic program for persons with amputation. (Courtesy NuStep Inc., Ann Arbor, Michigan.)

impact on postural control and functional ability in patients with partial foot or Syme amputation. However, it may have a significant impact on sitting balance, transitions between sitting and standing, and single-limb ambulation for persons with transtibial, transfemoral, or hip disarticulation amputation. An effective preprosthetic program incorporates activities that challenge patients to improve core stability, postural control, and equilibrium responses, learning how to control the repositioned COM effectively over an altered base of support. In sitting, this can be accomplished using a variety of reaching tasks including forward reaching, diagonal reaching across and away from the midline, reaching down to a lower surface or objects, reaching up and away from their center, and turning to reach behind them.[288] Anticipatory and reactive postural responses can also be practiced by throwing and catching games that require an automatic weight shift as part of the activity. The difficulty of the task can be advanced by progressively shifting the location of the catch or toss away from the midline of the patient's trunk; alternating locations from side to side or upward or downward; increasing the speed of the activity; increasing the weight of the object or ball that is being used; or performing the activity on a less stable seating surface (e.g., TheraBall, large bolster, or air-filled balance cushion).[288] Similar activities can be implemented in single-limb stance, initially within the parallel bars with physical guarding to insure safety. Such opportunity to practice anticipatory and reactionary postural control in single-limb stance lays the foundation for the postural control necessary for single-limb ambulation with an assistive device, as well as for eventual prosthetic use.

The effectiveness of postural responses is influenced by efficiency of the somatosensory system and visual systems, flexibility and strength of the trunk and limb girdles, and the length and power of the residual limb.[289,290] The prosthetic replacement of a missing limb increases the functional base of support in sitting; for some individuals the weight of the prosthesis serves as a stabilizing anchor during functional activity. For those with limited flexibility or strength, such a replacement might be essential for effective postural responses and the ability to reach, even if the potential for functional ambulation is small.

WHEELCHAIRS, SEATING, AND ADAPTIVE EQUIPMENT

Many patients with amputation rely on a wheelchair for at least some mobility needs during the postoperative, preprosthetic period.[291] Some patients with a short transfemoral amputation, hip disarticulation, or bilateral amputation prefer the relative energy efficiency of wheelchair mobility to ambulation with or without a prosthesis.[292,293] For others, comorbid cardiovascular or cardiopulmonary dysfunction precludes ambulation, and the wheelchair becomes their primary mode of locomotion.[294] The shift in COM after amputation has important implications for the choice of wheelchairs.

The design of many standard or traditional wheelchairs is based on the anthropomorphic characteristics of an "average" adult male with intact lower extremities. With the loss of a limb, the COM shifts in a posterior and lateral direction; when the patient is seated in a wheelchair, this moves the COM closer to the axis of rotation of the chair's wheels. If the patient with lower extremity amputation turns or reaches backward during a functional activity, the COM shifts even farther toward or beyond the wheel axis, and the chair may tip backward. Providing simple antitip devices reduces the risk of posterior tipping during functional activities. For those with transfemoral or bilateral amputation, a wheelchair with wheels that can be offset posteriorly is recommended. Patients with recent amputation must also be aware of altered dynamics when they reach forward while sitting in a wheelchair: High downward pressure on the wheelchair footplate by the intact limb when reaching forward is likely to lead to anterior tipping.

Specific wheelchair assessments and prescription are warranted for all individuals who will be using a wheelchair as their primary means of locomotion and mobility (see Chapter 16). This individual evaluation and prescription process ensures the wheelchair will provide adequate support of the thighs to increase seating stability and reach, adequate seating with an appropriate cushion for pressure distribution, and configuration of components that provides ease of wheelchair locomotion.

Wheelchair skills to be mastered by persons with new amputation and their caregivers include effective propulsion over level, carpeted, and uneven ground; turning and backing up; positioning of the wheelchair for safe bed, toilet, bathtub, furniture, and car transfers; ascending and descending thresholds, curbs, and ramps; and getting the wheelchair into and out of the family's motor vehicle. In addition, practice getting to and from the floor and the opportunity to react to a controlled fall (lowering backward to the ground) may ease concerns about the aftermath of falls. Readers are referred to textbooks on spinal cord injury rehabilitation, which contain chapters on wheelchair skill development that can be applied to persons with amputation.[293–295]

Along with a wheelchair, many persons with new amputation would benefit from the provision of adaptive equipment for their homes (e.g., tub benches, grab bars, toilet frames, raised toilet seats, handheld shower adapters) and the installation of temporary (or permanent) ramps to entrance/egress to the home. Consideration must also be given to access to sinks, as well as to using insulated coverings of exposed hot water and drain pipes. In some cases, if the individual is likely to use the wheelchair for a long period of time as primary means of mobility, modification of the home may be recommended for both safety and efficiency of function. Although these concerns are more typically addressed in inpatient and subacute rehabilitation settings, many patients with new amputation may be discharged to home to await sufficient healing prior to beginning prosthetic rehabilitation. Therapists in acute care must consider referral to home-care services if there is insufficient time to address wheeled mobility and accessibility during hospitalization. Once again, textbooks on spinal cord injury are good sources of information about durable medical equipment and home modifications for accessibility.[296,297]

BED MOBILITY AND TRANSFERS

In the acute care setting, PT intervention at the bedside includes instruction about optimal positioning of the residual limb and activities to assist the patient's ability to change position in bed and move to or from a seated position. Early mobility and activity significantly reduce the risk of atelectasis, pneumonia, and further physiologic deconditioning.[298] However, the therapist must be aware of the risk of postural hypotension and of postoperative complications, including deep venous thrombosis and pulmonary embolism. Assessment and monitoring of the patient's vital signs (i.e., pulse, respiratory rate, blood pressure, pulse oximetry) are recommended as bed mobility and out-of-bed activity begin.[299] Care must also be taken to minimize the risk of trauma to the newly amputated limb during activity, exercise, or transfers.

Many individuals with recent amputation can roll from supine to or from the prone position without great difficulty, although those with transfemoral amputation of the dominant limb may need to develop an adapted movement pattern or sequence. The strategies for transition into sitting are not substantially different from preferred preoperative strategies; however, efficiency of postural responses may be challenged by the alteration in body mass after amputation. Those who have become deconditioned by inactivity in the days and weeks before amputation may find bed rails, a trapeze, bed ladders, or other devices helpful early in rehabilitation. Strategic placement of a bed table or walker near the bedside at night serves as a reminder of the amputation for individuals who are likely to get up during the night to go to the bathroom (without otherwise fully awakening), reducing the risk of falling.

A primary goal of postoperative, preprosthetic rehabilitation is development of the ability to move between seating surfaces or from sitting to standing as safely and independently as possible. The majority of falls for persons with new amputation in acute care settings occur during self-transfer between wheelchair and bed or toilet.[300] Depending on the individual's preamputation level of activity, transferring between seating surfaces may require some degree of assistance or use of adaptive devices or may be accomplished relatively smoothly and easily. Those who are deconditioned or who have previous neuromuscular-related postural impairment may require a mechanical lifting aid, multiperson lifting, or some level of assistance in the early postoperative period. Others may benefit from a strategically placed transfer board as they develop their ability to perform a pivot transfer on their remaining limb.

Some persons require a walker or crutches for extra stability in single-limb stance in the midst of their pivot transfers. Still others quickly master scooting in sitting and pivoting on their remaining limb to become independent in transfers. Persons with single-limb amputation initially prefer transferring toward their remaining limb but should be encouraged to master moving in either direction. Individuals with bilateral limb loss or injury that precludes weight bearing on the remaining limb can scoot across a sliding board to a wheelchair or commode that is positioned diagonally from the bed. Those with bilateral transfemoral amputation (and those with bilateral transtibial amputation who have sufficient hamstring excursion) may prefer the surface-to-surface stability that is provided when the entire anterior edge of the wheelchair seat abuts the side of the bed, allowing them to scoot directly forward. Some individuals who require significant assistance to transfer without a prosthesis become nearly independent in pivot transfers when a prosthesis is worn: The sensory feedback that is provided to the residual limb within the socket when there is contact between the prosthetic foot and the floor enhances sitting balance during sliding board or pivot transfers. Persons with transfemoral amputation must learn that, although they can wear a prosthesis when seated, the prosthesis cannot be counted on for stability during transfers.

Mastery of single-limb or non–weight-bearing transfers in the postoperative period is the foundation for functional transfers whenever the person with amputation is not wearing his or her prosthesis. At times in the future, mechanical problems with the prosthesis, skin problems on the residual limb, or a medical problem (e.g., CHF or renal failure) may affect socket fit, temporarily precluding prosthetic use. Providing opportunities for patients to practice transferring between surfaces at different levels (e.g., wheelchair to stool to floor) in the postoperative, preprosthetic period is very important, especially if delayed prosthetic fitting is anticipated.

AMBULATION AND LOCOMOTION

Single-limb ambulation with an appropriate assistive device provides an opportunity to enhance postural control and to build strength and cardiovascular endurance, in addition to allowing patients with recent amputation to move about in their environment. A number of factors (e.g., safety, balance, and postural control, endurance, lower extremity muscle performance, fear of falling) must be considered in recommending an ambulator assistive device.[300,301] Although use of a standard or rolling walker may be appropriate in the initial PT sessions, many individuals with new amputation quickly master a two- or three-point swing-through pattern with crutches on level surfaces and are ready to build advanced gait skills on uneven surfaces, inclines, and stairs. Others are fearful of using crutches, preferring the stability provided by a walker to the mobility of crutches. A walker may be appropriate for patients with limited endurance and balance impairment who would otherwise be limited to wheelchair use. However, therapists must be aware of the potential long-term limitation in gait patterns imposed by walkers: The halting hop-to gait pattern interrupts forward progression of the COM. Individuals who have adapted to this pattern of motion before receiving a prosthesis may have difficulty developing a smooth step-through pattern or becoming comfortable with a less supportive ambulation aid once they are using their prosthesis. Walkers are also more difficult to use on inclines and are dangerous to use on stairs. Whenever possible, patients are encouraged to use crutches.[301] Table 20.5 summarizes the progressive single-limb ambulation skills for preprosthetic rehabilitation.

Individuals with limited endurance or poor balance spend much time practicing a hop-to or swing-through gait in the parallel bars before they acquire the confidence and motor skill necessary to move out of the parallel bars with a walker or crutches. Indeed, single-limb ambulation with an assistive device is often more energy intensive than walking with a prosthesis.[302,303] Achievement of functional single-limb ambulation is not a prerequisite for prosthetic fitting.[304] All individuals who can stand and use an assistive device to walk should be encouraged to ambulate as much as possible, even if they are walking for aerobic exercise rather than to accomplish a functional task. For those with single-limb amputation, wheelchair use should be reserved for long-distance transportation unless ambulation is not medically advisable. Wheelchairs are appropriate for patients with bilateral amputation; self-propulsion provides some aerobic conditioning and an energy-efficient means of locomotion.[301]

PATIENT AND FAMILY EDUCATION: CARE OF THE REMAINING LIMB

Patient and family education begins in the initial interview process and continues throughout the acute hospital stay, as illustrated in the preceding discussions of positioning, residual limb care, remaining/intact limb care, and enhancing motor performance and functional training.

Patient education about the risk of decubitus ulceration and strategies to reduce this risk are also key components of early postoperative care. Individuals with vascular disease and neuropathy are particularly at risk, with the heel and lateral border of the remaining foot most vulnerable.[246] Those with dysvascular limbs may have barely enough circulation to support tissue health in an intact or noninjured foot; once

Table 20.5 Comparison of Various Postoperative Options for Management of New Transtibial Residual Limbs Following Amputation

Outcomes

Strategy	Cost	Ease of Application	Wound Healing	Protection from Trauma	Degree of Postoperative Edema	Postoperative Pain	Knee Flexion Contracture Risk	Time to First Prosthetic Fitting
Soft gauze dressing without Ace wrap	Inexpensive	Not difficult	Little impact on primary or secondary healing	None	Significant	Often severe	Very high	Prolonged
Soft gauze with Ace wrap	Inexpensive	Figure-eight wrap requires skill, frequent reapplication	Little impact on primary or secondary healing	None	Significant	Often severe	Very high	Prolonged
"Shrinker" garment	Low-to-moderate cost	Requires UE strength, dexterity	Used after primary healing has occurred	Minimal	Moderate	Somewhat less	Very high	Slightly shortened
Rigid dressing (above knee cast)	Low cost	Requires training; MD or CP	Reduces time to primary healing	Excellent	Minimal	Minimized	Extremely low	Shortened
RRD (below knee)Plaster/custom	Low-to-moderate cost	Requires training; PT or CP	Reduces time to primary healing	Very good	Minimal	Minimized	Moderate	Shortened
RRD Prefabricated (thigh level)	Moderate cost	CP custom fits	Reduces time to primary healing	Very good	Minimal if worn consistently	Minimized if worn consistently	Extremely low	Shortened
IPOP Rigid dressing Plaster/custom	Low-to-high cost	CP applies in the OR, or fabricates	Reduces time to primary healing if protected WtB only	Very good when worn, protected WtB only	Reduced if worn consistently	Minimized if worn consistently	Low if worn consistently	Shortened
IPOP: pneumatic	Moderate-to-high cost	PT uses as part of rehabilitation	Less evidence about impact on healing available	Very good when worn, protected WtB only	Reduced if shrinker worn between IPOP use	Depends on options in place between IPOP use	Moderate if not in thigh RRD between use	Shortened

CP, Certified prosthetist; *IPOP*, immediate postoperative prosthesis; *MD*, physician; *OR*, operating room; *PT*, physical therapist; *ROM*, range of motion; *RRD*, removable rigid dressing; *UE*, upper extremity; *WtB*, weight bearing.

From Nawijn SE, van der Linde H, Emmelot CH, Hofstad CJ. Stump management after transtibial amputation: a systematic review. *Prosthet Orthot Int.* 2005;29(1):13–26; Smith DG, McFarland LV, Sangeorzan BJ, et al. Addendum 1: post-operative dressing and management strategies for transtibial amputations: a critical review. *J Prosthet Orthot.* 2004:16(S3):15–25; Walsh TL. Custom removable immediate postoperative prosthesis. *J Prosthet Orthot.* 2003;15(4):158–161.

a wound has occurred, circulation may be inadequate for tissue healing. An open wound on the remaining limb would preclude single-limb ambulation, increasing the risk of inactivity-related postoperative complications and making prosthetic rehabilitation even more challenging. Pressure-related wounds significantly delay rehabilitation, increase disability, and multiply healthcare costs for patients with amputation. Vulnerability to pressure increases with sensory impairment; altered mechanical characteristics of injured, calcified, or scarred tissues; poor circulatory status; microclimate of the skin; and (in combination with these factors) advanced age.[3,246] For those who have limited ability to change position, a pressure-distributing mattress and well-designed, carefully applied heel protectors can reduce the risk of decubitus ulcer formation. A routine of frequent position change, weight shifting, and exercise reduces weight-bearing pressures and enhances circulation to vulnerable tissues.

Before discharge, the rehabilitation team must ascertain how close to functional independence the individual and caregivers are in a variety of self-care activities, in mobility and locomotion, and performance of preprosthetic exercises (Fig. 20.23). As the program progresses, the ability of the individual and family in these areas is a key determinant of discharge readiness and placement (home with home care, home with outpatient follow-up, or to a rehabilitation or subacute facility).

Case Example 20.1b **Interventions for N.H., an 89-Year-Old Female With "Elective" Transtibial Amputation**

N.H. is now 4 days postsurgery, and her delirium is clearing. She is conversing with her typical sense of humor with family and staff. Her casted fiberglass rigid dressing was removed yesterday; the surgical wound is draining moderate amounts of serosanguineous fluid; the edges are closely approximate. An area of pressure-related abrasion and inflammation at the anterior distal tibia was noted when the cast was removed; granulation is now evident. N.H. can transfer to a bedside chair with moderate assistance of one person, with noted moderate impairment of postural control. N.H. tolerates being up in a bedside chair for 45 minutes. She rates her postoperative pain as 4 out of 10, except at dressing change, when it increases to 6 out of 10. She laughs but feels concerned that she feels mild cramping in the instep of the limb that is no longer there, wanting to stretch her foot and toes into dorsiflexion to relieve her discomfort. She is reluctant to look at or touch her residual limb but does not mind if nurses, physicians, or PT staff handle it during dressing changes or functional activities. She transferred from sitting to standing with a walker at bedside with moderate assistance of one person, complaining of dizziness after standing for more than a minute and requesting to return to sitting. She tells you that she is "ready to get going" and wants to return to her own home to use her wheelchair as soon as possible.

QUESTIONS TO CONSIDER

- Given her postoperative pain and phantom sensation, what PT interventions would be appropriate now for N.H.? Why would these be most appropriate from among available options? What are the pros and cons of each, concerning attention, memory, and ability to learn?
- Given the status of her wound and condition of her residual limb, what strategies for management of edema and limb shaping would you recommend? What pros and cons did you consider when deciding among options for compression and residual limb protection? Why do you think the option you selected is the most appropriate? How would this be similar or different if her amputation was at the transfemoral level?
- What strategies for intervention and patient-family education would you implement for skin care and scar management for N.H.? What issues or factors will assist or inhibit her ability to take responsibility for her skin care?
- What specific strategies for intervention and patient-family education aimed at ROM and flexibility do you recommend for N.H.? What impairments or functional limitations are you particularly concerned about for N.H.? What activities will you engage her in? What positions? For what period of time? With what equipment? What would you emphasize if her amputation was at a transfemoral level? What issues or factors will assist or inhibit her ability to take responsibility for exercises aimed at ensuring adequate ROM and flexibility in preparation for prosthetic use?
- What specific strategies for intervention and patient-family education to improve muscle performance do you recommend for N.H.? How do you address the strengthening of key muscle groups of extremities and trunk? How do you address power and muscle endurance? How do you address concentric, isometric, and eccentric control and performance? What issues or factors must be considered regarding exercise tolerance, intensity, frequency, and duration during her acute care stay? How will you address her concerns about her low aerobic fitness and conditioning level?
- What specific strategies for intervention and patient-family education aimed at improving static, dynamic, and reactionary postural control during functional activities do you recommend for N.H.? During which activities are postural control most likely to be problematic? What apparatus, equipment, and activities might you use to assist her postural control?
- What are your concerns about seating and wheelchair mobility for N.H.? Do you think a standard wheelchair will adequately meet her needs? Do you think she will be able to propel her chair? What tasks must she master if the wheelchair will be her primary source of mobility during the preprosthetic period?
- What types of bed mobility and transfer activities are important for N.H. and her family caregivers to master? What specific intervention and patient-family education strategies will you use to help her move toward safe and, hopefully, independent performance of bed mobility and transfer activities? How will you vary environmental conditions and task demands to ensure she can adapt her strategies and skills?
- What intervention and patient-family education strategies will you use to get her up and walking? What assistive or ambulatory device do you feel would be most appropriate? Why have you chosen this particular device from among available options? What gait pattern will she use? For what other dimensions or ambulatory skills (in addition to walking forward) will you provide instruction and opportunity for N.H. to practice? How will you address the likelihood that she will experience a fall at some point in her preprosthetic period? What is "functional distance" for ambulation for N.H. and her family?
- Are there any additional interventions that would be appropriate for N.H. at this point in her postoperative, preprosthetic rehabilitation?
- How will you determine her readiness for prosthetic fitting?

Case Example 20.2c Interventions for P.G., an Individual With Recent Amputation of Both Lower Extremities Following a Construction Accident

Now 3 days postoperation, P.G. is beginning his rehabilitation in preparation for discharge to home until there is adequate healing for prosthetic fitting and prosthetic training. Pain continues to be a serious concern, generally reported as 5 or 6 out of 10 on the visual analog scale. Postoperative agitation has cleared, although P.G.'s wife reports he is more subdued in affect than usual, and she is concerned about possible depression. Low-grade temperature persists, but white cell counts are within normal limits. P.G. can actively flex and extend both knees to within 10 degrees of full ROM, with effort and a "tight pulling sensation" behind the knee, when out of his SRD for dressing changes and wound inspection. Although he reports feeling "weak as a baby" and is quickly fatigued, P.G. can use upper extremity and body strength for contact guard sliding board transfers to and from bed to a bedside chair. Moving between sitting and supine is effortful and fatiguing, but P.G. manages these transitions with occasional standby assistance. He was previously involved in aerobic and strengthening exercises at the local YMCA, but he is unsure how to use the weights and equipment now that he has lost his limbs. Plans are being made to move temporarily to his parent's home on the first floor of a three-family house (although there are six steps to reach a front porch and entryway) because it is more accessible than his third-floor walk-up apartment. In the meantime, family and friends are apartment hunting for housing that will be less challenging for P.G. in the months ahead. P.G.'s major goal is to achieve independent mobility with a wheelchair before the birth of his child.

QUESTIONS TO CONSIDER

- Given his postoperative pain and phantom sensation, what PT interventions would be appropriate at this time for P.G.? Why would these be most appropriate from among available options? What are the pros and cons of each, concerning attention, memory, and ability to learn?
- Given the status of his wound and the condition of his residual limb, what strategies for management of edema and limb shaping would you recommend? What pros and cons do you consider when deciding among options for compression and residual limb protection? Why do you think the option you selected is the most appropriate? How would this change if his amputations were at the transfemoral level?
- What strategies for intervention and patient-family education would you implement for skin care and scar management for P.G.? What issues or factors will assist or inhibit his ability to take responsibility for his skin care?
- What specific strategies for intervention and patient-family education aimed at ROM and flexibility do you recommend for P.G.? What impairments or functional limitations are you particularly concerned about? What activities will you engage him in? What positions? For what period of time? With what equipment? How would these be similar or different if his amputations were at the transfemoral level? What issues or factors will assist or inhibit his ability to take responsibility for exercises to ensure adequate ROM and flexibility in preparation for prosthetic use?
- What specific strategies for intervention and patient-family education to improve muscle performance do you recommend for P.G.? How do you address the strengthening of key muscle groups of extremities and trunk? How do you address power and muscle endurance? How do you address concentric, isometric, and eccentric control and performance? How would this be similar or different if his amputations were at the transfemoral level? What issues or factors must be considered regarding exercise tolerance, intensity, frequency, and duration during his acute care stay? How will you address his concerns about low level of aerobic fitness and conditioning?
- What specific strategies for intervention and patient-family education aimed at improving static, dynamic, and reactionary postural control during functional activities do you recommend for P.G.? During which activities is postural control most likely to be problematic? What apparatus, equipment, and activities might you use to assist his postural control?
- What are your concerns about seating and wheelchair mobility for P.G.? Do you think a standard wheelchair will adequately meet his needs? Do you think he will be able to propel his chair? What tasks does he need to master if the wheelchair will be his primary source of mobility during the preprosthetic period?
- What additional bed mobility and transfer activities do you think are important for P.G. and his family caregivers to master? What specific intervention and patient-family education strategies will you use to help him move toward safe and, hopefully, independent performance of bed mobility and transfer activities? How will you vary environmental conditions and task demands to ensure he can adapt his strategies and skills?
- How will you address the likelihood that he will experience a fall at some point in his preprosthetic period?
- Are there any additional interventions that would be appropriate for P.G. at this point in his postoperative, preprosthetic rehabilitation to assist with his coping and adjustment to his limb loss?
- How will you determine his readiness for prosthetic fitting?

Preprosthetic Outcome Assessment

Current models of healthcare practice (and reimbursement) require assessment of the efficacy of intervention that has been provided, often by comparing information collected at initial and discharge examinations. Clinicians should emphasize the importance of establishing good therapeutic alliance, including open communication, collaborative goal setting, and promotion of self-efficacy, all of which can improve clinical outcomes.[305] Several tools and measures can be used to assess outcome of intervention in the preprosthetic period; Table 20.6 provides examples of such measures. The selection of the most appropriate tools from among those available can be challenging.[306] The first consideration is to determine which "population" the tool has been designed and validated for. Some measures have been evaluated for use with older adults who are hospitalized, and others have been evaluated specifically for persons with lower-limb amputation. The next concern is the domain the tool evaluates: outcomes can be assessed at the level of body

ACTIVITY	INDICATOR
Wound Inspection	____ Individual or caregiver is able to independently inspect status of incision and residual limb
	____ Individual or caregiver is able to describe signs of inflammation, infection, dehiscence, bleeding, orecchymosis requiring contact/visit with health professional
	____ Individual or caregiver is able to effectively inspect and care for intact limb
	____ Supervision or assistance by a health professional is necessary for wound inspection and care of either residual limb or intact limb
Residual Limb Care	____ Individual or caregiver is able to change wound dressings effectively, maintaining clean environment
	____ Individual or caregiver is able to appropriately cleanse and care for residual limb
	____ Individual or caregiver is able to safely effectively self-mobilize skin around incision site
	____ Individual or caregiver is able to apply appropriate compression strategy (circle: Ace wrap, removable rigid dressing or semirigid dressing, commercial shrinker garment, other)
	____ Individual with transtibial amputation is able to maintain limb in extended knee position
Mobility	____ Individual is able to move around in bed as needed Level of assistance ________ Equipment used ________
	____ Individual is able to transition from supine to sitting and return Level of assistance ________ Equipment used ________
	____ Individual is able to transfer from bed or chair to wheelchair and return Level of assistance ________ Equipment used ________
	____ Individual is able to transfer sit to single limb standing and return Level of assistance ________ Equipment used ________
	____ Individual is able to transfer to toilet and return Level of assistance ________ Equipment used ________
	____ Individual is able to transfer to shower or tub and return Level of assistance ________ Equipment used ________
Locomotion	____ Individual is able to ambulate on level surfaces using appropriate assistive device Level of assistance ________ Assistive/ambulatory device used ________ Gait pattern ________ Distance ________ Perceived exertion ________
	____ Individual is able to ascend/descend stairs using railing and appropriate assistive device Level of assistance ________ Assistive/ambulatory device used ________ Gait pattern ________ Number of steps ________ Perceived exertion ________
	____ Individual is able to ambulate on inclines and outdoor surfaces Level of assistance ________ Assistive/ambulatory device used ________ Gait pattern ________ Distance ________ Perceived exertion ________

Fig. 20.23 Example of checklist of key patient and family knowledge and skills after lower-limb amputation.

structure and function (e.g., wound healing, limb volume); activity ability or limitation (e.g., ability to ambulate, complete ADLs); or at the level of participation (e.g., quality of life, ability to participate in meaningful social roles).[307,308] There is no single "perfect" outcome measure for preprosthetic rehabilitative care; instead the rehabilitation team should collectively select those measures that best meet the needs of the patient, therapeutic goals, and expectations of the practice environment.[309,310]

What makes a good outcome measure for preprosthetic rehabilitation? The selection of measures should be based on the primary goals of the setting in which care is provided and the specific patient-centered goals that have been defined for the individual: What concepts, functions, or attributes need to be measured? In choosing an outcome measurement tool, we look for evidence of the following:

- *Reliability:* Can we trust the numbers the tool provides? Is the tool consistent in measurement over time? Do different raters tend to come up with similar scores? How much measurement error might be present in the "score"?
- *Validity:* How well does the tool measure what it intends to measure? Is it designed for patients like the ones that we provide care for? How well do scores on the measure discriminate between persons with and without the problem the measure attempts to examine?

____ Individual is able to ambulate on inclines and outdoor surfaces
Level of assistance________________
Assistive/ambulatory device used________________
Gait pattern________________
Distance________________
Perceived exertion________________

____ Individual/caregiver is able to safely propel wheelchair functional distances
Level of assistance________________
Distance________________
Perceived exertion________________

Self-Care Activities

____ Individual is able to manage clothing during activities of daily living and dressing activities
Level of assistance________________
Positions________________
Adaptive equipment needs________________
Perceived exertion________________

____ Individual is able to manage bathing and grooming activities
Level of assistance________________
Positions________________
Adaptive equipment needs________________
Perceived exertion________________

____ Individual is able to manage key instrumetal activities of daily living
Level of assistance________________
Types of activities________________
Adaptive equipment needs________________
Perceived exertion________________

____ Sufficient and safe transportation is available
Type of transportation________________
Level of assistance________________
Equipment used________________
Perceived exertion________________

Exercise Program

____ Individual and caregiver demonstrate mastery of stretching/flexibility component of program
Positions/activities ________________
Assistance required________________
Equipment used________________
Repetitions and frequency________________

____ Individual and caregiver demonstrate mastery of strengthening component of program
Positions/activities ________________
Assistance required________________
Equipment used________________
Repetitions and frequency________________

____ Individual and caregiver demonstrate mastery of aerobic conditioning component of program
Positions/activities ________________
Assistance required ________________
Equipment used________________
Repetitions and frequency________________

____ Individual and caregiver demonstrate mastery of balance/coordination components of program
Positions/activities ________________
Assistance required________________
Equipment used________________
Repetitions and frequency________________

Follow-Up Care

____ Plans for return to surgeon for post-op visit are in place
____ Plans for continued rehabilitation care are in place
____ Additional services are in place as appropriate
Nursing________________
Dietician________________
Counseling________________
Home health________________
Others________________

Fig. 20.23, cont'd

- *Responsiveness:* How well can this measure capture change? What is the minimal change in status or function that it can predict (MDC)? Do we understand what a clinically meaningful change might be (a minimal clinically important difference)?

Summary

Early rehabilitation in the postoperative, preprosthetic period lays the foundation for prosthetic rehabilitation. Initial emphasis is placed on wound healing and control of edema, essential prerequisites for prosthetic use. Early in the process, the individual with a new amputation and family caregivers become actively involved in the rehabilitation process and decision-making, assuming responsibility for limb compression, skin care, and desensitization. As early mobility begins, the therapist is alert for postoperative medical complications, such as postural hypotension or deep venous thrombosis. The therapist implements strategies to prevent secondary impairments and functional limitations, such as further deconditioning and contracture formation. Strengthening exercises targeting the residual limb and overall fitness begin in the acute or subacute setting and continue as an aggressive home program to prepare the individual for prosthetic training. Persons with new amputations

Table 20.6 Progressive Strategies for Preparing for and Mastering Single-Limb Mobility After Amputation

Phase	Purpose	Target	Examples of Activity Progression
Preparation	Strengthening		All activities: concentric, holding, eccentric contraction All activities: intact limb and residual limb
		Hip extensors Hip interior and exterior rotators Hip abductors	Bridging; uniplanar, diagonal antigravity, with resistance Gluteal sets Hip extension in prone, in standing, adding resistance, open chain, closed chain Hip abduction side-lying, in standing, adding resistance, open chain, closed chain
		Knee extensors	Quad sets, short arc quads Sit to stand at varying heights and speeds Progressive resistive exercise Low load, high repetition (endurance) High load, low repetition (strength)
		Ankle dorsiflexors	Toe raises in standing Manual resistance of active movement
	Flexibility	Hip flexor tightness Knee flexor tightness Tensor fascia lata/iliotibial band Plantar flexor tightness	Prolonged passive stretching, positioning antigravity Thomas test position or prone Proprioceptive neuromuscular facilitation: hold-relax/contract-relax followed by concentric exercise in new ROM Active stretching in various positions
Stability in standing	Rising to standing	Control of COM during transition	Part-to-whole practice progressing to serial practice of sit-to-stand transition Scooting to edge of seating surface Forward lean with trunk extension (anterior weight shift) Weight transfer onto foot Extension into upright position Achieving stability in upright position Controlled lowering back into sitting position Practice with varying speeds Adding appropriate resistance for sensory feedback and/or strengthening Practice with higher to lower seating surfaces Practice with various seating surfaces (firm to soft chair, toilet seat, tub seat) Practice with transfers into/out of car
	Postural control in single-limb stance	Discovering limits of stability Developing postural control	Static: standing in parallel bars Bilateral upper extremity support, single upper extremity support, no upper extremity support Anticipatory: directional reaching Forward, diagonal toward stance limb, diagonal away from stance limb Throwing activities: lightweight to heavier weighted balls; forward to diagonal directions; various distances Reactionary: gentle unexpected perturbations; catching activities; lightweight to heavier weighted balls; toward body center, away from body center; various speeds and distances All activities: initially standing on firm surface, progressing to compliant surface
Mobility	Ambulation	Forward progressionChanging directionBacking upSideward stepping	In parallel bars to over ground with appropriate assistive devices Over simple (tile) surface to more challenging (carpet, grass, etc.) surfaces In closed (predictable) environment, to open (unpredictable) environment Over level surfaces, inclines (ascend and descend)
		Stair management	Bilateral railings, to railing and one crutch Low to standard height steps Provide opportunity for family caregiver to practice guarding
		Managing environmental challenges	Opening doors: away from self, toward self, weighted doors, revolving doors Managing thresholds Managing curbs Environmental scanning: avoiding obstacles in walking path Home safety evaluation Crossing the street at times crosswalks
		Fall management	At least: demonstration/observation of chair to floor, stand-to-floor transition Discussion of risk factors for falls from wheelchair, from standing, on stairs Develop plan of action should fall occur Practice chair-to-floor and stand-to-floor transitions in controlled circumstances

COM, Center of mass; *ROM*, range of motion.

are encouraged to become as independent as possible in transfers, single-limb gait, and wheelchair mobility, depending on their medical status and functional capability. As the wound heals and edema subsides, the individual with new amputation, family caregivers, therapist, prosthetist, and physician begin discussing future prosthetic rehabilitation. The postoperative, preprosthetic period is a time of transition in which many individuals mourn the loss of their limb and question their future, yet are challenged and encouraged by the possibilities offered by prosthetic replacement of their limb. If the consensus is that prosthetic fitting is not viable, the emphasis shifts to the development of wheelchair mobility skills and adaptation of the patient's environment as rehabilitation continues. Suppose the consensus is that prosthetic fitting is likely. In that case, rehabilitation during this time focuses on building the physical and psychological resources that will ensure the person with a new amputation will become a successful prosthetic user.

References

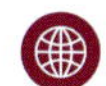

The complete listing of the References are available in the accompanying enhanced eBook version included with the print purchase of this textbook. Visit Elsevier eBooks+ (eBooks.Health.Elsevier.com) to access this content.

21 Understanding and Selecting Prosthetic Feet

MICHAEL K. CARROLL, KEVIN M. CARROLL, AND JOHN RHEINSTEIN

LEARNING OBJECTIVES

On completion of this chapter, the reader will be able to do the following:

1. Define the Medicare functional levels and how they relate to the provision of a prosthesis and prosthetic feet.
2. Explain key factors analyzed when selecting a prosthetic foot.
3. Define the fundamental characteristics of the different types of prosthetic feet.
4. Formulate a prescription recommendation for a prosthetic foot based on a person's needs.

Each person with a lower limb amputation or limb difference has unique needs that must be considered in the design of their prosthesis, especially their prosthetic foot. This selection should be made carefully because safety, performance, user satisfaction, and mobility can be impacted if the foot is not well matched to the unique needs of the user.[1] To make an effective foot selection among the multitude of choices, it is important to thoroughly consider each individual's current and potential abilities and needs. The rehabilitation team should carefully review each person's current and expected physical capabilities, prosthetic history, and goals while keeping in mind the performance, function, specifications, and appearance of available feet. Published research and evidence provide the basis for general clinical practice guidelines based on users' functional abilities and needs, but does not yet provide complete prescriptive pathways to individual foot selection.[2–4]

The aim of providing the optimal prosthetic foot is to maximize every person's rehabilitation potential so that they may reach their goals for their activities and function at a level comparable to their peers. Ideally, the function of a prosthetic foot should match that of a healthy anatomic human foot.[5] It should offer the level of shock absorption, compliance to uneven terrain, push-off, and ground clearance required by the user during the appropriate points in the gait cycle, all in a lightweight, low-maintenance package. Although modern prosthetic feet have many of these capabilities, in reality, no foot currently available matches the human foot in all these characteristics. The final choice is always a compromise because no prosthetic foot performs optimally for all activities and conditions with minimal weight and maintenance. The most appropriate foot is one that best serves the present and anticipated future unique needs of the individual. It is incumbent on the rehabilitation team to select the management strategies that (1) are consistent with each patient's needs, capabilities, and potential, (2) protect the patient from progressive overuse symptoms, and (3) avoid overuse and underuse of medical resources.

Once a foot model is selected, it must be tailored to meet the specific weight and activity level of each person so it will respond appropriately under load. If a person experiences significant changes in their weight or activity level, the foot should be replaced to match their new functional needs. For example, a weight gain of 20 or more pounds, and/or a substantial increase in activity, or loads carried may result in the foot being too compliant. Under these conditions the foot can no longer provide the necessary amount of support or energy return and may also result in catastrophic failure of the structural elements. On the contrary, decreases in weight may result in a foot that is too rigid or inflexible, creating undue forces on the user's residual limb. All the parts of a prosthetic system, especially feet, should be checked every 6 months for wear and tear, and for the presence of abrasive materials such as sand. Feet should be cleaned by the prosthetist and closely inspected for any visible cracks, splintering, or noises, as these are signs of structural failure and warnings that the foot should be replaced. It is difficult to predict the useful lifespan of a foot because of the wide range of users and the way in which they are used, but most feet have a manufacturer's warranty of 2 to 3 years covering structural components.

Factors in Selecting a Prosthetic Foot

When designing an appropriate prosthesis the rehabilitation team, in consultation with the user, should consider the following multiple factors that influence component selection. By understanding the function and features of the chosen foot, alignment and training can be targeted to maximize its functional benefits.

FUNCTIONAL LEVEL

Medicare guidelines define five functional levels (also known as "K levels") for unilateral lower limb amputees that are widely accepted by most payers. This classification system determines the medical necessity for feet and knees based on the patient's current and potential functional abilities.

Medicare policy states, *"A determination of the medical necessity for certain components/additions to the prosthesis is based on the beneficiary's potential functional abilities. Potential functional ability is based on the reasonable expectations of the prosthetist and treating physician, considering factors including, but not limited to:*

1. *The beneficiary's past history (including prior prosthetic use if applicable).*

2. *The beneficiary's current condition including the status of the residual limb and the nature of other medical problems.*
3. *The beneficiary's desire to ambulate.*

Clinical assessments of beneficiary rehabilitation potential must be based on the following classification levels:
Level 0: Does not have the ability or potential to ambulate or transfer safely with or without assistance and a prosthesis does not enhance their quality of life or mobility.
Level 1: Has the ability or potential to use a prosthesis for transfers or ambulation on level surfaces at fixed cadence. Typical of the limited and unlimited household ambulator.
Level 2: Has the ability or potential for ambulation with the ability to traverse low level environmental barriers such as curbs, stairs, or uneven surfaces. Typical of the limited community ambulator.
Level 3: Has the ability or potential for ambulation with variable cadence. Typical of the community ambulator who has the ability to traverse most environmental barriers and may have vocational, therapeutic, or exercise activity that demands prosthetic utilization beyond simple locomotion.
Level 4: Has the ability or potential for prosthetic ambulation that exceeds basic ambulation skills, exhibiting high impact, stress, or energy levels. Typical of the prosthetic demands of the child, active adult, or athlete."

The medical and prosthetic "records must document the beneficiary's current functional capabilities and their expected functional potential, including an explanation for any differences [between the current and expected level]. It is recognized, within the functional classification hierarchy, that bilateral amputees often cannot be strictly bound by functional level classifications."[6] It should also be noted that the use of a mobility aid is not a determinant in assessing functional level.

Ideally, the rehabilitation team examines and interviews the prosthetic candidate and reaches a consensus as to the potential functional level they are most likely to achieve. The key word in reaching such a decision is "potential," which challenges the team to predict future outcomes based on individual preamputation abilities, stated goals, and other unknowns. The choice of a prosthetic foot should not be based on a set formula, especially since, "Neither patient age nor amputation etiology should be viewed as primary considerations in prosthetic foot type."[2]

The user's functional classification level has real implications for the prosthetic user because it determines what type of foot they will be eligible to receive. Therefore if the rehabilitation team believes that a person currently performing at functional level K2 will reach level K3, the user should be provided with a level K3 foot. Not only does this allow the person to train with and use a foot that supports their higher activity level, but it will save cost over the long run by eliminating the need to purchase two different feet. In addition to the factors mentioned below, there are a number of performance-based and self-reported outcome measures that can assist in the determination of current and potential functionality.[7] For example, the Amputee Mobility Predictor instruments (AMPPRO and AMPnoPRO) are designed to measure ambulatory potential of lower limb amputees with or without a prosthesis.[8] The Prosthetic Limb Users Survey of Mobility is a self-report instrument for measuring mobility of adults with lower limb amputation and can also be used to compare an individual with other amputees and to monitor a person's progress and satisfaction over time.[9,10]

ACTIVITIES OF DAILY LIVING, VOCATIONAL, AND WORK REQUIREMENTS

It is rare that a single foot meets a person's needs in all situations. By determining the entirety of their current and future activities, a balance of performance features can be achieved. For example, for someone who works in an office during the week and who also plays golf on weekends, a foot with a multiaxial ankle would be recommended to accommodate uneven terrain.

BODY WEIGHT

Foot sizes and strengths are available for people ranging from infants to adults weighing up to 500 pounds. A small prosthetic foot for children is shown in Fig. 21.1. As the population becomes increasingly overweight, manufacturers are offering prosthetic feet for those heavier individuals.[11] A prosthetic foot expected to support heavier weights must be specially crafted for increased strength and durability; consequently, the prosthesis itself is larger and heavier because of the additional materials included in the foot, pylon, and socket required for structural integrity. The user's weight should be measured and recorded at every encounter to ensure that their foot is still appropriately matched.

Obesity makes prosthetic fitting more difficult, however, being overweight does not preclude the use of a prosthesis. While body mass is a contributing variable when predicting prosthesis user success, it alone should not be used as a predictor of failure for any outcome parameter.[12] Even people weighing more than 300 pounds should not give up hope. Although initially confined to a nursing home bed, rehabilitation teams that work with overweight individuals can fit them with a prosthesis, assist them with standing, begin therapy, and within just a few months have the same bedridden patients walking on their own. It is common for functional K1 level patients to progress to K2 level with

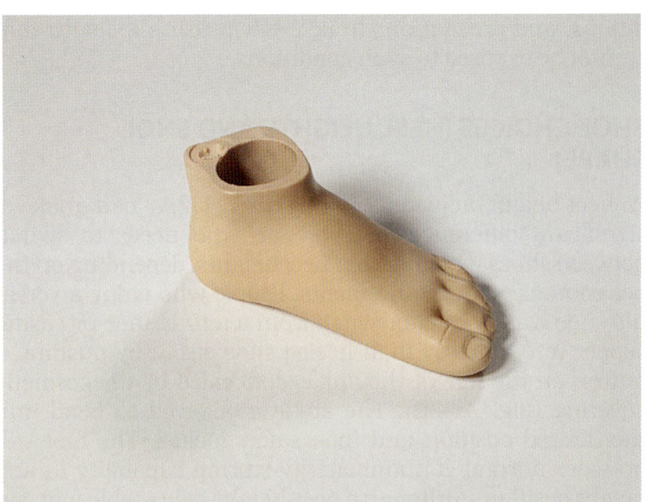

Fig. 21.1 A very small children's foot. (Courtesy Hanger Clinic, Austin, Texas.)

appropriate care and therapy. People are often deconditioned from the illnesses that precipitated their amputation and can make great strides as long as they are motivated to do the physical and occupational therapy needed to succeed.

RESIDUAL LIMB

Foot selection can bear directly on the health of the person's residual limb. Ground reaction forces that are transmitted through a person's body can be stressful or damaging to their residual limb, knee, hip, and/or back.[2] People with short or painful residual limbs are generally fit with feet that are softer to attenuate ground force transmission through the prosthesis. Choosing a foot with compliant heel action, vertical shock absorption, or articulating features can also reduce these impact forces.

COMORBIDITIES

Comorbid health conditions such as diabetes and peripheral vascular disease should be considered relevant only to foot selection to the degree to which they affect a person's functional abilities. Keep in mind that patients are often deconditioned from weight-bearing restrictions prior to amputation and can recover once they receive a prosthesis and physical therapy.

The deflection dynamics and alignment of a foot can affect the health and well-being of a person's joints. "Patients at elevated risks for overuse injury (i.e., osteoarthritis) to the sound side lower limb and lower back are indicated for an energy storage and return (ESAR) foot to reduce the magnitude of the cyclical vertical impacts experienced during weight acceptance."[2]

ENVIRONMENTAL EXPOSURE AND DURABILITY

People regularly in extreme environments need a foot that will not fail under harsh conditions. An additional, specially designed prosthesis with a solid foot or drain holes should be provided for water use if it is regularly needed for bathing, swimming, or water sports. Sand and dirt are especially destructive to feet. Users should be instructed on how to clean their prosthesis after exposure to abrasive or wet conditions, and precautions to take when using a device that cannot be exposed to such conditions.

SHOE CHOICES (HEEL HEIGHTS AND SHOE SHAPE)

A heel-height–adjustable foot (Fig. 21.2A) can make a significant difference for someone who needs to switch between shoes with different heel heights, depending on the occasion or work requirements. People who enjoy a versatile shoe wardrobe can switch from a tennis shoe or casual slipper into a dressy high-heeled shoe easily, by pushing a button on the side of the ankle, concealed by the cosmetic covering (Fig. 21.2B). The ankle is allowed to bend into the desired position and then safely locked. The foot still provides normal gait and energy-storing capability in any height position. Although a heel-height–adjustable foot can flatten for barefoot walking, the rubber foot shell will wear out quickly if it is used without a shoe. A prosthesis without

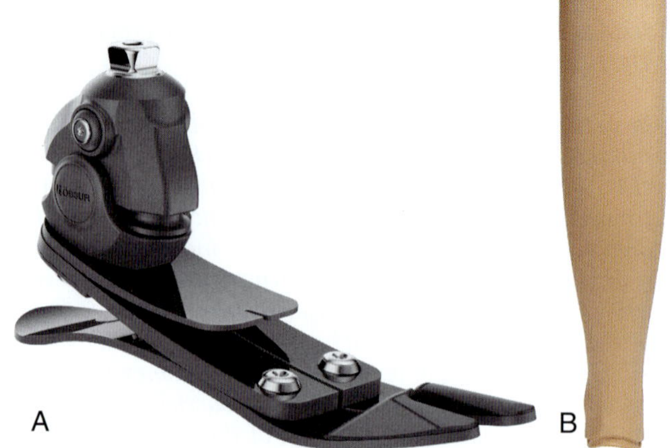

Fig. 21.2 (A) Heel height–adjustable foot. (B) Cover for foot. (© Össur.)

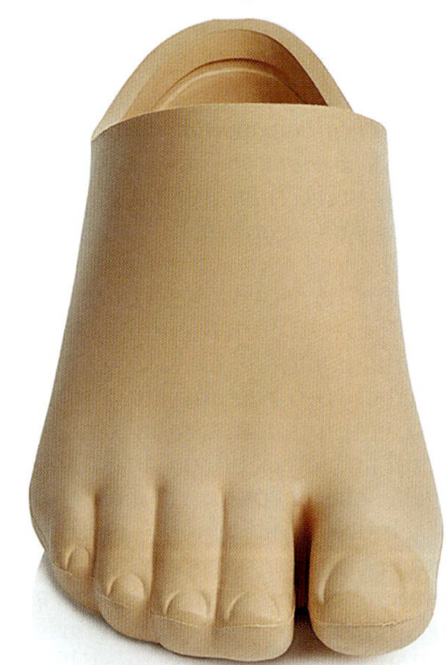

Fig. 21.3 Foot cover with split toes. (Courtesy Hanger Clinic, Austin, Texas.)

a heel-height–adjustable mechanism cannot be worn with shoes of different heel heights unless adjustment wedges are placed in the shoes to make the effective heel height the same among all the user's shoes. It is important to note, that when a heel wedge is added to the prosthetic side shoe, another must be added to the contralateral side to avoid changing the overall length of the prosthesis. However, a wedge may be added under the ball of the prosthetic foot with no effect on the overall length. Wedges >1.27 cm (0.5 in) should be avoided to ensure adequate footwear suspension and to limit rubbing on the contralateral heel.

Seasonal changes in shoes are also important; providing a split between the big toe and second toe may not seem important in the fall or winter but is very noticeable in the summer when the user wants to wear thong sandals (Fig. 21.3).

If a prosthetic foot is too wide, it may prove difficult to get into a shoe, and a foot that is too narrow may move around in the shoe causing instability. Asking the person to bring to the clinic all the shoes that they intend to wear can reduce uncertainty about foot size and shape. Individuals who have been prescribed a diabetic shoe should be encouraged to wear only those shoes.

INTERACTION WITH OTHER PROSTHETIC COMPONENTS

The foot is part of a closed chain in which ground reaction forces are transmitted through the prosthesis. The characteristics of the foot will affect the way a prosthetic or anatomic knee and hip joint respond to ground forces. For example, a foot with a stiff heel will send more flexion force to the knee at heel strike causing less knee stability. In addition, the anterior/posterior and medial/lateral placement, transverse rotation, and the dorsi-plantarflexion alignment of a foot relative to the prosthetic socket affect the way it feels to the wearer and the resulting gait. For example, moving a foot anterior relative to a prosthetic socket or plantarflexing it increases forefoot stiffness and support while simultaneously decreasing heel stiffness and support, which may lead to hyperextension of the knee. Alignment changes can cause shifts in socket pressures on a user's residual limb. Additionally, a prosthesis that is too short or long may cause back pain, a common ailment within the lower limb amputee community.[13] Prosthetic feet that have too high a category for the patient's weight will result in an inflexible foot. Excessive toe stiffness can cause the foot to behave similar to a poorly aligned foot system. Small alignment and component changes can produce dramatic shifts in the biomechanics of a prosthesis and should be undertaken with care under the guidance of a certified prosthetist.

PRIOR PROSTHETIC FEET AND GAIT HABITS

People who have become accustomed to the characteristics of a particular foot over many years may have difficulty adapting to a different one. Users using a broken foot often become acclimated to using an excessively flexible foot and when provided with a correctly functioning foot feel it is too rigid in comparison. When a change is warranted and implemented, a period of adjustment is expected. Users may benefit from physical therapy any time a new prosthesis, foot, or component is provided. Exercises and gait training for balance, weight transfer, and loading and releasing the forefoot should be tailored to the functional dynamics of the user's gait while using the prosthesis.[14]

PSYCHOLOGICAL INFLUENCES AND PERSONALITY TRAITS

The wearer's age has less to do with the choice of prosthesis than the wearer's attitude. For example, an 80-year-old might be running marathons, whereas a 45-year-old with less determination remains wheelchair bound. The difference may lie solely in their state of mind. A prosthesis wearer's personal preferences, practical goals, and lofty ambitions should all be considered when selecting a foot. Many people are able to expand their capabilities and motivation dramatically once they are fit with an appropriate prosthesis that allows them to improve their range of activities. Peer support can be an important element in helping to motivate someone who is not progressing to their potential.[15]

SKIN TONE

Most of the feet described in this chapter are available with a rubber cover, commonly referred to as a foot shell, that gives the appearance of an anatomic foot, while supporting and protecting the structural elements of the prosthetic foot. Current foot shells have a more natural appearance and greater durability than their predecessors, but they will still wear out faster than the structural element of the foot and thus should be checked every 6 months and replaced as needed. Most have toes and are available in three basic flesh tones. Flexible protective cosmetic covers can also be added over the prosthesis which closely approximate each person's skin tone.

COST

In general, higher-functional-level feet cost more; however, people with higher function and who fall less as a result of an appropriate prosthesis will likely incur less overall medical cost. Work by Dobson et al. found that those fit with a prosthesis "were more likely to receive extensive outpatient therapy," which significantly reduced the likelihood of "acute care hospitalizations, emergency room admissions, and ... facility-based care" almost eliminating the cost of the prosthesis after just 1 year.[16] More recently, researchers found that expeditious access to a prosthesis reduces reliance on emergency departments as well as the overall healthcare cost for users by approximately $25,000 after accounting for the cost of the prosthesis, indicating considerable savings.[17,18] Foot choices may be limited by insurance coverage and the person's ability to afford higher functioning feet.

BILATERAL LIMB LOSS

People missing both legs at the same amputation level generally receive a matched pair of feet. Outcomes for individuals with bilateral transfemoral amputations are improved if they are first trained to use very short prostheses with small rigid feet known as "stubbies."[19,20]

OSSEOINTEGRATION

Prosthesis users who use bone-anchored prostheses following an osseointegration surgery have similarly unique needs. Special attention must be given to ensure compliance with instructions from both the implant manufacturer and surgical team regarding foot selection, alignment, and the rehabilitation process.

Due to the direct nature of the prosthesis-skeletal attachment, there is no play between the foot and the rest of the prosthesis, as there is with a traditional socket. Because of this rigidity, many prosthetic feet do not have adequate transverse motion to prevent excessive forces on the osseointegrated implant. Users with these systems may benefit from the addition of a torsion element to their prosthesis or a prosthetic foot with integrated transverse rotation. Power-generating prosthetic feet and components should be avoided due to the potential force they generate, and to comply with implant manufacturer guidelines.[21]

All of the factors mentioned previously should be considered when narrowing the selection of appropriate prosthetic choices. It is important to thoroughly discuss with the person the choices available to them. Everyone on the rehabilitation team should understand the person's wishes and their plans for future or potential activities. Each person has different values as to what is important to them. Many manufacturers have short trial periods during which a foot can be returned if it is not working well for the wearer.

Performance Features and Appearance of Available Prosthetic Feet

FUNCTIONAL LEVEL K1 FEET

The solid-ankle, cushion-heel (SACH) (Fig. 21.4) foot is the most basic prosthetic foot commercially available. It is recommended only for those with limited functional ability and potential to ambulate. The SACH foot is provided primarily for transfers and limited ambulation. This foot's immovable ankle and soft heel give it the ability to absorb the impact of heel strike but provides minimal energy return and anterior support. There are numerous manufacturers who produce a version of the SACH foot that is simply crafted from a wooden or plastic block with a soft cushion under the heel segment and rubber toes. Because the SACH foot has no moving parts, little maintenance is required until the foot is worn out, at which time it should be replaced. However, no device is indestructible, and, with our increasingly overweight society, care should be taken to provide a foot with the appropriate category that matches the person's measured weight and activity level to avoid damage or failure. A carbon composite foot (see "Functional Level K3 Feet" later) may be required if a SACH foot cannot adequately support an extremely heavy-weight person. Single-axis feet with a pivoting ankle joint are also appropriate for functional level K1 ambulators. A recent Clinical Practice Guideline consolidated available evidence and recommended that, "For patients ambulating at a single speed that require greater stability during weight acceptance due to weak knee extensors or poor balance, a single-axis foot should be considered."[2] By moving quickly from heel strike to foot flat, less force is transmitted to the user's residual limb and to their knee, which makes their prosthesis more stable than with a SACH foot. Single-axis feet have moving parts and require periodic maintenance. Physical therapy training for patients using K1 feet should focus on taking short, controlled steps for safety.

FUNCTIONAL LEVEL K2 FEET

There is an array of different feet suitable for people with amputation at functional level 2, capable of walking inside their homes and outside in the community at a slow pace (Fig. 21.5). Most level 2 feet are lightweight, have a flexible keel and a multiaxial ankle, and provide some energy return. A full-length toe mechanism lends stability while providing smooth transitioning from heel strike to toe-off. These feet typically have foam-rubber cushions that assist the wearer with soft plantarflexion by providing a smooth transition from heel strike to midstance. The feet also allow for some transverse rotation. The flexibility of the ankle on most of these feet can be softened or stiffened by changing the rubber cushions. More features and adjustments also mean that more attention and maintenance must be provided. People at functional level K2 should be reassessed regularly by the rehabilitation team to determine whether they can progress to functional level K3. Additional physical therapy, peer support, or motivation may be all that is needed to push them to the next level. Physical therapy training for patients using K2 feet should focus on getting to foot flat early in the gait cycle as well as single leg standing for balance.

FUNCTIONAL LEVEL K3 FEET

Functional level 3 feet are appropriate for people with the ability or potential to perform daily activities beyond simple locomotion and to walk with variable cadence. Known as ESAR, these feet are fabricated from lightweight flexible materials such as carbon fiber and fiberglass, which are very responsive, lightweight, and extremely durable. Compared with a SACH foot, they reduce energy consumption, offer increased ankle motion, reduce sound side loading, and store and return more energy. ESAR feet should be considered for patients at elevated risks for overuse injuries. Individuals walking at faster speeds are subjected to higher

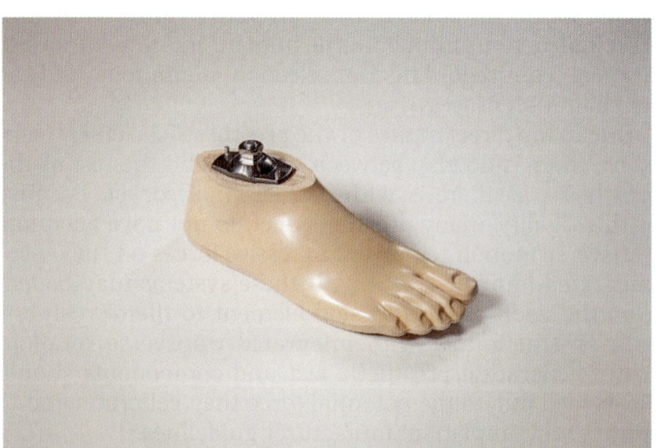

Fig. 21.4 K1 functional level foot: the solid-ankle, cushion-heel foot. (Courtesy Hanger Clinic, Austin, Texas.)

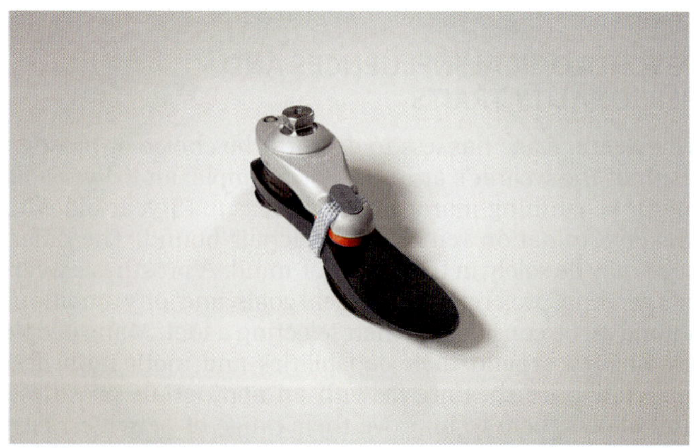

Fig. 21.5 K2 functional level foot. Ottobock 1M10. (Courtesy Hanger Clinic, Austin, Texas.)

ground reaction forces and can benefit from the way ESAR feet reduce the magnitude of the cyclical vertical impacts experienced during weight acceptance.[2] Initial studies indicate that fiberglass feet offer additional power generation over carbon fiber feet.[22] There are numerous designs available in this category, which vary based on the shape of the carbon fiber or fiberglass and the addition of other materials to absorb shock and rotational forces. They can be fitted with or without an integrated pylon. Although most are designed with no moving parts and need little maintenance, carbon fiber and fiberglass feet should be checked every 6 months for wear and tear, as well as to (1) clean out or replace the foot shell, (2) replace the inner protective spectra sock, and (3) determine if the foot still meets the needs, weight, and activity level of the wearer. Physical therapy training for patients using K3 feet should focus on loading the prosthetic toe at the end of midstance to get the maximum energy return from the foot.

The integrated pylon foot (Fig. 21.6) is the lightest of all foot prostheses. It is one continuous composite material unit from the toe to the top of the pylon, with a separate heel segment. Plantarflexion and dorsiflexion are achieved by deflection of the structural material of the foot. Some of these feet also provide inversion/eversion by way of a longitudinal split that bisects the foot, a urethane cushion, or a floating sole plate. These feet cannot be used for individuals with long residual limbs due to the extended build height. In addition, alignment capabilities are somewhat limited by the integrated pylon foot as adjustments can be made only just below the socket rather than at the ankle. Alignment wedges can be added to the foot or shoe to compensate for this shortcoming.

Energy-storing feet without the integrated pylon (Fig. 21.7) offer the same features as those described previously and are more likely to be indicated for those individuals with long residual limbs. They also allow the prosthetist to perform alignment adjustments at the ankle where the foot is joined to a separate pylon.

Feet with shock and torsion absorption are especially important for high-activity people, those performing repetitive motions, and those using osseointegrated prostheses. These features reduce the vertical and sheer forces that are transmitted to the residual limb by allowing these motions to take place in the foot rather than inside the socket (Fig. 21.8). Hydraulic damping is another ankle feature that permits increased fluidity of sagittal plane movement and is available in both level K2 and K3 versions (Fig. 21.9).

Microprocessor feet are the most recent development in prosthetic foot technology and have opened an exciting new spectrum of possibilities for many people with lower extremity amputation. In contrast to traditional prosthetic feet which are passive, microprocessor feet actively respond and adapt to changes in the environment such as changes in inclines, walking speed, and shoes. If the wearer ascends an incline, the foot automatically provides dorsiflexion and continues to do so for the extent of the incline. Similarly, the foot automatically responds with plantarflexion during the descent on a downhill grade. The Freedom Innovations—Kinex, Blatchford Élan, Össur Proprio, and Ottobock Meridium all perform these functions (Fig. 21.10A–D).

Microprocessor feet are heavier than most other feet. They are powered by an onboard battery that requires

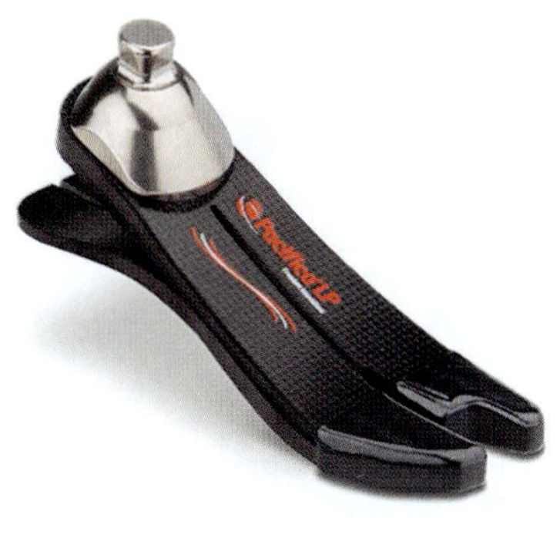

Fig. 21.7 K3 functional level foot with integrated pyramid—Össur LP Pro-Flex LP. (Courtesy Össur, Foothill Ranch, California.)

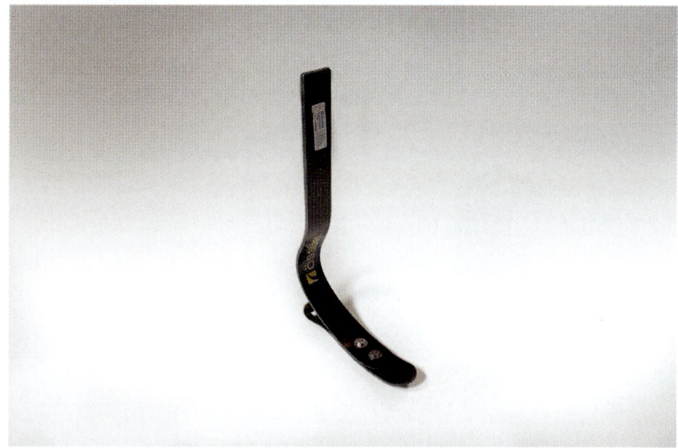

Fig. 21.6 K3 functional level foot with integrated pylon—Össur Variflex. (Courtesy Hanger Clinic, Austin, Texas.)

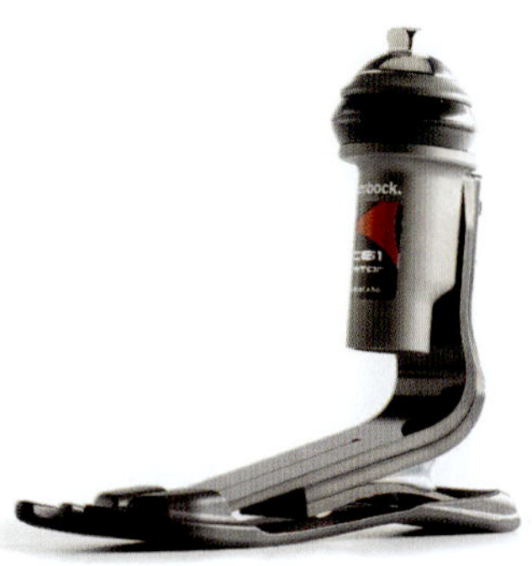

Fig. 21.8 K3 dynamic response foot with vertical shock and torque absorption—Ottobock Triton VS. (Courtesy Ottobock HealthCare, www.ottobockus.com.)

nightly recharging. The range of motion of microprocessor feet is thus far limited to this single-axis capability, though most feature a split toe design providing inversion and eversion flexibility that conforms to varied terrain. They are indicated for functional level 3 users who encounter inclines in their activities of daily living. Contraindications for microprocessor feet are very high activity, heavy body weight, and frequent exposure to dirt and extremes of temperature. Some of these feet offer a level of water resistance, but few are waterproof. This should be considered if the user frequently encounters aquatic environments.

While most microprocessor feet are adaptive in that they respond to varied terrains and gait, the Empower Ankle is the only available microprocessor foot designed to actively replace the propulsive function of the gastrocsoleus muscles (Fig. 21.10E). This foot generates power during plantarflexion, propelling the person forward. Research demonstrated a significant reduction in metabolic cost, which allows people with amputation to walk with less energy and better gait symmetry.[23] In spite of these benefits, adoption has been slow due to the high weight and cost of this foot. Additionally, some clinicians are reluctant to provide such feet out of a concern that the technology may be too arduous for some users, especially those who are older. Age should not be a limiter for access to these systems, but instead the user should be evaluated for their likelihood to accept and benefit from this technology.[24]

While not strictly impacting biomechanical functionality of the prosthetic foot, a number of feet feature integrated pumps designed to generate vacuum from the motion of walking for elevated vacuum sockets (Fig. 21.11). These sockets provide volume management and reduce movement between the residual limb and the socket.[25]

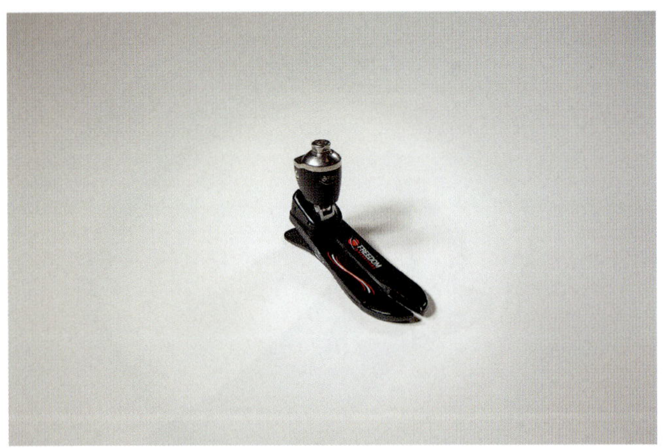

Fig. 21.9 Foot with hydraulic ankle—Proteor Kinterra. (Courtesy Hanger Clinic, Austin, Texas.)

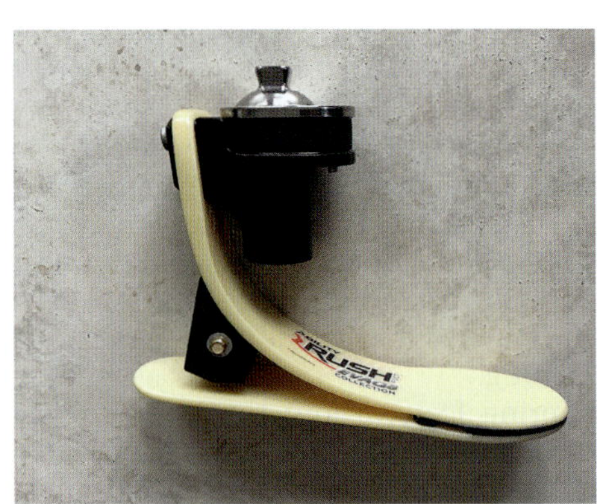

Fig. 21.11 Foot with integrated vacuum pump—RUSH—EVA. (Courtesy Hanger Clinic, Austin, Texas.)

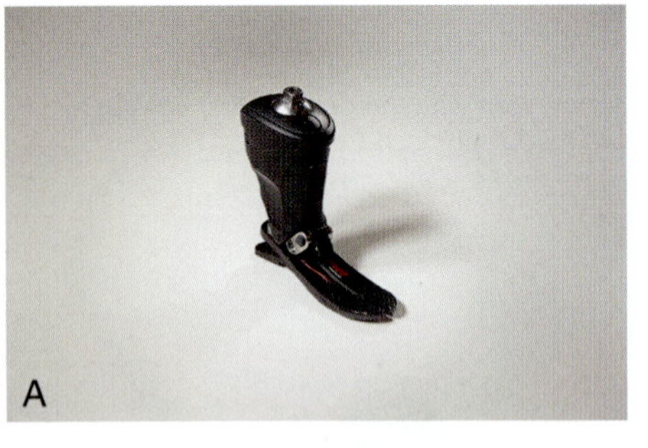
A

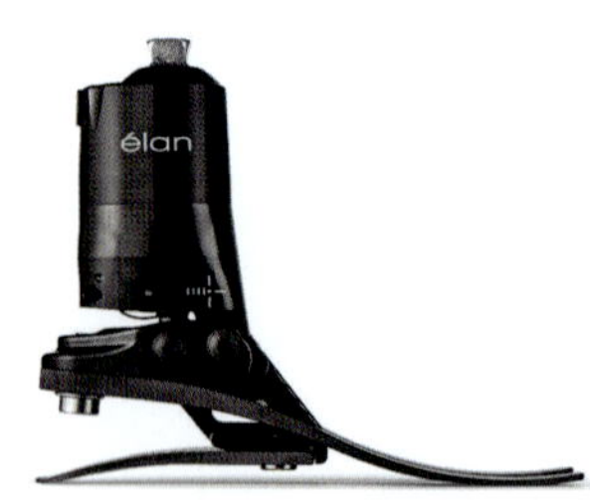

B

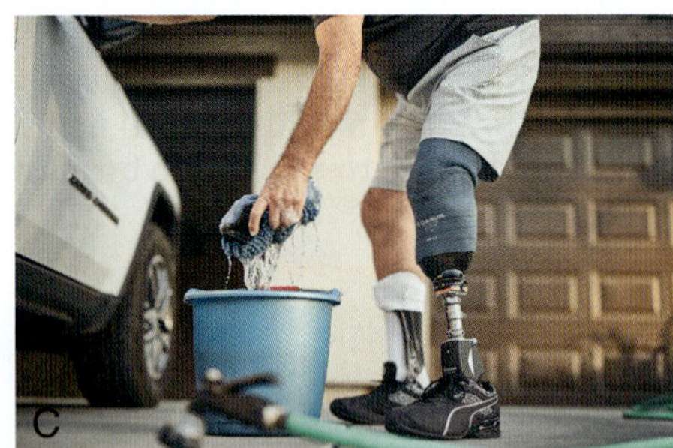
C

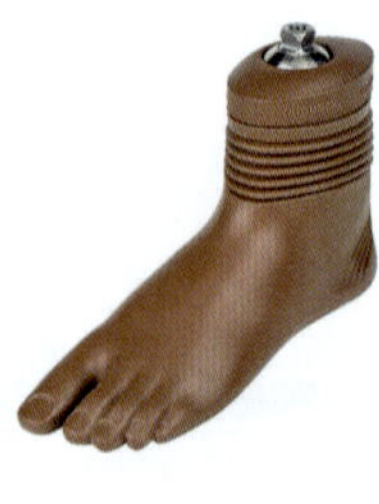
D

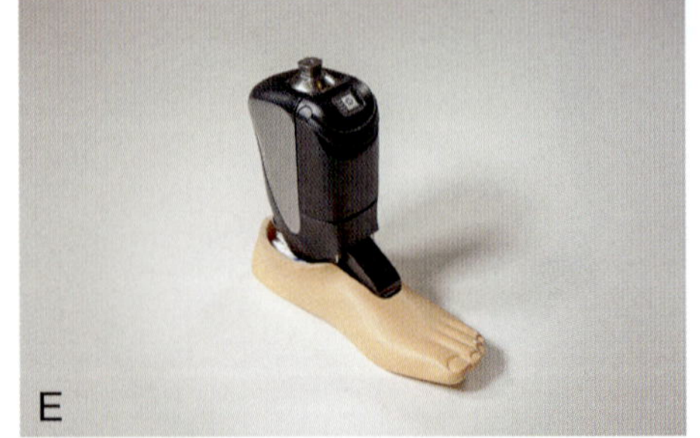
E

Fig. 21.10 Microprocessor feet. (A) Freedom Innovations—Kinex. (Courtesy Freedom Innovations, Irvine, California.) (B) Blatchford Élan. (Courtesy Blatchford, blatchford.co.uk.) (C) Össur Proprio. (© Össur, ossur.com.) (D) Ottobock Meridium. (Courtesy Ottobock HealthCare, **www.ottobockus.com**.) (E) Ottobock Empower Ankle. (Courtesy Ottobock HealthCare, **www.ottobockus.com**.)

FUNCTIONAL LEVEL K4: HIGH ACTIVITY AND SPECIALIZED FEET

A number of specialized prosthetic feet are available for the serious athlete and weekend warriors. Sprinting feet are designed for powerful bursts of speed, such as in a 100-m or 200-m race (Fig. 21.12). They do not have a heel component. Running feet are softer than sprinting feet for longer distance running up to marathon or half-marathon challenges and may have a heel (Fig. 21.13A and B). Choice of design depends on the person's activities and special interests. Running, sprinting, and activity-specific feet are not recommended for everyday wear, thus users will require a daily-use foot. Running feet are also available for children (Fig. 21.14). Specialized activity feet are available for a variety of sports (Fig. 21.15A–C). A swim foot is available that can be locked in plantarflexion for use with a swim fin. A short, rigid rock-climbing foot is designed for use with a specialized climbing shoe, and a skiing foot clips directly into the binding without a ski boot.

Summary

Selecting the most appropriate prosthetic foot can be a complex clinical decision because of a variety of factors, including a person's current and potential functional level, specific needs, the wide array of available choices, and cost. A miscalculation in the selection process can make a significant difference in outcome and level of success. Rehabilitation team professionals, together with the wearer, family members, and caregivers, should analyze and evaluate the best prosthetic options for advancing mobility that is functional, efficient, practical, and safe for people with lower extremity amputation. Advances in energy-storing materials and microprocessor technology offer people with lower extremity amputation improved function in daily activities as well as high-activity performance in sports, such as: running, swimming, golfing, biking, hiking, skiing, and rock climbing.

ACKNOWLEDGMENT

Thank you to Laura Rheinstein and Phil Stevens for their editorial assistance. Thank you to Elicia Pollard for her contributions to a previous version of this chapter.

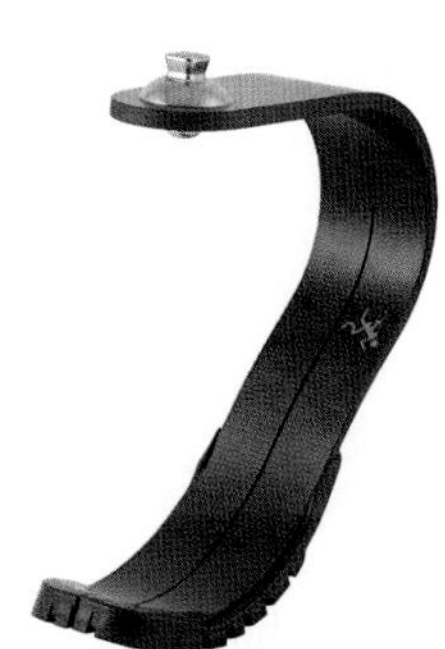

Fig. 21.12 Fillauer running blade. (Courtesy Fillauer Companies, Inc, Chattanooga, Tennessee.)

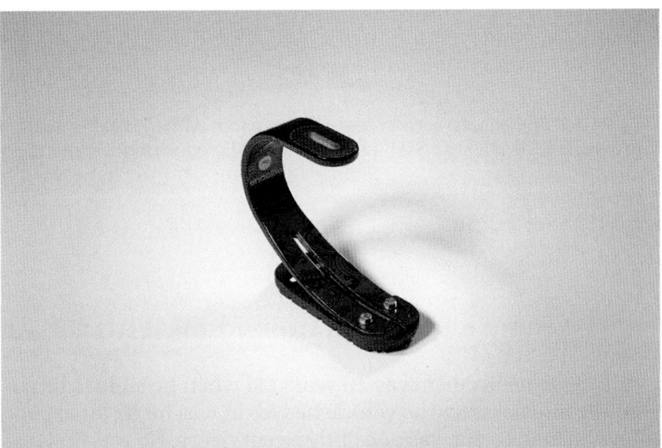

Fig. 21.14 Pediatric running foot. (Courtesy Hanger Clinic, Austin, Texas.)

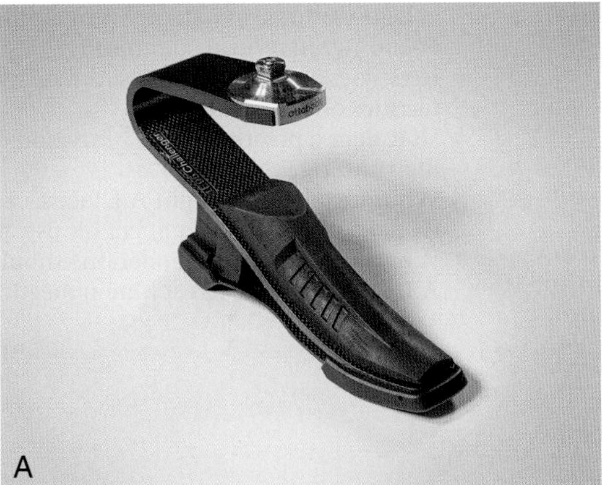

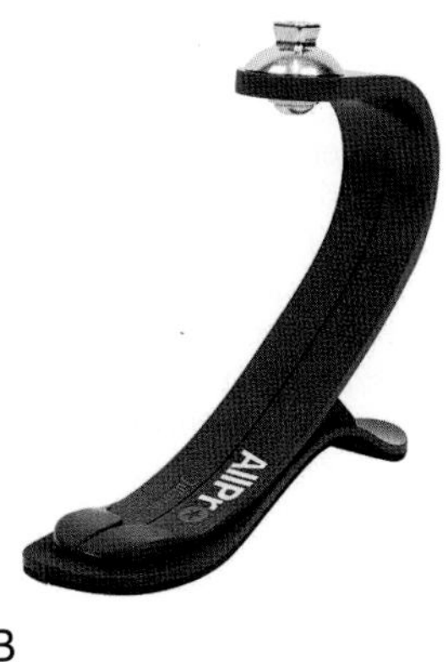

A B

Fig. 21.13 Running feet. (A) Ottobock Challenger. (Courtesy Ottobock HealthCare, www.ottobockus.com). (B) Fillauer allPro. (Courtesy Fillauer Companies, Inc, Chattanooga, Tennessee.)

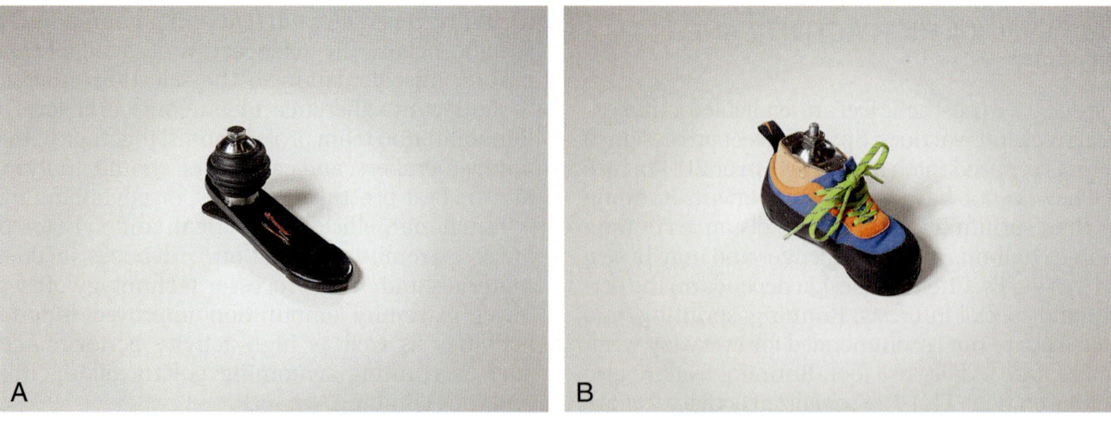

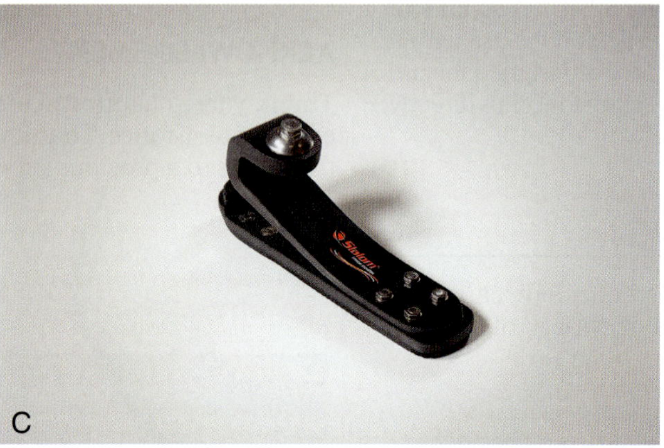

Fig. 21.15 **Specialized activity feet. (A) Swim foot with moveable ankle.** (Courtesy Freedom Innovations, Irvine, California.) **(B) Adult climbing foot.** (Courtesy TRS, Inc., Boulder, CO.) (C) Skiing foot. (Courtesy Freedom Innovations, Irvine, California.)

Case Example 21.1 **An Individual With a Transtibial Amputation**

A.J., a former soldier, was 20 years old when he endured traumatic injuries after the vehicle he was in was hit by an explosive ordnance. He was one of three survivors. He was flown to a hospital for emergency surgery and later transferred to a stateside medical and rehabilitation center. He severely injured his left leg, incurred damage to his right tympanic membrane, and lost his left thumb. After multiple surgeries, bone infection in his left leg, and months of rehabilitation, doctors decided to amputate his leg at the transtibial level. A.J. was offered an honorable discharge because of his injuries. He accepted the discharge and returned to his hometown where he continued rehabilitation.

In high school, he had been a competitive athlete for his track team, and he maintained an average weight of 180 pounds during his military service. One year after the accident, the 5-foot 11-inches-tall former soldier weighs 206 pounds and is ambulating independently with a transtibial prosthesis. A.J. has accepted the loss of his left leg and is ready to return to a "normal" life. He is determined to run again and plans to enroll at a local college. He currently lives with his mother in a small one-story house in a rural community and has not driven a vehicle since the accident.

QUESTIONS TO CONSIDER

- To what extent would A.J.'s age, height, weight, and lifestyle impact the selection and maintenance of a prosthetic foot?
- What prosthetic foot design would be most appropriate for athletic challenges?
- What environmental challenges might A.J. encounter on a college campus? What environmental challenges might he encounter in a rural community?
- How does a prosthetic foot simulate the functional characteristics of a human foot?
- How does a prosthetic foot's function during gait differ during running?
- What social issues might A.J. face as he enters college? How would a prosthetic foot affect his psychosocial health?
- What specific recommendations should be given to meet A.J.'s needs and to assist him in meeting his goals?

Case Example 21.2 An Older Adult With Amputation Due to Infected Nonhealing Neuropathic Ulcer

Mrs. R.T. is a 79-year-old female with long-standing diabetes and peripheral artery disease who developed a neuropathic ulcer at the first metatarsal head of her right forefoot 6 months ago. Despite conservative attempts to heal the wound using a total contact cast and subsequent vascular bypass surgery to restore blood flow to the distal extremity, the wound failed to heal and osteomyelitis developed. Mrs. R.T. underwent standard transtibial amputation 2 months ago and managed postoperatively with removable rigid dressing to protect the surgical site and control postoperative edema. Although the surgical incision was slow to heal, her surgeon has determined that it is now safe to begin prosthetic training, and she has been referred for prosthetic prescription.

Until the development of her neuropathic ulcer, Mrs. R.T. lived independently in a second-floor apartment of an urban retirement community in a small city, drove her own car to a nearby park to walk for exercise at least three times each week, and participated in many activities at her local senior center. Since her surgery, she has been living with her daughter in a nearby suburb, using a wheelchair (propelling it herself) for mobility, and receiving home care physical therapy to build her strength and endurance. She reports that she is able to transfer between bed and wheelchair independently but requires assistance to get into and out of the car. She looks forward to receiving a prosthesis but wonders if she will have the ability to return to community ambulation without the need of an assistive device.

Mrs. R.T. is 5 feet, 3 inches tall, and weighs 150 pounds. She admits that her memory "is not what it used to be" and has recently been diagnosed with mild cognitive impairment, but she has no clinical signs of dementia. She has significant osteoarthritis of her fingers and wrists, as well as in both of her hips.

QUESTIONS TO CONSIDER

- To what extent would Mrs. R.T.'s age, height, weight, and lifestyle impact the selection and maintenance of a prosthetic foot?
- What K level best reflects Mrs. R.T.'s functional potential? Why have you selected this K level?
- What prosthetic foot design would be most appropriate for Mrs. R.T.'s first prosthesis?
- What environmental challenges might Mrs. R.T. encounter if she is able to resume her preulcer activities? How might the challenges be similar or different in an urban versus suburban community?
- How does the prosthetic foot that you have chosen simulate the functional characteristics of a human foot?
- What are the effects of a prosthetic foot on gait?
- What specific recommendations should be given to meet Mrs. R.T.'s needs and assist her in meeting her goals?

References

The complete listing of the References are available in the accompanying enhanced eBook version included with the print purchase of this textbook. Visit Elsevier eBooks+ (eBooks.Health.Elsevier.com) to access this content.

22 Postsurgical Management of Partial Foot and Syme Amputation

STEVEN BROWN AND JONATHAN DAY

LEARNING OBJECTIVES

On completion of this chapter, the reader will be able to do the following:

1. Differentiate among the various joint disarticulation and transosseous surgeries used when amputation of the forefoot, midfoot, or rearfoot is necessary.
2. Describe gait performance and limitations of individuals with a partial foot and with Syme amputations.
3. Compare the advantages and disadvantages of prosthetic options for individuals with partial foot amputation.
4. Compare the advantages and disadvantages of the various prosthetic designs for persons with Syme amputation, including donning and pressure tolerance.
5. Compare how the various nonarticulating and dynamic response Syme prosthetic feet mimic the three rockers of gait.
6. Describe typical static and dynamic alignment variables or issues affecting gait for patients with a Syme or partial foot prosthesis.
7. Use knowledge of prosthetic options to suggest prosthetic prescriptions and plans of care for patients with partial foot and Syme amputation.

Partial foot and Syme amputations present advantages and challenges to the patient and the rehabilitation team. Preservation of the ankle and heel (in partial foot amputation) and most of the length of the lower limb (in Syme amputation) have an important advantage of distal weight-bearing capability: the individual with partial foot or Syme amputation is often able to ambulate without a prosthesis if necessary. However, the prosthesis provides protection for the vulnerable distal residual limb for patients with vascular compromise and neuropathy.

The length and shape of the residual limb present three challenges for successful fitting and prosthetic training for patients with partial foot or Syme amputation: suspension of the prosthesis on the residual limb, distribution of weight-bearing forces within the prosthesis, and attachment and alignment of the prosthetic foot. Improved communication combined with patient-centered care can have a positive influence on patient acceptance and adherence of prosthetic treatment.[1] This chapter defines the most common partial foot and Syme amputations and reviews the prosthetic management options currently available. Also identified are specific indications and contraindications for the various prosthetic designs.

Presurgical Considerations

Surgeons are tasked with the responsibility of determining the level of amputation based on each patient's specific circumstances and functional needs. Basic physics and biomechanics support a more distal amputation as functionally superior to a more proximal amputation. Therefore, surgeons must determine the most distal level of amputation with a reasonable expectation to heal after surgery. Vascular studies and clinical judgment are both used to select the most appropriate level of amputation. Additionally, several factors have been identified that are known to predict wound healing complications after amputation surgery. These factors include patient habits (smoking); comorbid status (poorly controlled diabetes); and metabolic factors (low albumin) among others.[2] Transmetatarsal amputations performed in patients with diabetes heal more predictably with a higher serum albumin.[3] Amputations performed without improving these factors have a predictably high failure rate and increased risk of readmission and revision amputation. Preoperative bloodwork should be used to optimize the patient's health and potential to heal prior to an elective amputation surgery.[2,4]

Pediatric Considerations

Skeletally immature patients present additional risks for predictable complications after amputation surgery. Preamputation surgical planning should consider the skeletally immature patient's increase risk for exostosis when bone is transected. A surgeon should try to incorporate disarticulation levels of amputation and avoid transecting bone when performing amputations in children. Surgeons should also consider the role epiphysiodesis could play in creating space for optimal prosthetic components over time while the child is still growing.[5] Additionally, amputation has a higher patient satisfaction rating compared to limb salvage for fibular hemimelia.[6]

Partial Foot Amputations

The incidence of partial foot amputation has been stable or increasing in developed countries worldwide. Partial foot amputation increased from 2006 to 2012 in one Philidelphia county.[7] National registry data in Sweden showed no change from 2008 to 2017 in the incidence of partial foot amputations.[8] Whereas, Germany and Finland data showed increases in partial foot amputations from 2015 to 2019 and 1997 to 2018 respectively.[9,10] Until the advent of antibiotics, disarticulation through the joints of the foot reduced the risk of sepsis and shock and improved the prognosis for healing compared with amputations that transected bone. The earliest partial foot amputation was recorded in 434 BCE by the Greek historian Herodotus,[11] who told of a Persian warrior who escaped death while in the stocks by disarticulating his own foot. He hobbled 30 miles to a nearby town, where he was nursed to health until he could construct a prosthesis for himself. Later he became a soothsayer for the Persian army but ultimately was recaptured by the Spartans and killed.

At present, distal partial foot amputations include a wide variety of ray resections, digit (phalangeal) amputations, and metatarsal transections (Fig. 22.1). Midfoot amputations include surgical ablation at the Chopart and Lisfranc levels (Fig. 22.2).[12] Chopart disarticulation involves the talocalcaneonavicular joint and separates the talus and navicular, as well as the calcaneus and cuboid.[13] Distal partial foot or minor amputations have higher complication and readmission rates compared to more proximal amputations.[14,15] The Chopart level of amputation has a high failure rate in adult patients with diabetes. Brodell and his colleagues reported 94% of the patients studied with a Chopart amputation developed wound complications and only 44% successfully used a prosthesis.[16] Lisfranc disarticulation separates the three cuneiform bones and the cuboid bone from the five metatarsal bones of the forefoot.

The three hindfoot amputations are the Pirogoff, Boyd, and Syme. The Pirogoff amputation is a wedging transection of the calcaneus, followed by bony fusion of the calcaneus and distal tibia with all other distal structures removed. In a Boyd amputation, the calcaneus remains largely intact rather than being wedged before arthrodesis with the tibia. Currently, the Pirogoff and Boyd amputations are infrequently performed on adult patients. Neither provides an easy fit with a prosthesis. The Boyd amputation has received positive clinical reviews when used in the management of congenital limb deficiencies in children in which the amputated limb is shorter than the sound limb.[17,18] In this case, there are usually fewer postoperative complications, such as scarring and heel pad migration, and less susceptibility to the bony overgrowth common in children with osseous transecting amputations. Heel pad migration remains a predictable complication of Syme amputation.[19] In children, the longer the remnant limb or foot, the better the functional outcome.[20] The Syme amputation is performed more frequently in adults because of the ease of prosthetic management at this level (Fig. 22.3). Because of the length of the residual limb in Pirogoff and Boyd amputations, the attachment of a prosthetic foot lengthens the limb when a prosthesis is worn. A heel lift on the contralateral sound limb is usually necessary to counteract this artificially long prosthetic limb.

Proximal partial foot amputations often result in equinus deformities because of muscular imbalance created by severed dorsiflexors and intact triceps surae.[21–23] Nevertheless, many individuals with a partial foot amputation function

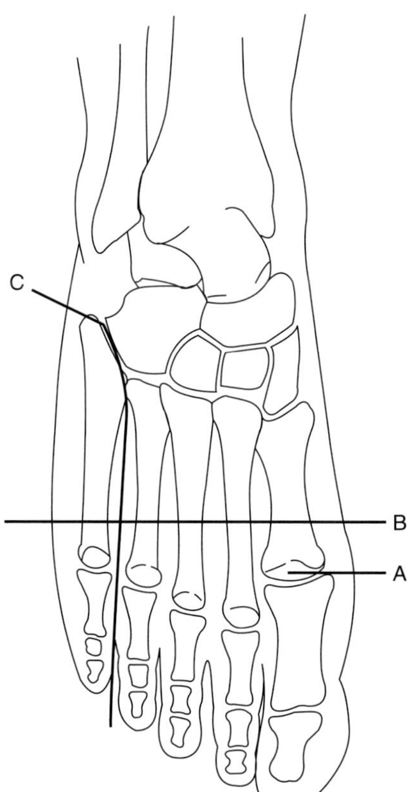

Fig. 22.1 Examples of amputations involving the forefoot. (*A*) This digit (phalangeal) amputation involves disarticulation of the phalanx at the metatarsal joint. More distal digit amputations remove either the distal phalanx or the middle and distal phalanges. (*B*) In this complete trans-metatarsal amputation, transection occurred just proximal to all five metatarsal heads. (*C*) Ray resections involve disarticulation of one or more metatarsals and their phalanges from the tarsal and neighboring metatarsals. Ray resections often require skin graft to achieve adequate tissue closure.

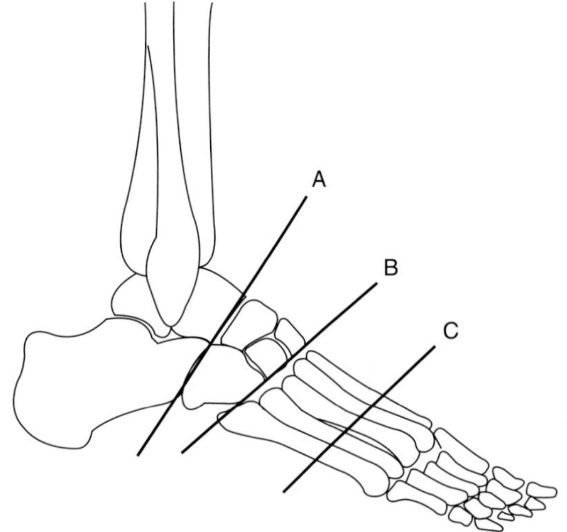

Fig. 22.2 In a Chopart amputation (*A*) there is disarticulation of the midfoot from the hindfoot at the level of the talus and calcaneus. In a Lisfranc amputation (*B*) there is disarticulation of the forefoot (metatarsals) from the midfoot (tarsals). (*C*) In a transmetatarsal amputation, there is transaction through the length of one or more metatarsals, usually just proximal to the metatarsal heads.

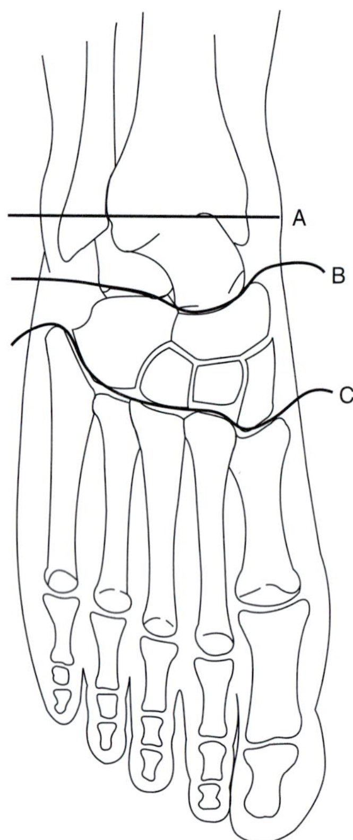

Fig. 22.3 *(A)* The Syme amputation involves removal of the inferior projections of the tibia and fibula and all bone structures distally while preserving the natural weight-bearing fat pad of the heel. *(B)* The Chopart amputation preserves the talus and calcaneus. *(C)* The Lisfranc amputation has disarticulation of metatarsals from the midfoot.

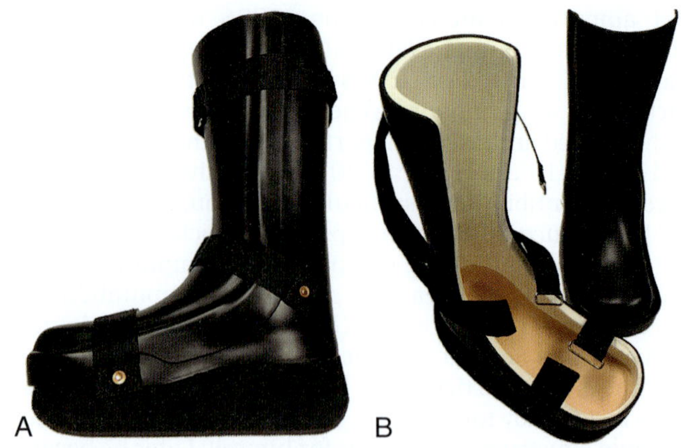

Fig. 22.4 The neuropathic walker, or CROW boot, provides maximum protection for the denervated foot at risk for amputation. The combination of custom-molded multidurometer liner, locked neutral ankle, and rocker bottom permits a rollover with minimal plantar pressure and shear. (A) Side view of custom CROW Walker. (B) Inside view of custom CROW Walker.

extremely well. In one survey, physicians and prosthetists reported that patients with partial foot amputation function better than those with the Syme amputation.[24] Although surgeons and prosthetists have long supported the Syme amputation in preference to the Lisfranc or Chopart amputations, many patients with midfoot amputation achieve high levels of function and long remnant limb durability.[25] For example, Jack Dempsey, a professional football player with a midfoot amputation, set several all-time field goal records wearing a custom-designed kicking boot.[26]

Patients with diabetes, particularly those with diabetic foot syndrome, have persistent high rates of limb amputation and mortality.[27] Minor amputations in patients with diabetic foot problems can be effective in limb salvage and can reduce morbidity and mortality.[28] Quality of life is influenced by age, time with diabetes, and presence of retinopathy—not level of amputation.[29] Functional benefits of partial foot amputation with a disproportionate risk of revision versus determining amputation level based on minimized risk of reulceration have to be considered prior to surgery.[30]

GAIT CHARACTERISTICS AFTER PARTIAL FOOT AMPUTATION

A person with a partial foot amputation typically has vascular insufficiency, is usually between the ages of 60 and 70 years, has compromised proprioception and sensation, and has weak lower limb musculature. After a Syme or partial foot amputation, a patient may be able to ambulate without a prosthesis but has a loss of the anterior lever arm in ambulation and an inefficient gait pattern. The primary need immediately after amputation is to protect the remaining tissue, which is vulnerable to vascular or neuropathic disease. The neuropathic walker developed at Rancho Los Amigos Medical Center locks the ankle in a custom-molded, foam-lined, thermoplastic ankle-foot orthosis (AFO) (Fig. 22.4). A rocker bottom is contoured to promote a smooth rollover as a substitute for the second and third rockers of gait, and the orthosis provides optimum protection for the insensate residual foot. For patients with adequate protective sensation, the risk of tissue breakdown is less and a custom shoe insert with in-depth or postoperative shoes often provides adequate protection.

A review of gait in partial foot case studies showed variations in single-limb support time directly related to the reduction of the forefoot lever arm of a partial foot and subsequent increase in the force concentration on the distal end during terminal stance (Fig. 22.5).[31] Uneven step lengths result from reduced single-limb support and occur as a consequence. In a person with a whole foot, a fully intact anterior lever arm preserves elevation of the center of mass at terminal stance. With normal quadriceps strength and eccentric control, slight knee flexion (15–20 degrees) provides shock absorption as weight is rapidly transferred onto the limb during loading response (Fig. 22.6). Some people with a dysvascular partial foot and a Syme amputation demonstrate significant weakness of the quadriceps. This functional weakness threatens eccentric control of the usual knee flexion angle that occurs during loading response. To compensate, the patient may keep the knee extended during loading response. This strategy shifts the ground reaction force vector to a position anterior to the knee joint axis, thus reducing the workload of the quadriceps. Although this compensatory strategy enhances early stance phase stability, it sacrifices the shock absorption mechanism at the knee and hip joints, increasing the likelihood of cumulative joint trauma at both joints (Fig. 22.6B). Neuropathic impairment of proprioception and sensation may further complicate control of the knee in early stance. In addition, compromised forefoot support increases center of gravity displacement, which results in higher energy expenditure.

A gait study of people with partial foot amputation included 18 patients with transmetatarsal amputations, 11 with one or more metatarsal amputations, 15 with ray resections, and 2 with either a Lisfranc or a Chopart amputation.[31–33] One portion of the analysis focused on the mechanics of the residual limb rockers. Partly because of a delay in the forefoot rocker, patients with all types of partial foot amputations walked with a significantly slower velocity than control subjects with healthy, intact feet (Fig. 22.7). Peak ankle dorsiflexion was also significantly delayed for all three partial foot groups compared with those with intact feet. Although the control group with intact lower limbs reached peak ankle dorsiflexion at a point 43% into the gait cycle, patients with partial foot amputation did not reach peak dorsiflexion angle until nearly the halfway point of the gait cycle (Fig. 22.8). This delay in reaching peak dorsiflexion subsequently delays forward progression over the shortened stance limb and the transition to double-limb support.

The rise rate of the vertical ground reaction force is the amount of force that occurs in 1% of the gait cycle and can be expressed as Newtons divided by the percent of the gait cycle. After controlling for variation in velocity, the rise rate

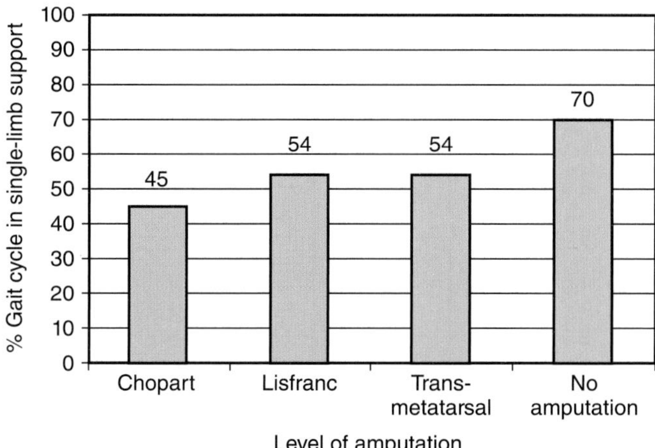

Fig. 22.5 Percent of the gait cycle spent in single-limb support for patients with midfoot Chopart or Lisfranc amputations and forefoot transmetatarsal amputation. Healthy older adults with intact feet typically spend between 65% and 75% of their gait cycle in single-limb support.

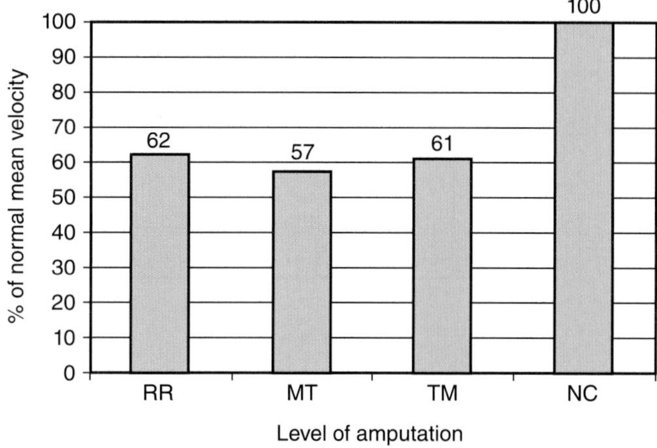

Fig. 22.7 Reduced gait velocity in patients with partial foot amputations. On average, patients walked at 62% of gait velocity of control subjects with intact lower limbs. *MT*, Metatarsal amputation of one to four rays; *NC*, normal control subjects; *RR*, ray resection; *TM*, complete transmetatarsal amputation.

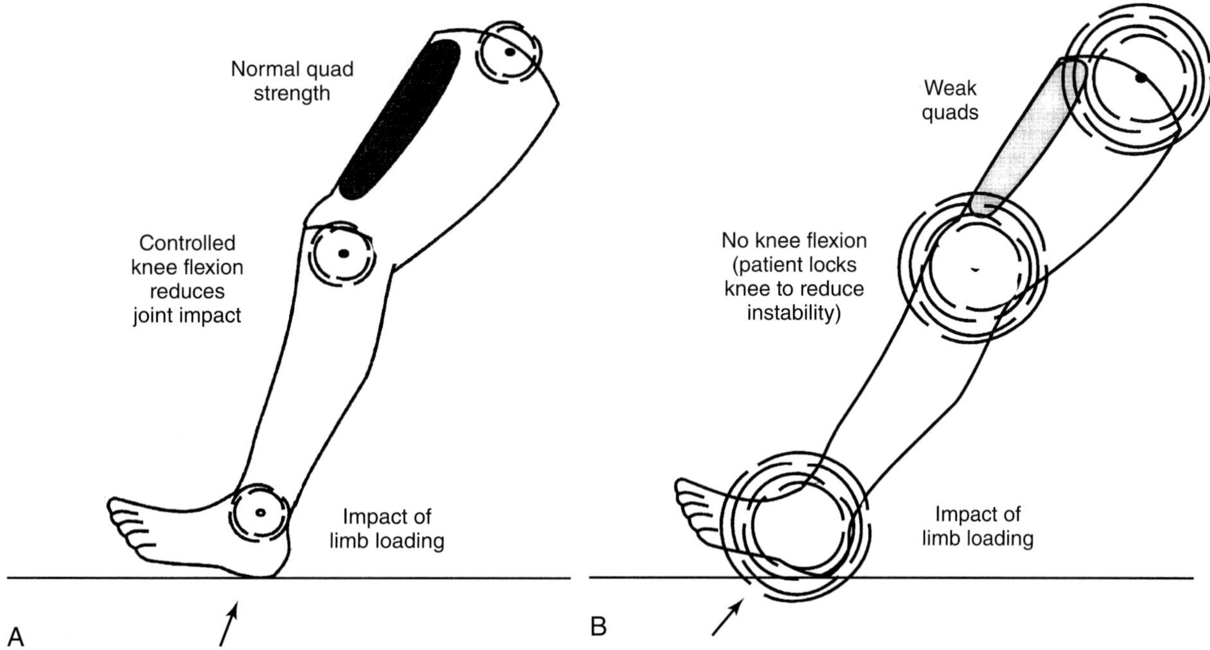

Fig. 22.6 (A) During loading in normal gait, knee flexion provides a significant shock absorption mechanism to protect the proximal joints. (B) The patient with weakness associated with dysvascular disease avoids knee flexion to increase stability, with a penalty of increased trauma to the proximal joints as a consequence of repeated higher impact loading.

of the vertical ground reaction force from midstance to terminal stance (as the force pattern nears its F2 peak) was significantly lower for all three amputation groups compared with the control group (Fig. 22.9). Peak vertical ground reaction forces were significantly higher for the sound limb than the affected limb, likely reflecting an abrupt unloading of the partial foot amputation limb.

The forefoot lever arm of the trailing limb typically provides anterior support and results in adequate terminal stance support time (Fig. 22.10). This results in appropriate step length of the advancing limb. By contrast, inadequate anterior support of the trailing limb with partial foot amputation reduces the lever arm, resulting in premature toe break and forefoot collapse. The step length of the advancing limb may be correspondingly reduced (Fig. 22.10B).

An inverse relation exists between surface area and peak pressure when body weight is loaded on the foot during stance. This relation is especially important for individuals with partial foot amputation during terminal stance. As the plantar surface area of the supporting forefoot is reduced, the magnitude of the pressure is increased.[31–33] The reduced forefoot lever arm also creates abrupt weight transfer to the contralateral side and can reduce step length, stride length, and velocity. Without prosthetic support, the advancing sound-side step length diminishes. Fear, insecurity, and

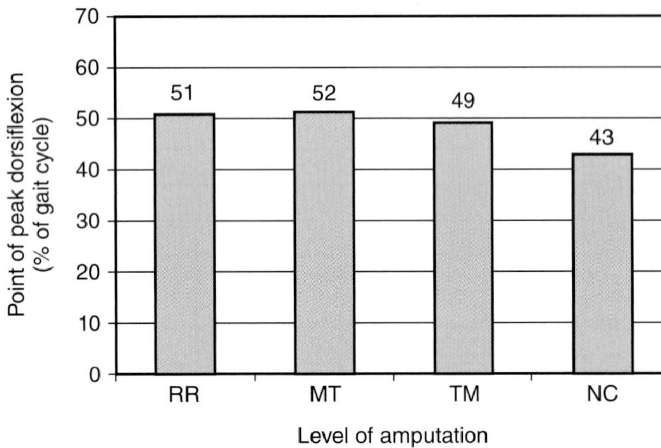

Fig. 22.8 For persons with partial foot amputations, maximum dorsiflexion is delayed during stance phase of the gait cycle. Although control subjects with intact feet achieved a maximum dorsiflexion angle at a point 43% into the gait cycle, those with partial foot amputation did not reach the maximum dorsiflexion angle until halfway through the cycle. The consequence of this delay is a slowed forward progression of the body's center of mass and transition to the subsequent period of double-limb support. *MT*, Metatarsal amputation of one to four rays; *NC*, normal control subjects; *RR*, ray resection; *TM*, complete transmetatarsal amputation.

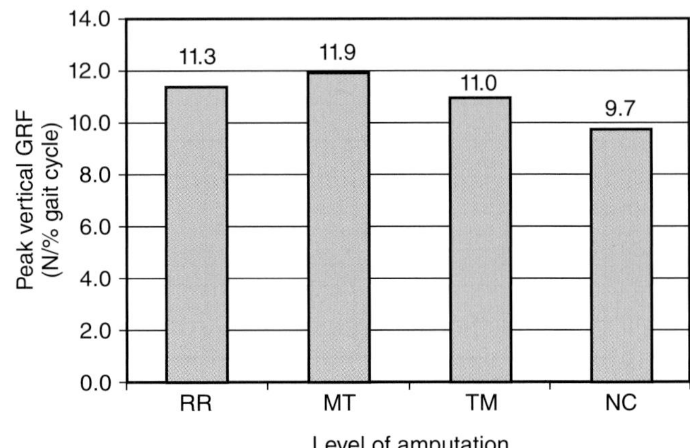

Fig. 22.9 Comparison of peak vertical ground reaction force (*GRF*) of the intact limbs of patients with partial foot amputations and persons without amputation, expressed as Newton (*N*) divided by percent of gait cycle. *MT*, Metatarsal amputation of one to four rays; *NC*, normal control subjects; *RR*, ray resection; *TM*, complete transmetatarsal amputation.

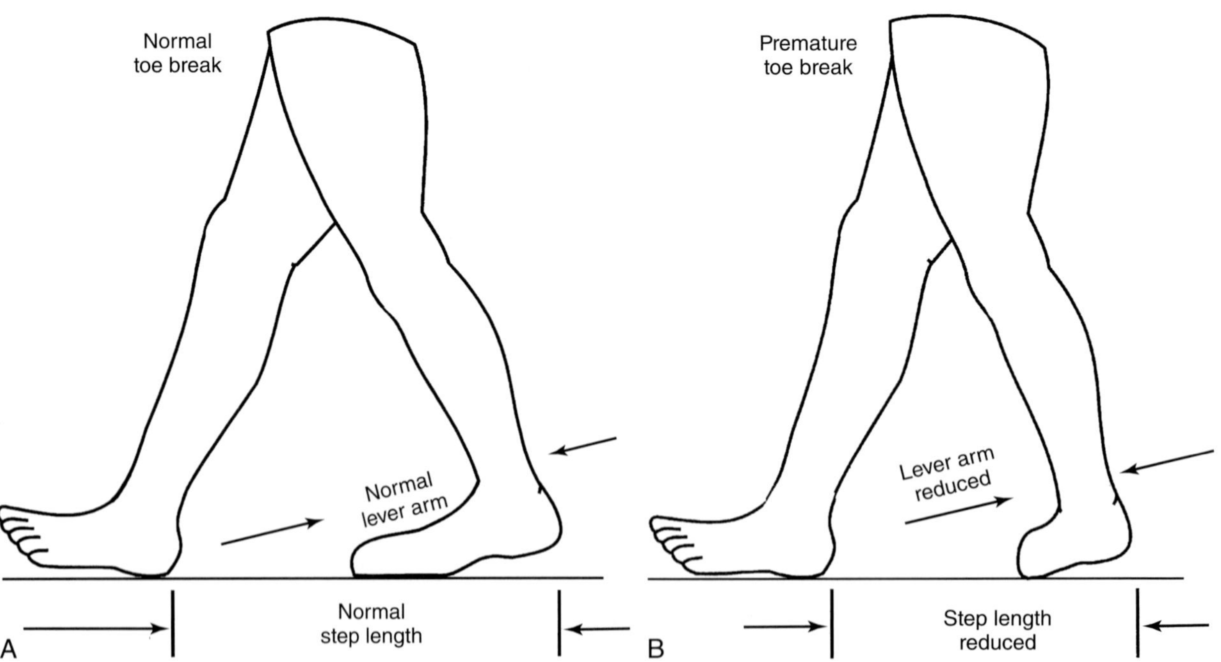

Fig. 22.10 (A) The forefoot lever arm contributes to a normal step length. (B) Reduction of the forefoot support after partial foot amputation produces a consequent reduction in contralateral step length.

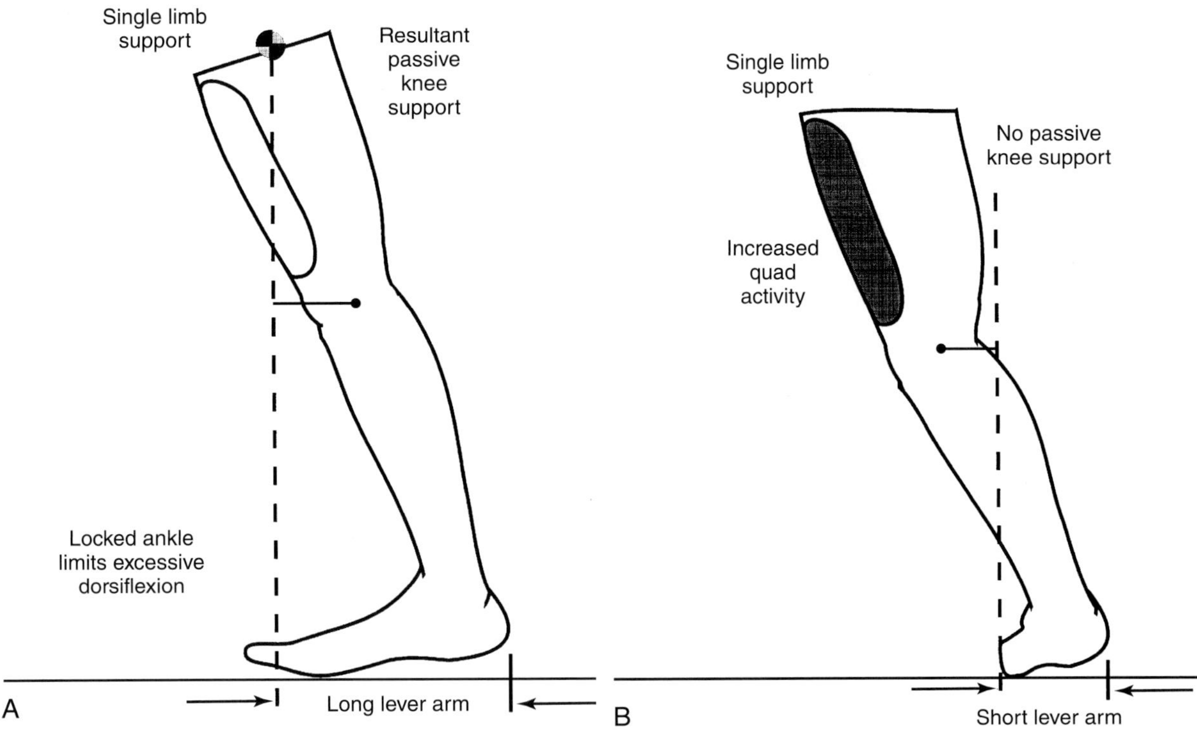

Fig. 22.11 (A) Normal energy-efficient passive knee support in late stance relies on a locked or rigid forefoot that limits further dorsiflexion at the ankle and a normal forefoot lever arm to maintain the ground reaction force anterior to the knee during late stance. (B) After partial foot amputation, the reduced forefoot lever arm often leads to increased quadriceps activity to compensate for reduced passive knee support and ensure stability in late stance.

pain aggravated by increased pressure near the amputation site collectively create an abrupt transfer of weight to the sound side, thus increasing the magnitude of the initial vertical force peak.[34]

In normal gait, the weight line is positioned more and more anterior to the knee joint as the gait cycle moves from midstance into terminal stance and preswing phases (Fig. 22.11). As a result, the limb is held in a passive, energy-efficient extended knee position, effectively supporting body weight and increasing stability in late stance. The length of the forefoot lever arm is one of the key determinants of this support. For persons with partial foot amputation, the lever arm of the foot is greatly reduced, leading to a less effective, premature loss of support at the end of stance phase. This shorter lever places the ground reaction force closer to or behind the knee in late stance (Fig. 22.11B). Because much of the passive stability provided by a normal forefoot lever in late stance is absent, the quadriceps must contract to maintain stance phase stability, contributing to an increased energy cost of walking for persons with partial foot amputation.

Pinzur and colleagues[35] described a functional relation between gait velocity and the level of amputation at the foot. As the amputation level becomes more proximal (as the length of the residual foot decreases), changes in temporal and kinetic gait characteristics include reduced sound-side step length, decreased velocity, increased energy cost, and increased vertical load on the sound side. An inverse relation exists between the length of the remaining portion of the forefoot and the time spent in single-limb support on the amputated side.[34] When the level of amputation is proximal to the metatarsal heads, medial support is lost at loading response. This may require orthotic "posting" to limit resultant valgus deformity. Patients with partial foot amputation frequently have plantarflexion contracture develop from muscle imbalance. Any plantarflexion contracture, in turn, increases pressure at the distal residual limb during terminal stance, causing discomfort, pain, and risk of ulceration.[36] A contracture is even more problematic for individuals with Hansen disease or diabetic neuropathy, because they already have compromised sensation.[37,38] Shoes worn without prosthetic replacement of the missing forefoot quickly become disfigured, collapsing at a displaced toe break, further endangering the vulnerable areas of the residual limb.[39] The areas of the residual foot most vulnerable to tissue damage during walking include the distal end, first and fifth metatarsal heads, navicular, malleoli, and tibial crest. The longitudinal and transverse arches, the heel pad, and the area along the pretibial muscle belly are pressure-tolerant areas for loading in a custom shoe or prosthesis.

PROSTHETIC MANAGEMENT

During the 1800s, digit amputations were fit using a wood or cork sandal with a leather ankle lacer.[40,41] Partial foot amputations were sometimes fit with a socket and keel fashioned from one piece of carefully chosen root wood, the grain of which followed the curve of the ankle. This was referred to as the *natural crook technique*. Another commonly used historical design incorporated steel-reinforced leather sockets.[42]

In recent decades, a wide variety of prosthetic options for individuals with partial foot amputation have emerged. The prescribing physician and patient care team must familiarize themselves with the broad array of options available in prosthetic components and design so that prescription considerations can best accommodate the patient's goals and functional needs Because of variability in level of amputation, sensitivity or insensitivity of the residual limb, concurrent foot deformity, and anticipated patient participation in community activities, no single prosthetic prescription can be used for all patients with foot amputation.[43] As the amputation level becomes more proximal and the length of the residual foot decreases, prostheses should incorporate supramalleolar-, AFO-, and patella tendon-bearing designs. This is especially true as a patient's activity level increases. Prosthetic treatment approaches include toe fillers placed inside the shoe, an arch support with a foam spacer, the University of California Biomechanics Laboratory (UCBL) shoe insert maximum-control foot orthosis with a toe filler, which provides better control of the heel position, and a boot or slipper made of flexible urethane resin (Smooth-On, Easton, PA). Cosmetic restoration of silicone and several variations of AFOs are also in common use.

The length and degree of flexibility of the prosthetic forefoot affect the anterior lever arm and consequently foot and ankle motion. The biomechanical goal of prosthetic treatment is to provide anterior support of the remnant limb and a controlled fulcrum of forward motion as the foot-ankle complex pivots over the area of the amputation level in the third rocker of late stance. An additional goal is to minimize pressure at the distal end and balance the weight-bearing forces on the remnant limb within the socket or shoe.

Toe Fillers and Modified Shoes

Historically, if a simple toe filler was prescribed, an extended steel shank or band of rigid spring steel was also placed within the sole of the shoe, extending from the calcaneus to the metatarsal heads. Currently, carbon fiber plates are designed in a variety of styles and degrees of stiffness that can be incorporated into prosthetic treatment. The challenge that faces the prosthetist is to match the appropriate degree of forefoot flexibility to the needs of each patient. For an energy-efficient and cosmetic gait, relative plantar rigidity should give way to at least 15 degrees of forefoot.

Flexibility distal to the metatarsal heads is critical to allow for toe break during late stance of the gait cycle. The steel shank (carbon plate) is helpful in providing a limited degree of buoyancy that substitutes for the lost anterior support of the foot.[45] Stiffening the sole with a spring steel shank (carbon fiber) increases the lever arm support but often at the expense of additional pressure on the distal end of the residual limb.[46]

For a patient with a more complex partial foot amputation, a rocker bottom shoe modification distributes force over a greater area and advances stance more quickly and efficiently. A curved roll or buildup on the plantar surface of the shoe encourages tibial advancement while minimizing weight-bearing pressures on the distal amputated end. For optimal function the plantar contour of a rocker bottom should follow a radius originating from the knee joint center but break or roll more abruptly just distal to the metatarsal heads. Although a rocker bottom assists rollover, it also compromises symmetry of gait. It is often prescribed for individuals with chronic pain or in conjunction with a custom-molded accommodative interface for those with a neuropathy-related risk of reamputation. Extra-depth shoes have 6 to 8 mm or more of space inside the shoe on the plantar surface to accommodate an orthotic insert or prosthesis and may be useful for patients with digit or ray amputations.[43]

Custom-molded shoes, when used in conjunction with a filler and carbon plate, improve the comfort level and reduce the risk of ulceration in many dysvascular patients with amputation. They are not as subject to forefoot collapse, provide major protection to the endangered foot, and may last longer than retail tennis shoes.[47]

Partial Foot Inserts and Toe Fillers

A custom-molded, flexible, plantar shoe insert is one of the options for individuals with amputation of the hallux or first ray. This partial foot prosthetic approach is typically used in combination with extra-depth shoes. The goals are to provide a flexible anterior extension to compensate for a missing or shortened first ray to improve the third rocker and to support and protect the amputation site during the simulated metatarsophalangeal hyperextension in late stance and preswing.[48] This provides some relief for metatarsal head pressure, supports the arch, and probably assists in normalizing the ground reaction force pattern during terminal stance and preswing. It may incorporate a toe filler to prevent premature forefoot shoe collapse and migration of remaining toes.[49–51] Partial foot inserts should be fabricated to support subtalar neutral to minimize remnant limb tissue stress.[52] Toe fillers consist of soft foam material such as room-temperature vulcanized elastomer, which fills the voids in the toe box of the shoe. They provide limited extension of the shoe life and a moderate degree of cosmesis. They also act as spacers, keeping adjoining toes properly positioned and reducing abnormal motion that can otherwise lead to ulceration. The toe filler alone provides limited mechanical advantage. An appropriately stiff carbon plate placed inside the shoe under the partial foot insert can further improve gait. An alternative to the spring steel shank and carbon plate is a longitudinal support built into a flexible custom insole. Either support device must end at the metatarsal heads or allow proper hyperextension of the metatarsophalangeal joints. A partial foot insert with arch support and filler is preferable to the simple filler because it can be used in different shoes and because it provides plantar support to an already compromised weight-bearing surface.[53] Custom partial foot insoles can also be made from a sawdust and epoxy resin instead of foams and thermoplastics as a base structure.

The UCBL orthosis, a foot orthosis that encapsulates the calcaneus, was developed at the UCBL during the 1960s and was comprehensively described in 1969.[54,55] The UCBL orthosis is designed to provide better control of subtalar and forefoot position than are custom-made shoe inserts, reducing motion and thus friction with a closer fit or purchase over the calcaneus and forefoot.[56] The UCBL orthosis design can be effectively incorporated into a custom partial foot prosthesis with toe filler for persons with partial foot amputation.

Case Example 22.1 **A Patient With a Unilateral Hallux (Great Toe), Second Toe, and Distal First Metatarsal Head Amputation With Rotated Skin Flap for Soft Tissue Coverage**

J. C. is an 84-year-old male with a 34-year history of type II diabetes. He has controlled his diabetes but has lost protective sensation due to neuropathy. On October 10, 2017, J. C. was working with his zero turn mower (ZTR) on his property. He left the engine and mower blades running and positioned himself in front of the mower, needing to move the ZTR only approximately 12 to 18 inches forward. The ZTR got stuck on a tree root and did not come straight forward; it wiggled and then broke free as J. C. fell. J. C. watched both feet go under the deck of the mower. His left foot ended up by the discharge chute, and his right foot got wedged and stalled the mower blades, preventing more extensive injuries as the mower deck came to rest on his right hip. J. C. was emergently taken to the operating room, and his right great toe, second toe, and distal first metatarsal head were amputated. A local skin flap had to be rotated for soft tissue coverage. By rotating this local skin flap, a split-thickness skin graft is not necessary (Fig. 22.12A–I). Partial foot amputations combined with split-thickness skin grafts usually require subsequent revision to a more proximal level.[44] The referring surgeon kept J. C. non–weight bearing on his right foot until mid-December, when he was released to begin the fitting of his partial foot prosthesis. There continues to be an area of healing on the dorsum of his right foot, which is expected to heal by secondary intention over time (Fig. 22.13).

QUESTIONS TO CONSIDER

- Considering his medical situation and awareness of his diabetic condition, what concerns might exist about the

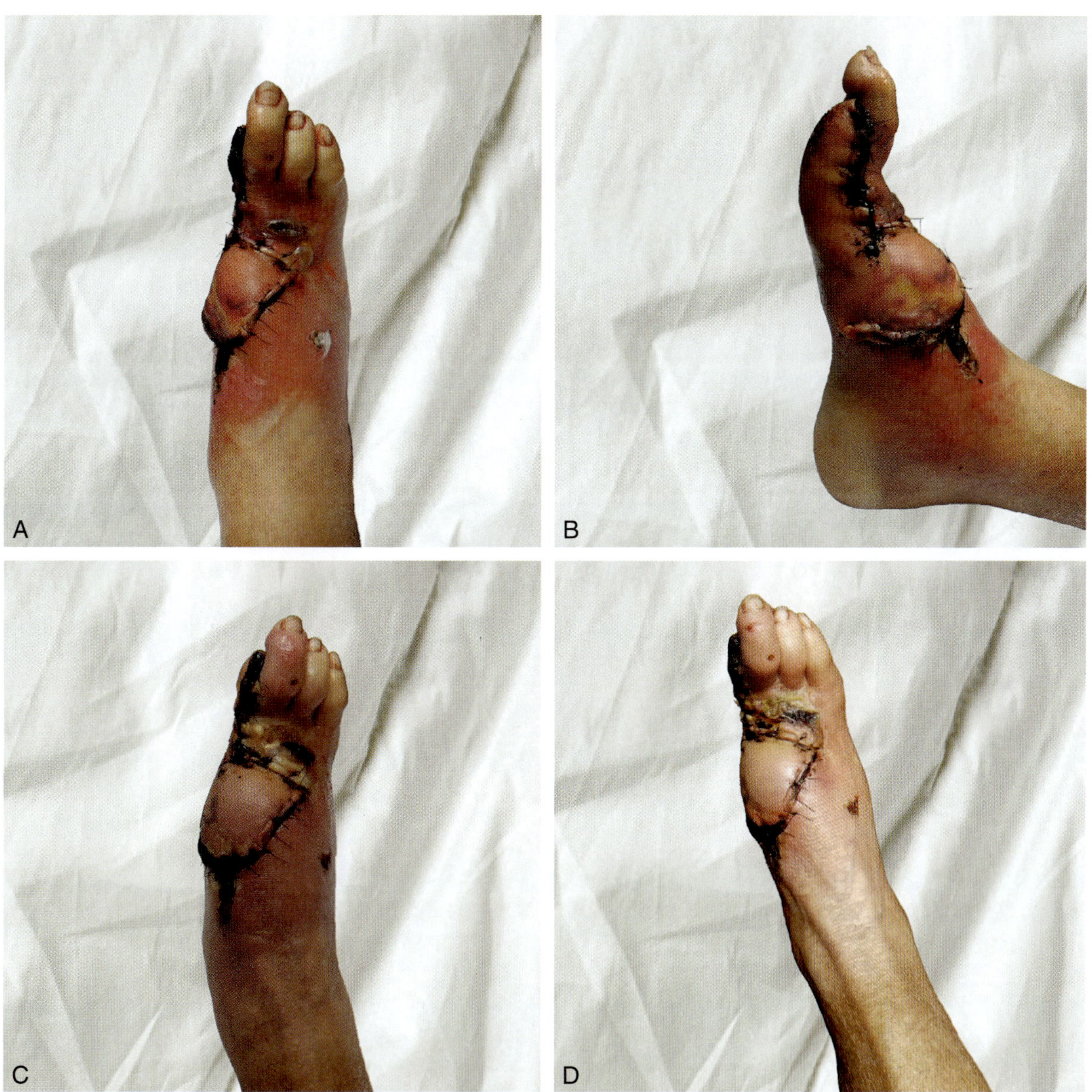

Fig. 22.12 (A–I) The progress of healing after J. C. suffered his traumatic partial foot amputation.

Case Example 22.1 A Patient With a Unilateral Hallux (Great Toe), Second Toe, and Distal First Metatarsal Head Amputation With Rotated Skin Flap for Soft Tissue Coverage—Cont'd

residual foot? Which part of the foot is most vulnerable to future complications?

- What is the primary mechanism for an increase in energy consumption with any digit amputation, and what is particularly concerning about a great toe (hallux) amputation?
- How will his shortened foot affect progression throughout the gait cycle with respect to each phase of gait and the specific three rockers of the foot?
- What would be the most optimal prosthetic recommendation? What are the primary goals of the prosthesis? How should the rehabilitation team assist him in caring for his new amputation, as well as in prevention of future more proximal amputations?

RECOMMENDATIONS

After obtaining all additional health information from J. C. and from all medical sources concerning J. C., it was noted that he had medically significant bilateral callusing of his heels and on the plantar surface of his feet over metatarsals 1, 3, and 5 on his left and 3 and 5 on his right. He had hammer toes bilaterally. His skin was thin, shiny, and frail. He was wearing appropriately sized tennis shoes. His right foot was considerably swollen relative to his left foot. After reviewing his medical history and completing his physical exam, the treatment team recommended a custom partial foot prosthesis with toe filler and carbon plate. The custom partial foot

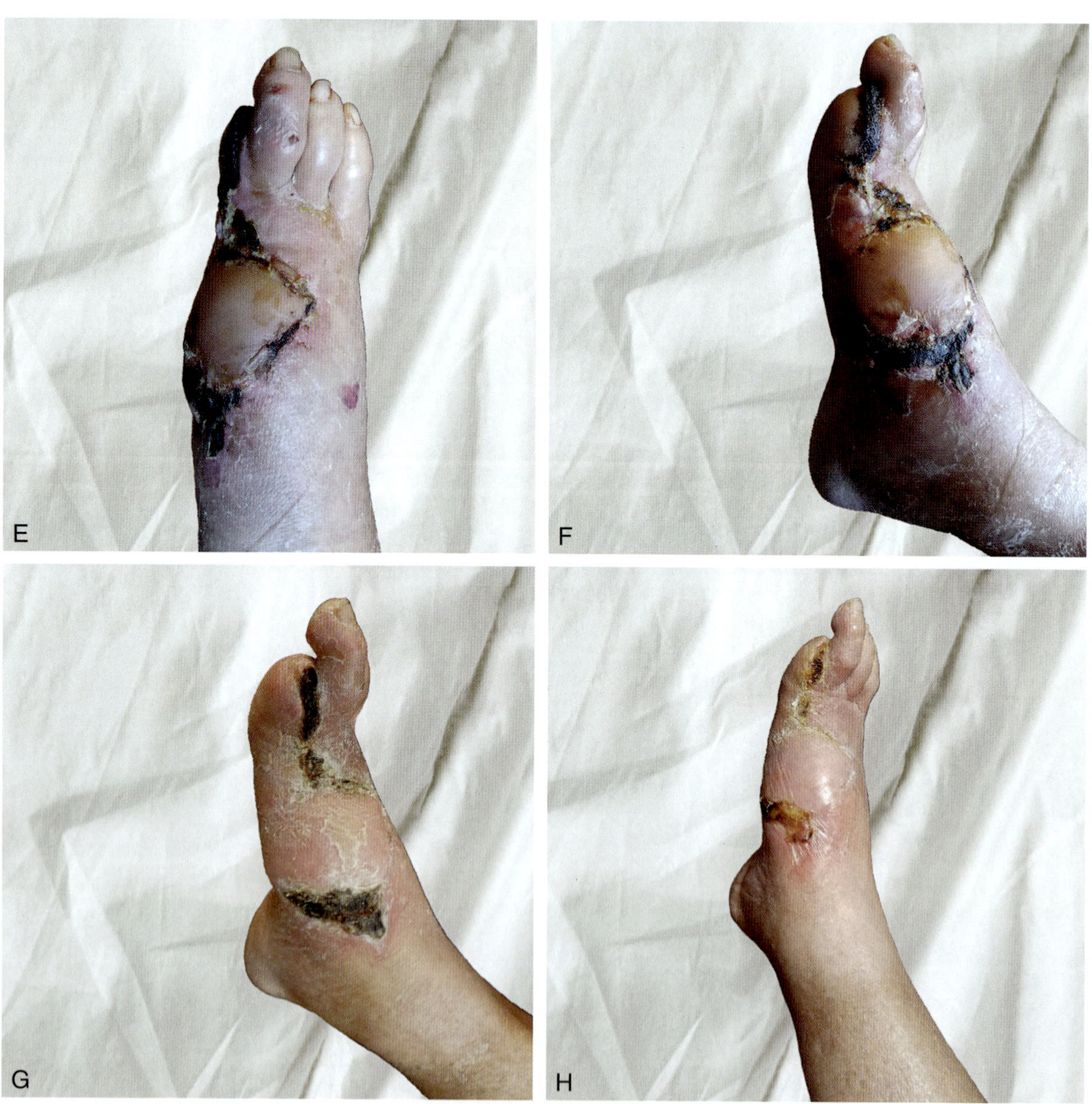

Fig. 22.12, Cont'd

(Continued)

Case Example 22.1 A Patient With a Unilateral Hallux (Great Toe), Second Toe, and Distal First Metatarsal Head Amputation With Rotated Skin Flap for Soft Tissue Coverage—Cont'd

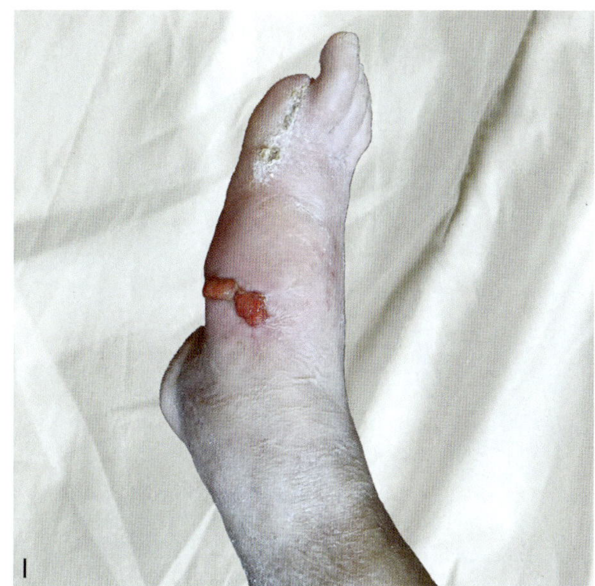

Fig. 22.12, Cont'd

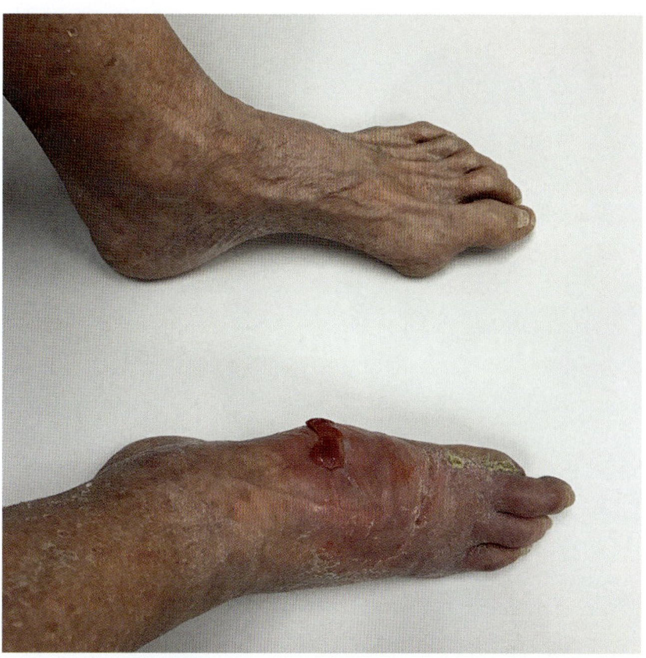

Fig. 22.13 The right remnant limb and intact foot of J. C. at delivery of his first prosthesis.

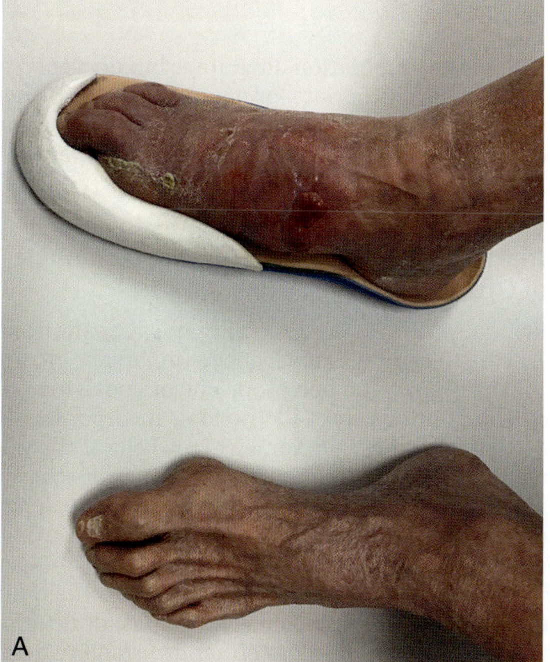

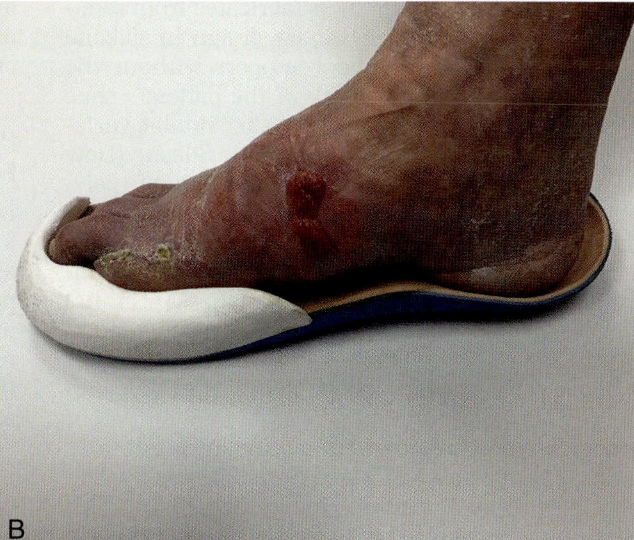

Fig. 22.14 (A and B) The right remnant limb of J. C. with his partial foot prosthesis and toe filler.

prosthesis consisted of a great, second, and medial foot filler, diabetic-compliant trilaminate foam, medial longitudinal arch support, and relief at the metatarsal heads (Fig. 22.14A and B). The carbon plate was left independent for use as needed to stiffen flexible shoes. After fitting him with his new shoes and right partial foot prosthesis, J. C. was able to ambulate with relatively equal step lengths. He stated, "I am glad to be walking again and not having to use the wheelchair." At his follow-up visit in January of 2018, J. C. had discontinued his use of the carbon plate because he felt he walked better and was more comfortable in these shoes without it (Fig. 22.15A and B).

Case Example 22.1 **A Patient With a Unilateral Hallux (Great Toe), Second Toe, and Distal First Metatarsal Head Amputation With Rotated Skin Flap for Soft Tissue Coverage—Cont'd**

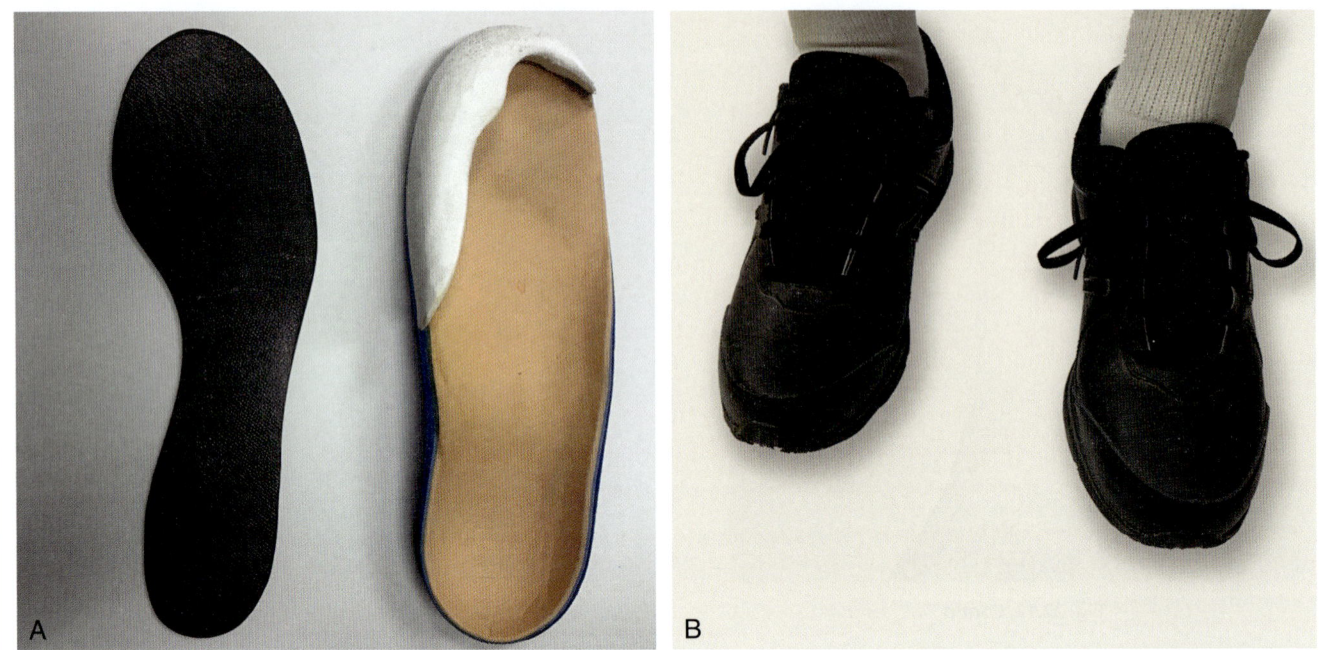

Fig. 22.15 (A) J. C.'s partial foot prosthesis with the carbon fiber foot plate. (B) J. C. wearing his prosthesis and shoes walking for the first time.

Cosmetic Slipper Designs

The slipper, one variation of which has been referred to as the *slipper-type elastomer prosthesis*, is fabricated from semi-flexible urethane elastomer.[57] A similar design in silicone may not provide adequate forefoot support without the addition of an extended steel shank in the patient's shoe or incorporation of a carbon plate. Another similar variation is made from a combination of silicone Silastic (Dow Corning, Midland, MI), polyester resin, and prosthetic (polyurethane) foam. These designs provide much of the support and control of the UCBL approach but with added cosmesis. These designs may be appropriate for individuals with transmetatarsal and metatarsal disarticulation (Lisfranc) amputations. They are ideal for swimming or water sports because most are water impervious, cosmetic, and capable of providing a flexible whip action, which is useful with swim fins.

Some slipper-type prostheses are cosmetic restorations made of silicone or vinyl and based on a "life cast" or on an alginate impression of a human model (Fig. 22.16). This prosthesis is made for patients who consider cosmesis paramount. This custom prosthesis is most often produced in a laboratory that specializes in manufacturing cosmetic silicone prostheses to restore limb loss. It can be ordered with hair and freckles and in a large variety of skin tones; however, it is most often a less-than-perfect match when compared with the intact contralateral foot. The patient should always share responsibility in the color swatch selection. The material itself is easily stained and changes color with time when exposed to sunlight. The cosmetic restoration provides little ambulation advantage but does increase shoe life. It may be appropriate for patients with transmetatarsal amputations who place a premium on cosmesis but is not always covered by insurance and may be the patient's financial responsibility.

Partial Foot Prostheses Incorporating an Ankle-Foot Orthosis

Individuals with reduced mobility may benefit from partial foot prostheses that extend above the ankle, incorporating an AFO design.[58] The polypropylene or copolymer shell supports the plantar aspect of the foot, incorporates the heel, and extends up the posterior leg to the belly of the gastrocnemius (Fig. 22.17). A circumferential anterior strap stabilizes the limb in the AFO. As an alternative, metal uprights may be attached to a shoe but have obvious cosmetic drawbacks. The AFO, whether metal or plastic, provides advantages of the arch support/UCBL orthosis and boot with maximum containment and a lever arm for support and substitution of the rocker mechanism. It offers enhanced stability and control because of its high proximal trim line. It has been an excellent solution for many patients with partial foot amputation and may be the prosthesis of choice for the active patient with a Chopart or Lisfranc amputation. Prefabricated carbon AFOs and custom-fabricated carbon AFOs can also be incorporated into partial foot prosthetic designs. Supramalleolar thermoplastic or laminated versions are fit with Tamarack (Blaine, MN) or Gillette (Gillette Children's Specialty Healthcare, St. Paul, MN) joints to provide free plantar and

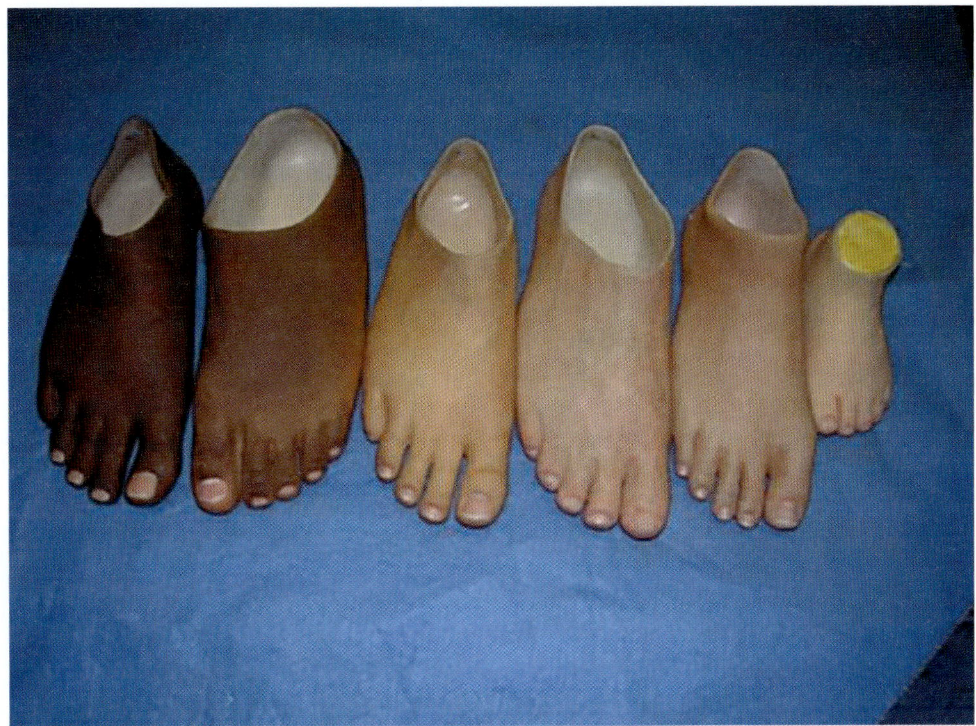

Fig. 22.16 The custom silicone partial foot prosthesis is available in a variety of skin tones to match each patient. Custom silicone partial foot prostheses provide psychosocial benefits along with restoration of functional ambulation. Stiffer silicone durometers can be incorporated to provide better biomechanical function. Photo provided by Life Like Laboratory.

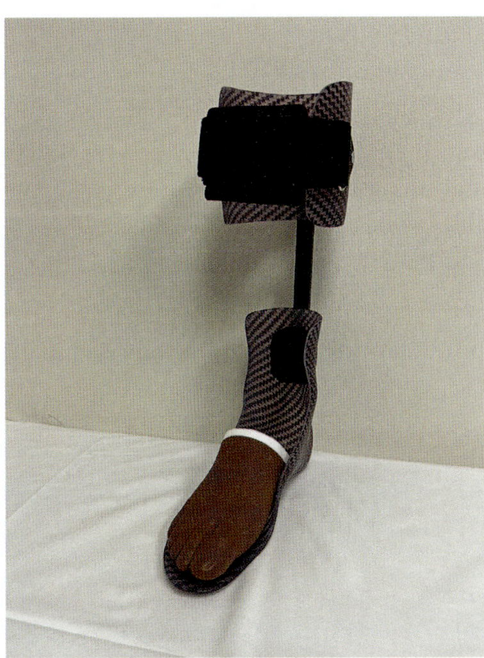

Fig. 22.17 A thermoplastic ankle-foot orthosis with posterior carbon strut can be utilized to restore biomechanical function for more proximal partial foot amputations.

dorsiflexion motion. This biomechanical solution is popular for the higher activity level of midfoot amputations. In the presence of acute ankle pain, a patient with a Chopart amputation was successful with a rear-entry ground reaction force AFO with a rigid solid ankle design.

AFO designs incorporating an interior tibial shell, clamshell, or panel distribute the toe lever forces during the terminal stance phase of gait.[59] Partial foot prostheses designed with a stiff forefoot and restricted dorsiflexion can manage the center of pressure of the remnant limb with less excursion.[59,60] This type of partial foot prosthesis, with articulated clamshell AFO, can affectively restore the foot length.[60]

Chopart Prostheses

Chopart socket designs are similar to Syme amputations, but there is no room for Syme prosthetic feet because the leg lengths of the patient remain the same after this level of partial foot amputation. A higher profile prosthesis with an anterior shell restores the anterior forefoot lever arm when compared to lower profile prostheses.[61] Prosthetic manufacturers have developed Chopart plates that can be directly laminated onto the plantar surface of the socket to minimize the leg length increase and to provide more dynamic function when compared with an AFO design. Otto Bock (Minneapolis, MN) has developed three Chopart plates; 1E80, 1E81, and 1E82 with heel heights of 0 (flat), 9, and 19 mm, respectively, and all three of these plates have a patient weight limit of 300 lb (136 kg). Ossur (Aliso Viejo, CA) has developed a Chopart plate that has a 10-mm heel height and a patient weight limit of 324 lb (147 kg). Proteor (France) designed a Chopart plate that has a 10-mm heel height and a patient weight limit of 360 lb (163 kg). All these plates are fixed once laminated to the distal socket and do not allow any alignment changes if the patient improves his or her strength, balance, and gait during rehabilitation.

Case Example 22.2 A 4-Year-Old With Traumatic Injuries Requiring Amputation of Right Foot

K. J. is a 29-year-old mother of two children with a 25-year history of right lower limb amputation. K. J. was run over by a lawn mower when she was 4 years of age. K. J. was a healthy, normally developing child without any medical comorbidities to consider when determining her optimal surgical and rehabilitative treatment. The limb-threatening injury ultimately required an amputation because the foot could not be salvaged.

QUESTIONS TO CONSIDER

- Given her pediatric medical history, what level of amputation would be best?
- Would you recommend a surgery that transects bone or disarticulates a joint?
- Would a Boyd, Syme, or transtibial amputation provide the best long-term outcome for a pediatric patient?
- Would a leg-length discrepancy be created by any of these amputation techniques? What is her risk for additional surgeries as she grows?
- Should an epiphysiodesis be performed at her initial amputation, later during her development, or not at all?
- How will her shortened lower extremity biomechanically progress through the gait cycle?
- Will she have functional compromise during any of the three gait rockers from initial contact through loading response, loading response through midstance, and midstance through terminal stance?
- What are the major goals for surgical and prosthetic intervention for K. J.?
- What specific recommendations should be made and why?
- What is her prognosis for functional ambulation?
- How should the efficacy of intervention be assessed?

RECOMMENDATIONS

At 4 years of age, K. J. underwent a Syme amputation. K. J. was treated with a Syme prosthesis almost annually due to growth, with a variety of functional prosthetic feet based on the available space or leg-length difference compared with the contralateral side. By age 8, the plantar calcaneal fat pad that was placed distal to her tibia and fibula during her amputation surgery had started to migrate. By age 12, the fat pad had migrated completely off the distal end of her remnant limb (Figs. 22.18–22.21). The uncovered distal end suffered recurrent callous and would not tolerate distal end bearing. The socket had to be elongated to reduce distal pressure, further limiting prosthetic foot options due to decreased space for her foot. In February 2012, K. J. underwent a transtibial amputation due to pain and recurrent distal remnant limb skin breakdown (Fig. 22.22). Her Syme amputation lasted through childhood and delayed surgical revision until she reached skeletal maturity and adulthood. Based on my clinical experience, a Boyd and epiphysiodesis would have been the preferred treatment originally. The Boyd amputation technique leaves the natural calcaneal attachment of the plantar heel fat pad, and the epiphysiodesis would provide remnant limb shortening over time to improve prosthetic foot options. Fat pad migration risk would have been reduced, decreasing the potential need for revision surgery (Figs. 22.19 and 22.20).

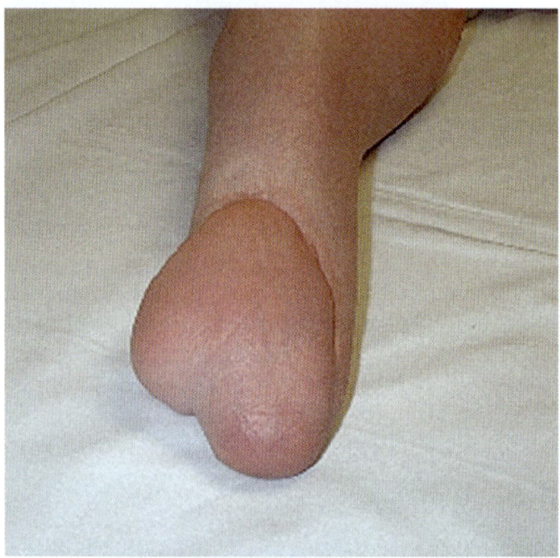

Fig. 22.19 Distal end of K. J.'s remnant limb.

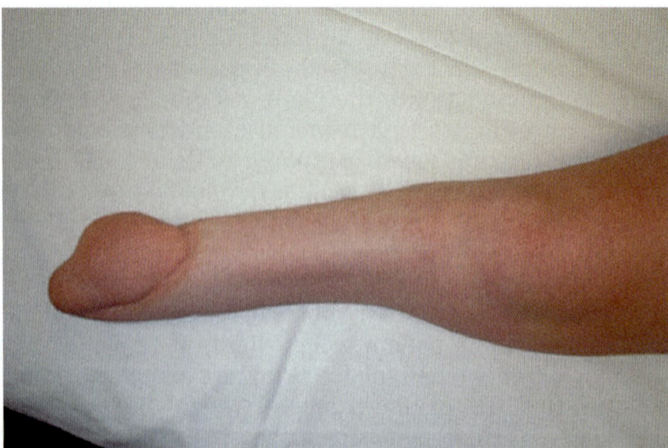

Fig. 22.18 K. J. right Syme residual limb showing the fat pad migration and tapper of her limb at 13 years of age.

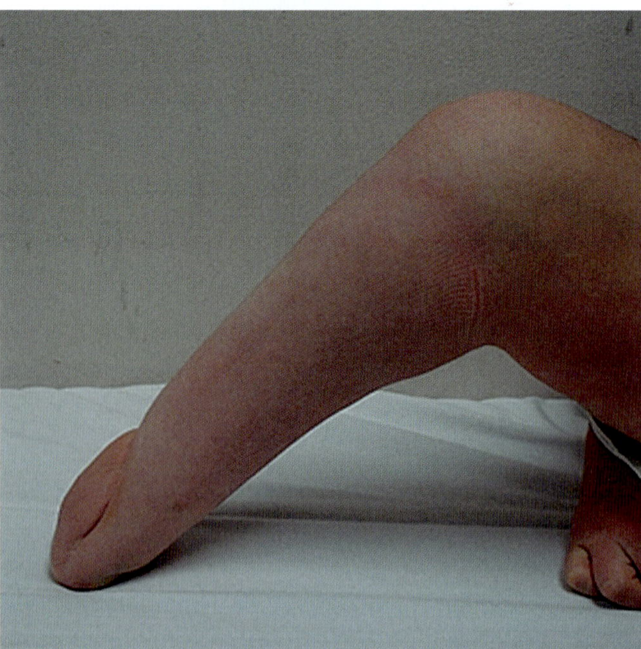

Fig. 22.20 K. J. demonstrating end bearing of her remnant limb into the exam table.

(Continued)

Case Example 22.2 A 4-Year-Old With Traumatic Injuries Requiring Amputation of Right Foot—Cont'd

K. J. has been an independent community ambulator with all her prostheses. Her prosthetic feet provided biomechanical function throughout her gait cycle. Growing up, K. J. participated in sports and continued her active lifestyle into adulthood. Her step lengths are equal, and her timing and gait symmetry approach normal. When K. J. is wearing jeans, public observers do not know she has any lower extremity impairment.

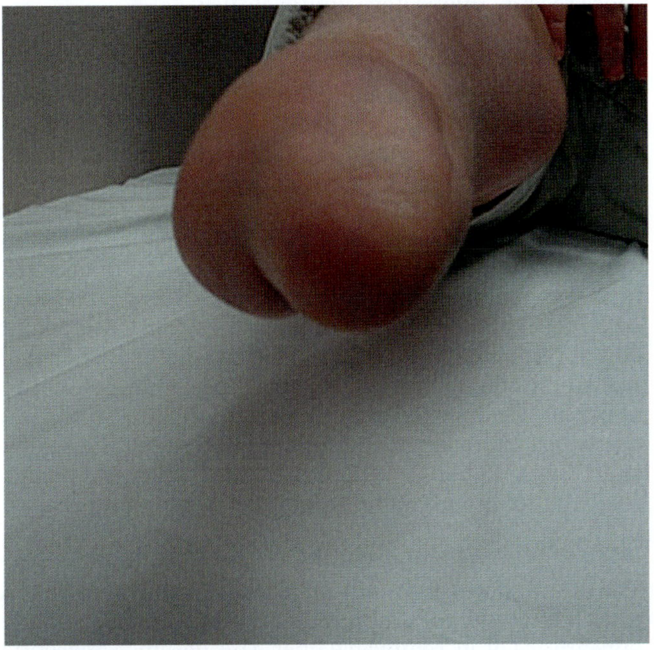

Fig. 22.21 K. J.'s distal remnant limb with skin over bone and no fat pad coverage to protect the bone during weight bearing.

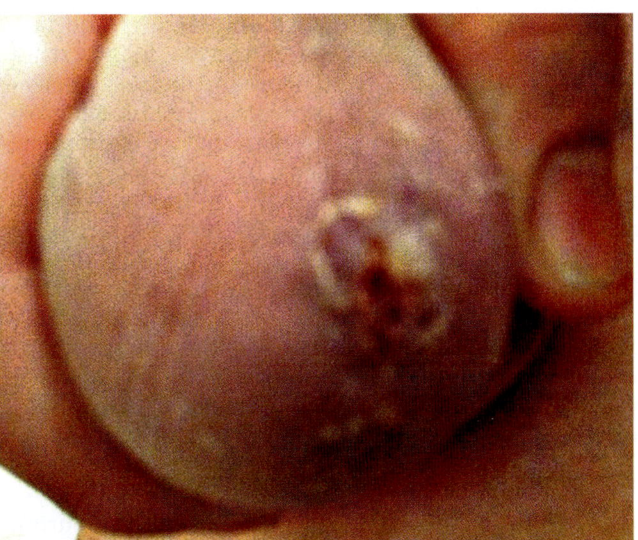

Fig. 22.22 K. J.'s distal limb with skin breakdown, which resulted in revision to the transtibial level during early adulthood.

Syme Amputation

In 1867 E. D. Hudson, the Surgeon General of the United States, described the Syme amputation with a litany of superlatives: "No amputation of the inferior extremity can ever compare in value with that of the ankle joint originated by Mr. Syme. Twelve years of experience with that variety of operation have afforded me assurance that it is a concept which is complete in itself and not capable of being improved in its general character."[62]

The Syme, or tibiotarsal, amputation is a disarticulation of the talocrural joint. The entire foot is completely removed, but the fat pad of the heel is preserved and anchored to the distal tibia. This allows distal end bearing and some degree of ambulation without a prosthesis (Fig. 22.3).[63] It gained popularity during the late 1800s primarily because the likelihood of survival with this technique was substantially greater than with other surgical choices, given the reduced degree of sepsis and shock that occurred when bone was not severed.[64]

Two possible problems exist in amputations at the Syme level: migration of the distal heel pad (which may be surgically avoidable) and poor cosmetic result (which can sometimes be partially addressed by decreasing the mediolateral dimension of the malleoli during surgery). For a positive outcome, the vascular supply must be adequate to ensure healing. The current resurgence of popularity of the Syme amputation is from an increased awareness of its energy efficiency in gait compared with transtibial levels, as well as improved vascular evaluation techniques and medical procedures that increase the likelihood of more distal primary wound healing.[65,66] In addition, the dramatic weight-bearing potential of a well-performed Syme surgery (with or without a prosthesis) has always been considered.[67] Pressure-sensitive areas of the Syme residual limb include the tibial crest, lateral tibial flair, fibula head, and the bony prominence around the distal expansion.[68,69] Pressure-tolerant areas include the midpatella tendon, medial tibial flair, and anterior tibialis (Fig. 22.29).

POSTOPERATIVE CARE: WALKING CASTS

To avoid migration of the heel pad in the postoperative period, gait training and other therapy that involve weight bearing should be encouraged only after delivery of the prosthesis. The prosthesis is designed to hold the prosthetic foot and bulbous distal tissue of the remnant limb in an appropriate alignment for ambulation. A fully mature residual limb is less likely to experience volume changes. Early prosthetic fitting may involve a preparatory prosthesis. Historically a temporary walking cast with a pattern bottom was utilized. The successful application of the Syme walking cast requires a more thorough knowledge base in prosthetics than might be readily appreciated, and the rehabilitation team all have to work together to prevent complications. Application of a walking cast should be done by a qualified medical professional.

PROSTHETIC MANAGEMENT

The prosthesis for the Syme amputation must be strong enough at the ankle section to withstand the forces of tension and compression that are produced by the long tibial lever arm throughout the gait cycle and at the same time provide an acceptable degree of cosmesis over the bulbous expansion at the ankle. All prosthetic designs strive to encompass the tibial section above the distal expansion firmly and still permit donning and doffing. Although prostheses designed for Syme amputations may be appropriate for Pirogoff and Boyd amputations, use of such prostheses may require that a lift be placed on the contralateral side to achieve bilateral limb length symmetry and a properly level pelvis during stance.

Before World War II, most patients with Syme amputations were fit with anterior lacing wooden sockets or leather sockets supported by a superstructure of heavy medial and lateral steel sidebars.[69,70] The prostheses most frequently fabricated today include the Canadian, medial opening, sleeve suspension, and flexible wall (bladder) designs.

Canadian Syme Prostheses

The *Canadian Syme prosthesis* design was introduced during the 1950s as the first major improvement over the traditional steel-reinforced leather.[71–74] When viewing the ankle in the coronal plane, no obvious buildups, windows, or hardware is present to increase the ankle diameter. The Canadian Syme prosthesis has a removable posterior panel to facilitate donning and doffing. This donning window extends from the apex of the distal expansion, moving proximal as far as necessary to provide clearance for the bulbous end.[75] Breakage may be higher than with other Syme prostheses because the ankle area, which undergoes the most compression and tension during ambulation, is weakened by the window cutout around the ankle in the posterior region. Modern carbon fiber and acrylic lamination materials and techniques have aided in meeting this challenge.[76,77] The Canadian prosthesis is a relatively cosmetic approach, but more recent options have limited its use.

Medial Opening Syme Prostheses

The *medial opening Syme prosthesis*, also known as the *Veterans Administration Prosthetic Center Syme prosthesis*, followed the introduction of the Canadian Syme prosthesis. Developed at the New York City Veterans Administration Medical Center in 1959, it has a removable donning door that extends proximally from the distal expansion to a level approximately two-thirds of the height of the tibial section on the medial side.[78,79] Like the Canadian design, the medial opening prosthesis is relatively cosmetic at the ankle and compares favorably with the Canadian design. The medial placement of the donning panel provides much more opportunity for anteroposterior strengthening of the prosthesis. All other factors being equal, this design is stronger than the Canadian design and is the approach of choice for many patients with Syme amputation.

Sleeve Suspension (Stovepipe)Syme Prostheses

The *sleeve suspension Syme prosthesis* is sometimes referred to as the *stovepipe Syme prosthesis* because of the cylindrical appearance of its removable liner. This design is appropriate for pediatric patients (Fig. 22.23A and B). It is constructed with an inner flexible insert or sleeve that has filler material in the areas just proximal to the distal expansion.[80,81] Before slipping into the outer shell or socket, the wearer first pulls on the flexible liner.[82] The outside sleeve then telescopes within the outer prosthetic shell (Fig. 22.24). In another version the

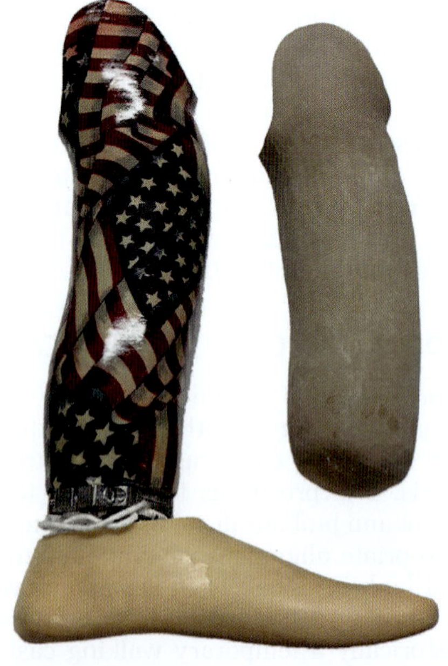

A

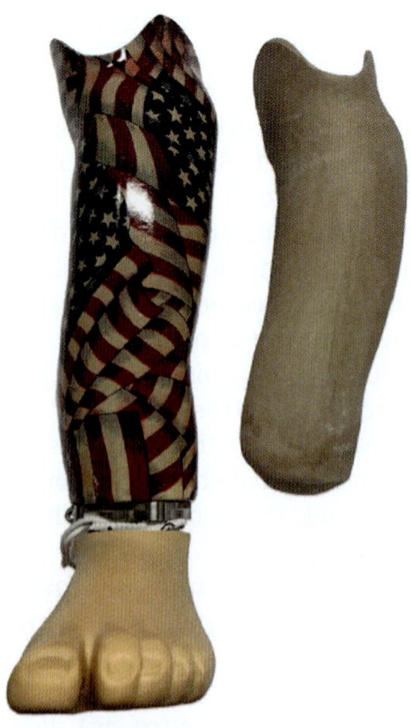

B

Fig. 22.23 (A and B) Two views of a Syme prosthesis showing the laminated socket and foam liner separately.

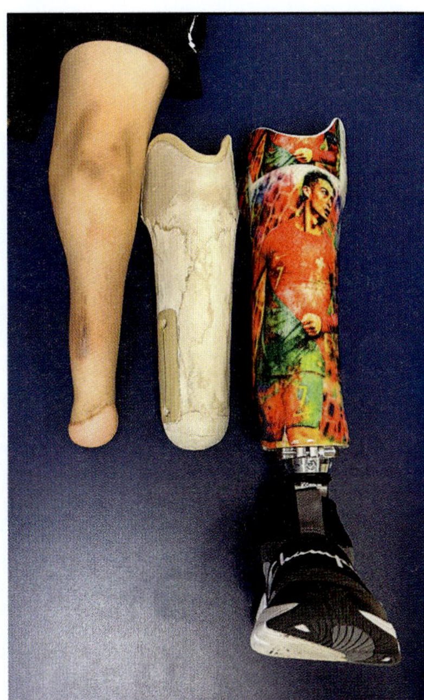

Fig. 22.24 Residuum, foam liner, and Syme prosthesis.

leather and foam inner sleeve does not cover the entire residual limb but wraps around the leg and fills up the void areas above the expansion.[83] The sleeve suspension prosthesis is bulky and not very cosmetic, but its strength is significantly better because no window is present to create a structural weakness. It is often chosen for the obese, athletic heavy-duty wearer, or for the patient with recurring prosthetic breakage of other designs. It is more adjustable and forgiving than the other Syme designs and is often chosen when the treating prosthetist anticipates major fitting problems.

Expandable Wall Prostheses

The *flexible, expandable wall,* and *bladder Syme prostheses,* of which several varieties are available, vary more by materials used than by mechanism of action. All are based on the concept of an inner socket wall just proximal to the distal expansion that is elastic or expandable enough to allow entry of the limb into the prosthesis and still provide a level of total contact around the ankle once donned.[84,85] This design normally requires a double prosthetic wall. The original bladder Syme prosthesis, described by Marx in 1969, obtained expansion by using flexible polyester resin in the neck area.[86] The more recent Rancho Syme prosthesis uses a flexible inner socket, supported by a frame or superstructure of laminated thermosetting plastic. The use of flexible thermosetting plastics and silicone elastomer for expandable wall sockets has gradually eclipsed the use of Surlyn (DuPont, Wilmington, DE) and other thermoplastics as a material of choice for the inner liner. Expandable wall Syme prostheses are slightly bulkier and less cosmetic at the ankle than their Canadian or medial opening counterparts because they require a flexible inner socket and a rigid exterior superstructure. The fabrication process is more involved, and fitting adjustments to the flexible inner socket can be difficult. Creating either a silicone elastomer or a Surlyn inner socket flexible enough for comfortable donning and doffing may significantly limit its durability. The Syme residual limb presents greater pressure distribution challenges to a prosthetist than do other types of lower-limb prostheses. A test socket is especially recommended for all Syme prostheses. Because the act of donning and doffing with this system is relatively simple, it may be the prosthesis of choice for patients with upper limb dysfunction or cognitive impairment.

Tucker-Winnipeg Syme Prostheses

The *Tucker-Winnipeg Syme prosthesis,* rarely seen in the United States, ignores the traditional requirement of comprehensive total contact by introducing lateral and medial donning slots.[87] The design is well suited for children. It is contraindicated for patients with severe vascular disease and for others who are prone to window edema. A loss of total contact can also affect proprioception and control of the prosthesis. In general, the method permits a prosthesis that is relatively cosmetic, easy to do, and not prone to the noises that are sometimes created by rubbing at the window covers of the medial opening on Canadian Syme prostheses.

Case Example 22.3 **A Patient With Bilateral Dysvascular Partial Foot Amputation**

L. P. is a 66-year-old man with a 23-year history of type II diabetes. He has comorbid history of diabetic retinopathy, hypertension, hyperlipidemia, peripheral neuropathy, stage III kidney disease, vascular complications associated with type II diabetes, bilateral foot ulcers, and vision changes. Five years ago, a right hallux amputation failed to heal and became infected, necessitating a right transmetatarsal amputation in 2013. After healing, he became proficient with a partial foot prosthesis, ambulating functional distances without assistive devices. In 2015 a large neuropathic wound developed under the metatarsal heads of his left foot. The wound failed to heal despite several attempted treatments. L. P. and his surgeon agreed that a transmetatarsal amputation on the left would allow him to heal, improve his functional status, and allow him to maintain his independence. The left transmetatarsal amputation failed to heal and became infected, leading to revision of his left partial foot back to a midtarsal level of amputation. His right residual limb is well healed, and the left is almost healed (Figs. 22.25A–C and 22.26A and B). The clinical team has agreed he is ready to return to prosthetic use and prescribes new prostheses.

QUESTIONS TO CONSIDER

- Given his medical history, what concerns exist about the condition of his residual feet?
- What areas are most vulnerable to pressures from repetitive loading during walking in prostheses?
- What types of muscle performance at his knee and hip are important to assess?
- What measures should be used to assess muscle function and strength?
- How will any impairments be addressed?
- How does the transmetatarsal and transtarsal amputation affect progression through the gait cycle?

Case Example 22.3 A Patient With Bilateral Dysvascular Partial Foot Amputation—Cont'd

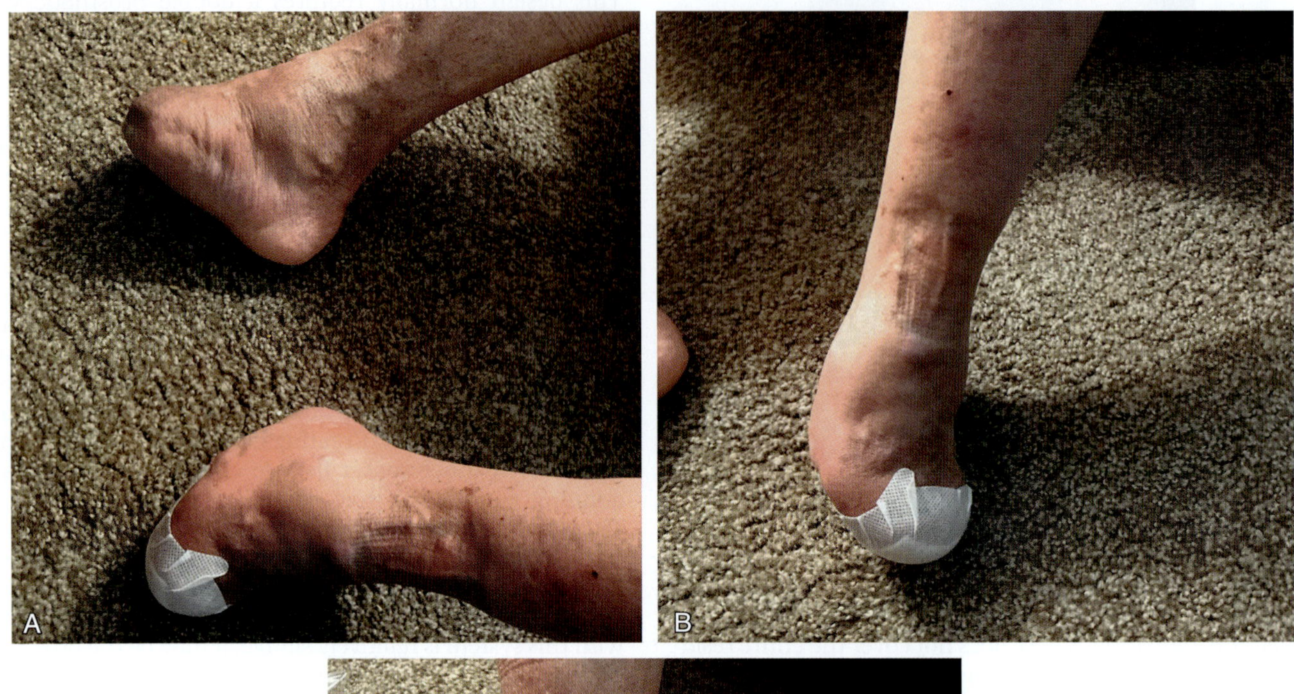

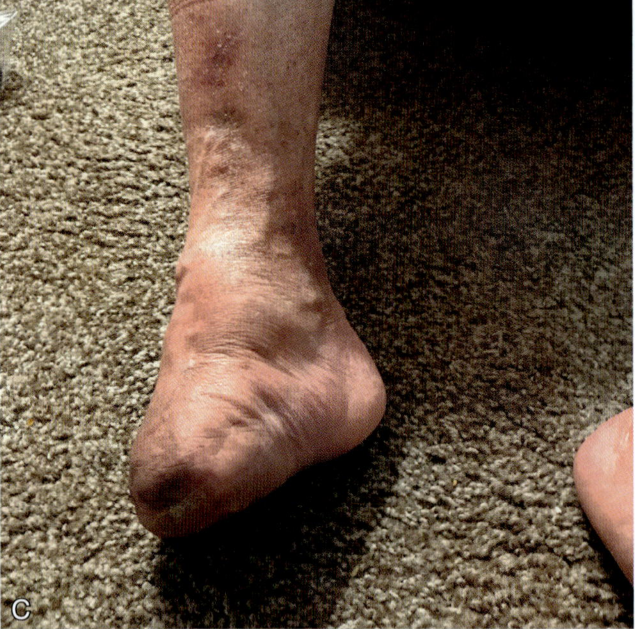

Fig. 22.25 (A) L. P.'s bilateral partial foot amputations. (B) Left transtarsal and (C) right transmetatarsal remnant feet.

- How might a prosthesis substitute for compromise of the three rockers of the gait cycle?
- How might these amputations affect step and stride length of the opposite swing limb?
- What are the major goals for prosthetic intervention for L. P.?
- What specific recommendations should be made for socket design, suspension, and biomechanical function?
- What options should be chosen from among those available?
- What is his prognosis for functional ambulation?
- Is an assistive device recommended for long-term use? Why or why not?
- How should the efficacy of intervention be assessed?

RECOMMENDATIONS

The clinical team determines L. P. is a candidate for bilateral limited motion, articulated ankle-foot orthosis style partial foot prostheses with toe fillers (Fig. 22.27A–C). L. P. currently ambulates with a rolling walker and is happy not to be using a wheelchair. He is receiving physical therapy and hopes to ambulate without any assistive devices again in the future. After delivery of the prostheses, L. P. reports immediate improvement of his balance and walking (Fig. 22.28A and B).

(Continued)

Case Example 22.3 A Patient With Bilateral Dysvascular Partial Foot Amputation—Cont'd

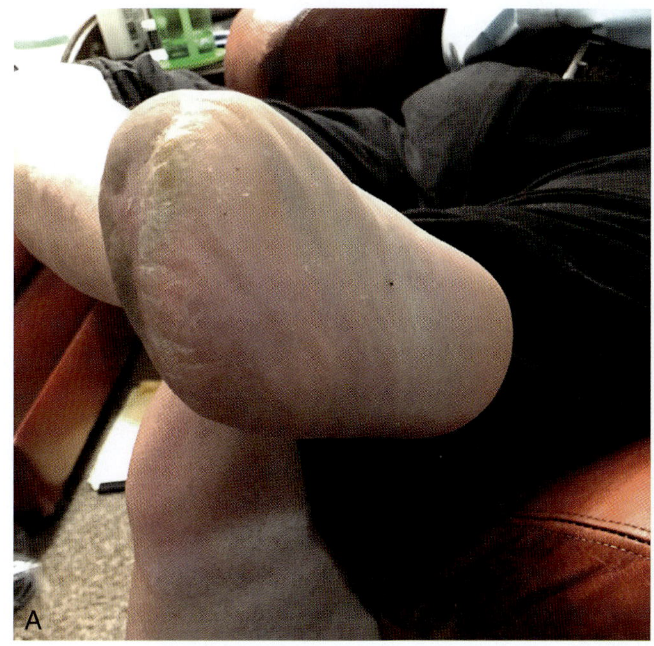

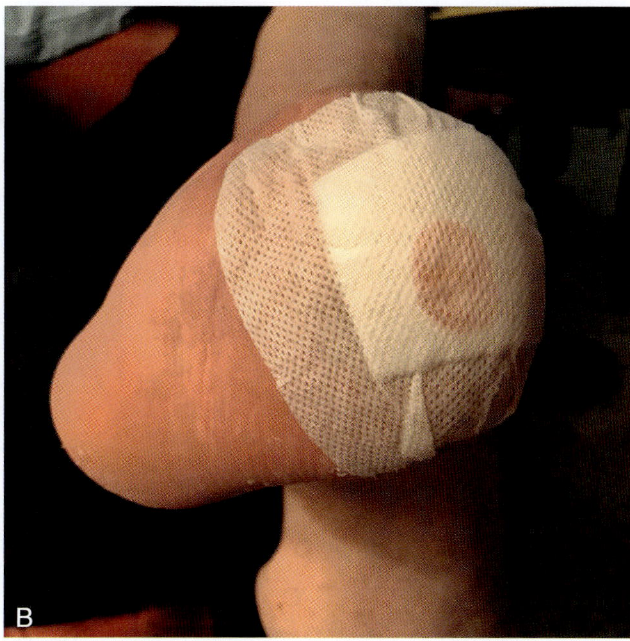

Fig. 22.26 (A) Right and (B) left plantar surface of L. P.'s remnant limbs.

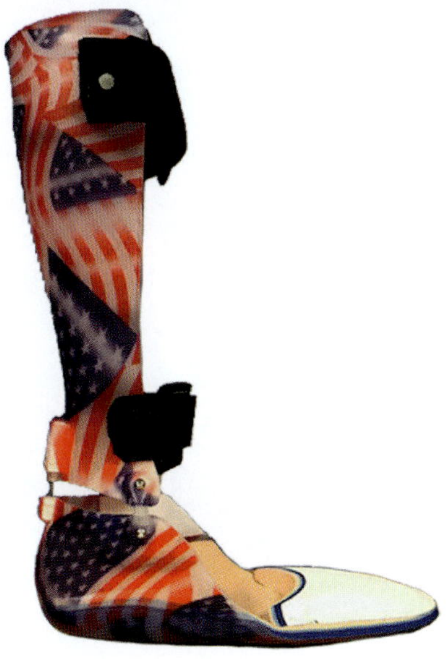

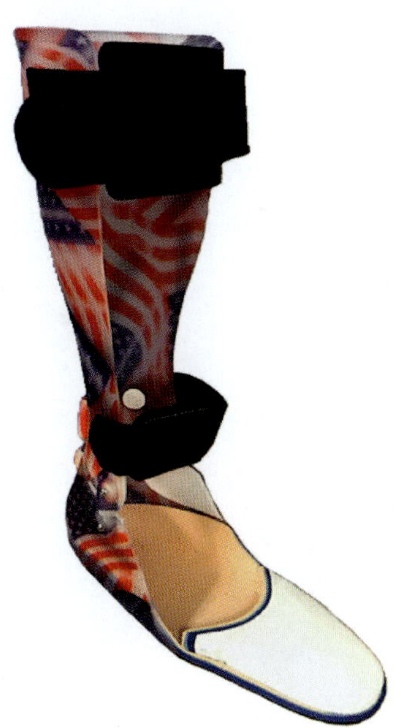

Fig. 22.27 (A–C) L. P.'s articulated ankle-foot orthosis design prostheses with toe fillers and dorsiflexion limiters.

Case Example 22.3 **A Patient With Bilateral Dysvascular Partial Foot Amputation—Cont'd**

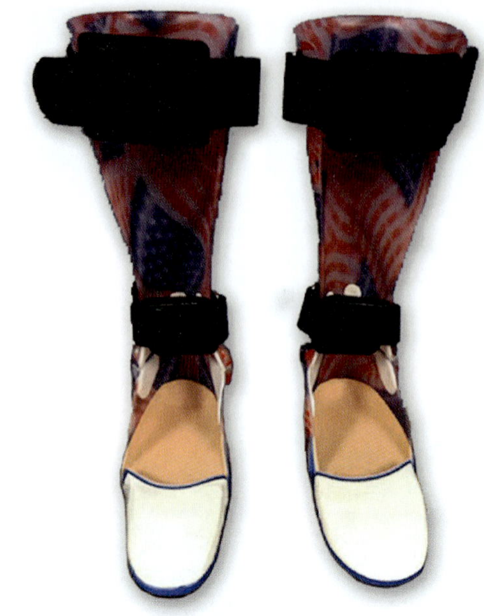

C

Fig. 22.27, Cont'd

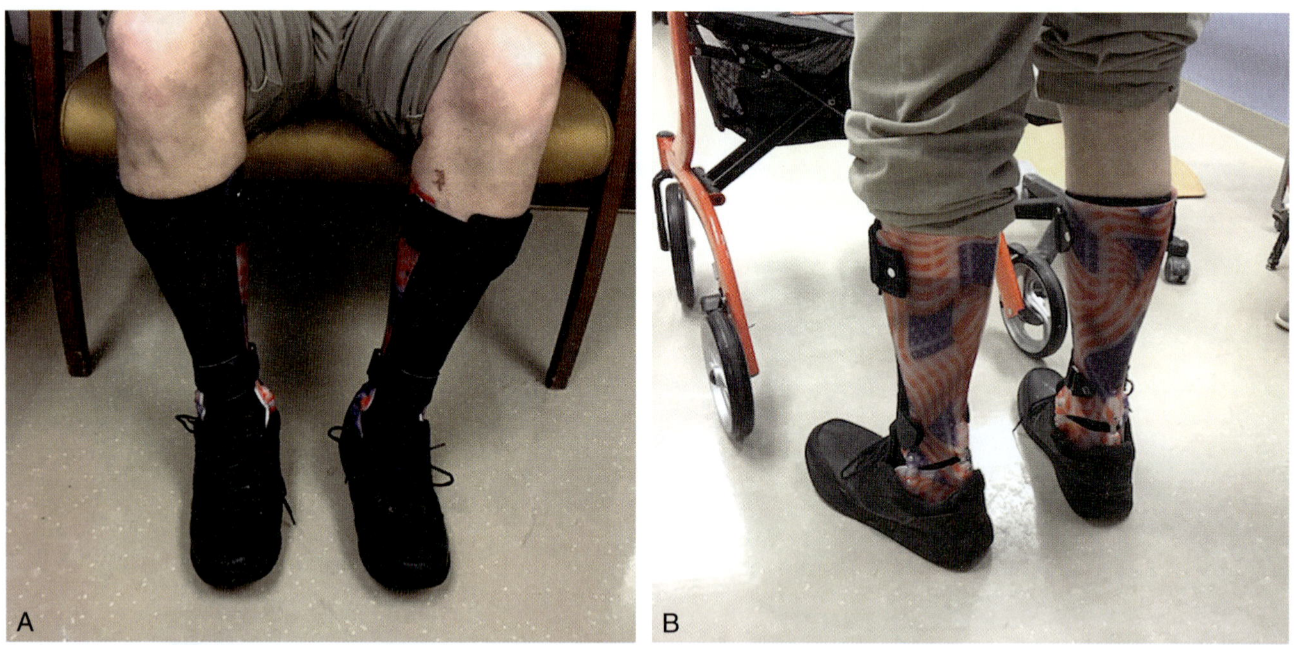

A B

Fig. 22.28 L. P. wearing his prostheses for the first time while sitting (A) and walking (B).

PROSTHETIC FEET FOR SYME PROSTHESES

One of the challenges in selecting prosthetic components for patients with a Syme amputation is fitting a prosthetic foot within the very limited space under the residual limb while still maintaining equal leg lengths and a level pelvis during standing. The rare exception to this is when bilateral ankle disarticulation has occurred; bilateral Syme amputation allows many more choices of foot designs to be considered for improved function. When there is unilateral Syme amputation, great care must be given to the minimal amount of space available between the distal residual limb and floor so that a heel lift on the contralateral side is unnecessary.

Determining the Prosthetic Clearance Value

In determining whether a particular Syme foot can accommodate a patient, the available space between the distal end of the residual limb and the floor is measured with the pelvis level and the anatomic clearance value is derived. Syme feet can be directly attached to the socket in the lamination by Syme nut (a threaded disk that is laminated into the socket) or using a variety of endoskeletal alignable lamination components. The nut, shaped to approximately match the contours of the distal residual limb, is approximately {5/8} inch tall, and this height must be considered when constructing the prosthesis. To determine the applicability of a particular foot for a patient, the space between the bottom of the heel of the foot and the top of the foot is added to height of the selected lamination component to ensure the prosthesis will not create a leg length discrepancy. This measurement is the prosthetic clearance value and should be less than or equal to the anatomic clearance value.

Nonarticulating Syme Feet

Many prosthetic feet used for transtibial amputation have been adapted for the Syme amputation. The first was the *SACH* foot, patented in 1863 by Marks and further developed at the University of California at Berkeley after World War II. It was introduced as a component of the Canadian Syme prosthesis in the 1950s.

The SACH foot design simulates plantarflexion as the patient rolls over a compressible heel, but because of a rigid wooden (typically maple) keel, it is neither flexible nor dynamic during the stance phase of gait. The SACH-type Syme foot was the historical foot of choice for patients with a Syme amputation in previous decades but is currently limited in use due to more functional options.

The *stationary-ankle flexible-endoskeletal* (SAFE) Syme foot has the advantage of providing a modest inversion and eversion component of motion through elasticity of the forefoot, and it is useful for uneven terrain ambulation. Not including the thickness of the Syme's nut, the SAFE II (Campbell-Childs, White City, OR) Syme foot requires 1⅜ inches of space between the distal end and the floor or shoe with pelvis leveled. The SAFE II was also used historically and is currently more limited in use due to lighter and more functional prosthetic feet options.

Dynamic Response Syme Feet

A variety of dynamic response foot designs have emerged for patients with syme amputation. The Impulse Syme's

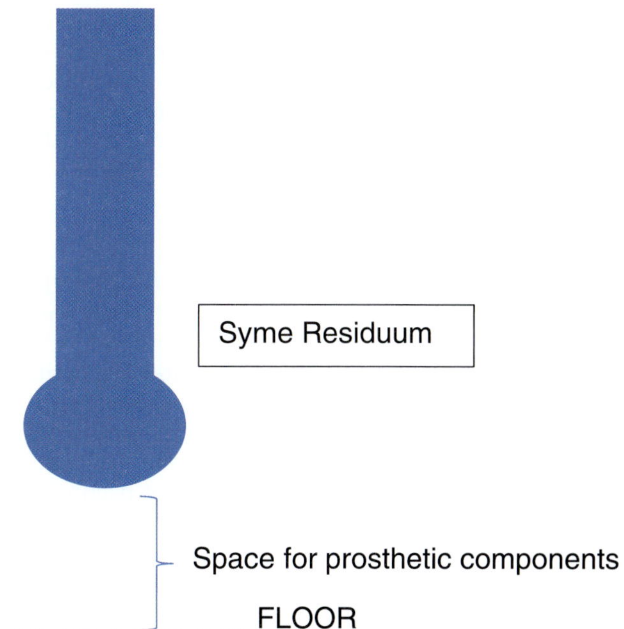

Fig. 22.29 Syme clearance for prosthetic components is calculated while the patient is standing with a level pelvis, the height difference between the amputated and contralateral leg provides the space for prosthetic design and foot clearance.

Foot (Ohio Willow Wood, Mt. Sterling, OH) has a Kevlar (DuPont, Wilmington, DE) keel with carbon deflection toe-spring plates and a weight limit of up to 250 lb (113 kg). The toe spring is a carbon-epoxy composite. A unique manufacturing technique allows carbon fibers to be optimally oriented and avoid wrinkling, buckling, and deformation. The most interesting part of the foot is alignment adjustability. Ohio Willow Wood also has a Carbon Copy II Syme foot available in two heel heights and with all the toe resistances and sizes of the standard (non-Syme) Carbon Copy II. The Carbon Copy II is available with a medium heel density for patient weights up to 250 lb (113 kg).

Ossur (Aliso Viejo, CA) offers a low-profile carbon Syme foot version for a very active prosthetic wearer weighing up to 285 lb (129 kg). The same foot can be worn by a low-activity level user weighing up to 365 lb (165.5 kg). The Ossur Low Profile requires 2 inches of clearance from the floor to the distal end of the socket and is designed with a flexible double-spring keel. It uses a fenestrated heel that allows greater compression, thus reducing shock. The upper spring bumper is coated with Teflon (DuPont), which reduces squeaks, a characteristic not uncommon to feet with more than one keel in the forefoot. Another Syme foot that may be used for patients up to 500 lbs (227 kg) is the Vari-Flex (Ossur), which requires only 1¾ inches of space under the socket and is attached using epoxy filler and lamination. Proteor (France) has developed the Pacifica (FS2) and LP Pacifica (FS4) with 10-mm heel height and build heights ranging from 1⅞ to 2½ inches depending on the foot size. Proteor (France) developed the Rush Rover with a unique design, moving the foot attachment to the socket more anterior, thus changing the biomechanics of the foot.

Another dynamic foot choice for the active individual is the Seattle Light Foot (Seattle Orthopedic Group, Seattle, WA).

Almost all prosthetic feet for Syme prostheses have ankles that are essentially locked. This characteristic results in increased work for the quadriceps for controlled knee flexion during loading response. Incorporation of several degrees of adjustable articulated plantarflexion (at the risk of increasing the weight of the prosthesis) might improve function for certain patients.

Alignment Issues

With most prosthetic feet, the small area between the distal residual limb and floor limits the prosthetist's ability to refine the relationship between the socket and foot in the dynamic alignment process. Chopart plates are laminated directly to the bottom of the socket and have no alignment adjustability (Figs. 22.30B, 22.31C, and 22.32A). Adjustable alignment devices, similar to those available for transtibial prostheses, have historically not been compact enough to fit in the available space between the prosthetic foot and the end of the socket. Two component options have been introduced with the goal of addressing this limitation.

The SL Profile and the Lo Rider Syme feet (Otto Bock, Minneapolis, MN) provide angular adjustability by a pyramid. Unfortunately, the height of the pyramid may preclude their use on many patients with a Syme amputation. The newest and very promising addition is the 1 C20 ProSyme's (Otto Bock), which can be fit on most patients and is a moderately dynamic urethane carbon fiber foot for patients with syme amputations weighing up to 275 lb (125 kg). It has a wide range of alignment adjustability, as well as heel height changes. Several alignable feet with various heel heights, weight limits, and functional benefits are currently being manufactured: Proteor makes the Rush Rover, Pacifica, and Pacifica LP; Ossur makes LP Vari-Flex and Pro-Flex LP; and Otto Bock makes Axtion, Lo Rider, Triton Low-Profile, and Triton K2 (Figs. 22.30–22.33).

Alignment can be significantly compromised when knee flexion contracture is present. To prevent breakage and premature wear from the anterior lever arm, the degree of anterior (linear) displacement of the socket over the foot is generally reduced from that of a transtibial prosthesis.

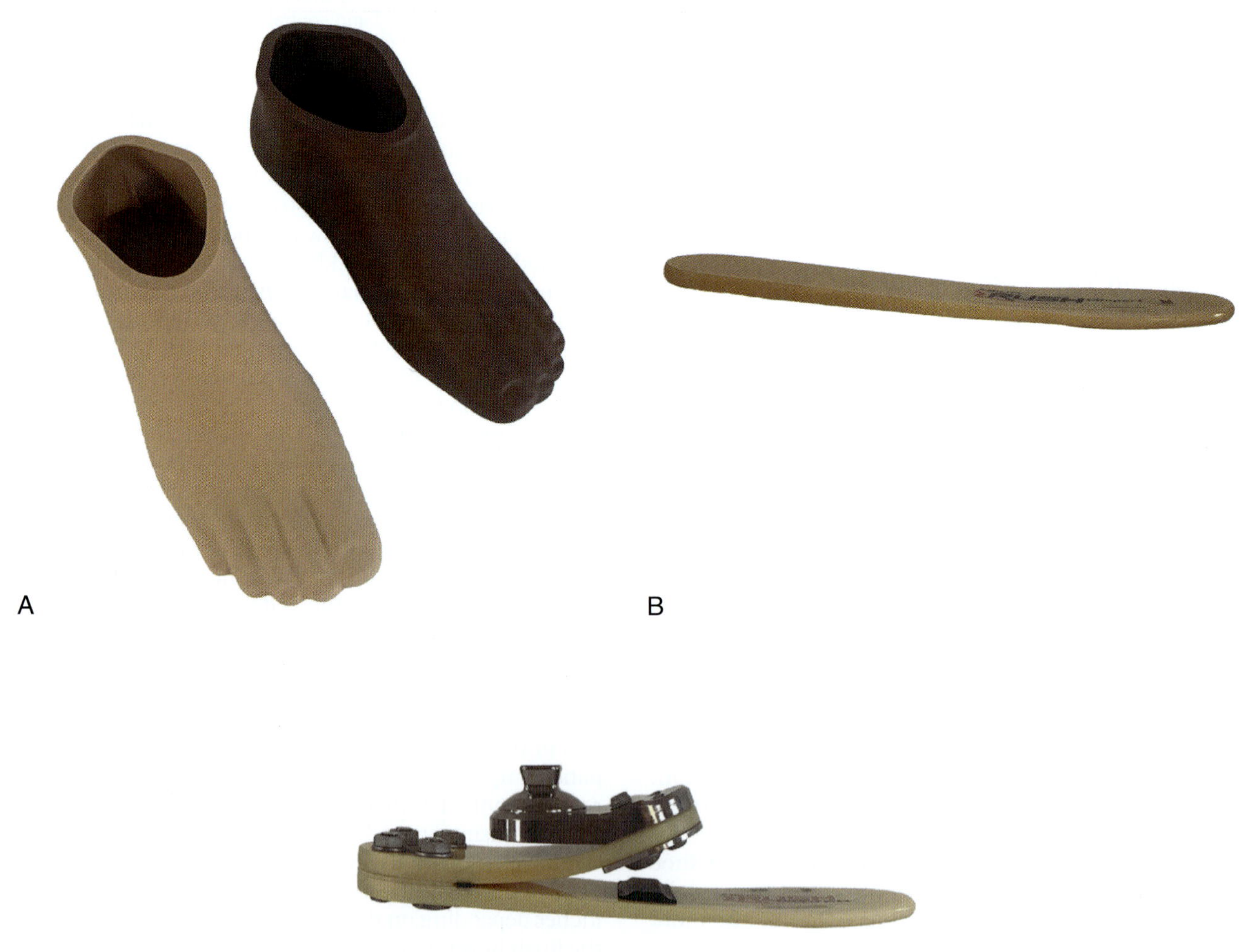

Fig. 22.30 (A) Proteorfoot shell examples with (B) Rush Chopart plate and (C) Rush Rover feet.

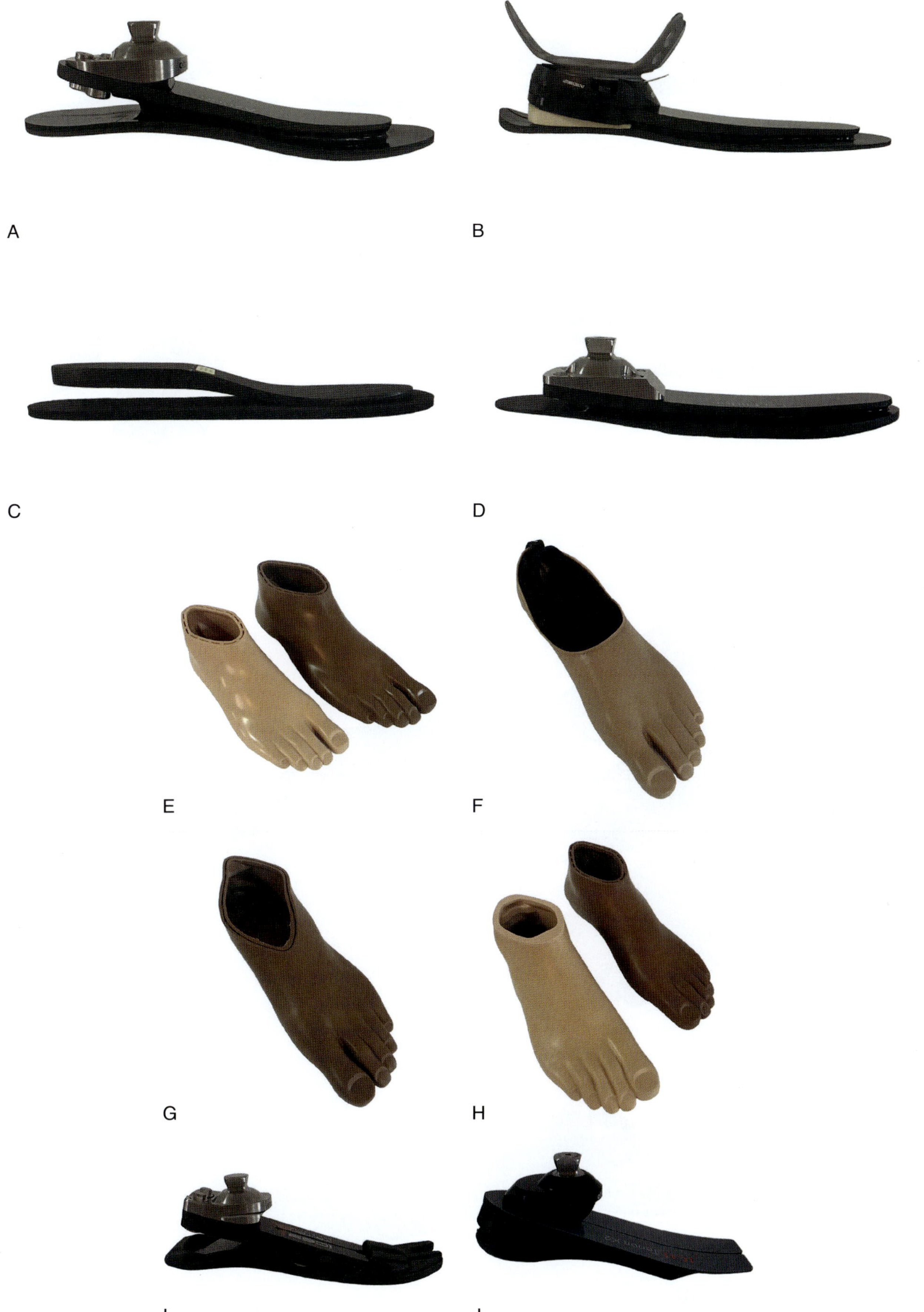

Fig. 22.31 Otto Bock feet and foot shell options. (A) Axtion. (B) ProSyme. (C) Chopart plate. (D) Lo Rider. (E) Split toe foot shells. (F) 2C66 foot shell. (G) ProSyme foot shell. (H) Foot shells. (I) Triton Low Profile. (J) Triton K2.

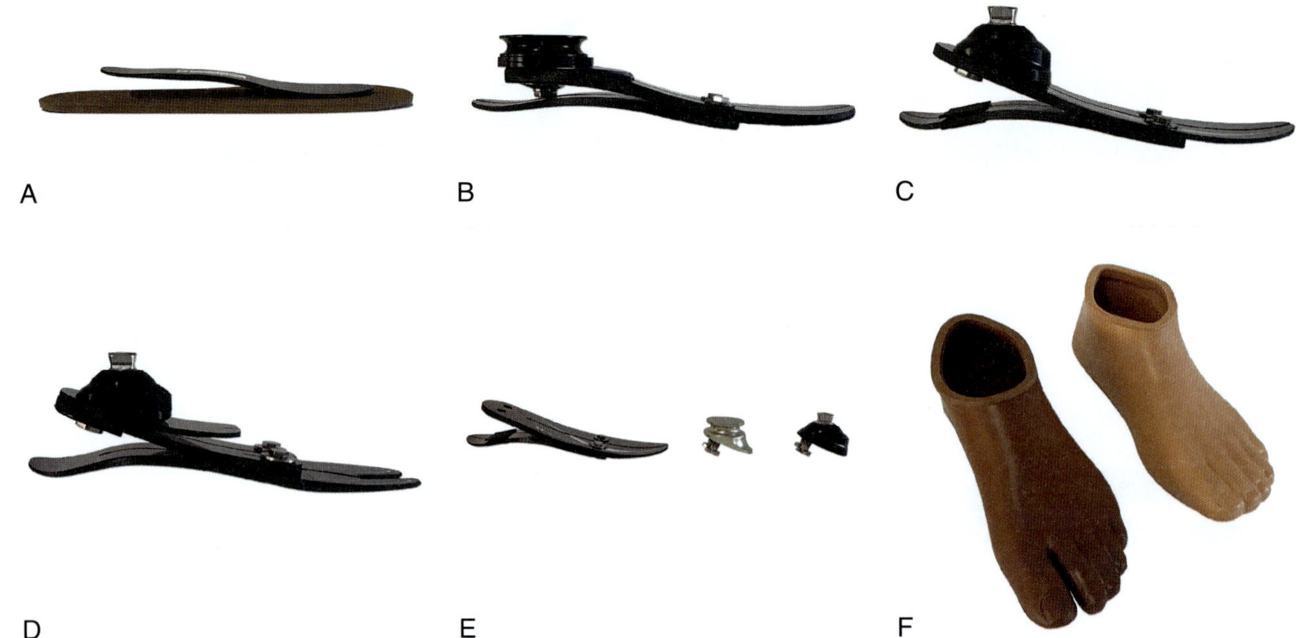

Fig. 22.32 Ossur feet and foot shells. (A) Chopart plate. (B) Flex Syme. (C) LP Variflex. (D) Proflex LP. (E) LP Variflex attachment options. (F) Foot shells.

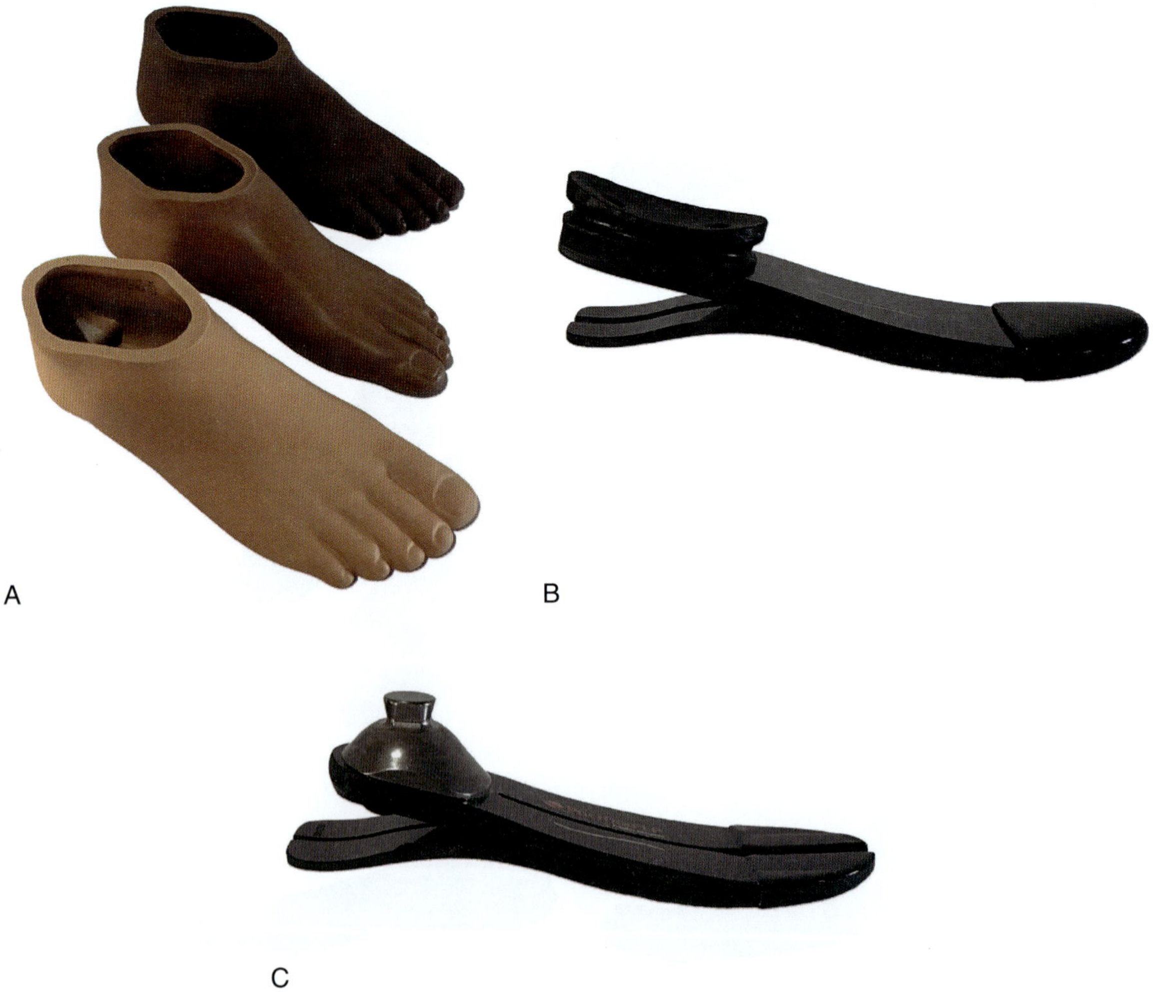

A

B

C

Fig. 22.33 Proteorfeet and foot shells. (A) Foot shell examples. (B) LP Syme. (C) Pacifica LP.

The Syme socket is positioned in an angle of adduction that matches the anatomic adduction angle of the tibia. The adduction of the socket should be positioned to create as smooth a transition as possible at the ankle and knee so that the prosthetic foot rolls over with the sole flat on the floor. The optimal spatial relation in the coronal plane is one that creates a slight varus moment. Socket adduction angle, foot eversion angle, and linear displacement affect the external varus moment at the knee during midstance. For an efficient and cosmetic gait, the knee must displace approximately 0 to 12 mm laterally at midstance, and should not collapse into valgus. Insufficient displacement implicates malalignment, most often at an inadequate eversion angle. Excessive displacement may be the result of malalignment or lateral collateral ligament laxity at the knee. The most successful strategy to address chronic weight-bearing ulceration at the knee that has not responded to a silicone liner, or to address major laxity of the collateral ligaments, is the addition of orthotic components (external knee joints and a thigh lacer) to provide extra support and protection.

Summary

This chapter explored the options for prosthetic management for patients with partial foot and Syme amputations. Because of the variability in surgical procedures, condition of the residual limb, and altered biomechanics of the residual limb in gait, no single best option exists for prosthetic design. More scientific research is needed to improve our understanding of biomechanics of ambulation after partial foot amputation to better guide the clinical judgment of the rehabilitation team.[88] For now, the characteristics of each patient (weight, skin condition, desired activity level, and length of residual limb) must be carefully considered in prosthetic prescription. The goal is to find the best match of the person's status and needs from the growing array of prosthetic design options for the partial foot and Syme amputations. This places an increasing demand on the knowledge base of prosthetists and other interdisciplinary team members involved in patient care for persons with amputation. More than ever, the physician, physical therapist, and prosthetist are challenged to function as a cohesive team, drawing on each other's strengths to achieve the best possible outcome for each patient.

References

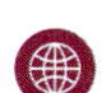

The complete listing of the References are available in the accompanying enhanced eBook version included with the print purchase of this textbook. Visit Elsevier eBooks+ (eBooks.Health.Elsevier.com) to access this content.

23 Transtibial Prosthetics

DANIEL G. MINER AND TODD DEWEES

LEARNING OBJECTIVES

On completion of this chapter, the reader will be able to do the following:

1. Define the goals of each phase of rehabilitation following transtibial amputation.
2. Identify key determinants for successful use of a transtibial prosthesis.
3. Describe the principles underlying current transtibial socket design and demonstrate a basic knowledge of key components of a transtibial prosthesis.
4. Identify key determinants of appropriate transtibial prosthetic alignment.
5. Identify key strategies for management of changes in residual limb volume and maintenance of residual limb health.
6. Recognize and differentiate patient-related versus prosthesis-related factors that may lead to transtibial prosthetic gait deviations.
7. Troubleshoot appropriate strategies to address transtibial gait deviations.
8. Identify evidence-supported outcome measures to evaluate strength, dynamic balance, mobility, and gait speed performance for transtibial prosthetic users.
9. Identify evidence-supported outcomes measures to determine fall risk for individuals with history of transtibial amputation.

Rehabilitation Following Transtibial Amputation

For individuals who require transtibial amputation, either due to trauma or vascular complications or cancer or other medical-related comorbidities, it is often a goal and priority to be able to be fit with a transtibial prosthesis and be able to return to activities that they enjoyed prior to their amputation. Chapter 20 highlights the early postoperative and preprosthetic fitting phases of rehabilitation, and Chapter 26 discusses prosthetic training considerations for individuals with lower-limb amputation due to vascular complications. Table 23.1 summarizes the guidelines for rehabilitation management of individuals with transtibial amputation from the Extremity Trauma and Amputation Center of Excellence, which was established in 2009 as a joint initiative between the US Department of Defense (DoD) and the Department of Veterans Affairs (VA) and in October 2022 was aligned with the US Defense Health Agency.

Determinants of Successful Use of Transtibial Prosthesis

Successful use of a lower-limb prosthesis following transtibial amputation requires intact cognitive function to learn the skills necessary to safely and appropriately manage and monitor residual limb health, to appropriately don/doff a lower-limb prosthesis and adapt to changes in residual limb volume to ensure appropriate fit and function of a prosthesis, and to safely manage the cognitive load during performance of mobility-related activities of daily living, which require individuals to utilize higher level executive cognitive functions to plan movement strategies, interpret sensory information to adapt, and anticipate adjustments that need to be made in real-time to maintain safety with mobility-related tasks.[4,5] A recent study of 22 participants with unilateral transtibial amputation demonstrated that better global cognitive function, assessed by the Montreal Cognitive Assessment (MoCA), and executive function, assessed by the Trail Making Test, was associated with faster walking speeds and greater functional mobility, assessed with an instrumented walkway and the L-Test respectively in both single-task and dual-task conditions.[4] However, better cognitive and executive function was not associated with improved dynamic balance, assessed with the Four-Square Step Test (FSST).[4] It is important to note that the FSST was modified with tape marking out the four quadrants as opposed to canes, which reduced the level of difficulty by not requiring participants to step over the canes.[4] Hunter and colleagues[5] reported on a study of 22 individuals with transtibial amputation in which lower cognitive functional scores on the Trail Making Test were associated with lower functional improvements in mobility performance, as assessed by the L-Test, 4 months after discharge from prosthetic rehabilitation.[5] However, it should be noted that 90% of the participants demonstrated improvements in single-task and dual-task mobility performance on gait speed and L-Test, which exceeded thresholds for minimum detectable change.[5] Cognitive assessments and screening tools such as the MoCA and the Trail Making Test may provide clinicians with valuable insight regarding cognitive and executive function to inform rehabilitation strategies to optimize outcomes for individuals with limb loss who have goals of using a lower-limb prosthesis.

Important considerations and predictors correlated with decreased participation with use of a prosthesis for individuals with limb loss include depression, chronic pain, and limited social support.[6] Additionally, issues related

Table 23.1 Summary of Unilateral Transtibial Amputation Rehabilitation Guidelines

Rehabilitation Phase	Guidelines	Goals	Milestones
Preoperative	■ Strengthening exercises to improve muscle tone and function ■ Strive for full/functional residual limb active/passive range of motion values ■ Improve cardiovascular fitness ■ Optimize medical management of any existing concurrent medical conditions ■ Optimize unilateral balance/proprioceptive training ■ Promote wellness, proper nutrition, tobacco cessation, and an optimal body weight ■ Educate patient on postoperative rehabilitation requirements to ensure an optimal functional outcome ■ Validate behavioral health and family support program is in place ■ Facilitate identification of any necessary assistive devices and/or durable medical equipment for procurement, use, and training if clinically indicated prior to surgery ■ Implement Vitamin D and Calcium supplementation, as per surgeon's recommendation	■ Achieve maximal hip and knee ROM with emphasis on hip and knee extension ■ Begin core/LE strength training with emphasis on quad/hip extension/ hip abduction strength	N/A
Protective Healing (Week 1–2)	■ Non–weight-bearing status of residual limb ×4–6 weeks postop ■ It is important to maintain knee extension while seated, use of limb support device or wheelchair residual limb attachment can assist in maintaining full knee extension ■ Physician may prescribe a residual limb protector postoperatively, to maintain knee extension and protect the limb (may or may not be worn during physical therapy session) ■ Avoid shear stress and protect incision site ■ Per physician's recommendation, patient can be fit with a shrinker or use Figure-8 wrapping for swelling management and shaping of the residual limb (timeline and wear schedule may vary per physician) ■ Range of motion as tolerated ■ Bed mobility ■ Transfer and appropriate assistive device training ■ Gait training (non–weight bearing on operative side) ■ Wheelchair mobility training ■ Aerobic conditioning (e.g., arm ergometer/rower) ■ Core and limb strengthening (e.g., mat therapy exercises to include closed kinetic chain bolster) ■ Neuromuscular reeducation (e.g., seated and standing balance activities) ■ Begin desensitization and mirror therapy for phantom limb and neuropathic pain ■ Monitor symptom responses for 24–48 hours after each exercise session. Pain should settle quickly post exercise with no significant increase in symptoms the next day (see pain monitoring model below)	■ Pain control, functional mobility ■ Protection of residual limb ■ Achieve knee extension to 0 degrees and hip extension to 10 degrees	N/A
Preprosthetic Training (Week 2–8)	■ Wound monitoring and assist with dressing changes as needed ■ Maintain/improve hip and knee ROM ■ Continue appropriate previous exercises with increased resistance and/or difficulty ■ Core strengthening exercises ■ Gait training on even and uneven surfaces with appropriate assisted device maintaining non–weight-bearing status on amputee limb ■ Suture removal depending on wound healing and surgeon preference (typically 2 weeks postop) ■ Liner fitting once cleared by Orthopedics, establish wear schedule (i.e., liner during the day and shrinker at night) ■ Once incision site is fully healed begin scar mobilization	■ Wound healing ■ Residual limb management ■ Desensitization and pain management	■ Tolerate liner wear 8 hours a day without skin issues ■ Maintain knee extension and quadriceps activation ■ Ambulate at a modified independence level with appropriate assisted device

Table 23.1 Summary of Unilateral Transtibial Amputation Rehabilitation Guidelines—cont'd

Rehabilitation Phase	Guidelines	Goals	Milestones
Prosthetic Training	▪ Socket fit typically occurs around 4–6 weeks postop to allow for adequate tissue healing ▪ Educated on prosthetic wearing schedule, skin inspection, management of limb volume changes, use of different ply socks, prosthetic fit, and hygiene instructions ▪ Gradually increase prosthesis wear time starting at 15 minutes intervals and increasing as tolerated with frequent skin checks ▪ Gait activities (e.g., weight shifts, step-ups, hurdles, level surfaces, ramps, curbs, stairs, grass, car transfers, etc.) focusing on equalizing step length, stance time, upright posture, equal reciprocal arm swing ▪ Balance activities (e.g., step-up, playing catch, rebounder with a weight ball, compliant surfaces, balance beam, etc.) ▪ Fall recovery training	▪ Pain control ▪ Independence with residual limb management (hygiene, skin care) ▪ Independence with prosthetic management (socket fit and use of sock ply for volume changes) ▪ Independence with mobility with prosthesis and least restrictive assistive device	▪ Wear prosthesis around 8 hours a day without any skin issues ▪ Full hip/knee ROM ▪ 5/5 MMT strength for hip and knee ▪ Score of ~30 on single leg bridge test (with 8-inch towel roll) ▪ Demonstrate fall recovery procedures training and floor to stand transfers ▪ Ambulate with modified independence with zero to minimal gait deviations on level and uneven surfaces over 1000 ft ▪ Amputee Mobility Predictor (AMPPRO) scores (normative values, see CPG): K0/K1 25±7; K2 35±7; K3 41±4; K4 45±2 ▪ 2 MWT or 6 MWT consistent with age rated normative values

CPG, Clinical Practice Guideline; *LE*, Lower extremity; *MMT*, Manual Muscle Test; *2 MWT*, 2-Minute Walk Test; *6 MWT*, 6-Minute Walk Test; *N/A*, not available; *ROM*, range of motion.
Adapted from Flint J, Pierrie S, Potter BK. *Unilateral Transtibial Amputation Rehabilitation Guidelines*. Extremity Trauma and Amputation Center of Excellence; 2021.

to self-esteem, amputation-specific body image, physical activity levels, and decreased balance confidence were correlated with decreased participation with use of prosthesis.[6,7] Physical activity level has been shown to be one of the strongest predictors of community participation following lower-limb amputation.[7] Comorbidities impacting the cardiopulmonary or integumentary systems impact participation for individuals with limb loss.[8] Individuals with limb loss who have diabetes mellitus or peripheral neuropathy also demonstrate decreased activity and participation.[7,9] To optimize activity and participation for individuals with limb loss, clinicians should focus on modifiable risk factors that may adversely impact activity and participation.[7,8]

Individuals with transtibial amputation often demonstrate impaired hip strength on the amputated side compared to the intact side.[10–12] For individuals with transtibial amputation the hip extensors play a critical role in producing forward momentum during ambulation. The hip abductors are important to stabilize the pelvis in the frontal plane.[10] Hip extension power and asymmetry of hip abduction power are important predictors of walking speed and performance in individuals with lower-limb amputation.[10,13] Impairments or deficits in hip extension and hip abduction strength and power will contribute to inefficient gait patterns and gait asymmetry and should be targeted for strengthening early in the postoperative phase of rehabilitation and throughout the prosthetic training phase.[10] A recent study by Seth and colleagues[12] utilized handheld dynamometry to assess sound limb and residual limb strength in hip extension, hip abduction, and hip adduction to identify cut-off scores, which may be used to identify individuals who are more likely to be sedentary, defined as walking <5000 steps/day.[12] Strength deficits following lower-limb amputation may contribute to asymmetric loading patterns during mobility-related activities and may contribute to secondary complications related to knee pain, hip pain, back pain, and associated degenerative changes.[11,14] For individuals with unilateral transtibial amputation strength deficits in knee extension have been associated with increased ratings of perceived exertion at slow and moderate walking speeds, increased heart rates at fast walking speed, and decreased distance on the 2-Minute Walk Test.[15] Strength deficits in knee flexion are associated with increased time required to ascend stairs for individuals with limb loss.[15] For individuals with limb loss who have goals of using a lower-limb prosthesis, these findings highlight the importance for rehabilitation programs to incorporate strength training to optimize functional performance, activity, and participation.

PROSTHETIC EVALUATION

When evaluating an individual for a transtibial prosthesis, a comprehensive physical examination including a detailed history interview is essential to understanding the goals and values of the individual patient. The comprehensive physical examination is described in more detail in Chapter 20; however, it is imperative that clinicians consider how an individual's medical comorbidities, cognitive and psychological status, and social support may impact their rehabilitation and the successful use of a prosthesis.

Medicare Functional Classification Level and Considerations for Selection of Components for Transtibial Prosthesis

As described in Chapter 20, it is critical to assess an individual's ability to perform simple mobility tasks following transtibial amputation. The amputee mobility predictor (AMP) is a useful tool to systematically evaluate performance of static and dynamic sitting and standing balance, anticipatory and reactive postural control in standing, ability to perform basic transfers, and ability to ambulate short distances and variable speeds and turn around safely.[16] The AMP can be performed prior to an individual being fit with a prosthesis (AMPnoPRO) or with a prosthesis (AMPPRO).[16] The use of objective, performance-based outcome measures is a useful strategy to identify individuals who have the ability or potential to perform at various Medicare Functional Classification Levels or MFCL K-Levels (K0–K4) (see Fig. 24.1 and Table 24.2).

An individual's performance on the Amputee Mobility Predictor, either AMPnoPRO or AMPPRO, may provide clinicians with insight regarding areas of functional mobility performance on which to focus their rehabilitation approach to optimize their patient's potential for successful use of a lower-limb prosthesis. Gailey and colleagues proposed an Evidence-Based Amputee Rehabilitation (EBAR) program that uses the findings of the AMP to inform recommendations for exercise prescription for individuals with limb loss and goals of improving mobility with a lower-limb prosthesis.[17] Clinicians must analyze the underlying impairments that led to deficiencies in performance of specific tasks on the AMP to devise targeted interventions to improve performance.[17] The EBAR program is an 8-week exercise-based program focused on the following five components, which are foundational to successful use of a lower-limb prosthesis: (1) cardiopulmonary endurance and flexibility, (2) trunk and lower-limb strengthening, (3) balance and coordination, (4) weight bearing and stance control, and (5) prosthetic gait training.[17] Following an initial warm-up, consisting of aerobic exercise and flexibility exercises, physical therapists design targeted exercise programs based on the foundational components discussed above.[17] Selection of specific exercises is guided by the physical therapist's analysis of the patient's performance on the AMP, targeting the underlying impairments associated with tasks on which the patient scored a 0 or 1 out of a full score of 2 points.[17] In a study of 18 individuals with unilateral transtibial amputation who completed the EBAR program (with mean age of 63.25 years and mean time of 8.1 years since amputation), the mean change in AMPPRO scores and 6-Minute Walk Test distances exceeded the minimum detectable change, 58.33% of participants improved by at least one MFCL K-level, and two participants improved by two MFCL K-levels.[17] An example of this program is provided in Fig. 23.1.

READINESS FOR PROSTHETIC FITTING

Postsurgical care and residual limb protection are critical in the postoperative phase of rehabilitation for individuals with limb loss. Postoperative care and preprosthetic rehabilitation is described in detail in Chapter 20, but successful prosthetic fitting for individuals following transtibial amputation will require management of postoperative residual limb pain versus phantom limb pain versus phantom limb sensation, edema and residual limb volume, wound healing, prevention of knee flexion contractures, and strength and mobility training.[18] Comorbidities such as diabetes mellitus with poorly controlled blood glucose levels, renal disease, and lifestyle choices such as smoking may delay the healing process and lead to delays in prosthetic fitting.[18]

Rigid removable dressings (RRDs) have been shown to be effective in minimizing knee flexion contracture development and protecting the residual limb during the postoperative healing phase.[19] The RRD keeps the knee in full extension to prevent contracture, protects the limb from exterior trauma, and controls swelling through total contact. This removable device is worn over at least one prosthetic sock and is held in place with Velcro straps (Fig. 23.2). It is also fenestrated to allow airflow and release moisture. The device can be worn 23 hours a day and can be removed easily for dressing changes and bathing. For more detail on postoperative care, refer to Chapter 20. Due to high incidence of falls, which may lead to trauma to the residual limb and potentially surgical revision, RRDs provide superior residual limb protection compared to soft dressings.[19,20] In 2018, Reichmann and colleagues[19] published a review that stated that RRDs should be considered as the treatment of choice for postoperative care for individuals recovering from transtibial amputation to minimize risk for injury to residual limb due to falls, to decrease residual limb pain, to minimize risk for knee flexion contracture development, and to decrease time for wound healing and prosthetic fitting.[19] However, Kwah and colleagues[21] suggest that the available evidence for rigid versus soft dressings is less certain due to methodological concerns and very high risk of bias and conclude that clinicians should exercise clinical judgment regarding use of rigid versus soft dressings based on individual patient risk factors.[21] A more recent randomized controlled trial demonstrated superior healing times and improved residual limb maturation with the use of RRDs.[22] Residual limb maturation was defined as the point when residual limb volume had stabilized (<10% change from previous assessment), soft-tissue atrophy had occurred, and residual limb had been molded into a cylindrical shape in preparation for prosthetic fitting.[22]

While immediate postoperative prostheses (IPOPs), as discussed in Chapter 20, provide the potential for early weight bearing for individuals following amputation, they may increase the risk of complications for wound healing for individuals with amputation due to complications related to vascular disease.[19] IPOP sockets are designed to allow some weight bearing on the medial tibial flare and patellar tendon, because these structures are proximal to the surgical site and are less likely to be impacted by postoperative edema. It is important to note that weight bearing, while in an IPOP, should be at the level of toe touch partial weight bearing. Full weight bearing is discouraged as there is generally not enough area to distribute the full body weight in a manner that the skin will tolerate for extended periods.

Definitions of healing and readiness for prosthetic fitting vary across different studies.[18] Some authors define healing as a painless, healed suture line enabling prosthetic fitting,[23] whereas others define healing as the absence of an open wound, drainage/discharge, or absence of need for a dressing,[24] or no need of more proximal revision of amputation within 6 months.[25] This discrepancy can make it difficult for rehabilitation clinicians to identify the optimal benchmarks to indicate readiness for prosthetic fitting.[18] Clinicians should consider the individual risk factors that may impact their patient's readiness for prosthetic fitting,

Amputee Mobility Predictor Evidence-Based Amputee Rehabilitation Exercise Guide[a]

AMP Task	Primary Construct/System	Exercises
Task 1: Sitting balance	Sitting balance, trunk stability, sitting endurance	☐Trunk rhythmic rotation ☐Resisted trunk flexion & extension ☐Dynamic surface sitting exercise ☐Sitting endurance progression
Task 2: Sitting reach	Sitting balance, trunk/hip extensor strength	☐Trunk rotations with cane ☐Trunk rotations with heavy ball ☐Dynamic surface trunk flexion & extension ☐Heavy ball catch and throw
Task 3: Chair to chair transfer	Dynamic balance, upper/lower limb strength	☐Organizational planning transfers ☐Seated prosthetic weight-bearing ☐Seated dips ☐Partial chair squats
Task 4: Arise from a chair	Dynamic balance, trunk/lower limb strength	☐Organizational planning standing ☐Seated forward weight shifts ☐Sit-to-stand progression ☐Partial to full wall squats
Task 5: Attempts to arise from chair	Dynamic balance, Trunk/lower limb strength	☐Dynamic stump exercises ☐Organizational planning standing ☐Dynamic surface trunk rotations with cane ☐Dynamic surface trunk flexion & extension
Task 6: Immediate standing balance	Dynamic standing balance, postural stability	☐Rhythmic stabilization in standing pelvis-trunk ☐Perturbation in standing: thighs-pelvis–trunk ☐Dynamic surface standing ☐Dynamic surface trunk rotations with cane
Task 7: Standing balance	Standing balance, postural stability, muscular endurance	☐Postural positioning and feedback with mirror ☐Frontal plane weight shift ☐Sagittal plane weight shifts ☐Diagonal weight shifts
Task 8: Single limb balance	Single limb balance, strength, endurance, postural stability	☐Bridging ☐Stool stepping ☐Single limb trunk rotations with cane ☐Ball rolls on prosthetic limb
Task 9: Standing reach	Standing balance, COM over BoS displacement, trunk extensor strength	☐Perturbation in standing: rapid flexion/extension ☐Sagittal plane weight shifts with arm swing ☐Standing heavy ball swings ☐Standing heavy ball throws
Task 10: Nudged	Ankle, hip, step strategies	☐Standing resisted trunk flexion ☐Rhythmic stabilization in standing ☐Standing rapid trunk perturbation ☐Standing heavy ball chest pass
Task 11: Eyes closed	Possible vestibular/balance impairment	Refer to vestibular specialist
Task 12: Picking up object off floor	Dynamic balance, postural extensor strength	☐Bridging ☐Squats ☐Lunges ☐Weighted ball lunges
Task 13: Sitting down	Dynamic balance, eccentric trunk, lower limb strength	☐Organizational planning standing ☐Seated forward weight shifts ☐Sit-to-stand progression ☐Partial to full wall squats

Fig. 23.1 Amputee mobility predictor evidence-based amputee rehabilitation exercise guide.

AMP Task	Primary Construct/System	Exercises
Task 14: Initiation of gait	COM displacement over BoS, prosthetic gait control	☐Level walking ☐Multi-directional stepping ☐Stop and go walking ☐Ramp decline walking
Task 15: Step length & height	Single limb balance, range of motion, prosthetic weight-bearing, prosthetic gait control	☐Stool stepping ☐Restoration of pelvic transverse rotation ☐Resisted gait training ☐Ball rolls
Task 16: Step continuity	Single limb balance, double support time, prosthetic gait control	☐Resisted gait training ☐Lateral walking ☐Braiding ☐Stop and go walking
Task 17: Turning	Dynamic single limb balance, lower limb strength	☐Restoration of pelvic transverse rotation ☐Prosthetic turning progression ☐Braiding ☐Forward/lateral cup-walking[c]
Task 18: Variable cadence	Dynamic single limb balance, prosthetic gait control, dynamic postural stability	☐Stool stepping ☐Restoration trunk rotation ☐Resisted walking, prosthetic foot late stance ☐Speed training: increased step frequency
Task 19: Stepping over an obstacle	Dynamic single limb balance, prosthetic gait control, dynamic postural stability	☐Stool stepping ☐Forward cup-walking ☐Obstacle course performance ☐Resisted elastic kicks
Task 20: Ascending and descending stairs	Dynamic single limb balance, lower limb strength, prosthetic control	☐Prosthetic stair ascent progression ☐Prosthetic stair decent progression ☐Wall squats ☐Lunges

[c]Courtesy Advanced Rehabilitation Therapy, Inc. Miami, Florida Copyright © 2016. AMP = Amputee Mobility Predictor, BoS = base of support; COM = center of mass.

Fig. 23.1, cont'd

MONITORING PAIN AND LOAD RESPONSE

Pain during exercise
0 = no pain 10 = worse pain imaginable

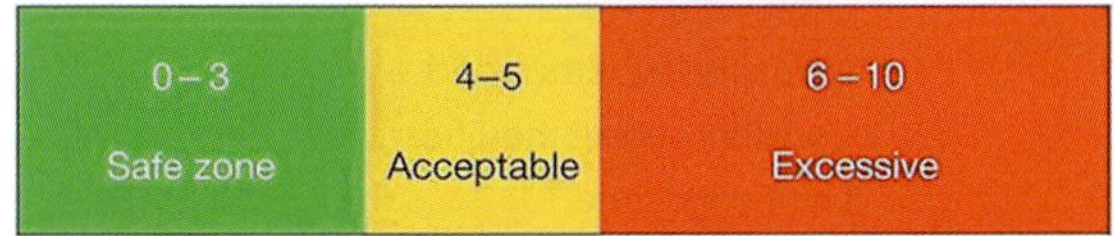

Monitor symptoms response for 24-48 h post exercise.
Pain should settle quickly post exercise with no increase in symptoms the next day

Fig. 23.2 Monitoring pain and load response with exercise.[1-3]

and decisions regarding prosthetic training, initial wearing time of prosthesis, and monitoring of the residual limb are important to minimize risks of complications to the residual limb. The most frequently identified predictive factors for wound complications were renal failure/dialysis and smoking/tobacco use, followed by individuals with sepsis/septic shock, those requiring emergency surgery or revascularization procedures, and individuals with elevated white blood cell counts, those using anticoagulants, and patients' alcohol abuse.[18]

Successful use of a lower-limb prosthesis requires individuals with limb loss to develop a daily routine of skin inspection of the residual limb and contralateral foot (for individuals with unilateral amputation), skin hygiene, care for the prosthesis and associated components including washing of liners, management of residual limb volume and monitoring of prosthetic fit, and recognizing and problem solving through issues related to prosthetic fit and function and identifying when to seek help of a physical therapist, prosthetist, or physician.[26] Table 23.2 provides an overview of important considerations for assessment and management of residual limb health from a clinician toolkit associated with the VA/DoD Clinical Practice Guidelines for Rehabilitation of Individuals with Lower Limb Amputation.[27] These important issues related to self-management are discussed in more detail in Chapters 20 and 26. Lee and colleagues[26] recently published an assessment to determine the understanding an individual with limb loss may have related to these important aspects of self-management to identify appropriate targeted educational interventions to increase long-term successful use of a lower-limb prosthesis.[26] The SMART system was found

Table 23.2 Management of Residual Limb Health

Management of Residual Limb

Problem	Look for	Assessment/Intervention	Refer to
Skin redness	Socket fit	Assess prosthetic alignment	Prosthetist for adjustment/ socket fit
	Suspension	Assess donning technique	
		Assess for proper sock ply	
		Limit wear time if redness does not resolve in 20 min	
Blister	Suspension	Assess donning technique	Physician for wound care
	Socket fit	Assess for proper sock ply	Prosthetist for adjustment/ socket fit
	Thermal	Assess prosthetic alignment	
		End wear time	
Rashes	Contact	Instruct pt in Liner hygiene	If severe or not resolving, physician referral
	Fungal	Instruct pt in skin hygiene	
	Bacterial	Assess suspension system	
Callosity		Identify only	Physician and prosthetist
Folliculits or epidermal cyst		Limit wear time	Prosthetist
		Instruct pt in liner hygiene	Dermatology referral for recalcitrant cases
		Instruct pt in skin hygiene	
		Consider socket modification	
Shape	Dog ears	Apply ace wrap/compression stocking	Prosthetist
	Bulbous	Apply shrinker	Therapist (PT/OT)
	Cylindical-oprimal *for TTA*	Consider custom gel liner Consider socket modification	
	Conical-optimal *for TFA*		
Volume	Abnormal volume that interferes with prosthetic fit	Review weight control	Dietitian
		Review positioning	Prosthetist
		Assess sock-ply management	PT/OT therapist
		Apply ace wrap/compression stocking	If bilateral edema physician
		Apply shrinker	
		Consider custom gel liner	
		Consider socket modification	
Bursae	Identify	Limit wear time	Prosthetics
		Modality ice/ultrasound	If recalcitrant, consider surgical referral
		Consider socket modification	
Heterotopic ossification	Identify	Limit wear time	Prosthetics
		Possibly NSAID during inflammatory phase	If recalcitrant, consider surgical referral
		Consider socket modification	
Infection	Warmth, erythema, discharge, fever, unexplained pain, poor glucose control	Identify only	Physician
Unstable bone/joint	Tibio/fibular	Consider socket/suspension change	Prosthetics
	Knee	Consult therapy to stabilize knee	Therapy (PT/OT)
			If recalcitrant consider referral to ortho
Scar formation	Excessive	Consider custom gel liner	Prosthetics
	Adherent	Perform scar massage	Therapy (PT/OT)
	Skin grafts	Slow, gradual progression of prosthetic use with frequent reexamination	If recalcitrant consider plastics/orthopedic
	Burns		

NSAID, Nonsteroidal antiinflammatory drug; *OT*, occupational Therapy; pt, patient; *PT*, physical Therapy; *TFA*, transfemoral amputation; *TTA*, transtibial amputation.

to be reliable and valid and includes a 14-item screening module, a 45-item comprehensive examination, a 10-item module focused on assessment of residual limb self-management, and a 15-item module focused on assessment of prosthesis self-management.[26]

Prosthetic Fitting and Residual Limb Volume

The most critical aspect of a lower-limb prosthesis is the quality of the fit of the prosthetic socket and its ability to distribute pressure to the pressure-tolerant regions of the residual limb while offloading pressure from pressure-intolerant regions of the residual limb.[28,29] One of the primary challenges to achieving a good fit between the prosthetic socket and residual limb are fluctuations in residual limb volume. Residual limb volume in individuals with limb loss may affected by an individual's level of activity, prosthetic wearing time, cardiovascular function, and renal function.[28,30,31] Prosthetic users who experience reductions in residual limb volume are instructed to add socks between their prosthetic liner and socket to improve the intimacy of their prosthetic socket and improve the distribution of pressures on the residual limb during weight-bearing activity (Fig. 23.3A and B).[28,30,32] Other prosthetic users may accommodate reductions in residual limb volume through periodic doffing of their prosthesis and liner.[30,31] It is estimated that there is significant fluid volume recovery within 30 minutes of doffing the prosthesis and liner.[30] Armitage and colleagues[33] have reported that the most reliable and valid methods for clinicians to evaluate residual limb volume for individuals with transtibial amputation include circumferential measurements of the residual limb and water displacement volumetry.[33] To ensure accuracy of circumferential measurements to evaluate for stability of residual limb volume, it is important that clinicians standardize the timing of measurements, patient position, residual limb position, and limb markings (e.g., bony landmarks).[33]

PROSTHETIC SOCKET DESIGN

Traditional socket designs for individuals with transtibial prosthetics have incorporated a combination of patella tendon bearing (PTB) and total surface bearing (TSB) designs.[34] Total contact socket designs distribute pressures across large pressure-tolerant regions of the residual limb, minimizing focal pressures in any single area.[35,36] The PTB socket has a patella tendon bar that is designed to apply pressure to the patella tendon and exert force on the residual limb, which is directed down and back during weight bearing; this force is countered by an anteriorly directed force applied by an inward bulge in the posterior wall of the prosthesis in the popliteal region.[36] The patellar tendon, calf musculature, and medial tibial flare are used for weight loading, while reliefs are made over bony prominences like the tibial crest and head of the fibula. The proximal trim line of the posterior wall should be located just proximal to the patellar bar to stabilize the limb in the anteroposterior direction and to prevent the limb from sliding too far down into the socket. The posterior trim line should be lower on the medial side to accommodate the insertion of the medial hamstring tendon during knee flexion. Anteriorly directed compression of the calf musculature maintains the patella tendon firmly against the bar and stabilizes anterior posterior motion of the residual limb within the socket.

The other major weight-bearing surface in the PTB socket is the medial flare of the tibia. The proximal end of the tibia broadens out medially and, when stabilized by pressure from the lateral wall of the socket along the shaft of the fibula, can effectively accept loading. However, it is necessary to simultaneously create a relief for the fibular head to avoid any pressure on the bony prominence or the fibular nerve. Pressure in TSB sockets is distributed more broadly to pressure-tolerant areas of the residual limb.[36] Strategic compression of soft tissue and relief for bony prominences are the tools used to direct more force into areas of the limb that can tolerate it and less force into areas that are prone to skin breakdown. Many TSB socket systems utilize different methods of vacuum-assisted suction suspension via mechanical or electrical pumps.[35,36] A recent literature review found that many studies fail to make a clear distinction between socket design and suspension systems and residual limb interfaces, which makes it difficult to draw conclusions based on socket design alone.[36] Newer socket designs incorporate mechanically adjustable sockets in which the tightness of the prosthetic fit can be adjusted with the turn of a knob.[35] These adjustable socket designs

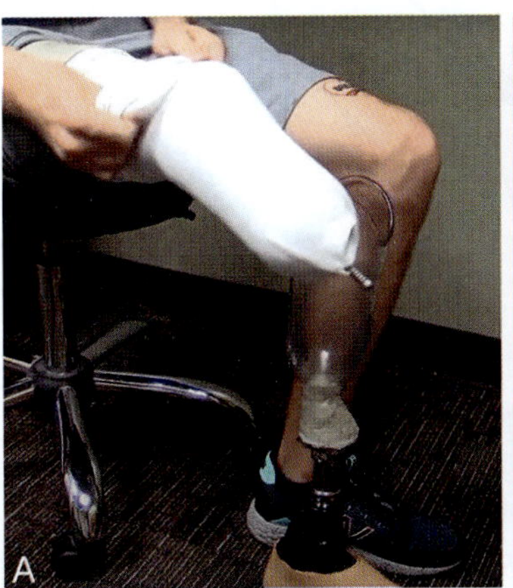

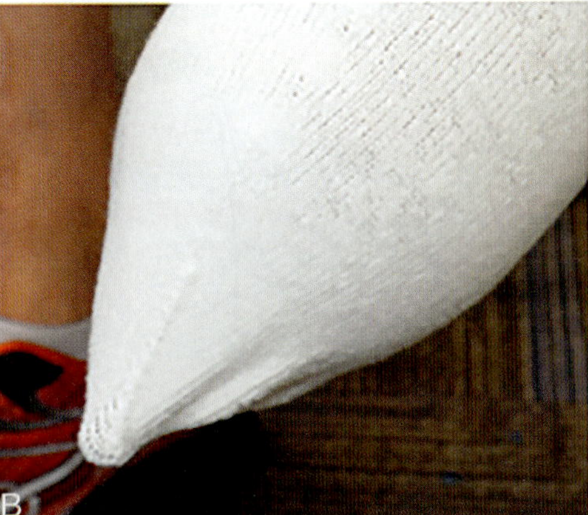

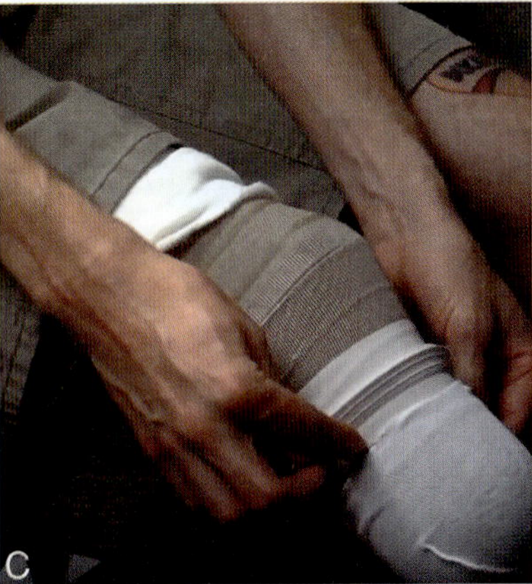

Fig. 23.3 Adding socks to accommodate changes in residual limb volume (A) Donning prosthetic sock over prosthetic liner with pin. (B) Prosthetic socks donned incorrectly. (C) Donning a half sock over a seal-in liner to accommodate for decreased volume in distal aspect of residual limb.

may allow prosthetic users to more readily adjust the fit of their prosthetic socket to accommodate for fluctuations or changes in residual limb volume.[29,35,37]

To fully accommodate the dynamic tissue loading that occurs in a prosthetic socket, the prosthetist must consider both the *shear* and the *normal* forces on the limb. Shear forces run parallel to the limb surface and are best mitigated through the use of a socket interface. Interface materials, such as socks, sheaths, flexible liners, and gel liners, offer a continuum of shear reduction on the skin surface. The best materials to minimize shear are those found in gel liners. Normal forces are those that are applied perpendicular to the surface of the limb. The socket walls should be contoured according to the type of tissue in the area and the anticipated loading patterns. There is no way to reduce the force on the limb without restricting the individual's activities; therefore the best way to reduce pressure is to distribute the forces over as broad a surface as possible. The actual forces on the limb are a combination of shear and normal forces that occur together in various proportions. Throughout the gait cycle the forces and moments on the socket and limb change continuously (Fig. 23.4). There is a flexion moment at the knee during loading response, which causes the knee extensors (e.g., quadriceps) to activate. For transtibial prosthetic users, activation of the quadriceps causes the anterior distal aspect of the residual limb to increase contact with the prosthetic socket; simultaneously there is increased pressure on the pressure on the residual limb from the posterior wall of the prosthesis in the popliteal region. At midstance, there is a varus moment at the knee which causes increased pressure from the prosthetic socket along the medial tibial flare. The pressure from the lateral wall of the prosthetic socket along the shaft of the fibula helps to stabilize the residual limb within the prosthetic socket and prevent the residual limb from bottoming out in the socket and helps minimize distal contact pressure. At terminal stance, an extension moment occurs at the knee, and as the knee flexes during preswing there is increased pressure on the posterior distal aspect of the residual limb against the posterior wall of the prosthetic socket. Simultaneously this creates increased pressure between the anterior proximal wall of the prosthesis and the residual limb. To tolerate ambulation with a transtibial prosthesis, a prosthetic user needs to be able to tolerate these force couples between the prosthetic socket and the residual limb as well as pressure related to rotational moments in the transverse plane (Fig. 23.5). The forces on the limb range from a compressive force of 1.2 times body weight in stance to a distractive force slightly higher than the weight of the prosthesis in swing phase.[38] A well-fitting prosthesis must provide tolerable pressure distribution in all of those varied loading conditions. Soft tissue, muscle tissue, and bone contours must each be accounted for in a specific way to achieve a good fit. Soft tissue can tolerate moderate compression so the prosthetist will precompress that tissue in the socket. Muscles can tolerate mild compression but should be encouraged to contract with each step so less precompression should be applied. The shape of muscle tissue changes when contracted. Flexible materials can be used over muscle bellies to allow for the geometric variability. Finally, bony prominences must be given extra volume within the socket so that when the tissue around them compresses during loading, the pressure will not exceed the tolerable limit. When evaluating patients who complain of socket discomfort during ambulation, clinicians should determine not only where the patient is experiencing pain on their residual limb, but at what point of the gait cycle the pain occurs. This information is helpful to determine whether the pain can be attributed to intolerance to the force couples encountered during normal ambulation and help inform discussions with the prosthetist regarding socket fit, socket/residual limb interface, and suspension considerations.

As socket fit, comfort, and satisfaction are critical to successful use of a lower-limb prosthesis, it is important that clinicians evaluate patient satisfaction and comfort of an individual's prosthetic socket. The Expanded Socket Comfort Score (ESCS) asks prosthetic users to rate the comfort of their prosthetic socket on a 0 to 10 scale (0 = most uncomfortable, 10 = most comfortable) when it is at its best and worst over the previous 7 days, on average over the previous 7 days, and at the moment.[39] However, the authors noted that scores on the ESCS were highly variable. Another useful tool to assess an individual's satisfaction with their prosthetic socket is the Comprehensive

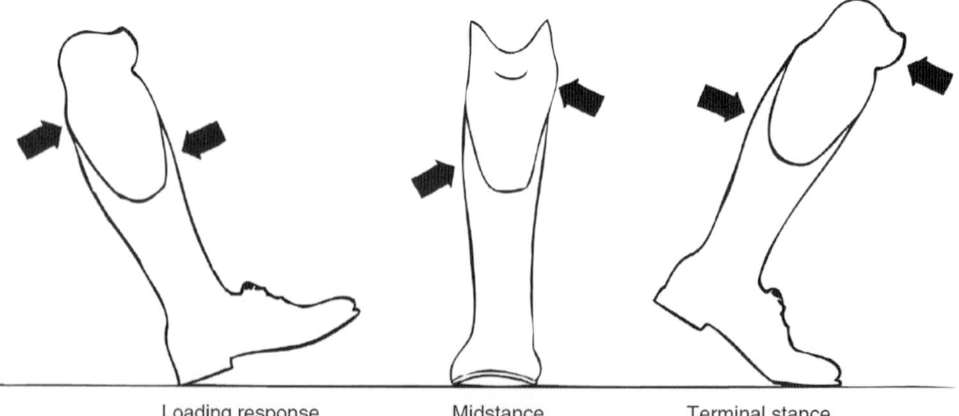

Fig. 23.4 The magnitude and direction of the forces on the socket change throughout stance phase, concentrating pressure in predictable areas. At initial contact and loading, there is an anterior force at the proximal posterior knee and distal anterior residual limb. At midstance, weight-bearing forces create proximal-medial and distal-lateral pressures. At the end of stance phase, the anterior force moves to the proximal-anterior knee and distal-posterior residual limb. (From Knee Prosthetics, Prosthetics-Orthotics Program, University of Texas Southwestern Medical Center, Texas, 1998.)

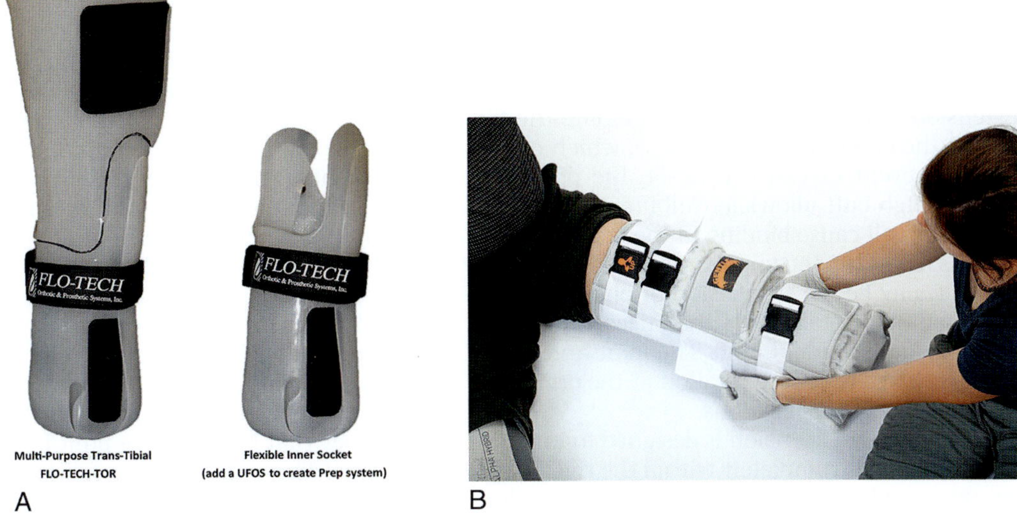

Fig. 23.5 Rigid removable dressings: (A) Flo-Tech TOR. (B) Rooke below-knee rigid protector.

Lower Limb Amputee Socket Survey, which is described in Chapter 24, and has been shown to have very good internal consistency.[40]

Residual Limb Health and Socket-Limb Interface

Approximately 75% of individuals with lower-limb amputation who use a prosthesis experience dermatologic conditions related to prosthetic use including skin blisters or ulcerations, skin irritation, folliculitis, and epidermoid inclusion cysts, which impact residual limb health.[41] These conditions may arise due to increased shear stresses at the interface between the skin of the residual limb and the prosthetic socket as well as compression and shear forces between the connective tissues of the residual limb and the surgically transected bone.[41] Residual limb health relies on optimizing the prosthetic socket fit for appropriate distribution of loads and optimizing suspension of the prosthesis to minimize the shear forces created due to excessive motion at the residual limb-socket interface.[41] However, one of the challenges in maintaining optimal residual limb health is that most traditional gel or silicone liners worn by prosthetic users have poor breathability and trap heat and moisture, which may lead to skin-related complications of the residual limb.[42] Hyperhidrosis and excessive sweating of the residual limb after amputation may also increase risk for complications related to skin irritation and impact use of a lower-limb prosthesis.[43] While use of nonscented antiperspirants are a recommended first-line approach for management of hyperhidrosis, a randomized placebo-controlled study on the impact of RimabotulinumtoxinB on hyperhidrosis for individuals with limb loss demonstrated a 50% reduction in sweat production 4 weeks after injection.[44] A recent case series showed promising results for the use of microwave thermoablation for long-term management of hyperhidrosis for individuals with limb loss who do not respond to antiperspirants or botulinum toxin.[45]

The material that separates the limb from the socket is referred to as an interface. Interfaces play an important role in lower-limb prosthetics. Interfaces can offer shock absorption, can mimic soft tissue to provide an extra layer of cushioning for those who are bony, and can help to mitigate shear forces on the limb, and wick away perspiration. Interfaces influence the hygiene, ease of donning, maintenance requirements of the prosthesis, and are often an integral part of prosthetic suspension.

SUSPENSION SYSTEMS

Suspension systems for transtibial prosthetics are critical for effective use of a transtibial prosthesis. Suspension refers to the method by which the prosthesis is held to the residual limb. When a prosthesis is suspended perfectly, there is no relative motion between the socket and the limb. When motion occurs because of a faulty or inadequate suspension system, the limb is subjected to an entirely different loading pattern. This motion is referred to as "pistoning," as it bears some resemblance to the motion of a piston in the cylinder of an internal combustion engine. Pistoning can lead to pain, skin breakdown, and reduced control of the prosthesis. Excessive pistoning can also lead to decreased function for the user, due to fear of the prosthesis coming off. Great care should be taken to minimize motion within the socket.

ANATOMICAL SUSPENSION SYSTEMS

The joints and corset suspension includes a skillfully molded corset over the smaller circumference of the thigh fitted over the femoral condyles just proximal to the knee joint. The stiff leather corset is fabricated with either straps or laces that can be tightened as the wearer dons the prosthesis. This permits the limb to pass through the corset and be held securely in position once the corset is tightened. The knee joints, which are typically made from steel, provide a secure connection to the socket. When the condyles are prominent, this can serve as the primary means of suspension, and a waist belt is not needed. As the prosthetic knee joints are positioned slightly posterior to the anatomical knee joint center, tension in the cuff decreases over the condyles as the knee flexes, thereby enhancing sitting comfort (Fig. 23.6). The joints and corset system can also include a posterior check strap that limits full knee extension. This can be used to eliminate the terminal impact at the end of the swing phase, which can be audible, and to prevent excessive wear on the prosthetic knee joints. The thigh cuff allows for full functional range of knee flexion but will cause binding in the popliteal fossa when the knee is flexed beyond approximately 110 degrees. Joints and corset may be the suspension of choice for persons with ligamentous instability of the knee, or for those who have a very short residual limb. The joint and corset system can also be used to reduce rotation of the prosthesis in certain activity-specific applications.

Supracondylar socket suspension is designed to incorporate the femoral condyles completely within the rigid transtibial socket. By extending the medial and lateral trim lines of the socket approximately 2 cm proximal to the adductor tubercle, the medial-lateral dimension of the top of the socket can be made narrower than the knee joint. This prevents the knee joint from moving upward out of the socket by capturing the femoral condyles. Supracondylar suspension also adds significant medial-lateral stability to the prosthesis by increasing the length of the lever arm proximal to knee center. Additionally, this increases the surface contact area, which can be helpful for short residual limbs. This technique, when combined with a PTB-style socket, is collectively referred to as "PTB-SC."

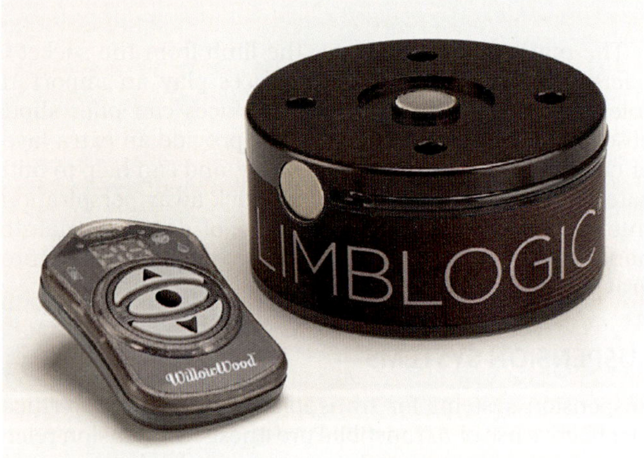

Fig. 23.6 Elevated vacuum suspension.

This type of socket can be difficult to don because the width of the proximal opening is smaller than the width of the condyles. This problem can be addressed in two ways: either by including the supracondylar wedge in a soft insert or by detachable medial wall. The first method uses a flexible liner that has a wedge built into it proximal to medial condyle. The rigid socket is fabricated over the liner such that the medial-lateral dimension of the proximal end of the socket is equal to the widest dimension of the knee. This allows donning of the flexible liner first, then with slight compression of the liner, the limb and liner together slide into the socket and are locked in place through pressure and friction (Fig. 23.7A). The second method uses a steel bar that is formed into the prosthesis. The entire medial wall of the prosthesis, along with the steel bar, can be removed for donning. Once the limb is in the socket, the bar slides back into a channel in the distal portion of the socket and locks into position with a ball detent (Fig. 23.7B).

It is necessary to have at least a 1-cm difference between the medial-lateral dimension of the knee joint and that of the thigh just proximal to the adductor tubercle so as to provide a secure supracondylar suspension. Widening the socket in the region just posterior to the condyles serves to loosen the grip over the condyles while seated in 90 degrees of knee flexion. It is noteworthy to mention that the high medial and lateral walls of this type of socket are apparent, even through long pants when the knee is flexed. Some individuals might find this unsightly and unacceptable.

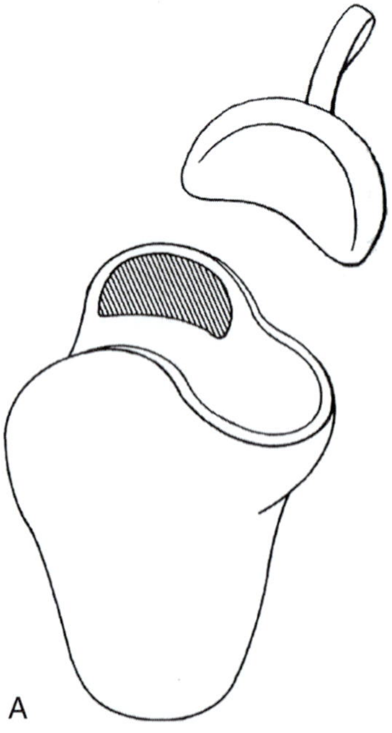

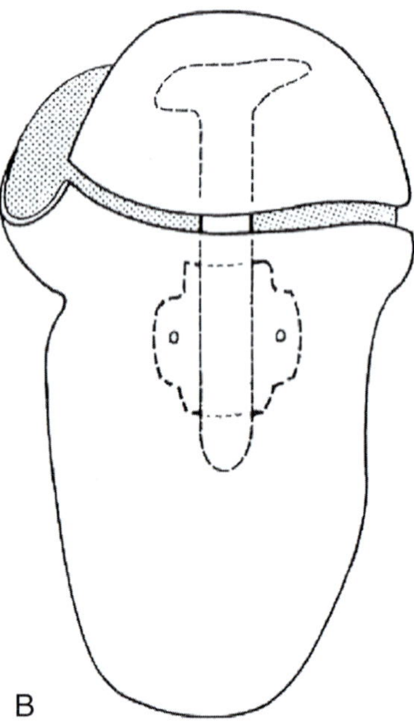

Fig. 23.7 (A) Supracondylar socket with removable wedge. (B) Supracondylar socket with removable medial wing.

SUCTION SUSPENSION

One-way air valves are commonly used in conjunction with sealing sleeves to allow air trapped during donning to escape from the socket. Sealing sleeves seal the proximal end of the socket against the skin so that no air can flow into, or out from, the socket. This creates a suction suspension. Sealing sleeves provide excellent suspension when combined with a TSB socket style. Once the socket is sealed, very little pistoning can occur as there are no voids between the limb and socket. For the sleeve to seal, the sleeve must touch the skin directly for at least the top 5 cm. The skin must be free from deep scars or invaginations in that area, as they would provide a path for air to enter under the sleeve. Because the sealing sleeves rely on an airtight seal to function, they are highly susceptible to failure as a consequence of leaks. Even a small hole in the sleeve can allow air to flow into the socket, defeating the vacuum and impairing suspension. Although sleeves are not very durable, they can be replaced without any special tools or equipment.

The soft tissue of the residual limb behaves like an incompressible fluid. For the limb to move within the sealed volume of the socket, the volume of the limb itself would have to change. This can only happen if fluid moves into or out from the limb through the bloodstream, a process that is too slow to be accomplished within the short interval of swing phase. Therefore the cyclic alteration between compression in stance and tension in swing slowly draws fluid into the limb and pushes it back out, assisting normal circulation. Suction suspension may provide a means for improving healthy circulation in the residual limb and controlling limb volume. Most modern suction suspension systems incorporate a cushion liner to increase comfort and protection of the residual limb (Fig. 23.8A and D).

LOCKING SUSPENSION

Locking suspension systems rely on gel liners that consist of three basic varieties: (1) silicone elastomers, which are highly crosslinked at the molecular level; (2) silicone gels that have a relatively low amount of crosslinking; and (3) urethanes. Silicone elastomers present the highest compressive stiffness values, so they are best suited to supporting loading without deformation.[46] Silicone gels have the lowest

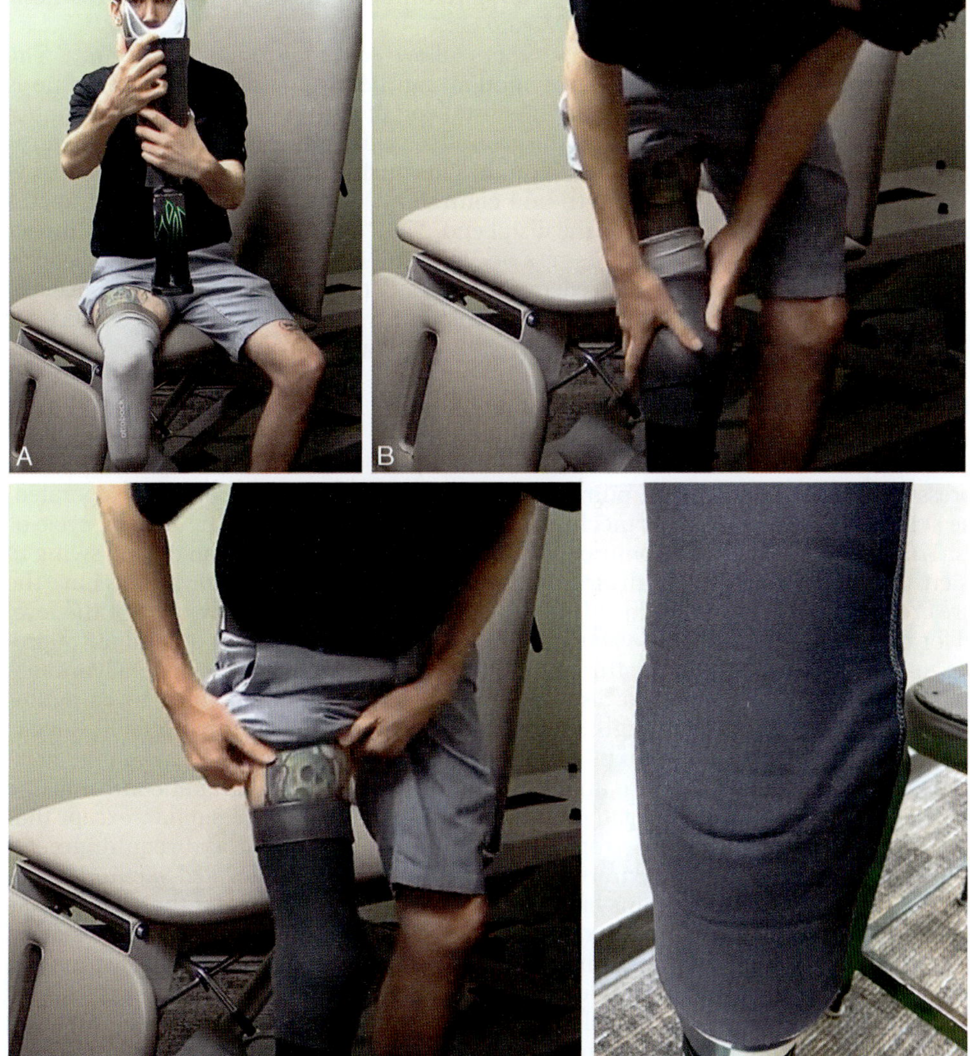

Fig. 23.8 Donning transtibial prosthesis with suction suspension with cushion liner and suspension sleeve. (A) Suspension sleeve below posterior wall of socket. (B) Introduce residual limb and ensure appropriate immersion in socket, roll up suspension sleeve. (C) Suspension sleeve should contact skin proximal to liner to ensure appropriate seal of suction. (D) Appropriate level of suction, contours of socket visible.

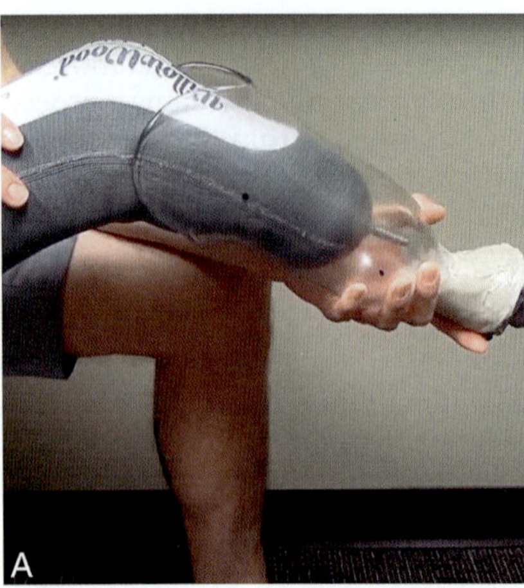
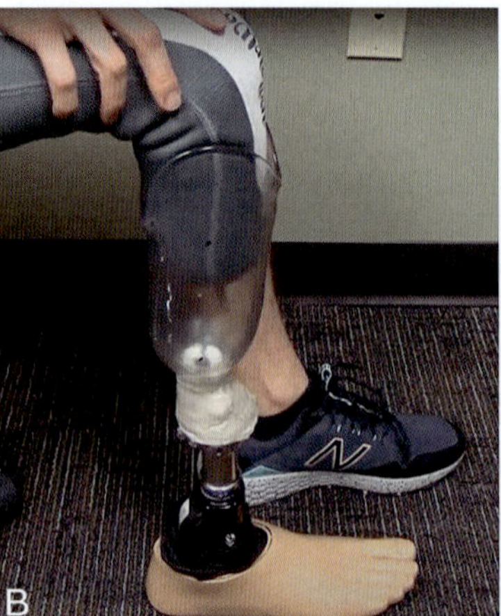
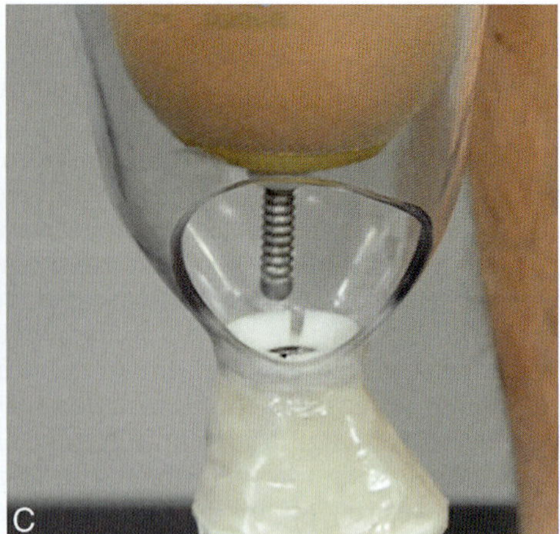

Fig. 23.9 Donning transtibial prosthesis with pin-lock suspension (A). (B) Pin not lined up with the lock. (C) Pin lined up appropriately with lock.

compressive and shear stiffness values.[46] This makes them useful in reducing compressive loading and limiting shear forces on the limb. Urethanes show the highest coefficient of friction with skin, a property that is useful for preventing localized skin tension and shear.[46] Gel liners have a high-friction inner surface where it is in contact with the limb, and a low friction outer surface where it meets the socket. This encourages whatever small amount of motion is present to occur on the outer surface of the liner and minimizes motion at the liner-skin interface. The colloidal nature of the gel absorbs the shear that is not dissipated by the liner-socket interface so that only a small percentage reaches the skin (Fig. 23.9A and C).

Incorporation of a locking pin at the distal end of the gel liner allows the liner to be used for suspension as well. This type of liner is referred to as a "locking liner" as opposed to a "cushion liner" that has no pin. The pin mates with a locking mechanism built into the socket to suspend the prosthesis. Locking liners may be used with other suspension systems such as lanyards. Roll-on gel liners should fit snugly, but not tightly. As the liner is stretched, a shear profile is established on the limb. A tighter fit creates higher frictional forces, and if the pressure distribution is not equal, the frictional forces on the skin will be uneven, leading to blisters and skin problems. This can occur with a very bony limb, unless the liner is custom made for the individual. Custom-made gel liners are created over a mold of the residual limb. This is indicated for unusually shaped limbs, those with deep invaginations, or those that need specifically located reliefs or cushions.

Most modern sockets use a pin-and-lock mechanism. This pin can range from approximately 3 to 10 cm in length. It works in conjunction with a locking mechanism built into the distal end of the socket that engages when the individual dons the prosthesis. Some wearers experience frustration with this as it can be difficult to align the pin so that it engages with the locking mechanism. To remove the prosthesis, the prosthetic wearer must disengage the pin manually while pushing the socket off with the other hand. There are several variants of locking mechanisms. Some offer an audible "click" to indicate that the pin has engaged, but will only lock in a limited number of positions. Others use a clutch mechanism or a smooth pin that allow for an infinite number of locking positions. Ideally, only one position should be needed (i.e., when the limb is positioned correctly in the socket). However, as an individual's limb volume varies throughout the day, it is not uncommon for there to be an additional "click" or two as they spend more time weight bearing in the prosthesis (Fig. 23.9A and C).

Locking liners allow some pistoning to occur.[47] The amount of motion can be dramatic when loose tissue is present at the distal end of the residual limb. As the limb is lifted off the ground in swing phase, the weight of the prosthesis pulls on the pin causing the liner and limb to elongate in length and contract in girth. This effect is most apparent at the distal end. This "milking" motion creates unnecessary stress on the distal end of the limb and can lead to ptain, edema, and skin breakdown.[48,49] This is especially problematic for limbs with adherent scar tissue, as the liner will attempt to pull the tissue away from the bone.

ELEVATED VACUUM

Elevated vacuum suspension systems incorporate the use of pumps which can be either electric (battery operated) or mechanical. Mechanical pumps use the natural cycle of compression during stance and distraction during swing to pull air from the socket during gait. Electric pumps have the added benefit of being able to accurately control the level of vacuum within the socket by turning on and off at preset thresholds (Fig. 23.6). Both systems have advantages and disadvantages. Mechanical pumps tend to be lighter weight, lower profile, and easier to maintain. Electronic pumps allow a more precise control of the negative pressure and some models allow for situational control of the negative pressure. The down sides are similar, except that electronic pumps need to be charged and require greater clearance under the residual limb. Elevated vacuum maintains limb volume by preventing fluid loss that occurs during prolonged weight bearing.[49,50] The elevated vacuum environment within the socket leads to decreased motion and therefore to fewer skin problems, improved prosthetic control, better balance, and enhanced comfort.[41] Elevated vacuum suspension has also been shown to improve oxygen perfusion of the amputated limb during gait[51] and has also been shown to have lower peak pressures and lower impact forces than traditional suction sockets.[52] During the swing phase of gait, elevated vacuum suspension has been shown to reduce axial motion of the socket relative to the limb as compared to passive suction suspension.[53] To achieve elevated vacuum, a sealing sleeve is required to prevent air from entering through the proximal end of the socket. Some wearers report a decrease in the amount of available knee flexion once the air has been evacuated from the socket. This is likely caused by tension in the sealing sleeve as it spans the entire knee joint. Additionally, any type of hole in the sealing sleeve will allow the negative pressure in the socket to equalize resulting in poor suspension.

Anatomical suspension systems such as supracondylar cuff/socket demonstrate the least stable suspension and allow the highest amount of movement at the residual limb-socket interface.[41] The least amount of movement at the residual limb-socket interface has been demonstrated by elevated vacuum suspension systems, followed by passive suction suspension with a sealing liner.[41] A study comparing suction suspension to pin-locking suspension indicated that prosthetic users reported improved socket comfort with suction suspension; however, self-reported mobility and balance confidence were similar.[54] Suction and elevated vacuum suspension has been shown to improve gait symmetry, reduce skin breakdown, and decrease distal residual limb pain compared to pin-lock and sleeve suspension systems.[49] A study investigating differences in residual limb volume management over a 5.5 hours activity protocol demonstrated that elevated vacuum suspension was associated with decreased change in residual limb volume compared to suction suspension with sleeve.[50] When considering the ease of donning and doffing a prosthesis and liner, it should be noted that older adults with limb loss and individuals with impaired hand function due to arthritis or stroke have an easier time managing prosthetics with pin-lock suspension compared to suction or elevated vacuum suspension.[49]

Accommodating Changes in Residual Limb Volume

Closed cell foam, used because it does not absorb moisture, can be molded over a model of the limb to create a soft insert. This insert lines the entire socket and terminates just proximal to the socket trim lines (Fig. 23.10). For increased protection, a distal end pad, which is an extra layer of soft material at the bottom of the insert, can be used to cushion the distal end of the tibia. Soft inserts provide an extra layer of cushioning that is needed for more mature limbs that lack adequate soft-tissue thickness. Soft inserts also allow the prosthetist a way to adjust socket volume and shape for a limb that is prone to change.

The sock also provides the individual with a method to control socket fit; as the residual limb matures and shrinks, additional sock ply may be required to restore the fit and comfort of the socket (see Fig. 23.11A and B). Prosthetic socks come in various ply thicknesses for convenience to the prosthetic wearer. For example, a person can wear one five-ply sock rather than having to don five individual single-ply socks. This is of particular importance since it has been shown that even within the same manufacturer three

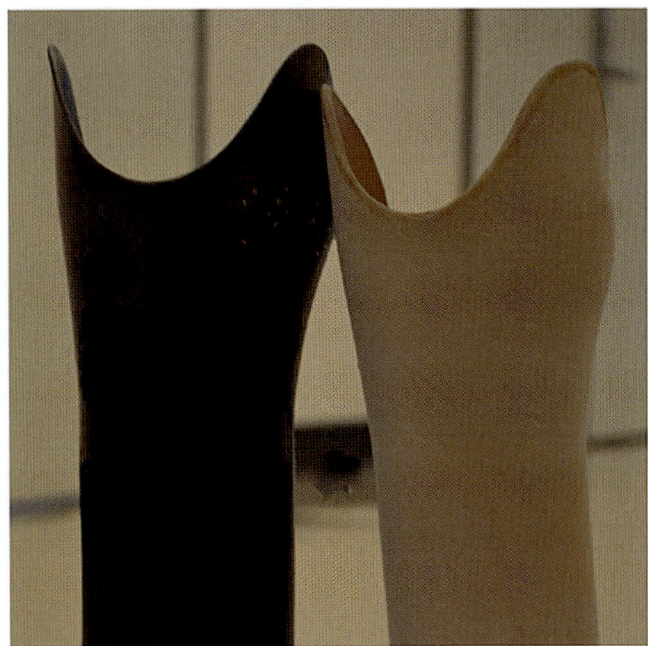

Fig. 23.10 Foam liner.

one-ply socks are not the same thickness as one three-ply sock.[32] It is important to educate the person wearing the prosthesis to use the fewest number of socks to achieve the proper number of ply. New prosthetic wearers are typically provided an assortment of one-, three-, and five-ply socks from which they can select. The socks can be layers one on top of the other to achieve the appropriate number of plies to optimize socket fit.

PROSTHETIC FABRICATION

The majority of follow-up visits to the prosthetist are for prosthetic users to be evaluated for concerns related to the fit and/or alignment of their prosthesis that impact their residual limb health and/or ability to perform mobility-related activities of daily living.[55,56] The first step in creating a well-fitting socket is capturing an accurate impression of the residual limb. This can be done in a variety of ways ranging from plaster bandages to noncontact optical scanners. Each technique has its own set of advantages and disadvantages, and there is no one best method for every limb. All methods share the common goal of capturing a model of the limb that accurately represents the location and geometry of each aspect of the limb. Capturing a static impression of the limb is quite simple and any method will suffice if done properly. The challenging task is to capture the dynamic nature of the biological tissue by compressing the soft tissues during the process to simulate the conditions that will be on the limb during weight bearing.

HAND CASTING

During hand casting, the limb is gently wrapped with either plaster or fiberglass bandage and the prosthetist applies pressure to key weight-bearing areas while the casting material is setting up. How much compression is needed and which areas to compress are determined based on

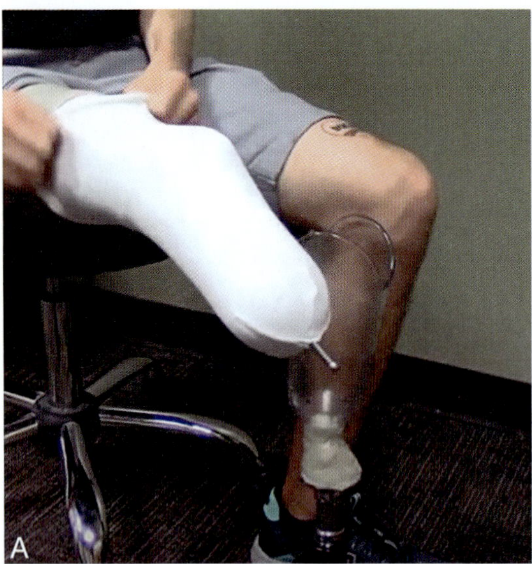

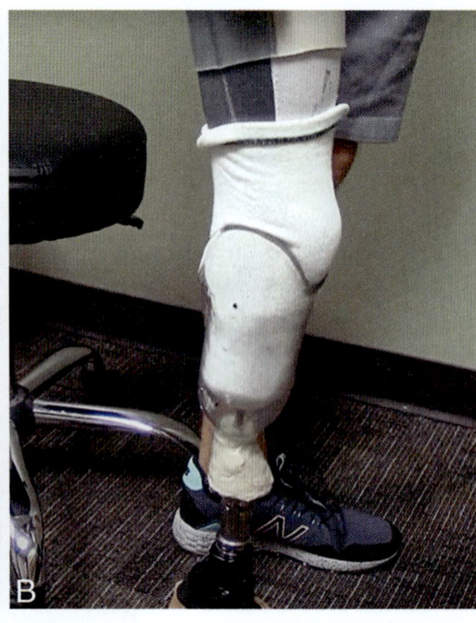

Fig. 23.11 (A) Adding prosthetic socks to accommodate for decreased residual limb volume. (B) Too many socks added, unable to engage pin-lock, tibial tuberosity contacting patella tendon bar.

bony anatomy and the prosthetist's individual knowledge, skill, and experience. Multistage casting procedures involve molding specific regions of the limb individually and joining them together once the individual sections have set up. This allows the prosthetist to position the limb in multiple postures during casting to capture unique features. The insertion of the hamstrings, for example, can be molded during active knee flexion when they are most prominent. For more details about casting, refer to Chapter 6.

PRESSURE CASTING

Another way to precompress the tissue is to use a pressurizing technique.[57] This involves placing the limb into a vacuum or pressure chamber while the plaster is setting up (Fig. 23.12). A vacuum chamber is typically a latex bladder pulled over the wet cast and sealed on the thigh. A vacuum pump attached to the distal end removes all air between the cast and bladder allowing the atmospheric pressure to compress the limb up to approximately 14 psi. A pressure chamber with a latex bladder attached inside is another option. The limb, wrapped with wet plaster, is placed in the bladder and air is pumped into the space between the cylinder and bladder. The pressure in the cylinder can be increased to 30 to 40 psi, providing additional compression. Alternatively, pressure casting can be done with the pressure casting technique (PCAST) method where pressure is provided by water in a closed cylinder. The full length of residual limb is wrapped in casting material. The limb is then placed on a flexible bladder inside a metal cylinder. The cylinder is filled with water creating a supportive environment on which the prosthetic user can weight bear. The prosthetic user then places equal body weight on each limb until the casting has set. This method allows for a weight-bearing mold to be taken of the residual limb.[58]

In all three methods, once the casting material has hardened, the pressure is released and the limb is removed from the chamber. Regardless of the casting method, differential pressure between the limb and the environment serves to apply uniform pressure over the entire surface of the limb. This leads to the most tissue compression in the softest areas and the least amount of tissue compression in the bony areas.

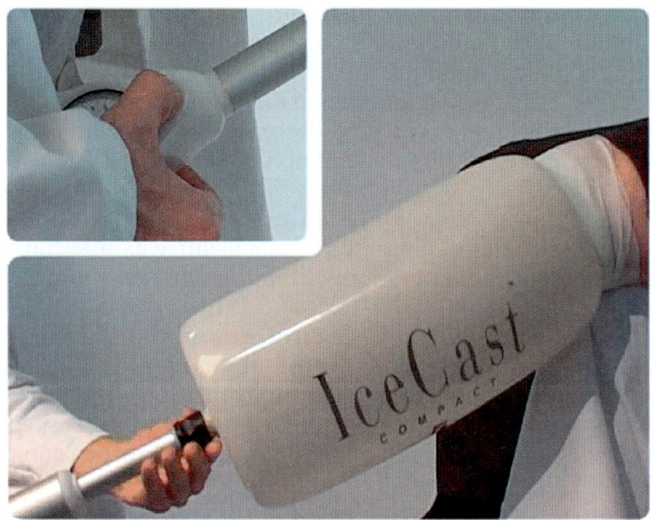

Fig. 23.12 Pressure casting provides uniform pressure on the residual limb as well as slight distraction, ensuring that the mold and residual limb match in length. (© Össur.)

The amount of differential pressure required will vary with the individual's weight, and the prosthetist should use the least amount of pressure required to achieve the optimal fit.

OPTICAL SCANNING

Optical scanners can be used to capture a three-dimensional external shape of the limb to within 1 mm of accuracy (Fig. 23.13).[59] They are quite useful in situations when hand casting is impossible or impractical, such as immediately following surgery or with bulbous limbs that cannot be removed from a plaster cast without cutting or distorting the cast. Digital markers and alignment lines can be attached to the virtual model to reference the location of bony landmarks and pressure-sensitive areas. Although it is not possible to compress the skin by hand while scanning, due to the hand blocking the view of the surface, compression of tissues and reliefs for bony landmarks can be accomplished using modification software.

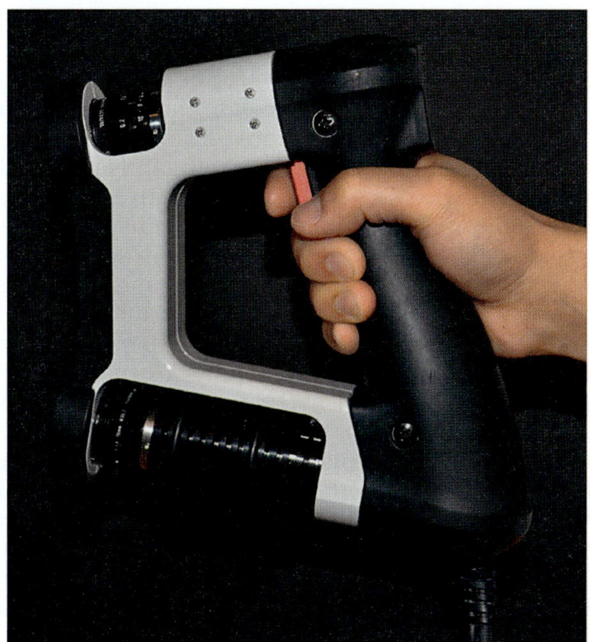

Fig. 23.13 Optical scanner.

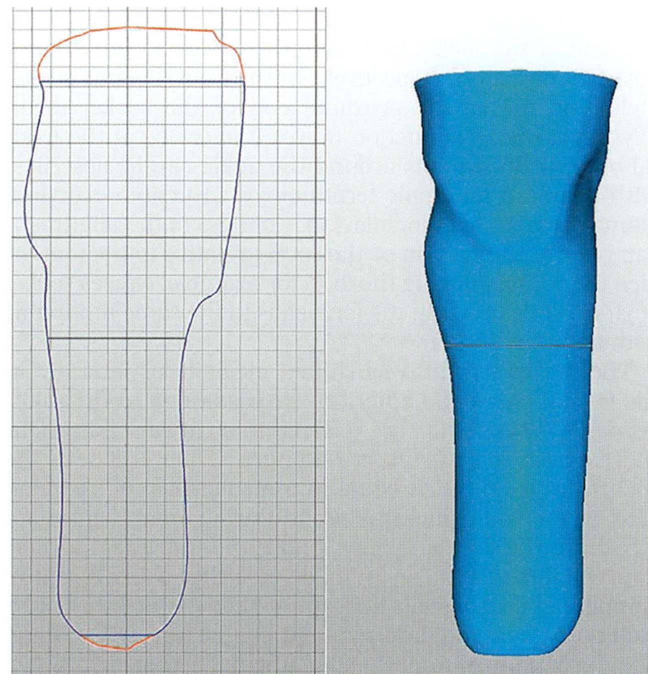

Fig. 23.14 Three-dimensional scan of residual limb.

Scanners used in prosthetic applications typically fall into one of two categories: (1) laser scanners and (2) structured light scanners (white or blue light). Laser scanners use triangulation of the beam reflecting off the surface of an object to determine its position in space. Since this process happens millions of times per second, the software is able to produce a map of the three-dimensional surface by connecting these points. Structured light scanners project a light pattern onto the surface of an object, and by measuring the distortion of that pattern, the software can calculate the precise measurements of the object being scanned. Both systems provide high accuracy and fast scan times, which makes them useful tools in the clinical setting.

The use of an optical scanning system to create a digital model of the residual limb, or computer-aided design (CAD) (Fig. 23.14), also requires a method of transferring that digital model to the real world, referred to as computer-aided manufacturing (CAM). CAD/CAM is a process used extensively in the manufacturing world, but in the O&P world, it is often closely associated with three-dimensional printing (additive manufacturing) and foam carvings of molds (subtractive manufacturing). While the use of three-dimensional printing of prosthetic devices is expanding, it has not yet become a standard tool for prosthetists. This is expected to change as advances in print materials, print methods, and print speeds are made. Currently three-dimensional printing in transtibial prosthetics is most prevalent in the production of check sockets and custom artistic fairings to provide shape to the prosthesis. More commonly, transtibial models are fabricated using a carver, which is computer guided and carves a foam block into the desired shape. The model produced in this method is then used to produce the prosthetic socket using traditional methods. Prosthetic sockets produced using CAD/CAM carver have been shown to improve quality of life parameters and reduce socket adaptation time in persons using them.[60] This system has the additional advantages of reducing fabrication time and maintaining objective data on socket shape and volume over the life of the prosthetic user.

ALIGNMENT

Alignment refers to the spatial orientation of the prosthetic socket relative to the foot. Alignment will influence the magnitude and direction of the ground reaction force throughout the gait cycle. There are four goals in prosthetic alignment: (1) facilitating heel strike at initial contact; (2) providing adequate single limb stability during stance phase; (3) creating smooth forward progression (rollover) during stance phase; and (4) insuring adequate swing phase toe clearance.[61] These goals are reached through dynamic alignment of the prosthesis, during which the person walks on a prosthesis that is fitted with an adjustable device that allows for alignment changes in all three planes. Although "normal" gait is not a goal, modern components do allow many persons with transtibial amputations to evade detection of gait abnormalities or deviations by all but the most skillful gait observers. Prosthetic alignment can also be used in conjunction with socket fit to address pressure issues within the socket. Because of this, socket fitting and dynamic alignment must occur simultaneously. Effective fitting and alignment require an iterative process as changing one aspect can affect many others. The end result is often a compromise. For example, the foot may require excessive dorsiflexion in order for the person to achieve sufficient swing clearance, even though this may contribute to a higher than optimal knee flexion moment during loading response. The prosthetist must understand biomechanics of the limb and gait cycle to weigh the factors appropriately to make the best decisions.

The modular components that connect the socket, pylon, and foot allow the prosthetist to make angular and rotational changes to the alignment. In the sagittal plane, socket flexion or socket extension refers to the tilting of the proximal end of the socket forward or backward in the anteroposterior direction, respectively. In the frontal plane, socket abduction moves the proximal end of the socket medially while socket adduction moves it laterally, in the frontal plane. Adjustments around the ankle can be described with standard anatomic terminology: inversion, eversion, plantar flexion, and dorsiflexion. Changes to the alignment can refer to the motion of the socket relative to the foot, or vice versa. Dorsiflexing the foot, for example, causes socket flexion; while everting the foot leads to the same motion as adducting the socket.

The socket can also be shifted medially or laterally in the frontal plane and anteriorly or posteriorly in the sagittal plane. These shifts are referred to as linear changes or slides. These, too, are relative changes. A lateral slide of the socket, for example, is equal to a medial slide of the foot. This type of adjustment is useful during static alignment to ensure the foot is directly under the individual's knee. Linear adjustments can be made by either using a special component that permits this type of slide (Fig. 23.15), or by using a pair of standard pyramid connectors and making equal but opposite angular adjustments.

A scoping review of 37 studies measuring prosthetic alignment indicated that optimal alignment was most frequently measured by the prosthetist's judgment and verbal or written patient report, while six studies incorporated gait analysis in assessment of alignment and five studies utilized sensor-based technologies to evaluate alignment.[55] Changes in alignment in one plane of motion impact socket reaction moments in other planes of motion. For example, externally rotating the prosthetic foot (increasing the amount of toe-out) has been demonstrated to increase the varus moment of the socket in the early stance phase of gait whereas internal rotation of the prosthetic foot (increasing the amount of toe-in) may increase the valgus moment of the socket in mid-to-late stance phase of gait.[62]A slight varus moment during stance phase of gait is preferred to provide prosthetic users with improved single-limb stance phase stability during ambulation.[63] Alignment changes in the sagittal plane impact the socket reaction moments in the sagittal and coronal planes; however, alignment changes in the coronal plane impact socket reaction moments in the coronal plane only.[62–65] Excessive extension of the prosthetic socket may cause prosthetic users to experience exaggerated knee extension or hyperextension and may report that they feel like they are "walking uphill."[63] This issue can be remedied by increasing the flexion of the prosthetic socket or by dorsiflexing the prosthetic foot.[63,65] Adduction or medial translation of the prosthetic socket may increase the valgus reaction moment of the prosthetic socket during stance phase of gait.[65] Significant challenges to prosthetic fitting and alignment are introduced in individuals with limb loss who have significant hip or knee flexion contractures. Prosthetic fitting becomes increasingly challenging when the severity of a hip or knee flexion contracture approaches or exceeds 25 degrees.[66] Accommodation of severe knee flexion contractures for individuals with transtibial amputation requires prosthetists to increase the flexion of the prosthetic socket, which may cause increased pressure on the anterior aspect of the proximal tibia or patellar tendon.[66] Given these challenges, it is imperative that clinicians educate individuals with transtibial amputation on strategies to prevent or minimize development of knee flexion contractures and advocate for early prosthetic fitting for those who are appropriate candidates for use of a lower-limb prosthesis.

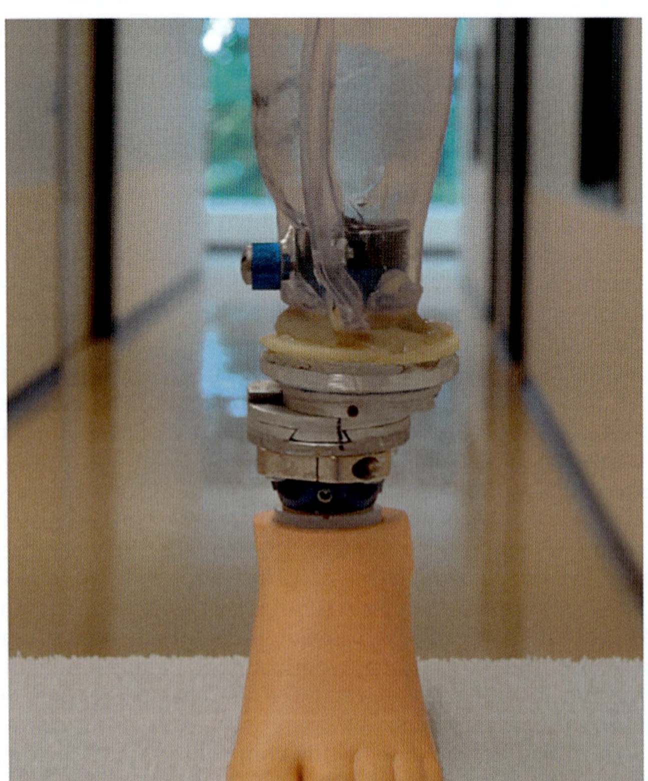

Fig. 23.15 Alignment adaptor.

BENCH ALIGNMENT

The first step in the alignment of a transtibial prosthesis is to position the socket in what is known as "bench alignment." This alignment serves as the starting point for the dynamic alignment process. In a standard bench alignment, the socket is set at 5 degrees of flexion and 5 degrees of adduction, while the top of the prosthetic foot is level in both the frontal and sagittal planes and the medial border of the foot is parallel to the line of progression. When viewed in the sagittal plane, a plumb line should fall from anatomic knee center and pass through the foot at a point one-third of the foot length from the back of the heel (Fig. 23.16). In the frontal plane, the line should go from mid-patella through the center of the heel. The reason for the 5 degrees of socket flexion is to elongate the quadriceps muscles slightly so that they are better prepared to accept the full weight of the body and to aid in shock absorption during loading response. The 5 degrees of adduction ensures that the foot is sufficiently inset to create the appropriate varus moment during stance. This properly loads the proximomedial and distolateral aspects of the limb that are best able to carry those forces. Standard bench alignment is not used when joint contracture or deformity is present; instead, the actual limb alignment is marked during the casting procedure and that alignment is used as the starting point in the dynamic analysis.

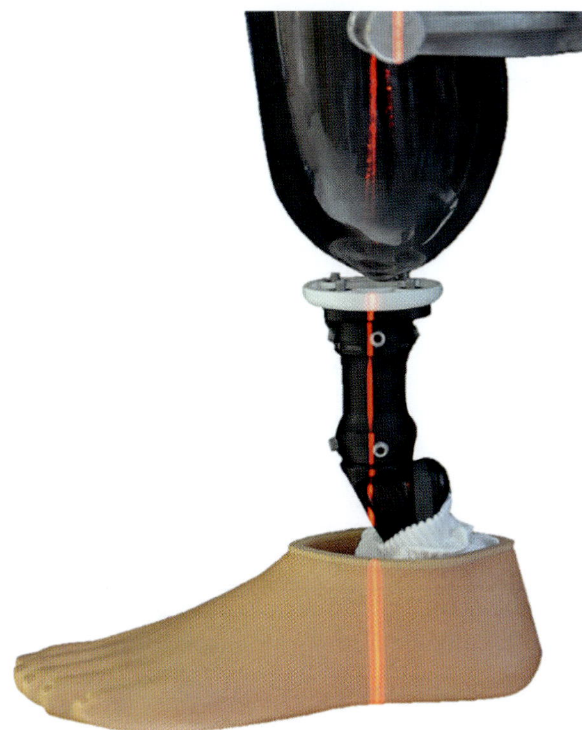

Fig. 23.16 Bench alignment.

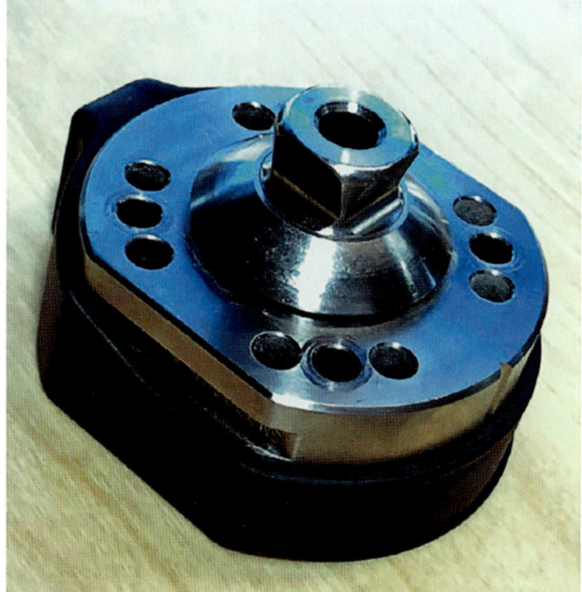

Fig. 23.17 Pyramid adaptor with computerized sensor.

HEIGHT

Once the prosthesis is bench aligned, the person dons the prosthesis and stands with equal weight bearing on both lower extremities. The first measurement examines the length of the prosthesis. The goal is to achieve relatively equal leg length, comparing the intact and prosthetic limbs. There are two accepted ways to assess the height: statically and dynamically. In a static assessment, the individual is asked to stand with feet shoulder-width apart, knees fully extended, and bearing equal weight on either limb. The distances from each iliac crest to the floor can be measured and compared. An alternative is to evaluate whether left and right iliac crests appear to be level. The measurement should not be taken in the supine position because the length of the prosthesis changes during weight bearing as a consequence of flexion of the dynamic components and compression of the interface material. In a dynamic assessment, the person is asked to walk and the entire body is observed, especially the head and torso. Many factors will affect the motion of the head and torso, so it is best to focus only on gross asymmetries that can be corrected by changing the length of the prosthesis. When the static and dynamic height measurements are different, a clinical decision is made to determine the optimal length for the prosthesis to provide the best function for the individual. It is not uncommon for the prosthesis to be up to 1 cm shorter than the sound limb under static conditions.

DYNAMIC ALIGNMENT

Alignment changes can be made with the standard modular connectors that are used to fasten the components of the prosthesis together. A standard pyramid connector (Fig. 23.17) can be set anywhere within an approximately 14-degree arc of adjustability. This means, for example, that the socket can be flexed up to 7 degrees or extended up to 7 degrees from the neutral starting position (Fig. 23.18). This is accomplished by loosening one screw and then tightening the opposite screw equally. Each pyramid permits adjustment in two orthogonal planes. For simplicity, the prosthetist will typically rotate the pyramid so that the adjustable planes are aligned with the frontal and sagittal planes. Transverse plane rotation is almost always infinitely adjustable; the standard connectors can accommodate any foot position. When the dynamic alignment differs greatly from bench alignment, it may be necessary to add a special alignable component to the prosthesis. This component will accommodate a larger window of adjustment and allows for linear changes in addition to angular changes. For example, the foot can be inset relative to the socket simply by sliding the foot medially and retightening the connector. This device is to be used during the dynamic alignment only and then removed during the final fabrication procedure. Small linear adjustments can also be made without the special component by performing equal but opposite angular adjustments on two adjacent pyramid connectors. This method will, however, simultaneously affect the height of the prosthesis.

During the dynamic analysis, the prosthetist will ask the individual to walk in a safe environment, typically within the parallel bars, and observe the motion of the prosthesis throughout the gait cycle. It is important for the prosthetist to employ a systematic approach, such as distal-to-proximal evaluation, to ensure efficiency in the process. Adjustments are made to minimize gait deviations and create a smooth, stable gait pattern. The prosthetist will attempt to create an energy-efficient stride by minimizing the horizontal and vertical displacement of the center of mass. Goals for the optimal alignment are stance stability, swing clearance, equal step length, and energy efficiency. Socket fit and suspension play an important role in providing stability, so final adjustments to both aspects are included as part of the dynamic

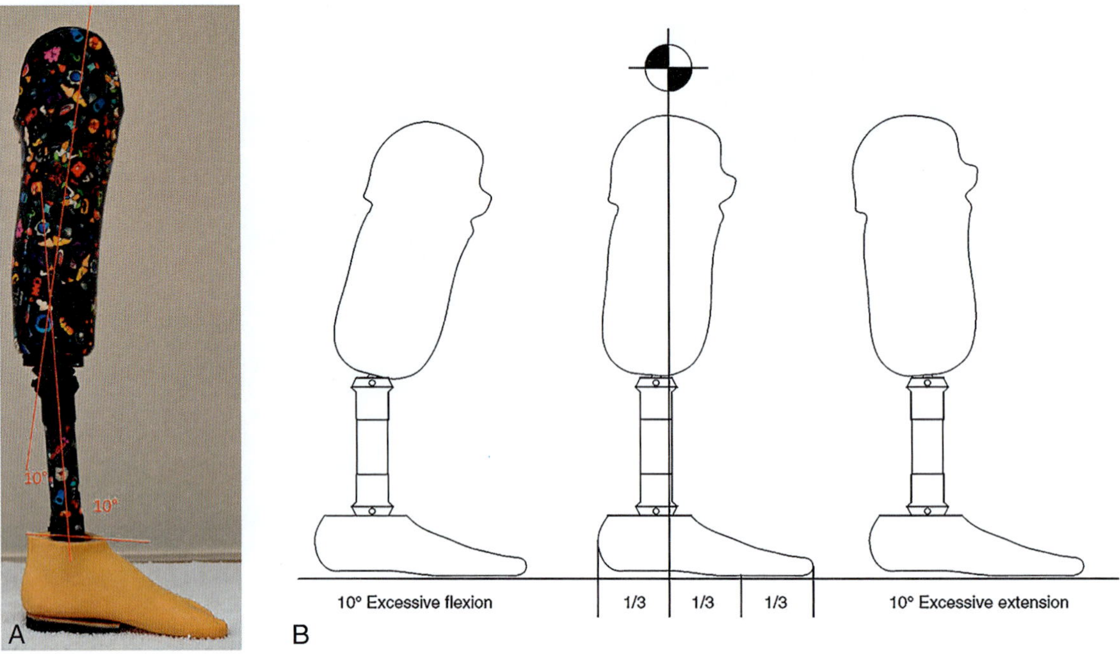

Fig. 23.18 (A) Alignment and socket angle. (B) Impact of socket angle.

analysis. Although dynamic alignment is typically done on a flat, level surface, many prosthetists will also attempt to simulate other terrains an individual will encounter in their daily lives. Ramps, stairs, and uneven surfaces all require slightly different alignments for optimal performance. It is very important to optimize prosthetic alignment as it has been shown to have significant clinical impact on gait kinetics and spatiotemporal parameters, including cadence and medial-lateral displacement of the socket.[67] Final alignment is often a compromise of function on the varied terrain an amputee will encounter.

As the question of whether or not optimal alignment of the prosthesis has been achieved is ultimately answered by the function and satisfaction of the person wearing the prosthesis, there is a fairly broad range of alignments that can be considered acceptable.[67] In an effort to standardize what is ultimately a subjective estimate of proper alignment, the concept of vertical alignment axis and alignment reference center has been proposed. The vertical alignment axis is a vertical line that passes through the geometric center of the socket at the level of the mid-patellar tendon. The alignment reference center is the point along the line from the center of the foot through the tip of the shoe, one-third of the way forward from the back of the heel. To align the prosthesis, the individual is asked to fully weight bear on the socket while the socket is supported on a padded stand. The person determines the socket axis based on the most comfortable weight-bearing position. When the socket is aligned with the socket axis in the most comfortable position and the vertical alignment axis goes directly through the alignment reference center (Fig. 23.19), the prosthesis is generally accepted to be well aligned.

ELECTRONIC ALIGNMENT

Technology has been developed to assist the prosthetist in making the alignment process a more objective process and thereby making prosthetic alignments more repeatable and predictable. Electronic sensors imbedded in the prosthetic components are capable of transmitting real-time gait data to a nearby computer (Fig. 23.17). The computer processes the data and superimposes a graph of the actual forces and moments for one complete gait cycle over a set of "normal" data (Fig. 23.20).[68] Displaying the otherwise invisible forces and moments on the prosthesis cues the prosthetist to focus in on specific variances and consider their possible causes. This can prevent undetected problems with alignment from causing long-term damage to the individual's limb. For example, an excessive varus moment at the knee can lead to premature medial compartmental osteoarthritis over a long period. This objective data can be captured and kept in the person's medical record to be referenced if problems arise or changes are necessary in the future.

Troubleshooting Issues Related to Prosthetic Fit

A common problem encountered by individuals with recent transtibial amputation is application of too few or too many sock ply. Sock-ply management is a skill that develops as the individual wears the prosthesis more and is conscientious about examining the limb after doffing the prosthesis. The number of socks will eventually become consistent, but early in the process of limb maturation, variability is common. The correct number of socks may vary from day to day, or even from hour to hour. There are a few basic cues that those new to prosthetic use must consider to ensure the limb is in the correct position within the socket.

The first cue is during donning—the limb should slide into the socket with some resistance. This is a subjective determination, and the person should be trained to recognize the amount of force needed to fully don the prosthesis with the correct number of socks. Too few socks allows the limb to

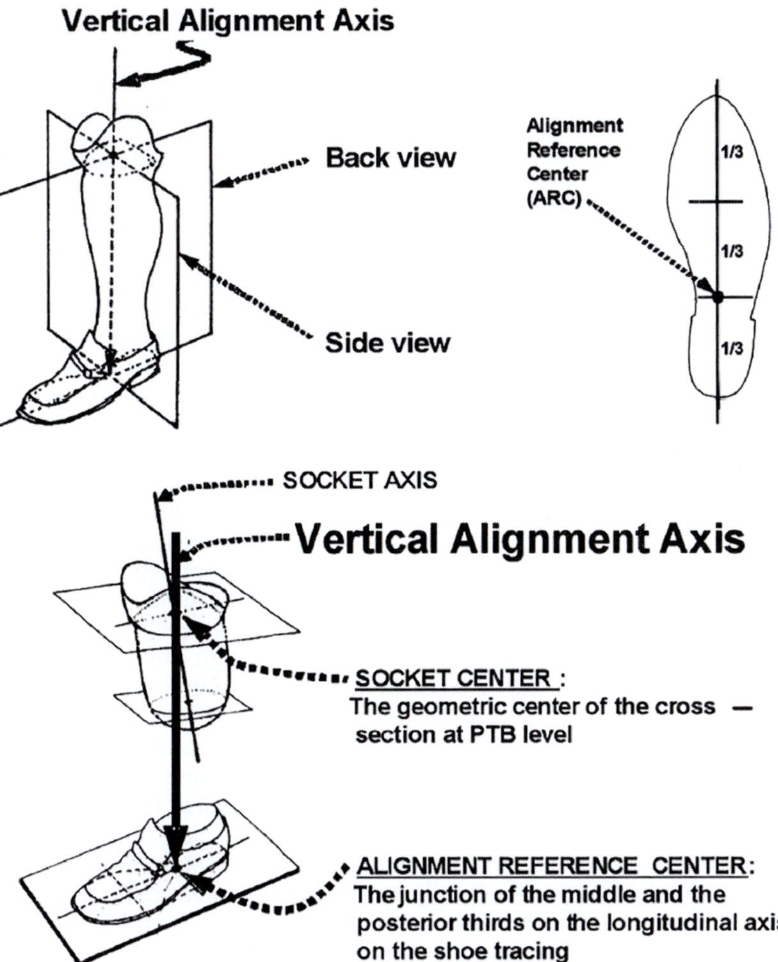

Fig. 23.19 Vertical alignment axis. *PTB*, Patella tendon bearing.

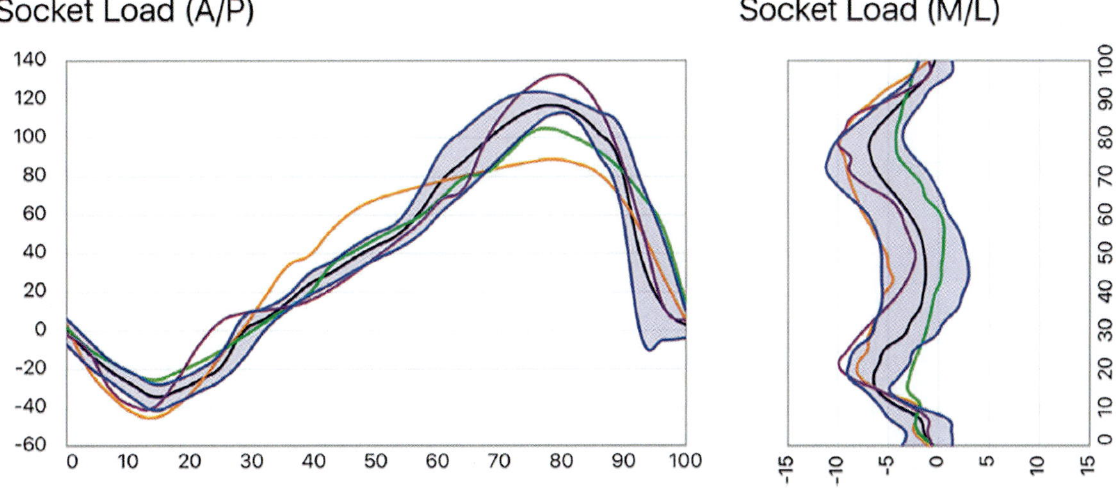

Fig. 23.20 Kinetic and kinematic data.

"bottom out" in the socket, where most of the weight bearing occurs on the distal end, leading to pain, instability, and increased pistoning. Conversely, too many socks prevents the limb from fully entering the socket (Fig. 23.11B), leading to loss of control and pressure on bony prominences. Too many ply of sock can also lead to hammocking, which is stress on the distal-end soft tissues as they are pulled tight over the distal tibia during weight bearing. For the person who has recently started using a prosthesis, this sensation may feel very much like the "bottoming out" sensation they feel with too few sock ply. It is important to educate the wearer on differentiating between the two conditions.

The second cue indicating the limb is not in the correct position within the socket is increased pistoning, anteroposterior, or medial-lateral motion within the socket when walking. This can be caused by an insufficient number of socks.

The final cue to incorrect position are signs of erythema while doffing the prosthesis. Erythema on the distal aspect of the fibular head or patella indicates the limb is too far in the socket and extra ply of socks are needed. If too many socks are being used, the erythema will appear on the tibial tubercle or the proximal aspect of the fibular head, as the limb is not far enough into the socket. In this case, there may also be signs of verrucous hyperplasia on the distal end of the limb as a result of the lack of distal contact.

Another common problem that can arise with prosthetic users is caused by inappropriate shoe wear. Although some prosthetic feet accommodate for the heel height of the shoe, most do not. Wearing a heel that is too high positions the limb in a way that creates a relative excessive flexion of the socket and actual excess flexion of the knee joint during stance. A heel that is too low or going barefoot tends to hyperextend the knee. Proper footwear is important for safe ambulation. The prosthesis can be checked by evaluating the top surface of the foot shell while the prosthesis is free standing on a level surface. If the top of the foot shell tilts posteriorly, the heel is too low (Fig. 23.21). Similar sagittal plane gait problems can occur by changing between footwear of similar heel height but differing stiffness of soling material. A stiff sole (leather sole) shoe will have similar effects as an increased heel height and a softer sole similar to barefoot. These changes will be most noticeable in the initial contact and loading response phases of gait.

In a well-fitting socket, the skin should appear uniform in color after wearing the prosthesis. Areas of erythema that fade after 20 minutes are not likely to be problematic. The skin should be soft and supple, especially on the distal end. Firm tissue associated with edema is a sign of poor contact and effort should be made to create some contact in the area of the firm tissue. The individual may not tolerate much pressure, but only a small amount of pressure is needed to push the extra fluid back into circulation. If erythema is observed over bony prominences, and the person's residual limb is properly seated in the socket, pressure in those areas needs to be relieved. Prosthetists can adjust the fit of thermoplastic sockets by heating and reshaping the areas needing adjustment. Thermoset sockets, like composites, can only be adjusted by cutting out fenestrations or by adding padding to the area around the prominent bone to shift it away from the socket wall. It is important to note that the addition of padding requires removal of some equivalent sock ply to maintain the same volume within the socket.

If skin irritation is present, especially over a bony prominence, placing a small mark on the affected areas with lipstick before donning the prosthesis will allow the lipstick to transfer to the socket during weight bearing. Once the prosthetic wearer removes the prosthesis, the lipstick will mark the areas of excessive contact. Alternatively, a thin flexible steel probe (a corset stay works exceptionally well) can be inserted between the socket and the interface to act as a feeler gauge to find areas of high pressure. The individual should be putting some weight through the socket during this evaluation. To assess distal contact in a finished socket, a ball of soft clay, about the size of a pea, can be placed into the bottom of the socket prior to donning. After the person dons the prosthesis and walks a few steps, the prosthesis should be removed and the clay examined. The clay should appear compressed. Postcompression clay thickness of 3 to 5 mm is considered ideal. Total contact in the socket can be assessed by lightly powdering the interior surface of the socket with a fine powder like cornstarch and having the individual carefully don the prosthesis and walk a few steps. Any powder that remains on the socket's surface after walking indicates that those areas are not in contact with the residual limb.

The amount of pistoning that is present in a socket depends on the socket design and the type of suspension

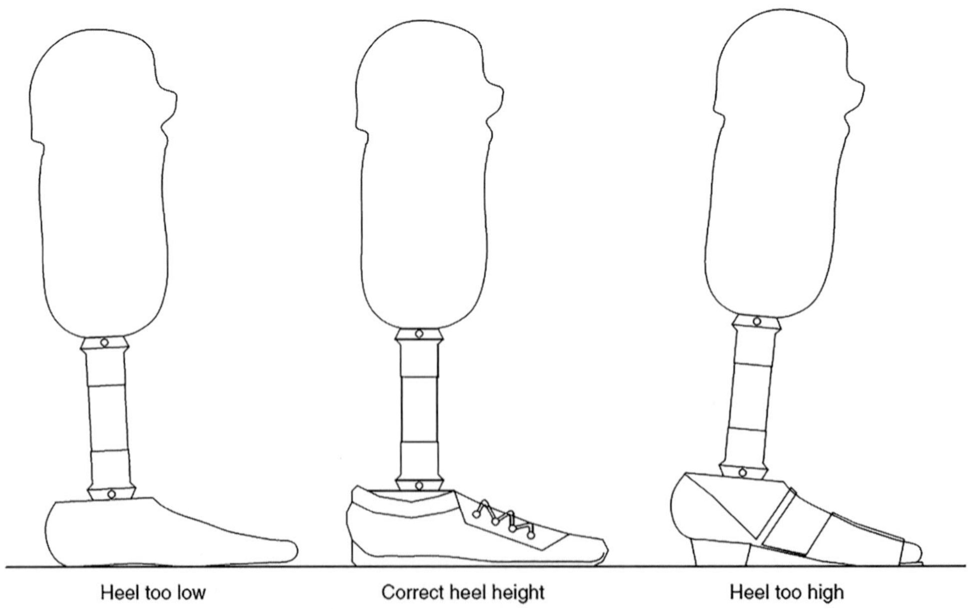

Fig. 23.21 Impact of different heel heights.

used. If the person is complaining of discomfort while ambulating but is comfortable while standing, pistoning is the likely cause of pain. Pistoning can be assessed by asking the individual to fully weight bear on the socket and then lift the prosthesis off the ground while the examiner is palpating the patella. Motion of more than 1 cm should be considered excessive. Faulty suspension and/or loose socket fit are generally responsible for pistoning. Wearing the correct ply of sock and ensuring that the suspension is functioning well should minimize motion within the socket to pain-free levels.

There are several patterns of erythema that indicate poor alignment of the prosthesis. Excessive varus moment on the limb is suspected when signs of pressure are observed on both the distolateral and the proximomedial aspects of the limb together. This pattern can be caused by excessive foot inset or too much socket adduction. When the erythema is observed on the distomedial and proximolateral aspects of the limb, an excessive valgus moment is likely. The foot may be too far outset or the socket may be excessively abducted. Anterior distal pressure accompanied by pressure in the posterior proximal aspect of the socket may be a result of an excessively long heel lever arm, excessive dorsiflexion, excessive socket flexion, or a heel that is too firm. This pattern can also be observed when an individual wears a shoe that has a higher heel than the prosthesis can accommodate. Conversely, if the person goes barefoot, the opposite pattern of pressure will be observed; erythema on the posterior distal end and the anteroproximal end of the residual limb. This same pattern can be caused by a toe lever arm that is too long, an overly plantarflexed foot, or an excessively extended socket.

Case Example 1 **A Male With Traumatic Transtibial Amputation**

PROSTHETIC PRESCRIPTION

Let us consider the case of J.W., a 37-year-old male whose left leg was amputated below the knee following a motorcycle accident. He has since recovered from all injuries and is now medically stable. He was recently approved for weight bearing as tolerated on his left limb. He is 5′8″ tall, weighs 175 lb (79.5 kg), and his residual limb measures approximately 20 cm from knee center to distal end. J.W. has significant amounts of scar tissue on the surface of the residual limb including a skin graft from his thigh. The skin on the distal end of the limb is adhered to the distal end of the tibia. He was very active prior to his injury and would like to return to that lifestyle as soon as possible. He arrives at the clinic on crutches.

QUESTIONS TO CONSIDER

- Is the individual a good prosthetic candidate?
- What type of interface, suspension, and socket design are appropriate?
- What other components are recommended?
- Who are the other members of the rehab team?

RECOMMENDATIONS

The first decision is to determine whether or not J.W. is a prosthetic candidate. His entry into the clinic on crutches indicates that his balance, upper extremity strength, and contralateral limb are all sufficient for gait. The only factor jeopardizing his prosthetic candidacy is the condition of the soft tissue of his residual limb. In the past, soft-tissue condition may have prevented successful use of the prosthesis, but with modern techniques and materials, a successful fitting is likely.

The interface with the skin should be determined next. Two conditions need to be considered: the adherent tissue on the distal end and the fragile skin graft. Gel liners are most efficient at eliminating shear forces on the limb. This will be a major factor in preventing skin breakdown of the adherent skin. The skin graft would benefit from a soft durometer gel, rather than a silicone elastomer or urethane liner. The selection of the right interface will be critical to J.W.'s outcome. The decision to use an off-the-shelf size or a custom-made liner will depend on the shape of the limb and how well he could be fitted with a standard liner size.

The suspension for J.W. should be the system that will lead to the least amount of pistoning. Elevated vacuum will maintain the limb volume by drawing fluid back into the tissues between weight-bearing cycles. This is important for J.W. as the tissues of his limb will be subjected to a large amount of strain once he reaches his goal of readopting an active lifestyle.

PROSTHETIC FITTING AND ALIGNMENT: VISIT 1

J.W. is seen today for the initial fitting of his first prosthesis. The gel liner is donned directly on the skin and a single-ply sock is worn over the liner. The limb is then placed into the socket and a sealing sleeve is rolled up to mid-thigh to seal off the proximal edge of the socket. J.W. is then asked to stand up in the parallel bars, keeping all his weight on the sound limb. As tolerated, J.W. will then slowly transfer weight over to the prosthesis. Once he is comfortable bearing his full weight on the prosthesis, he can begin to take his first steps.

As he begins to walk and feel more confident in the prosthesis, J.W. begins to let go of the bars and walk hands-free. Once he does this, his knee begins to rapidly flex during loading response and the foot starts slapping the floor.

QUESTIONS TO CONSIDER

- Is the alignment of the prosthesis adjusted properly? Is the foot making an appropriate heel strike? Has the heel height of the shoe been properly accommodated?
- Is the socket stable on his limb? Are there signs of pistoning? Is there excessive medial shift of the prosthesis during stance?
- Are his knee extensors strong enough to eccentrically control knee flexion during full weight bearing?

RECOMMENDATIONS

A plumb bob through the midline of the socket falls between the posterior one-third and anterior two-thirds of the foot when the shoe is donned, and the top of the foot shell is level with the ground. This indicates that the alignment is appropriate. Muscle strength testing reveals that the quadriceps of the residual limb are 2 out of 5. Due to the lack of strength in the quadriceps muscle group, he is unable to regulate knee flexion during loading response. A rehabilitation protocol for quadriceps strengthening should be implemented that includes ambulation with the prosthesis. At the same time, the prosthesis can be altered to improve his gait pattern as he regains his strength. The foot should be moved anteriorly, relative to the socket. This will decrease the mechanical advantage of ground reaction force to flex the knee by shortening the heel lever.

Case Example 1 A Male With Traumatic Transtibial Amputation —cont'd

It will simultaneously increase the length of the toe lever, which will provide more stability in midstance. The potential downside is that the knee extension moment in terminal stance will also be increased, so there is potential for the knee to hyperextend. The individual should be asked to monitor posterior knee pain and report any as soon as it is recognized.

Because his muscle weakness is expected to resolve relatively quickly, the alignment of the prosthesis should be monitored on a regular basis so that the foot can be gradually shifted back to the appropriate position and normal gait can be restored.

PROSTHETIC FITTING AND ALIGNMENT: VISIT 2

J.W. has done well with rehabilitation and use of his lower-extremity prosthesis. His limb has healed well and his strength is generally good. He has good balance and endurance for walking with the prosthesis. He has gradually increased his prosthesis wear time and activity level. He works a 5-hour day in agriculture. Today he returns to therapy for a scheduled follow-up appointment. He complains of discomfort in the distal end of his residual limb and loss of stability in the socket. While observing his gait, the prosthesis appears to be a little short. Assessment of the residual limb reveals erythema on the distal end and on the distal aspect of the patella.

QUESTIONS TO CONSIDER

- What changes have occurred since his last visit? Has he made changes to sock ply or footwear? Has he gained or lost weight?
- Is this an alignment- or fit-related issue? When does the pain occur in the gait cycle? Does the pain increase throughout the day?
- Is the interface worn out? How old is the interface now? How long should it be expected to last? Are there thin areas in the interface that might indicate excessive pressure and premature wear?

RECOMMENDATIONS

J.W. reports his weight and footwear have not changed. He is wearing the same single-ply sock with which he began his prosthetic use. His gel liner is still in excellent condition and should be expected to last for about a year of constant wear. Consideration of all the information indicates that the limb has changed since the initial fitting. As his pain is worst at midstance and increases proportionally with his time spent weight bearing, the conclusion is that the limb is too far distal in the socket. He should increase the number of socks he is wearing, one ply at a time, until the limb is seated correctly in the socket. This will also address the length of the prosthesis, which had appeared too short.

In experimenting with sock ply, J.W. went from initially wearing a single sock to six plies, but he found this number of socks created a new set of problems. He is feeling excessive pressure on the tibial tubercle and proximal aspect of the fibular head. During loading response, he is unable to regulate his knee flexion because of pain on the anterior distal aspect of the tibia. Despite good suspension, he is also starting to scuff his toe during swing phase. All these symptoms indicate that he is now too far out of the socket. This position decreases the control of the tibia and allows the socket to flex and extend beyond the position of the limb, leading to excessive pressure on the ends of the bones. It also positions the bony prominences of the limb in areas that do not have adequate reliefs. Removal of several sock plies is the correct intervention, as this will allow him to seat further in the socket and increase comfort and stability. When J.W. wore four-ply socks, the comfort and control of the prosthesis were restored.

Case Example 2 An Older Female With Amputation Related to Vascular Disease

PROSTHETIC PRESCRIPTION

G.R. is a 76-year-old female with type 2 diabetes and peripheral vascular disease. G.R. sustained an abrasion at the lateral malleolus of the right leg. The skin abrasion failed to heal and developed into a stage 4 nonhealing wound. Circulation at the lower leg was markedly impaired. After several months of multiple failed therapies to improve circulation and promote wound healing, the right leg was amputated below the knee 2 months ago. G.R. is 5′4″ tall and weighs 204 lb (92.5 kg). Prior to the problems with her leg, she was living independently and caring for her husband, who is significantly disabled. The transtibial amputation wound site has completely healed. Her physician is recommending that she begin bearing weight on the limb as tolerated. She has been using a wheelchair for mobility in the house, but she is able to stand on her left leg with support of a standard walker. She is concerned that she will not be able to do her chores around the house and the shopping even after she receives her prosthesis.

QUESTIONS TO CONSIDER

- What are G.R.'s goals for the prosthesis? Will she be a functional ambulator? Will the prosthesis be used only for standing and transfers?
- Will she require assistance with activities of daily living and care for her husband?
- What are the main design goals for her prosthesis? What system will allow her to don the prosthesis independently? Which will require the least maintenance and most reliable function?

RECOMMENDATIONS

Evaluating G.R.'s candidacy for a prosthesis will involve assessing her risk-to-benefit ratio as a bipedal ambulator against the negative health effects of prolonged sitting. Her motivation to ambulate is clear in her expressed desire to continue to care for her husband. Her ability to stand on one leg is a fortuitous sign, even if her balance is impaired at this point. Her knee ROM is within normal limits. If her skin integrity is good and her right knee extensors are 4/5, she will likely be a good prosthetic candidate.

Her prosthesis should be easy to put on, as she will not have assistance available. Her limb has ample soft tissue based on her weight and etiology, although her diabetes puts her at risk for fragile skin and delayed healing. The most appropriate interface for her will be one that most effectively reduces shear. A silicone elastomer cushion liner in a TSB socket will work

(Continued)

Case Example 2 An Older Female With Amputation Related to Vascular Disease—cont'd

well for her. A sealing sleeve and expulsion valve will utilize suction as a means of suspension, thus minimizing pistoning. This prosthesis should allow her to wear a cotton sock that is easily laundered as she loses limb volume. The trim lines should be set higher proximally to gain as much control as possible for her prosthesis.

PROSTHETIC ALIGNMENT AND FITTING: VISIT 1

G.R. is seen for delivery of her preparatory prosthesis. She is instructed on donning the device and is able to roll on the gel liner and place her limb into the socket, with moderate effort. Her limb is seated correctly all the way in the socket. After she rolls the sealing sleeve into position, she stands at her walker and slowly begins to load the prosthesis. She is comfortable in the socket and a small amount of air is heard as it is expulsed from the socket through the valve. The sleeve is rolled down so that a corset stay can be inserted between the gel liner and the socket. As no areas of excessive pressure are found, the corset stay is removed and the sleeve is rolled back up. Her first steps are tentative, and she is bearing the majority of her weight through her arms during stance on the prosthetic side. After some guidance from her therapist, she begins to bear more weight through the prosthesis. Her strides are asymmetric, with a very large step on the prosthetic side and a truncated step on the sound side.

QUESTIONS TO CONSIDER

- Why is her step length shorter on the sound side? Is the prosthesis aligned properly? Is her range of hip flexion and extension within functional limits? Is she stable in stance?
- What are her goals for ambulation? Does she have sufficient stance stability? Does she have adequate clearance in swing? Is her gait pattern energy efficient?

RECOMMENDATIONS

The gait pattern she uses is typical of the individual with recent amputation who is uncertain about weight bearing through a mechanical device. The feeling of instability on the prosthesis causes her to limit stance time on that side, thereby shortening swing phase on the sound side. Alternately, the individual is accustomed to bearing weight unilaterally on the sound side, so the stance time is increased allowing the prosthesis to move ahead excessively. Weakness of the quadriceps and gluteus minimus and medius will also impair stance stability. She should be encouraged to take smaller steps with the prosthesis and larger steps with her sound limb. She may need further conditioning of her knee extensors and hip abductors to completely eliminate this asymmetry.

Excessive socket flexion can increase prosthetic step length, but it also tends to increase the step length on the sound side as well. Extending the socket makes it more difficult to advance over the foot during stance and will tend to shorten step length on the contralateral side.

PROSTHETIC FITTING AND ALIGNMENT: VISIT 2

G.R. returns for therapy and is complaining about discomfort in her socket. Inspection of her skin reveals excessive pressure, as evidenced by erythema, on her femoral condyles and fibular head. She has been doing a good job managing her sock ply and is now seated correctly in the socket wearing eight ply. She explains that the tightness she feels does not get worse during weight bearing.

QUESTIONS TO CONSIDER

- What changes may have taken place since her last visit? As her activity level increases, what is the effect on limb volume? Which areas of the limb are most susceptible to volume loss?
- What is the source of the erythema? Is there swelling of the knee? Does the redness appear anywhere else on the limb? Does it appear to be an allergic reaction like contact dermatitis? Is her liner clean and in good condition?

RECOMMENDATIONS

After discussing good hygiene and prosthetic care with G.R., it is clear that she is washing her gel liner daily with a mild soap and then rinsing thoroughly, and that she is washing her limb every day and patting it dry. She is not using any lotions that may create buildup in the liner or an allergic reaction when confined in the warm moist environment of the liner. The fit of the socket is assessed next by probing between the liner and socket with a thin metal corset stay. This is done in the non–weight-bearing state, as that is when the pressure is occurring. The corset stay encounters great resistance when passing over the fibular head and is completely stuck when trying to pass over the femoral condyles. This indicates excessive pressure over those bony structures. Although she is wearing the appropriate number of socks, they are creating the extra bulk that makes the socket too tight in those areas. A referral should be made to her prosthetist so that the socket can be modified. It is likely that pads can be added in strategic areas that are more prone to volume loss, such as the area over the calf muscle and on either side of the tibia. This will take up volume in the socket and require her to reduce the number of sock ply she wears. Following that adjustment, G.R. is feeling more comfortable in the socket and her skin is free from irritation.

PROSTHETIC FEET

As discussed in Chapter 21, most individuals at the K1 functional level will use either a solid-ankle-cushion heel (SACH) foot or a single-axis foot; multiple-axis or flexible-keel prosthetic feet are typically used by individuals functioning at a K2 level; Energy Storing and Returning Feet (ESAR), dynamic response, or microprocessor feet are typically used by individuals functioning at a K3 level.[69] Any prosthetic foot is appropriate for individuals with the ability or potential to function at a K4 level.[69] With selection of prosthetic componentry, clinicians should be aware of the benefits associated with specific components and the potential tradeoffs or limitations of those components (see Table 23.3). A randomized, controlled cross-over study of 45 participants compared the outcomes related to balance performance, quality of life, and patient satisfaction between a standard energy storage and return (ESAR) prosthetic foot and a microprocessor-controlled foot and found that individuals with the microprocessor-controlled foot demonstrated improved balance, quality of life, and patient satisfaction without any significant differences in energy expenditure.[70] It should be noted that the microprocessor-controlled foot utilized in this study, the Proprio-Foot, incorporates features of an ESAR foot with the addition of a microprocessor-controlled ankle, which allows it to better adapt to changes in terrain.[70]

Table 23.3 Benefits and Limitations/Tradeoffs Associated With Prosthetic Feet

Prosthetic Foot Classification	Benefits	Limitations/Tradeoffs
SACH	■ Minimal maintenance required	■ Minimal energy return
Single Axis	■ Increased limits of stability compared to SACH foot for forward weight shift[73]	■ May disrupt forward progression of center of pressure through stance phase[74]
	■ More sagittal plane motion than multiple axis or ESAR feet[74]	■ No increase in backwards limits of stability[73]
	■ Improved stability in loading response[74]	■ Minimal energy return
	■ Achieve foot flat earlier shifting ground reaction force anterior to minimize knee flexion moment during weight acceptance[74]	■ May limit ability to ambulate at faster or variable walking speeds[74]
	■ May be helpful for individuals with transfemoral amputation having difficulty controlling a prosthetic knee[74]	■ Limited ability to accommodate to uneven terrain
Multiple Axis	■ Provide range of motion in multiple planes to accommodate to uneven terrain	■ Increased mobility at the expense of energy storage and return
Flexible Keel	■ Provides some energy return	■ Insufficient energy return for individuals capable of walking at faster gait speeds
	■ Smooth transition from heel strike initial contact to toe-off at terminal stance/preswing	
ESAR	■ Increase prosthetic-side propulsion[74]	■ Limited ability to adapt to nonlevel surfaces or inclines[75]
	■ Faster walking speeds[74]	■ May require postural compensation to adapt to terrain due to limited adaptability of ESAR feet[75]
	■ Improved stair ascent compared to SACH foot[74]	
	■ Decrease fatigue compared to single-axis and multiple-axis feet[74]	
	■ Reduced energy cost and increased gait efficiency[74]	
	■ Better shock absorption resulting in reduced pain, skin problems, shock & stress at low back, hip, and knee[74]	
	■ May be used for jogging or sports-related activity	
Microprocessor Feet	■ Increased adaptability and adjustability to accommodate to inclined surfaces[75]	■ For individuals with transfemoral amputation, the prosthetic knee plays a more significant role for walking on inclines than the foot[75]
	■ May improve ambulation on uneven terrain[75]	■ Not appropriate for running
	■ Decreased residual and sound side loading[75]	■ Requires battery charging
	■ Increased toe clearance during swing phase, especially at faster walking speeds[76]	■ Increased weight
	■ Improved range of motion for sit to stand, stair negotiation, and retrieving objects from the floor[76]	
	■ During ramp descent, rapid plantar flexion reduces flexion moment at the knee providing improved perceived safety/stability[76]	

ESAR, Energy storage and return; *SACH*, solid-ankle-cushion heel.

The impact of different types of prosthetic feet on energy costs of walking have significant importance to individuals with limb loss as the energy cost of self-selected or comfortable walking speed is between 12% and 36% greater for individuals with transtibial amputation than those without limb loss.[71,72] Evidence suggests that individuals functioning at higher MFCL K-levels, especially K3 and K4, would be most affected by differences in the energy cost associated with different categories of prosthetic feet. There is evidence to suggest that prosthetic feet with powered dorsiflexion decrease energy costs of ambulation compared to dynamic response feet when walking down declines, ramps, and hills, and for slow walking speeds on a treadmill and possibly with over ground ambulation.[72] Dynamic response feet have not been shown to reduce energy cost during walking on level terrain compared to ESAR, flexible keel, or SACH feet.[72] For limited community ambulators functioning at a MFCL K-level 2, preliminary evidence suggests that energy cost of walking on level terrain may be reduced with multiaxis feet compared to SACH feet.[72] Running-specific feet do not significantly reduce energy cost of running on level terrain compared to dynamic response feet.[72]

Gait and Mobility Performance

Objective performance-based measures of gait performance are important to provide clinicians with insight related to functional capacity and mobility performance of individuals with lower-limb amputation who use a prosthesis for mobility. Gait speed can be measured via the 10 Minute Walk Test or the 2-Minute Walk Test and is useful to classify individuals performing at different MFCL K-levels, especially the higher levels (e.g., K3 vs. K4).[77,78] It has been suggested that the 2-Minute Walk Test is highly predictive of performance on the 6-Minute Walk Test.[79] The distance covered on the 6-Minute Walk Test provides clinicians with insight related to an individuals' capacity for community distance ambulation and is a measure of walking endurance.[80] Measures such as the Timed Up and Go Test or the L-Test are measures which inform not only walking speed but incorporate turns and sit to stand and stand to sit transitions associated with real-world mobility tasks and may be useful to identify individuals at risk for falling.[81–85] However, one key limitation of these performance-based assessments is that they do not provide clinicians with insight regarding the underlying determinants of gait performance or help clinicians identify key impairments on which to focus targeted rehabilitation interventions to improve mobility performance.

It has been suggested that gait asymmetry may contribute to worse walking performance for prosthetic users with lower-limb amputation.[86,87] Gait asymmetry and impaired dynamic balance during walking increases the energy cost of walking for individuals with lower-limb amputation.[71] For individuals with transtibial amputation due to nonvascular causes energy cost of ambulation is 12% greater than for those without limb loss, for individuals with transtibial amputation due to vascular causes the energy cost increases by 36%.[71] Further insight regarding gait symmetry can be gained through gait analysis on instrumented walkways or by having prosthetic users wear sensors to measure gait kinematics, however, these assessments are more routinely performed in a laboratory setting and may be underutilized in a clinical setting.[86,87] Most clinicians, physical therapists and certified prosthetists, utilize observational gait analysis to identify gait deviations for prosthetic users to identify impairments which may be contributing to gait asymmetry and inefficiency.[88] Skilled observation is required to determine whether the observed gait deviations are related to patient-related causes versus prosthetic-related causes to inform treatment decisions to address the underlying determinants of gait dysfunction and optimize walking performance. Most available tools for observation gait analysis for individuals with limb loss either do not report their psychometrics or are associated with limited reliability.[88,89] Gailey and colleagues recently described a new observational gait analysis screening tool for individuals with limb loss who use a lower-limb prosthesis, the Functional Lower-Limb Amputee Gait Assessment (FLAG), which focuses on the assessment of six components of gait while observing for eleven common gait deviations for lower-limb prosthetic users which have been identified in the literature (Fig. 23.22.).[88] This tool provides clinicians with observable signs for each gait deviation of interest and provides an evidence-based list of the most likely patient-related and prosthesis-related causes of each gait deviation.[88] A recent reliability assessment of the ability of physical therapists and certified prosthetists to utilize the FLAG for video-based observational gait analysis demonstrated moderate to near perfect intra-rater reliability.[88] The inter-rater reliability of the FLAG for physical therapists exceeded the clinically acceptable level of agreement (kappa ≥0.41) for four gait deviations, with kappa ≥0.41 for six gait deviations among certified prosthetists.[88] Common gait deviations seen in lower-limb prosthetic users which were not included in the FLAG include: hip hiking, circumduction, and contralateral vaulting.[88] The authors explained that these gait deviations are compensatory postural adjustments for the prosthetic side being functional too long to clear the floor during swing

Gait action	Observed deviation	Expected normative observation	Plane of observation	Gait task	Observable signs	Possible causes
Step width	1. Intact limb foot at midline ☐	5–10 cm (2" to 4")	Coronal	Weight acceptance	• *Primary.* Heel placed directly under intergluteal cleft • *Secondary. Intact limb externally rotated*	• Poor balance on prosthesis • Habit of relying more on intact limb
	2. Prosthetic limb abducted ☐	5–10 cm (2" to 4")	Coronal	Weight acceptance	• Step width > 5–10 cm (2–4") • Prosthetic limb abducted beyond natural line of progression	• To increase stability • Weak/improperly trained prosthetic side hip abductors
Step length and time	3. Intact limb step shorter ☐	Minimum 30 cm (12") from trailing limb toes to leading limb heel	Sagittal	Weight acceptance	• Distance between prosthetic toes and intact heel < 30 cm (12") • Intact limb step length shorter than prosthetic step length	• Poor balance on the prosthesis • Pain or discomfort • Decreased confidence
	4. Intact limb step faster ☐	Temporal symmetry between prosthetic and intact step time	Sagittal	Single limb support	• Prosthetic single limb support time, less than intact single limb support time	• Poor balance on the prosthesis • Pain or discomfort • Decreased confidence
	5. Prosthetic limb step shorter ☐	Minimum 30 cm (12") from trailing limb toes to leading limb heel	Sagittal	Weight acceptance	• Distance between intact toes and prosthetic heel < 30 cm (12") • Prosthetic limb step length shorter than intact step length	• Habit of spending too much time on intact limb

Forefoot load	6. Decreased prosthetic forefoot load ☐	Forefoot break or rocker	Sagittal and coronal	Late single limb support and early swing limb advancement	• Primary:
					  • Absence of forefoot crease
					  • Insufficient time spent on forefoot
					• *Secondary (intact):*
						• Poor balance over the prosthetic forefoot

Fig. 23.22 Functional lower-limb amputee gait assessment (FLAG).

Gait action	Observed deviation	Expected normative observation	Plane of observation	Gait task	Observable signs	Possible causes
					• *Vaulting* • *Shorter step length* • *Secondary (prosthetic):* • *'Lift' and 'kick'* • *Circumduction* • *Hip hiking*	
Knee flexion	7. Less than expected knee flexion ☐	30°–40° at pre-swing 60° at initial swing	Sagittal and coronal	Swing limb advancement	• Primary: • <30° flexion during pre-swing • <60° flexion during initial swing • *Secondary (intact):* • Vaulting • *Secondary (prosthetic):* • *Circumduction* • *Hip hiking*	• Decreased pelvic transverse rotation • Prosthesis too short • Too much knee flexion resistance
Pelvic transverse rotation	8. Reduced prosthetic limb forward pelvic transverse rotation ☐	5° forward and backward rotation on both sides	Sagittal and coronal	Swing limb advancement	• Primary: • Forward motion of anterior superior iliac spine • *Secondary (intact):* • *Weight remains back on heel* • *Toe extension during prosthetic swing limb advancement* • *Toe flexion during prosthetic weight acceptance* • *Vaulting* • *Secondary (prosthetic):* • *'Lift' and 'kick'* • *Circumduction* • *Hip hiking*	• Inadequate pelvic and hip biomechanics • Prosthesis too short

Gait action	Observed deviation	Expected normative observation	Plane of observation	Gait task	Observable signs	Possible causes
Trunk and arm motions	9. Decreased trunk rotation ☐	5° rotation in opposition to pelvis	Sagittal	Swing limb advancement	• Primary: • Lack of shoulder rotation in opposition to pelvis • *Secondary:* • *Abducted arms*	• Poor balance • Use of assistive device
	10. Asymmetrical arm swing ☐	Symmetrical arm swing	Sagittal and coronal	Swing limb advancement	• Asymmetrical arm motion	• Poor balance • Use of assistive device
	11. Lateral trunk lean ☐	Neutral, upright alignment	Coronal	Single limb support	• Trunk leans laterally past vertical line of prosthetic limb	• Prosthesis too short • Weak/improperly trained prosthetic side hip abductors • Pain or discomfort • Habit
	None of the above gait deviations ☐					

Fig. 23.22, cont'd

limb advancement and are typically attributable or caused by other gait deviations already included in the FLAG, for example, less than expected knee flexion or reduced prosthetic limb forward pelvic transverse rotation during swing limb advancement.[88]

In 2017 the VA and DoD released the VA/DoD Clinical Practice Guideline for Rehabilitation of Individuals with Lower Limb Amputation to provide a framework for rehabilitation management of individuals with lower-limb amputation.[27] As part of this initiative a VA/DoD Amputation

System of Care was formed and resources were developed to help clinicians implement the recommendations of the clinical practice guidelines. Among these resources is a clinician toolkit which provides clinicians with valuable clinical pearls for pain management, management of the residual limb, and analysis and treatment of abnormal gait for individuals with transtibial and transfemoral amputation. The recommendations for evaluation and management of gait deviations for individuals with transtibial amputation is provided in (Table 23.4).[27]

Table 23.4 Common Gait Abnormalities and Patient-Related Versus Prosthetic-Related Causes

Gait Analysis—Abnormalities in Transtibial Amputation

	Patient Related			Prosthetic Related	
Gait Abnormality	**Possible Causes**	**Additional Evaluation**	**Interventions**	**Prosthetic Causes**	**Additional Evaluation**
1. Vaulting An attempt to lengthen the stance phase on the intact limb by knee extension and ankle plantar flexion during midstance phase	Inability to adequately flex the knee on the prosthetic side	Test knee ROM (all other causes are excluded)	Step-ups with prosthetic leg	Prosthetic limb too long	Evaluate pelvic height in standing with equal weight through both limbs
	Habit gait pattern	None	Repetitive Step forward-step back with prosthetic leg (sound leg remains stationary)	Poorly suspended prosthesis	Evaluate pistoning and/or a socket that is too loose
				Excessive ankle plantar flexion of the prosthetic foot	Posterior leaning prosthesis when observed off of the patient
2. Circumduction The prosthetic limb travels in an a lateral arch during swing phase	Inability to adequately flex the knee on the prosthetic side	Test knee ROM	Step-ups with prosthetic leg	Prosthetic limb too long	Evaluate pelvic height in standing with equal weight through both limbs
	Habit Gait Pattern	None	Repetitive Step forward-step back with prosthetic leg (sound leg remains stationary)	Poorly suspended prosthesis	Evaluate pistoning and/or a socket that is too loose
	Weak hip flexors	Perform manual muscle test	Traditional exercises for hip strengthening	Excessive ankle plantar flexion of the prosthetic foot	Posterior leaning prosthesis when observed off of the patient
3. Abducted Gait Pattern The prosthetic limb is carried in an abducted position throughout the swing and stance phase	Adaptation for medial compartment knee pain	Knee joint evaluation	Weight shifting activities over prosthetic limb	Outset prosthetic foot can give an apparent abducted gait pattern	Evaluate iliac crest height in standing
	Adaptation for focal residual limb pain	Inspect residual limb integrity	Refer for management of residual limb problems	Prosthesis is too long	Evaluate iliac crest height in standing
	Balance impairment/ fear of falling	Evaluate balance and stability	Advanced balance activities	Medially placed foot	Evaluate static prosthetic alignment
4. Knee Instability Excessive knee flexion on prosthetic side in early stance	Knee flexion contracture	Test knee ROM	Stretch accordingly	Excessive foot dorsiflexion	Evaluate static prosthetic alignment
	Quad weakness	Perform manual muscle test	Closed-chain strengthening exercises while wearing prosthesis	Excessive socket flexion	Evaluate static prosthetic alignment
				Posterior translation of the foot/pylon	Evaluate static prosthetic alignment assess heel
				Excessively hard heel cushion or prosthetic heel keel	Evaluate compression during manual loading
5. Genu Recurvatum The knee on the prosthetic side hyperextends during mid to late stance phase	Inadequate knee flexion range of motion	Test knee ROM	Stretch accordingly	Excessively compliant prosthetic heel cushion or too rigid forefoot keel	Assess heel compression during manual loading

Table 23.4 Common Gait Abnormalities and Patient-Related Versus Prosthetic-Related Causes—cont'd

Gait Analysis—Abnormalities in Transtibial Amputation

	Patient Related			**Prosthetic Related**	
Gait Abnormality	**Possible Causes**	**Additional Evaluation**	**Interventions**	**Prosthetic Causes**	**Additional Evaluation**
	Quad weakness	Perform manual muscle test	Closed-chain strengthening exercises while wearing prosthesis	Inadequate socket flexion	Evaluate static prosthetic alignment
	Hip flexion contracture	Test hip ROM	Stretch accordingly	Excessively plantar flexion of the prosthetic foot	Evaluate static prosthetic alignment
				Anterior translation of prosthetic foot/pylon	Evaluate static prosthetic alignment
6. Reduced Toe Clearance Prosthetic toe drags or catches during swing phase	Muscle weakness of the hip and/or knee flexors	Perform manual muscle test	Knee flexion plus bridging with ball Traditional exercises	Prosthetic limb too long	Evaluate iliac crest heights in standing with equal weight bearing on the prosthetic limb
	Reduced range of motion in hip flexion or knee flexion	Test ROM	Stretch accordingly	Inadequate suspension/pistoning	Evaluate adequacy of suspension
	Contralateral hip abductor weakness	Perform manual muscle test	Sidestepping with prosthesis with or without the Theraband Traditional exercises	Residual limb not getting into prosthetic socket all the way	Evaluate the relationship of the residual limb to the distal end of the prosthetic socket
				Excessive plantar flexion of the prosthetic foot	Evaluate static alignment of the prosthetic limb
7. Excessive Valgus Moment at the Knee Abnormal valgus moment at the knee of the residual limb during prosthetic stance phase	Short residual limb may cause poor stabilization of the prosthetic socket	Evaluate residual limb length in conjunction with adequacy of socket	No intervention for structural deformity	Excessive lateral translation of the prosthetic pylon/foot	Evaluate static prosthetic alignment
	Ligamentous instability may contribute to this abnormality	Evaluate ligament integrity using typical manual testing techniques	None	Excessive valgus angulation at the prosthetic socket pylon junction	Evaluate static prosthetic alignment
8. Deceased Prosthetic Stance Time The total duration of stance phase on the prosthetic limb is reduced	Residual limb pain	Examine residual limb to identify source of pain	Appropriate modality for pain and gait training	Poorly fitting prosthetic socket	Identify possible signs of poor prosthetic socket fit
	Musculoskeletal pain in proximal structures	Musculoskeletal evaluation to identify source of pain	None	Prosthetic foot alignment	Ensure that there are no underlying alignment abnormalities that contribute to a sense of instability
	Reduced confidence in the prosthesis		Forward/back with sound limb (prosthesis stationary)		
	Balance impairment	Evaluate balance function	Advanced balance activities		
9. Pelvic Drop The pelvis on the prosthetic side drops on initial contact as if "stepping into a hole"	Contralateral hip abductor weakness	Perform manual muscle test	Sidestepping with prosthesis with or without the theraband Traditional exercises	Prosthetic limb too short	Compare iliac crest heights in standing
				Residual limb has shrunk relative to the socket	Evaluate adequacy of residual limb volume to the socket and sock ply
				Excessively compliant heel cushion or prosthetic heel keel	Assess heel compliance during manual loading

ROM, Range of motion.

GAIT DEVIATIONS

Gait deviations can be caused by improper socket fit, misalignment of the prosthesis, or by weakness or other musculoskeletal pathologies of the individual. They can be quite common in persons with transtibial amputations; one study has shown deviations in nearly 20% of the 60 kinetic, kinematic and temporospatial parameters of gait.[90] Such deviations are known to increase metabolic cost due to excessive displacement of the center of mass.[91]

Careful evaluation is essential to determine the cause of deviations and what can be done to correct them (readers refer to Chapter 5 for a review of the biomechanics of normal gait). Variations in limb volume or shoe type can introduce deviations in a prosthetic wearer's gait that had not been exhibited before. It can be very productive to ask the person if there have been any changes in their routine recently. Changes in diet, medications, shrinker wear, or activity level can all effect limb volume. If a shoe with a higher or lower heel is placed on the prosthesis, it will change the orientation of the socket to the ground. Unless there is a component that will accommodate the new heel height, the patent's gait will be adversely affected. Common gait deviations will be reviewed as they occur in the gait cycle in each individual plane.

INITIAL CONTACT

Sagittal Plane

Initial contact should be made with the heel (Fig. 23.23). If the user makes contact at the midfoot/forefoot first, there may be either excessive plantar flexion of the prosthetic foot or limitation of the person's knee extension range of motion (i.e., knee flexion contracture). Both of these circumstances contribute to an increased knee extension moment during loading response that causes the knee to move posteriorly. This motion negatively impacts efficiency and can damage the knee joint over time. Every effort should be made to create a heel strike at initial contact. Interventions include therapeutic exercises to increase knee ROM and knee extensor strength, prosthetic alignment changes to accommodate knee flexion contractures, and proper height and suspension of the prosthesis. If the prosthesis is too long or does not suspend well, the prosthesis may hit the ground early, shortening swing phase.

Frontal Plane

Excessive inversion or eversion of the foot at initial contact indicates misalignment of the prosthesis. The heel of the prosthetic foot should be level when it meets the ground. The lateral border of the heel may contact the surface first; this is related to the transverse plane alignment of the foot to accommodate a normal toe-out angle of 5 to 10 degrees. This lateral heel contact sets up the standard progression of the ground reaction force up the lateral border of the foot and then crossing to the medial aspect of the forefoot during stance phase.

Transverse Plane

The rotation of the prosthesis is fairly consistent throughout stance phase. The medial border of the foot should be relatively parallel to the line of progression. Transverse plane rotation at initial contact is an indicator that the limb is fitting too loosely in the socket, or that the foot is not directly under the limb. External rotation of the prosthesis may be seen with an inset foot, while internal rotation could be a result of an outset foot.

Loading Response

Sagittal Plane

Excessive knee flexion moment during loading response is caused by a foot that is set too far posteriorly, is too dorsiflexed, or has a heel that is too rigid. The transition during loading response should be smooth and controlled. The knee should bend to approximately 15 degrees of flexion as the forefoot meets the ground. This advances the limb and aids in shock absorption. Insufficient knee flexion moment can be caused by a heel that is too soft or a foot that is positioned too far anteriorly. This can cause the knee to hyperextend, leading to pain and inefficiency. Adjustment of the heel lever length, stiffness, and orientation should be made to provide the appropriate degree of knee flexion. When accommodating for the heel stiffness, the soling material of the shoe should also be considered since an excessively stiff or soft heel material can exaggerate this tendency.

Frontal Plane

Rapid loading of the foot during this phase would produce significant moments at the knee if the foot were not parallel to the ground at initial contact. The plantar surface of the

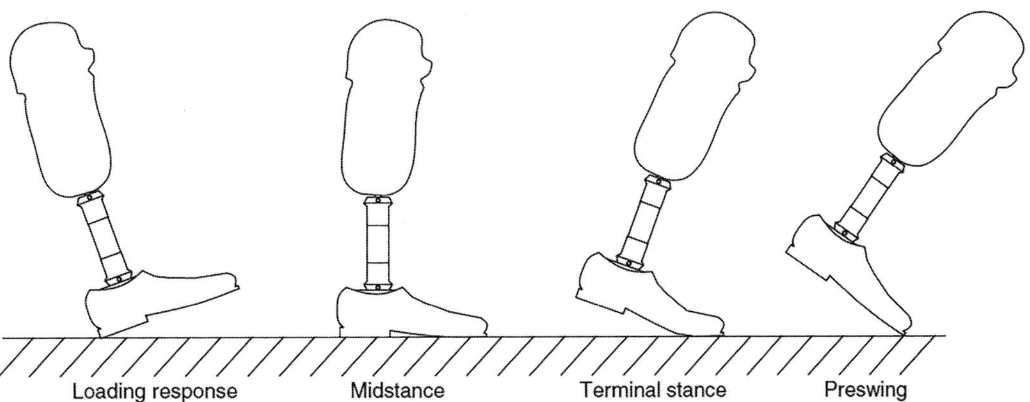

Fig. 23.23 Phases of gait cycle.

foot should be level during this phase as viewed in the frontal plane. Some modern prosthetic feet have rearfoot inversion and eversion capabilities and can adapt to the surface upon weight bearing, making them useful for uneven surfaces. Be sure to observe the motion as the loading occurs. When there is motion while ambulating on a flat surface, the alignment of the foot should be changed to eliminate that motion.

Transverse Plane

Any rotation of the foot during loading may indicate an excessively loose socket or faulty torsion adapter. Rotary moments can be generated by excessive toe-in or toe-out, and the torsion adapters can allow that motion to occur uncontrolled.

MIDSTANCE

Sagittal Plane

A choppy or segmented midstance is caused by differences in the dynamic characteristics between the prosthetic heel and the prosthetic toe, indicating a lack of stability. The heel and toe lever arms are adjustable by shifting the socket anteriorly to shorten the toe, or posteriorly to shorten the heel. The optimal foot position is one where the forward velocity of the knee is consistent between loading response and midstance. The prosthetic foot must accommodate smooth transition of the ground reaction force from the heel to the forefoot during midstance. Over this period, the moment at the knee changes from a flexion moment to an extension moment. A steady increase in dorsiflexion should be observed as the knee moves over the foot.

Frontal Plane

There is a normal and desirable varus moment during midstance. To maximize energy efficiency during gait, the body's center of mass does not shift all the way over the stance foot. The knee should move laterally approximately 1 cm during midstance. Shift of the knee greater than 2 cm indicates an excessive varus moment and will lead to stress on the medial compartment and lateral ligaments of the person's knee. This stress can be reduced by adducting the socket or shifting it medially. If the socket does not move or shifts medially during midstance, the socket is too far inset (or the foot is too outset), or the socket is excessively adducted. Lateral gapping is a condition where a large gap occurs during loading between the limb and the lateral wing of the socket. If a gap larger than 2 cm is observed, the socket may be too loose and an additional ply of sock should be added.

Transverse Plane

Rotation that occurs during midstance is typically seen between the limb and socket and is almost always attributable to poor socket fit. If motion occurs, the person may complain of patellar impingement on either the medial or lateral aspects of the patella. Often, the remedy is to tighten the socket by adding a ply or two of socks. In cases in which socks are insufficient to stabilize the rotation, the socket should be adjusted by the prosthetist. Pretibial pads that provide pressure on either side of the tibial crest a pad over the posterior calf are effective solutions to limit rotation.

TERMINAL STANCE

Sagittal Plane

Drop off is the excessive descent of the center of mass during terminal stance caused by a toe lever that is either too short or too soft. It is often characterized by diminished heel rise. This compromises energy efficiency of walking. It occurs at a point when the body's center of mass is already near the bottom of its sinusoidal path. The toe lever of the prosthetic foot must have sufficient stiffness to resist dorsiflexion when the person's entire weight is placed on the ball of the foot. In terms of energy efficiency, this is a critical phase of gait. Proper loading of the forefoot promotes knee stability, maintains altitude (i.e., level pelvis), and stores energy in the ligaments that can be released during swing phase to assist with limb advancement.

Early heel off is an indication the foot is too plantarflexed or the toe lever is too stiff. The heel should come off the ground at the point when the swing foot has already passed anterior to the stance limb. Forward momentum of the body is impeded by early toe-off and may force the individual into an anterior lean with the trunk to maintain forward progression. The ankle should be set to dorsiflex until the swing limb reaches terminal swing, so that the heel remains on the ground until the center of mass has progressed sufficiently forward. This will preserve step length and enhance stability.

Frontal Plane

The heel should rise off the ground with the knee breaking over the point on the foot between the first and second toes. Any large variance from this position will create instability and consequently shorten step length. The knee should travel in a straight line as it flexes; any lateral motion during this phase will lead to a whip in swing.

Transverse Plane

The toe load is highest during this phase of gait; therefore there is potential for rotation of the prosthesis due to suboptimal alignment or socket fit. External rotation can be caused by a foot that is too far outset or having excessive toe-out. Internal rotation is caused by an excessively inset or internally rotated foot.

PRESWING

Sagittal Plane

As the body weight transfers rapidly to the contralateral limb, the prosthesis should roll forward over the toe and lift off the ground. Toe-drag may result from a foot that is excessively plantarflexed or from a faulty suspension system.

Frontal Plane

The knee should not move medially or laterally during preswing. An externally rotated foot can cause a valgus moment that pushes the knee medially as weight is transferred off the prosthesis. A valgus moment can also be caused by an outset foot or an excessively adducted socket. Lateral motion during preswing can be caused by an internally rotated foot, an excessively inset foot, or an excessively abducted socket.

Transverse Plane

Many of the same factors that lead to instability in the frontal plane can lead to instability in the transverse plane. Appropriate attention to transverse plane alignment throughout stance phase should help to avoid issues in pre-swing as well.

SWING PHASE

Sagittal Plane

The transtibial prosthesis swings passively forward during swing phase. If sufficient ground clearance is not obtained, the amount of knee flexion should be noted. In cases where appropriate knee flexion is observed, the suspension of the prosthesis should be evaluated. A faulty suspension or a plantarflexed foot will reduce swing clearance. The amount of pistoning varies with the type of suspension used. Motion exceeding 1 cm should be considered excessive. If insufficient knee flexion is observed during swing phase, active and passive motion should be assessed. Weakness or contracture of the knee can limit knee motion, as can a tight suspension sleeve or an aggressive supracondylar wedge. Although suspension and knee flexion are often adversarial, a balance should be attainable that permits enough foot clearance for safe ambulation; otherwise, the prosthesis may require shortening.

Frontal Plane

Socket instability during swing is typically caused by either a faulty suspension or a loose-fitting socket. The weight of the socket pulls the prosthesis into varus during swing if the limb is not well seated in the socket. Increasing sock ply and implementing an improved suspension should remedy any swing phase instability.

Transverse Plane

Rotation during swing phase is often caused by a prosthetic "whip." A medial whip is when the heel of the prosthetic foot moves medially in initial swing and then laterally during midswing. A lateral whip follows the opposite pattern. Whips can be caused by misalignment of the knee axis at the onset of swing or by irregular loading of the limb in terminal stance. Alignment of the knee axis in a person using a transtibial prosthesis is determined by the function of the hip, and should be addressed by strengthening and ROM exercises. Prosthetic remedies must examine the loading of the prosthesis. Medial whips can be caused by a foot that is too far inset or externally rotated. Both medial and lateral whips can be caused by a foot that is too plantarflexed or a toe lever that is too stiff.

Outcome Measures for Individuals With Transtibial Amputation

GAIT SPEED, STRENGTH, AND DYNAMIC BALANCE

For individuals with transtibial amputation, the mean distance walked on the Two-Minute Walk Test is 152.9 ± 43.0 m (range = 49–259) at an average gait speed of 76.7 ± 21.6 m/min (range = 25–130 m/min).[77] This gait speed equates to 1.28 ± 0.36 m/s (range = 0.42–2.17 m/s). It should be noted that the participants of this study had an average age of 50.9 ± 14.3 years, 46% of the participants had a history of transtibial amputation, and 40% of the participants had amputations due to nontrauma-related conditions.[77] Another study by Batten and colleagues[78] also evaluated gait speed for individuals with lower-limb amputation; however, their study included a sample with an average age of 63 years old with 71% of participants with transtibial amputation and 70% due to vascular causes. Batten and colleagues[78] reported a median gait speed for individuals with transtibial amputation on the 10-Minute Walk Test of 0.63 m/s (range = 0.46–0.83 m/s).[78] Not only gait speed, but the ability or potential to ambulate at variable cadences is required to provide medical justification for advanced prosthetic componentry for individuals at higher levels of mobility performance (e.g., MFCL K-Level 3 or higher). A recent study demonstrated that self-selected walking speed on the 10 Walk Test, L-Test, and Figure-8 Walk Test were good indicators of the potential to ambulate at variable cadences to enable clinicians to differentiate between individuals classified at the MFCL K2 versus K3 level.[92]

STRENGTH AND DYNAMIC BALANCE

One of the primary performance-based outcome measures for lower-extremity strength and power recommended for individuals with limb loss is the 5× Sit to Stand Test.[93,94] The 5× Sit to Stand Test has demonstrated the ability to distinguish between individuals functioning at different MFCL K-levels, especially K3 versus K4.[92,94] Recently however, it has been proposed that modifying the 5× Sit to Stand Test by allowing lower-limb prosthetic users to use the upper extremities to assist with the sit to stand may allow clinicians to distinguish between individuals at a broader range of MFCL K-levels.[94] Table 23.5 provides reference values for 5× Sit to Stand Test performance for each MFCL K-level.

Fig. 23.24 provides an example of the layout for several of these performance-based outcome measures.[96]

When selecting outcome measures to utilize in the clinic to monitor a patient's progress and response to rehabilitation interventions, clinicians must analyze outcome measure performance in the context of the responsiveness of the selected measure to detect change in performance over time. Minimum detectable change scores provide clinicians with insight into how much improvement a patient would need to demonstrate to increase their confidence that true change has occurred, beyond the level of error inherent in the measurement. Table 23.6 provides minimum detectable change scores for common outcome measures utilized in rehabilitation for individuals with limb loss.[97]

Fall Risk Assessment

There is limited agreement in the literature regarding the most significant factors that may increase risk of falling in individuals with lower-limb amputation.[99–103] A recent

Table 23.5 Strength, Dynamic Balance, Mobility, and Gait Speed Performance and Medicare Functional Classification K-Levels (MFCL)

Test	MFCL K1	MFCL K2	MFCL K3	MFCL K4
5× Sit to Stand[93]			8.85 s (8.07–9.63 s)	8.06 s (7.17–8.94 s)
Modified 5× Sit to Stand[94]	22.1 s	17.0 s (8.6–48.7 s)	13.5 s (7.5–29.9 s)	10.7 s (6.0–20.8 s)
Figure-8 Walk Test[93]			6.39 s (5.94–6.83 s)	5.80 s (5.29–6.30 s)
360° Turn Time—Prosthetic Side[93]			2.35 s (2.13–2.57 s)	2.14 (1.90–2.39 s)
360° Turn Time—Sound Side[93]			2.31 s (2.08–2.54 s)	2.02 s (1.76–2.28 s)
Modified Four-Square Step Test[93]			8.82 s (8.30–9.34 s)	7.80 (7.21–8.38 s)
TUG[95]			12.82±0.54 s (11.74–13.89 s)	9.45±0.76 s (7.92–10.98)
10 Walk Test—Self-Selected[95]			0.88±0.04 m/s (0.80–0.96 m/s)	1.21±0.05 m/s (1.11–1.32 m/s)
10 Walk Test—Fast[95]			1.12±0.05 m/s (1.02–1.22 m/s)	1.56±0.07 m/s (1.41–1.70 m/s)
AMPPRO[95]			40.4±0.4 (39.6–41.2)	44.9±0.6 (43.7–46.0)
6-Minute Walk Test[95]			311.30±18.98 m (273.05–349.55 m)	427.42±26.94 m (373.13–481.70 m)

AMPRO, Amputee mobility predictor; *TUG*, Timed Up and Go Test.

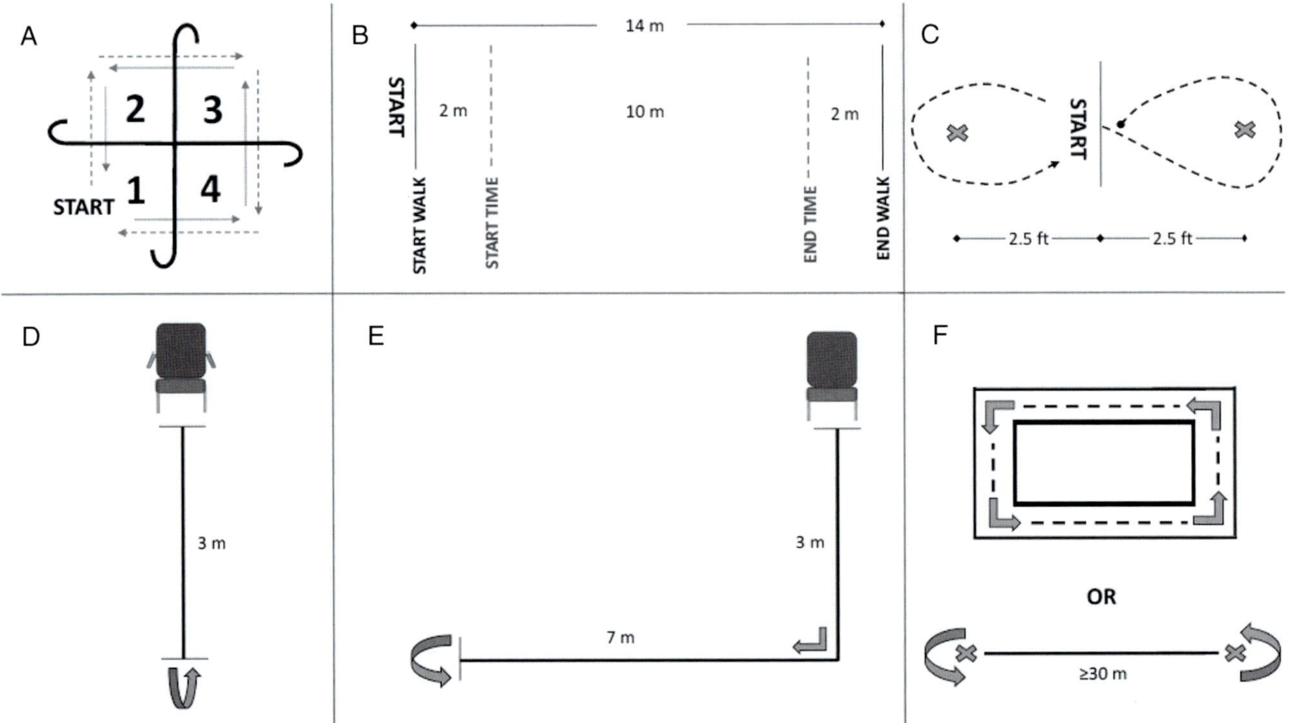

Fig. 23.24 Course layout for common performance-based outcome measures.[96] (A) Four-square Step Test; (B) 10 Walk Test; (C) Figure-8 Walk test; (D) Timed Up and Go Test; (E) L-Test of functional mobility; (F) 2-Minute Walk Test or 6-Minute Walk Test.

scoping review found that the literature has not identified the optimal clinical outcome measure or gait parameter to identify individuals with limb loss who are at increased risk for falls.[104] Recent studies designed to better understand falls in individuals with lower-limb amputation have utilized a Fall Type Classification system to better understand the cause of falls for lower-extremity prosthetic users by examining the location of the destabilizing force, the source of destabilization, and the ensuing fall pattern.[99,100,105,106] Fig. 23.25 provides a description of this classification system.[105] Evidence suggests that many, if not most, falls for prosthetic users occur while walking on level surfaces and that clinicians may consider focusing interventions to mitigate falls

Table 23.6 Minimum Detectable Change for Common Outcome Measures

Test Instrument	Minimum Detectable Change
2-Minute Walk Test[83]	MDC(90) = 34.3 m
6-Minute Walk Test[83]	MDC(90) = 45 m
Activity-Specific Balance Confidence Scale[98]	MDC(90) = 49% MDC(95) = 58%
AMPPRO[83]	MDC(90) = 3.4
L-Test of Functional Mobility[81]	MDC(95) = 6.2 s; MCID = 4.5 s
Timed Up and Go Test	MDC(90)[84] = 1.28 s;MDC(90)[83] = 3.6 s

AMPPRO, Amputee mobility predictor; *MCID*, minimal clinically important difference; *MCD*, minimum detectable change.

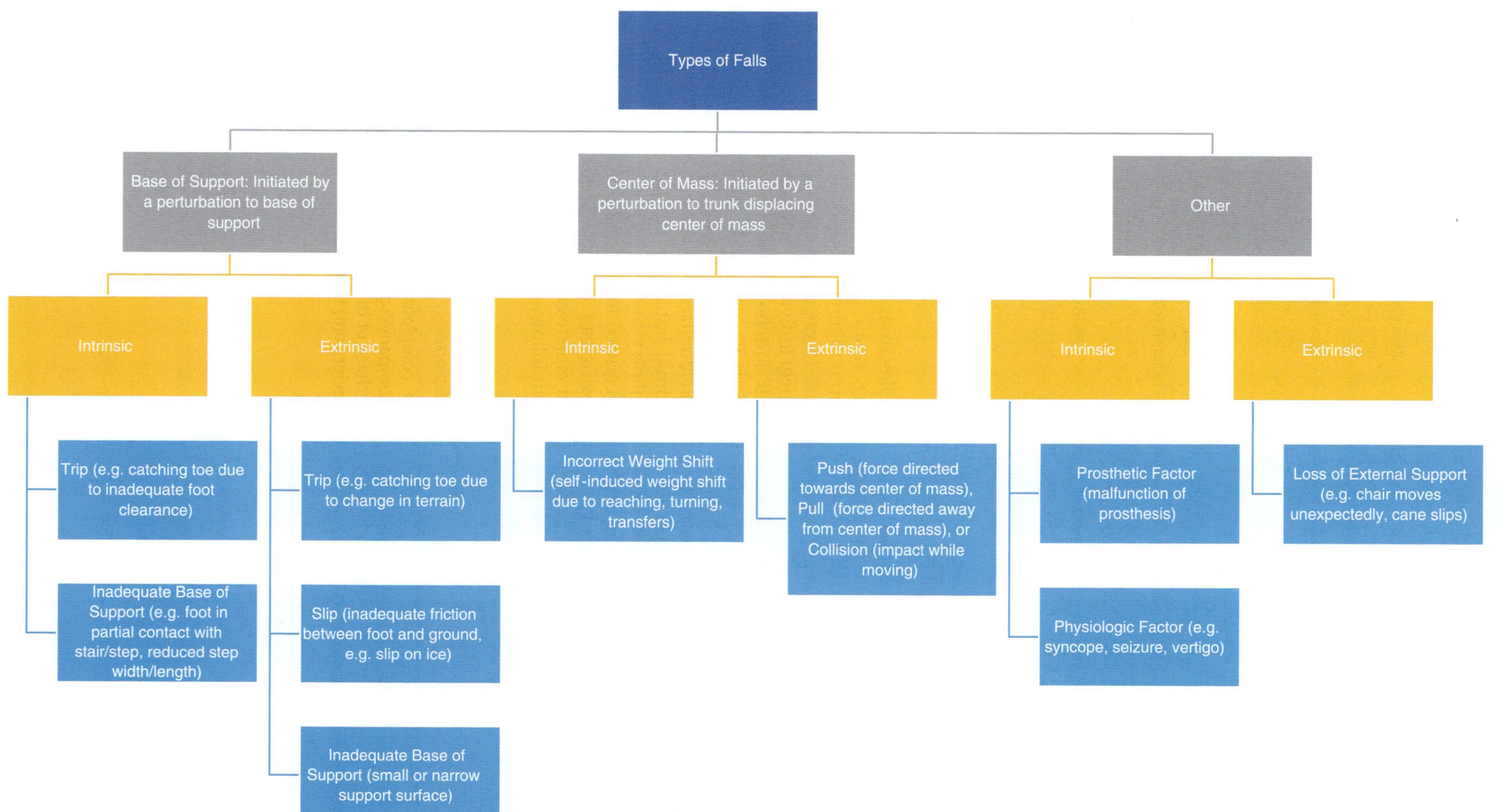

Fig. 23.25 Fall type classification system. (Modified from Kim J, Major MJ, Hafner B, Sawers A. Frequency and circumstances of falls reported by ambulatory unilateral lower-limb prosthesis users: a secondary analysis. *PM&R.* 2019;11(4):344–353.)

Table 23.7 Psychometric Properties of Performance-Based Clinical Balance Tests for Fall Risk Assessment[85]

Test	Cut-Off Score	Sensitivity (95% CI)	Specificity (95% CI)	LR+ (95% CI)	LR− (95% CI)
≥1 FALL (ANY FALLS)					
NBWT	≤0.43	73% (53%–90%)	76% (54%–96%)	3.0 (1.5–6.9)	0.36 (0.19–0.77)
TUG	≥8.17 s	83% (68%–98%)	68% (46%–92%)	2.6 (1.3–5.6)	0.24 (0.13–0.56)
FSST	≥8.49 s	74% (58%–92%)	68% (46%–92%)	2.4 (1.1–5.2)	0.36 (0.17–0.78)
BBS	≤50.5	67% (48%–86%)	62% (39%–86%)	1.8 (0.89–3.6)	0.53 (0.27–1.1)
ABC	≤80.2%	50% (30%–70%)	74% (54%–96%)	1.9 (0.78–5.1)	0.67 (0.41–1.1)
Model 1 (NBWT; FSST; PLUS-M; Amputation Level)	n/a	80% (64%–96%)	73% (51%–96%)	3.0 (1.3–7.1)	0.27 (0.12–0.63)
≥2 FALLS (MULTIPLE FALLS)					
NBWT	≤0.43	88% (73%–100%)	79% (65%–92%)	4.2 (1.7–6.9)	0.16 (0.042–0.60)
TUG	≥9.25 s	82% (64-100%)	83% (67%–98%)	4.7 (1.9–11.9)	0.21 (0.075-0.61)
FSST	≥8.71 s	94% (83%–100%)	74% (60%–92%)	3.6 (1.8–7.3)	0.08 (0.012–0.54)
BBS	≤50.5	88% (73%–100%)	70% (51%–88%)	2.9 (1.5–5.5)	0.17 (0.045–0.64)
ABC	≤80.2%	65% (42%–87%)	78% (61%–95%)	3.0 (1.3–7.0)	0.45 (0.23–0.89)
Model 2 (NBWT; TUG; PLUS-M; K-Level, Amputation etiology)	n/a	76% (56%–97%)	83% (67%–98%)	4.4 (1.7–11.3)	0.28 (0.12–0.68)

ABC, Activity-Specific Balance Confidence Scale; *BBS*, Berg Balance Scale; *CI*, confidence interval; *FSST*, Four-Square Step Test; *n/a*, not available; *NBWT*, Narrow Beam Walking Test; *TUG*, Timed Up and Go Test.

due to perturbations of an individual's base of support while walking.[105,107] Balance activities that promote improved single-limb stance control, dynamic changes to base of support, and reaction time for anticipatory and reactive postural control may help decrease risk for falls.

A recent study of various performance-based outcome measures for fall prediction concluded that balance tests alone were not able to predict future falls for lower-limb prosthetic users. However, a predictive model for falls based on fall history in the previous 12 months in combination with performance-based outcome measures (TUG and FSST) was able to predict incidence of falls for prosthetic users with unilateral transtibial amputation. Table 23.7 presents the psychometric properties and cut-off scores of the performance-based outcome measures recommended for fall risk assessment in individuals with lower-limb amputation.

Summary

Current prosthetic technology along with recent advances have expanded options for individuals with transtibial amputation to return to levels of activity and participation similar to age-matched peers without limb loss. Currently only small percentages of individuals with lower-limb amputation are referred to or receive physical therapy services. Physical therapists should be the providers of choice to help individuals with lower-limb amputation to optimize their functional recovery and quality of life. Successful prosthetic rehabilitation requires physical therapists to incorporate their patient's values and goals to develop an individualized, evidence-informed plan of care to achieve optimal outcomes. An understanding of prosthetic componentry and how to assess appropriate fit and function is required for therapists to coordinate care with certified prosthetists to enable patients to realize their full potential and empower them with skills necessary for self-management following limb loss.

References

The complete listing of the References are available in the accompanying enhanced eBook version included with the print purchase of this textbook. Visit Elsevier eBooks+ (eBooks.Health.Elsevier.com) to access this content.

24 Transfemoral Prostheses

DANIEL G. MINER AND KEVIN K. CHUI

LEARNING OBJECTIVES

On completion of this chapter, the reader will be able to do the following:

1. Describe how surgical decisions impact use of transfemoral prosthetics.
2. Identify goals of all phases of rehabilitation following transfemoral amputation.
3. Identify outcome measures that help to distinguish individuals who meet criteria for various Medicare Functional Classification Levels to justify selection of componentry for transfemoral prostheses.
4. Compare the design, fit, and function of transfemoral socket designs and suspension systems.
5. Describe the functional characteristics, advantages, and limitations of the components of transfemoral prostheses.
6. Indicate how the alignment of the transfemoral prosthesis influences comfort, stability, and ease of walking with transfemoral prostheses.
7. Describe common gait abnormalities for prosthetic users with transfemoral amputation and identify common patient-related and prosthetic causes of gait dysfunction.
8. Identify strategies for further evaluation and intervention to address common gait abnormalities for prosthetic users with transfemoral amputation.
9. Describe strategies for selection of appropriate outcome measures to evaluate progress with rehabilitation for prosthetic users with transfemoral amputation.

Surgical Considerations

Surgical procedures for individuals with transfemoral amputation are discussed in Chapter 19. Surgical decisions that impact prognosis for successful use of a transfemoral prosthesis include residual limb length, myodesis versus myoplasty, wound closure, need for skin grafting, and amount and distribution of soft tissue of residual limb. Residual limb length directly impacts how much hip extension torque an individual is able to generate, which has implications for the ability to control a prosthetic knee unit for stability during the stance phase of gait. Longer residual femur length is associated with more efficient gait and is less susceptible to the development of hip flexion and hip abduction contractures that negatively impact gait performance with a transfemoral prosthesis.[1] According to expert opinion from prosthetists, it is easier to achieve optimal fit and alignment of a prosthesis for an individual with a longer residual limb.[1] If the residual limb is too long, however, or for individuals with knee disarticulation, the knee center of the prosthetic side will not be aligned with the sound side, which may impact cosmesis and may limit options for various prosthetic knee units.[1] Myodesis involves securing the fascia of amputated muscles directly to bone tunnels in the distal end of the femur which helps to stabilize the femur for more efficient use of a prosthesis.[2] In myoplasty the posterior muscles are sutured to the anterior muscles to provide coverage for the distal end of the femur, but the femur is not stabilized.[2] There is no evidence that the stability of the femur contributes to more stable residual limb volume.

Rehabilitation Management of Individuals With Transfemoral Amputation

The goal for many individuals following transfemoral amputation is to be able to walk again with a transfemoral prosthesis. Successful future use of a transfemoral prosthesis depends on many factors including the etiology of amputation (discussed in Chapter 17) and education and compliance with guidelines for rehabilitation beginning in the preoperative phase and continuing through the prosthetic training phase into long-term follow-up. In 2009 the Extremity Trauma and Amputation Center of Excellence (EACE) was legislated by Congress to enhance partnerships between the Department of Defense (DoD) and the Department of Veterans Affairs (VA) to optimize outcomes of service members, veterans, and beneficiaries with extremity trauma or amputation. The EACE developed rehabilitation guidelines to provide rehabilitation of individuals with unilateral transfemoral amputation and knee disarticulation and identify goals for each phase of rehabilitation and important milestones and goals for individuals with limb loss who have goals of using a prosthesis (Table 24.1).[3]

Table 24.1 Summary of Transfemoral Amputation Rehabilitation Guidelines

Rehabilitation Phase	Guidelines	Goals	Milestones
Preoperative	■ Strengthening exercises to improve muscle tone and function ■ Strive for full/functional residual limb active/passive range of motion values ■ Improve cardiovascular fitness ■ Optimize medical management of any existing concurrent medical conditions ■ Optimize unilateral balance/proprioceptive training ■ Promote wellness, proper nutrition, tobacco cessation, and an optimal body weight ■ Educate patient on postoperative rehabilitation requirements to ensure an optimal functional outcome ■ Validate behavioral health and family support program is in place ■ Facilitate identification of any necessary assistive devices and/or durable medical equipment for procurement, use, and training if clinically indicated prior to surgery ■ Implement vitamin D and calcium supplementation, as per surgeon's recommendation	■ Achieve maximal hip ROM with emphasis on hip extension ■ Begin core/LE strength training with emphasis on hip extension and abduction strength	N/A
Protective Healing	■ Non–weight-bearing status of residual limb x 4–6 weeks postoperative ■ It is important to maintain hip extension, complete prone lying multiple times a day ■ Avoid shear stress and protect incision site ■ Per physician's recommendation, patient can be fit with a shrinker or use Figure-8 wrapping for swelling management and shaping of the residual limb (timeline and wear schedule may vary per physician) ■ Range of motion (ROM) as tolerated (focus on maintaining presurgical hip extension ROM) ■ Bed mobility ■ Transfer and appropriate assistive device training ■ Gait training (non–weight bearing on operative side) ■ Wheelchair mobility training ■ Aerobic conditioning (e.g., arm ergometer/rower) ■ Core and limb strengthening (e.g., mat therapeutic exercise to include closed kinetic chair bolster) ■ Neuromuscular reeducation (e.g., seated and standing balance activities) ■ Begin desensitization and mirror therapy for phantom limb and neuropathic pain ■ Monitor symptom responses for 24–48 h after each exercise session. Pain should settle quickly postexercise with no significant increase in symptoms the next day	■ Pain control, functional mobility ■ Protection of residual limb ■ Achieve hip extension to ~10 degrees ■ Normalize pelvic coordination	N/A
Preprosthetic Training	■ Wound monitoring and assist with dressing changes as needed ■ Maintain/improve hip ROM ■ Continue appropriate previous exercises with increased resistance and/or difficulty ■ Core strengthening exercises ■ Gait training on even and uneven surfaces with appropriate assisted device maintaining non–weight-bearing status on amputee limb ■ Suture removal depending on wound healing and surgeon preference (typically 2 weeks postop) ■ Liner fitting once cleared by physician, establish wear schedule (i.e., liner during the day and shrinker at night) ■ Once incision site is fully healed begin scar mobilization ■ Fall recovery training	■ Wound healing ■ Residual limb management ■ Desensitization and pain management	■ Tolerate liner wear 8 h a day without skin issues ■ Hip extension ~10 degrees ■ Ambulate at a modified independence level with appropriate assisted device

Table 24.1 Summary of Transfemoral Amputation Rehabilitation Guidelines—cont'd

Rehabilitation Phase	Guidelines	Goals	Milestones
Prosthetic Training	■ Socket fit typically occurs around 4–6 weeks postop to allow for adequate tissue healing ■ Educate on prosthetic wearing schedule, skin inspection, management of limb volume changes, use of different ply socks, prosthetic fit, and hygiene instructions ■ Gradually increase prosthesis wear time starting at 15 min interval and increasing as tolerated with frequent skin checks ■ Balance activities (e.g., step up, playing catch, rebounder with a weight ball, compliant surfaces, balance beam, etc.) ■ Activities that master control of prosthetic knee flexion and extension to optimize confidence in stability ■ Gait activities (e.g., weight shifts, step ups, hurdles, level surfaces, ramps, curbs, stairs, grass, car transfers, etc.) focusing on equalizing step length, stance time, upright posture, equal reciprocal arm swing ■ Fall recovery training	■ Pain control ■ Independence with residual limb management (hygiene, skin care) ■ Independence with prosthetic management (socket fit and use of sock ply for volume changes) ■ Independence with mobility with prosthesis and least restrictive assistive device	■ Wear prosthesis around 8 hours a day without any skin issues ■ Full hip ROM ■ 5/5 MMT strength for hip ■ Score of ~30 s on single leg bridge test (with 8-inch towel roll) ■ Demonstrate fall recovery procedures training and floor to stand transfers ■ Ambulate with modified independence with minimal gait deviations on level and unlevel surfaces over 1000 ft ■ Ascend and descend four steps with least restrictive device and modified independence ■ AMPPRO scores (normative values, see CPG): K0/K1 25 ± 7; K2 35 ± 7; K3 41 ± 4; K4 45 ± 2 ■ 2 MWT or 6 MWT consistent with age-rated normative values

2 MWT, 2-Minute Walk Test; *6 MWT*, 6-Minute Walk Test; *AMPPRO*, Amputee Mobility Predictor; *CPG*, clinical practice guideline; *MMT*, muscle strength test.
Adapted from Extremity Trauma and Amputation Center of Excellence. *Unilateral Transfemoral Amputation and Knee Disarticulation Rehabilitation Guidelines*; 2022.

Medicare Functional Classification Level and Considerations for Selection of Components for Transfemoral Prosthesis

As described in Chapter 20, it is critical to assess an individual's ability to perform simple mobility tasks following transfemoral amputation. The Amputee Mobility Predictor (AMP) is a useful tool to systematically evaluate performance of static and dynamic sitting and standing balance, anticipatory and reactive postural control in standing, ability to perform basic transfers, and ability to ambulate short distances and variable speeds and turn around safely.[4] The AMP can be performed prior to an individual being fit with a prosthesis (AMPnoPRO), or with a prosthesis (AMPPRO).[4] The use of objective, performance-based outcome measures is a useful strategy to identify individuals who have the ability or potential to perform at various Medicare Functional Classification Levels (see Chapter 21), or K-levels (K0–K4), with use of a transfemoral prosthesis (Fig. 24.1).[5]

Table 24.2 provides a summary of various performance-based outcome measures that may be useful to distinguish between individuals who have the ability or potential to function at various K-levels.

Eligibility for and selection of prosthetic componentry is largely determined through documentation of an individual's Medicare Functional Classification Level or K-level but is also based on historical factors including age at limb loss, level of amputation, etiology of amputation, comorbidities related to safe use of prosthesis, cognitive ability, prior level of function, current level of function, patient goals, social situation including caregiver support and home environment (e.g., steps to enter); and physical examination findings including cardiopulmonary status, skin integrity/wounds, residual limb length/shape and readiness for prosthesis, range of motion and strength, upper extremity function, sitting and standing balance, and transfer and ambulation ability.[5]

Prosthetic Socket and Suspension Systems

The fit and comfort of a prosthetic socket is critical for individuals with transfemoral amputation to be successful prosthetic users and be able to perform mobility-related activities of daily living and return to work.[9] Optimal fitting of a prosthetic socket and selection of an appropriate suspension system requires a skilled prosthetist and an individualized approach to facilitate weight bearing and utilize force couples and appropriate suspension to minimize movement between the residual limb and prosthetic socket.[10] Appropriate fitting of prosthetic socket and suspension system selection will depend on several individual factors including residual limb length and shape, skin integrity, scar tissue location and mobility, body mass index, soft tissue (redundancy and coverage of bony prominences), stability versus fluctuation of residual limb volume, muscle strength, activity level, hand function, and cognitive status.[9] One reliable tool that may be helpful for clinicians to evaluate an individual's satisfaction with their prosthetic socket and suspension is the Comprehensive Lower-Limb Amputation Socket Survey (CLASS) (Fig. 24.2).[9]

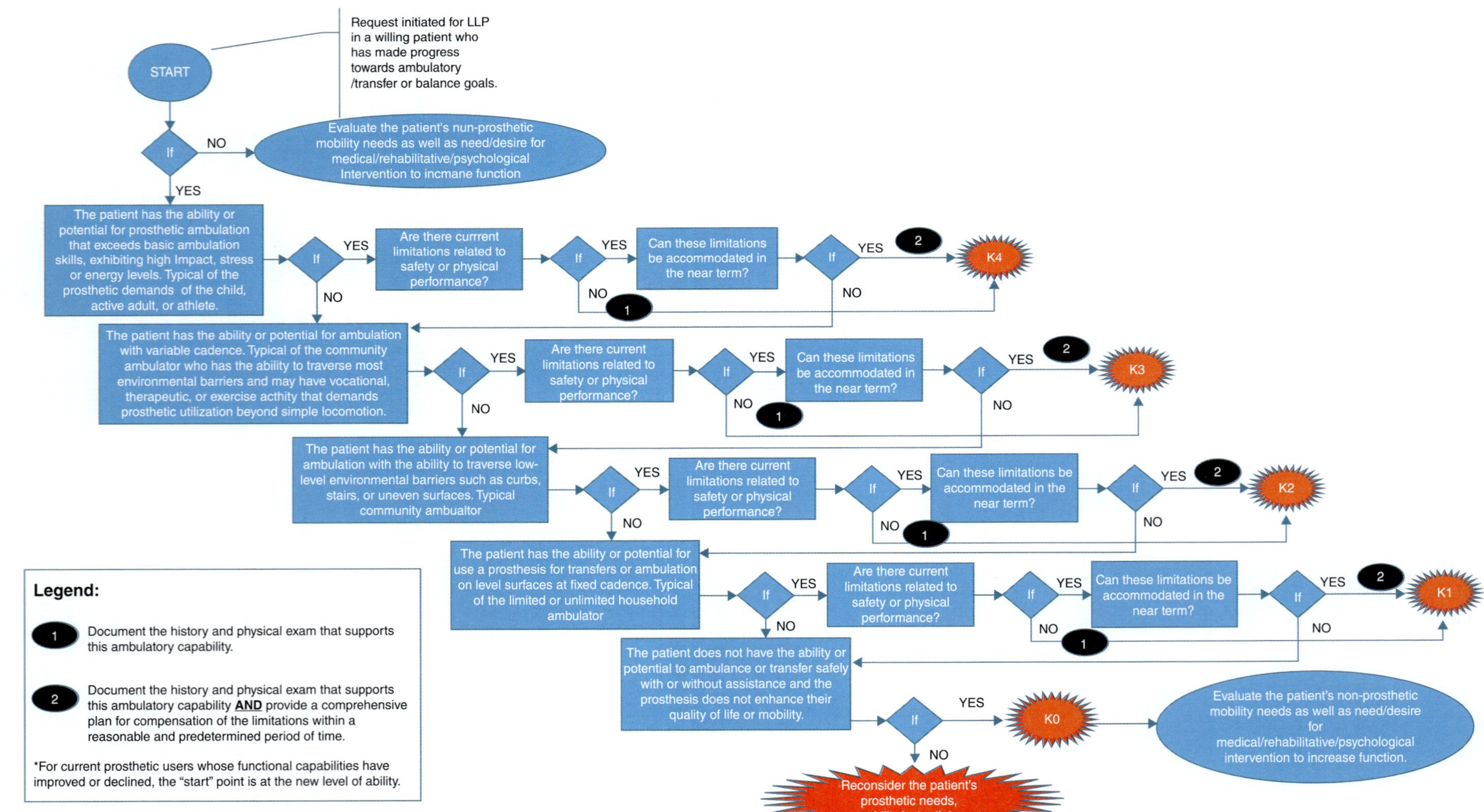

Fig. 24.1 **Algorithm for determination of K modifiers for initial lower-limb prosthetic.** From Centers for Medicare & Medicaid Services Health Technology Assessment. *Lower Limb Prosthetic Workgroup Consensus Document*; 2017. Available at: **https://www.cms.gov/Medicare/Coverage/DeterminationProcess/downloads/LLP_Consensus_Document.pdf.**

Table 24.2 Performance-Based Outcome Measures and K-Levels

K-Level	AMPnoPRO[4]	AMPPRO[4,6]	2-Minute Walk Test[7] (m)[a]	6-Minute Walk Test[4,6] (m)	10 m Walk Test[8] (m/s)[b]	Self-Selected Walking Speed[6] (10 mWT in m/s)	Fast Walking Speed[6] (10 mWT in m/s)	Timed Up and Go Test[6] (s)
K1	9.67 ± 9.51	25.0 ± 7.37[4]	n/a	49.86 ± 29.82[5]	0.17 (0.15–0.19)	n/a	n/a	n/a
K2	25.28 ± 7.32	34.65 ± 6.49[4]	81.7 ± 26.9	189.9 ± 111.3[5]	0.38 (0.25–0.54)	n/a	n/a	n/a
K3	31.36 ± 7.38	40.5 ± 3.9[5] 40.4 ± 0.4[6]	138.4 ± 28.5	298.64 ± 102.37[5] 311.3 ± 18.98[6]	0.63 (0.50–0.71)	0.88 ± 0.04	1.12 ± 0.05	12.82 ± 0.54
K4	38.49 ± 3.03	44.67 ± 1.75[5] 44.9 ± 0.6[6]	177.9 ± 31.1	419.46 ± 86.15[5] 427.42 ± 26.94[6]	1.06 (0.95–1.18)	1.21 ± 0.05	1.56 ± 0.07	9.45 ± 0.76

[a]Mean 2-Minute Walk Test distance for individuals with transfemoral amputation is 135.6 ± 30.1 m.[7]
[b]Median gait speed for individuals with transfemoral amputation is 0.35 m/s (0.23–0.51).[8]
n/a, Not available.

Comprehensive lower-limb amputee socket survey (CLASS)

Instructions. We would like to know how well your current socket fits. For each of the following 15 items, please read the question and select the single "best" response that describes your prosthetic socket within the past day or when you last performed the activity. Select "Not applicable" only if the activity does not pertain to you.

Please select one response for all items.

Stability **I feel stable and balanced in my socket when I:**	**Strongly disagree**	**Disagree**	**Agree**	**Strongly agree**	**Not applicable**
Sit	(1)	(2)	(3)	(4)	(0)
Stand	(1)	(2)	(3)	(4)	(0)
Walk	(1)	(2)	(3)	(4)	(0)
Ascend or descend stairs	(1)	(2)	(3)	(4)	(0)
Suspension **I feel secure in my socket with no excessive movement when I:**	**Strongly disagree**	**Disagree**	**Agree**	**Strongly agree**	**Not applicable**
Sit	(1)	(2)	(3)	(4)	(0)
Stand	(1)	(2)	(3)	(4)	(0)
Walk	(1)	(2)	(3)	(4)	(0)
Ascend or descend stairs	(1)	(2)	(3)	(4)	(0)
Comfort **My socket is comfortable when I:**	**Strongly disagree**	**Disagree**	**Agree**	**Strongly agree**	**Not applicable**
Sit	(1)	(2)	(3)	(4)	(0)
Stand	(1)	(2)	(3)	(4)	(0)
Walk	(1)	(2)	(3)	(4)	(0)
Ascend or descend stairs	(1)	(2)	(3)	(4)	(0)
Appearance **I like the appearance of my socket when I:**	**Strongly disagree**	**Disagree**	**Agree**	**Strongly agree**	**Not applicable**
Sit	(1)	(2)	(3)	(4)	(0)
Stand	(1)	(2)	(3)	(4)	(0)
Wear tight pants	(1)	(2)	(3)	(4)	(0)

Stability _/16=_% Suspension _/16=_% Comfort _/16=_% Appearance _/12=_%
For a percentage valve of "socket fit," add the total points for each item and divide the total score by 16 or 12 as shown. Subtract 4 points from the denominator value for each item that was marked "Not applicable."

Fig. 24.2 Comprehensive Lower-Limb Amputation Socket Survey (CLASS).

SOCKET SHAPES/DESIGNS

In theory, minimizing or limiting motion between the bony anatomy of the residual limb and the prosthetic socket should improve patient comfort and optimize function.[10]

Different socket designs have been described, including a quadrilateral socket design, which was more prevalent in the 1950s, and the ischial containment socket, which has been the standard of care for the last 30 years.[11–14] However,

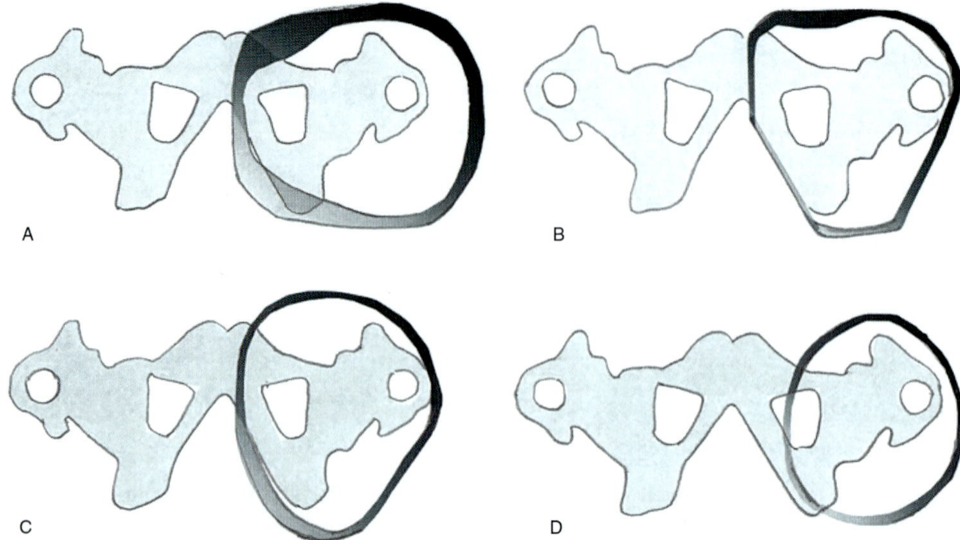

Fig. 24.3 Cross-section views of transfemoral sockets. The quadrilateral socket has a narrow anteroposterior dimension (A); ischial containment socket (B) and Marlo-Anatomical Socket (C) have narrow mediolateral dimensions. The subischial socket (D) has a more oval shape.

these socket designs have been criticized for restricting the motion of the hip through their contact with the pelvis.[12] Advances in technology for prosthetic suspension systems have allowed newer prosthetic socket designs including the Marlo-Anatomical Socket and subischial sockets to prioritize lowering the trimlines to allow increased hip range of motion without sacrificing control/stability or suspension.[12]

QUADRILATERAL SOCKET

Quadrilateral sockets were more common in the 1950s and have been criticized for limiting hip range of motion.[12] This shape has four walls fashioned to contain the thigh (Figs. 24.3 and 24.4A). A flat posterior shelf is the primary weight-bearing surface for the ischial tuberosity and adjacent gluteal muscles. The anterior wall creates a posteriorly directed force to stabilize the ischial tuberosity on its seat. The anterior wall has a convexity (buildup), the Scarpa bulge, which increases the area contacting the tender femoral triangle. The medial wall has a concavity (relief) for the adductor longus tendon and is approximately level with the posterior brim. The lateral wall is approximately as high as the anterior wall; it has a relief for the greater trochanter. The anterior-posterior dimension is narrower than the medial-lateral dimension. Customized muscle channel contours are critical to maintain rotation stability with a quadrilateral socket design.[12,15] This design is not appropriate for individuals with excessive soft tissue, significant fluctuations in residual limb volume, or individuals with a short residual limb length.[15]

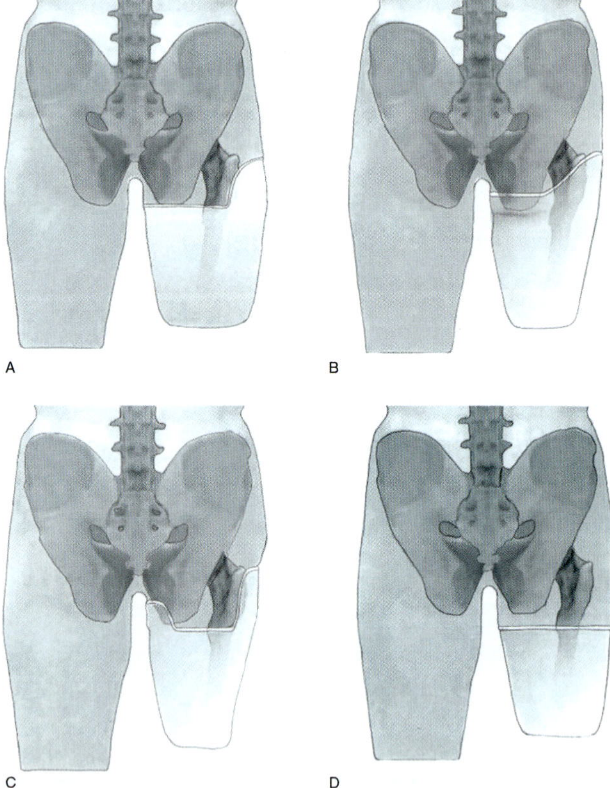

Fig. 24.4 Posterior views of quadrilateral socket (A) with the ischial tuberosity on the posterior brim; ischial containment socket (B) with ischial tuberosity inside the socket; Marlo-Anatomical Socket (C) with the ischial tuberosity within the socket; and subischial socket (D) with the socket trim line considerably below the ischium.

ISCHIAL CONTAINMENT SOCKET

Ischial containment sockets have been the standard of care for transfemoral socket design since the 1980s.[12,15–17] The ischial containment socket (see Figs. 24.3B and 24.4B) covers the ischial tuberosity. The socket is thus wider anteroposteriorly than mediolaterally to resist lateral shifting of the socket during weight bearing and to maintain the femur in as much adduction as possible. The relatively wide anteroposterior dimension is intended to provide more room to accommodate muscle contraction. The ischial containment socket has relatively high medial and posterior walls and a lower anterior wall than the quadrilateral socket. The lateral wall is approximately the same height on both the ischial containment and quadrilateral designs. Compared to quadrilateral sockets, ischial containment sockets may provide needed stability for higher-level activities and sports and are more likely to be a successful option for individuals with shorter residual femur length or those with excessive soft tissue or fluctuations in residual limb volume.[15]

Maikos and colleagues recently investigated the movement of the residual femur relative to the prosthetic socket using dynamic stereo x-ray and found that ischial containment sockets allow less proximal-distal translation of the residual femur relative to the socket.[18] However, there was no difference in anterior-posterior or medial-lateral translation of the femur compared to the compression/release stabilization socket.[18]

MARLO-ANATOMICAL SOCKET

A variation of the ischial containment socket is the Marlo-Anatomical Socket (see Figs. 24.3C and 24.4C). The Marlo-Anatomical Socket allows for increased hip range of motion by lowering the trimlines on the anterior and posterior walls of the socket, but increasing contact with the medial ischial ramus with the medial wall.[12] Its lower posterior trimlines allow the user to sit directly on the buttock instead of on the posterior socket.[19] Additionally, the increased hip range of motion allowed by this socket design helps to minimize dysfunctional gait kinematics and may help reduce the energy cost of walking compared to ischial containment socket designs.[19]

SUBISCHIAL SOCKET

Unlike the quadrilateral and ischial containment designs, the subischial socket terminates several inches below the pelvis (see Figs. 24.3D and 24.4D). Preliminary evidence suggests that wearers are more comfortable and have greater hip mobility and stability while wearing this socket.[11,12,20,21] The transverse contours of the sockets also differ (Fig. 24.3D). Due to the lower trimlines associated with subischial sockets, prosthetic fit and suspension can pose a challenge. Advances in vacuum suspension technology have made it possible to lower the proximal trimlines without sacrificing stability or suspension.[11–14]

One example of a subischial socket design is the Northwestern University Flexible Subischial Vacuum Socket (NU-FlexSIV).[12] Not all individuals with transfemoral amputation are appropriate for a subischial socket design. Appropriate candidates for a subischial socket have well-healed residual limbs with minimal fluctuation in residual limb volume. To be successful with use of a transfemoral prosthesis with a subischial socket, individuals need to be compliant with residual limb management and hygiene of their residual limb and liners, and must have a residual limb that can tolerate significant circumferential compression and vacuum suspension. Individuals with redundant soft tissue that may bunch up or scar tissue with deep invaginations may result in loss of total contact with the prosthetic liner or trap air between the residual limb and liner, which may increase risk for skin breakdown with use of vacuum suspension.[12] A recent randomized crossover trial of 30 participants with transfemoral amputation found that the subischial socket design did not change gait kinematics related to hip range of motion or frontal plane socket stability (lateral trunk flexion and step width), but participants reported greater socket comfort and satisfaction with the subischial design compared to the ischial containment socket design.[13,14]

Compression/Release Stabilization Sockets

A newer design of prosthetic socket, first described for individuals with transhumeral amputation,[22] utilizes alternating areas of longitudinal compression through rigid struts to provide stability and open windows for release to provide relief for soft tissues. In theory, the compressed tissue allows for more efficient transfer of torque from the prosthetic user to the socket and prosthesis.[22] In practice, achieving appropriate levels of "precompression" to stabilize the residual femur in the socket for individuals with transfemoral amputation poses a logistical challenge with axial loading.[18] Adequate levels of precompression to stabilize the residual femur may not be well tolerated, and insufficient precompression results in increased proximal-distal translation of the residual femur during stance phase compared to use of ischial containment socket designs.[18]

FLEXIBLE SOCKETS

Flexible sockets are vacuum formed from flexible thermoplastics. Examples of this design include the Scandinavian flexible socket and the Icelandic-Scandinavian-New York socket.[23] The socket is encased in a rigid frame, which provides support during weight bearing. Cutouts or windows can be made in the rigid material to offload sensitive areas of the residual limb. The socket accommodates to changes in muscle contour as the wearer moves and can be easily modified by heat.[17] Users report that flexible sockets are more comfortable, especially when sitting, because the wearer contacts the chair with a pliable interface. Flexible sockets can be made with either a quadrilateral or ischial containment design.[23]

SUSPENSION SYSTEMS

Appropriate socket fit and choice of prosthetic suspension system are critical considerations that impact prosthetic user's satisfaction with their prosthesis and directly impact mobility performance and comfort with mobility-related activities of daily living.[24] Inadequate prosthetic suspension may allow the prosthetic limb to lose contact with the residual limb during swing limb advancement contributing to a functionally long limb, which may impact swing limb clearance and contribute to compensatory circumduction, hip hiking, or contralateral vaulting to clear the prosthesis during swing. This is more of a concern for individuals using transfemoral prosthetic limbs than transtibial prosthetic limbs because the increased weight of a transfemoral prosthesis creates greater distraction forces, which increases the demand for adequate suspension.[17] The loss of contact between the residual limb and the prosthesis may also contribute to rotational instability with a medial or lateral whip at late stance and or excessive vertical translation of the residual limb in the socket due to "pistoning."[24] Excessive pistoning between the residual limb and the prosthesis may cause individuals discomfort and may increase risk for skin breakdown of the distal residual limb. There are advantages and disadvantages to different types of suspension systems and clinicians need to understand the benefits and limitations of different suspension options to identify the best option for their individual patient's needs.

Suction

Suction suspension requires snug proximal socket fit and an air-expulsion valve that allows air to exit but prevents air from entering the socket. Donning may be accomplished by drawing tubular cotton stockinet (or an elastic bandage) over the thigh to the inguinal ligament, then passing the distal end of the stockinet through the valve hole. Usually, the patient stands and pulls down on the stockinet while flexing and extending the opposite hip and knee until the entire stockinet is withdrawn. This process requires considerable agility and balance. The valve is then installed in the socket. A second option is to apply a lubricant to the thigh to enable sliding the limb into the socket that already has the valve installed. After the thigh is inside the socket, the valve is pressed to release any trapped air.

Intimate fit required for suction suspension enhances prosthetic control and proprioception.[17,25] Suction suspension is inappropriate for patients with a recent amputation whose limb volume will continue to decrease or for those with fluctuating edema or unstable weight. High shear force associated with donning may preclude its use for patients with fragile or sensitive skin, painful trigger points, significant scarring, adhesions, or upper-limb weakness.

TOTAL ELASTIC SUSPENSION BELT

The total elastic suspension (TES) belt is made of an elastic neoprene. The distal sleeve of the TES belt fits snugly around the proximal half of the socket. The TES belt encircles the waist and attaches in front with hook and loop tape. The TES belt is easy to don, comfortable to wear, and an excellent auxiliary suspension system. It is often chosen for the person who has had recent surgery whose amputation limb has not yet matured to stable size, for older patients unable to use suction or liners, and for those with tender skin or adhesions. It is also secondary suspension for athletes. The TES system has limited durability, especially for active people, and tends to retain heat.

Liners

Suspension with liners as an interface between the residual limb and the prosthetic socket was introduced in the 1980s and significantly improves suspension, stability, and user comfort compared to suction suspension.[17] Donning is simple and can be accomplished while seated. However, liners become worn or torn and must be replaced several times a year depending on the wearer's activity level. Liners may increase skin temperature and perspiration. A few people develop dermatitis. Liners must be cleaned daily to prevent accumulation of perspiration and bacteria. Different mechanisms are used to secure the suspension with liner interfaces.

ROLL-ON LINERS

Roll-on liners are made from silicone, polyurethane, or other elastomers.[17] Worn against the skin, roll-on liners are donned by being turned inside-out, then rolled over the residual limb. Prosthetic users need to exercise caution in ensuring appropriate distal contact of the liner with their residual limb and avoid letting any air enter between their skin and the liner as this may increase risk for skin irritation or breakdown. The roll-on liner creates negative pressure and is somewhat adhesive. The liner can be used for suspension with a shuttle lock, lanyard, seal-in liner, or air-expulsion valve or as part of an elevated vacuum socket. Suspensions with air-expulsion valves or elevated vacuum may also require use of a suspension sleeve to help maintain the seal of negative pressure to maintain adequate suspension. Although liner use facilitates donning, sitting, walking, and comfort, problems with durability remain.

Cushion Liner With Air-Expulsion Valve

A resilient liner (Fig. 24.5A) is put on the amputation limb, which is then pushed into the socket, creating negative pressure environment by expelling air through an expulsion valve (Fig. 24.5B). This system allows prosthetic users to add additional socks over their liner to adjust the fit of their prosthetic socket as needed with changes in residual limb volume to assist with pressure redistribution throughout the residual limb and minimize focal pressure at the distal aspect of the residual limb, which may be caused by "bottoming out" in the socket due to decreased residual limb volume. This method of suspension typically requires the addition of a suspension sleeve over the prosthetic socket to maintain negative pressure for adequate suspension. The proximal aspect of the suspension sleeve should contact the user's skin and not the prosthetic socks or liner.

PIN/SHUTTLE LOCKING LINER

The liner has an external cap. In the center of the cap a serrated pin protrudes approximately 1½ inches (Fig. 24.6). The pin engages a shuttle lock inside the bottom of the socket, when the wearer stands and pushes the amputation limb down into the socket. To remove the prosthesis, one disengages the serrated pin by depressing a release button on the medial aspect of the socket exterior. The pin/shuttle lock liner allows prosthetic users to add additional socks over their liner to adjust the fit of their prosthetic socket as needed with changes in residual limb volume to assist with pressure redistribution throughout the residual limb and minimize focal pressure at the distal aspect of the residual limb, which may be caused by "bottoming out" in the socket due to decreased residual limb volume.

Lanyard

The prosthetic user dons a liner on the bottom of which is a lanyard (strap or cord). The lanyard is routed through a hole in the distal socket. As the prosthetic user dons the

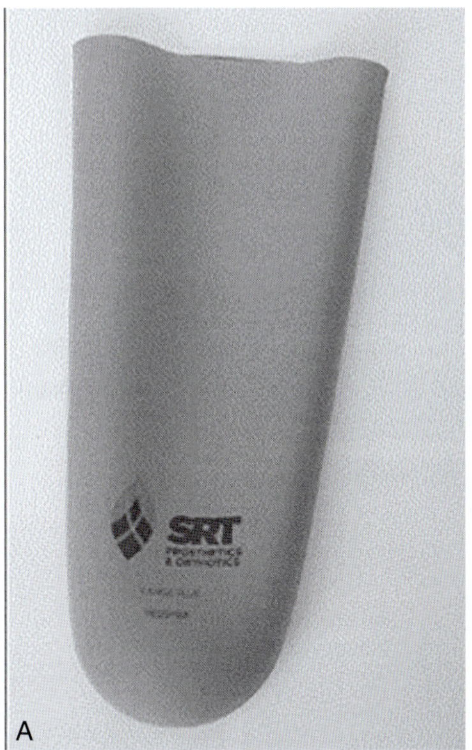

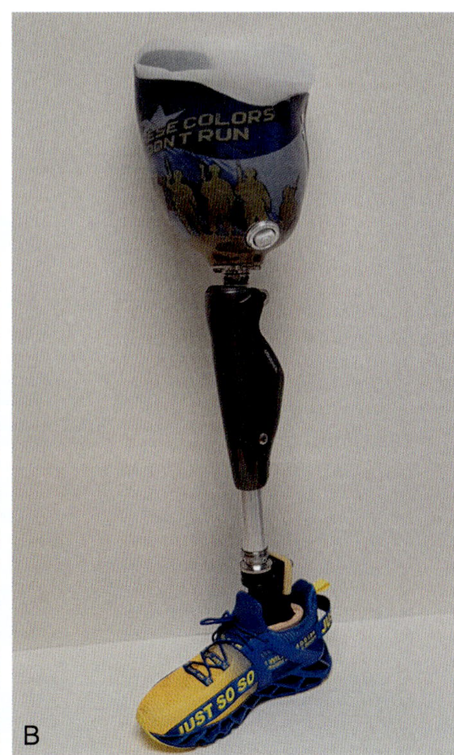

Fig. 24.5 (A) Cushion liner. (B) Air expulsion valve on transfemoral prosthesis.

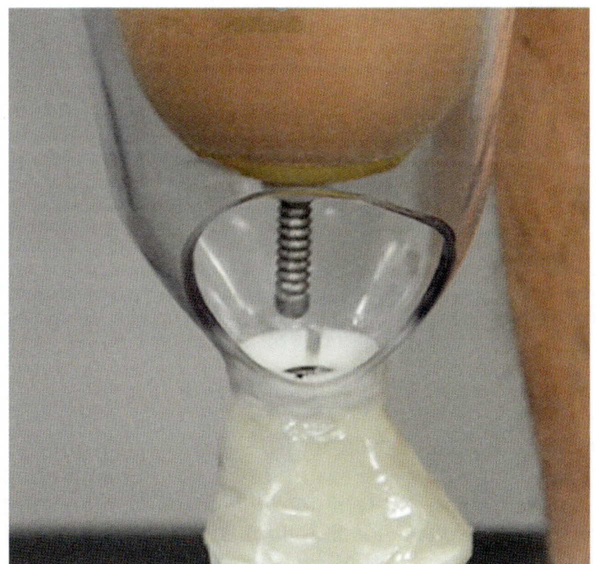

Fig. 24.6 Prosthetic liner with pin/shuttle lock mechanism.

prosthesis while pulling the lanyard (Fig. 24.7A and D) up the lateral exterior of the socket and typically threaded through and D-ring and secured with hook and loop tape or another mechanism. Lanyard suspension can improve prosthetic user's ability to don a transfemoral prosthesis, especially if they have difficulty consistently aligning and engaging a pin/shuttle lock suspension.

Seal-In Liner

Seal-in liners incorporate a hypobaric sealing membrane around the distal aspect of the liner to create a vacuum seal between the liner and prosthetic socket.[24] The sealing membrane is typically lubricated with hand sanitizer to allow the residual limb to slide into the socket; air in the socket escapes through a one-way valve at the distal end of the socket, the hand sanitizer evaporates, and the prosthetic user is left with a well-suspended prosthesis (Fig. 24.8A and B). Seal-in liners are not an ideal option for individuals whose residual limb volume fluctuates widely. There is limited ability to accommodate for fluctuations in residual limb volume with this suspension system. The seal-in system was found to be easier for prosthetic users to don/doff compared to traditional suction sockets.[24]

ELEVATED VACUUM SUSPENSION

Elevated vacuum suspension systems incorporate an active vacuum system that maintains a negative pressure environment between the prosthetic liner and the socket.[26] Suction suspension allows air to exit through the valve when the amputation limb moves in swing phase, whereas elevated vacuum suspension uses a pump to continuously remove air between the liner and socket to create a constant pressure differentiation.[26] Consequently, suspension is more secure and the socket can have a lower trim line.

With elevated vacuum suspension, negative pressure is maintained when the prosthesis is offloaded during swing

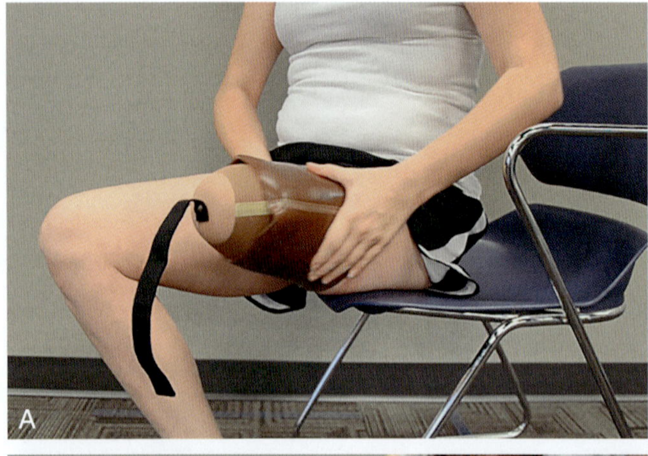

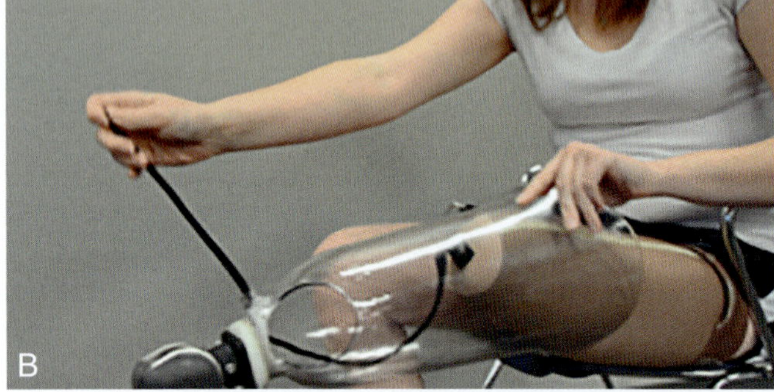

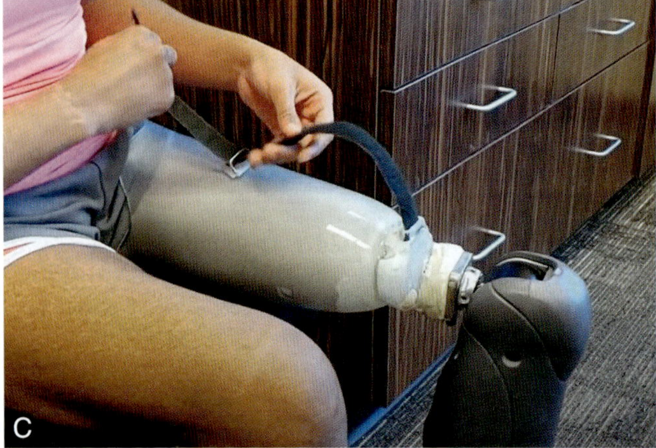

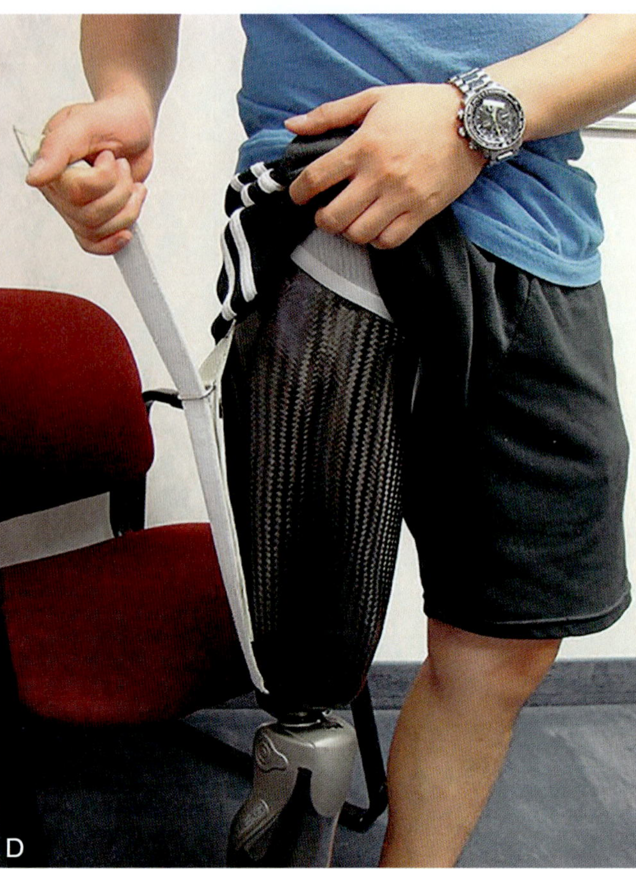

Fig. 24.7 (A) Donning roll-on liner with lanyard. (B) Passing lanyard through distal opening in socket. (C) Threading lanyard through D-ring to secure prosthesis in preparation for sit to stand. (D) Readjusting tension on lanyard in weight bearing position to ensure good distal contact of residual limb in socket.

limb advancement, which minimizes movement between the prosthesis and residual limb and liner.[25] Shear forces are reduced with elevated vacuum, which helps to protect the skin of the residual limb, and pistoning between the limb, liner, and socket is virtually eliminated. Users report greater proprioception, security, comfort, and a sense that the prosthesis feels lighter.[25] Fluctuations in residual limb volume are reduced with the use of elevated vacuum.[25] Elevated vacuum improves blood circulation and may help to heal wounds. Potential limitations of this type of suspension include need for battery charging and maintenance.[25]

OSSEOINTEGRATION

Osseointegration involves direct skeletal fixation of a surgical implant into the medullary canal of the distal residual femur.[27] On December 18, 2020, the US Food and Drug Administration approved a two-stage surgical procedure for the Osseoanchored Prostheses for the Rehabilitation of Amputees Implant System (manufactured by Integrum AB in Mölndal, Sweden) for individuals who were not able to successfully use a prosthesis with a socket. The first stage of the surgery involves implanting (anchoring) the intermedullary implant and the second stage is a percutaneous procedure in which an abutment attachment is placed to allow for prosthetic fitting.[28] Surrounding soft tissues are closed, but the distal aspect of the abutment remains exposed to facilitate direct attachment of the transfemoral prosthesis, thereby eliminating the need for a socket.[27] Implantation is performed after the amputation limb has healed from the initial amputation surgery.

Appropriate candidates for consideration of osseointegration procedures are transfemoral prosthetic users who have had problems with traditional socket prostheses due to

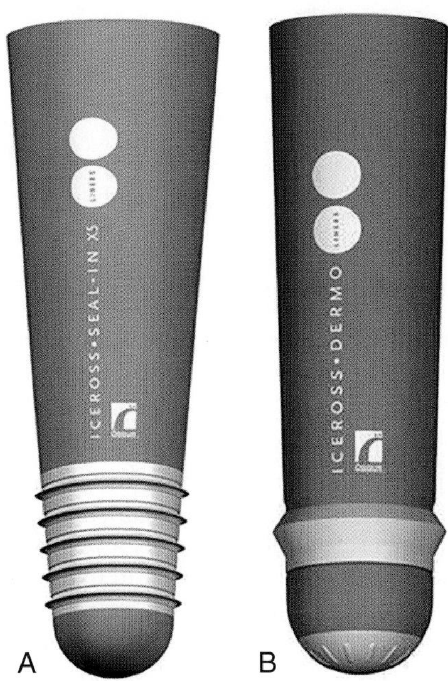

Fig. 24.8 (A and B) Seal-in liner.

discomfort/pain, inadequate suspension, or issues that may limit the ability to successfully use a prosthesis with a socket including extensive soft tissue scarring, extensive areas of skin grafting, or a short residual limb.[27] Contraindications to osseointegration include severe peripheral vascular disease; diabetes; current chemotherapy; corticosteroid use or immunosuppressant drugs; limb exposure to radiation; pregnancy; mental illness or psychiatric disorder; smoking (smoking cessation encouraged); osteoporosis; body weight >220 pounds; infection; skin disease involving residual limb; and ability to use conventional socket technology.[27] Complications that have been reported include infection, failure or breakage of the intramedullary implant, or femur fracture.[29,30] Mild infections have been effectively management nonoperatively, and failed implants can potentially be revised.[29,30]

The primary outcomes reported by those who successfully use osseointegrated prosthetics include improved quality of life,[31,32] improved walking distance on the 6-Minute Walk Test,[31,32] improved mobility performance on the Timed Up and Go Test,[31,32] reduced oxygen consumption during walking,[32,33] normalized gait kinematics,[34] improved sitting comfort,[32,35] increased use of prosthesis,[32] easier and more efficient don/doff of prosthesis,[32,36] and improved osseoperception.[32]

TRANSFEMORAL PROSTHETIC COMPONENTRY

Prosthetic componentry can have a significant impact on walking performance. In a study by Gailey,[37] use of a formula based on AMPnoPRO score, age, and comorbidities is proposed to predict the functional value of providing upgraded prosthetic technology. Utilizing this formula, two different scenarios were presented:

Example 1: A healthy 25-year-old with unilateral transfemoral amputation and no comorbidities scored a 38 on the AMPnoPRO, which would be consistent with a K3–K4 functional level. With K1 level componentry this individual walked 233 m on the 6-Minute Walk Test (6 MWT). Based on the predictive formula, it is anticipated that this individual would walk 330 m on the 6 MWT with a cadence responsive knee and a multiaxial foot (K2 componentry), and 349 m with a cadence responsive knee and an energy-storage-and-return (ESAR) foot (K3 componentry).[37] Appropriate componentry is predicted to contribute to a 49.7% improvement in walking distance and an improvement in walking speed of 0.32 m/s.[37]

Example 2: A 75-year-old with unilateral transfemoral amputation and multiple comorbidities scored a 25 on the AMPnoPRO, consistent with a K2 level of function. With K1 level componentry this individual walked 76 meters on the 6 MWT.[37] Based on the predictive formula, it is anticipated that this individual would walk 173 m with a cadence responsive knee and a multiaxial foot (K2 componentry), and 192 m with a cadence responsive knee and an energy-storage-and-return (ESAR) foot (K3 componentry). Appropriate componentry is predicted to contribute to a 152.6% improvement in walking distance and an improvement in walking speed of 0.32 m/s.[37]

The actual functional value of upgrading prosthetic componentry has not been established, and though improved walking distance and walking speed are important markers of function, they do not tell the whole story. It has been reported that only 25% of individuals with transfemoral amputation receive a prosthesis and many of these individuals rely on a wheelchair as their primary mode of mobility.[38] This predictive model does not factor in the therapeutic benefits of walking and prosthetic use on general health and wellness. This is particularly important to consider for individuals with dysvascular transfemoral amputation. There is a fourfold increased risk of cardiac events following transfemoral amputation in individuals with vascular disease.[38] Physical inactivity is one of the greatest and most modifiable risk factors for development of cardiovascular disease.[39] Provision of a prosthesis that decreases energy cost, improves gait efficiency, decreases residual limb and sound-side loading, increases safety and assists with stumble recovery, and decreases stress on the low back, hips, and knees is likely to facilitate increased levels of activity for individuals with transfemoral amputation. However, appropriate education and rehabilitation management across the continuum from the postoperative and preprosthetic phase through prosthetic training and long-term follow-up are critical to successful lifelong prosthetic use.

PROSTHETIC FOOT CATEGORIES

Descriptions of various types of prosthetic feet are provided in Chapter 21. Prosthetic feet can be categorized into six different classifications: solid-ankle-cushion-heel (SACH), single-axis, multiple-axis, flexible-keel, energy-storage-and-return (ESAR), and microprocessors.[40] As discussed in Chapter 21, most individuals at the K1 functional level will use either a SACH foot or a single-axis foot; multiple-axis or flexible-keel prosthetic feet are typically used by individuals functioning at a K2 level; ESAR, dynamic response, or microprocessor feet are typically used by individuals functioning at a K3 level.[37] Any prosthetic foot is appropriate for individuals with the ability or potential to function at a

K4 level.[37] With selection of prosthetic componentry, clinicians should be aware of the benefits associated with specific components and the potential tradeoffs or limitations of those components (see Table 23.3).

PROSTHETIC KNEE CATEGORIES

Prosthetic knee units have traditionally been categorized under the following classifications: manual-locking knees, weight-activated stance control (safety knees), single-axis or polycentric knees (constant friction), hydraulic or pneumatic knees, and microprocessor-controlled knees. Prosthetic users with transfemoral amputation with ability or potential to perform at a K1 functional level will typically use a manual-locking knee or a weight-activated stance control (safety knee); single-axis or polycentric and constant friction knees with or without stance control are typically appropriate for those at the K2 functional level; cadence responsive knees with hydraulic or pneumatic resistance mechanisms are indicated for individuals at the K2–K3 functional level; and microprocessor-controlled knees are typically indicated for individuals at the K3 functional level.[5,41,42] Any prosthetic knee is appropriate for individuals with the ability or potential to function at a K4 level.[42]

Prosthetic knee systems are designed to perform two major tasks: (1) to provide stability during stance phase of gait to reduce risk for falls and (2) to provide shock absorption on loading to protect joints and reduce pain and risk for development/progression of osteoarthritis.[42] Most mechanical prosthetic knees used by individuals at the K1–K2 functional level are locked into extension during stance phase to provide more stability and reduce risk for falls. However, this stability comes at the expense of shock absorption provided by allowing early stance flexion.[42] Some prosthetic systems attempt to provide increased shock absorption by incorporating a vertical shock pylon to dissipate the force of impact at early stance (initial contact into loading response); however, the shock absorption provided comes at the expense of energy loss requiring increased work at the residual hip joint for forward propulsion at push-off.[43] Prosthetic knee units that allow early stance flexion provide improved shock absorption without compromising knee stability during stance phase of gait and provide a more smooth transition from swing phase into stance phase of gait. However, early stance flexion is not recommended for prosthetic users at lower functional levels (K0–K2) due to risk for knee buckling, which may increase risk for fall-related injury.[42] There is a growing body of evidence to support the benefits of microprocessor-controlled knees for individuals at the K2 functional level due to safety features that may decrease incidence of stumbles and falls.[41,44–47]

MANUAL-LOCKING KNEE UNITS

Manual-locking knee units are designed to be locked in extension throughout the entire gait cycle. The pin automatically locks with an audible click when the knee is fully extended. The prosthetist will often set up a prosthesis with a manual-locking knee to be slightly shorter than the sound-side limb to facilitate foot clearance during swing limb advancement of the prosthesis. Depending on the length of the prosthesis, individuals who ambulate with a prosthesis with a manual-locking knee may demonstrate a compensatory hip-hike or circumduction pattern to facilitate swing limb clearance. With the knee locked in extension, there is significantly reduced demand on the prosthetic user's hip extensors to control the knee extensor mechanism during stance phase of gait.[42] In order for the prosthetic user to unlock the knee to return to sitting, the lock release mechanism (Fig. 24.9) is typically attached to the proximal prosthetic socket and can only be released when the prosthesis is not being loaded.[42] There are several different designs of manual-locking knee units, but most locking mechanisms will automatically engage once the knee is fully extended. Manual-locking knees provide maximum stability and safety during standing at the expense of mobility and efficiency of gait. This knee design is primarily intended for individuals who are less active and primarily use a prosthesis for transfers and limited distance household ambulation consistent with a K1 functional level.

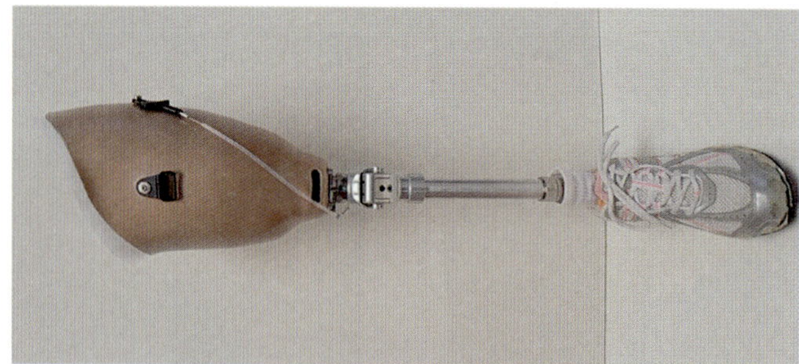

Fig. 24.9 Transfemoral prosthesis with manual-locking knee unit.

WEIGHT-ACTIVATED KNEE UNITS

Weight-activated knee units are designed to engage a frictional brake during early stance to stabilize the knee in extension for stability in stance (Fig. 24.10). As weight is transferred to the sound side at preswing the braking moment is reduced allowing the prosthetic knee to flex in preparation for swing limb advancement.[42]

Single-Axis Knee Units

The single-axis knee has a transverse hinge that allows the shank to swing in flexion and extension. This knee is lightweight and durable. Stability of the knee is achieved by alignment of the parts of the prosthesis with or without additional mechanism. Appropriate alignment helps to minimize the demand on the hip extensors to control the prosthetic knee during stance phase of gait.[42]

Polycentric Knee Units

The polycentric knee has two or more pairs of bars connecting the upper and lower portions of the unit. The bars pivot at both ends thus creating a moving center of rotation (Fig. 24.11A and B). As the wearer bends the knee, the bars cross proximally and posteriorly, thereby changing the center of rotation. The polycentric knee will shorten as it flexes, which facilitates swing limb clearance; however, the changing center of rotation during flexion may compromise

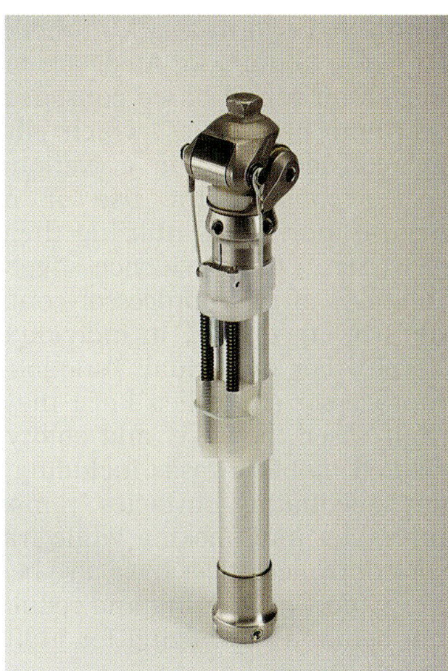

Fig. 24.10 Stance control/weight-activated knee.

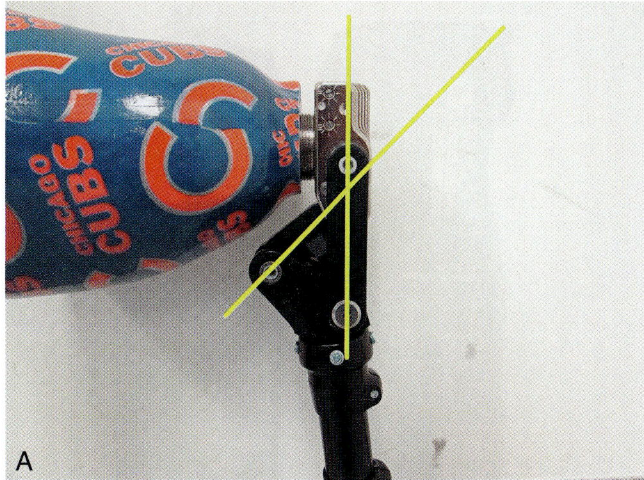

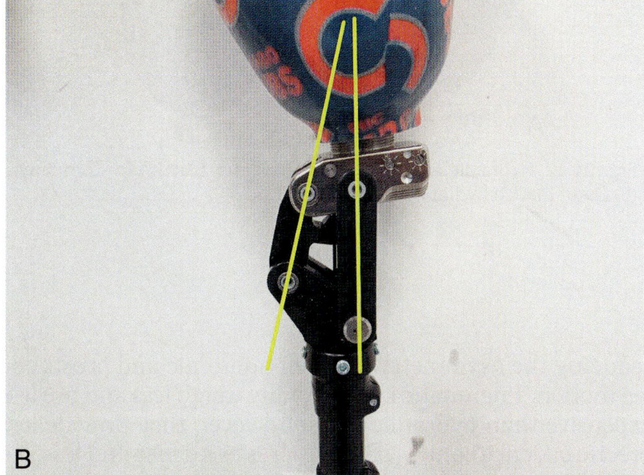

Fig. 24.11 Polycentric knee unit. (A) Flexed. (B) Extended. (Courtesy Shriners Hospital Portland, Oregon.)

stance phase stability if full knee extension is not achieved prior to heel strike at initial contact.[42] Polycentric knee units can be adjusted to move the initial center of rotation more posteriorly to provide a "hyperstabilized" knee, which performs similarly to a manual-locking knee.[42] The knee can also be adjusted to allow users more voluntary control for stability on rough terrain, and inclines and when taking shorter steps.[42] Polycentric knee units have generally been shown to improve stability during stance phase, but prosthetic users need to ensure the polycentric knee swings into full extension prior to loading, otherwise the ground reaction force will be posterior to the knee center of rotation and cause the prosthetic knee to buckle. Adequate strength and motor control of their hip extensors is required to maintain stability of the polycentric prosthetic knee through stance phase.[42]

SWING PHASE CONTROL

Hydraulic Knee Units

Hydraulic knee units regulate the swing of the shank according to the walker's speed. The unit has an oil-filled cylinder attached to the knee axis, whether single-axis or polycentric. A piston from the axis to the cylinder interior descends during early swing; this action forces oil to flow through narrow channels to provide frictional resistance. The faster the knee swings, the greater the resistance. Variable resistance permits a swing phase that simulates normal gait. The amount of resistance can be adjusted by the prosthetist who widens or narrows the channels through which the oil flows. The narrower a channel, the greater the resistance. Variable resistance is useful for active individuals and those with mobility impairment. However, hydraulic units are heavier and more expensive than other units.

Some hydraulic knee units also have stance control provided by a braking mechanism that markedly increases resistance to knee motion at early stance when the knee unit is subjected to a flexion moment of force (Fig. 24.12A and B). This feature allows the individual to walk with greater confidence over uneven surfaces and use a step-over-step pattern when negotiating hills and descending stairs. Some hydraulic knee units are equipped with a mode selector switch that allows the user to change the function of the knee from a normal gait mode to a high hydraulic resistance or "locked" mode for maximum stability or to a low hydraulic resistance or "free-swing" mode that can be utilized for cycling exercise. Hydraulic knee units are cadence responsive and allow users to walk at variable gait speeds with improved speed and symmetry.[41] However, the range of speeds available is limited compared to microprocessor-controlled knees.[42]

Pneumatic Knee Units

Pneumatic knee units have an air-filled cylinder into which a piston descends during early swing and ascends during late swing. Because air is also a fluid, the amount of resistance is directly proportional to the speed of motion; the faster the person walks, the greater the resistance thereby

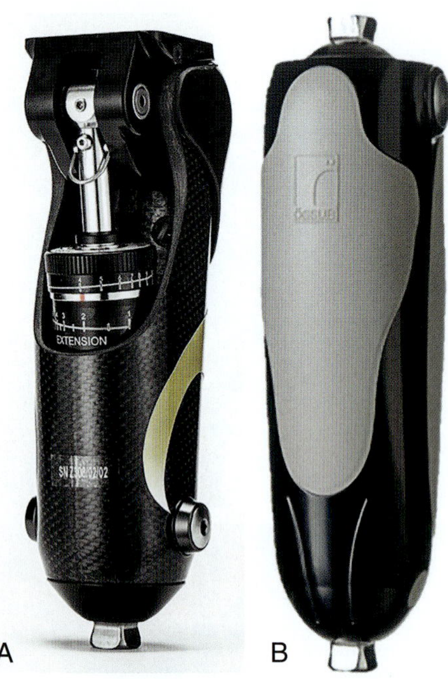

Fig. 24.12 Hydraulic knee unit. (A) Endolite a Blatchford Company. (B) Össur mauch hydraulic knee.

reducing the asymmetry between anatomic and prosthetic leg motion. Pneumatic knees usually weigh less and are less expensive than hydraulic units; however, they provide less precise cadence control because air is less dense and less viscous than oil. Pneumatic knee units are cadence responsive and allow users to walk at variable gait speeds; however, the range of speeds available is limited compared to microprocessor-controlled knees.

Microprocessor-Controlled Knee Units

Most microprocessor-controlled knee units have a single-axis design with a hydraulic system that provides controlled early stance flexion and stance stability, which is under adaptive control based on real-time microprocessor analysis of movement data from accelerometers, gyroscopes, and inertial sensors integrated into the knee unit. The amount of resistance on knee extension during swing phase can also be regulated on microprocessor-controlled knees. Real-time data analysis allows microprocessor-controlled knees to automatically adapt to changes in walking speed, terrain, or obstacles encountered by the user. Many microprocessor-controlled knees are also equipped to identify a trip or stumble and increase knee extension resistance to assist with stumble recovery and prevent knee buckling to reduce risk of fall-related injury. Chapter 27 provides a comparison of various types of microprocessor-controlled knee units and the implications for rehabilitation.

Historically, reimbursement for microprocessor-controlled knees has only be available to individuals with the ability or potential to perform at a K3 functional level or higher. In 2017, the Centers for Medicare and Medicaid Services developed an expert-based consensus statement regarding lower-limb prosthetics, which advocated that "CMS strongly consider opening a National Coverage Determination to consider the use of microprocessor knees in those individuals utilizing their prostheses at the K2 level (page 16)."[5] Evidence suggests that the added safety features of microprocessor-controlled knees may reduce falls by up to 80% in individuals functioning at a K2 level.[41] For individuals functioning at a K2 level, a microprocessor-controlled knee may contribute to improved gait speed, balance, and ability to perform community-related mobility tasks including walking on uneven terrain; negotiating obstacles, ramps, hills, and stairs; and improving multitasking while walking.[41,45–48] Microprocessor-controlled knees have also been shown to reduce the energy cost of walking and reduce the cognitive/attentional demand of walking for individuals with transfemoral amputation.[41]

TRANSFEMORAL ALIGNMENT

Appropriate prosthetic alignment normalizes joint contact forces to minimize excessive joint loading and decrease risk for joint injury, and facilitates stance limb stability to control the prosthesis against ground reaction forces.[49] The prevalence of hip and knee pain on the intact side due to osteoarthritis has been shown to be higher in individuals with transfemoral amputation than transtibial amputation.[49] Shock absorption during normal gait is provided by the natural pronation of the foot and ankle and controlled knee flexion during the loading response. Shock absorption during the loading response for individuals who use transfemoral prostheses depends on the shock-absorbing functions of the prosthetic foot design and whether or not the prosthetic knee provides early stance flexion. As a result of having fewer muscles available to control the prosthesis, transfemoral prosthetic users often demonstrate decreased confidence and stability during stance phase on the prosthetic side and compensate by increasing their stance time on the sound side (Box 24.1). Stance time is relatively decreased on the prosthetic side and transfemoral users often demonstrate a rapid offloading of the prosthetic side at late stance with an abrupt weight shift to the intact side, which increases sound-side loading and may predispose individuals to increased risk for osteoarthritis of their sound side.[49]

SAGITTAL ALIGNMENT

The most important goal in transfemoral prosthetics is to obtain knee stability during stance phase. A prosthetic knee that is unstable could lead to a fall. Alternately, a knee that is difficult to flex interferes with swing phase clearance and increases the likelihood of tripping.

Optimum alignment allows the wearer to control prosthetic movement. If the knee axis is positioned slightly posterior to a vertical line from the greater trochanter to the ankle, the weight line passes anteriorly to the knee axis resulting in an extension moment, which provides alignment stability, and thus, minimal hip extensor power is

Box 24.1 The ability for transfemoral prosthetic users to control the prosthesis during stance phase of gait depends on the following factors:

1. Length of the residual limb
2. Range of motion available into hip extension
3. Motor control and strength of hip extensors and abductors
4. Alignment of the prosthetic socket, knee, and ankle
5. Mechanical stability of the knee unit

required. However, stable alignment increases the effort required to initiate knee flexion in late stance phase. If the knee axis is positioned at or slightly in front of the vertical line, the weight line passes behind the knee axis and stance phase is less stable and greater motor control and/or hip extensor power is required to maintain stability; however, this alignment enhances the ability to flex the knee to initiate swing phase (Fig. 24.13).

An individual's ability to control the prosthetic knee is determined by the strength of hip extensors and by the length of the amputation limb. An inverse relationship exists between length of amputation limb and amount of muscular force necessary to control the prosthetic knee.

Voluntary control of the prosthetic knee may be compromised by a hip flexion contracture or weakness of hip extensors. It is critical that preprosthetic training for individuals with transfemoral amputation focus on minimizing the development or progression of hip flexion contractures and emphasize the importance of maintaining hip extension range of motion and develop motor control and strength of hip extensors and abductors. Historically, it has been advised that individuals with transfemoral amputation with hip flexion contractures >25 degrees not be fit with a prosthesis due to challenges with alignment to provide adequate knee stability during stance phase of gait.[50] Prosthetists make an effort to accommodate hip flexion contractures with the alignment of the prosthesis. To do this, it is important to measure the degree of hip flexion contracture via the Thomas Test for hip flexor length.[51] The prosthetist will typically align the prosthesis by flexing the socket of the prosthesis to match the degree of hip flexion contracture and then add 5 degrees of flexion in the socket to give prosthetic users at least 5 degrees of hip extension range of motion to control the prosthetic knee unit. More severe hip flexion contractures may require significant amounts of socket flexion. To provide more stability for the prosthetic knee, a posterior offset plate (Fig. 24.14A and B) may be used to better align the weight line relative to the knee axis to provide an appropriate balance of stability and mobility to meet the prosthetic user's needs.[51] If the prosthetic knee is aligned too far anteriorly, prosthetic users may compensate by exerting more hip extension torque to stabilize the knee and/or decrease their step length, and/or increase trunk flexion during stance, and/or decrease prosthetic loading, and/or decrease their stance time.[51] Aligning the socket in slight flexion elongates hip extensors, thereby

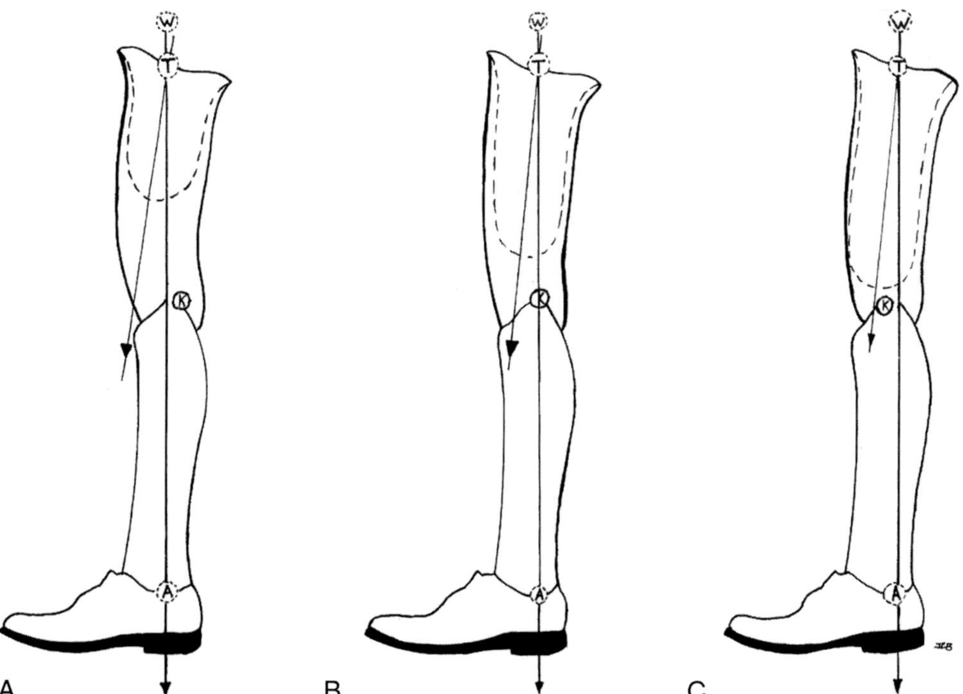

Fig. 24.13 (A) Maximum alignment stability when the weight line (W) passes anteriorly to the knee axis. (B) Minimum alignment stability when the weight line passes through the center of the knee axis. (C) No alignment stability when the weight line passes behind the knee axis. Stability must be achieved by a mechanism within the knee unit.

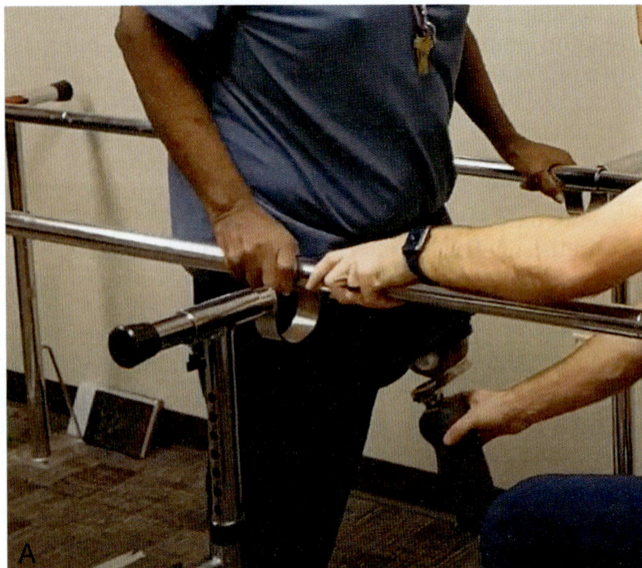

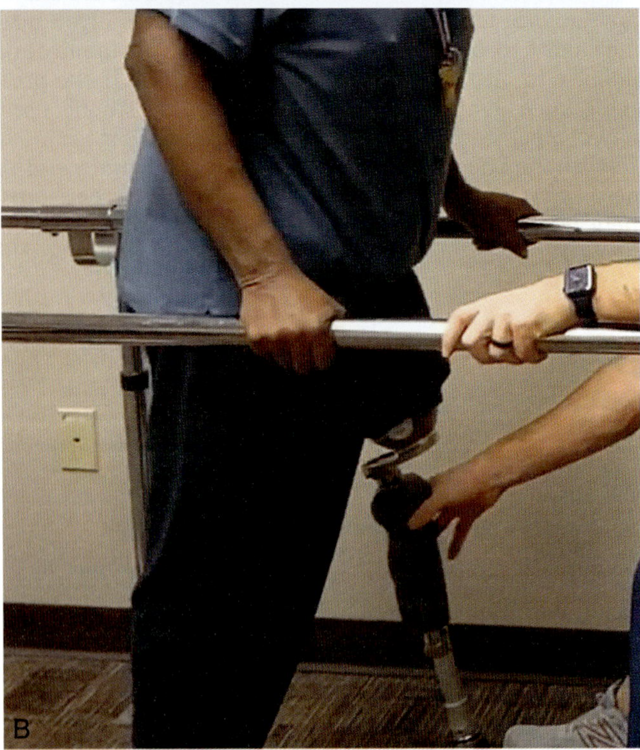

Fig. 24.14 (A) Posterior offset plate to facilitate improved knee stability in stance phase of gait. (B) Therapist preparing to provide knee extension assist as needed during loading response.

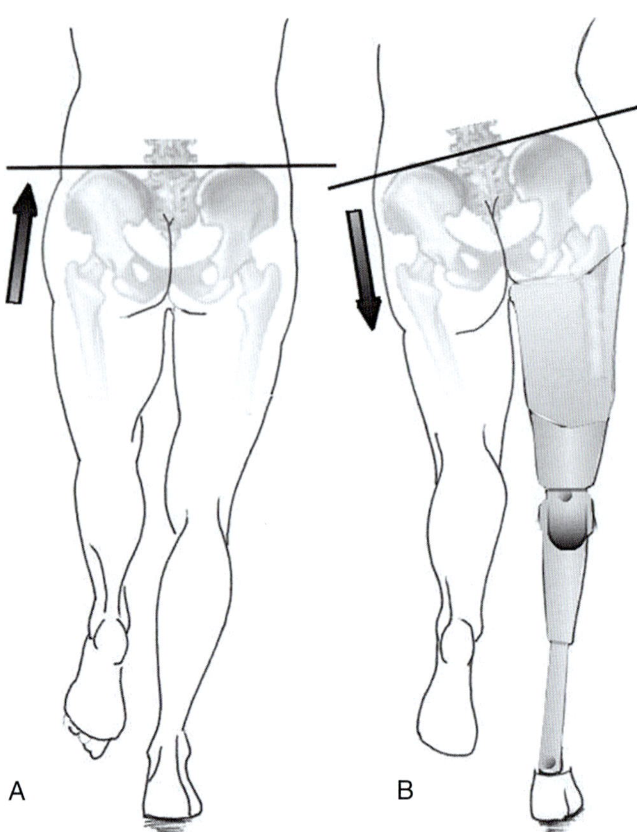

Fig. 24.15 (A) In the intact leg, when weight is borne on the stance limb, gravity causes the pelvis to dip to the swing side. Contraction of the gluteus medius on the stance side prevents excessive dip. (B) Amputation removes the distal attachment of the femur to the knee; consequently, the femur tends to move laterally within the socket during weight bearing. Adduction of the lateral socket wall helps to counteract lateral femoral displacement.

enhancing their contractile ability. Prosthetic sockets that fail to accommodate hip flexion contractures may result in prosthetic users compensating with increased anterior pelvic tilt and lumbar lordosis, which may alter gait kinematics and loading patterns and contribute to increased low back pain.[52]

FRONTAL ALIGNMENT

Following transfemoral amputation, hip or femoral adduction in the frontal plane is compromised due to loss of the distal attachment of the adductor muscles, which decreases the ability of the adductor muscles to counteract the influence of the hip abductor muscles during stance phase (Fig. 24.15).[53] The loss of femoral adduction is more pronounced the shorter the residual limb.[53] This muscle imbalance and loss of frontal plane stability often results in compensatory lateral trunk bending over the prosthetic side during stance phase of gait and contributes to higher loading in the thoracic and lumbar region, which may contribute to increased complaints of back pain.[53] In an effort to reduce compensatory postural adjustments due to muscle imbalance, the transfemoral prosthetic socket is adducted in an effort to facilitate frontal plane stability. A recent study demonstrated that adduction of the transfemoral prosthetic socket successfully reduced lateral trunk lean to the prosthetic side during stance phase, and an socket adduction angle of 6 ± 1 degrees appeared adequate for prosthetic users with a medium residual limb length.[53] Rehabilitation strategies for individuals should focus on developing strength and motor control of hip abductors to maintain pelvic stability in the frontal plane, which may help reduce the energy cost associated with compensatory lateral trunk bending and minimize risk for secondary complications such as low back pain.[54]

Case Example 24.1

J.T. is a 35-year-old male Marines Corp veteran with history of right transfemoral amputation following a traumatic injury due to a motorcycle accident 1 year ago. J.T. is otherwise healthy with no significant past medical history or comorbidities. J.T.'s transfemoral residual limb required split thickness skin grafting for management of severe wounds sustained in the accident. J.T.'s residual limb has healed; however, he has had difficulty tolerating use of a prosthesis due to complaints of socket discomfort at his skin grafting sites and due to adherent scar tissue along the incision line at the distal aspect of his residual limb. J.T.'s goal is to get a well-fitting prosthesis that will allow him to be more active and to go hiking with his wife and young children.

QUESTIONS TO CONSIDER

- What outcome measure(s) would be best to evaluate J.T.'s current level of satisfaction and mobility with his prosthesis?
- What would be the benefits versus concerns of various types of prosthetic sockets and suspension systems? Which option might be best for J.T. and why?
- Would J.T. be a candidate for consideration for revision of his residual limb for an osseointegrated prosthesis? Why or why not?
- What would be the benefits versus potential risks/concerns of an osseointegrated prosthesis?
- What type of prosthetic componentry (e.g., prosthetic knee and foot) would be most optimal to help J.T. achieve his goals of increasing his activity level and being able to go hiking?
- Which mobility assessments and performance-based outcome measures would be most useful to provide justification that J.T. has the ability or potential to perform at a functional level that would warrant use of the prosthetic componentry identified above?

PROSTHETIC HEIGHT

The height of the prosthesis is evaluated when the wearer stands with weight equally distributed on both feet. The iliac crest height of the pelvis should be level (Fig. 24.16A and B). The initial prosthesis may be ¼ inch shorter than the sound side to facilitate clearance of the prosthetic foot during swing phase of gait. The prosthetic socket must fit comfortably when the patient stands with symmetrical weight bearing and during walking and sitting without undue pressure from its margins. Increased pressure or discomfort from the medial wall of the prosthetic socket may exacerbate lateral trunk flexion during stance phase of gait in an effort to reduce pressure in the groin area.

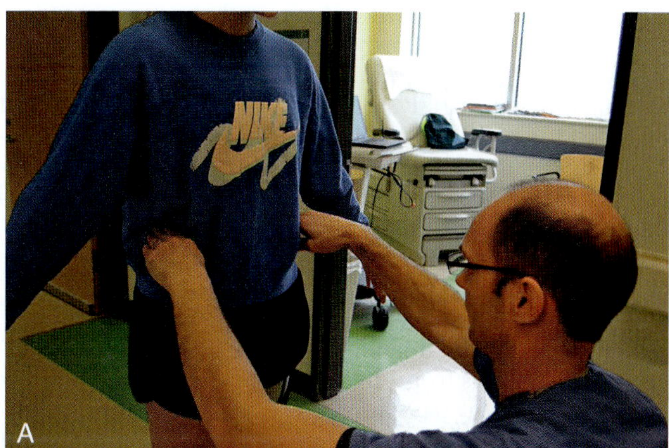

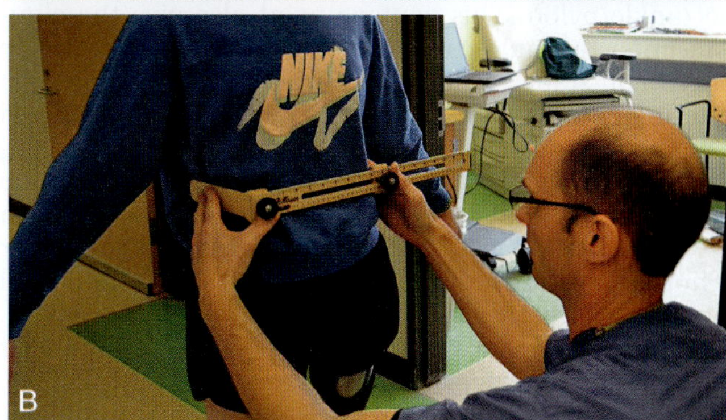

Fig. 24.16 Height of the prosthesis should approximate that of the sound limb. (A) Compare the heights of the iliac crests. (B) Checking the pelvis using a leveling device. (Courtesy Shriners Hospital Portland, Oregon).

GAIT-TRANSFEMORAL PROSTHETIC MOBILITY

Energy Costs

The energy cost of ambulation with a transfemoral prosthesis has been reported to be 20% to 60% greater than that of individuals without limb loss.[55,56] Even military service members with transfemoral amputation and high levels of preinjury fitness were reported to demonstrate a 44% to 47% increase in metabolic rate and cost of walking at a self-selected speed when compared to active duty controls without limb loss.[56] It has been suggested that individuals self-select a step length, step width, cadence, and walking speed that minimizes their energy cost of ambulation.[57] Asymmetrical gait with increased sound-side loading compared to loading of the prosthetic limb may increase the energy costs of walking and place increased demand on the sound side to generate more work in an effort to maintain stability and preserve forward momentum during walking.[58] A recent study has shown that sound-side quadriceps strength was associated with increased 6-Minute Walk Test distance, but sound-side isokinetic quadriceps power was associated with improved walking distance and decreased metabolic cost.[58] Rehabilitation programs for individuals with transfemoral amputation may consider prioritizing development of improved sound-side quadriceps strength and power to minimize energy cost and improve walking performance.[58]

OBSERVATIONAL GAIT ANALYSIS

When performing an observational gait analysis it is important to take a systematic approach to assessing the critical events of the gait cycle: weight acceptance (initial contact and loading response); single-limb support (midstance and terminal stance); and swing limb advancement (preswing, initial swing, midswing, and terminal swing).[59] The prosthetic user's gait should be evaluated in the sagittal plane (viewing from the side) as well as the frontal plane (viewing from the front and rear) to identify gait deviations that may impact an individual's safety, stability, and/or efficiency of gait. Once a gait deviation has been identified, clinicians need to develop a hypothesis-oriented approach to develop a targeted evaluation strategy to determine the most likely cause of the gait deviation and identify the most appropriate intervention. Clinicians should consider both patient-related and prosthetic-related causes of the observed gait deviation.[60] In 2017 the VA and the DoD released the VA/DoD Clinical Practice Guideline for Rehabilitation of Individuals with Lower Limb Amputation to provide a framework for rehabilitation management of individuals with lower-limb amputation.[60] As part of this initiative a VA/DoD Amputation System of Care was formed and resources were developed to help clinicians implement the recommendations of the clinical practice guidelines. Among these resources is a clinician toolkit that provides clinicians with valuable clinical pearls for pain management, management of the residual limb, and analysis and treatment of abnormal gait for individuals with transtibial and transfemoral amputation. The recommendations for evaluation and management of gait deviations for individuals with transfemoral amputation are provided in Fig. 24.17.[60]

SAGITTAL PLANE GAIT DEVIATIONS

When viewing an individual ambulating with a transfemoral prosthesis from the side, the clinician should look for deviations in trunk flexion/extension, hip flexion/extension, knee flexion/extension, and progression of foot/ankle/pylon. This vantage point also give the clinician important information regarding symmetry of step length and stance time, stance limb stability, swing limb clearance (contralateral vaulting), trunk lordosis, and adequacy of suspension (limb clearance). If knee instability is observed early in stance phase, in addition to the patient-related and prosthetic-related cause identified in (Fig. 24.18A and C), clinicians should consider whether or not the knee was fully extended prior to heel first initial contact and whether the individual took too big of a step. Clinicians should also consider the design of the prosthetic knee (e.g., mechanical/nonmicroprocessor controlled vs. microprocessor controlled) to determine whether or not the problem may be addressed by fine tuning the prosthetic knee unit.

FRONTAL PLANE GAIT DEVIATIONS

When viewing the patient from the front or rear clinicians are able to best identify the following common gait deviations seen in prosthetic users with transfemoral amputation: lateral trunk lean over prosthesis, abducted gait, circumduction/hip hiking, external rotation of prosthesis, medial/lateral whip, increased stride width, and adequacy of suspension (pistoning) (Fig. 24.19A and D).

SELF-REPORTED OUTCOME MEASURES

The Prosthetic Limb Users Survey of Mobility (PLUS-M) is a self-reported outcome measure that was developed to measure mobility in individuals with lower-limb amputation.[61,62] The intended use of this tool is to measure changes in mobility for prosthetic users over time and to establish mobility-related classifications for prosthetic users. The PLUS-M was found to have convergent construct validity with performance-based outcome measures for prosthetic mobility and is able to discriminate between prosthetic users according to Medicare Functional Classification K-levels.[61,63] The PLUS-M includes a 12-item survey and a 7-item survey (Fig. 24.20A and B), but also includes a larger item bank to allow it to be customized to the individual and minimize the impact of a ceiling effect, which limits the utility of several other self-report outcome measures.[61] All PLUS-M instruments were found to have excellent psychometrics with excellent reliability and validity, and are available (https://plus-m.org) to use in clinical practice and research.[61,63] It should be noted that one of the main limitations of self-reported outcome measures is that they reflect an individual's perception of their own level of function and may not be reflective of their true capacity for activity/mobility or their actual performance of mobility-related skills. The responsiveness of the PLUS-M for the 12-item Short Form is reported through minimum detectable change (MDC) scores with MDC(90) = 4.5, MDC(95) = 5.36; the responsiveness of the 7-item Short Form is reported as MDC(90) = 4.69, MDC(95) = 5.59.[64]

Functional Performance-Based Outcome Measures

BALANCE AND FALL RISK ASSESSMENT

The literature suggests that over 50% of prosthetic users with lower-limb amputation report falling at least once per year and as many as 39% report history of multiple recurrent falls each year.[65] Interestingly, and perhaps contrary to conventional wisdom, it has been reported that individuals with lower-limb amputation with better balance performance on the Berg Balance Scale are at greater risk for falling than those with more impaired balance.[66] It has been suggested that individuals with greater balance and mobility impairment may limit their activity and avoid activities that may expose them to increased risk for a fall-related injury.[67]

In a recent study of transtibial and transfemoral prosthetic users, cut-off scores were used to identify those at greatest risk for falling. Timed Up and Go Test (TUG) scores ≥8.17 seconds identified individuals with one or more fall with a sensitivity of 83% (negative likelihood ratio = 0.24) and specificity of 68% (positive likelihood ratio = 2.6). A cut-off score of ≥9.25 seconds on the TUG identified those with two or more falls with a sensitivity of 82% (negative likelihood ratio = 0.21) and specificity of 83% (positive likelihood ratio = 4.7).[65] The Four-Square Step Test times of ≥8.49 seconds identified those with one or more fall with a sensitivity of 74% and specificity of 68%, but, a cut-off score of ≥8.71 seconds improved the sensitivity to 94%

Gait Analysis – Abnormalities in Transfemoral Amputation

Gait Abnormality	Patient Related			Prosthetic Related	
	Possible Causes	Additional Evaluation	Interventions	Prosthetic Causes	Additional Evaluation
1. Lateral trunk lean over prosthesis Trunk bends laterally over the prosthesis (compensated Trendelenberg) during stance	Weak hip abductors	Perform manual muscle test	Side stepping with prosthesis	Inadequate adduction of the socket	Check socket fit
	Painful residual limb	Examine residual limb to identify source of pain	Appropriate referral	Prosthesis too short	Check length at iliac crest
	Gait habit	None	Gait retraining	Outset foot	Adjust prosthesis
				Medial wall too high causing pain	Check socket fit
	Hip abduction contracture	Assess ROM	Appropriate stretching	Gapping at lateral wall of socket	Evaluate socket fit
2. Abducted Gait Abduction of prosthetic limb with unilateral widened base of support on prosthetic side during stance	Abduction contracture	Assess ROM	Appropriate stretching	Prosthesis is too long	Check leg length at iliac crest
	Weak adductors	Perform manual muscle testing	Side stepping with prosthesis	Medial wall too high	Check fit in full weight bearing
	Fear or habit, or insecurity with knee control		Traditional exercises Weight shifting activities over the prosthesis Gain confidence through increased wear time and gait training	Adductor roll	Assess for proper shrinkage device/ application Evaluate socket fit
				Outset foot	Adjust prosthesis
				Improperly aligned pelvic band	Check socket fit
				Improper relief for proximal medial trim line	Check fit in full weight bearing
3. Circumduction of prosthesis Abduction of the prosthetic limb in swing with to normal base of support in stance	Weak hip flexion	Perform manual muscle test	Traditional exercises Teach proper use of prosthetic knee	Excessive knee friction	Adjust prosthetic knee function
	Insufficient muscle activation	Perform manual muscle test Biofeedback	Weight shifting activities Rhythmic stabilization on residual limb while standing without prosthesis	Prosthesis too long	Check leg length at iliac crest
				Foot set in excessive plantar flexion	Evaluate static alignment of prosthetic limb
	Excessive soft tissue	Assess for proper shrinkage device	Review wrapping technique or use of shrinker	Inadequate suspension	Modify suspension
	Gait habit		Gait training	Socket too large	Check height/shape of medial brim Check sock ply

Fig. 24.17 Analysis and treatment of abnormal gait for individuals with transfemoral amputation. (From VA/DoD Clinical Practice Guideline. *Rehabilitation of Lower-Limb Amputation—Clinician Tool Kit*; 2017.)

Gait Analysis – Abnormalities in Transfemoral Amputation

Gait Abnormality	Patient Related			Prosthetic Related	
	Possible Causes	Additional Evaluation	Interventions	Prosthetic Causes	Additional Evaluation
4. External Rotation of Prosthesis Toe out on prosthetic side; Knee rotated outward in both swing and stance	Poor residual limb muscle control (decreased stability)	Perform manual muscle tests of hip external rotators and abductors	Strengthen hip external rotators and abductors Resistive gait training	Heel cushion or plantar-flexion bumper is too stiff	Evaluate heel compression during manual loading
				Too much toe-out	Check static alignment
	Improperly donned	Evaluate alignment of prosthesis in full weight bearing	Teach proper donning of prosthesis	Too much heel lever	Check static alignment
				Anterior or medial brim pressure	Evaluate alignment of knee under socket
5. Pelvic Drop Off Stepping in a hole Initial Contact	Weak abductors on the opposite side	Test strength of opposite abductors	Strengthening exercises	Prosthesis too short	Check leg length at iliac crest
				Excessively compliant prosthetic heel	Assess heel compliance during manual loading
6. Knee Instability (flexion) Prosthetic knee buckles in stance phase	Weak hip extensors	Test hip extensor strength	Strengthening exercises	Knee axis too far ahead of TKA line	Evaluate static alignment of the prosthesis
	Severe hip flexion contracture	Test hip ROM	Stretching exercises	Insufficient socket flexion	Evaluate alignment while wearing the prosthesis
	Heel height of shoes	Evaluate shoes	Change shoes to proper height	Heel keel or plantar flexion bumper too stiff	Evaluate heel compression during manual loading
	Poor weight shift	Evaluate weight shifts	Weight shifting activities with prosthesis	Too much dorsiflexion Too long heel lever	Check static alignment
7. Increased Knee Extension (terminal impact) Excessive impact with heel strike in terminal swing	Vigorous hip fl xion followed by strong hip extension	Listen to the heel strike	Balance activities Weight shifting activities	Insufficient friction of the prosthetic knee	Adjust prosthetic knee function
	Lack of prosthetic trust	Evaluate balance function	Single limb stance Resistive gait training		
8. Medial/Lateral Whip Abrupt medial or lateral movement of the prosthetic heel during swing	Improperly donned	Evaluate socket position	Teach proper donning of socket	Excessive external or internal rotation of socket	Evaluate alignment of the knee axis
	Excessive soft tissue	Assess for proper shrinkage device	Review wrapping technique or use of shrinker	Socket too tight	Assess for proper shrinkage device/application Evaluate socket fit
	Insufficient or poor timing of muscular activation	Biofeedback	Rhythmic stabilization at hips	Inadequate suspension	Modify suspension
				Excessive valgus of prosthetic knee	Evaluate static prosthesis alignment

Fig. 24.17, Cont'd

Gait Analysis – Abnormalities in Transfemoral Amputation

Gait Abnormality	Patient Related			Prosthetic Related	
	Possible Causes	Additional Evaluation	Interventions	Prosthetic Causes	Additional Evaluation
9. Increased Stride Width Wide based gait pattern during stance	Poor balance or poor weight-shifting	Check standing balance	Standing balance Weight shift activities	Prosthesis too long	Check leg length at iliac crest
	Hip abduction contracture	Evaluate hip ROM	Stretching exercises	Outset foot	Adjust prosthesis
	Adducted sound limb	Evaluate hip ROM	Stretch adductors and strength abductors	Socket too abducted	Check static alignment
	Gait habit		Gait training	Medial wall pressure	Check static alignment
				Medial leaning pylon	Check static alignment
10. Increased Knee flexion (excessive heel rise) Heel of prosthesis rises higher than the sound foot in toe off	Strong hip flexors	Test hip extensors strength	Strengthen hip extensors	Insufficient knee friction	Adjust prosthetic knee function
	Hip flexion contracture	Test hip ROM	Stretching exercises		
11. Increased Stride Length Long prosthetic step (decreased stance time on prosthesis)	Lack of confidence in prosthesis, inadequate weight bearing/shift, poor balance or pain	None	Weight shifting activities over the prosthesis Gain confidence through increased wear time and gait training Balance Exercises	Painful socket	Evaluate socket fit
	Hip flexion contracture on prosthetic side	Evaluate ROM of the hip	Stretching exercises	Prosthesis too long	Check leg length at iliac crest
	Compensate for decreased stride with sound limb	Measure stride length	Resisted walking Theraband exercises Step-ups Training in forward weight shift of hips		
	Knee flexion contracture on sound side	Evaluate Knee ROM	Stretching exercises		
12. Trunk Lordosis Increased lumbar arch during stance	Tight hip flexors	Evaluate hip ROM	Stretch hips	Insufficient socket flexion	Check TKA line for excessive knee stability
	Weak hip extensors	Check strength of hip	Strengthening exercises	Posterior wall promotes anterior pelvic tilt	Adjust socket
	Weak abdominal muscles	Check abdominal muscles	Core strengthening		
	Gait habit		Gait training		

Fig. 24.17, Cont'd

Gait Analysis – Abnormalities in Transfemoral Amputation

Gait Abnormality	Patient Related			Prosthetic Related	
	Possible Causes	Additional Evaluation	Interventions	Prosthetic Causes	Additional Evaluation
13. Decreased Toe Clearance Prosthetic toe drags or catches during swing phase	Muscle atrophy	Check hip and knee strength both sides	Strengthening knee exercises	Prosthesis too long	Check leg length at iliac crest
	Improperly donned	Evaluate socket position	Teach proper donning of socket	Pistoning Poor socket fit Change in the residual limb	Observe side view alignment Check socket fit, socket ply, and suspension
	Insufficient pelvic rotation	Evaluate resisted pelvic rotation	Assisted pelvic rotation in parallel bars	Prosthetic foot set in excessive plantar flexion	Evaluate static alignment of prosthetic limb
	Weak hip or knee fl xors	Evaluate strength of hip and knee	Strengthening knee and hip exercises		
14. Vaulting Lengthen sound side by rising on toes during stance of sound limb	Fear of not clearing prosthetic toe	None	Weight shifting activities with prosthesis Gain confidence through increased wear time and gait training	Prosthesis too long	Check leg length at iliac crest
	Weak hip flexors	Check hip strength	Stepping practice	Excessive knee friction	Adjust knee function
	Insufficient pelvic rotation	Check appropriately donned socket	Assisted/resisted pelvis rotation exercises	Inadequate suspension/ pistoning	Check socket fit, socket ply, and suspension
				Foot set in excessive plantar flexion	Evaluate static alignment of prosthetic limb

Fig. 24.17, Cont'd

(negative likelihood ratio = 0.08) for individuals with two or more falls.[65] A cut-off of ≤50.5 points on the Berg Balance Scale identified those with two or more falls with 88% sensitivity (negative likelihood ratio = 0.17).[65]

WALKING ABILITY

The 6-Minute Walk Test has been used to help discriminate between individuals of different Medicare Functional Classification K-Levels (MFCL) and is a test that is commonly used to evaluate the ability to walk community distances.[4] The 2-Minute Walk Test has been shown to be predictive of 6-Minute Walk Test distance in individuals with lower-limb amputation.[68] The 2-Minute Walk Test has also demonstrated the ability to discriminate walking performance of prosthetic users based on cause of amputation, amputation level, health risk classification, MFCL K-level, and age.[7] The average 2-Minute Walk Test Distance for individuals with transfemoral amputation is 135.6 ± 30.1 m, with a gait speed of 68.0 ± 14.8 m/min or 1.13 ± 0.25 m/s.[7]

The L-Test is another performance-based outcome measure of mobility performance and is a modification of the TUG that, in addition to walking speed, incorporates evaluation of sit to stand, 90-degree turns to the right and left, two 180-degree turns, and stand to sit.[69,70] The L-Test has been shown to have excellent reliability and validity for individuals with lower-limb amputation.[69] An improvement of 4.5 seconds on the L-Test has been estimated to reflect a minimum clinically important difference (MCID) on mobility performance.[70]

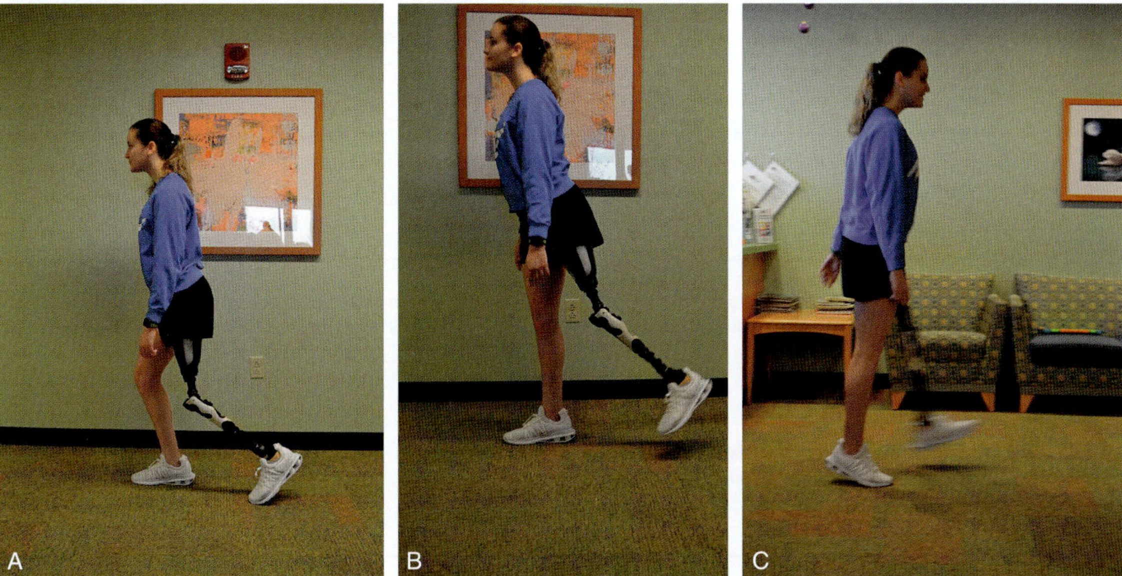

Fig. 24.18 Sagittal plane gait deviation examples. (A) An unstable prosthetic knee during stance phase often results in a quick, short step taken by the sound limb. The problem may be caused by hip extensor weakness, hip flexion contracture, or anterior displacement of the prosthetic knee. (B) Excessive knee flexion/heel rise in early swing delays the extension of the knee, which is necessary to prepare for the next initial contact. (C) Vaulting describes exaggerated plantar flexion of the intact ankle, which provides clearance for the prosthesis during swing phase. (Courtesy Shriners Hospital Portland, Oregon.)

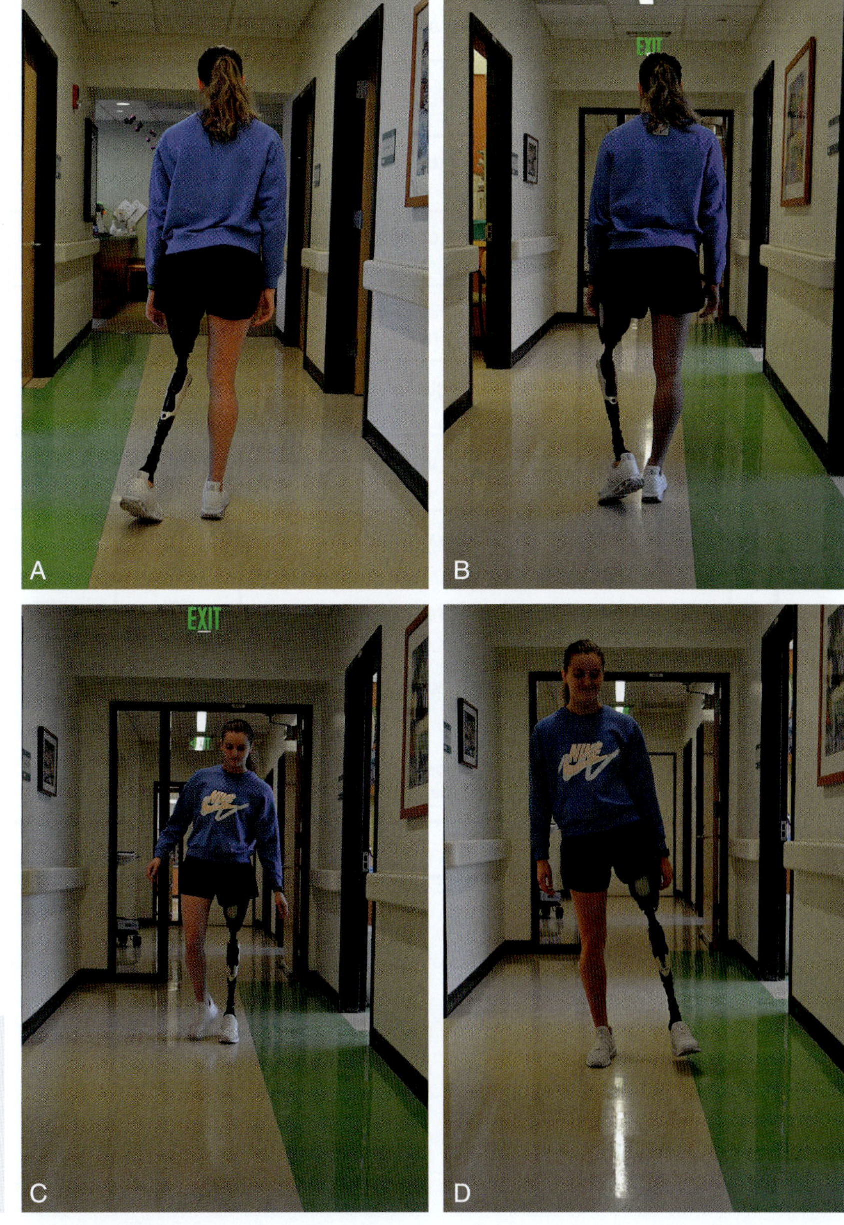

Fig. 24.19 Frontal plane gait deviation examples. (A) A lateral whip describes the shank and foot swinging in a lateral arc. (B) A medial whip describes the opposite movement. (C) Lateral trunk bending over the prosthesis is typically the result of discomfort in the perineum. (D) With circumduction, the prosthesis swings in a wide lateral arc to facilitate toe clearance in swing. (Courtesy Shriners Hospital Portland, Oregon.)

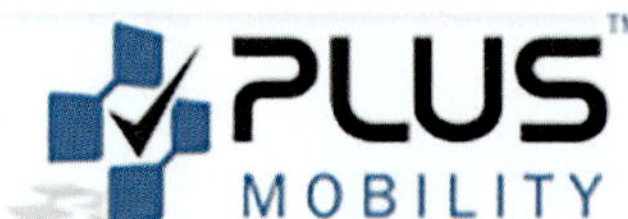

Name: ______________________ **Date:** ______________

Instructions: Please respond to all questions as if you were wearing the prosthetic leg(s) you use most days. If you would normally use a cane, crutch, or walker to perform the task, please answer the questions as if you were using that device.

Please choose "unable to do" if you:

- Would need help from another person to complete the task,
- Would need a wheelchair or scooter to complete the task, or
- Feel the task may be unsafe for you

Please mark one box per row.

Question	Without any difficulty	With a little difficulty	With some difficulty	With much difficulty	Unable to do
1. Are you able to walk a short distance in your home?	☐ (5)	☐ (4)	☐ (3)	☐ (2)	☐ (1)
2. Are you able to step up and down curbs?	☐ (5)	☐ (4)	☐ (3)	☐ (2)	☐ (1)
3. Are you able to walk across a parking lot?	☐ (5)	☐ (4)	☐ (3)	☐ (2)	☐ (1)
4. Are you able to walk over gravel surfaces?	☐ (5)	☐ (4)	☐ (3)	☐ (2)	☐ (1)
5. Are you able to move a chair from one room to another?	☐ (5)	☐ (4)	☐ (3)	☐ (2)	☐ (1)
6. Are you able to walk while carrying a shopping basket in one hand?	☐ (5)	☐ (4)	☐ (3)	☐ (2)	☐ (1)
7. Are you able to keep walking when people bump into you?	☐ (5)	☐ (4)	☐ (3)	☐ (2)	☐ (1)
8. Are you able to walk on an unlit street or sidewalk?	☐ (5)	☐ (4)	☐ (3)	☐ (2)	☐ (1)
9. Are you able to keep up with others when walking?	☐ (5)	☐ (4)	☐ (3)	☐ (2)	☐ (1)
10. Are you able to walk across a slippery floor?	☐ (5)	☐ (4)	☐ (3)	☐ (2)	☐ (1)
11. Are you able to walk down a steep gravel driveway?	☐ (5)	☐ (4)	☐ (3)	☐ (2)	☐ (1)
12. Are you able to hike about 2 miles on uneven surfaces, including hills?	☐ (5)	☐ (4)	☐ (3)	☐ (2)	☐ (1)

www.plus-m.org PLUS-M™ 12-item Short Form (v1.2)

A

Fig. 24.20 (A) Prosthetic Limb Users Survey of Mobility (PLUS-M) 12-item. (B) Prosthetic Limb Users Survey of Mobility (PLUS-M) 7-item.

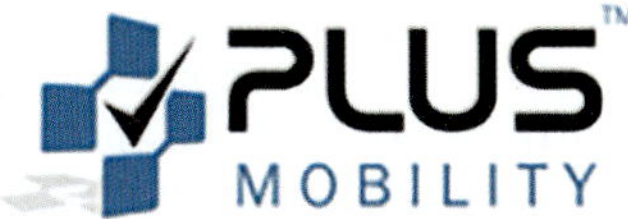

Name: ______________________ **Date:** ____________

Instructions: Please respond to all questions as if you were wearing the prosthetic leg(s) you use most days. If you would normally use a cane, crutch, or walker to perform the task, please answer the questions as if you were using that device.

Please choose "unable to do" if you:

- Would need help from another person to complete the task,
- Would need a wheelchair or scooter to complete the task, or
- Feel the task may be unsafe for you

Please mark one box per row.

Question	Without any difficulty	With a little difficulty	With some difficulty	With much difficulty	Unable to do
1. Are you able to walk a short distance in your home?	☐ (5)	☐ (4)	☐ (3)	☐ (2)	☐ (1)
2. Are you able to step up and down curbs?	☐ (5)	☐ (4)	☐ (3)	☐ (2)	☐ (1)
3. Are you able to walk while carrying a shopping basket in one hand?	☐ (5)	☐ (4)	☐ (3)	☐ (2)	☐ (1)
4. Are you able to keep walking when people bump into you?	☐ (5)	☐ (4)	☐ (3)	☐ (2)	☐ (1)
5. Are you able to keep up with others when walking?	☐ (5)	☐ (4)	☐ (3)	☐ (2)	☐ (1)
6. Are you able to walk down a steep gravel driveway?	☐ (5)	☐ (4)	☐ (3)	☐ (2)	☐ (1)
7. Are you able to hike about 2 miles on uneven surfaces, including hills?	☐ (5)	☐ (4)	☐ (3)	☐ (2)	☐ (1)

www.plus-m.org PLUS-M™ 7-item Short Form (v1.2)

B

Fig. 24.20, Cont'd

COGNITIVE FUNCTION

A systematic review found that for individuals with lower-limb amputation due to vascular pathology, cognitive ability was a significant predictor for successful use of a prosthesis.[71] However, the systematic review found that there was a lack of consistency in how cognitive ability was defined and evaluated.[71] There is limited agreement on the optimal tool for assessment of cognitive function to predict successful use of lower-limb prostheses; however, those with dementia, impaired memory, and/or impaired attention are more likely to have worse outcomes related to prosthetic use.[71] A recent study also found that cognitive impairment and increased depressive symptoms on the Hospital Anxiety and Depression Scale were associated with worse perceived physical function for individuals with lower-limb amputation.[72]

Responsiveness of Outcome Measures

The selection of appropriate outcome measures is critical to enable clinicians to more objectively assess the outcomes of rehabilitation for prosthetic users with lower-limb amputation. Clinicians should select outcome measures that not only have established validity to measure the outcome of interest, but that are also reliable and reproducible to monitor and individual's progress with rehabilitation over time. Responsiveness of an outcome measure describes the ability of an outcome measure to detect change over time and is a critical psychometric property for clinicians to consider to objectively measure the efficacy of a therapeutic intervention.[73] MDC scores are reported to inform clinicians that an observed change or improvement in performance is reflective of true change beyond that which could be explained by error or variability in the measurement.[73] MCID is the threshold of change beyond which an individual will perceive therapeutic benefit or functional improvement.[73] Table 24.3 provides a summary of MDC and MCID values for select outcome measures for prosthetic users with lower-limb amputation.

Table 24.3 Summary of Responsiveness for Select Outcome Measures for Individuals With Lower Limb Amputation

Outcome Measure	Minimum Detectable Change (MDC)	Minimum Clinically Important Difference (MCID)
Amputee Mobility Predictor	MDC(90) = 3.4[74]	
Activity-Specific Balance Confidence Scale	MDC(90) = 0.49[64] MDC(95) = 0.58[64]	
2-Minute Walk Test	MDC(90) = 34.3 m[73,74]	MCID = 37.2 m[75]
6-Minute Walk Test	MDC(90) = 45 m[73,74,76]	
L-Test	MDC(95) = 6.2 s[69,76]	MCID = 4.5 s[70]
TUG	MDC(90) = 1.28–3.6 s[74,76,77]	
PLUS-M	12-item Short Form[64] MDC(90) = 4.5 MDC(95) = 5.36 7-item Short Form MDC(90) = 4.69 MDC(95) = 5.59	
CHAMP	MDC(95) = 3.74[78]	

CHAMP, Comprehensive High-Level Activity Mobility Predictor; *PLUS-M*, Prosthetic Limb Users Survey of Mobility; *TUG*, Timed Up and Go Test.

Case Example 24.2

R.L. is a 47-year-old female with history of right transfemoral amputation due to complications of a nonhealing right transtibial amputation. R.L. has history of type 2 diabetes mellitus, obesity, hypertension, hyperlipidemia, peripheral arterial disease, and stage 2 chronic kidney disease. R.L. has been using a transfemoral prosthesis for the last 18 months. She was initially fit with a prosthesis with the Össur Total Knee 2000, a polycentric knee equipped with adjustable stance flexion, hydraulic swing control adjustment, and an adjustable extension promoter. R.L. is referred to outpatient physical therapy for prosthetic training because her prosthesis has recently been upgraded to a microprocessor-controlled knee. During observational gait analysis R.L. is demonstrating a hip-hike/circumduction pattern during swing limb advancement on the right, decreased right knee flexion during swing limb advancement, and increased trunk flexion during stance phase of gait on the right. R.L. complains that she is unable to walk longer distance due to complaints of gradually increased pain in her left leg with activity. She reports that the pain resolves with rest.

During the physical therapy assessment R.L. achieves the following scores:

- 2-Minute Walk Test = 284 ft (gait speed = 0.72 m/s)
- Timed Up and Go Test = 14.3 s
- Four-Square Step Test = 15.8 s

QUESTIONS TO CONSIDER

- What are the most likely patient-related causes of the gait deviations observed above?
- What are the most likely prosthesis-related causes of the gait deviations observed above?
- What are the benefits versus tradeoffs of a polycentric/hydraulic prosthetic knee compared to a microprocessor-controlled prosthetic knee?
- What would be appropriate exercise-based interventions to address the gait deviations observed?
- What is your overall interpretation of R.L.'s performance on the outcome measures performed during the physical therapy assessment? Does she need skilled PT intervention? Provide rationale to support your answer.
- Based on R.L.'s history, what is the most likely cause of her left lower extremity pain? What would you need to evaluate further?

DAILY WALKING

Many performance-based outcomes in rehabilitation literature are focused on assessment of the capacity for activity compared to improvements in activity performance in daily life, or what people actually do on a day-to-day basis.[79] Individuals with limb loss are at increased risk for health complications including arthritis, low back pain, obesity, diabetes, peripheral artery disease, heart disease, lung disease, depression, and premature mortality; and the risk is amplified by lower levels of activity following amputation.[80] A recent scoping review found that individuals with unilateral transfemoral amputation average 3553 steps per day, and those with bilateral transfemoral amputation average just 1387 steps per day, which is significantly below the recommended daily target of 10,000 steps per day for general health and wellness.[80] This suggests that steps per day may be a valuable outcome measure to assess actual activity performance for individuals with transfemoral amputation, which may also help promote development of habits for general health and wellness in this population.[80]

RETURN TO RUNNING

Athletic options for persons with limb loss are addressed in Chapter 28, but some individuals recovering from transfemoral amputation may have goals for return to running. The DoD EACE has given recommended criteria for individuals with unilateral transfemoral amputation or knee disarticulation with goals for return to running (Box 24.2). Clinicians can use these criteria as therapeutic targets and goals for a prerunning program for individuals with goals for return to running.

Return to running and sports requires a combination of strength, power, static and dynamic balance, prosthetic control, agility, ability to move in multiple planes of motion, and cardiovascular endurance. The Comprehensive High-Level Activity Mobility Predictor (CHAMP) is a reliable and valid performance-based assessment tool to determine readiness for return to running and higher-level sports, recreation, and vocational activities following lower extremity limb loss.[78,81–83] Recently, it was reported that the 2-Minute Walk Test is highly correlated with performance on the CHAMP and may be a reasonable alternative assessment of high-level mobility capability for prosthetic users with lower-limb amputation.[83]

Box 24.2 Recommended Criteria for Return to Run Programming

- No earlier than 4–6 months postamputation
- DEXA, scan at the discretion of the physician.
- Wear prosthesis throughout the day without skin breakdown
- Walk a mile without an assistive device
- Score of ~40 s on single-leg bridge test (with 8-inch towel roll)
- Single-leg stance greater than 3–6 s (prosthetic side)
- Single-leg step up on residual limb x10 on 6-inch step without UE support
- AMPPRO ≥K3 (≥40.5 ± 3.9)

DEXA, Dual-energy X-ray absorptiometry; *UE,* upper extremity.

References

The complete listing of the References are available in the accompanying enhanced eBook version included with the print purchase of this textbook. Visit Elsevier eBooks+ (eBooks.Health.Elsevier.com) to access this content.

25 Prosthetic Options for Persons With High-Level and Bilateral Amputations

CAROL ANN MILLER, WILLIAM HOLBROOK, AND MILAGROS JORGE

LEARNING OBJECTIVES

On completion of this chapter, the reader will be able to do the following:

1. Discuss the incidence and prevalence of high-level and bilateral lower limb amputations.
2. Describe the etiology of high-level and bilateral lower limb amputations.
3. Identify primary biomechanical limitations of hip disarticulation and higher-level prostheses.
4. Estimate the relative energy cost of ambulation with high-level or bilateral lower limb loss.
5. Describe the prosthetic and rehabilitation needs of persons with high-level and bilateral lower limb amputations.

High-level amputation including transpelvic, hip disarticulation, and bilateral amputations of the lower extremity are most often the result of traumatic accident or disease pathology such as malignant tumor of the limb or pelvis, peripheral vascular disease associated with complications from diabetes, malignant tumors, or limb infection. Hip disarticulation and transpelvic amputation is most often necessary due to invasive tumors of the bone and soft tissue of the femur or pelvis or from significant lower limb infection.[1] In the 21st century, increased incidence and prevalence of traumatic high-level and bilateral lower limb amputations is associated with war injuries sustained from the use of land mines, improvised explosive devices (IEDs), and combat fire.[1,2] Advances in military body armor have saved the lives of many soldiers, which would otherwise perish, at the cost of high-level amputations of the extremities.[3] High-level amputation whether the result of disease or traumatic accident presents unique challenges for prosthetic function and fit due to the extent of musculoskeletal and soft tissue involvement.[1–5] Additionally, for those requiring transpelvic amputation there is greater potential for pelvic organ involvement, which can create significant challenges for prosthetic fit.[5]

Peripheral vascular disease—either primary or diabetes related—is the leading cause of bilateral lower limb amputations in the United States.[4,6] Dysvascular symptoms are generally most pronounced in the distal limb, leading to nonhealing ulceration, infection, gangrene, and ablation. Vascular disease sometimes, although rarely, leads to higher-level transpelvic and hip disarticulation amputations.[7,8] The trunk and upper thigh are usually spared even in the presence of severe peripheral vascular disease. The assumptions about healing, cardiovascular limitations, and tolerance of activity derived from experience with dysvascular amputations do not apply to patients with traumatic high-level amputations. Most of the latter occur in individuals who are relatively healthy and have reasonable cardiopulmonary reserves, excellent cognition, and a strong desire to attempt the use of a prosthesis.

High-level and bilateral lower limb loss, especially when the result of disease creates substantial challenges to the patient, the prosthetist, and other rehabilitation professionals. Individuals with high-level and bilateral limb loss require sufficient aerobic capacity to meet the increased cardiovascular demands of walking, good core/trunk muscle strength, effective motor coordination and balance, and the ability to control the weight of the prosthesis for optimal function and community participation. As such, many individuals with high-level and bilateral transfemoral amputation may benefit from a well-fitted wheelchair as the primary assistive device for community mobility.[9,10]

Although successful fitting of a prosthesis can often be time-consuming and difficult for many individuals with high-level or bilateral lower extremity amputations, prostheses can enhance functional independence and mobility. The purpose of this chapter is to summarize key concepts for the prescription and fabrication of prostheses in individuals with high-level transfemoral and bilateral lower extremity amputations and provide an overview of rehabilitation guidelines, which are based on clinical factors, research evidence, and expected outcomes.

High-Level Lower Limb Loss

The first part of this chapter focuses on options for patients with a unilateral high-level lower limb loss, which is an amputation at or above the hip joint. Hip disarticulation, transpelvic and translumbar losses have been estimated to comprise fewer than 2% of all amputations in the United States.[11] As a result, only those clinicians associated with specialty centers, such as major trauma hospitals, have the opportunity to see significant numbers of such cases. Most prosthetists, therapists, and physicians see only a handful of patients with such high-level loss in a practice lifetime. One result of treating each high-level patient on such an individualized basis is that many different prosthetic and rehabilitation approaches can be found in the literature.

CAUSES OF HIGH-LEVEL AMPUTATION

Hip disarticulation and transpelvic amputation, high-level amputation, is a relatively rare with the incidence being reported at 0.5% to 3.0%.[11,12] Causes of high-level amputation include malignancy, end-stage vascular disease, infection, and trauma. Causes for transpelvic amputation are similar. The most common indications for transpelvic and hip disarticulation are malignancy or locally aggressive and destructive tumors of the bone and soft tissue of the femur, pelvis, and adjacent muscles.[1] Reportedly, the 1-year mortality rate is significant, 35% to 40%, most often due to postoperative infections and readmission for medical conditions related to the severity of the cause for high-level amputation.[13–15]

Although limb-sparing techniques are improving for individuals who have amputation due to sarcomas, there are significantly more medical and postoperative complications, greater postoperative pain, and increased morbidity and mortality associated with high-level amputation.[1,15–18] Fortunately, the frequency of tumor-related high-level amputation is decreasing with advances in limb salvage procedures and more effective chemotherapy and radiation therapy.[19–22]

Other indications for high-level amputation include soft tissue infection, such as necrotizing fasciitis of the lower limb with or without sepsis, periprosthetic infection following total hip joint replacement, and significant peripheral vascular disease resulting in limb gangrene; both infection and peripheral vascular disease are also associated with higher mortality.[14,22,23] These serious medical conditions necessitate immediate surgical intervention and aggressive medical management following high-level amputation to achieve successful outcomes.

In civilian life, work-related and motor vehicle traumatic accidents are rare causes of high-level lower extremity amputation. Globally, however, the use of land mines in many developing nations throughout the 20th and 21st centuries has contributed to an increase in high-level limb loss. Military conflicts in Iraq and Afghanistan and the use of IEDs have created numerous wounded warriors who survived significant trauma and were transported to military hospitals for extensive medical care and rehabilitation.[3,5,24–26] Because of these war conflicts, there are now a greater number of individuals with hip disarticulation living in the United States.[5,24] Hip disarticulation and other high-level lower limb amputation from traumatic injury often necessitate lifesaving emergency medical and surgical interventions.

Whether the result of disease or trauma, high-level amputation results in high morbidity and decreased self-reported quality of life—physically and mentally. Morbidity is more often associated with cause of the amputation, depression, increased phantom and residual limb pain, greater dependency in activities of daily living (ADLs), and decreased community mobility.[15,16,25,27–29]

To address issues related to morbidity, recent advances in surgical management are focusing on reducing soft tissue issues due to trauma, phantom and limb pain, and prosthetic limitations associated with socket use for high-level amputation. For example, for individuals with significant damage from trauma, pelvic floor reconstruction using longer lower limb residual muscles, such as the hamstring, is able to provide improved soft tissue coverage, which can allow for more optimal prosthetic fitting.[5] Targeted muscle reinnervation, a nerve transfer technique redirecting a major peripheral nerve into an intact nerve, is associated with reduction in phantom and residual limb pain.[13,30] In addition, skeletal transcutanous osseointegration (OI) for hip disarticulation is found to be effective in improving physical function for a young individual who was "intolerant to a traditional socket following a traumatic war-related "blast inury."[31]

A multidisciplinary rehabilitation team experienced in the management of persons with high-level amputations is essential to assure the most desirable outcomes for individuals with high-level amputation.[32,33] Most patients with high-level amputation should be offered the opportunity to be fitted with a prosthesis and for rehabilitation. The benefits of early prosthetic fitting are well established and offer benefit both physically and psychologically.[19] Patients who require amputation because of tumor can be divided into two groups: those with benign or fully contained tumors who require no further oncologic intervention and those undergoing chemotherapy and radiation after amputation. Persons with benign or fully contained tumors are typically in excellent physical condition after their amputations, eager to return to their former lives as much as possible, and ready for early fitting of a prosthesis. High-level amputation as a result of vascular disease, especially in those with preoperative coronary artery disease, is associated with unsuccessful prosthetic fitting.[28] Successful prosthetic rehabilitation is possible in these cases, but will require careful medical monitoring throughout the continuum of rehabilitation (Case Example 25.1).

Early rehabilitation should focus on mobilization, and single-limb gait training on the contralateral limb with an appropriate assistive device is recommended to reduce the risk of deconditioning, which occurs even after a few days of hospitalization following high-level limb loss.[32,33] The rehabilitation and management of patients requiring chemotherapy or radiation therapy, or undergoing extensive antibiotic treatment to resolve infection, may have to be adapted or delayed depending on the patient's physical condition, energy level, tolerance of activity, and stage of healing. Physical therapists working with individuals with high-level amputations are encouraged to initiate discussion with the prosthetist for immediate postoperative fitting, which will facilitate mobility and gait training as soon as possible.[34]

Biomechanical Principles

Although, historically, loss of the entire lower limb assumed the use of locked joints in the prosthesis, ample clinical evidence indicates that locked prosthetic joints are seldom necessary. Since the 1950s, free-motion hip, knee, and ankle joints for hip disarticulation and transpelvic prostheses have become the norm. The Canadian design hip disarticulation prosthesis was introduced by Colin McLaurin,[35] and its biomechanics were clarified by Radcliffe in 1957.[36] These same biomechanical principles also apply to the functional design of prostheses for patients with higher-level amputation.

In essence, the high-level prosthesis is stabilized by the ground reaction force (GRF), which occurs during walking.[37] For example, when standing quietly in the prosthesis, the person's weight-bearing line falls posterior to the hip joint, anterior to the knee joint, and anterior to the ankle joint. The resultant hip and knee extension moments are

Case Example 25.1 A Patient With Traumatic Hip Disarticulation

J.S. is a 20-year-old male with a traumatic hip disarticulation amputation caused by a motorcycle accident 2 weeks earlier. His residual limb is healed but complicated by multiple skin grafts and insensate areas in the abdominal region from the amount of trauma. He is eager to return to college as quickly as possible to avoid having to repeat this semester's courses but must walk several blocks to various buildings on the small, hilly campus. He has a lean, athletic build and demonstrates excellent balance and strength when ambulating on his remaining limb with bilateral forearm crutches.

QUESTIONS TO CONSIDER

- What additional information might be gathered to help determine J.S.'s potential to use a hip disarticulation prosthesis? How does his medical history and reason for amputation affect his rehabilitation prognosis?
- How should J.S.'s readiness to be fitted with a prosthesis be determined? What tests and measurements should be used?
- What major concerns or challenges will J.S., his prosthetist, and his rehabilitation team face in fitting his hip disarticulation prosthesis?
- What options for socket and suspension will the team likely consider for J.S., given his functional needs and prognosis?
- What factors will influence the choice of knee unit for J.S.'s prosthesis? What type of knee should be recommended? Why?
- What factors will influence the choice of a prosthetic foot for J.S.'s prosthesis? What type of foot should be recommended? Why?
- How should J.S.'s rehabilitation goals be prioritized as he begins his prosthesis training? How should his rehabilitation progress? How should the efficacy of intervention be assessed to determine how well these goals have been met?
- How should the International Classification of Function Core Set for persons following amputation be applied to this patient?

RECOMMENDATIONS

On the basis of findings during the evaluation and discussion with J.S. about his current functional needs and ultimate goals for the use of a prosthesis, the team recommends an initial endoskeletal prosthesis with a flexible silicone inner socket with a composite external frame socket that includes additional gel padding in the region of the tender grafted skin, a microprocessor-controlled stance and swing-control hydraulic knee, dynamic-response foot, and torque absorber. The clinical team considered first providing a less complex knee but decided against that option because it would require training to use a less responsive prosthesis followed by retraining with the microprocessor knee more appropriate for his projected functional abilities, thereby increasing the duration of his rehabilitation.

Intensive in-patient therapy should be focused on intensive core training, aerobic conditioning exercises without the prosthesis, and gait training first within the parallel bars and then with his forearm crutches to facilitate J.S.'s return to campus. He will continue with outpatient therapy until his gait has matured and will most likely learn to ambulate with no balance aids. When his socket no longer fits because of normal postoperative atrophy, he will receive a socket replacement and protective covering for the prosthesis but will continue to use the same functional components originally provided for as long as they remain functionally appropriate for his needs. Based on his past medical history, he has excellent potential to participate in both recreational and advanced sports activities with and without a prosthesis. If this is a goal for him, he would need to be reevaluated and fitted with a sports specific prosthetic.

resisted by mechanical hyperextension stops of the prosthetic hip and knee joints, and the dorsiflexion moment is resisted by the stiffness of the prosthetic foot (Fig. 25.1).

Ambulation with a high-level prosthesis also relies on the GRF (Fig. 25.2). When an experienced prosthetic wearer walks with an optimally aligned hip disarticulation or transpelvic prosthesis, the dynamic gait is surprisingly smooth and consistent. The basic functions of the GRF during ambulation with one type of high-level prosthesis can be summarized as follows: At initial contact, as the prosthetic heel touches the ground, the GRF passes posterior to the ankle axis, the heel cushion compresses, and the foot is lowered to the ground. At the same time an extension moment is created at the prosthetic knee as the GRF passes anterior to the knee joint axis (see Fig. 25.2A). By midstance, alignment stability is maximal as the GRF passes posterior to the prosthetic hip joint axis and anterior to the prosthetic knee joint axis, just as it does during quiet standing (see Fig. 25.2B). As forward progression continues into preswing, the GRF moves posterior to the knee joint axis, allowing the knee to bend passively and facilitate swing-phase foot clearance while weight is being shifted onto the opposite limb (see Fig. 25.2C).

Two major biomechanical deficits are inherent with hip disarticulation and transpelvic prostheses. First, the prosthetic limb is always fully extended at midswing because of the loss of active hip flexion. As a result, the length of the prosthesis is typically shortened slightly compared with the length of the remaining limb to assist in toe clearance during the swing phase of gait. The consequence of this strategy, however, is a second biomechanical deficit—limb-length discrepancy.[38] However, due to many advances in prosthetic knee and foot componentry, these deficits are greatly reduced.

Socket Design and Suspension

A variety of socket designs have been described in the clinical literature; however, there is lack of high-quality evidence supporting the benefits of the various socket types and prosthetic components on gait, user satisfaction, and energy expenditure.[10] The most critical factors for their successful use are careful fitting and secure suspension regardless of which socket design is selected. For patients with hip disarticulation, encapsulation of the ascending pubic ramus may add stability, although not every patient is able to tolerate a proximal trim line in the perineum. Suspension is achieved by carefully contouring the socket just proximal to the iliac crests whenever possible. The socket should provide stability from front to back, side to side, and top to bottom. The interior of the hip disarticulation socket is fabricated from

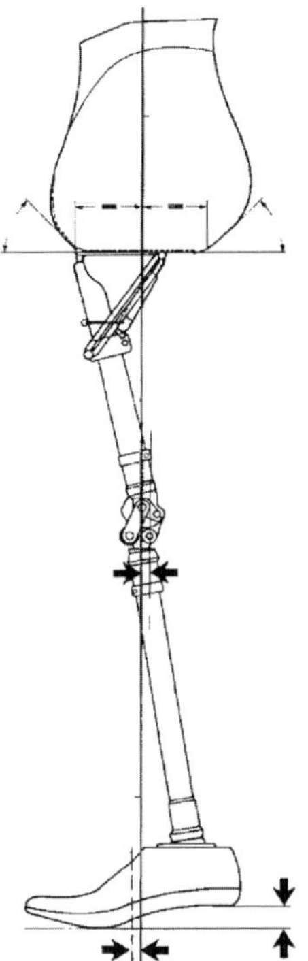

Fig. 25.1 Static balance with a high-level lower limb prosthesis is achieved when the ground reaction force passes posterior to the hip joint and anterior to the knee and ankle joints. The resulting extensor moments at the hip and knee and dorsiflexion moment at the ankle make the prosthesis stable. Mechanical stops in the prosthetic joints prevent further movement and the patient is able to stand without exertion. (Courtesy Ottobock Orthopedic Industry, Inc., Minneapolis, Minnesota.)

either flexible silicone rubber (Fig. 25.3A) or thermoplastic material (see Fig. 25.3B). The socket contour prevents a pistoning action within the socket; however, the use of a silicone system can create a very warm, moist environment. A recent case study report revealed that using custom-fit shorts with permeable and elastic fabric (moisture wicking) can help mitigate some of the issues with socket comfort and excessive perspiration with the use of silicone.[39]

The prosthetic socket is statically aligned with the knee and foot components (see Fig. 25.3B and C). Prosthetic alignment is adjusted to ensure proper posture in static stance (Fig. 25.4A) and following dynamic gait assessment. When the patient is obese or has no ileum, shoulder straps may be necessary to minimize swing-phase pistoning of the prosthesis. Custom silicone design are prosthetic options that allow for improved comfort and fit and may be beneficial for patients with fluctuating volume changes, irregular shaped limb, extensive scarring, and skin graft.

The transpelvic socket must fully enclose the gluteal fold and perineal tissues and completely contain the soft tissues on the amputated side. Full enclosure provides comfortable weight bearing on the residual tissues despite the absence of a hemipelvis. Failure to contain the transpelvic residuum adequately results in obvious protrusion where the trim lines are insufficient. Prosthetists modify the positive plaster model of the transpelvic residuum to incorporate a diagonally directed compressive force in the socket design to support and contain transpelvic tissues and eliminate the risk of perineal shear and tissue breakdown.

For patients with transpelvic amputation, weight bearing is achieved with a combination of soft tissue compression and thoracic rib support (see Fig. 25.4B and C). Despite the loss of more than half of the body mass in this amputation, weight-bearing tolerance is better than might be expected.

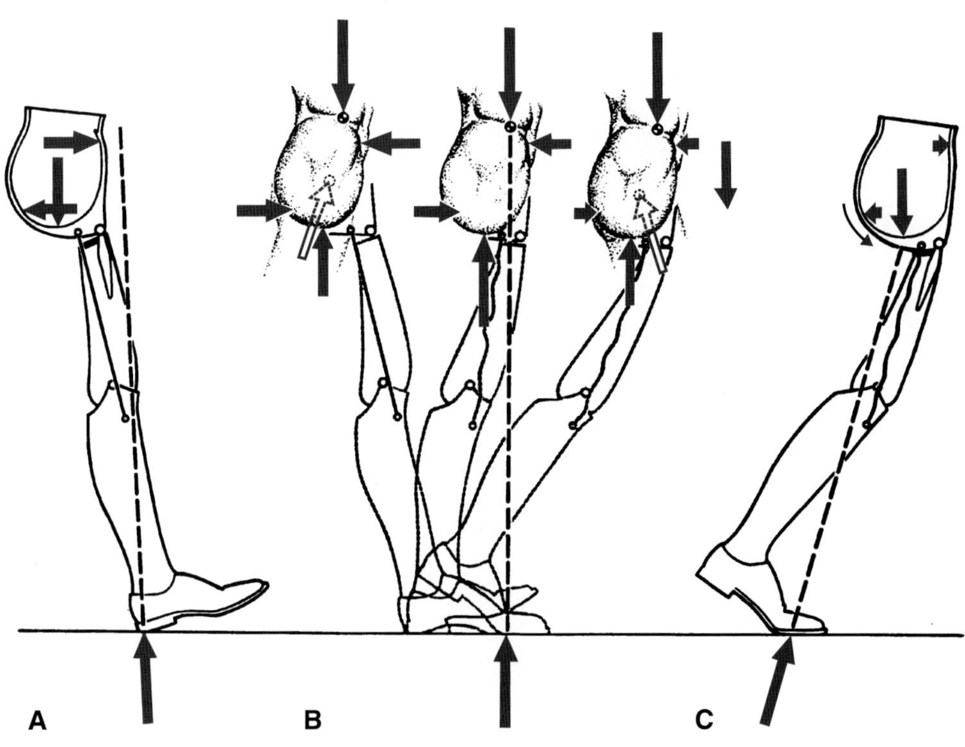

Fig. 25.2 The ground reaction force at initial contact. From loading response through midstance (A) and terminal stance (B) and just prior to preswing (C) of the gait cycle for patients using a unilateral high-level prosthesis. Once properly aligned, the prosthesis will move in a consistent, predictable fashion and permit slow but steady ambulation. The patient uses trunk motion to initiate and control prosthetic movements. (From Van der Waarde T, Michael JW. Hip disarticulation and transpelvic management: prosthetic considerations. In: Bowker JH, Michael JW, eds. *Atlas of Limb Prosthetics: Surgical, Prosthetic, and Rehabilitation Principles*. Second ed. Mosby-Year Book; 1992:539–552.)

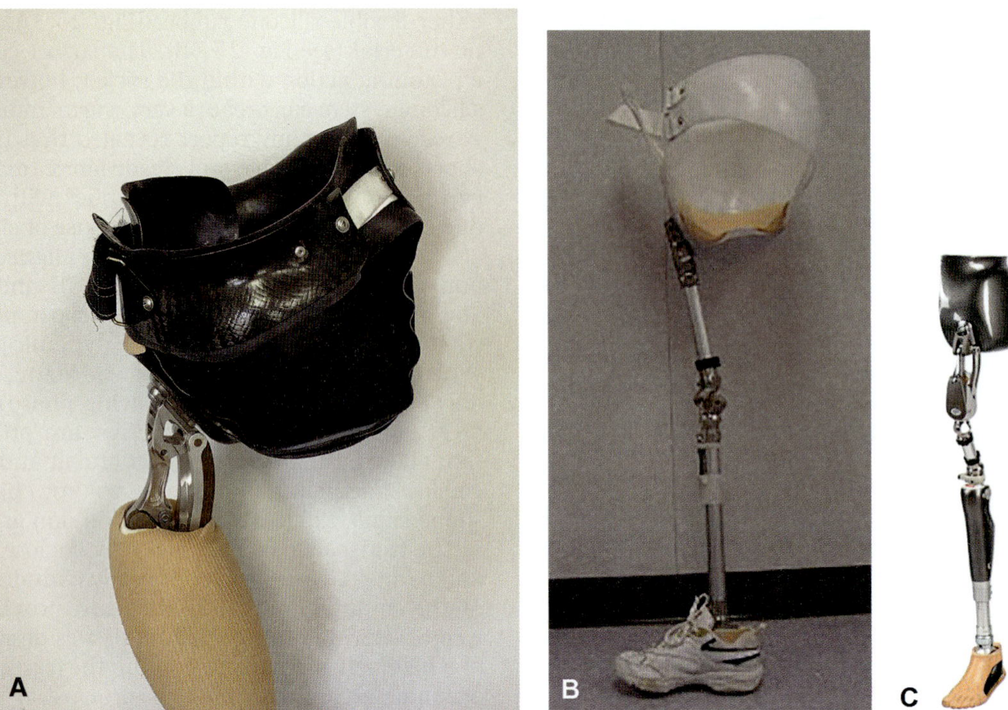

Fig. 25.3 (A) The interior of a hip disarticulation socket fabricated from flexible silicone rubber. Note the contouring of the proximal brim to encase the crest of the ileum. (B) Hip disarticulation thermoplastic socket. (C) Hip disarticulation prosthesis with components: socket, hip joint, upper pylon, rotator, knee joint, lower pylon, and foot. (A, Courtesy Fourroux Prosthetics, Atlanta, Georgia; B, From Kelly BM, Spires MC, Restrepo JA. Orthotic and prosthetic prescriptions for today and tomorrow. *Phys Med Rehabil Clin N Am*. 2007;18(4):785–858, Copyright © 2007 Elsevier Inc.; C, Courtesy Ottobock HealthCare, **www.ottobockus.com**).

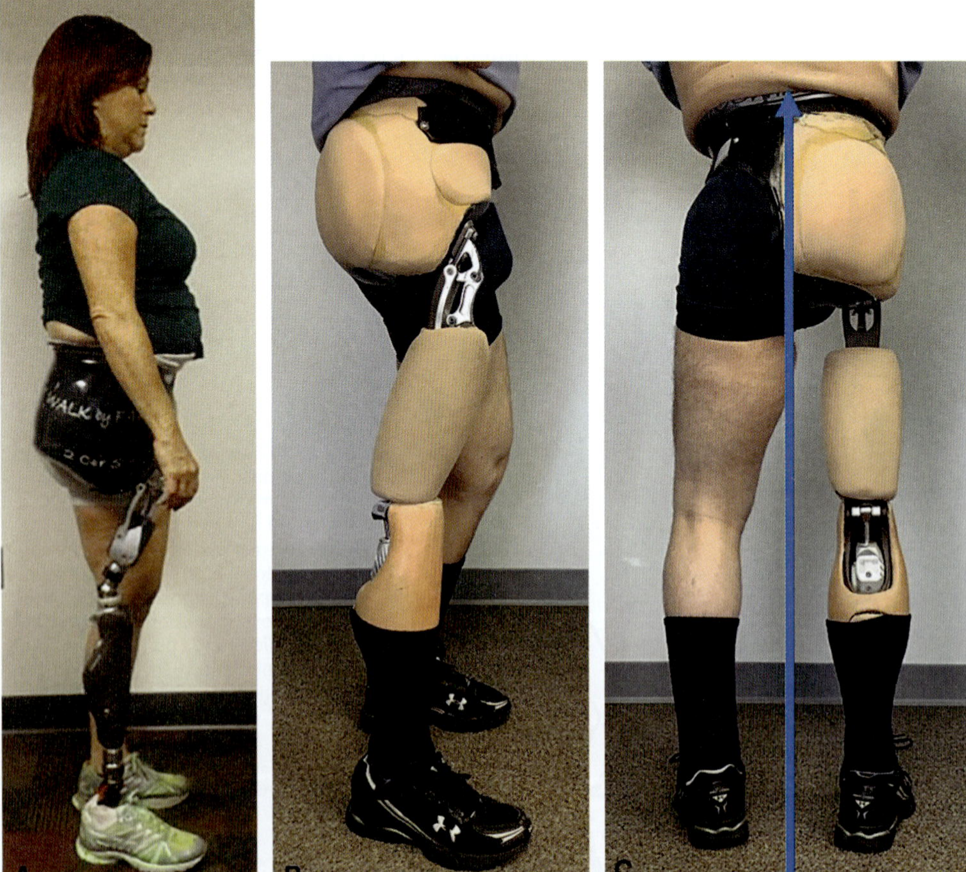

Fig. 25.4 (A) Prosthetic alignment with ground reaction force (GRF) for patient with hip disarticulation. (B) Prosthetic alignment with GRF for patient with transpelvic amputation. Note: weight bearing for transpelvic amputation is achieved with a combination of soft tissue compression and thoracic rib support (C). (Courtesy Fourroux Prosthetics, Atlanta, Georgia.)

Designs that allow the patient to vary the compression by adjustable straps are often useful. Many patients with transpelvic amputation successfully progress to ambulation for short distances with a prosthesis and may choose to wear prosthetic limbs to enhance their cosmetic appearance and self-image (Fig. 25.5). Cosmetic covering will allow the prosthesis to look anatomically correct in clothing as well as protect the componentry from the environment, such as excess moisture, dirt, and debris. Use of a cover, however, can increase the overall weight of the prosthesis and reduce ease of access to the components for servicing.

Long-term follow-up demonstrates positive outcomes; return to work or school is usually a realistic goal. To reduce the potential for postural spinal deformities with sitting and to optimize participation in the community, however, many patients with transpelvic and translumbar amputations may require a socket system for effective seating and wheeled mobility such as a pelvic leveler[40] (Fig. 25.6 A–C). Additionally, for most patients, polycentric knees provide sufficient stability for the household ambulation typical of this population, making locking joints unnecessary. The development of hip-knee-ankle systems such as the Helix 3D system from Ottobock (see Fig. 25.3C), which incorporates a microprocessor knee and ankle systems to dynamically react to the patient's gait and thus improve efficiency and safety, have dramatically improved the quality of gait obtainable by persons with high-level amputation. However, the cost may be prohibitive; these components are generally reserved for those individuals with a higher level of daily function.[41]

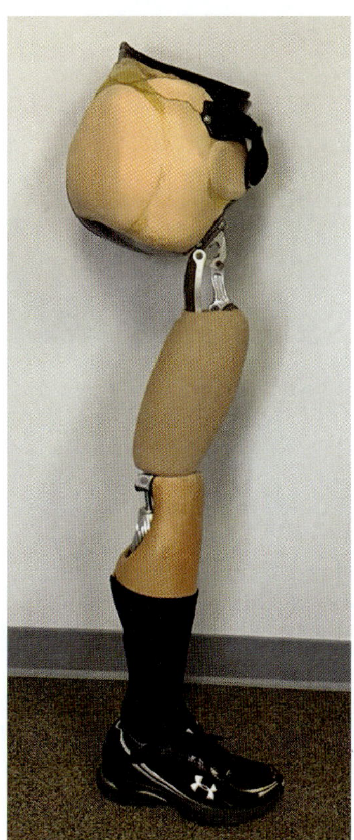

Fig. 25.5 Prosthetic cover for transpelvic amputation allows the prosthesis to look anatomically correct in clothing as well as protect the componentry from the environment, such as excess moisture, dirt, and debris. (Courtesy Fourroux Prosthetics, Atlanta, Georgia.)

Component Selection

In recent years, a strong consensus has emerged that, to meet the patient's functional needs and goals fully, components for patients with hip disarticulation and transpelvic amputations should be selected for the same reasons and with the same criteria as for those with transfemoral and transtibial amputation.[38,41–43] The assessment of components such as a passive microprocessor-controlled knee versus an active powered microprocessor-controlled knee for level walking is evaluated for each individual.[44] For individuals who had OI, the principles for biomechanical alignment of the prosthetic and the type of components selected for the hip, knee, and ankle/foot would follow a prescription that is similar for those who are prescribed a socket.[45]

CHOOSING A PROSTHETIC FOOT

All prosthetic feet have been successfully used for transpelvic and hip disarticulation high-level amputations. Nonarticulating designs are often chosen because of their dependability, durability, and low maintenance; these designs rarely require servicing as a result of wear and tear. Single-axis feet (which allow the patient to quickly attain a stable foot-flat position) are used when enhanced knee stability is a concern. Multiaxial and dynamic-response designs are usually reserved for higher-activity individuals who appreciate the added mobility of such components. Microprocessor-controlled hydraulic and externally powered prosthetic foot/ankle systems such as the Elan, Meridium, and Proprio are additional options to assist in gait, but are generally avoided due to their additional weight.[46]

CHOOSING A PROSTHETIC KNEE UNIT

The prosthetist selects a particular knee unit on the basis of the patient's functional needs. Because of the biomechanical stability of these prostheses, locked-knee designs are rarely necessary. They have two additional drawbacks: they must be unlocked before sitting and they may increase the risk of injury in the event of a fall. When stability is a primary concern, stance control or polycentric knees may be most appropriate. When properly aligned, single-axis knees also work well. The prosthetist might choose a pneumatic or hydraulic knee unit to provide fluid swing-phase control for patients who are active and want the ability to change cadence.[38,42,43,47] Most recently, quite encouraging clinical results have been reported with a microprocessor-controlled hydraulic stance- and swing-control knee, allowing active individuals to descend stairs foot over foot with a hip disarticulation prosthesis for the first time.[48,49] As with prosthetic foot/ankle systems, powered knee systems such as the Ossur Power Knee are available to provide the user with not only stance stability and free swing but also propulsion; the additional weight can prove cumbersome for many individuals. This type of knee has been found to drastically reduce energy expenditure during ambulation for younger and healthier individuals.[46]

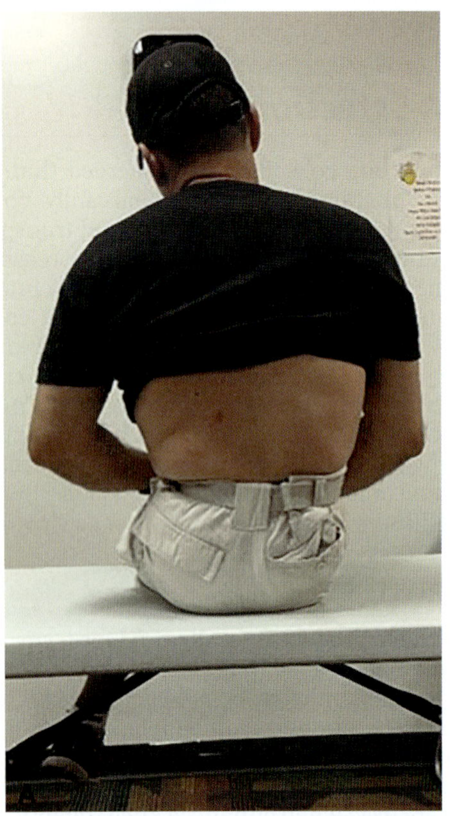

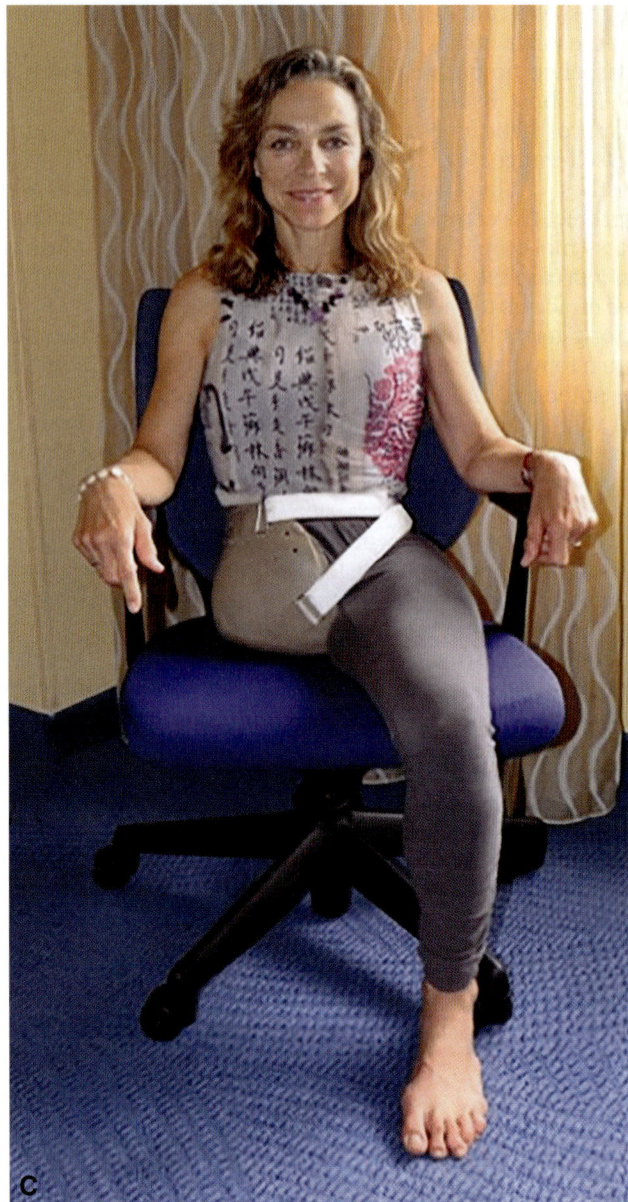

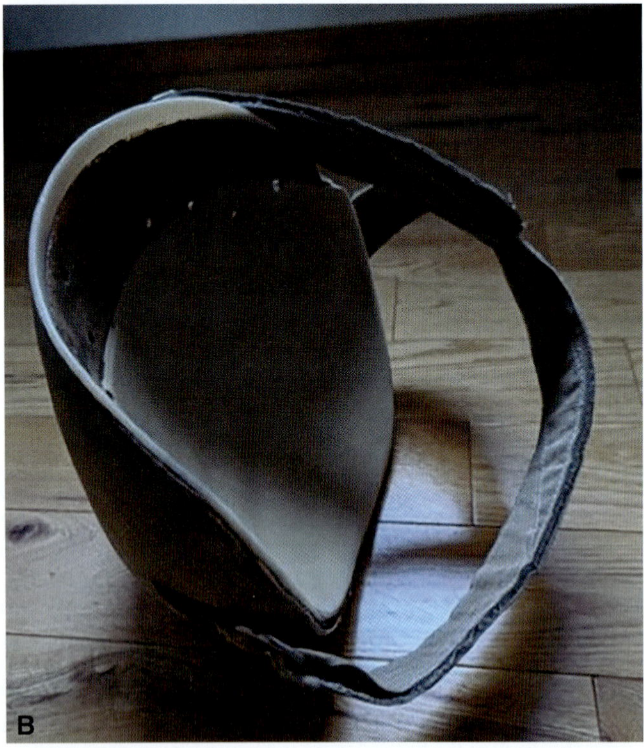

Fig. 25.6 (A) Transpelvic patient sitting posture without pelvic leveler illustrating negative effect on spinal alignment. (B) Pelvic leveler insert. (C) Pelvic leveler with lumbar sacral corset orthosis. (A, Courtesy Fourroux Prosthetics, Atlanta, Georgia; B, From Skoski C. The Pelvic Leveler an alternative to a sitting socket. *InMotion Magazine*. 2005; 15(1). Available at: **https://www.amputee-coalition.org/resources/the-pelvic-leveler/**).

CHOOSING A PROSTHETIC HIP JOINT

The majority of patients with hip disarticulation benefit from a free-motion hip joint, although locking joints are still sometimes chosen for those with limited ambulation capabilities. Great effort has been made to provide some measure of active hip flexion motion in these prostheses because that would reduce or eliminate the key biomechanical deficits previously noted. In prior decades, modification of the hip joint by adding a coil-spring mechanism that induced hip flexion when the prosthesis was unweighted was tried with some success, but maintenance and breakage of the spring precluded widespread acceptance. More recently, a flexible carbon fiber thigh strut that functions as a leaf spring has been used clinically with good success. Initial reports suggest that this approach increases cadence and that the improved swing clearance achieved by better prosthetic hip and knee flexion eliminates the need to shorten the prosthesis.[28] The use of vertical shock-absorbing shin elements and knees with stance flexion features is also being explored, with encouraging clinical acceptance. More advanced options, such as the Ottobock Helix system, also exist, providing dynamic stability and triplanar motion control, making it easier to extend the leg and clear the toe during gait.[50–52]

TORQUE ABSORBERS

With the loss of three major biologic joints of the lower limb, a corresponding loss of the body's ability to compensate for the rotary motions inherent in gait occurs. For this reason, many prosthetists strongly recommend that a torque-absorbing device be included in these high-level prostheses. Torque absorbers typically improve both stride length and comfort by absorbing rotational forces that would otherwise be transmitted to the socket as skin shear. Incorporation of a lockable turntable (*rotator*) above the prosthetic knee is also suggested to facilitate common daily activities such as dressing and entering a vehicle (Fig. 25.7).

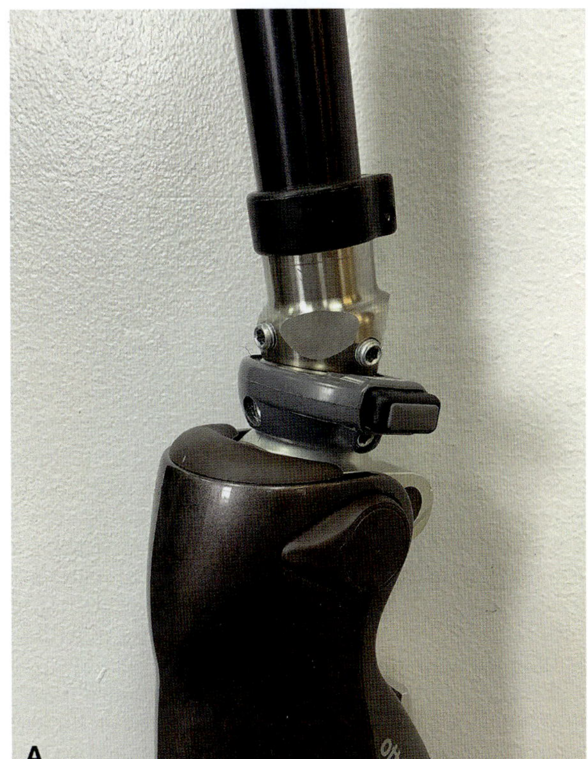

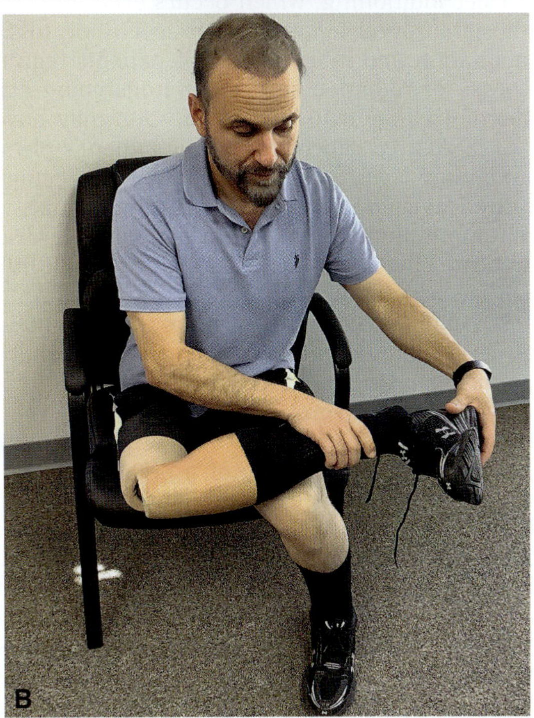

Fig. 25.7 A lockable turntable (A) positioned in the prosthesis above the prosthetic knee makes dressing, entering a vehicle, and similar daily tasks much easier for individuals with high-level amputation. (B) Additional components, including lockable turntables and torque absorbers, should always be considered for patients with high-level amputation. (A, Courtesy Ottobock Orthopedic Industry, Inc., Minneapolis, Minnesota; B, Courtesy Fourroux Prosthetic, Atlanta, Georgia.)

Energy Consumption and Cost

The major unresolved drawback to prosthetic use in those with high-level amputation is the tremendous increase in effort required to control a prosthetic limb with passive joints. Walking with a hip disarticulation or transpelvic prosthesis is energy consuming as it requires increased use of core abdominal muscles, which are not physiologically designed for quick "phasic" movement.[53] The weight of the prosthesis is also a contributing factor to the energy needed to be ambulatory. The concentration and energy required to ambulate makes short-distance ambulation much more practical than distance walking for all but the most vigorous adult wearers. Researchers investigating energy consumption during prosthetic walking and the relationship to physical fitness have reported that older persons with hip disarticulation who have good physical fitness were able to use the prosthesis successfully in community settings.[27,28,52,53]

Most rehabilitation professionals believe that any patient with an amputation who is physically and mentally capable of using a prosthetic device should, if interested, be fitted with an initial prosthesis. Recent case reports and studies illustrate successful prosthetic use, even if limited in mobility, for older adults,[54,55] and for adults with increased body mass index, advancing age, history of depression, and other comorbidities.[27,28] Although patients may opt to only use the prosthesis for limited activities, having the prosthesis available gives the user the ability to employ it situationally as needed. For example, wearing the prosthesis can be helpful especially when needing to stand for long periods of time or when needing to use both hands for manual tasks without crutches. Additionally, when the patient wishes to appear symmetric, cosmetically, wearing the prosthesis may promote greater participation in social situations. Younger patients with transpelvic and hip disarticulation surgery due to trauma are capable of intensive rehabilitation training and can become proficient users of prosthetic devices.[56] Patients that are fit with prosthetic devices and use them on a regular basis will decrease the changes of overuse of their shoulder, wrist, and elbow. Overuse of the upper extremities is a major concern, which often results from relying on increased arm propulsion while using a wheelchair, walker, crutches, etc.

Rehabilitation Outcomes After High-Level Amputation

Individuals with hip disarticulation or transpelvic amputations who have sufficient balance and strength can learn to walk without any external aids, although the use of a cane is common. Most patients with hip disarticulation or transpelvic amputations will not advance past using a cane when ambulating in large open areas or places with uneven terrain. Use of a cane gives the patient better stability and security in these situations.

Early rehabilitation should focus on mobilization, and single-limb gait training on the contralateral limb with an appropriate assistive device is recommended to reduce the risk of deconditioning, which occurs even after a few days of hospitalization following high-level limb loss.[32,33] The rehabilitation and management of patients requiring chemotherapy or radiation therapy or undergoing extensive antibiotic treatment to resolve infection may have to be adapted or delayed depending on the patient's physical condition, energy level, tolerance of activity, and stage of healing. Physical therapists working with individuals with high-level amputations are encouraged to initiate discussion with the prosthetist for immediate postoperative fitting, which will facilitate mobility and gait training as soon as possible.[34] Despite the obvious challenges that face patients with high-level amputations, a substantial percentage are able to manage a prosthetic device with appropriate training and long-term follow-up.

Although the rate of prosthesis use varies, the trend is toward increasing functional use of a prosthesis.[34,57] The use of a multidisciplinary team approach and fitting by an experienced prosthetist are believed to enhance the likelihood of success and to improve functional outcomes. In the rehabilitation of persons with lower extremity amputations, a primary functional goal is ambulation with a prosthetic device. Because these devices are very expensive and lower extremity amputations often occur in the elderly, insurance providers are faced with the task of determining who would best benefit from prosthetic equipment and how to best utilize the available resources.

There are number of outcome measures that can be implemented by physical therapists and prosthetists to determine an individual's potential for use of a prosthesis versus nonuse of the prosthetic equipment ordered.[58–63] In the United States, Medicare established K Levels or Medicare Functional Classification Levels as a structured approach to quantifying need and potential benefit of prosthetic devices for patients after lower limb amputation and are widely used to determine the predictability of persons with amputations to be effective users of prosthetic equipment[59] (Table 25.1).

Table 25.1 Medicare Functional Classification Levels

Level 0	Does not have the ability or potential to ambulate or transfer safely with or without assistance; a prosthesis does not enhance quality of life or mobility
Level 1	Has the ability or potential to use a prosthesis for transfers or ambulation on level surfaces at fixed cadence; typical of limited and unlimited household ambulators
Level 2	Has the ability or potential for ambulation with the ability to traverse low-level environmental barriers such as curbs, stairs, or uneven surfaces; typical of the limited community ambulator
Level 3	Has the ability or potential for ambulation with variable cadence; typical of the community ambulator who has the ability to traverse most environmental barriers and may have vocational, therapeutic, or exercise activity that demands utilization of a prosthesis beyond simple locomotion
Level 4	Has the ability or potential for ambulation that exceeds basic ambulation skills, exhibiting high-impact, stress, or energy levels; typical of the demands of the child, active adult, or athlete

From https://www.ncbi.nlm.nih.gov/books/NBK531517/table/ch2.tab1/

The Amputee Mobility Predictor (AMP) without a prosthesis and with the prescribed prosthesis is often implemented by physical therapists to assess functional potential. The AMP is a well-known, reliable, and valid instrument[60,61] that can be used to predict the functional classification level for those with high-level amputation. Minimal clinical difference in AMP scores have been reported,[62] which can reflect change in functional performance over time and thus support the need for future prosthetic modifications. Today, there are many validated outcome instruments that can be used to assess prosthetic potential. Implementing in practice a standardized performance-based instrument, such as the 10 m Walk test, or Timed-Up and Go, and/or self-report instrument, such as Orthotic and Prosthetic User's Satisfaction survey, will provide clinicians with effective means for determining initial abilities and for monitoring future progress.[61–63]

Lastly, detailed information on the rehabilitation of persons with amputations is covered in Chapter 26. For persons who have undergone hemipelvectomy, hip disarticulation, or multiple amputations, the rehabilitation process varies based on the precipitating events that led to the limb loss—for example, in the instance of limb loss due to IEDs, burn care may be the priority.[22] The outcomes vary based on health-related circumstances, the patient's age, and his or her motivating factors. Persons with high-level amputation should be assessed by the prosthetist and physical therapists considering the International Classification of Function model. Incorporating and documenting all data collected from a detailed examination with specific limb loss outcome measures should support the recommended prosthetic prescription for achieving the highest functional levels possible.[27,61,64]

Bilateral Lower Limb Loss

In the United States, the major cause of bilateral lower extremity limb loss is dysvascular disease with and without associated complications from diabetes. Vascular disease affects both limbs, thus individuals who have had single-limb dysvascular amputation have significant risk of eventual bilateral limb loss, which is most often the result of disease progression in the nonamputated limb.[7,12] Following amputation of a single lower limb due to peripheral artery disease with or without diabetes, contralateral limb amputation has been reported to occur at a rate of 15% over the following 2 to 3 years[65] and as high as 50% over 5 years.[66,67] Having end-stage renal disease and atherosclerosis with or without diabetes were most predictive of contralateral limb loss[65] and were also associated with greater morbity.[68]

The medical history, disease cause for necessitating bilateral amputation, and the level of amputation of each limb will present different challenges for the rehabilitation team. Whenever feasible, preservation of the knee joint on one limb offers greater potential for improved function with less extensive rehabilitation needed.[68] Individuals with bilateral above-knee amputation due to disease will require significantly greater prosthetic and physical therapy management and may not benefit from being fitted with prosthetics.[68,69] Clinical follow-up suggests that successful use of a unilateral prosthesis, for those with disease, increases the likelihood of success with bilateral artificial limbs.[70] For this reason early fitting after initial amputation is strongly advocated, even when amputation of the opposite limb seems imminent (Case Example 25.2).

In the United States, simultaneous bilateral loss is infrequent; such cases are typically the result of traumatic

Case Example 25.2 A Patient With Bilateral Lower Extremity Amputations Caused by Chronic Dysvascular/Neuropathic Disease

R.W. is a 72-year-old female who recently underwent an elective right transtibial amputation because of infection associated with diabetic neuropathy. Her residual limb is well healed and not unduly edematous, and she is eager to return to the condominium she shares with her daughter. Five years previously, R.W. underwent left transfemoral amputation after failed femoral-popliteal bypass surgery; she had been a successful full-time prosthesis wearer until she was hospitalized for her second amputation.

QUESTIONS TO CONSIDER

- What additional information might be gathered to help determine R.W.'s potential to use prostheses for her new right transtibial and existing left transfemoral residual limbs? How will her medical history and reason for amputation affect her rehabilitation prognosis?
- How should R.W.'s readiness to be fitted with a transtibial prosthesis be determined? What tests and measurements should be used to make this determination?
- What major concerns or challenges will R.W., her prosthetist, and her rehabilitation team face in fitting the new transtibial prosthesis?
- Given her functional needs and prognosis, what options for socket and suspension will the team likely consider for R.W.'s new transtibial and transfemoral prostheses?
- What factors will influence the choice of knee units for R.W.'s transfemoral prosthesis? What type of knee should be recommended? Why?
- What factors will influence the choice of prosthetic feet for R.W.'s transtibial and transfemoral prostheses? What type of foot should be recommended for each prosthesis? Why?
- How should rehabilitation goals be prioritized as R.W. begins her training?
- How should rehabilitation be assessed?
- Should R.W.'s wearing schedules for her new transtibial limb be similar to or different from her transfemoral limb? Why or why not?
- How should the efficacy of intervention be assessed to determine how well the goals have been met?
- How should the International Classification of Function Core Set for persons following amputation be applied to this patient?

RECOMMENDATIONS

Although her age and comorbidities make the use of two artificial limbs challenging, R.W. is a good candidate for bilateral fitting because of her motivation and proven success with a prior prosthesis. Her existing transfemoral prosthesis is well worn and no longer fitting optimally, so the rehabilitation team recommended that two new prostheses be prescribed.

The transtibial prosthesis will provide primary balance and propulsion and enable R.W. to rise from a seated position, applying significant forces to her residual limb. Her initial transtibial prosthesis will include a roll-on locking liner for suspension and gel spot inserts as needed to protect the residual limb and provide mediolateral stability at the knee through its supracondylar contours. She will use lightweight, solid-ankle dynamic-response prosthetic feet on both artificial limbs because she prefers these components and has found them both stable and functional with her unilateral prosthesis.

R.W.'s new transfemoral prosthesis will be similar to what she has successfully worn, with a roll-on locking liner for suspension and a flexible ischial containment socket within a rigid frame for weight bearing and rotational stability. The roll-on suspension permits donning from a seated position, which is particularly advantageous for people with bilateral amputations. Initially R.W. will wear an auxiliary elastic suspension belt for added security and rotational control.

R.W.'s unilateral prosthesis incorporated a single-axis knee with pneumatic swing control, but she will require a more mechanically stable design for bilateral stability. Because of cardiopulmonary restrictions and the loss of her second leg, the clinical team believes that she will not vary her walking pace as widely henceforth, so the weight of a pneumatic swing-control unit is no longer necessary. R.W. will receive a stable polycentric knee in her new prosthesis and undergo gait training for several weeks.

Although she is eager to have her endoskeletal prostheses finished with protective covers that make them appear more lifelike, this fabrication step will be deferred until after she has completed gait training and mastered the use of bilateral artificial limbs. R.W.'s prosthetist will see her periodically to reevaluate the alignment of both prostheses as her gait pattern matures, making small changes in alignment in response to her changing needs and balance. Once her gait pattern has stabilized, the final fabrication will be completed.

For traversing long distances, R.W. will also be prescribed a wheelchair with a posteriorly offset axle. Training in wheelchair transfers and mobility will also be an important part of her rehabilitation.

transportation or industrial accidents or electrocution. In areas of armed conflict and postwar zones, however, simultaneous limb loss is more frequent secondary to the nature of and the extent of blast injuries from roadside bombs and land mines.[56,71] Fortunately, most patients with traumatic amputations are healthy and strong and generally have a good prognosis for the successful use of prostheses.[56]

When both limbs are lost simultaneously from traumatic accident, there is greater potential for significant soft tissue damage, which often requires extensive tissue grafting. Scar tissue has significantly less extensibility resulting in skin breakdown, which can greatly affect socket comfort and fit. Additionally, there is an increased risk for developing heterotopic ossificans with associated increased limb pain, which can alter the anatomic structure of the residual limb and potentially complicate prosthetic fit. Although less commonly performed in individuals with bilateral transfemoral traumatic amputation, OI is shown to be effective in ameliorating factors associated with increased morbidity.[72] For individuals who cannot tolerate traditional socket use, a recent 10-year follow-up retrospective report illustrated that bone-anchored prosthetics was found to improve sitting comfort and increase time in everyday use of the prosthetics for function and locomotion.[72]

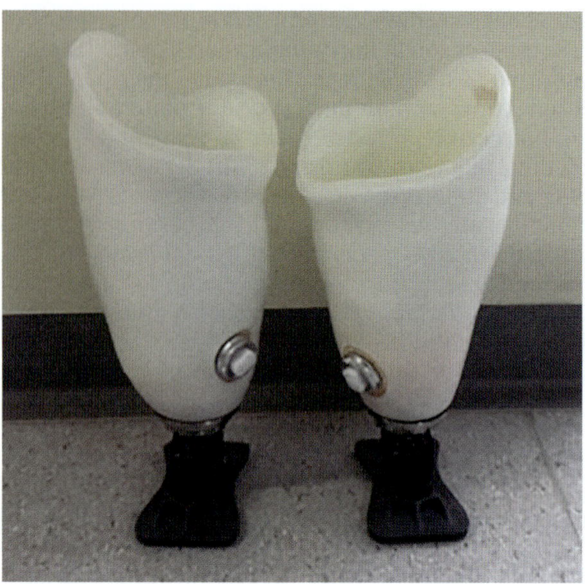

Fig. 25.8 A pair of shortened prostheses, sometimes called *stubbies*, for early gait training in patients with bilateral traumatic transfemoral amputations. In these prostheses, patients can develop postural control without having to worry about the stability of prosthetic knee units. (From Devinuwara K, Dworak-Kula A, O'Connor RJ. Rehabilitation and prosthetics post-amputation. *Orthop Trauma.* 2018;32(4):234–240. Copyright © 2018. Elsevier.)

Socket Design and Suspension

The person with bilateral lower limb loss is constantly bearing full weight on artificial limbs while walking or standing. All options to increase skin protection and comfort should be actively considered, and suspension must be as secure as possible. A soft insert and flexible sockets may be used to enhance comfort during wear and reduce the likelihood that shear forces will be problematic for the skin. Suction and/or elevated vacuum suspension—with silicone sleeves or inserts minimizing pistoning during swing phase—should be considered for those individuals who present with the appropriate characteristics, limb girth, shape, and integrity that could benefit from that suspension method. Although rarely used today, cotton or wool prosthetic socks may be used as an interface between the residual limbs and the sockets when suction suspension is not feasible. In that case, suspension would include use of a sleeve overlying the socket and rolled on the thigh for transtibial or with a belt for transfemoral. Because most patients with bilateral amputations use a pair of prostheses, suspension belts can be integrated into a single assembly. Because thigh corsets with metal side joints, hip joints, pelvic bands, and waist belts can be cumbersome for donning and doffing, they are typically avoided unless absolutely necessary.

Ischial containment sockets are as effective for patients with bilateral amputation at the transfemoral level (of one or both limbs) as they are for patients with a single transfemoral amputation. Patients who have previously worn a quadrilateral transfemoral socket and those who are limited ambulators may be satisfied with a traditional quadrilateral design. Total contact of the residual limb in the socket is important for both ischial containment and quadrilateral socket skin integrity.

The loss of both feet and both knees makes the use of bilateral transfemoral prostheses quite challenging. For many adults with acquired limb losses, an initial fitting with sockets attached to special rocker platforms may be advocated to facilitate initial gait training. These "stubbies" (Fig. 25.8) lower the wearer's center of gravity considerably and therefore require less energy and balance than full-length prosthetic limbs, giving the patient the best chance for successful ambulation. Once the patient is able to balance effectively on the stubbies, the prostheses can be converted to use artificial feet with solid pylons, which are gradually lengthened to increase the height of the prostheses. If the patient is able to manage full-length prostheses, prosthetic knees are incorporated and a definitive prosthesis with full components is provided.

Not all patients with bilateral transfemoral amputation choose to pursue ambulation with prostheses. Some are unable to build the necessary muscle strength or postural control for a safe gait. Others find the energy cost of ambulation with prostheses excessive. In these cases, patients choose wheelchair mobility as a much less strenuous means of mobility and willingly adopt wheelchair use for the independence it provides.

Many patients with bilateral transfemoral amputations find a wheelchair most practical for long-distance mobility and use their prosthetic limbs for walking short-to-moderate distances at home and work. Some patients accept the stubbies for long-term use, particularly if these devices allow them to remain independent in the home setting. Others choose to use their stubbies at home because they take less effort, but they wear full prostheses in public.

Component Selection

The selection of components for patients with bilateral lower limb amputations is made by the same guidelines as for unilateral limb loss. There are no unique or distinct components specifically designed or intended for use in bilateral prostheses. The prosthetist should consider both prostheses together rather than simply generate a "right-side" and a "left-side" prescription recommendation. Prosthetists generally recommend that the same ankle-foot device be used on both sides so that gait mechanics will be consistent, but this is not an absolute necessity. Some patients ambulate best with different prosthetic feet depending on the level of their amputations, the length and condition of their residual limbs, the nature of their preferred activities, and other individual characteristics.

The range of physical differences between two patients with bilateral lower limb loss makes each patient and each prosthetic fitting a unique challenge. During the dynamic alignment procedure, a brief clinical trial with the recommended components is often helpful in confirming suitability for a specific individual before the prescription details are finalized. This trial is particularly helpful for experienced ambulators, who commonly develop strong preferences for specific components after walking with them for many years.

BILATERAL TRANSTIBIAL AMPUTATION

For individuals with bilateral transtibial amputation due to dysvascular disease, a solid-ankle cushion-heel prosthetic foot is often chosen because such feet offer predictable standing balance. Many patients with bilateral amputation are concerned about falling backward; therefore the prosthetist often chooses to use a slightly stiffer heel resistance to minimize this risk. When there is concern about forward falls, the prosthetist may also choose to use a slightly stiffer keel to offer additional resistance to falling forward. Patients classified as limited ambulators, those with poor postural responses, and those who walk with a very slow cadence often find this approach useful.

Those with traumatic bilateral amputation and active individuals are able to walk well with elastic-keel and dynamic-response feet or with multiaxial designs as long as they have sufficient strength and postural responses to manage these flexible components. Theoretically single-axis feet are designed to generate an abrupt hyperextension moment at midstance, which loads the cruciate ligaments of the residual limb. In practice there is little evidence that this loading is harmful; some patients with bilateral transtibial amputations prefer single-axis feet, choosing them over solid-ankle or dynamic-response designs. Patient preference is an important consideration in prosthetic prescription. If a patient expresses definite dissatisfaction with a particular foot during the fitting process, an alternative component should be tried before proceeding further.

The consideration of ancillary components, such as torque absorbers or shock-absorbing pylons, is important for all patients with bilateral amputations. Because such patients must bear all their body weight on prosthetic devices all the time, components that increase comfort or protect the skin are particularly appropriate. Lessening the weight of the prostheses, particularly at the ankle-foot area, is also important, because lighter-weight prostheses are easier to control and are more likely to be accepted. Whenever possible, heavier components should be placed as close to the socket as possible.

BILATERAL TRANSFEMORAL AMPUTATION

Postural responses are compromised in patients with bilateral transfemoral amputations because of the loss of both anatomic ankles and knees. For this reason, a primary goal of prosthetic prescription is stability in the stance phase of gait. One of the most effective prosthetic components for stance-phase stability during level walking is a polycentric knee unit. For those patients who have the potential to walk at varying speeds, the addition of fluid swing-phase control is recommended. Hydraulic stance- and swing-control units are also quite successful for this population. In recent years, microprocessor-controlled hydraulic knees offering both stance- and swing-phase control have been well received clinically, and many experts believe that this technology offers more reliable stability and better mobility under real-world conditions than strictly mechanical knee mechanisms. The risk of injury in a fall is greater if locking or stance-control knees are used in both prostheses. For patients with significant stability issues, such a knee may be used on one side. Because single-axis knees are stabilized by muscle control and postural responses at the hip, older adults with dysvascular amputations often find bilateral single-axis knees difficult to use safely. Bilateral single-axis knees may be appropriate for small children because their short stature reduces the balance required to manage adult-size components.

Ankle-foot components that emphasize stability and standing balances are typical for the group with bilateral limb loss. Solid-ankle designs predominate. Articulating designs are used less often; only individuals with very long transfemoral residual limbs and good muscle strength are typically able to control the added mobility provided by articulating ankle components. Many patients with bilateral transfemoral amputations use crutches or canes to assist with balance and postural control. Single-axis or multiaxial feet become easier to control if the patient leans forward slightly, shifting the center of gravity forward, so that the weight line falls anterior to the ankle axis at all times, thus eliminating the risk of falling backward.

Ancillary components, such as torque absorbers, often make walking easier and more comfortable for patients with bilateral transfemoral amputations. There is some evidence that including components that permit controlled transverse rotation improves the gait kinematics of patients who wear two lower limb prostheses. Locking rotation devices make many ADLs easier to accomplish. Because the weight of such ancillary components must be considered, the perception of the artificial limb feeling heavy is minimized if the devices are positioned as far proximally within the prosthesis as possible.

TRANSFEMORAL AND TRANSTIBIAL AMPUTATION

For patients with one transfemoral and one transtibial amputation, the preservation of one biologic knee makes prosthetic use much easier and successful ambulation more likely. For most patients, the transtibial side is the propulsive and balance limb and the transfemoral side supplements these functions. On the basis of these functional differences, the prosthetist may choose to use different prosthetic feet. When the transfemoral amputation is relatively short, for example, a single-axis foot and stance control knee might be recommended for the transfemoral prosthesis whereas a dynamic-response foot might be used in the transtibial prosthesis.

Energy Consumption and Cost of Bilateral Limb Loss

The effort required to use a unilateral prosthesis increases in direct proportion to the level of amputation: the longer the residual limb, the lower the energy cost of walking with a prosthesis.[73] Saving as much functional limb length as possible is therefore an axiom in amputation surgery. Although preservation of the anatomic knee joint is important for patients with unilateral amputations, it is a critical consideration in cases of bilateral limb loss. When at least one biologic knee joint remains, the chances for practical ambulation increase significantly.

In general patients with dysvascular amputations have lower energy reserves and expend more effort in walking than do those with traumatic amputations.[13] Individuals with bilateral transtibial amputations tend to do well with prostheses regardless of the reason for the amputation. A significant number of those with traumatic bilateral transtibial amputations successfully use prostheses long term.[74] Interestingly, bilateral transtibial prostheses require less effort than a unilateral transfemoral prosthesis; this finding emphasizes the importance of retaining biologic knee function whenever possible.

Long-term and community use with bilateral transfemoral prostheses is uncommon due to energy cost, but not impossible for older adults with dysvascular amputations. In a comparative study on energy expenditure and select gait parameters, however, it is important to recognize that even in younger individuals with bilateral traumatic amputation significantly slower walking speeds and >60% greater energy expenditure when compared to age-matched healthy controls are evident.[75] For bilateral transfemoral amputation, stubbies are often used for training and long-term prosthetic use to reduce energy expenditure during ambulation; however, the speed of walking is found to be below the threshold for most functional activities and ambulation.[9,76] In a single subject comparative study, findings revealed that the full-length prosthesis with a microprocessor knee unit improved walking speed, while only minimally increasing energy cost when compared to the stubbies. At the conclusion of the study, the subject reportedly preferred to use a wheelchair for community mobility to "reach his destination more rapidly and efficienctly"[76] (p.1716). When considering functional ability, full-length users rated their abilities to complete functional skills, such as stair descent and sit-to-stand tasks, as reported on the Prosthesis Evaluation Questionnaire—Mobility Scale.[9] Further research is clearly needed to better understand factors that optimize prosthetic function following bilateral lower limb amputation.

Rehabilitation Outcomes After Bilateral Limb Loss

Rehabilitation for individuals with bilateral lower extremity limb loss is similar to the rehabilitation of persons with unilateral amputation; however, the additional loss of muscle and limb joints result in increased energy consumption and marked changes in balance control during ADL and walking. Thus the pace of advancement is slower and treatment must be individualized according to the patient's aerobic capacity, strength, balance, and ability. Fortunately, most patients with traumatic amputations are healthy and strong and generally have a good prognosis for the successful use of prostheses.[56]

Breaking down complex skills into small incremental tasks that can be more readily mastered is generally useful. Without the benefit of a sound limb, patients with bilateral loss can be expected to walk slowly and cautiously, often with a relatively wide-based gait that maximizes their sense of balance. Bilateral transfemoral amputees face even greater energy demands and lower rates of full-time prosthetic use for functional ambulation.[32]

The use of balance aids such as canes is common but not universal in the gait training and mobility rehabilitation process for persons with bilateral amputations. Environmental barriers such as ramps, hills, irregular surfaces, and curbs or stairs present special challenges that must be identified and overcome. The ability to sit, rise from a chair, fall in a controlled manner, and recover from a fall are all important tasks to be mastered. Transfer with and without artificial limbs is also an important skill to foster independence. Persons with bilateral lower limb amputations require a wheelchair for mobility for independent toileting in the night and for times when the prosthetic legs need repair.

Rehabilitation for individuals with bilateral lower limb amputations occurs in various phases, including a preoperative phase if time permits, an immediate postoperative phase, and an acute rehabilitation phase. The Bilateral Amputee Mobility Predictor (BAMP) was created to assess functional prosthetic potential for individuals with various types of bilateral amputation without a prosthesis and later with the prescribed prosthesis to document change.[77] Similar to research evidence and support for the AMP, the BAMP has been found to be a reliable and valid instrument and can be used to predict the functional classification level.[72]

The rehabilitation process is patient-centered and should be individualized for each one, taking into account his or her physical condition, biomechanical loss, and need for a prosthesis. The reason for the amputation influences the pace and level of rehabilitation. An otherwise healthy individual who sustained traumatic limb loss may be able to advance rapidly unless there is skin trauma on the residual limb. Early fitting is a critical factor in attaining a long-term successful outcome.[78]

Summary

Individuals with high-level or bilateral lower limb amputations are rare in the developed world. In the United States, fewer than 5% of all persons with amputations have high-level amputation. Given these statistics, most prosthetists and therapists have limited opportunity to work with patients with such significant levels of limb loss. Although successful prosthetic training and rehabilitation for these patients are challenging, a large body of clinical information about managing such cases is available in the literature. This chapter highlighted the key principles involved in rehabilitation of the individual with high-level or bilateral lower limb amputations.

Surgical technique during the amputation largely determines the potential for long-term ambulation. Today, advances in surgical technique such as targeted muscle reinnervation show promise for reducing common postoperative complications related chronic residual limb and phantom pain. Additionally, techniques that address improved handling of soft tissues and careful preservation of all functional joints and bone lengths, especially following traumatic accident, optimize socket fit. Anchoring functioning muscles to bone (myodesis) at their normal resting length, whenever possible, is strongly encouraged and effective for improving prosthetic control.

The socket design and suspension methods chosen for patients with high-level or bilateral amputations should incorporate strategies to protect the skin and maximize patient comfort, especially for individuals with bilateral amputations. Components reflect each individual's need for stability and responsiveness at the ankle-foot, knee, or hip-joint level. Ancillary components to make the prosthesis more comfortable and easier to manage are advocated.

Although patients with bilateral transfemoral amputation caused by vascular disease often have difficulty mastering dual prosthetic devices, long-term use of functional prostheses is a realistic goal for patients with traumatic or tumor-related amputation who are otherwise healthy. With appropriate fitting and rehabilitation, many patients with hip disarticulation and transpelvic amputations continue to use their prostheses definitively. Even patients with translumbar amputation are able to return to productive education or work activities with an appropriate prosthesis for sitting or limited ambulation.

Despite the obvious physical and psychological challenges faced by patients with high-level or bilateral lower limb amputations, prosthetic rehabilitation must always be considered and is often successful, especially when offered by an experienced multidisciplinary team in a supportive setting. Although the sequelae from amputations of this magnitude present significant challenges, advances in surgical technique, prosthetic design and components, and rehabilitation contribute to successful outcomes for patients with high-level and bilateral amputations.

References

The complete listing of the References are available in the accompanying enhanced eBook version included with the print purchase of this textbook. Visit Elsevier eBooks+ (eBooks.Health.Elsevier.com) to access this content.

26 Early Rehabilitation in Lower Extremity Dysvascular Amputation

DANIEL J. LEE, KELLY J. NEGLEY AND JULIE D. RIES

LEARNING OBJECTIVES

On completion of this chapter, the reader will be able to do the following:

1. Understand the special needs of persons with lower extremity limb loss due to dysvascular etiologies.
2. Organize each component of a comprehensive physical therapy examination for the individual with transtibial or transfemoral amputation and synthesize this information.
3. Establish diagnosis, prognosis, and treatment plan of care for rehabilitation.
4. Implement a well-defined and focused treatment plan that addresses the needs of the individual with transtibial or transfemoral amputation as related to participation restrictions, activity limitations, and impairments.
5. Prioritize issues about which transtibial or transfemoral amputees and their caregivers must be educated and execute a reasonable education plan.
6. Identify appropriate outcome measures for use with transtibial or transfemoral amputees.
7. Provide a justification for the clinical decision-making associated with each phase of the comprehensive physical therapy rehabilitation of dysvascular amputees.

Persons who undergo amputation secondary to dysvascular etiologies are in many ways uniquely different from those who have had amputations due to a traumatic event. Dysvascular etiologies are those typically related to peripheral vascular disease, diabetes, or a combination of both.[1] Thus the individual who has undergone amputation for reasons related to the vascular system will likely also have involvement of the cardiopulmonary, neuromuscular, integumentary, and other bodily systems.[2] Unlike the individual who has a traumatic amputation, individuals who have experienced a dysvascular amputation are more likely to be older, functionally impaired, and have a higher risk of reamputation and mortality following the initial amputation.[3] Therefore when providing care to those with limb loss due to dysvascular disease, a comprehensive interdisciplinary approach must be taken to ensure high-quality care to this vulnerable population.

While this chapter discusses early rehabilitation for those with dysvascular limb loss, the focus is on the older adult (age >65 years). Despite declining rates of age-adjusted amputations nationally, there is an increase in the number of amputations experienced in older adults due to demographic shifts, with approximately 20% of the US population expected to be 65 or older by the year 2030.[4,5] The highest rates of lower limb amputation occur in males who are older than 75 years old, with a median age estimated to be 67 years old.[6,7] Minor amputations (distal to the ankle) are the most common, followed by transtibial and transfemoral amputations, respectively.[7] Medicare Functional Classification Levels (K-levels) in those with dysvascular limb loss are typically lower than those with traumatic limb loss at a comparable amputation level.[8]

Multiple body systems are impacted when an individual has had an amputation secondary to dysvascular disease. For those with diabetes, damage to the visual, sensation, and cardiovascular systems are typically pronounced, resulting in greater difficulty donning the prosthesis.[9] Mobility limitations secondary to musculoskeletal conditions like osteoarthritis are commonly found in older adults without amputation,[10] but in those with limb loss the prevalence of chronic pain, especially of the lumbar spine, is even greater.[11] Considering that low back, knee, and hip pain are commonly experienced complications from prosthesis use, an older adult with preexisting pain is more likely to have functional impairments as a result of the pain.

Cognitive impairments are also common in those with dysvascular disease. Since donning, doffing, self-managing, and utilizing a prosthesis requires problem-solving and decision-making, deficits in cognition can be a significant factor influencing the ability of the individual to rehabilitate after amputation.[4,12] Those with cognitive impairments are less likely to receive a prosthesis, and for those that do receive one, they are less likely to use it in a functional manner.[13]

Given the complex biological, psychological, and societal nature of living with limb loss due to dysvascular disease, the interdisciplinary team must be considerate of the biopsychosocial interactions at play, which may necessitate multiple care settings. Changes in reimbursement for the provision of healthcare services have necessitated a transition in how postamputation rehabilitation care is provided in the United States. Postamputation rehabilitation, which historically was performed in the inpatient rehabilitation environment, is now more often provided in home-care or outpatient clinics, with stringent limits to the number of physical therapy (PT) visits. Due to the relatively fragile nature of a person with dysvascular limb loss, any lapse in high-quality care can result in preventable complications like infection, skin breakdown, or injury.[14] It is imperative that therapists working with this population have an excellent understanding of the "big picture" progression of care, the need for appropriately intensive training, and a mechanism for follow-up over time. The goal of this chapter is to provide a foundation for evidence-based practice in the management of dysvascular transtibial or transfemoral amputees regardless of the practice setting.

This chapter also provides a range of interventions for persons with new transtibial or transfemoral amputations, from early PT treatment ideas that focus on preparing the limb for the use of a prosthesis to building tolerance to prosthesis exposure. As the person with limb loss develops basic mobility skills, interventions progress to more complex, higher-level bipedal activities. This chapter focuses primarily on strategies for initial and intermediate-level rehabilitation, including a short discussion of more advanced training. Anticipated functional outcomes for prosthesis users who have undergone a transtibial or transfemoral amputation are addressed.

Components of the Physical Therapy Examination

Effective PT management for persons with limb loss begins with a thorough and comprehensive initial examination. The PT examination may occur before or after the amputation, at the time the prosthesis is fitted, or after the individual has already obtained their prosthesis; it may also occur in any practice setting. The purpose of the examination is to collect the patient's history, conduct a systems review, perform tests and measures, and determine the functional status of the patient. The data collected should represent all levels of the World Health Organization's International Classification of Functioning, Disability, and Health (ICF) model, including impairments, activity limitations, and participation restrictions, with consideration of contextual factors (environmental and personal modifiers). Timely reassessment is necessary to track the patient's functional progress over time, and may also be required after any changes in medical status, including prosthetic componentry.

HISTORY

The patient's history comprises the health-related, personal, and social factors that give context to the individual's current situation and informs the plan of care and prognosis. Table 26.1 provides the relevant components for

Table 26.1 Important Patient-Client History Components of the Physical Therapy (PT) Examination

Component	Topics for Consideration
Social history	■ Cultural beliefs and behaviors
	■ Family and caregiver resources
	■ Social interactions, activities, and support systems
	■ Amenability to peer/mentor support
	■ Insurance/reimbursement
Employment/work/leisure	■ Current and/or prior work
	■ Current community/leisure activities and goals related to community/leisure activities
	■ Family/work roles
Living environment/equipment	■ Prior use of, or need for new assistive devices and adaptive equipment
	■ Home set up (e.g., stairs, bathroom set up)
	■ Projected discharge destination if acute
General health status	■ General health perception
	■ Cognition
	■ Biopsychosocial function
Social health habits	■ Health risks (e.g., smoking, alcohol, or drug abuse)
	■ Level of physical fitness and exercise habits and desires
Family history	■ Relevant family medical history and health risks
Medical/surgical history	■ Prior hospitalizations, prior amputations, surgeries
	■ Preexisting medical and other health-related conditions (e.g., visual impairments, neuropathy, coronary artery disease, dysvascular conditions, diabetes complications, kidney disease)
	■ Weight-bearing or mobility restrictions on residual or contralateral limb
Chief complaint/current condition	■ Concerns that led the person or caregiver to seek PT services
	■ Current medical or therapeutic interventions
	■ Mechanism of injury/disease including date of onset and course of events
	■ Client/caregiver/family expectations and goals
	■ Client/family/caregiver's perceptions of the person's emotional response to the current situation
	■ Previous therapeutic interventions for this problem
Activity level	■ Current and prior level of function in mobility, self-care, activities of daily living, and home management
	■ Current and previous functional demands in work and community/leisure activities
Medications	■ Medications for current and/or other coexisting conditions (prescription and over the counter)
Review of available records	■ Laboratory and diagnostic tests if applicable

Adapted from https://guide.apta.org, with permission.

the therapist to consider when taking the client's history, with specific considerations given to the client with lower extremity dysvascular amputation.

The subjective component of the examination provides valuable insights about the person's communication ability, emotional status, cognitive status, coping strategies, and preferred learning style as well as the availability of emotional and instrumental support systems (assistance with activities of daily living [ADLs]). It is important to consider the person's perspective of their illness, functional limitations, and disability, as these have a powerful influence on the rehabilitation process and the person's adaptation to limb loss.[15] High resilience, self-efficacy, and social support are also noted to play a role in the functional outcomes and level of disability after lower limb amputation.[16–19] Therefore the therapist should consider asking questions or using an outcome measure (Table 26.2) to gauge the patient's ability to demonstrate constructive coping, cognitive flexibility, and acceptance of the amputation, as these may influence the rehabilitation outcome.

There are a number of important areas that must be explored while the patient's medical history is being taken. Although all areas provide important information, several are integral to the establishment of the PT diagnosis, prognosis, and plan of care. The person's age, general health status and presence or stage of vascular, renal or endocrine comorbidities may affect their rehabilitation outcomes and biopsychosocial functions.[18] Discussion of the current condition/chief complaint gives the therapist a sense of the individual's concerns, previous interventions, and course of events. It is important to understand the individual's goals and aspirations and to gauge whether they appear to be over- or underambitious. The therapist can then address these issues, with education and interaction with peer mentors as possible interventions.

Information about the person's preamputation and/or preprosthetic level of activity and mobility is also important to gather to establish a realistic prognosis. Patients with amputation who were functionally ambulatory prior to and/or immediately following amputation surgery are more likely to recover at least a modest degree of ambulation ability with a prosthesis; specifically, the ability to stand on one leg and higher levels of fitness are associated with prosthetic success.[20,21] Focused and probing interview questions are often helpful in obtaining clear and accurate information. Although many individuals are excellent historians, others may have an incomplete understanding or imprecise memory of what has happened. It is always advisable to confirm information when possible.

Lastly, many individuals with limb loss do not have a clear understanding of what to expect during rehabilitation or how their comorbidities or disease process might affect rehabilitation outcomes. Every individual benefits from being well educated about his or her condition and treatment. For many, the events that brought them to rehabilitation may be a blur of disjointed experiences and medical jargon or a laundry list of conditions that seem unrelated or independent. The physical therapist can help them to place their history and experience into a meaningful context, which, in turn, assists them in forming realistic expectations and may decrease the likelihood of complications or a second amputation.

SYSTEMS REVIEW

The systems review is a gross, limited review of the anatomic and physiologic status of the patient's cognitive, cardiopulmonary, musculoskeletal, vascular, integumentary, neuromuscular, endocrine, gastrointestinal, and urogenital systems. This screening process aids in focusing and prioritizing the tests and measures portion of the examination. Careful attention should be paid to the assessment of vital signs, given the large proportion of cardiovascular comorbidity in adults with dysvascular amputation.[22] A thorough cognitive screen should also be a top priority in the older adult population with dysvascular amputation, as higher rates of altered cognition are noted in the general older adult population, and impaired cognition can impact the success of the rehabilitation outcome.[12,23] While a gross screen of strength and range of motion (ROM) of all extremities are indicated in this phase, special attention should be placed on hip extension ROM and hip abduction strength, as both play a critical role in functionally utilizing the prosthesis.

TESTS AND MEASURES

Tests and measures are deliberately prioritized to elicit the most relevant objective data for a given individual. Components of functional status will always be a top priority (this may include tests and measures associated with balance, gait, and mobility). Some categories of tests and measures may be revealed as unwarranted if the systems review "clears" the system (e.g., integumentary, musculoskeletal, and cognitive screenings may effectively eliminate the need for immediate further testing in these areas). Combining collected data with findings from the history and systems review, the physical therapist establishes a working diagnostic hypothesis related to the movement system dysfunction the individual is experiencing. The physical therapist chooses, from an array of possible tests and measures, those that will best confirm or deny the developing diagnostic hypothesis. Data collected will funnel the therapist's thought process to prioritize problems and formulate the most appropriate plan of care. It is important to note that some assessments, such as strength testing or joint play motions, might require modification of technique because limb loss necessitates a change in the lever available for applying therapeutic forces.

Table 26.2 provides specific considerations for the tests and measures that are appropriate to administer during the PT examination after dysvascular lower extremity amputation. Decisions about specific areas included in the assessment are driven by many factors, including clinical setting, time since amputation, and whether or not the individual has received a prosthesis. An inpatient assessment on postoperative day 2 will include different priorities than those associated with a home-care assessment for an individual who is 1 month postamputation and ready to be fitted for a prosthesis. And here again the priorities will differ from those associated with the outpatient clinic visit of an individual who has recently received a prosthesis and is ready to learn how to use it. Regardless of the clinical setting, therapists should use a documentation strategy that will provide insurers with a vivid picture of the person's functional baseline, and allow them to track progress over time.

Table 26.2 Data Gathered During the Initial and Follow-Up Physical Therapy Examinations

Objective	Considerations (Variable Depending on Clinical Setting and Length of Time Since Amputation)	Outcome Measure (If Applicable)
Motor function	■ Strength	
	■ Hand function and dexterity (relevant to prosthetic donning/doffing)	
	■ Muscle power and endurance	
	■ Motor control: timing, coordination, and agility	
Balance	■ Supported and unsupported static/dynamic sitting/standing balance with/without prosthesis	■ TUG
	■ Supported and unsupported static/dynamic sitting/standing balance with/without prosthesis	■ Berg Balance Scale
		■ ABC Scale
Mobility	■ Transfer status with/without prosthesis	■ 10-Meter Walk Test
	■ Wheelchair mobility	■ Amputee Mobility Predictor (AMPPRO, AMPnoPRO)
	■ Ambulation with/without prosthesis (need for assistance, type of assistive device, distance, terrain)	■ L Test
	■ Prosthetic gait deviations from observational gait analysis	■ PLUS-M
	■ Stair negotiation with/without prosthesis	■ CHAMP
	■ High-level functional activities (e.g., running, sport-specific)	■ PEQ-MS
	■ Floor-to-stand transfers	■ LCI
Integumentary: residual limb inspection	■ Size (length, girth), shape (cylindrical, conical, bulbous), redundant tissue ("dog ears" or adductor roll), edema (characteristics of edema)	■ SMART
	■ Integument status: incision line (indications of healing vs. concern/infection); scar (general appearance, tissue mobility vs. adhesions)	
	■ Color and integrity of skin	
	■ Type of postamputation dressing	
	■ Tolerance to prosthetic wear	
Integumentary: remaining limb inspection	■ Circulation: assessment of color, temperature, trophic changes, pulses, responsiveness to position changes	■ Doppler Ultrasound ■ Monofilament Testing
	■ Integument: overall status and integrity of skin, presence of ulcers, lesions, calluses; status of nails, protective sensation	
	■ Neurologic: peripheral nerve integrity (motor and sensory testing), reflex integrity, protective sensation	
	■ Footwear assessment	
Prosthesis assessment	■ Ability to don/doff: based on client report and/or observation	■ SMART
	■ Socket fit	■ OPUS
	■ Socket comfort	■ Houghton Scale
	■ Prosthesis alignment: based on observation in static standing and during gait	■ Socket Comfort Score
	■ Prosthesis function based on componentry	■ CLASS
	■ Hours/days of use	
	■ Satisfaction	
	■ Cosmetic appearance	
Aerobic capacity/ endurance	■ Cardiovascular and pulmonary response to exertion	■ 2-Minute Walk Test
		■ 6-Minute Walk Test
Cognition	■ Cognitive function	■ MOCA
	■ Observations related to individual's ability to comprehend instructions, attend to task, solve problems, show safety awareness and judgment	■ Connor Davidson Resilience Scale
	■ Preferred learning strategies	■ Mini-Cog
	■ Self-efficacy, resilience, and coping ability	
Pain	■ Somatic residual limb pain	■ NRS
	■ Phantom pain	■ SF-MPQ-2
	■ Pain with/without prosthesis	■ VAS
	■ Pain elsewhere from residual limb	■ Socket Comfort Score
	■ Current regimen for management of pain and its effectiveness	■ CLASS
ROM and joint integrity and mobility	■ Hip extension, adduction, internal rotation	
	■ Knee extension for those with transtibial amputations	
	■ Lumbar spine mobility	
Environment	■ Recommendations for environmental modifications (e.g., additional handrails, grab bars, ramps)	

ABC, Activities-specific Balance Confidence; *AMPnoPRO*, Amputee Mobility Predictor without prosthesis; *AMPPRO*, Amputee Mobility Predictor with prosthesis; *CHAMP*; Comprehensive High Level Amputee Mobility Predictor; *CLASS*, Comprehensive Lower limb Amputee Socket Survey; *LCI*, Locomotor Capabilities Index; *MOCA*, Montreal Cognitive Assessment; *NRS*, Numerical Rating Scale; *OPUS*, Orthotics and Prosthetics Users Survey; *PEQ-MS*, Prosthetic Evaluation Questionnaire—Mobility Subscale; *PLUS-M*, Prosthetic Limb Users Survey of Mobility; *ROM*, range of motion; *SF-MPQ-2*, Short-Form McGill Pain Questionnaire-2; *SMART*, Self Management Assessment of the Residuum and prosThesis; *TUG*, Timed Up and Go; *VAS*, visual analog scale.

This ensures continuity of care within and across clinical settings, allows patients to take advantage of insurance benefits for reimbursement of therapy services, and is an important component of the person's assigned Medicare Functional Classification Scale (K-level), which determines prosthesis eligibility.

THE EVALUATION PROCESS

The process of evaluation requires the physical therapist to interpret and integrate the information obtained from the history, systems review, and tests and measures to identify the primary areas of participation restriction, activity limitation, and impairment. The physical therapist uses professional judgment to predict the likely functional outcome and time required for effective preprosthetic and/or prosthetic rehabilitation. The evaluation must include a summary of the individual's major problems and the presumed underlying causes. Problems are prioritized, with those that have the most significant functional implications receiving top priority. This is done within the personal and environmental context of the individual, as the same problem may affect different people in different ways. For instance, poor sensation of the residual limb in an individual who is cognitively intact may be easily resolved with education about compensating for the sensory deficit with visual inspection, effectively reducing the risk of compromising skin integrity. Another person with the same sensory deficit who also has cognitive impairment may present with a higher risk of skin complications and require a more extensive educational intervention focused on residual limb care with the assistance of others who can help monitor skin integrity. Physical therapists must also be skilled in determining the functional implications of specific findings from the evaluation. For instance, a slight knee flexion contracture can be accommodated for in transtibial socket alignment, whereas a significant knee flexion contracture prohibits fitting with a conventional prosthesis. Prosthesis prescription and PT intervention may be different for two individuals with similar amputations but different degrees of contracture. Evaluation also includes understanding the limitations and capabilities of their current prosthesis, which may involve research into the prosthesis via the manufacturer's educational materials.

Establishing a Physical Therapy Diagnosis and Prognosis

The establishment of the PT diagnosis for a patient with lower extremity amputation is related to the movement system and must be put into a functional context; for instance, a documented PT diagnosis might be: "difficulty in walking" or "abnormality of gait and mobility." The physical therapist uses data from the history and test findings in the context of knowledge from the literature to predict each person's rehabilitation potential and probable functional outcome. Based on the individual's prognosis, measurable short-term and long-term goals are defined to guide intervention planning. These goals are used to inform outcomes assessment as rehabilitation progresses. An important component of the prognosis is determining the likely time frame for achievement of the optimal outcome. Younger individuals with transtibial dysvascular amputation, void of postoperative complications, are likely to progress through rehabilitation programs more quickly than the medically frail and/or deconditioned older adults after transfemoral amputation. Research findings indicate several prognostic indicators of functional use of a prosthesis following rehabilitation. All of the following have been found to negatively affect functional use despite rehabilitation efforts: advanced age,[20,21,24] the presence of comorbidities,[20,21,24,25] level of amputation (transfemoral vs. transtibial),[20,21] cognitive and/or memory impairment,[12,20,21] and lower levels of functioning prior to amputation rehabilitation as indicated by fitness, mobility, ADLs, and/or functional tests.[20,21,24] This information is *not* intended to suggest the exclusion of individuals with any of these predictors from rehabilitation efforts; in fact, there is some evidence of training success in those 80 years of age and older,[26] but therapists must be realistic in assessing the challenges facing each individual user of a prosthesis. An efficient and useful predictor of functional prosthesis use is the level of preamputation mobility. Persons with amputation who were ambulatory before surgery and/or after amputation prior to receiving a prosthesis are much more likely to be able to use a prosthesis for ambulation.[20,21] Consideration of all of these factors should be reflected in the plan of care, along with specific goals and the anticipated rate at which those goals will be met.

Plan of Care

The PT plan of care includes information about the frequency, duration, location, and specific PT interventions and is directly related to the goals delineated by the evaluation/prognostic process. Little is known about dose-response relationships in PT generally and in amputation rehabilitation specifically,[27] although underdosing in rehabilitation is a consistent issue.[28] The prioritized problem list provides a foundation for functional short- and long-term goals that direct rehabilitation activities. If independent donning and doffing of a prosthesis is the primary short-term goal, the associated treatment plan must include education strategies, opportunities to practice this skill, and remediation or adaptation of any movement components that, if missing, would compromise the individual's ability to perform this necessary task (e.g., the person may need to improve grip strength or intrinsic hand strength to manipulate prosthetic suspension). The plan includes information about equipment to be ordered, referrals to be made, and the ultimate PT discharge plan. Lastly, to maximize postamputation outcomes, the therapist should utilize a patient-centered communication approach to create a strong therapeutic alliance and collaboratively establish the plan of care with the patient.[29]

Preprosthetic Interventions

Successful use of a prosthesis involves having functional ROM of the hip and (if applicable) knee; functional strength of muscles at the hip and (if applicable) knee; adequate motor control and balance; sufficient aerobic capacity and endurance; effective edema control, skin and soft tissue management of the maturing residual limb; and sensory integrity of the residual limb. It is crucial to address these areas early in the rehabilitation process. Inability to achieve a certain status or level of performance in one area does not prohibit a good rehabilitation outcome; however, difficulties in multiple areas have an impact on prosthetic candidacy and use. Each of these areas should be carefully evaluated throughout the person's clinical course and appropriate interventions undertaken to achieve at least minimal requirements for functional prosthesis use if not an optimal level of performance. However, even when persons with dysvascular amputations are deemed not to be candidates for the use of a prosthesis, they should be given the opportunity to benefit from rehabilitation interventions and learn how to safely navigate their environments in the context of their new amputation. People with dysvascular amputation and cardiac comorbidity are also at increased risk for hospital readmission,[30] and those with renal dysfunction are at a high risk for contralateral limb amputation.[31] Therapists can focus early rehabilitation efforts on education for the prevention of complications from the amputation, as well as on minimizing the sequelae of their comorbidities that led to the amputation.

RANGE OF MOTION

Early achievement of functional ROM of the involved lower extremity is of paramount importance. Assessment and treatment of ROM of the intact limb is also important, as loss of ROM of either limb has an impact on the quality and energy efficiency of functional mobility and gait. The flexor withdrawal pattern of hip flexion, abduction, external rotation, and knee flexion is a position associated with lower extremity pain and is often a position of choice for the residual limb after surgery. Elevation of the extremity on pillows serves to reinforce this undesirable posture and puts these individuals at risk for contracture formation (especially hip and knee flexor contractures), which can have a negative impact on the ultimate use of a prosthesis.[32] Maintaining or increasing available ROM at the hip for persons with a transfemoral residual limb and at the hip and knee of the transtibial residual limb continues to be a primary treatment goal as the person moves from preprosthetic into prosthetic rehabilitation. The prevention of loss of ROM is much easier than efforts to regain lost motion. Prone positioning is an excellent strategy to combat contracture formation of the hip flexors. The Veterans Affairs, Department of Defense clinical practice guidelines suggest the initiation of prone lying as early as possible for bouts of 30 minutes, twice a day.[33] Those people with significant contractures may not be able to tolerate prone initially or for a full 30 minutes, and variation in prescription might be necessary; a pillow or wedge under the abdomen may minimize discomfort while still achieving a stretch. Low-load long-duration stretch is safe and can lead to significant elastic and plastic changes in soft tissues.[34] Side-lying hip extension or the Thomas test position are options for those unable to achieve a prone position at all, such as those with cardiovascular or pulmonary comorbidity and/or elevated BMI. Persons with limb loss should understand the difference between hip joint extension and the substitution of increased anterior pelvic tilt or lumbar lordosis. Full-functional hip active ROM into flexion, extension, and adduction is critical to achieving efficient ambulation and functional mobility with a prosthesis. Typical gait on level surfaces requires the hip to move from 30 degrees of flexion to 10 degrees of extension and requires adduction slightly beyond neutral.[35] More extreme ranges of hip flexion are required for transitioning from sit to stand and reaching forward from a seated position; hip abduction range is required for sidestepping in a functional context. Although alignment of the transfemoral socket will decrease the need for the typical amount of hip extension required during walking or abduction during side stepping (due to the slight flexion/posterior tilt and adduction/lateral tilt of the transfemoral socket), it is advisable to work toward functional ROM in all planes of motion and to balance strength and ROM around the hip joint.

To avoid or minimize the progression of existing knee flexion contractures after a transtibial amputation, a postoperative rigid dressing or knee-extension splint or board (e.g., transfer board extending from under a seating cushion) can be an effective technique while the person with amputation is in the seated position. Full knee extension ROM is required in typical ambulation on level surfaces[35] and for exploiting passive stability at the knee joint in static standing; however, prosthetic alignment of the typical transtibial socket (slight flexion/anterior tilt) eliminates the need for full knee extension during gait. Nonetheless, maintaining or regaining full knee extension in individuals with recent transtibial amputations should be encouraged with the use of strategic positioning, a knee-extension splint, and/or frequent active quadriceps exercises ("quad set"). If the person is using a splint or positioning board, they must also be taught to check the integrity of the residual limb's skin regularly so as to minimize the risk of pressure-related skin damage, which would delay use of the prosthesis. For individuals with transtibial amputations, achieving knee flexion ROM is sometimes overlooked early in rehabilitation. Typical gait on level surfaces generally requires approximately 60 degrees of knee flexion,[35] and more than 90 degrees is required for efficient step-over-step stair ambulation, rising from a seated position, and high-level mobility activities such as kneeling or rising from the floor.

Table 26.3 summarizes potential mobility problems associated with loss of functional ROM. Physical therapists may utilize active and passive stretching, joint mobilization, manual therapy techniques, and other modalities to facilitate ROM recovery. ROM should be emphasized in individual education and home positioning and exercise routines. All exercises started during the preprosthetic phase are generally appropriate to continue as prescribed or to be progressed as tolerated during the prosthesis training phase. Once full-functional ROM is achieved, the person should be educated on how to maintain this level.

STRENGTH

There are several factors that may contribute to the strength deficits of people with lower limb loss. The disease process that led to the amputation may predispose someone to deficits in strength, as compared to someone with a traumatic amputation. In addition, the length of the residual

Table 26.3 Implications of Range of Motion Limitations for Prosthesis Users

Range-of-Motion Limitation	Potential Functional Limitation	Implication
AFTER TRANSTIBIAL AMPUTATION		
↓ Knee flexion	Inability to place foot flat on the floor when sitting	Inability to weight bear through prosthesis during sit-to-stand transfers
	Inability to climb or descend stairs step over step	Limited to step-to-step method, which may be less efficient and slower
↓ Knee extension	Limb functionally shorter	Gait deviations associated with leg-length discrepancy
	Inability to take advantage of extensor moment at knee	Quadriceps fatigue, decreased midstance stability during gait
	Knee extensors firing continually to maintain knee stability	
↓ Hip extension	Inability to achieve upright posture in stance and inability to take advantage of extensor moment at hip	Fatigue of hip and low back extensors
	Hip and low back extensors firing continually to maintain upright, resulting in anterior pelvic tilt	Risk for low back pain
		Instability during stance phase of gait
	Compensatory knee flexion	Decreased step and stride length of contralateral limb in gait
	Body cannot progress beyond prosthetic leg during gait	Increased falls risk due to anterior trunk lean
↓ Hip adduction	Abducted stance in gait (wide base of support)	Increased lateral excursion of center of mass (abductor lurch)
		Lateral trunk lean during stance phase on ipsilateral side, decreasing gait efficiency
↓ Internal rotation	Toe-out stance and gait	Knee joint pain and/or pathology of knee joint due to lack of anterior/posterior orientation
	Pelvic progression over stance limb in gait may be limited (contralateral pelvis rotates anteriorly from fulcrum of weight-bearing hip; if limited internal rotation, this will impede pelvic rotation on fixed femur)	Decreased step and stride length of contralateral limb during gait
AFTER TRANSFEMORAL AMPUTATION		
↓ Hip Extension	Inability to achieve upright posture in stance and inability to take advantage of extensor moment at hip	Increased falls risk
		Risk for back pain
	Disengagement of knee friction mechanisms of prosthesis	Suboptimal programming of microprocessor knee
↓ Hip adduction	Abducted stance in gait	Lateral trunk lean during stance phase

limb as well as surgical approach and ability to secure a good length/tension relationship on the muscles may alter strength.[36] Beyond the strength of the residual limb, therapists should consider that people with dysvascular amputations often go through protracted periods of inactivity before and after amputation, and may present with a generalized loss of strength. They may also have experienced intermittent or extended periods of time that required offloading of a limb, further contributing to the strength deficits in the lower extremities and core muscles. Therefore an accurate strength assessment and a comprehensive strengthening program should address not solely the residual limb, but also the uninvolved limb, trunk, and upper extremities, as the full-body strength demands will be increased during preprosthetic and prosthetic training.

Strength assessment of the lower extremity after amputation may present some challenges. The standard lever arm for providing resistance on the amputated lower extremity has been altered by the amputation, and will require the therapist to adjust their hand placement to accurately assess strength. Additionally, many people are unable to assume the standard muscle testing positions after amputation due to limited functional mobility and/or comorbidities, and so the therapist must be mindful of this when selecting the testing positions. The therapist should also recognize that the peak strength of the amputated lower extremity during strength assessment is decreased when compared to age-matched peers without amputation, and that this reduced strength is often not observed until the person attempts to functionally use the prosthesis.[37] For these reasons, therapists may choose to assess the functional strength of the lower extremity muscles with concentric and eccentric closed-chain activities instead, as these reflect the muscle activity during normal gait and functional activities. And once the user receives the prosthesis, the therapist should reassess strength with the device on, using standardized positions and hand placements when possible. Isokinetic instrumentation or handheld dynamometry[37,38] may also be used to more objectively evaluate muscle strength, although these are utilized more in research settings versus clinical practice and the psychometric properties of these tests are still under investigation.[39] The optimal strengthening protocol will depend on the characteristics of the individual person, including his or her general health, mobility status, current strength levels, and goals. The following sections will describe some additional considerations for strengthening each of the key areas: lower extremities, upper extremities, and trunk. Table 26.4 highlights some exercises that may be helpful in strengthening the residual limb after transtibial or transfemoral amputation.

Lower Extremities

There is abundant evidence of a significant strength difference between the muscles of the residual limb compared with those of the sound limb after transtibial and transfemoral amputation,[40–42] as well as evidence that the residual

Table 26.4 Examples of Therapeutic Exercises for Strengthening During Preprosthetic and Prosthetic Training

Suggested Exercises[a,b,c]	Targeted Areas
Bridging: place residual limb over ball, bolster, foam wedge, or padded stool; start bilateral and progress to unilateral with focus on pelvic stability	Core, hip/pelvic girdle
In quadruped: ■ Hip extension ■ Hip abduction ■ Shoulder extension and/abduction ■ Pairing contralateral hip/shoulder extension	Core, hip/pelvic girdle, shoulder girdle
In tall kneeling: ■ Static/dynamic balance activities: trunk rotation, ball toss, upper extremity resistance exercises	Core, hip/pelvic girdle, shoulder girdle
Resistance training with or without machines or exercise bands: ■ Leg press (intact limb) ■ Upper extremity: seated lat pulldowns, bicep/tricep pulls, scapular retraction ■ Lower extremity: hip IR/ER rotation, hip extension, hip abduction, knee extension (TF)	Hip/pelvic girdle, shoulder girdle, upper extremities
Proprioceptive neuromuscular facilitation (in supine, sidelying and standing): progression from passive to active with resistance ■ Pelvis ■ Shoulder ■ Lower extremity ■ Upper extremity	All patterns can target major muscles of lower extremities/upper extremities as well as core

[a]All exercises that require weight bearing through the residual limb should occur once complete wound healing has occurred. Routine skin checks should confirm patient tolerance to weight bearing through the newly healed residual limb
[b]Exercises can be progressed with the use of resistance through resistance bands and/or weights where appropriate
[c] For transfemoral amputation, pillows or Airex pads can be placed under the healed residual limb to account for the leg-length discrepancy between the residual limb and the intact limb.
ER, External rotation; *IR*, internal rotation; *PNF*, proprioceptive neuromuscular facilitation; *TFA*, transfemoral amputation; *TTA*, transtibial amputation.

limb shows strength deficits compared with the limbs of age-matched peers without amputations.[36] Although direct relationships between strength impairment and activity limitations cannot be assumed, there is evidence to support the impact of weakness on gait and mobility in those with limb loss.[37,43]

Strengthening programs should address all muscles of the residual and sound limbs, but prioritizing exercises that address hip extensor and abductor strength on the amputated side—and knee extensors for those with transtibial amputations—is imperative, as these muscle groups will be pivotal for stance stability during prosthetic gait.[44–46] Hip extensor strength on the amputated side is the most critical contributor to knee stability in the sagittal plane during prosthetic gait[46] and a useful predictor of functional outcomes (e.g., performance on the 6-minute walk test). Hip abductor strength in people with lower extremity amputation is correlated with improved weight bearing on the prosthetic limb in quiet stance and stability in the frontal plane during gait.[45] Preamputation weakness of proximal muscles is often subtle with little to no observable abnormality in preamputation gait patterns; however, these impairments of strength (and likely muscle endurance) may be magnified in gait with a prosthesis. The combination of proximal muscle weakness, the loss of distal musculature, along with the increased external torque demands created by the weight of a prosthesis can magnify impairments with gait and balance.

Hip and pelvic control in single-limb stance is inherently important to stability and to the effective forward progression of the body over the prosthesis. The strength requirements for ambulation with a prosthesis are similar but not identical to those of normal gait. Both the involved and intact lower extremities display increased muscle activity during their respective stance phases. Several studies examining prosthetic gait provide evidence of increased and prolonged activity of the hip abductors and extensors on the amputated side and, if present, the knee extensors.[36] Studies also confirm increased ground reaction forces and demand on the intact limb, presumably as a result of the absence of the normal foot and ankle mechanism on the prosthetic side. This results in increased hip abductor, hip extensor, and, if present, knee extensor muscle activity and power generation of the intact limb.[36]

A comprehensive strengthening program targeting the lower extremity muscle groups should be initiated early and progressed appropriately. Utilization of closed- (e.g., residual limb on bolster or gymnastic ball, or individual in kneeling position if tolerated) and open-chain exercise techniques, with both concentric and eccentric muscle contractions, is appropriate and effective once the residual limb is appropriately healed and able to tolerate weight-bearing activities.

Trunk

Strengthening of the abdominals, paraspinals, and other trunk muscles is an essential component of the preprosthetic and postprosthetic exercise program, as a stable core is essential for mobility training, transfers, and gait. As an individual's strength improves, exercises should become more functionally oriented as well as more intense. Closed-chain exercises can take on greater emphasis as individuals transition to prosthetic training from the preprosthetic phase, and core strengthening may occur in the context of upright functional activities.

Upper Extremities

Preprosthetic gait with axillary crutches or walkers requires significant upper extremity strength. Strengthening of the rotator cuff and shoulder depressors should be a key component of the early strengthening program, both for successful preprosthetic gait and also protection of the shoulder joints. Hand strength and dexterity may be a prerequisite to independent prosthetic donning and should be addressed as needed.[47] People with dysvascular amputation may have distal weakness in their hands from peripheral neuropathy and physical therapists should make appropriate referrals to occupational therapists, as this may influence the person's ability to properly don and doff the prosthesis.

Progressive resistance protocols are often used to improve strength and muscle endurance. Resistance may be applied manually (e.g., proprioceptive neuromuscular facilitation [PNF] techniques are desirable, as they strengthen multiple joints and planes simultaneously) or with equipment (e.g., cuff weights, elastic bands, pulley weights). Resistance is generally not applied at or near the suture line until the surgical wound is well healed. Using body weight is an effective way to introduce resistance training (e.g., bridging or planks with modifications as needed). Basic physiologic principles of strengthening (e.g., overload principle, specificity of training) are employed in the design of an appropriate resistance program, and exercises should specifically target muscles identified as weak in the examination and muscles that are functionally required in gait, transfer, and mobility activities. Strengthening within the context of functional activities is ideal. Correct exercise techniques are important for achieving the desired strength gains, and the physical therapist's expertise in movement analysis is important in helping individuals understand how to perform their exercises properly and how to self-critique performance.

Therapists should also ensure that people with limb loss engage in a regular home exercise program to maintain strength, as functional mobility with the prosthesis alone is not sufficient to maintain strength. Maintenance of strength and endurance is important for the prevention of secondary impairments (e.g., back pain, skin breakdown) that may develop over time as an individual performs ADLs and instrumental ADLs.

BALANCE AND POSTURAL CONTROL

Effective postural control during functional tasks has two fundamental components: (1) controlling the body's position in space for purposes of stability (maintaining center of mass over base of support) and (2) orientating the trunk and limbs in space (appropriate relationship between body segments and between body and environment).[48] The normal balance mechanism relies on visual, vestibular, and somatosensory input. Visual and vestibular information add awareness of position in space with respect to objects in the environment and to gravity, and somatosensory input provides information about the positions of the joints of the lower extremity and the pressures through those joints. Balance mechanisms function both proactively and reactively. With loss of the distal limb to amputation, somatosensory and proprioceptive input can no longer provide direct information about the position of the limb and its interaction with support surfaces.

Balance deficits as well as falls are well documented in people with lower extremity amputation,[49–52] as is diminished balance confidence.[53] Balance, as assessed with a variety of different measures, is associated with prosthetic ambulation outcome.[20,21,49] Table 26.2 provides the recommended outcome measures for balance assessment in people with lower extremity amputation.[20,21] Risk factors for falls in individuals with dysvascular amputations are consistent with those for the general older adult population (i.e., lower extremity weakness, increased age, multiple comorbidities, and/or polypharmacy),[49,54] but people with preexisting sensory deficits from peripheral neuropathy on both the residual and intact limbs may be at an even higher risk. Moreover, it has been found that after amputation some individuals with lower balance confidence have poorer performance on balance tests, have decreased walking ability on year post-amputation, and have increased need for an assistive device (AD).[53,55,56] This probably reflects the self-limiting mobility of those who lack confidence in their balance, yet it serves as an excellent reminder that overconfidence in balance performance can be dangerous. The incidence of falls in people with lower limb amputation is higher than that in age-matched peers without amputation, and risk factors for falls seem to vary across different phases of recovery (acute care vs. rehabilitation vs. community dwelling).[50,52,54] Early on, individuals may fall when getting out of bed due to referred sensations of the limb. As mobility progresses, falls are noted to occur in the context of transitional movements such as transfers to and from a wheelchair, gait, stair navigation, and performance of ADLs, thus highlighting the importance of education regarding safe transfer strategies.[57]

Balance assessment and training should begin in the immediate postoperative phase, and continue throughout the remainder of the rehabilitation process. Training programs should be tailored to meet the needs of the individual and be modified as the individual progresses throughout their rehabilitation. In the immediate postoperative phase, therapists should consider that some individuals will have difficulty adjusting to changes in sitting balance and bed mobility following lower extremity amputation. In addition to the changes in the center of gravity after amputation, the loss of the weight of the amputated lower extremity diminishes the stabilizing potential of the lower body for supine-to-sit transitional movements; this is abundantly evident in individuals with bilateral lower extremity amputations who struggle to achieve sitting from a side-lying or supine position. Such individuals must rely more on upper extremities and trunk musculature for position changes. In sitting, lack of a second foot on the floor and, in the case of transfemoral amputation, loss of the surface area of the thigh on the seating surface alter the base of support, and loss of the mass of the lower extremity elevates the body's center of gravity, making sitting more precarious. Most individuals adjust fairly quickly, developing competence and confidence in static sitting; but the inability to shift weight onto the missing foot can challenge dynamic sitting, especially with reaching tasks requiring movement anterior and ipsilateral to the amputated side. For this reason, seated reaching ability is evaluated during the initial examination and is addressed in treatment as necessary. Once an individual is training with a prosthesis and again has two feet on the floor, dynamic sitting balance often need not be a focus of treatment.

In the preprosthetic phase, standing balance focuses on single-limb stance to prepare the person for mobility with a prosthesis. This might include single-limb standing in the parallel bars or alternate support surface with decreasing the person's reliance on upper extremity support. The ability to stand on the sound limb without upper extremity support has been associated with better prosthetic gait outcomes in individuals with unilateral lower extremity amputations,[20,21] making this an important skill to assess and train as early as possible.

The therapist should also creatively seek ways to challenge the person's limits of stability during early upright balance training. In people with transtibial amputations, if the individual can tolerate a kneeling position over the healed surgical site, exercises can be performed in quadruped with progression to high kneeling (Table 26.4). In those with transfemoral amputations, if they can tolerate some pressure to the healed distal end, the individual may kneel with the intact limb on the mat and the residual limb resting on a foam block or wedge, progressing exercises from static to dynamic. Another progression might be to stand with the sound limb on the floor and rest the residual limb (transtibial or transfemoral) on an elevated surface (e.g., mat, gymnastic ball, or foam block), providing balance support but minimal weight bearing. Preprosthetic gait training with an appropriate AD is another useful and functional approach to upright balance training. It is important to realize that weight bearing through the distal end of the residual limb must be allowable per the surgeon performing the amputation, and the time frame for a noncomplicated residual limb to heal varies between 6 and 10 weeks.

Because sensory and proprioceptive input from the distal segment is absent after amputation, individuals must learn to compensate for this lack of important postural information. Given underlying vascular pathology and comorbidity of diabetic neuropathy in people with dysvascular amputation, the somatosensory mechanisms that inform balance cannot be presumed to be intact on the remaining limb. In addition to the loss of sensory input (due to loss of limb and compromised sensory status of remaining limb), the loss of muscles of the amputated foot and ankle will compromise existing motor plans for postural control. Balance reactions are considered to result from the combination of preprogrammed synergistic muscle activity as well as a continuous adaptive feedback system gleaning information from lower extremity joints.[48] Ankle, hip, and change in support/stepping strategies are used to ensure that the center of mass stays within the base of support in response to anteroposterior perturbations, and these postural strategies are evident during functional activities. The ankle strategy requires intact ROM and strength of the ankle. After amputation, this strategy is no longer available to the involved limb and the person may not be able to resolve the balance perturbation using intact limb response only; thus he or she may have to rely on a hip strategy (movement of the trunk over the base of support) or a change in support strategy (stepping or hopping to move the base of support under the center of mass).

Therapeutic balance challenges during preprosthetic rehabilitation provide opportunities to address environmental demands during various functional tasks in anticipatory (feedforward) and reactive (feedback) modes. For example, successfully catching and throwing a ball or batting a balloon requires the person to anticipate postural demands in an effort to throw and react to postural challenges in an effort to catch. This task can be progressed through a series of postures (e.g., seated, straddling bolster on mat, kneeling on mat with amputated side on foam block, standing in parallel bars with amputated side on foam block, standing in parallel bars in unilateral stance, decreasing reliance on upper extremity support in bars). Reaching activities in standing help individuals develop skill and confidence in their anticipatory postural responses and, should the reach distance be excessive, their reactive postural responses as well. Therapists must consider the person's ultimate likely functional requirements and design a variety of balance tasks to help the person achieve levels of functioning commensurate with his or her potential. To facilitate improved balance and success in the self-identification of limits of stability, individuals must experience loss of balance in the context of training. This can be achieved safely with excellent guarding technique and can be facilitated by the use of harness systems (e.g., Zero G, Biodex, LiteGait) if available. It is also advised that therapists provide education and training on how to fall safely, and recover from a fall prior to the completion of the rehabilitation program, as this may minimize the adverse events related to a fall.

Once the person has been fitted with a prosthesis, the therapist can revisit the same balance activities performed preprosthetically and the focus of balance training becomes the equal distribution of weight between the intact and prosthetic sides. In the context of integration of sensory information within the balance systems, individuals may learn to substitute for lost somatosensation and deduce the position of the prosthetic foot and contact with the support surface by the angle of the hip or, in the case of the person with a transtibial amputation, the knee, and pressures felt within the prosthetic socket.

CARDIORESPIRATORY FITNESS

Physical therapists should be mindful that persons with lower extremity dysvascular amputation are likely to have comorbidities that negatively affect cardiorespiratory fitness, and recognize that periods of immobility that often precede the amputation can further contribute to decreased aerobic capacity. Aerobic capacity of persons with lower extremity dysvascular amputation has also been demonstrated to be lower than that of age-matched peers without amputation.[24,58] Taking these into consideration, with the increased energy requirement of prosthetic gait, therapists must thoroughly assess and prescribe aerobic exercises that are appropriate and seek to improve cardiorespiratory fitness.[59] Some additional key physiologic considerations for prosthetic gait, as evidenced in literature reviews,[24] may also inform the exercise prescription:

- The energy cost of walking is greater in individuals with amputations than those without.
- Higher-level amputations are associated with higher energy costs of gait than lower level amputations.
- Persons with dysvascular amputations demonstrate greater energy cost of gait than those with traumatic amputations.
- Customary or self-selected gait speed decreases with higher levels of amputation.

- The average rate of oxygen consumption during self-selected gait speed may not be significantly greater than normal, especially for transtibial prosthetic users, as individuals decrease their self-selected speed to mitigate rising oxygen consumption.
- It is generally more efficient for an individual with a prosthesis to ambulate with the prosthesis (with or without an AD) than it is to ambulate without the prosthesis using an AD. An exception to this may be the person with a dysvascular transfemoral amputation, where energy expenditure may be similar with and without a prosthesis if the individual is highly dependent on the AD.

Energy expenditure for over-ground walking in people with unilateral dysvascular amputations has been noted to be increased for higher gait speeds and more proximal amputations when compared against healthy controls.[60] It is important to consider that many individuals are deconditioned on entering the rehabilitation course and, given that fitness correlates with the successful use of a prosthesis,[20,21] aerobic training is an essential component of the preprosthetic and early prosthetic rehabilitation phases. It is well documented that peak oxygen consumption (VO_{2max}) in individuals with dysvascular amputations is significantly less than in healthy age-matched peers without amputation.[61,62] The VO_{2max} is decreased, but the energy cost of gait is increased, thus simply walking can consume a much larger percentage of VO_{2max}[58,62] and cause individuals to be functioning closer to their aerobic threshold.

Preprosthetic aerobic conditioning may be in the form of wheelchair propulsion, single-limb ambulation with an appropriate AD, bilateral upper and/or unilateral lower extremity ergometry, circuit training, or swimming. These activities often continue as therapy progresses to the prosthetic phase of rehabilitation. As the condition of the residual limb and wearing tolerance permit, ambulation with the prosthesis can be used as a cardiorespiratory endurance activity, but the therapist needs to be mindful of monitoring the patient's heart rate to ensure they are working at enough intensity to exert cardiorespiratory changes.[59] Individuals who are taught to monitor their own pulse, respiratory rate, and/or rate of perceived exertion are able to participate more confidently and independently in aerobic training. Training programs are individually prescribed by the therapist based on the person's past medical history and current cardiovascular, pulmonary, and musculoskeletal status utilizing standardized guidelines for older adults as a goal.[63] For maximal impact, the therapist must introduce the appropriate level of challenge within the context of an activity that is agreeable and motivating to the person. For individuals with few cardiovascular restrictions, once they are tolerating prosthetic wearing, brisk walking, and/or the use of exercise equipment (e.g., treadmill, stationary bicycle, NuStep, stair climber, elliptical machine, circuit training), these constitute excellent endurance training activities for the appropriate person. An amputation need not prevent individuals from participating in health and wellness exercise programs during and following their rehabilitation. However, the prosthesis itself must be considered during activities, as not all prostheses can function for all demands.

EDEMA CONTROL OF THE RESIDUAL LIMB

The reduction of postsurgical edema is critical in the early postoperative rehabilitation phase. Use of standard or removable rigid postoperative dressings (e.g., cast or prefabricated polyethylene dressing) after transtibial amputation appear to be superior to soft dressings (including elastic bandages) in controlling the volume of the residual limb, and are associated with a shorter time from amputation to initial fitting of the prosthesis.[64,65] Removable rigid dressings seem to be the optimal choice for postoperative dressings because they offer the same benefits as standard rigid dressings (e.g., edema control, limb shaping, and protection) but also offer the opportunity to inspect the surgical site and monitor wound healing; however, this type of postoperative care is not routinely used in the United States, perhaps because of the debate among payers regarding who is responsible for reimbursement (hospital vs. insurance). When the more common soft dressings are used, elastic bandages for compression are applied over the residual limb dressing. Elastic bandages should be applied in oblique angles (not circumferentially, so as to avoid a tourniquet effect), with a gradual increase in pressure from distal to proximal, and always extending above the knee, as the transtibial prosthetic socket engulfs the medial and lateral aspects of the knee.

The transfemoral residual limb does not lend itself to rigid postoperative dressings and is more challenging to wrap with elastic bandages, as it requires anchoring over the pelvis, and it may be difficult for a person to elevate their pelvis after amputation for wrapping. Nevertheless, techniques for postsurgical compression wrapping should be a part of the treatment plan. In addition, people with amputation and their family members should be instructed in the correct wrapping technique, as the elastic bandage typically has to be reapplied several times a day, and inaccurate application can disrupt healing, lead to infection, and delay prosthetic fitting.[66]

After the staples or sutures have been removed, use of a commercial pressure garment ("shrinker") is suggested for persons with either transtibial or transfemoral amputations. Residual limb edema plays a big role in determining when initial prosthesis fitting will take place—if the prosthesis is fitted too early and the residual limb is still substantially shrinking, this will affect the intimacy of prosthetic socket fit, making training more difficult and increasing the risk of complications caused by a poorly fitting socket. Prerequisites for initial prosthesis fitting include sutures removed, surgical wound healed or healing, and edema controlled, with distal measurements less than or equal to proximal measurements. The importance of continued shrinking efforts, even after prosthesis training has begun, should be emphasized. Individuals must usually continue to wear a shrinker when they are not wearing their prosthesis, at least during early training efforts, to reduce the likelihood of insidious edema when the prosthesis is not being worn. If people allow the edema to return to the limb, the socket may no longer fit and aggressive efforts to reduce the limb volume will have to precede any further prosthesis training. Individuals prone to fluctuations in fluid volume (e.g., those with kidney dysfunction or congestive heart failure) will likely have to use a shrinker indefinitely. For others, whose residual limb ultimately reaches a stable size and shape, a shrinker may not be necessary once the prosthesis is consistently being used. The decision to discontinue the use of a shrinker permanently is based on two factors: (1) consistency in the number of sock layers worn during the day and (2) the ability to don the prosthesis without decreasing the usual number of sock layers after a night's sleep without the shrinker. Significant changes in body weight can also dramatically affect socket fit. All people with amputation should be educated regarding the importance of contacting the prosthetist and/or therapist if their weight changes significantly over time.

SOFT TISSUE MOBILITY OF THE RESIDUAL LIMB

Soft tissue and bony adhesions that limit tissue mobility around the incision scar and the surrounding area may have an impact on tolerance, comfort, and use of the prosthesis. Surgical amputation can include muscle-to-muscle (myoplasty), muscle-to-fascia (myofascial), and/or muscle-to-bone (myodesis) surgical fixations to stabilize the remaining muscle.[67] Scarring or adhesions can occur in any or all of these tissues. The normal stresses and shearing forces of cyclic loading and unloading during gait require that soft tissue throughout the residual limb be mobile. If the soft tissue is not able to move independently of the scar tissue or skeletal structures, the resulting stress can lead to tissue breakdown and/or discomfort. Soft tissue mobilization techniques early in the rehabilitation process can help to establish appropriate tissue mobility in the residual limb. Once the surgical incision is well healed, soft tissue massage can be an effective tool for maintaining tissue mobility. It may also be helpful in managing scar tissue along the incision. Individuals can be instructed in the use of this modality with specific guidelines for proper technique. Appropriate technique is essential to minimize the risk of damaging the fragile skin around the incision site, as too much friction generated between the fingers and skin results in irritation, blistering, or breakdown and can delay the use of a prosthesis until adequate healing has occurred.

SENSORY STATUS OF THE RESIDUAL AND REMAINING LIMBS

Sensation of the residual limb and sound limb should be formally assessed during the initial PT examination. Standard sensation testing guidelines may be used to assess all sensory modalities (e.g., pain, temperature, light touch, deep pressure, proprioception, vibration). Semmes-Weinstein monofilament testing may be used to assess for protective sensation of the sound limb. Several commonly occurring postamputation sensory phenomena can have implications for functional outcome in persons with amputations. These include hyposensitivity, residual limb pain, phantom limb sensations, and phantom limb pain.

Hyposensitivity

Hyposensitivity is most often encountered among those with a history of diabetes, neuropathy, traumatic nerve damage, or vascular disease. People who have impaired sensation are at high risk for skin breakdown because they may not recognize discomfort associated with skin irritation resulting from repetitive stresses and pressures. Inclusion of education about the preventative need for visual inspection for signs and symptoms of soft tissue lesions and supervised practice of this task can reduce the risk of skin breakdown. Adaptive equipment, such as mirrors, or the assistance of caregivers may be necessary for people with concurrent limitations in cognition, flexibility, and/or visual impairment.

Residual Limb Pain

Early in rehabilitation, it is not uncommon for people to encounter somatic and neuropathic forms of residual limb pain.[68,69] Common in the immediate postoperative phase, somatic and surgical pain may be present, and they usually subside over time.[70] Ongoing complaints of residual limb pain should prompt careful inspection of the residual limb, as the therapist may pick up on signs of the formation of heterotopic ossification,[71,72] infection, or small cutaneous/subcutaneous problems that could manifest as pain. This careful inspection and follow-through is especially important in individuals with renal and vascular disease, as data suggest that those who have an initial distal amputation at any level are at a substantial risk of revision of amputation to a higher level,[73] and have higher mortality[74] and increased risk of readmission to the hospital,[30,75] all of which increase the persons mortality risk[76] and delay a successful rehabilitation outcome. The therapist should also be mindful that residual limb pain is often confused with prosthesis-related pain, and in some cases a simple fix (e.g., adjustment of prosthesis or number of socks) can provide relief.[77]

Generalized hypersensitivity of the residual limb may also exist and this is thought to be a consequence of nerve damage from the amputation surgery itself.[78] Hypersensitivity can be effectively managed by employing a tactile desensitization program, which involves bombarding the residual limb with tactile stimuli using a variety of textures and pressures.[70] Strategies for reducing hypersensitivity include gently tapping with the fingers, massaging with lotion, touching with a soft fabric (e.g., flannel or towel), rolling a small ball over the residual limb, and implementing a specific wearing schedule for shrinkers and removable rigid dressings. Intensity of intervention is based on the individual's tolerance to the sensory stimulation. The techniques can be progressed in intensity, type of modality used, and duration of stimulus (e.g., touching the limb with a rougher fabric and increasing wearing time for the shrinker). It is strongly encouraged that these techniques be performed independently as part of the home program. Over time these techniques should help to reduce the hypersensitivity, with the ultimate goal of tolerance to normal sensory input without discomfort. Physiologically, overloading the nervous system with sensory stimuli is thought to encourage habituation via downregulation of neural receptors.

Localized hypersensitivity may be an indication that a troublesome neuroma has developed at the distal end of a surgically severed peripheral nerve.[79] A neuroma is suspected when localized tapping sends a shock sensation up the leg (the Tinel sign). If conservative clinical treatment is unsuccessful in reducing hypersensitivity and pain caused by a neuroma, injection of a local anesthetic directly into the region or surgical removal may be necessary. Targeted muscle reinnervation is a surgical technique that can be both preventative and corrective for cases of acute and chronic postamputation neuroma pain, hypersensitivity, and phantom limb pain (described subsequently).[80–82] Although this technique was initially developed to facilitate intrinsic control of upper extremity prostheses, it appears that it also has the added benefit of reducing neuroma formation and decreasing postamputation pain after lower extremity amputation.[80,81,83] The procedure involves transferring the cut ends of peripheral nerves to targeted motor units of the remaining limb (e.g., tibial nerve to a motor branch of the semitendinosis),[81] creating specific electromyographic signals detectable by a myoelectric prosthesis. Targeted nerve reinnervation is another similar technique that also demonstrates success at reducing neuroma formation at the time of amputation. It may be more appropriate for those individuals who are ineligible or uninterested in using myoelectric prostheses because the procedure is less concerned with the rearrangement of the muscle-nerve units following amputation and generally allows for more distal nerve transfers.[84] Although slightly different in approach, both procedures are documented to minimize neuroma formation as well as residual limb and phantom limb pain by reducing the aberrant sprouting of the severed nerves.[80,83,84]

Phantom Limb Sensations and Pain

Phantom limb sensations are quite common after amputation.[85–87] Many individuals report experiencing feelings of pain, itching, tingling, numbness, or sensations of heat and cold in the toes or foot of the limb that has been amputated. Although the sensation can include the entire missing extremity, proximal sensation often fades, leaving only distal perceptions, a phenomenon known as "telescoping," presumably related to the large area of somatosensory cortex dedicated to the distal extremity.[88] While phantom limb sensations (if painful) may negatively impact someone's quality of life, it also has the potential to provide a semblance of proprioceptive feedback from the prosthesis. Be alerted, however, as to the importance of educating individuals of the potential danger of phantom limb sensations: nighttime falls are not uncommon when, half asleep, an individual attempts to stand and walk to the bathroom, expecting the phantom foot to make contact with the floor.

Phantom limb pain occurs in 50% to 80% of all persons with amputation and has wide variability in presentation.[82,86–88] The incidence of phantom limb pain has been demonstrated to be greater with proximal as compared with distal amputations, and people who experience phantom limb pain typically report that it decreases over time.[78] When phantom pain occurs, it is most often described as a cramping, squeezing, aching, or burning sensation in the part of the limb that has been amputated. The spectrum of complaints may vary from occasional mild pain to continuous severe pain. The absence of observable abnormalities in the residual limb is common. Although the etiology of phantom pain is not definitively understood, changes in the peripheral nervous system, spinal cord, and maladaptive reorganization at the level of the cerebral cortex may all be involved in the perception of phantom limb pain.[88–91] It is uncertain if phantom limb pain is associated with preamputation limb pain. The relationship of amputation etiology with the presence of phantom limb pain is also unclear, but recent data support that the incidence of phantom limb pain is higher in those with vascular and infection causes, as compared to oncologic.[78]

Whatever the etiology and predisposing factors, phantom limb sensations and pain are challenging to manage and can limit the success with a prosthesis if the pain is severe. There are several therapies that are documented to alleviate the sensations: mirror therapy, graded motor imagery, and visual virtual feedback.[92,93] Mirror therapy involves strategically placing the sound limb in front of an angled mirror to create the illusion that the amputated limb is intact; the individual watches the reflection in the mirror as he or she performs exercises of the sound limb and imagining the movement of the phantom limb. The individual receives visual feedback (in the mirror) confirming the "movement" of the phantom limb (the residual limb is concealed behind the mirror). This pairing of *thinking* about moving the phantom limb and *seeing* it move is aimed to help resolve the mismatch of information that exists in phantom limb pain (i.e., feeling pain in an extremity that does not exist is a conflict between the sensory experience and the visual experience).[93] Graded motor imagery[92] has also been used in treating phantom limb pain. Intervention components include a series of left/right limb orientation tasks directed toward limb laterality (distinguishing the phantom from the intact limb), explicit motor imagery tasks (imagining moving the amputated limb through a series of exercises), and mirrored visual feedback tasks. Although the mechanism by which these strategies minimize pain remains unknown, it is thought that both mirror therapy and graded motor imagery influence neural networks and cortical reorganization to combat the maladaptive neural plasticity caused by phantom limb pain. Other strategies used to address phantom limb pain include medications (e.g., antidepressants, anticonvulsants, analgesics); neural blockade; transcutaneous electrical nerve stimulation; heat and cold modalities; acupuncture, biofeedback; firm pressure applied to the residual limb (e.g., massage, compression or prosthetic socket); exercises of the phantom limb; psychologic treatment; and education.[87,94–97]

CARE OF THE SOUND LIMB

Ongoing assessment of the intact lower extremity should be the responsibility of the patient with support from the physical therapist and, if necessary, caregiver. Individuals with diabetes, peripheral neuropathy, or peripheral vascular disease who have undergone lower extremity amputation as a result of the disease process are likely to have changes in the protective sensation and vascular supply on the sound limb. There is also an increased functional demand on the remaining limb after amputation and the added burden to the remaining limb extends beyond the preprosthetic period. Once ambulatory with a prosthesis, individuals will preferentially initiate level surface walking with the prosthetic limb, placing a larger burden on the sound limb for stability and propulsion.[98] As an ambulatory individual makes adjustments to increase walking speed and distance and navigate uneven surfaces, demands continue to increase on the sound limb.[99,100]

Contralateral limb amputation is a very real threat to those with diabetes, renal and/or vascular compromise.[31,101,102]

Special consideration should be given to those people who are Black and/or Hispanic and those who receive dialysis, as current literature suggests that these are the highest risk factors for contralateral limb loss.[31] To minimize the risk of loss of the remaining limb, close monitoring of limb condition (especially for subtle or insidious trophic, sensory, or motor changes) and optimal foot care are essential. Ongoing, systematic and frequent assessment of pulses, edema, temperature, and skin is suggested. Education about the importance of a daily routine of cleansing, drying, and closely inspecting the foot (including the plantar surface and between the toes) is crucial. Podiatric care of nails, corns, and plantar calluses, appropriately fitting footwear or accommodative foot orthoses, and avoidance of barefoot walking are three additional imperatives for the longevity of the remaining foot. If unable to perform daily foot inspection independently because of disease or visual impairment or decreased agility, individuals must be able to direct a caregiver in inspecting the foot. Even if individuals are physically incapable of performing certain tasks for their own health and safety, they are ultimately responsible for their own care. Developing or improving on a person's skill at directing assistance is a useful and realistic PT treatment goal.

Candidacy for a Prosthesis and Prescription

Determining candidacy for a prosthetic device should be a team-based approach due to the multifactorial nature of the intrinsic and extrinsic factors that can influence the prescription of the prosthesis.[103,104] Generally, older age, higher amputation level, lower physical activity level, and presence of multiple comorbidities are negative predictors for a successful prosthesis fitting.[2] Conversely, younger age, vascular patency, and good physical function were positive predictors for success with a prosthesis.[105] Considering older adults with dysvascular amputations being fit for a prosthesis are estimated to be as low as 36%, numerous factors must be considered when determining candidacy.[106]

INTRINSIC FACTORS

Biological Systems

The integrity of the body systems plays a key role in determining whether a person with limb loss is a candidate for a prosthesis. In general, a prosthesis can be fit to an individual regardless of medical condition, but certain medical conditions can make prosthesis use prohibitively difficult or impractical. For example, an individual with bilateral transfemoral amputations who has clinically significant cardiopulmonary disease may not benefit from, or be able to withstand, the rigorous rehabilitation following the amputation.[107] A history of cerebrovascular accident with hemiplegia on the side opposite the amputation may limit functional use of a prosthesis, though not necessarily prohibit the prescription, especially if the prosthesis can assist with transferring.[108] Therefore medical condition in and of itself is not the determining factor for prescription of the prosthesis, rather it is the individual's ability to functionally utilize the prosthesis. Since exposure to a prosthetic device raises the incidence of secondary complications, biological system integrity must be sufficient enough to withstand the rigors of prosthesis use.[47,109]

Musculoskeletal system: It should be no surprise that lower limb strength is needed to properly use a prosthesis. Depending on the level of the amputation and prosthesis type, strength of the lower extremities can be a limiting factor for functional prosthesis use. For transtibial-level amputations, knee extension and flexion strength are less on the residual limb, with extension torque being up to 70% less than the intact limb, which can contribute to knee instability during gait and increased risk of falls.[36,50] For transfemoral prosthesis users, hip flexion and extension strength on the residuum is approximately 25% less than the intact limb, while hip abduction and adduction is nearly 50% less.[36] Lack of hip strength, specifically hip abduction and extension, can cause gait abnormalities and compensatory postures, which in turn can contribute to development of secondary complications like low back pain.[37,109] Beyond the lower extremities, strong core musculature (abdominals and spinal) have been shown to improve spinal mechanics and improve gait mechanics in those using a prosthesis.[110] One must also look at the strength of the hands, particularly in those with dysvascular amputations, as hand dexterity and strength can be a limiting factor for the individual's ability to don or doff a prosthesis.[47] Shoulder strength and integrity will be needed to prevent overuse, especially during the initial training progression when the patient may be less comfortable weight bearing through the prosthesis and is dependent on the upper extremities for support.[111] Joint contractures can render prosthesis use untenable, with hip or knee flexion contractures greater than 25 degrees being considered the clinical limit for functional everyday use, although it is still possible.[32]

Cardiopulmonary: The amount of energy needed to ambulate a distance with a prosthesis typically exceeds the same distance for a person without a prosthesis, demanding more from an already impaired system.[112] Circulatory issues can result in nonhealing of the residuum if a wound is due to friction or improper management of the residual limb socket interface.[14,113] This can lead to nonuse of the prosthesis, or in certain circumstances an increase in risk of infection or reamputation. Edema that occurs as a result of heart failure or cardiovascular issues can make the process of suspending a prosthesis cumbersome and onerous, limiting the wearing time or requiring modifications to the socket.[114]

Neuromuscular: The effect of diabetes can be found in nearly all organic tissue, but especially the small blood vessels of the eyes and distal extremities. This can result in decreased sensation of the intact limb, further putting it at risk for infection. Neurological tone can impact the ability of the prosthesis wearer to functionally utilize a prosthesis, especially when combined with a contracture of the residual limb. Significant coordination impairments like those associated with cerebellar infarcts or ataxic conditions can make use of the prosthesis unwieldy and hazardous. Of great impact to the likelihood of receiving a prosthesis is cognitive function. Those with diminished cognitive function are less likely to receive a prosthesis when compared to their noncognitively impaired counterparts.[12]

Other systems: While function of the systems above make up the majority of considerations for prescription, other biological systems must be taken into account as well. The genitourinary system, including kidney function, may be impaired due to the influence of diabetes, vascular disease, or a combination of both. Since many medications utilize the genitourinary pathways to excrete excess fluid to manage blood pressure, a candidate may have to urinate frequently. As such, the act of urinating may be impeded by the suspension system used to attach the prosthesis, requiring a sometimes complex process of doffing the prosthesis to urinate, then redonning again to ambulate. This process can be impractical for many persons with limb loss, especially those who don their prosthesis in a supine position.

Function: While not a specific biological system, prior functional status will likely have great bearing on the determination to be prescribed a prosthesis. An individual who required substantial assistance for functional mobility before amputation may have limited ability to use a prosthesis. Preamputation ambulation ability is predictive of walking ability with a prosthesis,[21] although it is important to consider how far back to measure walking ability; a series of toe or forefoot amputations may precede transtibial or transfemoral amputation, and individuals may have had limited walking mobility for months prior to the final surgery.

Psychological Aspects

Depression: In the case of an amputation due to dysvascular disease, the lead-up to the surgery is typically longer than that of a traumatic amputation. Due to this longer lead-up time, individuals will generally be debilitated due to the prolonged limb-salvaging process, and as a result have less engagement in avocational and vocational activities. For many, this can lead to depression, which is estimated to have a prevalence of 40%, due both to the prolonged periods of inactivity but also to the adjustment to loss of limb.[115] Those with higher depressive symptoms also report an increase in pain and lower quality of life.[115] Since low motivation is a sign of depression, and learning to use a prosthesis requires a high degree of motivation, depression can be a barrier to success with a prosthesis.[116]

Anxiety: The anticipation of having an amputation would naturally increase anxiety in most people. Both before and after the amputation there is a heightened level of anxiety.[117] The anxiety may be anticipatory in nature, looking to what their future function may look like. Others may fear the reality of living with limb loss, and as a result may be apprehensive about the rehabilitation process. High levels of anxiety can be detrimental to successfully adjusting to life without limb; therefore a consideration for prescription would be the patient's ability to manage anxiety in the rehabilitation process and beyond.[118]

Social Factors

Support at home: Those with low function prior to the amputation will likely require assistance from family members, significant others, or caregivers to help with one or more tasks. The potential to be a limited household ambulator with a prosthesis may be important in reducing the burden on caregivers and may allow a person to remain at home with a caregiver as opposed to living in an institution.

Support in the workplace: For many individuals, workplace accommodations can be made to support effective participation in occupational demands. However, for more physically demanding occupations, the prosthesis itself is a consideration if the individual can go back to their prior level of function. Since most individuals who have amputations secondary to dysvascular disease typically have lower levels of function, the prosthetic components will be designed to efficiently match their functional needs. Therefore a consideration for prosthetic device candidacy will be the occupational needs and ability to accommodate in the workplace.

Avocational interests: Since many dysvascular amputations occur later in life, there may be a large number of avocational interests that are important to persons with limb loss. Some may not be impacted significantly because of the amputation, others may not be feasible or may be impractical. Candidacy for a prosthesis considers these avocational interests, and prescription would need to find a balance between everyday demands and the occasional specialty demand.

EXTRINSIC FACTORS

Insurance: The type of insurance can determine what prosthetic device the patient will receive, regardless of the patient's desires and availability of technologically advanced componentry. While we know that certain components can decrease fall risk and improve function in persons with dysvascular amputations, the cost barrier can preclude the prescription of more expensive and advanced prostheses in favor of simpler and more affordable options, despite evidence showing that microprocessor knees can reduce falls by 2.5-fold.[119]

For those with economic means to pay for their own prosthesis, this is not an issue, but given that the cost of a lower limb prosthesis is 12 to 15 times higher than the gross national income of many lower-middle income countries, this excludes a large proportion of the limb- loss population.[120]

Environment: Not all prosthetic devices are appropriate for all environments. For example, an individual who ambulates primarily in rugged terrain and navigates uneven terrain will need a different device than a person who will only use the device for transfers in a controlled environment on stable surfaces. While more technologically advanced componentry may offer benefits to users, they also have the trade-off of having restrictions to certain environmental and atmospheric conditions. For example, a microprocessor knee can be more susceptible to environmental contamination from sand, dirt, or water, thus making it an impractical consideration for certain terrains.

MEDICARE FUNCTIONAL CLASSIFICATION LEVEL

The Medicare Functional Classification Level (known as the K-level) consists of five categories (K-levels 0–4) and is used to determine which prosthesis components are appropriate based on the amputee's level of function and rehabilitation potential.[121] The considerations for determining the K-level are made by the multidisciplinary team, and are based on the patients' prior, current, and perceived future level of function. Note, the K-level classification only applies

Table 26.5 Description of Medicare Functional Classification Levels and Prosthetic Componentry

K-Level	Description	Transtibial Component	Transfemoral Component
0	This does not imply the ability or potential to ambulate or transfer safely with or without assistance, and such a prosthesis does not enhance the individual's quality of life or mobility.	N/A	N/A
1	This enables the ability or potential to use a prosthesis for transfers or ambulation on level surfaces at a fixed cadence; it is a household ambulator.	■ SACH ■ Single axis	■ Single axis
2	A prosthesis at this level enables the ability or potential for ambulation with and to traverse low-level environmental barriers such as curbs, stairs, and uneven surfaces; it is a limited community ambulator.	■ Flexible-keel ■ Multiaxial	■ Polycentric
3	Such a prosthesis can facilitate the ability or potential for ambulation with variable cadence; it is an advanced community ambulator, enabling the amputee to traverse most environmental barriers. It may also enable vocational, therapeutic, or exercise activity that demands utilization of the prosthesis beyond simple locomotion.	■ Dynamic response ■ Multiaxial ■ Microprocessor	■ Hydraulic/ pneumatic ■ Microprocessor
4	This type of prosthesis implies an ability or potential for ambulation that exceeds basic ambulation skills, exhibiting high-impact, stress, or energy levels; it is useful to active children, young adults, and older adults engaged in recreational activities and sports.	Any system	Any system

to lower limb prosthetic devices. See Table 26.5 for further descriptions of K-level classifications.

It is important for physical therapists to understand the role they play in determining the K-level. Because physical therapists spend a great deal of time working with people one-on-one, they often have a clearer idea of the individual's prior, current, and perceived future level of function. The therapist may gain insight or information that is important in the decision-making process. If he or she is familiar with the components of prostheses and the K-levels under which those components are covered, the therapist may begin to form an opinion about the best prosthetic prescription for a given amputee during the early rehabilitation phase. This makes the physical therapist a key stakeholder in the determination of the prosthetic prescription, but the ultimate responsibility will be shared among the prosthetist and prescribing medical doctor.

It is imperative that individuals be assigned the appropriate functional level, as assignment into a lower K-level may hinder optimal mobility. For instance, classification as K-1 will result in a SACH foot, whereas a K-2 is eligible for a multiaxis foot and a K-3 for a dynamic response foot; those rated K-2 or K-3 will have greater ease in walking over uneven surfaces compared with those classified as K-1.[121] Use of higher K-level knee componentry appears to reduce falls risk and improve mobility, reminding therapists to suspend biases that higher-tech equipment should be reserved only for younger individuals.[119,122–124]

The process of K-level determination is not consistent across clinicians, prosthetists, and physicians. A survey of 213 US prosthetists by Borrenpohl et al. in 2016 found that 47.3% of prosthetists assign K-levels alone; 42.9% of prosthetists collaborate with other healthcare providers (e.g., physical therapists); and 7.3% reported that K-levels were assigned by the physicians.[121] In the same study, it was also concluded that a standard method for K-level determination does not exist; some prosthetists and clinicians reported using performance-based measures such as the Amputee Mobility Predictor (AMP), Berg Balance Scale (BBS), or the 2-minute walk test; others used self-report measures such as the Orthotics and Prosthetics Users Survey (OPUS) or Activities-Specific Balance Confidence (ABC) Scale.[121] Some literature suggests that the AMP may be the ideal outcome measure to determine K-levels, especially in differentiating between K-levels 3 and 4.[125] Recently, a study found that scores on the Prosthetic Limb Users Survey of Mobility (PLUS-M), age, body weight, and cause of amputation are predictive in classifying functional class when entered into a classification tree prediction model.[126]

Prosthetic Device Considerations

ALIGNMENT OF THE PROSTHESIS

This is evaluated by the prosthetist and/or physical therapist in quiet standing (statically) and during gait activities (dynamically). *Static alignment* refers to the relationships between the socket, prosthetic knee joint (if applicable), pylon, prosthetic ankle/foot, and floor; the length of the prosthesis; and the overall fit of the socket on the residual limb. Information gleaned from this assessment can provide clues regarding pressure distribution on the tissues of the residual limb within the socket. Improper alignment effect not only pressures within the socket but also the biomechanics of gait and the translation of forces from the prosthetic foot up the kinematic chain. The assessment of dynamic alignment includes all components of static alignment but in the context of movement and also the assessment of suspension and symmetry of gait. Both static and dynamic alignment must be evaluated from anterior, posterior, and lateral (prosthetic and sound side) views. Table 26.6 provides a basic rationale for standard transtibial and transfemoral static alignment, which is important for therapists to understand given the close association of prosthetic alignment with the biomechanics of gait. Note: only the prosthetist is qualified to adjust the prosthesis, and the physical therapist should not adjust screws related to alignment without explicit permission. For a thorough review of prosthetic alignment, see the chapters on the relevant components.

TEMPORARY PROSTHESIS

For those with dysvascular amputation, initial fitting typically occurs when the surgical incision is healed and the

Table 26.6 Static Alignment of Prosthesis and Rationale

Alignment	Rationale for Alignment
POSTERIOR VIEW	
Prosthesis height (symmetric leg length)	Prevents gait deviations associated with leg-length discrepancy
	Provides optimal weight bearing through the socket to prevent pain and skin issues
	Prevents sound limb orthopedic deformity associated with leg-length discrepancy
Plumb line: midsocket to slightly lateral to midheel	In the transtibial prosthesis, creates slight varus moment during stance, as in normal gait
	In the transtibial socket, directs compressive forces to pressure-tolerant areas at medial proximal (medial tibial flare, medial femoral condyle) and lateral distal (fibular shaft) residual limb and minimizes compressive forces on nontolerant areas at lateral proximal (fibular head) and medial distal residual limb
	In the transfemoral socket, directs forces onto the residual lateral femoral shaft
Slight adduction of transfemoral socket	Adduction of the transfemoral socket serves to improve length tension relationship and efficiency of the hip abductors in maintaining a level pelvis during unilateral stance
LATERAL VIEW	
Transtibial socket in 5–10 degrees of flexion (anterior tilt of socket, encouraging slight knee flexion) when in a midstance position	Distributes weight-bearing forces to anterior pressure-tolerant aspect of transtibial residual limb
	Limits vertical displacement of center of mass at midstance to decrease energy cost of gait
	Allows for controlled knee flexion in loading response and late stance, as in normal gait
	Prevents abnormal hyperextension of the knee in midstance
Transfemoral socket in 5 degrees of flexion (posterior tilt of socket, encouraging hip flexion) with the knee in full extension at the midstance position	Serves to improve length tension relationship and efficiency of the hip extensors during stance phase of gait
	Distributes weight-bearing forces to posterior pressure-tolerant aspect of transfemoral residual limb
Plumb line: midsocket to anterior edge of heel	In transtibial alignment, allows for knee flexion from mid- to terminal stance
	In transtibial alignment, prevents hyperextension of the knee in stance
Assessment of trochanter-knee-ankle line	In transfemoral alignment, provides assessment of the location of the center of rotation of the knee joint in the transfemoral prosthesis relative to hip and ankle, which dictates the stability of prosthetic knee extension during stance and the ease of prosthetic knee flexion in preparation for swing

patient is medically stable. The time from surgery to initial fitting with the temporary prosthesis in uncomplicated scenarios generally ranges from 6 to 12 weeks. The temporary prosthesis is the first prosthetic device fitted to the patient, and may or may not contain the components of their permanent prosthesis (the device they will use for the next 3 years). The purpose of the temporary prosthesis is to allow the patient to learn how to functionally utilize their device, but the socket will need to be reduced in volume to accommodate the rapidly shrinking residual limb. The temporary may also have more rudimentary componentry, like a single-axis knee and SACH foot, but serves as a platform for the patient to demonstrate their functional abilities. If their abilities exceed that of the prescribed K-level, the designation can be modified to elevate the K-level and allow the prosthesis user access to higher grade componentry when appropriate.

SUSPENSION

Suspension occurs between the residual limb and the prosthesis, and is a critical component of achieving a proper fit of the prosthesis. Those with dysvascular amputations are at a heightened risk for skin breakdown from exposure to the prosthesis, therefore there are specific considerations when suspending a prosthesis for this population. Vacuum-assisted socket systems (VASS) have been shown to improve pressure distribution, balance, transfers, gait, and fear of falling, while not increasing the risk of skin breakdown.[127,128] However, VASS are heavier and more costly than some other suspension types. Gel liners, which serve as intermediate between the residuum and socket, help reduce load concentration, thus decreasing the risk of pressure-sensitive areas breaking down.[128] The thicker the liner, the more comfortable it is, but the trade-off is a sensation of instability during gait.[129] Other forms of suspension include lanyard/straps, shuttle locks, and various forms of suction. While all have their benefits, the choice of suspension type is determined by the patient's functional needs, physical capabilities of the user, ease of donning/doffing, and the physiological integrity of the residuum.

PROSTHETIC SOCKS

Prosthetic socks are used to modify the fit between the socket and the shrinking residual limb. Proper use of prosthetic socks enhances residual limb weight bearing in pressure-tolerant areas, decreases the likelihood of skin breakdown in pressure-sensitive areas, and increases comfort within the socket. Wool or cotton prosthetic socks are available in a variety of different sizes, configurations, and ply. Uniform thickness socks are commonly found in either 1, 3, or 5 ply. Some socks have a split thickness, where the top or bottom has a different ply thickness than the bottom, which can be useful for an individual who is shrinking in a nonuniform manner or who has a more bulbous distal residuum. An antimicrobial sheath may be worn under the socks to minimize friction and wick moisture away from the skin.

Depending on the suspension system, socks may or may not be used, but are typically utilized during the initial year of prosthesis use as the residual limb volume decreases. Socks are applied over the liner (if being used) prior to the limb being placed in the socket. Socks are combined to create a snug fit that uses the fewest socks to achieve the appropriate sock thickness. Once a sock ply of approximately fifteen is achieved, the fit of the prosthesis can suffer, thus requiring modifications to the socket to accommodate the now reduced residual limb.[130]

PRESSURE-TOLERANT/SENSITIVE AREAS

Persons with limb loss should understand where weight-bearing pressures are best tolerated on the limb and where pressure sensitivity is likely to occur. Sockets are designed to distribute weight-bearing forces across pressure-tolerant areas, while decreasing pressure along sensitive areas. For the transtibial residuum, tolerant areas include the patellar tendon, anteromedial and anterolateral surfaces of the residual limb, and the medial tibial flare. Sensitive areas include hamstring tendons and the bony prominences of the residual limb. The transfemoral residual limb is tolerant along the muscular bulk of the thigh and ischial tuberosity, but sensitive along the bony prominences of the pelvic brim and greater trochanter.[131]

SELF-MANAGEMENT

Self-management is a term used for many chronic medical conditions that require the individual to make purposeful behavioral modifications to their daily routines to prevent secondary complications. For example, in the case of an individual with diabetes mellitus, monitoring of blood sugar, adjusting diet, and responding to glycemic crises are all forms of self-management. In the case of limb loss, self-management includes problem-solving the fit of the prosthesis, maintaining the integrity of the residual limb, and preventing secondary complications like skin breakdown or infection.[132]

Problem Solving the Fit

The most commonly reported issue reported by prosthesis users is the comfort of the prosthesis, and difficulty problem solving the fit is frequently reported as a barrier to success.[133]

A close fit between the residual limb and the socket is a key component of achieving a comfortable fit. A comfortable fit translates into improved function and decreased risk of developing secondary complications associated with limb loss.[134] The optimal prosthetic fit is intimate, allowing the muscular forces of the residual limb to translate efficiently through to the ground via the prosthesis. Because the immature residual limb undergoes volume fluctuations, both daily and over time, the process of problem solving the fit between the limb and the prosthesis becomes a critical component of patient education. The temporary prosthetic socket will be shaped to initially fit the residual limb, but it may take a few weeks for the prosthesis to arrive after measuring, which may result in significant shrinking of the residuum volume. Since total contact within the socket is very important, and skin problems can occur when total contact is not achieved, problem solving the fit is part of the intervention starting day one.

The residual limb will undergo decreases in volume as it matures. Shrinkage of the residual limb in early training is accommodated by the addition of layers of socks to maintain a snug residual limb-prosthesis interface. Fluctuations in limb volume associated with edema in the first weeks and months after amputation often mean that the appropriate number of sock layers must vary from day to day and often within a given day. Because of the potential for rapid fluctuations in limb size, choosing and monitoring the correct number of socks may be challenging for those new to the use of a prosthesis. Therapists and prosthetists work with new users to assist in the development of problem-solving skills and strategies to determine the appropriate number of socks to use.

The suspension system utilized can assist the prosthesis user in achieving a proper fit. For example, the speed and number of pin "clicks" for a shuttlelock liner can indicate that the fit is proper. If the clicks are rapid and exceed the expected number (typically the pin should never be completely engaged into the socket, rather the middle-bottom third of the pin), it indicates to the wearer that they may need additional ply of socks. For those using a lanyard or strap system, a line drawn on the strap can indicate if the fit is appropriate based on the length of strap exposed/unexposed from the socket. Another indication would be the phenomena of pistoning during ambulation, which occurs when the prosthesis slips downward when unweighted and upward on weight bearing. If pistoning is suspected, close observation will reveal that excessive superior/inferior motion is occurring, which can be mitigated by donning additional sock layers.

Although pistoning is usually an indication of too few layers of socks, paradoxically it can also be seen in a person wearing too many layers because the residual limb is never fully situated in the socket and therefore never gains good purchase, causing the socket to move up when weight bearing and down when unweighted. Indications that too many layers of socks have been donned may be complaints that the prosthesis is difficult to don, fits too tightly, or feels slightly longer during gait.

When the transtibial prosthesis and socks are taken off to inspect the skin, reactive hyperemia (redness) is seen at the proximal patellar tendon and the inferior border of the patella as well as at the distal anterior residual limb. Redness may also be present on the fibular head, which has contacted the socket below its intended relief area. These are all signs that the residual limb is sinking too deep into the socket and that additional sock layers should be added. Too few socks in a transfemoral socket may lead to increased weight bearing and hyperemia on the distal residual limb and complaints of pressure in the groin as the socket rides up higher than intended.

In the transtibial amputee, if inspection of the skin after ambulation reveals reactive hyperemia on the distal patellar tendon, tibial tubercle, and/or head of fibula, these landmarks may be contacting the socket above their intended reliefs (i.e., too many socks prohibits the residual limb from being well positioned in the socket).

Since problem solving the fit can be so problematic, there are numerous forms of education available. Since the process has more similarities than differences between most prosthesis users, a decision tree approach can be useful. A decision tree can walk the user through the various steps needed to achieve an intimate fit of the residual limb in the prosthesis. While there are published decision trees that can be used for a patient, specific and personalized decision trees can be made by the practitioner for the person with limb loss that are specific to a unique suspension system or set of circumstances.[14,134] An example decision tree is shown in Fig. 26.1.

Hygiene

Residual limb hygiene involves proactive maintenance of the integrity of the skin coupled with responsive interventions if hygiene issues present.[133] Skin problems are a frequent issue, with estimates of nearly 75% of prosthesis users experiencing integumentary issues within the last month.[135] Older adults, who statistically have a greater preponderance of dysvascular amputations, have a higher risk of skin issues despite generally having a lower functional level than younger counterparts.[136] The hostile environment created by the prosthetic socket promotes sweating and bacterial growth due to the increased heat generated from both friction and the insulation from the surrounding material.[137] This can create dermatologic conditions like contact dermatitis or superficial fungal infections.[33] Therefore the prosthesis user must become adept at self-managing the hygiene of their residuum if they are to be successful with life after limb loss.

Daily hygiene routines entail cleaning of the residuum using hypoallergenic soap and warm water, inspecting the skin for breakdown or irregularities, and maintaining the

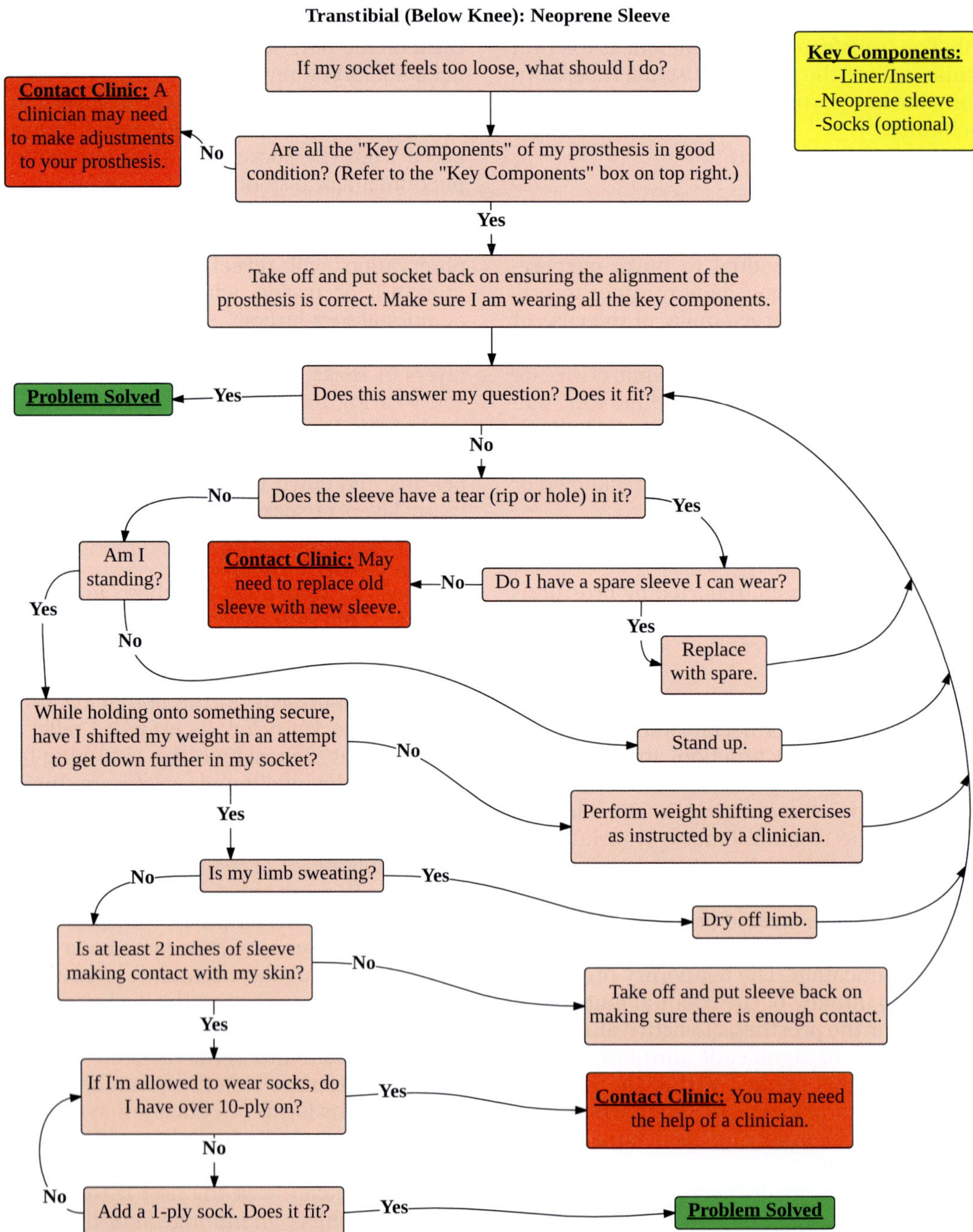

Fig. 26.1 The SMART (Self Management Assessment of the Residuum and prosThesis) decision tree,[132] designed to assess the self-management knowledge of persons with limb loss.

integrity of the skin through moisturizing. While these steps are simple in nature, it can be an area of issue for many with limb loss. Since those with dysvascular amputations may have peripheral neuropathy due to diabetic complications, hot water can result in a burn to the residuum. Therefore warm water is more appropriate and less likely to cause thermal injury to tissues. Skin inspection should be done with a mirror, ideally handheld, so that all aspects of the residuum can be visualized. If an area of concern is identified in an individual with dysvascular etiologies of amputation, it is best to not wear the prosthesis until a medical professional can evaluate due to risk of further injury. Moisturizing of the residual limb should be done daily, but typically not within 30 to 60 minutes of donning the prosthesis. The rationale is that for individuals using a silicone liner, the lotion may impede the skin friction necessary to gain purchase and form an intimate fit. Lotion should be water based and hypoallergenic, and the residual moisturizer should not feel oily. Defer to the skin product manufacturer's recommendations.

Besides cleaning of the residual limb, the prosthesis itself should be cleaned according to the manufacturer's suggestions. Typically, this involves simply wiping down the exterior and interior with a damp lint-free cloth. Persons should be cautioned to avoid using any harsh cleaners or products that may potentially degrade the materials used to formulate the socket. The liners should be cleansed daily, again with a lint-free cloth and soap and water. Drying the liner can be done on a liner tree or laid flat with the cloth side of the liner (not the one that touches the skin) facing outward to prevent accumulation of contaminants. Inspection of the prosthesis and components should be performed during the cleaning process, identifying any areas of poor form or function and addressing the issue with a healthcare professional.

Red Flag Recognition

Common red flags related to prosthesis exposure are skin breakdown, infection, and pressure injury. It is imperative that the prosthesis user identify the presence of such complications early and intervene if they are to prevent secondary complications due to residual limb injury.[132] Because prolonged wound healing and the development of skin irritation can delay training and significantly affect daily functioning,[138,139] the prevention and management of skin problems are important components of treatment. The prevalence of skin problems on the residual limb in prosthesis users has been reported to be between 36% and 63%.[140–142] Especially vulnerable to skin issues are very active users and those with impaired hand function.[47,143] Thermal discomfort and sweating within the socket is a complaint shared by up to 53% of prosthesis users.[139,144] Pressure, friction, and shearing forces are the primary causes of skin breakdown related to prosthetic wear. If during weight bearing, external pressure exceeds capillary refill pressure (25–32 mm Hg) for an extended time, the delivery of oxygen and nutrients and the removal of waste products from active tissues are interrupted.[145] If relief of pressure is provided, this local ischemia is followed by a reactive vasodilation or hyperemia. This is the mechanism that produces the redness over weight-bearing areas that is observed in new users of prostheses. A blanchable area of redness over weight-bearing areas, which returns to normal skin coloration within 10 minutes, is expected in early training and indicates normal reactive hyperemia.[146] If redness persists or the skin does not blanch on firm palpation, tissue damage has likely occurred and the risk of skin breakdown will increase significantly.

It is important that therapists and persons with limb loss recognize the implications of redness over pressure-tolerant versus pressure-sensitive areas of the residual limb. If a pressure-tolerant area shows evidence of excessive pressure, socket fit and alignment may be appropriate but the amount of weight bearing or duration of wearing may have to be decreased. If pressure-sensitive areas are showing signs of too much pressure, it is more likely that socket fit or alignment must be adjusted. When excessive redness is observed, successful problem solving dictates changing a single variable at a time and assessing the effect of this one change on the problem. If multiple changes are made at the same time (e.g., wearing time, alignment, and socket fit are all altered), it will be unclear which change solved the problem if indeed the problem is solved. If the problem is not solved, there will be no way of knowing if the interventions may have been more successful independent of one another.

If localized increased pressure is determined to be the cause of tissue breakdown, pressure relief is the goal and socket modification by the prosthetist may be necessary. Certain methods of pressure relief are inappropriate and should be avoided. The use of "donut" padding around an area of breakdown or potential breakdown is counterproductive for three reasons. A donut pad (1) increases pressure to the area surrounding the lesion when the limb is placed in the socket, (2) increases the ischemic effect of weight bearing, and (3) potentially leads to edema or extrusion of the vulnerable tissue through the "hole" of the donut. Dressings should be used sparingly inside a prosthetic socket as the socket fit is designed to be snug, and any padded dressing increases pressure over the affected area, which is counterproductive to the goal of wound healing. There are multiple options for thin, self-adherent, nontextured dressings (e.g., Tegaderm, Second-Skin) that can be used within the prosthesis's socket to effectively provide another "tissue" layer to an area that is threatening to break down or is in the process of healing.

Assessing Self-Management

Since hygiene, problem solving, and red-flag recognition are critical in preventing secondary complications associated with limb loss and prosthesis use, it behooves the therapist and healthcare team to first assess the individual's self-management knowledge early on in the rehabilitation process. Much like in the case of diabetes mellitus, where self-management knowledge is assessed as a routine component of individual care, the same should be done for those with limb loss. The only validated measure designed to assess self-management knowledge in those with limb loss is the Self-Management Assessment for the Residuum and prosThesis, or SMART.[132] The SMART is a knowledge assessment tool that can quickly determine whether or not the individual has gaps in their knowledge in all the major domains of self-management. Once a gap in knowledge is identified, targeted educational interventions can be applied to the individual's specific situation to address the knowledge gap. See Fig. 26.1 for an example of the SMART system.

WEARING SCHEDULE FOR THE PROSTHESIS

It is vital that new users of a prosthesis understand the importance of the gradual progression of wearing time and are compliant with their personalized wearing schedule. Constant reassessment of socket fit and comfort and diligent assessment of the skin of the residual limb after bouts of wear are necessary during the entire training phase. Amputees and/or their care providers should be well educated on residual limb inspection. Rapid and significant changes in residual limb shape and size are common in early prosthetic training due to weight bearing, compression within the socket, and the muscle pumping action that occurs with walking. As a result, socket fit may become less intimate, which can lead to skin issues. The duration of early wearing time is usually conservative, especially for individuals with a history of skin integrity problems. Initial weight-bearing activities are closely supervised, lasting no longer than 5 to 10 minutes in between skin inspections. Inspection of the residual limb after the first few minutes of weight bearing should reveal redness of the skin in predictable load-bearing regions. Because both the transtibial and transfemoral sockets are designed to be in total contact with the residual limb, the entire limb may develop a mild reactive hyperemia (redness) that is apparent when the socket is first removed.

Once an individual is spending 30 to 60 minutes in the prosthesis without problems, total time in the prosthesis is gradually increased, often in increments of 15 to 30 minutes as tolerated. The therapist works with the amputee to determine how much of the wearing time he or she should spend up and walking. People with no history of skin integrity problems (e.g., traumatic amputation or revision of congenital limb anomaly) often progress quickly with wearing activities, whereas those with sensory impairment or peripheral vascular disease may have to progress more cautiously. An individualized written schedule should be provided to guide prosthetic wearing of the prosthesis and prevent misunderstandings about the time permitted for its use and the suggested amount of upright weight-bearing activity per bout of wear.

DONNING AND DOFFING THE PROSTHESIS

Donning the prosthesis will become second nature—just another component of getting dressed each day—but early in rehabilitation it must be deliberately taught through a series of specific steps that will be dictated by the prosthesis's components. A common suspension system for a transtibial prosthesis is a roll-on silicone liner with a pin-lock suspension system. Donning of this type of prosthesis is represented in Fig. 26.2. This procedure requires the individual to attend to the orientation of the distal pin when rolling the liner onto the residual limb so as to anticipate appropriate need for socks for optimal fit, to orient the pin into the ring-lock mechanism in a seated position, and to stand and bear weight for the final engagement of the suspension mechanism. On weight bearing, the pin will depress into the ring, which is confirmed by a predetermined number of audible clicks to indicate appropriate fit (too many or too few clicks point to a need to reassess alignment and prosthetic socks). Other types of suction/vacuum suspension systems (e.g., a roll-on seal-in ring for transtibial or transfemoral prostheses or double-wall vacuum system or classic valve system for transfemoral prostheses) have distinctive requirements for optimal donning technique and usually require cleaning of the residual limb and/or application of a lubricant prior to donning. Balance and hand strength and dexterity may be prerequisites to independent donning; they are therefore addressed in the preprosthetic phase. The chapters on prosthetic components elucidate further the donning

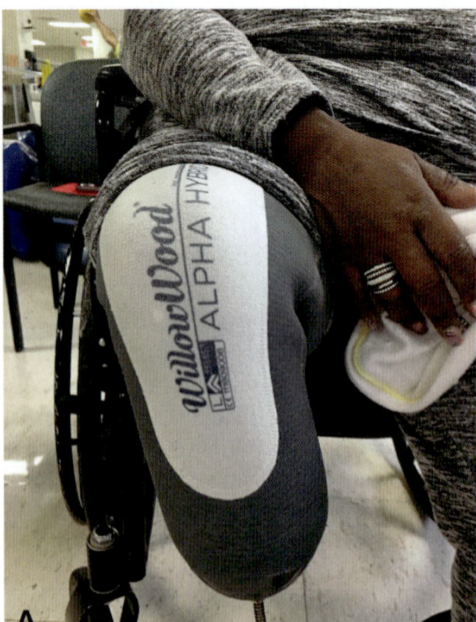

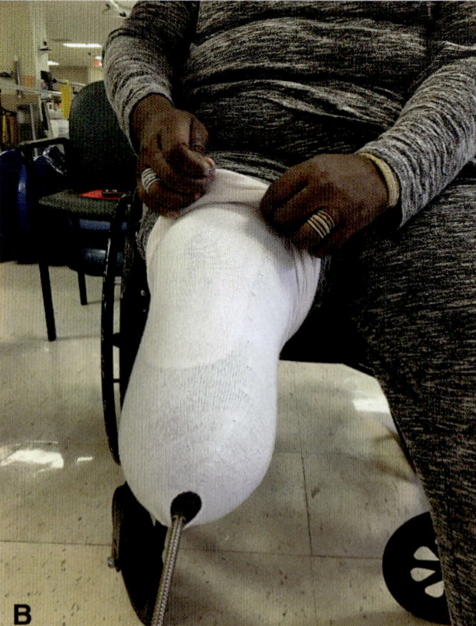

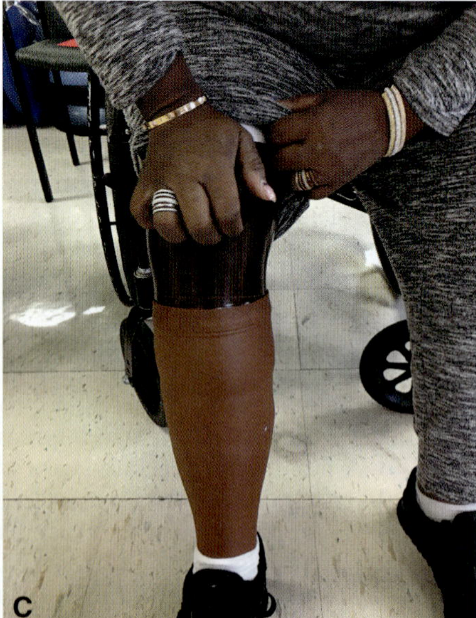

Fig. 26.2 This person with a recent transtibial amputation demonstrates the correct sequence for donning her prosthesis. (A) First, she applies the silicon liner, attending to the orientation of the pin. (B) Once the liner has been positioned, prosthetic socks are added, one at a time, and carefully adjusted for a smooth fit until the desired number of layers is reached. (C) The final step is to insert the residual limb with socks and liner into the prosthesis. The prosthesis is donned in the seated position, gradually increasing weight bearing to achieve the desired total contact fit.

requirements for specific types of prostheses, and therapists can rely on their prosthetist colleagues to answer questions about specific donning needs related to any device with which they are not familiar.

Whereas donning technique is specific to socket and suspension type, there are some universal themes in donning that should be taught to all users. For instance, individuals are taught to dress the prosthesis first (i.e., for ease of dressing, put the prosthesis through a pant leg and place a shoe on the prosthetic foot prior to donning the limb). Additionally, all users must learn to pay close attention to the orientation of the socket in the horizontal plane. The contours of the socket are precisely designed to accommodate the residual limb's anatomy. In a person with a sensate residual limb, this may be constructive in assuring proper alignment, as the socket will not "feel right" unless it is oriented correctly. In the person with impaired sensation in the residual limb, vision and palpation of the residual limb structures may be used to assure proper alignment. Often individuals use the prosthetic foot as a reference for horizontal plane alignment; static prosthetic alignment often places the foot in slight out-toeing in standing, and the individual can use this visual cue as affirmation of proper prosthetic alignment.

Early instruction and assessment of donning and fit of the transfemoral socket often requires the therapist to palpate the ischial tuberosity and potentially other structures (e.g., pubic rami, adductor tendons) for optimal positioning within the socket. This requires clear and professional communication and education to clarify the purpose and process of palpation that would otherwise be considered a serious invasion of personal space.

PROSTHETIC GAIT TRAINING

Functional ambulation involves moving the body through space effectively and efficiently while meeting environmental and task demands. For the prosthesis user, this has many prerequisites, including (1) achieving the necessary baseline of flexibility, strength, and endurance; (2) building tolerance to prosthesis wear and weight bearing through the residual limb; (3) controlling dynamic weight shifting through the prosthetic foot in all planes of movement; and (4) reintegrating postural control and balance despite the missing sensory/proprioceptive input, muscle activity, and ROM from the amputated limb. The skilled physical therapist will shepherd the person with limb loss through the training process, helping him or her to build proficiency and confidence along the way. Of interest, there is conflicting evidence on whether exercises or gait training yield the best outcomes on prosthesis-related mobility, with specific exercises improving gait speed and walking distance but not necessarily balance.[147] An individual's fears and concerns influence determination and motivation and are powerful determinants of community ambulation.[148,149] Mobility apprehension can also be related to pain, with fear avoidance and pain catastrophizing leading to poorer functional outcomes.[150] Additionally, the absence of peripheral neuropathy and an increase in self-confidence, self-reported physical activity, and prosthesis use explained greater than 50% of the variance in those who participate at a community level.[151] Those with greater per-person step counts are also shown to have lower falls, consistent with community ambulators being less likely to fall when compared to non-community ambulators with lower limb loss.[152]

Initial Training

For the new user of a prosthesis, the initiation of gait training typically begins with ambulation on level surfaces with few environmental demands. The parallel bars are an excellent starting point, offering a stable, secure, protected environment with minimal challenges. Individuals are encouraged to use a relaxed, open-handed grip when they train in the bars, as the tendency to pull and rely heavily on the secure bars is a difficult habit to "untrain" when transitioning to a less protected environment (Fig. 26.3). Progressing from weight bearing and gait activities with significant bilateral upper extremity support to minimal or no support is a common early goal in the rehabilitation process of both transtibial and transfemoral prosthesis users. However, transtibial and transfemoral rehabilitation trajectories may be different due to the knee component requiring greater physiological demands, with transfemoral prosthesis users having more gait deviations than the transtibial counterparts.[153] In the beginning, the therapist must remain cognizant of the need for frequent skin checks for signs of pressure intolerance and skin irritation. Once the threat of skin breakdown has been alleviated, less frequent checks are needed. Another component of gait training is how feedback is provided. Feedback can be provided in a variety of different fashions, but it is typically performed with verbal cueing. While verbal cueing can be effective to improve motor learning, evidence suggests that feedback is typically focused internally, rather than externally, which may limit the effect of the intervention.[154] Auditory, visual, and proprioceptive forms of feedback can also be used, but age, level of amputation, intensity, and timing of feedback may influence its effectiveness.[155]

A typical progression of early prosthetic training activities might include the following:

1. Static weight bearing with decreasing dependence on upper extremity support (e.g., progressing from bilateral open-handed upper extremity support to contralateral open-handed upper extremity support to ipsilateral open-handed upper extremity support to no upper extremity support).
2. Standing reaching activities that require the person to reach to a variety of heights and directions within a functional context. These activities are progressed by decreasing upper extremity support, increasingly challenging reaching limits in all directions, and varying foot position. Therapists should carefully observe and critique weight shifting and weight bearing during reaching tasks. Reaching excursion in the direction of the prosthetic limb should be significantly greater with the prosthesis than it is without. If reaching distances are similar, this is likely an indication that the individual is not truly using the prosthesis to broaden his or her base of support; this is required to promote a larger shift of center of mass in reaching. These early reaching activities are prerequisites to later more progressed functional goals such as reaching to high shelves, lifting something of substantial weight, and picking objects up from the floor.

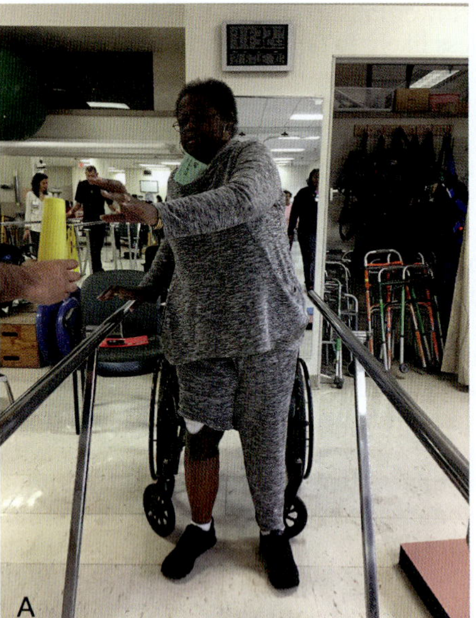

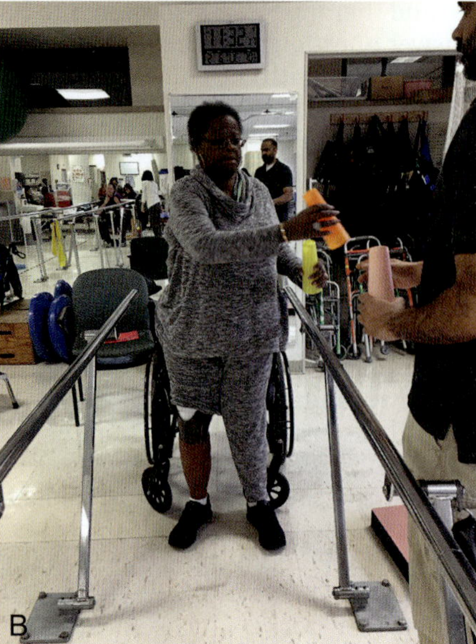

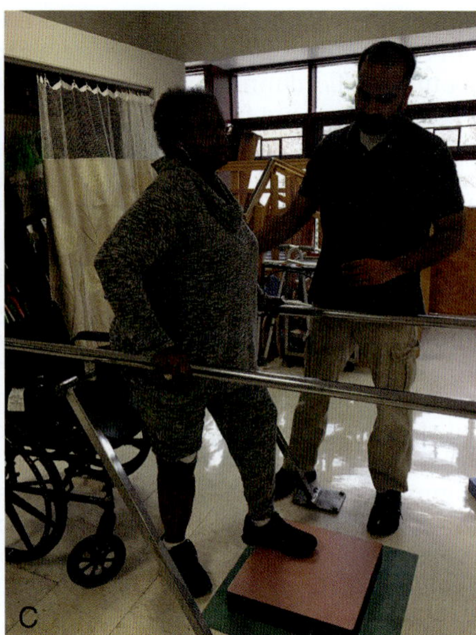

Fig. 26.3 Weight-bearing, weight-shifting, and balance activities in early prosthetic training. (A) A new prosthetic user practices loading weight onto the prosthesis by performing a trunk rotation and reaching activities in the parallel bars. Note full weight bearing through the prosthesis, demonstrating good prosthetic alignment and erect trunk and head posture, with a gentle open-handed grip on the parallel bars. (B) Rotation to the sound limb facilitates weight shifting on and off the prosthesis and can challenge balance and postural control. (C) Stepping up a low step can increase weight bearing through the prosthesis in the early stages of rehabilitation.

3. Simple dynamic weight-shifting activities, consisting of loading and offloading body weight through the prosthesis in multiple directions (anterior/posterior, medial/lateral, and diagonal patterns) as is required in gait and functional activities. These tasks are progressed by decreasing upper extremity support and/or varying foot positions (parallel stance, step stance, tandem stance). It may be helpful to cue the individual to think about the weight going through the "ball" or "heel" or the medial or lateral surface of the prosthetic foot as he or she shifts weight in different directions. This heightened awareness of what is happening distally may help to correlate sensations within the prosthesis's socket with former somatosensory experiences of the foot. Another strategy during weight-shifting activities is to have the individual focus proximally on pelvic position. The focus on the pelvis is important for several reasons: (a) There is clear evidence of asymmetries in pelvic stability and control during gait in amputees.[156] (b) The pelvis is key to stability in upright posture, so the individual is cued in to this important locus of control. (c) By focusing on the pelvis, the individual is being directed to control a part of the body that is intact and "whole." Although he or she may never have focused on pelvic awareness prior to rehabilitation, this takes the focus off the prosthesis and the "new" challenges the amputee is facing. (d) Awareness of pelvic position in early weight-shifting activities may make later gait demands, such as emphasizing pelvic protraction or rotation, easier for the individual to grasp. In controlling the pelvis during weight-shifting activities, the prosthesis user might envision the pelvis as a tabletop with a tall vase centrally located on the table, so if the pelvis tips in any direction, the vase will fall and break; or they may imagine a ball on that table and—regardless of the direction of the weight shift—they must not let the ball roll off of the table. These cues are intended to encourage anterior, posterior, and lateral translational movements of the pelvis without substantial anterior, posterior, or lateral tilting of the pelvis.
4. Repeated stepping activities (e.g., breaking down the gait cycle into its component parts, varied stepping patterns in different directions) with decreasing upper extremity support. The focus here is in loading and offloading the prosthetic limb with good proximal/pelvic control. Repetitive loading of the prosthesis is an appropriate task, even without full translation of weight over the foot, as it requires repetitive and appropriate positioning of the prosthetic limb (as required for the initial contact phase of gait) and initiation of the transfer of weight (as required for the transition from initial contact into loading response). The progression to full weight bearing and the single-limb support phase of gait is an intuitive next step, as is the integration of loading and offloading the prosthesis within the full gait cycle. Although the use of weight-bearing and stepping strategies outside of the functional context of walking may seem contrary to fundamental tenets of motor learning (i.e., encouraging action-directed/whole-task performance), practicing the component parts and integrating them into functional gait and mobility skills is a reasonable and acceptable motor learning principle.[48] Regardless of the focus of the intervention (weight bearing, balance, postural control, or coordination and sequencing), the activity can and should be integrated into the gait cycle or the functional task within the same treatment session.
5. Stepping with the uninvolved limb onto an elevated surface (begin with a low surface and progressing to height and/or beginning with a stable surface, such as a step-stool or thick book, and progressing to a less stable surface, such as an air disc or small ball) forces increased

weight bearing through the prosthetic limb with progressively decreasing upper extremity support. The focus is on slow and controlled motions of the sound limb without substantial proximal instability on the weight-bearing prosthetic limb. Activities might include stable standing on the prosthetic limb while performing toe tapping with the sound limb on a stool or manipulating of a ball on the floor (rolling the ball forward and back under the foot) (see Fig. 26.3).

6. Many prosthetic knees rely on the translation of weight bearing over the prosthetic forefoot in terminal stance and preswing to generate the knee flexion required to forward the limb in swing phase and this may require focused practice. These loading and offloading techniques can be practiced in pregait stepping drills or repetitively in early gait training.

Some individuals may have difficulty aligning themselves symmetrically over their feet in stance when initially training with the prosthesis. They may appear hesitant to weight bear on the prosthetic limb and their perceived line of gravity may strongly favor the sound limb with the prosthetic-side hip appearing abducted and the sound hip adducted. Ironically, individuals who have been especially active and functional during the preprosthetic phase, ambulating with crutches or a walker, may find weight bearing through a prosthesis difficult. During the preprosthetic phase, the sound limb often gravitates to a more central location under the individual so that their center of gravity is directly over their single-foot base of support. These individuals must work to reorient their lower extremity positioning and line of gravity to center themselves over their "new" two-footed base of support. Fig. 26.4 illustrates this concept.

Individuals who are hesitant to bear weight through the prosthesis due to fear or weakness or habitual pattern may be tempted to use the prosthesis as an "AD" for ambulation rather than as a true replacement limb. These individuals maintain the prosthetic limb in an abducted posture and struggle to decrease reliance on upper extremities and the sound lower extremity during standing and ambulation activities. It is important for both therapist and new prosthesis wearer to recognize that improved weight bearing allows for decreased mechanical stresses on the sound limb, which inevitably has vascular compromise. Clinical strategies used to encourage optimal alignment and weight shifting over the prosthesis may include stepping on a bathroom scale to provide objective data regarding weight bearing through the prosthesis, use of a mirror for visual feedback to self-assess alignment, and biofeedback in the form of virtual reality.[157]

Progressing prosthetic training requires increasing challenges to postural control and balance. Ultimately, dynamic therapeutic activities without (or with limited) upper extremity support and activities that require both anticipatory and reactive balance strategies (e.g., playing catch, kicking a ball with a partner) can be used to prepare the prosthesis user for more open, unpredictable real-world environments (Fig. 26.5). Coordination, sequencing, and timing of gait may be facilitated by auditory or visual cues. Use of a metronome or musical beat to time steps or a floor ladder or spaced targets to drive step length can be integrated into gait training.

The focus on pelvic awareness and control (as introduced in the context of weight shifting, discussed earlier) can be further emphasized in training with the integration of PNF techniques in standing and during pregait and

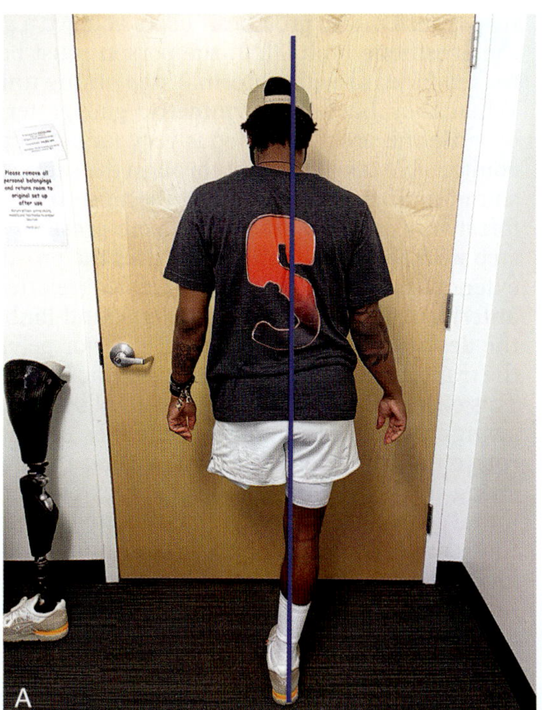

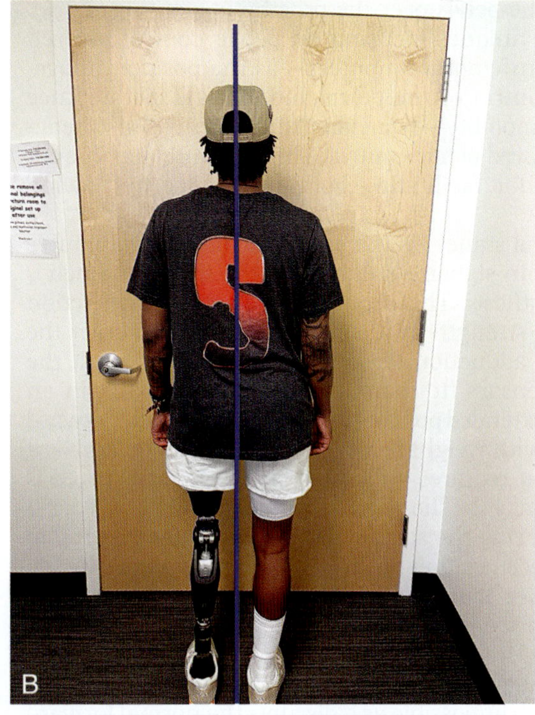

Fig. 26.4 Line of gravity with and without the prosthesis. (A) During the preprosthetic phase, the line of gravity shifts to directly over the sound limb. (B) Individuals must work to reorient their lower extremity positioning and line of gravity to fall midline when wearing their prostheses.

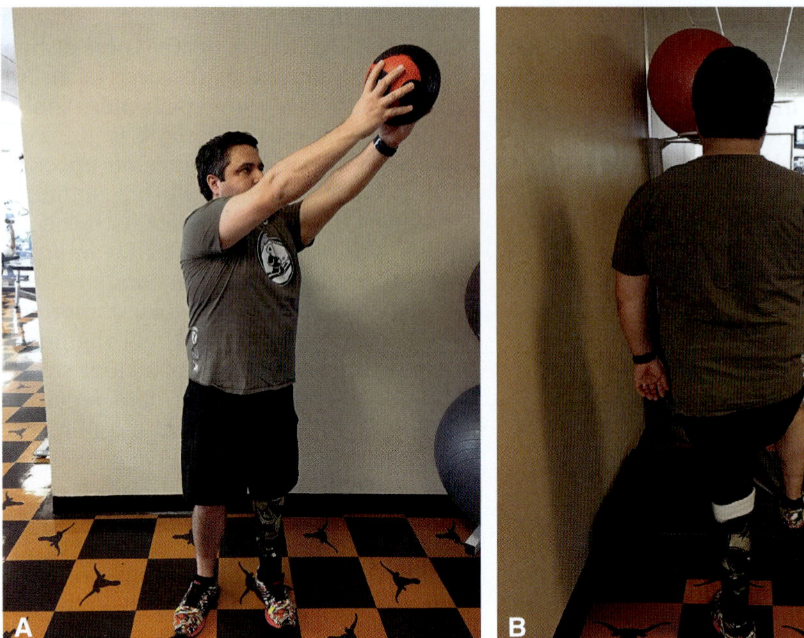

Fig. 26.5 Progression of weight shifting and balance activities in prosthetic training. (A) Trunk rotation outside of the parallel bars, using all planes of movement and decreasing reliance on upper extremities. (B) Stepping up to a higher surface outside of the parallel bars to increase the challenge and translate into community mobility.

gait activities.[158] Facilitating muscle activation via joint approximation, using rhythmic stabilization (i.e., having the individual hold pelvic position against resistance in varying directions) to strengthen and improve pelvic control, and providing mindful and deliberate verbal, tactile, and/or manual cues to facilitate control and movement of the pelvis are all PNF strategies. The therapist's hand placed on the anterolateral aspect of the involved pelvis to cue movement into the hand can facilitate anterior progression of the pelvis over the prosthetic foot (Fig. 26.6). Although techniques focusing on pelvic control are relevant for transfemoral amputees—as the position, movement, and control of the pelvis and hip will dictate knee stability and mobility—transtibial amputees will also benefit from improved pelvic control. These manual techniques are relevant for facilitating both the stance and swing phases of gait.

In unilateral stance on the prosthetic limb, the amputee must be able to stabilize and control the trunk and pelvis over the prosthesis. This requires adequate reverse-action function and strength in hip abductors (to counteract the gravitational adduction torque in the frontal plane at the hip) and extensors (to maintain the hip and trunk in an upright and extended position in the sagittal plane). Forward progression with weight bearing on the prosthetic limb is a challenge that requires a focus on pelvic control. There is often a tendency for the prosthetic limb to rotate or "drift" posteriorly during the stance phase (sometimes referred to as a "retracted" position of the pelvis), accompanied by hip flexion/anterior trunk lean; the swing-side pelvis should be rotating forward at this time, but the stance-side pelvis should not actively rotate posteriorly. This posterior pelvic rotation and hip flexion makes smooth transition over the prosthetic limb impossible as it disrupts the normal forward translation of body weight over the prosthetic foot.

The therapist can facilitate forward pelvic progression during stance using principles of PNF with deliberate application of hand position and input to muscles (e.g., resistance, quick stretch).

Swing phase likewise requires training to facilitate the correct motion. An effective swing will allow for correct step length and facilitates a smooth transition into stance. Symmetric step lengths are conducive to a fluid and energy-efficient gait pattern. There are two specific cues that may help transfemoral prosthesis users achieve a good swing of the prosthetic limb. First, the person must be encouraged to step forward with a normal step on the uninvolved side. When they have an asymmetric gait pattern, it is often because the prosthetic step is very large (because they are comfortable taking weight through the sound limb) and the sound limb step is very small (because they are not comfortable taking weight through the prosthesis). A full-size step with the sound limb step leaves the prosthetic-side hip extended and pelvis posteriorly rotated (relative to the active anterior rotation of the swinging sound limb). Because of the design of many prostheses, anterior pelvic rotation in the transverse plane at preswing will facilitate "knee break." This effectively shortens the limb to allow clearance during swing phase. Transfemoral amputees should be cued to rotate the pelvis forward while flexing the hip, which will swing the prosthetic limb forward, extending the knee for initial contact. Early gait training with a transfemoral prosthesis might involve practice and perhaps facilitation of this forward pelvic translation to help the person get the feeling of the knee break and initial swing. The same types of PNF techniques that are used to facilitate stability of the pelvis during weight bearing can be used to facilitate active movement of the pelvis for optimal swing. Forceful hip flexion in the absence of pelvic rotation to advance the prosthesis prohibits normal step length. Likewise vaulting, hip hiking,

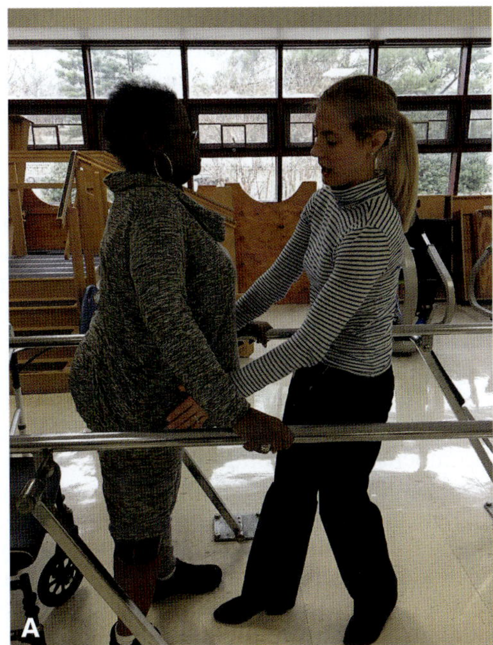

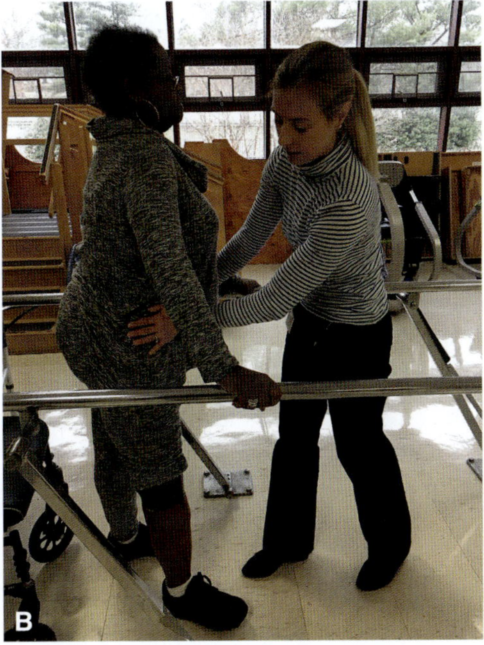

Fig. 26.6 Facilitation of forward pelvic motion for efficient prosthetic gait. (A) The therapist can use manual techniques to cue pelvic position. (B) The therapist can use proprioceptive neuromuscular facilitation at the pelvis and appropriate resistance, asking the patient to move the pelvis upward and forward as he or she steps with either limb.

and circumduction are not efficient methods of forwarding the prosthesis during swing phase. These are common gait deviations that should be mitigated as quickly as possible.

Gait training with a harness system (with or without body-weight support) either over ground or on a treadmill has become a popular treatment strategy in many PT clinics, perhaps because it offers a safe environment to challenge and progress walking ability and increase walking confidence. Finding a consensus in the literature on optimal gait training methods to advance distance, speed, and other time/space parameters is challenging owing to the heterogeneity of the research literature as it relates to subject population (traumatic vs. dysvascular), training techniques, and varying levels of amputation.[159] A preliminary study of "seasoned" community users found no significant difference between body-weight support and conventional treadmill training in improving endurance and falls risk as measured by the 6-minute walk test and the Timed Up and Go.[160] Self-selected comfortable gait speed on the treadmill has been demonstrated to be significantly slower than over-ground walking at the same energy cost, which suggests a higher energy cost in walking on the treadmill than over ground.[161] A small case series suggests that movement strategies may also be altered in walking on a treadmill versus over ground,[162] although some authors attribute this to the constraints of the treadmill.[163] Therapists who have harness systems and/or treadmills available should use their clinical reasoning skills to determine the individualized potential benefit of these modalities as a component of gait training activities.

The use of mental imagery of successful motor mastery of prosthetic training activities may be an appropriate adjunct to PT,[164] although recent research efforts to demonstrate its effectiveness are not without methodologic flaws.[165] Virtual reality and video gaming have become more common in the rehabilitation of older adults[166] after lower limb amputation but are not yet well studied. A small Canadian survey study demonstrated therapists' positive perceptions about the use of commercial gaming (e.g., Nintendo Wii Fit) in improving weight shifting and walking abilities in amputees undergoing rehabilitation.[167] Therapists could consider gaming as a potentially fun and motivating treatment modality within their treatment tool kit. There is limited evidence that treadmill walking in a virtually depicted environment via a Computer Assisted Rehabilitation Environment (CAREN) system may translate to over-ground walking,[163,168] but this limited research involves young participants with traumatic amputation, and this technology is not readily available.

ASSISTIVE DEVICES

ADs can provide help with balance (i.e., single-point cane or quad cane) or with weight bearing and balance (i.e., standard walker, rolling walker, axillary crutches, or Lofstrand crutches). The goals of AD use are to provide only the amount of support that is necessary to reduce the risk of falling without hampering the individual's willingness or ability to load the prosthesis. It may be prudent to spend time on prosthetic weight-bearing and weight-shifting activities in the protected environment of the parallel bars or at a stable surface to allow the person to progress directly to an AD that aids in balance only. Optimally, the prosthetic limb can tolerate 100% weight bearing, so that upper extremity weight bearing through an AD is unnecessary. Individuals who demonstrate good weight bearing, strength, and balance may progress directly from the parallel bars to the use of a single-point cane or no AD at all. For those who are unable to achieve early full weight bearing through the prosthesis and require a weight-bearing AD, the devices of choice are crutches or rolling walkers. Crutches allow individuals to progress to a two-point gait using a step-through gait pattern. Individuals may begin with bilateral support and progress to unilateral support with crutches as prosthetic weight bearing improves. Rolling walkers are preferred over standard walkers, which impede a reciprocal gait pattern, limiting forward progression to a "step-to" rather than "step-through" movement strategy. This limitation, imposed by the walker's cross bar, hampers smooth forward progression of the center of mass over the base of support and precludes effective terminal stance and pre-swing. A wheeled walker can minimize interruptions to the gait cycle if it is advanced between each step or if the person is instructed to push the walker continually while walking (like a grocery cart).

PROSTHETIC GAIT

An understanding of the biomechanics of normal gait is crucial for physical therapists, as it provides the standard by which prosthetic gait is measured.[169] An important objective of prosthetic fit, alignment, and PT intervention is to achieve a gait that is safe, comfortable, energy efficient, and cosmetically agreeable. Although some may demonstrate a near-normal symmetric gait pattern that is free of significant deviations without the use of ADs, this may not be a realistic goal for all. In fact, review studies support a definite asymmetry in gait in both traumatic and dysvascular amputees, with those having higher-level amputations demonstrating greater asymmetries.[100,156,170,171] Although therapists often strive for symmetry in gait activities, a truly symmetric gait pattern is not necessarily required for the person with limb loss to have efficient and functional gait. It is also well documented that the gait speed of amputees is slower than that in age-matched peers without amputation.[62,172]

Biomechanically there are several well-documented changes in comparing prosthetic gait to gait of able-bodied individuals. In transtibial amputees, the lack of plantarflexors is thought to be the most influential component driving gait changes[170,171,173]; this is compensated for by increased activity and power of the muscles around the hip of the prosthetic limb, most notably the hip extensors. In transfemoral prosthesis users, the strength, endurance, and power demands on the musculature of the hip are higher still, as the hip must also compensate for the missing knee.

Prosthetic devices are often marketed as improving efficiency, biomechanics, and quality of prosthetic gait. Systematic reviews do not provide statistically convincing evidence of these benefits when microprocessor- and non-microprocessor-controlled knees are compared (e.g., pneumatic, hydraulic, and mechanical)[174] or dynamic response/energy-storing feet are compared with articulating feet (e.g., single axis, multiple axis). However, there is some evidence of improved gait efficiency with energy-storing feet as compared with SACH feet in transtibial amputees.[175] There is also some limited evidence of componentry positively affecting balance in dysvascular older adult amputees (e.g., microprocessor knee, vacuum-assisted socket).[106,176]

Despite the lack of evidence supporting objective benefit of more advanced prosthetic componentry, individuals often perceive benefits related to efficiency and confidence in their gait.[174] Power or robotic knees and feet and the introduction of bionics to prosthetic components are not yet well studied, so their benefits and drawbacks have yet to be identified. A broader discussion of prosthetic componentry is beyond the scope of this chapter, but the therapist should work closely with the prosthetist in identifying the best prosthetic prescription for amputees based on their ambulation and functional goals.

As movement system experts, physical therapists typically perform observational gait analysis to determine gait deviations and their causes. Commonly observed prosthetic gait deviations have many different potential contributors. Deviations may be a product of intrinsic factors (pertaining to the individual using the prosthesis) or extrinsic factors (pertaining to the prosthesis and/or environmental factors). The observed problem may be a primary gait deviation, caused directly by an intrinsic or extrinsic factor, or a compensatory/secondary deviation, a result of the individual's attempt to avoid a primary deviation.

During initial gait training, prosthetic alignment issues may not be immediately evident. Hesitancy to fully load the prosthesis and upper extremity weight bearing through the parallel bars or AD will affect the resulting gait pattern. As the individual becomes more willing to bear weight through the residual limb, a "truer" gait pattern will emerge and the function of the prosthesis will become more critical. The therapist, along with the prosthetist, must be attentive to the need to correct prosthesis alignment as the individual improves in weight bearing and as impairments improve (i.e., changes in strength, ROM, or balance might warrant changes in the alignment of the prosthesis).

When occupied in solving problems, the clinician must think about why certain gait deviations might occur and whether they are primary or compensatory. Answers to these questions allow the therapist to focus treatment on the most salient issues. For example, if a transfemoral prosthesis user is observed to ambulate with a forward-leaning trunk throughout the stance phase of gait. This may be a primary gait deviation resulting from a hip flexion contracture that limits the individual's ability to achieve upright posture, or it could be the direct result of weak hip extensors. This may also be a compensatory strategy of the person who is fearful of knee instability during stance. By using a forward-leaning trunk, the individual modifies the ground reaction force vector during stance phase to stay significantly anterior to the knee joint, thus improving stability at the knee by creating an extensor moment at that joint. If this is deemed to be the issue, the therapist must determine if it is related to an intrinsic (e.g., weakness, lack of confidence) or extrinsic issue (e.g., prosthetic alignment). Table 26.7 describes some of the more common prosthetic gait deviations and their most likely potential causes.

Notably, low back pain is a common complaint among people with both transtibial and transfemoral amputation, with a recent study reporting a prevalence of back pain as high as 82% following the amputation, and 70% within the last year.[177] Back pain may be associated with lumbopelvic asymmetries in the movement strategies of the individual with amputation.[156,178] Acasio et al. reported that pelvic ROM decreased by over 50%, along with an increase of 48% spinal load when comparing those with unilateral lower limb loss and those without.[179] These alterations in biomechanical strategy are hypothesized to accelerate muscular fatigue, which in turn may result in the development of

Table 26.7 Prosthetic Gait Deviations

Gait Deviation	Phase of Gait	Category[a]	Possible Causes
GAIT DEVIATIONS COMMON TO TRANSTIBIAL AND TRANSFEMORAL AMPUTEES USING PROSTHESES			
Lateral trunk lean toward prosthetic side	Loading response through terminal stance	Intrinsic	Lacking hip abductor strength and/or timing on prosthetic side (compensate with lateral lean to avoid Trendelenburg)
			Abductor contracture on prosthetic side
			Hip joint pain on prosthetic side
			Very short transfemoral residual limb (poor purchase in socket, poor leverage)
		Prosthetic (extrinsic)	Prosthesis too short
			Foot too outset
			Transfemoral socket medial wall trim line too high
			Transfemoral socket places femur in abduction
			Transfemoral socket lateral wall fails to provide adequate femoral support/stabilization
		Environmental (extrinsic)	Uneven terrain
Anterior trunk lean	Loading response through terminal stance	Intrinsic	Hip flexion contracture
			Lacking knee extensor strength and/or timing in individual with transtibial amputation (compensate with forward lean to create extensor moment at knee)
			Fear of instability of physiologic or prosthetic knee
			Insufficient hip extensor strength or lumbar extensor strength making maintenance of an upright trunk difficult
		Prosthetic (extrinsic)	Transtibial socket set too posterior (forcing knee hyperextension)
			Transtibial socket lacks anterior tilt
			Transfemoral prosthetic knee positioned too anterior (TKA line not providing stability)
		Environmental (extrinsic)	Walking up incline
Insufficient weight bearing through prosthesis	Loading response through terminal stance	Intrinsic	Residual limb pain or hypersensitivity
			Excessive upper extremity weight bearing on assistive device
			Instability of the physiologic or prosthetic knee joint
			Decreased muscle strength of residual limb
			Fear of falling/lack of confidence in prosthesis
		Prosthetic (extrinsic)	Prosthesis is too long
			Poor socket fit
		Environmental (extrinsic)	Walking uphill
			Walking on rugged terrain
Inadequate prosthetic foot clearance[b]	Throughout swing phases	Intrinsic	Poor hip stabilization on sound limb (pelvic drop on prosthetic side during swing)
			Lacking active anterior pelvic rotation (strength and/or timing issue) to initiate prosthetic swing
			Lacking hip flexion (strength and/or timing issue) to initiate prosthetic swing
			Lacking knee flexion (strength and/or timing issue) to contribute to prosthetic swing in transtibial amputation
		Prosthetic (extrinsic)	Prosthesis too long
			Transfemoral prosthetic knee too "stiff"
			Prosthetic foot/ankle too plantarflexed
		Environmental (extrinsic)	Uneven terrain with unexpected elevations
Pistoning (downward translation of prosthesis on residual limb when unloaded)	Throughout swing phases	Intrinsic	Error in sock application (too few or too many layers)
		Prosthetic (extrinsic)	Inadequate suspension
			Poor socket fit
		Environmental (extrinsic)	Muddy or flooded environment can create pull on prosthesis
GAIT DEVIATIONS COMMON TO TRANSTIBIAL AMPUTEES USING PROSTHESES			
Excessive knee flexion/knee instability	Initial contact or loading response to midstance	Intrinsic	Knee or hip flexion contracture
			Lacking knee or hip extensor strength and/or timing
			Anterior distal residual limb pain

Table 26.7 Prosthetic Gait Deviations—cont'd

Gait Deviation	Phase of Gait	Category[a]	Possible Causes
		Prosthetic (extrinsic)	Excessive dorsiflexion of the prosthetic foot
			Excessive transtibial socket flexion (anterior tilt)
			Transtibial socket positioned anterior to prosthetic foot
			Excessive heel cushion stiffness (SACH foot)
			Prosthesis too long
		Environmental (extrinsic)	Walking down inclines
Excessive knee extension (no shock absorption)/ hyperextension	Initial contact or loading response to midstance	Intrinsic	Lacking knee extensor strength and/or timing (hyperextend knee as compensation)
			Cruciate ligament insufficiency
			Lacking hip extensor strength and/or timing
			Posterior distal residual limb pain
		Prosthetic (extrinsic)	Excessive plantarflexion of prosthetic foot
			Lacking appropriate socket flexion (posterior tilt of socket)
			Excessively soft heel cushion (SACH foot)
			Socket positioned posterior to prosthetic foot
			Prosthesis too short
		Environmental (extrinsic)	Ascending inclines/walking uphill
Genu valgus moment at knee	Midstance	Intrinsic	Medial collateral ligament insufficiency
			Coxa vara at hip
			Medial distal residual limb pain
		Prosthetic (extrinsic)	Excessive outset of prosthetic foot
			Tilt of transtibial socket in frontal plane
		Environmental (extrinsic)	Walking on uneven surfaces
Excessive genu varus moment at knee	Midstance	Intrinsic	Lateral collateral ligament insufficiency
			Coxa valga at hip
			Lateral distal residual limb pain
		Prosthetic (extrinsic)	Excessive inset of prosthetic foot
			Tilt of transtibial socket in the frontal plane
		Environmental (extrinsic)	Walking on uneven surfaces
Early heel rise/early knee flexion or "drop off"	Midstance to preswing	Intrinsic	Hip and/or knee flexion contracture
			Weakness of hip extensor muscles
			Anterior/distal residual limb pain
		Prosthetic (extrinsic)	Excessive dorsiflexion of prosthetic foot
			Socket positioned anterior to prosthetic foot
			Too much socket flexion (anterior tilt)
			The opposite prosthetic problems (plantarflexed foot, socket positioned posteriorly, not enough socket flexion) can all cause this same gait deviation if the person is working to "overcome" being forced into hyperextended knee position by the prosthesis
		Environmental (extrinsic)	Walking down inclines or hills
Delayed heel rise/delayed knee flexion	Terminal stance to preswing	Intrinsic	Knee hyperextension as compensation for instability or weakness earlier in stance makes transition to knee flexion difficult
			Decreased anterior weight shift (weight through heel of prosthesis)
			Posterior/distal residual limb pain
		Prosthetic (extrinsic)	Excessive plantarflexion of prosthetic foot
			Socket positioned posterior to prosthetic foot
			Insufficient socket flexion
			Excessively long keel of prosthetic foot
		Environmental (extrinsic)	Walking up inclines/hills
GAIT DEVIATIONS COMMON TO TRANSFEMORAL AMPUTEES USING PROSTHESES			
Excessive anterior pelvic tilt/ lumbar lordosis	Initial contact through preswing	Intrinsic	Hip flexion contracture
			Weak hip extensors and/or abdominals
			Effort to shift center of gravity anteriorly for stability at prosthetic knee
		Prosthetic (extrinsic)	Insufficient flexion (posterior tilt) of socket
			TKA line does not provide adequate knee stability
		Environmental (extrinsic)	Walking up inclines/uphill

(Continued)

Table 26.7 Prosthetic Gait Deviations—cont'd

Gait Deviation	Phase of Gait	Category[a]	Possible Causes
Abducted gait	Initial contact through preswing	Intrinsic	Hip abduction contracture
			Adductor tissue roll/redundant tissue
			Impaired balance (compensatory widened base of support)
			Distal femur pain
		Prosthetic (extrinsic)	Prosthesis too long
			Socket alignment places femur in abduction
			Medial socket wall too high
		Environmental (extrinsic)	Uneven terrain
Delayed prosthetic knee flexion	Terminal stance to preswing	Intrinsic	Lacking active anterior pelvic rotation (strength and/or timing issue) to offload prosthesis
			Lacking hip flexion (strength and/or timing) to initiate swing of prosthesis
		Prosthetic (extrinsic)	TKA line providing excessive knee stability
			Excessive plantarflexion of prosthetic foot or excessively soft heel cushion (SACH foot)
		Environmental (extrinsic)	Walking up inclines
Medial heel whip	Preswing to early swing	Intrinsic	Loose residual limb tissue that rotates freely around femur
			Improperly donned socket in internally rotated position
		Prosthetic (extrinsic)	Prosthetic knee oriented in external/lateral direction
			Prosthetic foot oriented laterally
			Prosthetic foot toe break oriented laterally
		Environmental (extrinsic)	Rugged terrain
Lateral heel whip	Preswing to early swing	Intrinsic	Loose residual limb tissue that rotates freely around femur
			Improperly donned socket in externally rotated position
		Prosthetic (extrinsic)	Prosthetic knee oriented in internal/medial direction
			Prosthetic foot oriented medially
			Prosthetic foot toe break oriented medially
		Environmental (extrinsic)	Rugged terrain
Terminal swing impact (prosthetic knee extension thrust)		Intrinsic	Excessive anterior pelvic rotation and/or hip flexion to assure knee extension in swing
		Prosthetic (extrinsic)	Insufficient knee stiffness, excessive extension aid
		Environmental (extrinsic)	Environment demands rapid movement

[a]Intrinsic problems are due to personal factors. Extrinsic problems are associated with prosthetic issues (alignment or fit) or environmental issues (best understood by analyzing the specific condition or activity in which they are observed).
[b]Possible compensations for inadequate prosthetic swing-phase clearance include a lateral lean of the trunk toward the sound limb, vaulting on the sound limb, hip hiking or circumduction of the prosthetic limb, and, in the case of transtibial amputation, a steppage gait.
SACH, Solid ankle cushioned heel; *TKA*, trochanter-knee-ankle.

pain.[180] Chronic back pain has been linked to strength and endurance deficits of low back extensors in individuals with amputation.[181] Those with lower limb loss demonstrate decreased multifidi activity and increased intramuscular fat, potential modifiable contributing factors to low back pain.[53,182] Studies have demonstrated pain-relieving benefits of a strengthening program that improved strength and endurance of lumbar extensors and strength of abdominal muscles in long-term prosthetic users.[110] Therapists should be prepared to utilize manual therapy techniques and exercise interventions as appropriate to address complaints of back pain.

GAIT TRAINING ON ALTERNATE SURFACES

To adapt to and meet environmental demands, the individual using a prosthesis must be able to adjust his or her step length and cadence while ambulating in response to environmental conditions or circumstances. The PT program might begin with practice opportunities until the person is able to achieve a nonvariable cadence. It might then progress to activities that demand an increased or decreased cadence, stops and starts, and transitional gait movements, such as sidestepping, turning, walking backward, and obstacle avoidance. These skills can initially be practiced in the clinic with minimal environmental demands. They can be progressed to situations in which the environment presents a challenge, such as crossing a street in a timely manner, getting on and off an elevator or escalator, walking through a crowded corridor in a busy store, or walking to a seat in the middle of an auditorium. Successful community ambulation also requires management of many different ground surfaces, including steps, curbs, ramps, and varied terrain. In providing therapeutic practice opportunities for a person who is new to the use of a prosthesis, the therapist considers the following important extrinsic variables:

1. Level of physical assistance required for safe performance.
2. The specific demands of the environment, such as depth or height of steps and curbs or degree of slope of a ramp.
3. The need for an AD or railing.
4. The optimal technique for performing the task safely.
5. The ability to superimpose an additional activity while walking or moving in the environment (dual and multitasking).
6. Facilitators and barriers presented by the prosthesis.

An initial goal might be to decrease the level of assistance (physical assist or AD) on these alternative surfaces. This can be accomplished by simplifying one or more of the variables of the task, such as decreasing the depth of the step/curb, allowing the use of sturdy rail versus crutch or cane, and/or allowing the sound limb to "lead" or dominate the task. As skill improves, the task demands are increased. Early skills in stair climbing are generally developed in a step-to gait pattern with the sound limb leading in ascent and the prosthetic limb leading in descent. Advanced gait training activities may instead require the person with amputation to use the sound limb first in descent, placing the weight bearing eccentric control demand on the prosthetic limb, or require ascent with the prosthetic limb leading. These step-over-step stair ascent/descent strategies are possible for transtibial and transfemoral amputees who have the appropriate knee componentry (e.g., microprocessor knees allow for descent, power knees allow for ascent/descent). Step-over-step stair descent requires placement of the prosthetic forefoot off of the step to allow for the forward progression of the prosthetic shank, mimicking the ankle dorsiflexion required in lowering the body weight to the next step.

The management of slopes, inclines, and ramps is challenging. The loss of sensory information in the prosthetic limb (and possibly the sound limb) limits the ability to know where the foot is in space and the relative stiffness of the ankle (depending on type of prosthesis) does not allow for the fully functional dorsiflexion or plantarflexion that is required for adaptability to the slope of the surface.[183] In the person with a transfemoral prosthesis, the loss of the knee joint and accompanying quadriceps control compounds the challenge. Most people with transfemoral prostheses navigate inclines, declines, ramps, and slopes using one of two methods (or some combination of the two). They will either shorten the step length of the involved limb to help compensate for the lack of quadriceps contraction and ankle mobility and continue with an asymmetrical step-to-step pattern or they will turn partially sideways and employ a sidestepping pattern leading with the uninvolved limb going up and prosthetic limb going down. By reorienting the axis of rotation for knee motion in this manner, there is less risk of the slope directly affecting knee position or stability. The method used is generally determined by personal preference and the grade of the slope. As in stair descent, if the person has a microprocessor-controlled knee, angled surfaces are more easily managed by the computer control of the knee, especially in descending. New technology has focused on the design of an "intelligent" ankle prosthesis that allows for real-time adaptability when walking over uneven surfaces and also provides some plantarflexion power during push-off.[183,184] Literature also suggests that these types of ankles allow increased gait speed and toe clearance when walking over uneven surfaces as compared with those using nonpowered prosthetic ankles[183] and to some extent help improve dynamic balance in stance when walking down a slope.[185]

Curtze demonstrated that when transtibial prosthesis users were faced with the challenge of rough terrain versus smooth surfaces, arm swing speed increased (presumably to assist with balance) and gait speed decreased slightly, but other gait parameters were not significantly altered.[186] Vrieling and colleagues concluded that specific training for prosthetic gait initiation, termination, obstacle crossing, and incline and decline management should be a purposeful component of the rehabilitation regime, as movement strategies of these functional tasks are different than those of able-bodied individuals,[100,187–189] and addressing these tasks in rehabilitation has the potential to impact safety and confidence.

Superimposing functional activities on gait during therapeutic treatment prepares individuals for the daily "real world" challenges they are sure to encounter. The variety of functional tasks practiced by the individual should be driven by the goals specific to that person. Safe ambulation while carrying objects of varying weights and sizes is an important functional skill and an appropriate PT activity. The individual's specific goal may be to carry a full laundry basket down the hall or a cup of hot coffee from the kitchen to the living room. As individuals become functional users of prostheses, household tasks and leisure or work activities may guide their therapeutic needs. Safe ambulation while dual-tasking, such as texting, is another very likely goal, as those with limb loss demonstrate a higher degree of difficulty and less safety than healthy controls.[190]

FUNCTIONAL ACTIVITIES

A comprehensive rehabilitation program includes a variety of other functional activities, such as transfer training from a variety of surfaces, reaching and picking up objects from different levels and surfaces, kneeling, management of falls, and rising from the floor. Motor learning theory supports that prescriptive instruction on different functional tasks such as these may not be the most effective way to assist individuals in developing these skills; rather, encouraging individuals to solve their own motor problems and figure out how to best perform a given functional task allows them to "own" the task and to better generalize to other related tasks.[48] Specific functional tasks should also be designed to address unique goals as they relate to ADLs, job-related activities, or recreational activities. Occupational therapists have excellent knowledge of adaptive devices and skill in environmental adaptation and may also screen for return to driving, thus working with these team members is of great benefit.

For many, there is a strong desire or need to return to work and leisure activities. A review of international studies on return to work after lower extremity amputation identified a return to work rate of 66% for persons with lower extremity amputation (inclusive of changes in job responsibilities and transition to part-time work), but this was for all amputation etiologies, and many studies represented young adults with traumatic amputations.[191]

Factors found to be associated with success in returning people to work after lower extremity amputation include younger age at the time of amputation, lower level of amputation, higher education level, good prosthetic comfort, and higher gross annual income.[191,192] Conversely, those who work full time and have greater self-efficacy are more likely to be functionally mobile.[18] Functional tasks that simulate job activities would be appropriate to incorporate into the plan of care. A small study of return to leisure activity in older adults with limb loss demonstrated that after surgery, their participation in leisure activities decreased, but their satisfaction with the activities remained high.[193] In progressing functional, vocational, and leisure activities, therapists should design interventions that are specific to the individual's needs and desires, are task-oriented, and provide opportunities for creative problem-solving. Table 26.8 describes some more advanced rehabilitation activities that can help to prepare individuals to take part in their chosen activity.

OUTCOME ASSESSMENT

Measuring the effectiveness of PT interventions on the function and quality of life of a person with limb loss is an important component of the plan of care for both prognosis and reimbursement.[194] The documentation of change over time is important to determine functional K-levels to assist with prosthetic prescription and eligibility. The ICF framework reminds us that it is important to assess performance at different levels of the ICF paradigm: the body-function level (impairments); the activities level (activity limitations); and the participation level (participation restrictions). Some of the outcome measures that have been used in limb loss rehabilitation are population specific (e.g., Amputation Mobility Predictor with and without prosthesis [AMP and AMPnoPRO], Houghton Scale, or the Prosthetic Evaluation Questionnaire); others are broader rehabilitation outcome measures that have been used with this population (e.g., BBS, ABC Scale, Functional Independence Measure). Standardized walking tests that have been used in limb loss rehabilitation research include 2-minute walk test, 6-minute walk test, Timed Up and Go, and 10-minute walk test. Reid et al. recently demonstrated that the 2-minute walk test predicts the 6-minute walk test in lower extremity amputees and therefore may be used to save the time and energy of those evaluated.[195] Although normative values for these outcome measures in amputees have not been well established, norms are available for the older adult, and these can be useful in monitoring change over time and assessing performance relative to age-matched peers without amputation. Gait speed has been routinely linked to function and overall health status in the older adult; therefore it is important to assess baseline gait speed and monitor change over time.[196] Self-selected gait speed is slower in those with dysvascular versus transfemoral limb loss versus those with traumatic transtibial prosthesis users.[197,198] A 2016 study by Wong et al. presented gait speed data from 180 users of prostheses (about half of whom were dysvascular) as calculated from the 2-minute walk test.[199] Independent community ambulators walked at 1.06 ± 0.32 m/s (range: >0.8–1.2 m/s); limited community ambulators/household ambulators walked at 0.59 ± 0.29 m/s (range: 0.5–0.8 m/s); and limited household ambulators walked at 0.41 ± 0.29 m/s (range < 0.5 m/s). These benchmarks may be useful in considering the functional implications of gait speed findings.

Table 26.8 Advanced Functional Exercises After Lower Extremity Amputation

Standing balance activities	Standing activities on compliant surface (foam, Bosu ball) or mobile surface (rocker board, Biomechanical Ankle Platform System board); can progress to superimpose tasks while standing (ball catch/throw)
	Catching and throwing balls of different shapes, sizes, and weights and throwing variable distances; can progress with altered base of support (staggered stance, tandem stance)
	Prosthetic single-limb stance, with stool stepping with sound limb, progress to stepping on less stable surface (foam, Bosu ball); can progress to superimpose tasks while standing (ball catch/throw)
	Elastic band UE and/or LE strengthening activities while standing without UE support (i.e., band affixed to wall or door and individual works against resistance in diagonal or straight plane patterns); this requires balance and stability of the core and LEs when performing UE exercise and stability of the opposite LE and core when performing LE exercises
Dynamic balance activities with progressively superimposed speed and agility requirements	Dynamic ambulatory tasks: functional multidirectional walking; starts, stops, and turns in rapid progression; obstacle avoidance (over, around); figure-eight walking; head turns while walking; progressively more narrow base of support with goal of line/beam walking
	Altered terrain walking: a string of yoga mats laid out over towels on floor at unpredictable intervals makes a nice indoor rugged terrain; outdoor walking on grass, sand, or gravel. Other environmental challenges: steps, curbs, ramps, elevators, escalators
	Picking up objects of different weights and sizes from floor: carrying objects while walking
	Dual-tasking: superimposed motor task on gait (ball catch/throw), superimposed cognitive task on gait (serial subtractions, naming items in a category)
	Floor transfers: reasonable to train with all individuals (not reserved for only high-level training), but can work toward less reliance on external support and getting onto and off of floor in timely and safe manner
	Progressing to task-specific goals: fast-walking; sport/leisure-specific goals (gardening, bowling)
Cardiovascular activities	Swimming, cycling, treadmill walking, stepper

LE, Lower extremity; *UE*, upper extremity.

Summary

The rehabilitation of those with dysvacular limb loss is both challenging and rewarding. Early in the rehabilitation process, functional mobility, ROM, strengthening, and aerobic conditioning are prioritized as the residual limb is prepared for the fitting of a prosthesis. On receipt of the prosthesis, a gradual wearing schedule in the context of a comprehensive rehabilitation program[200,201]—including weight-bearing activities, gait training, resistive training in gait, balance training, and functional task training—is introduced and strategically progressed. Emphasis is on gait safety, comfort, quality, and efficiency (with or without an AD) and on safe and independent functional mobility with the prosthesis. Training progresses to include varied functional activities under many environmental conditions. Physical therapists may work with these individuals in acute care, inpatient rehabilitation, or long-term care, home care, or another outpatient environment. The diversity of those with limb loss requires the therapist to carefully consider individual circumstances to guide the education and practice strategies of the rehabilitation program.

References

The complete listing of the References are available in the accompanying enhanced eBook version included with the print purchase of this textbook. Visit Elsevier eBooks+ (eBooks.Health.Elsevier.com) to access this content.

27 Advanced Rehabilitation for People With Microprocessor Knee Prostheses

CHRISTOPHER K. WONG AND DANIEL J. LEE

LEARNING OBJECTIVES

On completion of this chapter, the reader will be able to do the following:

1. Provide a chronology for the development of prosthetics research leading to the microprocessor knee (MPK) prosthesis.
2. Compare knee control function for a variety of MPK prostheses.
3. Explain functional ambulation skills and activities of daily living that are challenging for users of transfemoral prosthesis or higher that do not have MPK.
4. Describe the Medicare K-level requirements when considering MPK prostheses for patients.
5. Explain the similarities and differences of MPK prostheses.
6. Describe how an MPK unit can benefit the user during gait, stair climbing and ramp negotiation, transfers, and stumbling.
7. Discuss prosthetic and training solutions for common gait deviations from which MPK prostheses can significantly benefit.
8. Evaluate physical therapy interventions that can be applied when rehabilitating individuals with transfemoral amputation who use MPK prosthesis.
9. Describe the evidence to support the use of MPK prostheses.

Historical Development

Since Ambroise Paré's 16th-century articulated transfemoral prosthesis,[1] surgeons, patients, and engineers have attempted to imitate the function of the human leg. In the United States, scientific prosthetics development began in 1945 with the establishment of the Prosthetic Appliance Service of the Veterans Administration and the research and development program of the National Academy of Science.[2] Early versions of sophisticated knee units include the 1942 Filippi hydraulic stance control unit[3] and the hydraulic swing and stance control knee unit patented by engineer Hans Mauch and radiologist Ulrich Henschke in 1949.[4] The Veterans Administration approved the first hydraulic swing-phase control mechanism in 1962; the component linked a hydraulic knee unit to a single-axis ankle.[5]

Research beginning in the 1970s led to the 1993 introduction by Blatchford (Basingstoke, England) of the first commercially available microprocessor-controlled prosthetic knee: the Endolite Intelligent Prosthesis. The Intelligent Prosthesis required a wired connection to program the variable swing-phase control. The Adaptive Prosthesis followed in 1998, allowing wireless programming and featuring an onboard processor that controlled adjustment of the hybrid pneumatic/hydraulic microprocessor knee (MPK); Endolite's latest generation MPK is the Orion 3 (Fig. 27.1).[6] Since introduction of the Intelligent Prosthesis, at least six other companies have joined the marketplace in offering MPK prostheses. Ottobock (Duderstadt, Germany) initiated the hydraulic C-Leg MPK in 1997.[2,7–10] Other manufacturers presented comparable units. Össur (Reykjavik, Iceland) launched the Rheo Knee in 2006 and the Power Knee in 2009.[11] In the United States, Freedom Innovations of Irvine, California (now Proteor) introduced the Plié MPK unit.[12] The Nabtesco Corporation of Japan also offers MPK units.[13]

The purpose of this chapter is to (1) discuss the unique features of MPKs that are increasingly available and (2) provide prosthetic and training solutions for persons with common gait deviations that can be reduced by using an MPK.

Overview of Non-Microprocessor Knee Prostheses

After amputation that includes the knee joint, people face significantly more difficulty in mobility tasks than those whose knees remain intact. Without the knee and the muscles that control it, the prosthesis user must control knee flexion in new ways to avoid falling. The simplest way to remain stable is to use a mechanically locked knee unit. Some older first-time prosthesis users prefer the security of a locked knee to one that is unlocked.[14] If the knee is not locked, knee stability can be maintained simply through alignment of the joint axes combined with significant residual limb gluteal muscle power. However, many prosthesis users who wish to walk in the community with additional stability benefit from more sophisticated non-microprocessor knee (non-MPK) units.

Weight-activated friction-brake knees are non-MPK units that control knee flexion on initial loading and through most of stance phase. Weight bearing on the prosthesis activates strong braking resistance to knee flexion even when the knee is slightly bent. If the knee is flexed more than 20 degrees, no flexion resistance is provided, making stair descent or stumble recovery difficult. Hydraulic non-MPK units provide sufficient resistance to weight-bearing knee

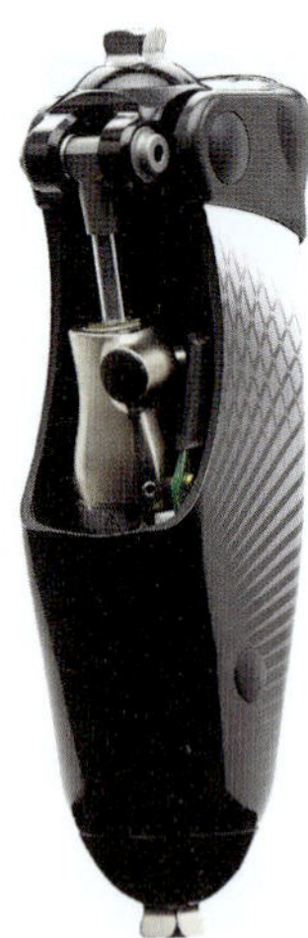

Fig. 27.1 Orion: a pneumatic microprocessor knee unit with stance and swing-phase control. (Courtesy Blatchford, blatchford.co.uk.)

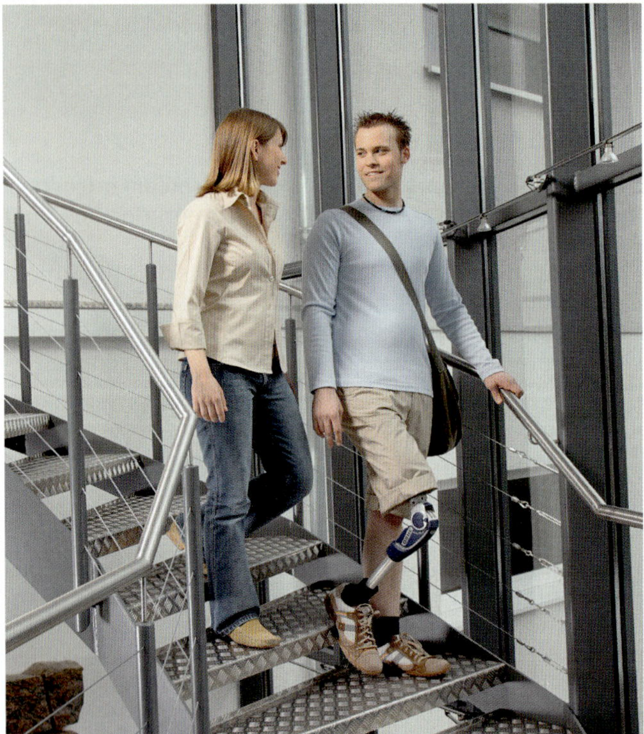

Fig. 27.2 Prosthetic and sound foot placement for stair descent. (Courtesy Ottobock HealthCare, www.ottobockus.com.)

flexion beyond 20 degrees to allow step-over-step descent of stairs or curbs (Fig. 27.2).[15] Hydraulic or pneumatic knees also provide variable levels of resistance to knee flexion during swing phase to minimize asymmetry between sound and prosthetic knee flexion at different gait speeds.

The two different resistance modes in hydraulic knees make these units ideal for those who are able to move at different speeds and traverse a variety of surfaces such as encountered in the community. However, these knees require specific motions during gait to provide the mechanical cue, such as a firm knee hyperextension force of at least 0.1 second in terminal stance phase,[11] to switch between the two different levels of resistance required for weight-bearing stance phase and non–weight-bearing swing phase. If a sufficient cue is not achieved at the end of swing phase, the appropriate resistance to support the weight-bearing limb will not be applied and a fall may occur. Alternatively, if the cue is not achieved at the end of stance phase, the leg may remain stiff in swing phase, leading to an awkward gait pattern. As a result, the user must be careful to move with adequate hip action to prevent stumbles.

Users of non-MPK prostheses must use compensatory techniques for other activities. For instance, to go from sit to stand, the wearer generally places more weight on the sound limb and depends on that leg, and arms as needed, to raise themselves to standing. When sitting, unweighting the prosthetic leg is required in order for the knee to bend easily. Such basic activities place extra stress on the sound limb, which can contribute to the frequent reporting of low-back and sound-limb pain among prosthesis users.[16] Another example is descending slopes, a difficult activity for users of transfemoral prostheses. A step length matching that of the sound limb often results in a prosthetic knee angle that exceeds the approximately 20-degree safety range of a hydraulic stance phase control or a weight-activated knee unit. Thus most prosthesis users learn to take very short steps. Finally, ascending stairs step-over-step is very difficult for any transfemoral prosthesis user, generally requiring use of a bannister if the step is of standard height.

Introduction to Microprocessor Knee Prostheses

Unlike non-MPK prostheses that use alignment, locked knees or weight-activated friction brakes, and hydraulic or pneumatic mechanisms, MPK prostheses incorporate an onboard microprocessor to compute data from various electronic sensors and provide real-time adjustments during the user's activities. The computer's processor enables rapid adjustments in knee resistance during both swing and stance phase control, usually with pneumatic or hydraulic components. The speed of microprocessors allows data sampling from sensors in the MPKs at speeds of faster than 50 times per second[17] to provide more responsiveness to individual movements than can be offered by non-MPK pneumatic and hydraulic knee prostheses. Based on input from various combinations of joint position and motion sensors, pressure sensors, and gyroscopes, proprietary software algorithms determine the phase of gait or function of the leg to provide real-time adjustment of resistance within the MPK unit to facilitate the optimal walking pattern.

The prosthetist performs the initial MPK calibration for the wearer's typical use patterns with software specific to the MPK manufacturer. Calibration requires that the wearer walk at slow, normal, and fast speeds for about 12 m (40 ft). Then the wearer negotiates stairs and ramps so that the appropriate knee resistance levels can be set. At times, additional adjustments may be necessary as the user bears more weight on the prosthesis and participates in more activities.

MPKs offer a variety of swing and stance phase control functions, including resisted swing-phase knee extension

Table 27.1 Microprocessor Knee Prostheses Offer a Variety of Knee Control Functions

	Manufacturer				
Gait Phase Controlled	**Endolite**	**Proteor**	**Nabetsco**	**Ottobock**	**Össur**
Swing only	SmartIP		Intelligent Hybrid		
Stance only				Compact	
Swing and stance	Orion 3, Smart Adapt	Plie 3.0	Allux 2	C-Leg, X3, Genium	Rheo Knee, Power Knee
Stair ascent (powered assist)					Power Knee

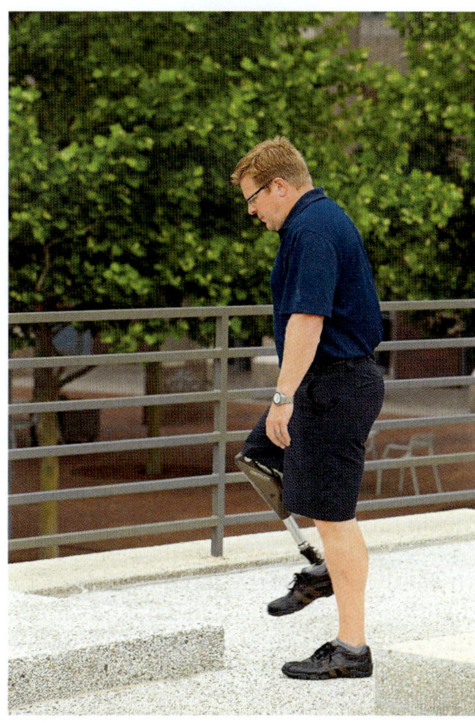

Fig. 27.3 Genium microprocessor knee with gyroscope, accelerometer, and angle sensors responds to movement in all directions. (Courtesy Ottobock HealthCare, www.ottobockus.com.)

Table 27.2 Medicare Functional Levels for People With Unilateral Transtibial and Transfemoral Amputation

Level	Typical User Profile	Functional Abilities With Prosthesis
K1	Household ambulator	Has ability or potential to transfer and ambulate on level surfaces at slow speeds with fixed cadence. Time and distance severely limited.
K2	Limited community ambulator	Has ability or potential to ambulate and traverse common environmental barriers such as curbs, stairs, or uneven surfaces. Time and distance often limited.
K3	Community ambulator	Has ability or potential to ambulate at faster speeds with variable cadence and traverse most environmental barriers. Can undertake vocational, therapeutic, or exercise activity that demands use beyond ambulation. Time and distance still somewhat limited.
K4	Active user (child, active adult, athlete)	Has the ability or potential for prosthetic use that exceeds ambulation, including high impact, torsion, or energy levels common to sport. Time and distance essentially unlimited.

and knee flexion, resisted stance phase knee flexion, powered stance phase knee extension, locked or unlocked (free) knee motions, and various combinations for specific functional applications. MPKs typically offer stance phase knee resistance within a 0- to 35-degree range, though some provide resistance through an even greater range for static activities (Table 27.1).[6]

As with the non-MPK units that have both swing and stance phase control functions, the MPK must switch between different functions. MPK units receive data from various sensors, such as force and angle sensors, accelerometers, and gyroscopes, that indicate the portion of stance phase, especially initial loading. Some MPKs, like the C-Leg and the Rheo Knee, allow controlled knee flexion on initial loading to reduce vertical shock impact and normalize gait. Angle and velocity of the knee indicate the oncoming of terminal swing. An MPK like the Genium has a gyroscope, which senses the direction of movement and determines when the user lifts the leg to ascend stairs or to step over an obstacle (Fig. 27.3).

In general, manufacturers suggest that MPKs with stance phase control be prescribed for Medicare K2 to K3 level users (Table 27.2) whereas MPKs with both stance and swing-phase control be prescribed for K3 to K4 level users who will utilize different walking speeds.[11,17] However, most available MPKs are designed for low- to moderate-impact activities.[11,17] Processor and actuator speeds are typically insufficient for high-speed activities and, as with all electronic devices, MPKs are vulnerable to overheating. While a few new entries into the market such as the Ottobock Genium X3 have been designed to support high-speed and impact activities, most prosthesis users at the K4 level who engage in high-impact activities, such as running or jumping, are more suited to hydraulic non-MPK designs.[11]

In addition to different combinations of swing and stance phase control, the commercially available MPKs have other options. For instance, the Plie 3.0 knee utilizes a pneumatic mechanism that the user pumps regularly to adjust resistance levels (Fig. 27.4).[12] The pneumatic Hybrid is available with both single and multiaxial knee joints that allow up to 160 degrees.[13] MPKs, however, generally provide knee flexion range from 120 to 140 degrees, which exceeds that of most non-MPKs. MPKs generally dampen knee extension to minimize terminal knee extension impact as well as to adjust the arc of shank swing to the speed of walking, but not early swing-phase knee flexion. The C-Leg and Genium

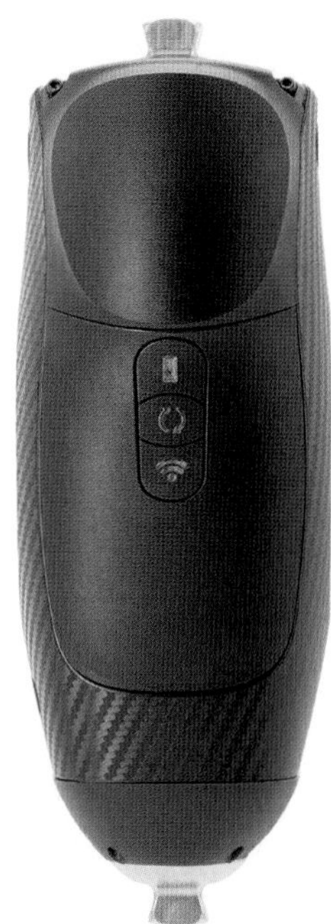

Fig. 27.4 Plie 3.0: a water-resistant pneumatic microprocessor knee unit. (Courtesy PROTEOR.)

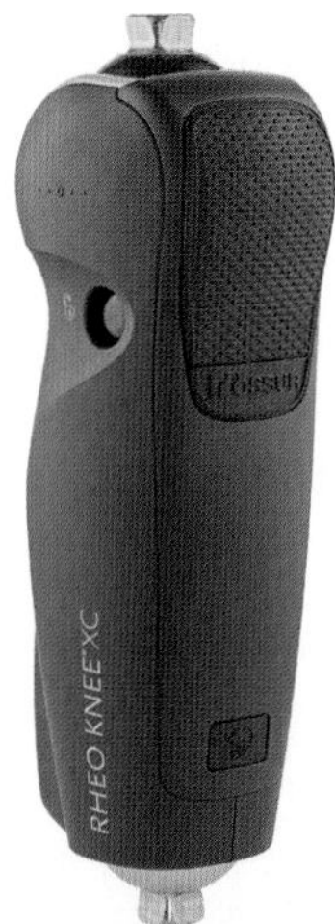

Fig. 27.5 Power Knee provides assisted knee extension. (© Össur.)

have dampened swing-phase knee flexion to approximate the 60 degrees normal in level walking.[17,18] The Power Knee offers powered robotic assistance in sit-to-stand and stair ascent functions (Fig. 27.5).[11]

All MPKs have some common characteristics. Although individual MPK technical specifications vary, all are powered by batteries that must be charged 4 to 14 hours for use limited in general to 1 to 5 days. The Power Knee, the only MPK to provide robotic assistance to movement, maintains its charge for up to one day depending on use.[11] Depending on use intensity, most MPKs can maintain charge for 2 days with an industry maximum of 3 days.[6,11–13,17] The battery and hydraulic mechanisms do not function in all environments and are limited to operating temperatures ranging from −10 to 60°C (14–140°F) for the C-Leg,[17] sufficient for most people's requirements. As with other electronic devices, such as laptop computers, MPKs are also vulnerable to sand, debris, and water—especially saltwater. The degree of environmental hardiness is measured by the Ingress Protection rating (IP rating). The numerical value associated with the IP rating (i.e., IP67) indicates the prosthetic component's ability to withstand solid and water exposure. For example, the Plie 3 is rated IP67, which means it can withstand occasional (<30 minutes) submersion in shallow water (<1 m), while the Ottobock Genium X3 is rated IP 68 and can operate underwater (up to 3 m) for an hour, as well as being saltwater resistant (see Fig. 27.4).

Electronic signals such as repeated beeps or vibrations warn the user of impending shutdown due to computer or hydraulic overload or other malfunction, as well as changes in mode of function. The wearer must learn the meaning of the different signals to assure proper use. On shutdown, either in the case of malfunction or battery depletion, the MPK will default to various states, including a safety mode. Most default to swing-phase control, which allows knee bending in swing phase, but can also permit collapse in stance phase. The C-Leg and Power Knee default to stance phase resistance, which causes the knee to lock and protects against falls if the microprocessor receives abnormal input that can occur during a stumble or step onto an obstacle or uneven surface. A stance phase resistance default setting, however, requires circumduction, hip hiking, or vaulting in swing phase until normal MPK function is restored.

The battery and other electronic components add weight, causing MPKs to be heavier than hydraulic non-MPK units. Weights for MPK units range from 1145 g (2.5 lbs) to nearly 6 lbs for the more complex Power Knee, compared with the hydraulic non-MPK units such as the SR95[17] that weighs 360 g (12.6 oz) or the Mauch Knee that weighs 1140 g (2.5 lbs).[11] Although the Mauch Knee Plus can accommodate high-impact use by users weighing up to 166 kg (366 lbs),[11] MPKs are generally designed for low- to moderate-impact use by individuals who weigh <125 kg (275.6 lbs). The Genium X3 can support people up to 150 kg (330.7 lbs).[17]

Typical MPK units cost US$20,000 to US$50,000 with total cost of the prosthesis and prosthetic work higher.[19] Costs for a prosthesis outfit with an MPK now exceed US$120,000 for the Ottobock Genium X3.[20] Standard warranties run 2 to 3 years with some companies offering extended 5- to 6-year warranties.[17] Cost to provide the prosthesis can be 2 to 3 times the cost of a non-MPK unit. However, patient and family expenses such as housekeeping and decreased work productivity for non-MPK users can offset the cost to acquire a MPK prosthesis. When direct and indirect healthcare costs associated with falls and osteoarthritis over 10 years were included in cost effectiveness models, overall quality adjusted life years increased with MPKs.[21] While MPKs are more commonly provided to higher functioning people without chronic diseases, people with diabetes using MPK had greater incremental cost effectiveness due to fewer falls and fall-related hospitalizations.[21,22]

Any MPK can be integrated with many other prosthetic components with the exception of microprocessor feet. Endoskeletal construction is typically employed to save weight and provide space for componentry. Each company recommends integrating its MPK with an energy-storing foot selected from its catalog. The difference between feet may not make a substantial difference[23] and can be individually determined based on the judgment of the prosthetist, patient, physician, and therapist.

When integrating an MPK into a hip disarticulation prosthesis, some shank, feet, or hip joint units may provide functional benefits. Particularly useful are shank devices that provide transverse plane rotation, such as the Delta Twist, which can dampen rotation and can be combined with most MPKs. The Ceterus foot,[11] for instance, may also help provide transverse plane rotation accentuated by the longer step lengths that sometimes result when using an MPK.[24] The Helix3D hip joint provides transverse plane rotation unlike other prosthetic hip joints.

Microprocessor Knee Prostheses Control Mechanisms

The MPK works by sensors transmitting input to the microprocessor, which converts the data so that the appropriate output can be provided. In some cases, artificial intelligence allows the MPK to adapt to the user's movements in different activities. Two types of mechanisms provide input to the MPK, namely computational and interactive.[25]

Computational control mechanisms use sensors to detect movement and forces and send this information to a computer that processes the information and adjusts the resistance provided by the knee mechanism to accommodate for variations determined by the data. For instance, 70% of body weight borne through the weight-bearing foot will be interpreted as occurring during stance phase leading to full resistance to knee flexion. This intrinsic mechanism is so-called because the sensory information and decision-making process is intrinsic to the knee unit sensors and microprocessor, which prompts an automatic reaction. It is the most common form of input mechanism.

Interactive control mechanisms, more common to upper-limb myoelectric prostheses, integrate the user's conscious initiation. Pattern recognition or electromyographic signal sensors detect the movement initiation. Upper-limb prosthetic function is distinctly different from lower-limb function. Arm movement is modulated primarily by the cognitively variable central nervous system to perform complex acts like grasping a variety of foods. In the lower limb, most everyday function involves walking, which is modulated by the spinal cord and central pattern generators without many fine motor variations.

While the transfemoral prosthesis user would not want to think about each of the average 3500 steps taken each day,[26] the future may bring interactive control of the prosthesis through myoelectric input. Preliminary experiments with people with lower-limb amputations using myoelectric technology in a virtual environment demonstrate that electrodes embedded in muscles of the residual lower limb can be used to facilitate specific movements, as is typically done in myoelectric upper-limb prostheses. However, the time to complete simple tasks like extending and relaxing the knee in sitting exceeded 1.5 seconds.[27] Perhaps myoelectrically driven intrinsic control mechanisms may eventually assist slow and deliberate non–weight-bearing tasks for people with leg amputation.

Commercially available MPK's and microprocessor feet currently on the market are displayed with important characteristics in Table 27.3. The first microprocessor foot available to the market was the Proprio foot, which debuted in 2006[11] and was designed with an accelerometer, joint sensor, and motorized actuator, can plantarflex and dorsiflex the foot in non–weight-bearing positions on receiving the correct cues (by heel tap or wireless remote control) enabling the user to sit or don trousers more easily (Fig. 27.6). Powered microprocessor feet like the Ottobock Empower can actively plantarflex during terminal stance to propel the lower extremity forward, mimicking the actions of the plantarflexor muscles.[17] Other functions for the transfemoral prosthesis user, such as rotating the leg to place it on the knee to don shoes and socks, would be the kind of action such an interactive control system may perform in the future.[11] Currently, microprocessor feet and knees cannot be used together.

Once the sensor data has been input and the microprocessor has determined what function is occurring, the MPK can provide two types of knee movement output: resistance or powered assistance. Most commonly, MPKs resist movement, which can be thought of as an eccentric force such as knee function in gait that resists knee flexion in early stance or resisting knee extension in terminal swing phase. By providing the appropriate amount of resistance through the required range of motion, the MPK can assist the wearer to walk at varied speeds and descend stairs and ramps with less difficulty.

Powered MPKs can also assist movement, comparable to a concentric force. Such a force can be helpful in ascending stairs and rising from a chair, especially for those with bilateral limb loss or a weak intact limb. While powered assistance provides the potential for the most complete replication of normal leg function, this potential is limited by actuator technology and electromechanical speed. For instance, the human knee moves over 300 degrees/s in walking[28] and can increase to over 600 degrees/s in running.[29] It would be difficult for actuators that have activation times only as fast as 10 ms[12] to create such high velocities, without overheating when maximum speeds are maintained. User adaptation and acceptance of a powered MPK improves over time[30] and has led to improvements in functional walking tests. However, active control can restrict mobility for middle-age and older adults,[31] perhaps due to the complexity even though most adjustable parameters are not required for common functions.[32]

Artificial intelligence is used in MPKs to varying degrees. Standard setup includes initial programmed learning while the wearer walks with the MPK at various speeds and negotiates ramps and stairs. Setup programming prepares the prosthesis for normal function but may not provide sufficient information for the knee to respond appropriately during unexpected events, such as stepping into a divot. Though technically possible, most MPKs do not use real-time accommodation, as it is unnecessary for ordinary use. For instance, even unexpected situations such as stumbles cause predictable inputs that are anticipated by default settings.

Table 27.3 Characteristics of Microprocessor Knee and Feet Prostheses

Knees	Manufacturer	K-Level	Maximum Body Weight (lbs)	Battery Life	Max Knee Angle (Degrees)	Powered Assist	Weight (lbs)	Protections	Target User	Link
C-Leg 4	Ottobock	2–4	300	2 days	130	No	2.75	IP67	Community ambulator	https://www.ottobock.com/en-us/product/3C88-3~23C98-3
Kenevo	Ottobock	2	275	1 day	124	No	2	IP22	Household or limited community ambulators. Lightweight. Not for sustained outdoor use.	https://www.ottobock.com/en-us/product/3C60
Genium X3	Ottobock	3, 4	330	5 days	135	No	3.77	IP681 hour submersion at <3 m depth	Active individuals who want limited submersion abilities. Running mode	https://www.ottobock.com/en-us/product/3B5-3
Genium	Ottobock	3, 4	330	5 days	135	No	3.3	IP67	Similar to X3 but without submersion abilities or running mode.	https://www.ottobock.com/en-us/product/3B1-3
Power Knee	Össur	2, 3	256	1 day	120	Yes	5.8	IPX54	Actively assists the user into standing or when negotiating elevations. Heavy and not for athletes.	https://www.ossur.com/en-us/prosthetics/knees/power-knee
Rheo Knee	Össur	3	300	3 days	120	No	3.5	IP34		https://www.ossur.com/en-us/prosthetics/knees/rheo-knee
Rheo Knee XC	Össur	3, 4	300 (moderate impact), 243 (high impact)	3 days	120	No	3.5	IP34	Same as Rheo but allows for high impact activity.	https://www.ossur.com/en-us/prosthetics/knees/rheo-knee-xc
Allux 2	Proteor	3, 4	275 (K3), 220 (K4)	4 days	180	No	3.33	IP44		https://us.proteor.com/knee-portfolio/allux-2/
Plie 3	Proteor	3, 4	275 (K3), 220 (K4)	1 day (can use external battery packs)	117-125	No	2.7	IP67	Submersible for 30 min at a depth of 1 m.	https://us.proteor.com/knee-portfolio/plie-3/
Quattro	Proteor	3, 4	300	2 days (can use external battery packs)	135	No	3.65	IP67	Submersible for 30 min at a depth of 1 m.	https://us.proteor.com/knee-portfolio/proteor-quattro/
Orion 3	Blatchford	2–4	275 (K3), 220 (K4)	3 days	130	No	3.5	NA		https://www.blatchford-mobility.com/en-us/products/knees/orion3
SmartIP	Blatchford	2–4	275 (K3), 220 (K4)	NA	140	No	2.8	NA		https://www.blatchford-mobility.com/en-us/products/knees/smartip

Table 27.3—cont'd

Foot/ Ankle System	Manufacturer	K-Level	Maximum Body Weight (lbs)	Battery Life	Max DF/ PF Angle (Degrees)	Powered Assist	Weight (lbs)	Protections	Target User	Link
Elan	Blatchford	3	275	2 days	3/6	No	2.63	NA		https://www.blatchford-mobility.com/en-us/products/feet-ankles/elan
ElanIC	Blatchford	3	275	2 days	3/6	No	2.7	IP67	Submersible for 30 min at a depth of 1 m.	https://www.blatchford-mobility.com/en-us/products/feet-ankles/elanic
Meridium	Ottobock	3	275	1 day	14.5/22	No	3.27	IP54		https://www.ottobock.com/en-us/product/1B1-2
Empower	Ottobock	3	287	8 hours	22 plantarflexion	Yes	4.73	NA	Powered assist into plantarflexion	https://www.ottobock.com/en-us/product/1A1-2
Proprio Foot	Össur	3	275	2 days	33 degrees total	Yes	4.65 with battery pack	IP67	Submersible for 30 min at a depth of 1 m. Actively DF for elevation negotiation and for improved foot clearance.	https://www.ossur.com/en-us/prosthetics/feet/proprio-foot
Kinnex 2.0	Proteor	3	275	1 day	10/20	No	3.3	IP67	Submersible for 30 min at a depth of 1 m.	https://us.proteor.com/ankle-portfolio/kinnex-2-0/

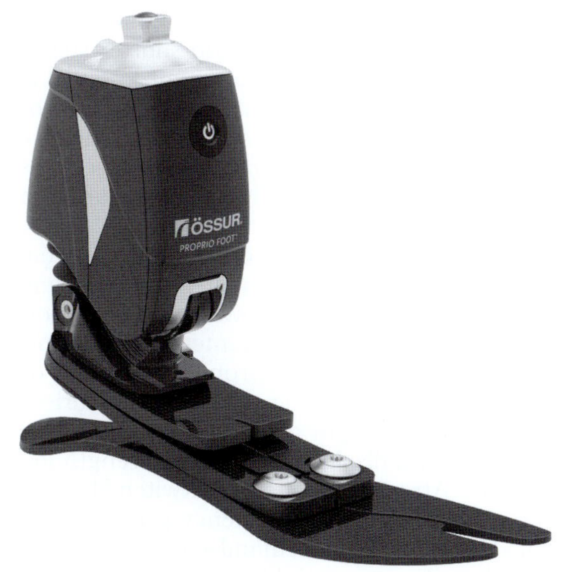

Fig. 27.6 Proprio foot. (© Össur.)

Common Mobility Problems and Potential Solutions

Despite sophisticated technology, prosthesis users face a variety of problems in moving around the community. Some problems can be significantly improved by MPK use, although users who are transitioning from non-MPK prostheses may have developed habits that must be unlearned. To illustrate how an MPK unit can benefit the user, common problems in gait, stair, and ramp negotiation, transfers, and stumbling will be presented.

People with lower-limb loss using an MPK demonstrate improved gait symmetry.[33,34] Few studies have focused on physical therapy training to improve prosthetic walking function, but various approaches including functional training, balance training, and exercises for specific muscle groups have shown promise.[35] Despite rigorous training and dedicated practice, some gait deviations persist.[15,36] The most common deviations from which MPK users can significantly benefit are discussed here with prosthetic and training solutions.

STANCE PHASE

Loading response: A common stance phase deviation is decreased prosthetic knee flexion during loading response. Decreased knee flexion develops because amputation of the knee robs the lower limb of the eccentric function of the quadriceps, which typically absorbs impact shock as the knee flexes approximately 15 degrees during initial loading.[37] Knee buckling in loading response is a primary concern in early prosthetic training. The experienced non-MPK user may prevent collapse and potential falls by keeping the knee extended in loading response. Decreased prosthetic knee flexion, however, diminishes shock attenuation and transmits stress up the kinetic chain to the hip, pelvis, and spine.[38] Weight-activated friction brakes stabilize the knee when in the safe 0- to 20-degree knee flexion range. Hydraulic units provide graded resistance to knee flexion within the 0- to 20-degree range for descent of stairs, but will buckle readily beyond this range. Although this range of support is usually adequate for level walking, more range is required when descending a ramp, stepping on uneven surfaces, or when missteps occur. Lacking graded eccentric knee flexion control on initial loading, the user learns to walk with a habitually extended knee.

Prosthetic solutions: Some MPKs, like the C-Leg and Rheo Knee, allow knee flexion on loading to provide the normal shock-absorbing function of the anatomic knee on heel strike. For experienced prosthesis users who have learned to walk with the prosthetic knee extended on initial contact, this function may seem strange. Indeed, the transfemoral amputation limb generates substantial hip extension power in the initial loading phase of gait particularly on the amputated side to push the thigh posterior and maintain the knee extended as well as to power the body forward over the stance limb.[39] The new MPK user transitioning from a non-MPK unit must unlearn old habits and let the knee bend on initial contact to benefit from the MPK's capacity for greater shock absorption. The prosthetist can adjust the level of resistance as the user adapts.

Training solutions: Whether learning to walk with a prosthesis for the first time or transitioning to an MPK that allows dampened knee flexion on initial contact, prosthetic training should develop both movement ability and trust in the leg. Although strengthening the gluteus maximus is always beneficial to increase eccentric motor control that can support knee flexion control, the major factor is developing the trust in the MPK to allow knee flexion. Initially standing in parallel bars to provide security, the MPK user can step forward onto the prosthesis, perceiving the resistance to knee flexion and posterior thigh pressure on the socket as their weight progresses from the heel to the toe. Repeatedly leaning on the prosthetic foot to rock from heel to toe as the knee bends gives the MPK user awareness of the strength of knee resistance and proprioceptive feedback that helps foster trust in the leg (Fig. 27.7). Training can progress to practice stepping performed with knee flexion on heel contact as the body advances over the prosthetic foot, causing knee extension, similar to an able-bodied gait. This can be practiced independently at home with hands on a wall in front of the person, in the parallel bars, and later advanced to walking with initial knee flexion on heel contact, guarded by the physical therapist, who can ensure that the knee unit will progress into extension as in normal gait. Training proceeds to ramp descent, best begun using a railing with therapist assistance. Developing the confidence to descend ramps while the MPK flexes through initial loading can seem like a leap of faith at first. Making the transition from walking with a hyperextended prosthetic knee to allowing the knee unit to flex during loading response can be difficult. Nevertheless, as little as 10 weeks has been needed to acclimate to the MPK.[40]

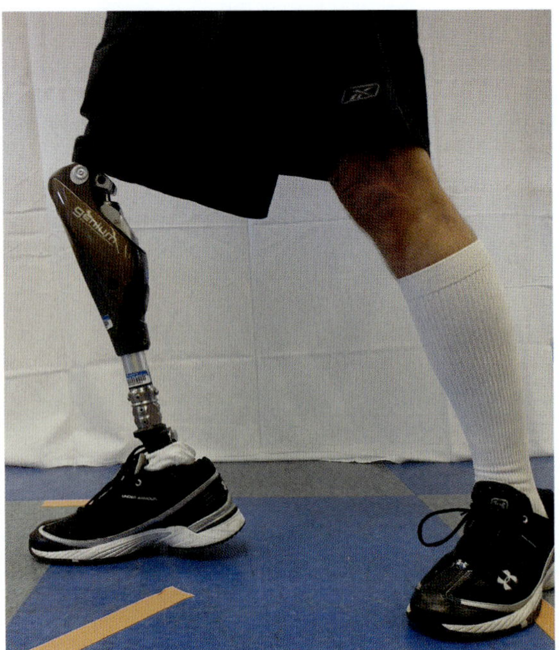

Fig. 27.7 Rocking onto toes to feel the microprocessor knee flexion resistance.

Asymmetric step length: Various physical impairments make asymmetric step length a common deviation for prosthesis users. The sound-limb step is typically shorter than that of the prosthesis. Amputated side hip extensor weakness, uncertain balance, and limited hip extension range of motion further restricted by the 10-degree hip flexion built into the transfemoral socket bench alignment all cause a briefer sound-limb swing time and shorter step length. Decreased hip rotation and concomitant lessened contralateral pelvic rotation also contribute to shorter prosthetic steps. Increasing hip extension range of motion and hip strength improves balance and facilitates longer prosthesis stance time. Practice walking with shorter sound-limb step lengths can also reduce asymmetry.[24]

Gluteus maximus strength is critical during initial loading to generate the hip extension force in early stance that lifts the center of gravity from lowest to highest point and converts stance limb torque from internal to external rotation. Extensor strength is the strongest predictor of prosthetic walking speed.[41] In the absence of quadriceps and with the inevitable atrophy of the hamstrings,[42] hip extension and abduction display the greatest strength loss after amputation.[43] Atrophy of gluteal fast twitch fibers explains the slower gluteal contraction latency periods observed in amputated limbs.[44] Greater demand and slower contractions on the weakened amputated side hip extensors decrease the user's ability to quickly raise the center of gravity from the lowest point in dual limb stance to the highest point by midstance,[41] particularly if long prosthetic steps are emphasized early in the rehabilitation process when gluteal strength is weakest. As a result, prosthetic stance time is significantly briefer than on the sound side, leading to shorter sound-limb swing-phase duration and step lengths.[45,46]

Hip abductor weakness reduces the ability to maintain the body in prosthetic limb stance. This leads to a similar scenario in the frontal plane that also contributes to shorter sound-limb steps.[47] Insufficient gluteus medius strength also diminishes the confidence to maintain single-limb stance long enough to complete the normal lateral weight shift. The prosthesis user compensates by placing the sound foot farther from the midline, widening the base of support. The wide base shortens the gluteus medius length-tension relationship, further impairing hip abduction strength while simultaneously requiring a larger lateral weight shift. Hip abductor weakness also plays a role in step length asymmetry, with weakness correlating with slower gait, shorter steps on both sides, and decreased weight bearing on the prosthesis.[47] Those with shorter amputation limbs have more abductor weakness, demonstrated in midstance by faster and/or greater pelvic drop.[48,49] In both situations, longer and/or wider steps are a disadvantage to the gluteal muscles.

In terminal stance, decreased prosthetic side hip extension range of motion restricts the body's advance over the prosthetic foot causing the sound limb to take a shorter step forward. Lack of sufficient hip extension due to hip flexor contracture occurs with able-bodied people but is more prevalent among people with lower-limb amputation. Prolonged sitting during the rehabilitation process that can continue at home due to decreased activity is common after amputation.[26] The standard flexed bench alignment of the transfemoral socket can accommodate mild hip flexion contractures but reduces hip extension excursion.[46]

In the presence of limited hip extension range of motion, users attempt to advance the body over the prosthesis by exaggerating anterior pelvic tilt[48,49] with accentuated lumbar paraspinal muscle use, leading to greater lumbar extension compared with able-bodied people.[50] Such compensation may lead to lower back strains; people with both amputation and low-back pain had weaker back extensors.[51] Increased demand for hip and lumbar extension strength and range of motion might be met with extra training to guard against low-back pain. Abdominal and hip flexor strength is also critical to maintain hip stability and protect end-range lumbar extension in double support phase of gait.[52]

In normal gait, stance phase hip extension occurs with rotation around the stance hip.[37] Although often observed as contralateral forward pelvic rotation, the rotation occurs primarily at the hip. After amputation, hip extension and contralateral forward rotation around the prosthesis are greatly reduced compared with the sound limb,[48] because transection through the femur minimizes transverse plane bony leverage. As a result, translation of rotary forces from the limb to the socket is greatly reduced because the femur rotates within the soft tissues of the thigh. Any looseness in socket fit reduces the translated forces even more. In fact, unlike sound side- or able-bodied individuals, prosthetic stance phase is marked by internal, rather than external, torque,[49] which decreases trunk counterrotation and arm swing. Less trunk rotation is needed to counterbalance pelvic rotation when the individual wears a prosthesis. Nevertheless, when pelvic rotation is decreased, trunk rotation for prosthesis users is also diminished by limited joint mobility, weaker abdominal strength, incoordination between pelvis and trunk, and habit.

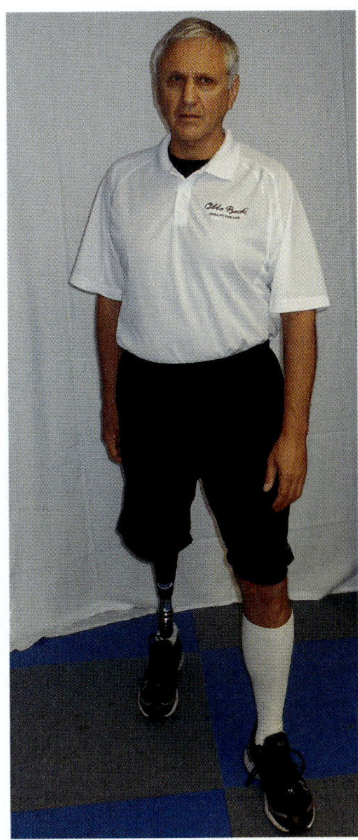

Fig. 27.8 Reduced prosthetic side arm swing provides a hip extension moment but causes gait asymmetry.

Lessened trunk rotation decreases the alternating forward momentum that normally drives arm swing, leading to decreased shoulder movement. The ipsilateral upper limb may be unconsciously held posterior to the hip axis to maintain a hip extension moment for enhanced stability (Fig. 27.8).

For more experienced and usually healthier users who have more confidence in the prosthesis and have striven to walk faster, prosthetic steps may be shorter than those of the sound limb.[18,53] Multiple years of hip flexor stretching increases hip extension range.[51] However, iliopsoas often atrophies and weakens,[52] providing insufficient power to protect the hip and lumbar spine and to enable uniform step lengths. Increased lumbar rotation that compensates for limited hip rotation after amputation may exacerbate low-back pain.[50] Regardless of which step is shorter, coordination of trunk and pelvis is important to stabilize the lumbar spine dynamically and produce sufficient trunk and pelvic rotation to achieve symmetrical step length.

Prosthetic solutions: The enhanced stance phase stability of an MPK obviates the need to use the arm to maintain a hip extension moment throughout stance and allows the user to spend more time on prosthetic single-limb stance, thus equalizing step lengths and restoring the normal external rotation torque in stance phase. A torque adapter in the shank can augment the limited contralateral pelvic rotation around the prosthesis. Regardless of the type of knee unit, significant hip abductor strength is required for single-limb stance on the prosthesis without contralateral pelvic drop or ipsilateral trunk lean.

Training solutions: Developing symmetry in prosthetic gait requires a comprehensive approach that reduces underlying

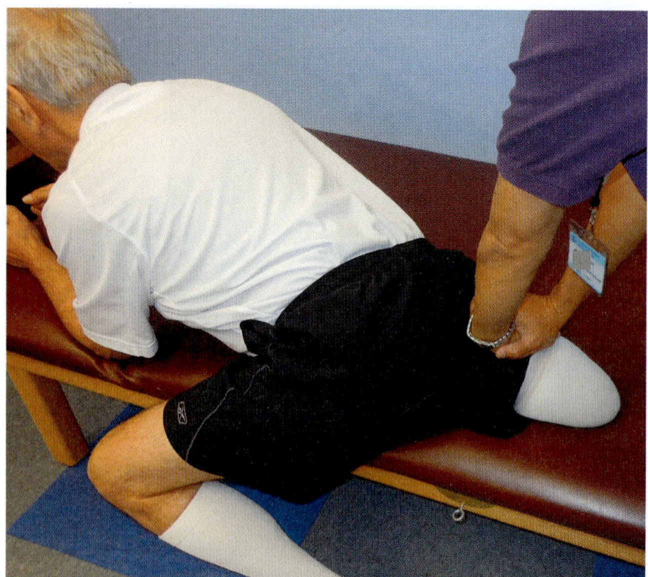

Fig. 27.9 Anterior hip joint capsule mobilization.

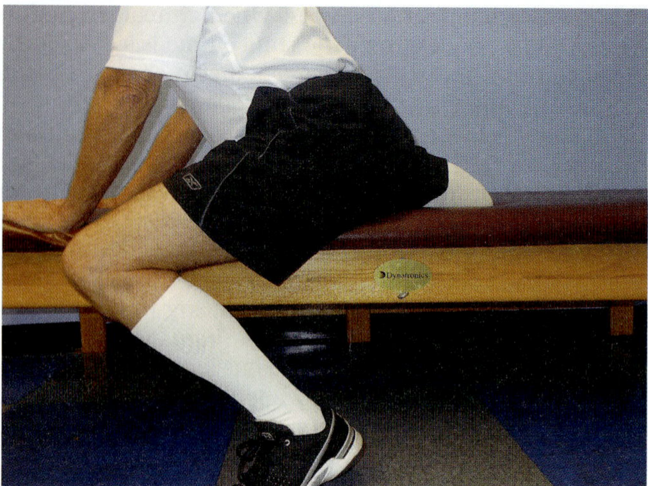

Fig. 27.10 Hip flexor stretch.

joint and muscular impairments to optimize body structure/function capability and contribute to functional outcomes.[54] Starting by optimizing potential capability via minimizing spinal and peripheral joint mobility that can be built on with strengthening exercises and neuromotor training is a logical and orderly approach to rehabilitation.[54] To enable the user to walk with as much symmetry as possible, the person should have normal range of motion throughout the lower limb, particularly the hip. Anterior hip capsular tightness limiting hip extension range is common due to prolonged sitting. Anteriorly directed hip mobilization can help restore hip extension and rotation range (Fig. 27.9).[55] Additional mobilization of the sacroiliac and lumbar joints may also show improvement and yield short-term immediate strength gains by minimizing myotomal inhibition,[56] an approach that has been used for both community- and household-level walkers after unilateral amputation.[57,58] Soft tissue mobilization for the iliopsoas and tensor fascia lata followed by stretching can help maintain hip flexor flexibility[57,59] and can be performed in the prone position or with the patient lying prone with the sound foot on the floor to help maintain or increase hip range (Fig. 27.10).

Once joint motion is optimized, weight-bearing gluteal strength must be increased. These muscles minimize lumbar extension and frontal plane gait compensations that typically result from hip weakness. In addition to residual limb hip abduction exercise performed side-lying against a bolster,[60] the person can wear the prosthesis to perform closed-chain exercises. Forward step-ups are a challenge; however, lateral step-ups on a low platform activate the gluteus medius.[61] To progress a user's efforts, increase the step height gradually. Activities involving sustained stance on the prosthesis also develop prosthetic side hip strength, especially hip abductors. Standing on the prosthesis while pushing in the opposite direction against a wall is an example (Fig. 27.11A and B). More dynamic activities include standing on the prosthesis while using the sound limb to roll a ball on the floor, kicking against Theraband,[62] reaching in different directions around a circle like the star excursion balance test,[63] or maintaining the sound limb on a stool or unstable surface while throwing a ball (Fig. 27.12). Using one hand to lightly maintain balance is important for safety; however, if both hands are required, the activity is probably too difficult and should be modified.

In addition to unilateral trunk bridging that focuses on gluteus maximus strengthening and control, hip extensor strength can be developed wearing the prosthesis while standing or simulating gait positions. One method to activate the gluteus maximus is to stand with hands in front pushing forward against a wall or kitchen counter, while leaning forward far enough to lift the prosthetic heel off the floor. As the trunk shifts forward over the forefoot, a hip flexion moment is created that must be maintained with hip extensors to keep the heel high (Fig. 27.13). Promoting forefoot loading facilitates gluteus maximus activation and trains the user to activate MPK functions. Developing sufficient prosthetic side hip power to take long sound-limb steps can be performed by standing with the prosthetic foot ahead of the intact foot facing a low stool. The wearer steps forward with the sound limb progressing to higher steps. This activity exaggerates the demands on the gluteus maximus and can be used to develop the power needed for more challenging activities (Fig. 27.14).

Strengthening the gluteus maximus, the primary external rotator of the hip, is also vital in transforming the leg torque from internal to external rotation after initial loading. Activities described above such as the sound-limb star balance excursion test or exaggerated step lengths to ever higher steps increase gluteal strength and develop pelvic rotation around the prosthetic stance limb. Exercises that emphasize hip rotator strength include pressing the contralateral arm or leg back against a wall to promote isometric contralateral trunk rotation (see Fig. 27.11B). Active rotation around the prosthesis can be performed by turning the pelvis to point the sound foot as far around as possible in each direction and then maintaining the position, using the hands of a clock as a visual cue (Fig. 27.15A and B). Rotational activities can be progressed by pivoting on both heels to turn the toes in and out. Even more challenging is weight bearing through the forefeet while turning first one then both heels medially and laterally (Fig. 27.16A and B).

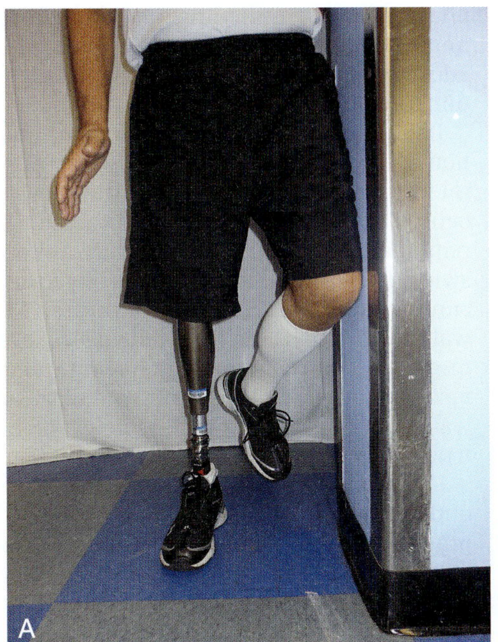

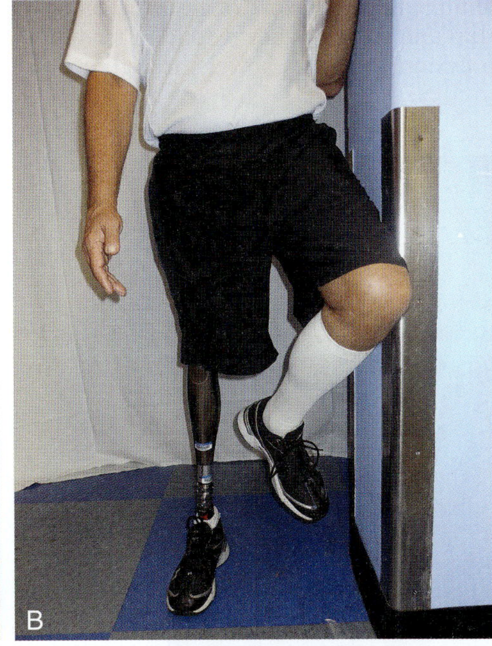

Fig. 27.11 (A) Isometric hip abduction and (B) isometric hip external rotation against a wall.

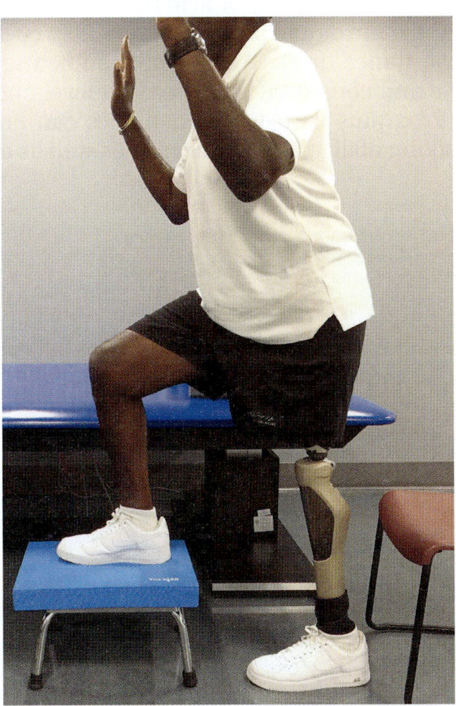

Fig. 27.12 Step standing with sound limb on an unstable surface.

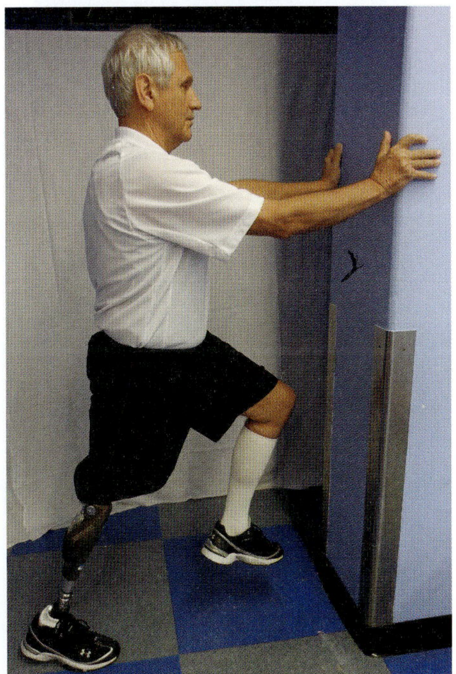

Fig. 27.13 Pushing forward against a wall while rising onto the forefoot for hip extension and external rotation.

Pivoting with weight on the toes develops hip strength and assists functional use of the MPK during turns and side-steps. For effective neuromuscular reeducation and activation of the hip rotators, the therapist may use cueing or apply resistance through the sound limb (Fig. 27.17). Pelvic rotation contributes to the overall goal of uniform step length with faster gait speeds although specific pelvic motions may become less symmetrical.[48]

More advanced gluteal strengthening activities can integrate trunk and upper extremity function through exaggerated elements of gait. One method is to face a wall, then press only the ipsilateral hand against the wall while simultaneously lifting the prosthetic heel off the floor and flexing the sound hip as high as possible (see Fig. 27.13). Avoid lumbar hyperextension to protect the back. Maintaining this position with spinal stability activates the abdominal muscles and helps promote contralateral pelvic rotation around the prosthesis with upper trunk counter-rotation and arm swing often impaired in gait. Spinal stabilization exercises increase prosthetic step length and gait speed.[53] Strengthening the hip flexors of both limbs also helps protect the hip and spine as they extend in terminal stance phase. Hip flexion generates power through swing phase. Hip strengthening and functional proficiency are important for both legs because sound-limb hip rotation adds impetus to prosthetic swing phase, trunk counterrotation, and arm swing.

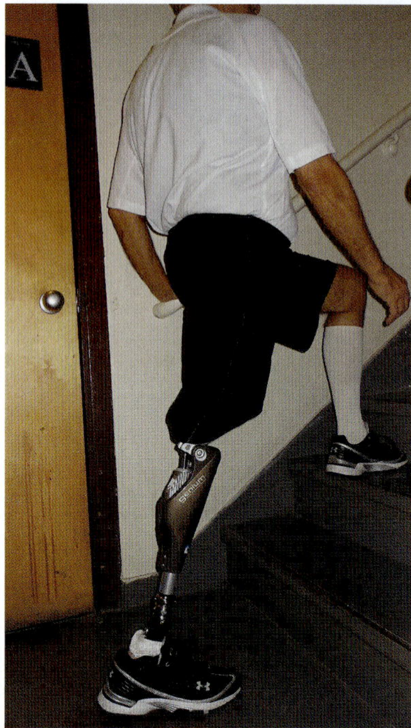

Fig. 27.14 Sound limb to high step.

In addition to pelvic and trunk rotation training, additional practice may be necessary to make arm swing natural. For the experienced wearer, the habit of keeping the arm behind the hip is likely to be ingrained. Focused training is required to restore normal trunk counterrotation and arm swing. Facilitating arm swing through the shoulders or with canes held in each hand by both user and therapist while walking in synchronicity can help. Pelvic and trunk rotation in gait can be progressed by having the user and therapist face each other while the user walks forward as the therapist walks backward resisting the pelvis or hands to integrate trunk counterrotation and arm swing (Fig. 27.18).

Functional activities to develop transverse plane rotation and gait symmetry can eventually be used for independent practice by highly functioning individuals include tandem balancing (Fig. 27.19) and walking or grapevine walking to encourage rotation around each hip as well as decrease the base of support. Floor markers placed evenly apart can serve as visual cues for uniform step lengths, and a full-length mirror at the end of a walkway allows the prosthesis user to check the symmetry of arm movements and general symmetry. A metronome provides an audible cue to rectify asymmetric stance times. A treadmill can be used to train progressive and consistent gait speed on level and inclined surfaces. Programs with varied activities can build confidence, walking ability, and endurance as well as awareness

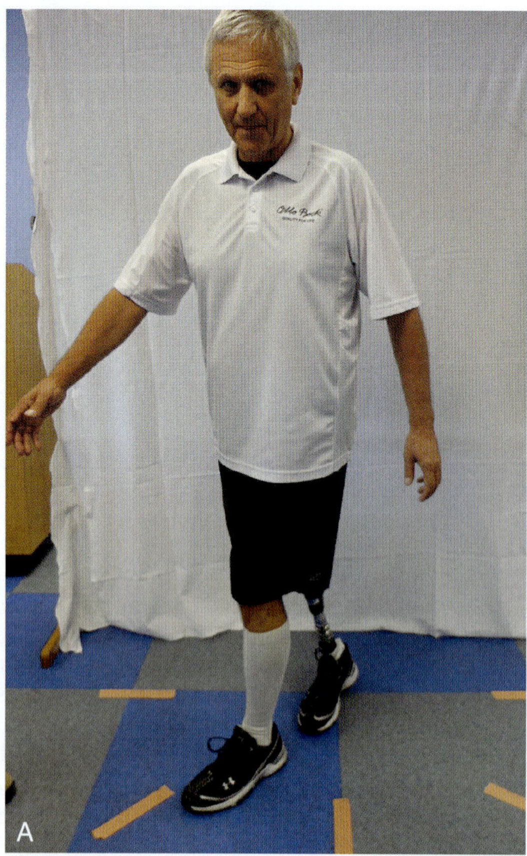

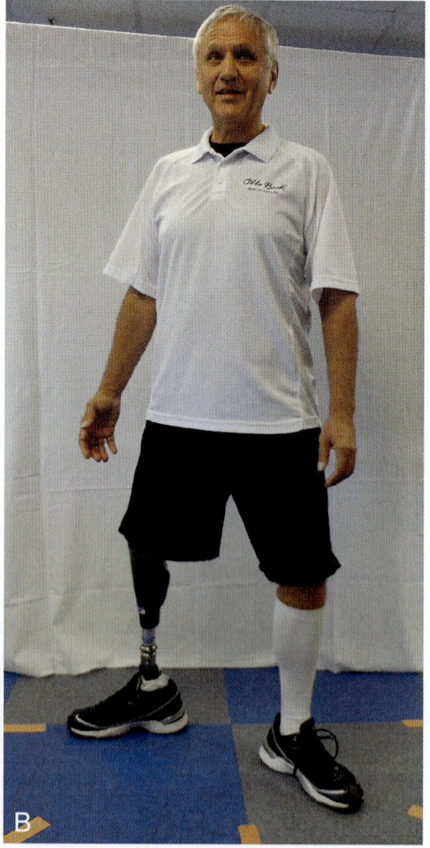

Fig. 27.15 Stepping and holding in hip rotation: (A) internal and (B) external.

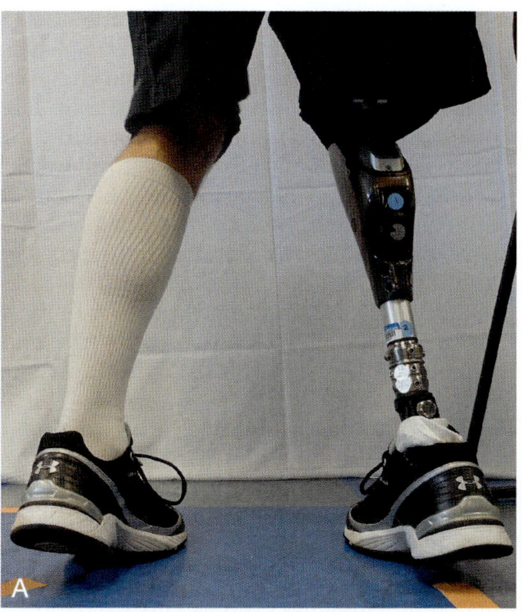

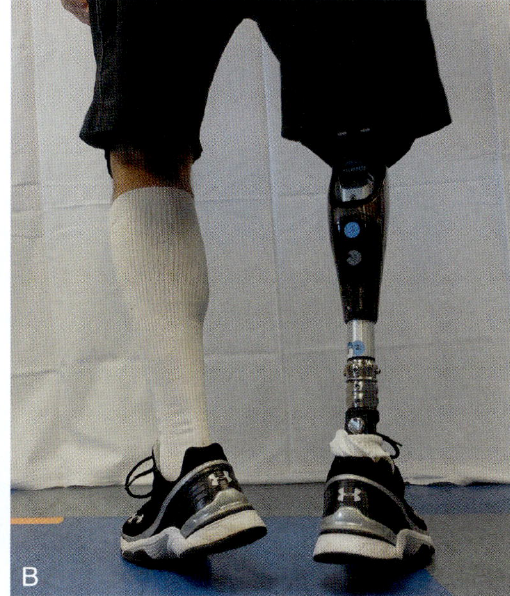

Fig. 27.16 Pivoting on both heels (not pictured) and toes from (A) internal to (B) external.

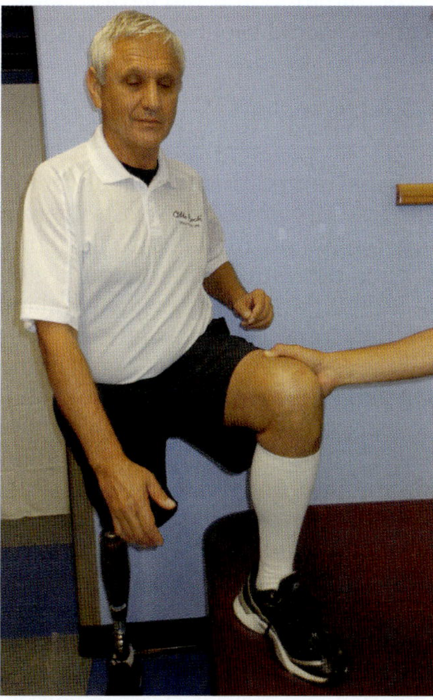

Fig. 27.17 Resisted hip external rotation by therapist through the sound knee.

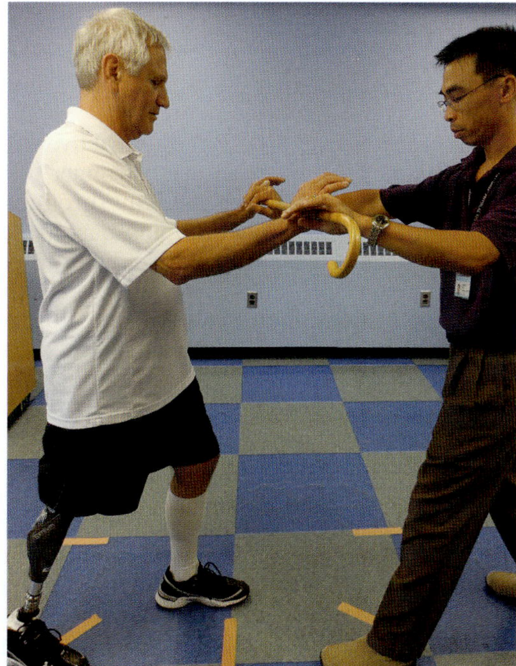

Fig. 27.18 Resisted gait with cane.

of muscle function and the limit of stability.[64,65] As ability increases, additional challenges can be designed, such as stepping onto unstable surfaces.

Other stance phase deviations discussed elsewhere in this text, such as wide base of support and lateral trunk lean or Trendelenburg, are unlikely to be affected specifically by MPK use but may benefit from the proposed training solutions. Regardless of prosthetic components, training is required to minimize gait deviations and maximize function.

Swing phase: Gait asymmetry can be affected by the difficulty transitioning from stance to swing phase. For able-bodied individuals, ankle plantarflexion prior to swing phase raises the body, providing much of the propulsive power.[37] Hip flexors contract to decelerate end-range hip extension, then initiate swing phase with the adductors. The flexing hip and the forward propulsion of the body create momentum that first passively flexes the knee from heel off to early swing then extends the knee through terminal swing when hip flexion is reversed by the hip extensors. When momentum is reduced, as in slow gait, the hamstring muscles flex the knee to assure toe clearance augmenting foot dorsiflexion.

Amputation eliminates active ankle plantarflexion. Work shifts to the iliopsoas muscle increasing power derived from

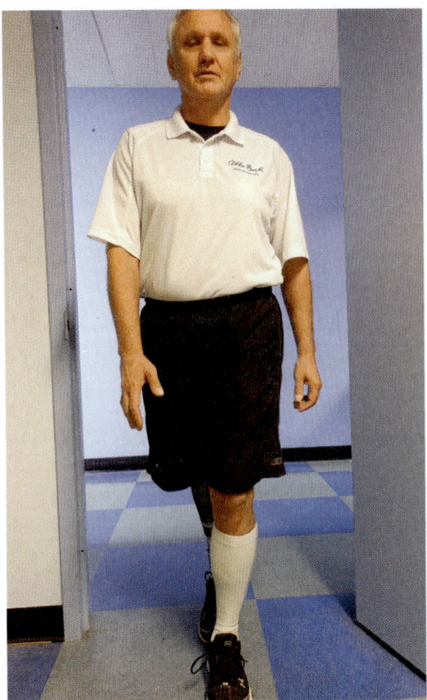

Fig. 27.19 Tandem stance in a doorway.

the hip flexor group by over 50%.[39] Without active knee flexion, the hip flexors must contract even stronger to supply sufficient momentum to advance the limb through swing phase. Unfortunately, the ipsilateral iliopsoas atrophies.[52] Developing hip flexor strength can be difficult, especially with shorter amputation limbs. The new user can have difficulty advancing the limb, leading some to exaggerate hip flexion by kicking the leg laterally to initiate swing. Exaggerated kicking can lead to swing-phase deviations like steppage (exaggerated hip and knee flexion) that can linger long after sufficient strength is restored.

Non-MPK hydraulic knee users must also switch their knees from stance phase control knee flexion resistance to swing-phase resistance. While unnatural at first, prosthesis users learn to perform the knee extension motion without much thought.[66] However, swing phase is delayed and stance times asymmetric.[45] When momentum is not directed forward, such as when turning or side stepping, transition between stance and swing-phase knee resistance can be ineffective resulting in occasional circumduction, hip hiking, or vaulting if adequate swing resistance is not activated. Knee collapse and falling may occur if stance resistance is not activated.

Prosthetic solutions: For the MPK user, transition between resistance phases is initiated intrinsically in response to electronic sensors. In the C-Leg the user must achieve knee extension for 0.1 second with 70% body weight forefoot loading to disengage stance control and allow swing-phase knee flexion. The amount of body weight required can be adjusted depending on the user's needs. Default settings of the specific MPK determine what happens if the criteria are not met. For instance, the C-Leg defaults to stance phase control to protect the wearer from knee collapse, a significantly improved safety feature compared with non-MPK prostheses. Other MPK units like the Rheo Knee default to swing phase control to avoid toe drag in swing phase.

Training solutions: To ensure that the user is comfortable bearing weight through the prosthetic forefoot, activities involving forefoot loading are critical. Pivoting can be practiced with weight on both forefeet to allow rapid swing-phase action during turns (see Fig. 27.16B). Lateral weight shifts onto the toes with one or two quick bounces can help prepare for side stepping. Forefoot bouncing can also be useful, and some MPKs like the Power Knee use forefoot bounces as mechanical cues to change knee resistance modes. Pushing off the forefoot to kick into swing-phase can assist forward walking or the quick transition into swing phase necessary for a brief jog.

For those with decreased pelvic and trunk motion, abdominal muscles may be recruited to assist swing phase, particularly for people with amputation limbs shorter than 57% of the sound length where hip flexors are weaker. Shorter limb length correlates with increased pelvic tilting during gait even after traumatic amputation.[67] Core abdominal mobility exercises are even more important after hip disarticulation or higher amputations that deprive the user of all active hip motion. In addition, rapid stepping can improve the coordination and hip flexion power necessary to increase gait speed and avoid obstacles.

Stairs and Ramps

Descents: Stairs and ramps remain difficult for even for experienced users. Descents and ascents pose different problems. As in walking, limited prosthetic knee flexion is a particular problem when descending stairs and declines. Limited shock attenuation is particularly evident on landing on the prosthetic limb when descending stairs, curbs, or declines. Because the wearer descends stairs onto the heel, not the forefoot as able-bodied individuals do, more shock is transmitted to the extremity; the user commonly feels a jolt on landing. Although the prosthetic limb is subjected to less vertical force than a normal limb on landing, this force is more poorly attenuated without normal knee flexion and ankle dorsiflexion on loading. The hip on the prosthetic side must exert greater extension force to help control the knee. On the sound limb, the relative lack of prosthetic knee flexion results in about 50% greater vertical impact forces as the body lowers from a greater height.[68,69] In fact, all sound-limb joints experience increased stress in gait, exposing the sound side to more risk of injury.[30] As a result, most people with transfemoral or higher amputations instinctively take smaller steps of shorter duration to decrease ground reaction forces and muscle demand on ramps whether descending or ascending.[70] The new wearer usually takes short prosthetic steps to prevent accidental collapse and compensates with longer sound-limb steps to maintain speed, making gait asymmetrical.

Non-MPK hydraulic stance control knees provide graded resistance to knee motion beyond 20-degree flexion, giving time for the sound limb to alight onto the next lower step in a step-after-step pattern. Nevertheless, most users still have noticeably decreased prosthetic stance time when descending stairs.[69] Descending ramps is more difficult than stairs because in order to place the prosthetic foot flat on the ground without the normal ankle plantarflexion range, the prosthetic shank must be thrust forward downhill, creating a rapid, sizeable knee flexion moment. Knee flexion resistance in a non-MPK hydraulic stance control unit can be adequate on shallow ramps, but knee flexion resistance is not always sufficient on steeper ramps. Prosthetic users often hesitate when descending ramps.

Prosthetic solutions: As in level walking, MPK sensors provide data used to adjust the real-time resistance needed for descent. For the typical MPK, full knee extension at terminal swing combined with prosthetic heel weight bearing triggers knee flexion resistance to match the individual's body weight, angle of descent, and gait speed through a greater range of motion (30–35 degrees) than provided by non-MPK units.[24] Slow, interrupted, or unsteady stair descent may cause insufficient momentum to create full knee extension, thereby leaving MPKs with swing-phase resistance default settings unready to provide stance phase stability; this deficiency can lead to knee collapse. Collapse is less of a problem for the C-Leg, which defaults to stance phase knee resistance, even in knee flexion ranges of 36 to 55 degrees.[68] Prosthesis users functioning at the Medicare K2 or K3 levels (see Table 27.2) performed better on stairs and declines with MPK compared with non-MPK hydraulic knees.[71] After the MPK software is adjusted and the user develops confidence and balance through training, the wearer can descend steep declines with significantly longer prosthetic steps that promote less asymmetry and faster speeds.[24]

Training solutions: To descend stairs, the MPK user must learn to place only the rear foot on the lower step and load substantial body weight through the heel (see Fig. 27.2). This foot placement triggers the graded knee flexion resistance needed while leaving the toes to angle down and progress to the next step as the knee bends. To step down stairs onto the heel in this manner can be anxiety producing for the new MPK user and should be practiced initially on the bottom step using a bannister with guarding.

The prosthesis user can mitigate some of the impact shock to the residual limb by reaching the prosthetic leg down toward the next step so the foot meets the lower stair with less impact. This motion, referred to as pelvic anterior depression,[72] can be practiced on level ground or by standing on a low platform to reach the heel forward and down with a pelvic motion before returning to the starting position.

Taking long prosthetic steps when descending a ramp is unnatural to the person who has habitually used a non-MPK prosthesis. This habit may be overcome by training the MPK user to (1) utilize pelvic anterior depression in terminal swing, (2) activate the hip extensors to advance the body forward during initial loading, (3) rotate the contralateral pelvis around the stance hip in midstance, and (4) maintain weight bearing through the prosthetic forefoot in terminal stance. Training can include practice placing the prosthetic heel on targets placed on the floor around the individual. A banister provides safety during the training process until the new wearer develops confidence to progress to resisted training and finally unassisted declines.

Ascents: Most people with transfemoral amputation ascend stairs in a step-to fashion. A similar gait pattern is used for steep inclines. When ascending, the wearer typically flexes the sound limb more to make up for the lack of prosthetic side elevation normally provided by ankle plantarflexion.[70] In the community, some people ascend stairs two steps at a time with the sound limb to maintain the same speed as companions. Greater knee flexion, however, increases forces on all sound-limb joints when climbing stairs.[69] In the stance phase of ramp ascent, the prosthetic shank is thrust backward making it difficult to advance the body forward and causing a short step on the intact side.

Prosthetic solutions: When ascending ramps, forefoot weight-bearing causes the shank to be thrust backward, exerting a strong knee extension moment. An MPK in the stair ascent mode gives less swing-phase resistance to knee flexion to help the foot clear the edge of the next step. Software can be adjusted to the user's needs. Once the foot is on the next step, however, the user must exert considerable hip extensor power to lift the body onto the next step, which is typically accomplished with the assistance of a hand on a bannister. In the absence of a bannister, step-over-step stair ascent is very difficult for most users.

The Power Knee provides powered assistance to ascent. The user must stop at the bottom stair for 3 seconds to default to the standing state before ascending. Initiating knee extension activates the assisted knee extension function. Data sent wirelessly from sensors strapped to the sound leg help match prosthetic movement to the sound limb. At the top of the stairs, the user must pause again for 3 seconds to reset the MPK before walking. The powered mechanism makes sounds noticeable to passersby; the noise bothers some users.

The Genium uses a gyroscope and accelerometers to recognize that the user is ascending a step. A quick hip extension movement to drag the foot off the ground followed by quick hip flexion in a whipping motion lifts the foot to the next step with prosthetic hip and knee flexion. Once the foot is on the next higher step, the Genium provides maximal resistance preventing further knee flexion in the bent-knee weight-bearing position. Use of the Genium has shown to improve step-over-step ability, though significant effort is still required by the opposite lower limb to raise the body and upper limbs to pull up on a bannister.[73–75]

Training solutions: Due to hip flexor weakness, the prosthesis user may have to elevate or tilt the pelvis posteriorly, using the abdominals to gain sufficient elevation and to compensate for limited prosthetic ankle dorsiflexion on stairs and inclines. If the user stops on a step, restarting swing phase up the stairs is difficult. Turning diagonally allows space for the foot to clear after a stop on the stairs without excessive hip hiking. Ascending step-over-step requires great hip extensor strength and usually the assistance of a bannister. Recent MPK designs, including the Power Knee and Genium, meet this challenge. The Power Knee only requires the user to initiate knee extension with the hip extensors. Step-over-step ascent with the Genium requires significant hip extensor strength and is recommended only for active users at the K3 to K4 levels (see Table 27.2).

Sitting and squatting: Although navigating stairs can be difficult for people using prosthetic knees, knee bending and straightening activities like rising from a chair or squatting demand compensatory movements, which impose added stress to the sound limb. Many prosthetic knees require unloading the prosthesis to allow the knee unit to bend so that the user can sit at a speed similar to able-bodied individuals. As a result, many prosthesis wearers stand with 10% to 30% more body weight on the sound limb than on the prosthesis.[47,76] Squatting with both legs can be useful. For instance, the prosthesis user may want to squat to reach down to a child or pick up something from the floor without bending from the waist to avoid low-back pain, which occurs in more than 80% of people using transfemoral prostheses.[52] After 30 degrees of knee unit flexion, most MPKs provide insufficient flexion resistance to prevent collapse.[68] Thus for many users, sit-stand transitions and especially squatting become single-limb activities that place substantial stress on the sound limb. Potential solutions for sit-to-strand transitions and squatting follow.

Prosthetic solutions: When the wearer begins to sit down, MPKs like the C-Leg and Rheo Knee provide controlled resistance to knee flexion activated by prosthetic weight bearing. MPKs allow symmetrical distribution of weight between the feet to reduce stress on the sound limb; resistance settings can be adjusted to the needs of the user. Whether using non-MPK or MPK, wearers continue to bear weight asymmetrically and sit slower than able-bodied individuals.[76] To sit rapidly without adjusting the resistance, MPKs that have swing-phase default settings can be off-loaded; this shifts stress to the sound limb as with non-MPKs.[38] Although MPKs allow symmetrical weight bearing during stand-to-sit transitions, the user must be trained to bear more weight on the prosthesis by pressing the thigh against the inner posterior socket wall with a hip extension force to off-load the sound limb.

Most MPKs do not assist sit-to-stand activity; the user depends greatly on sound-limb strength to rise. The Power Knee, however, assists user-initiated knee extension. A push up from the chair armrests activates the assisted sit-to-stand function. As compared with those wearing unpowered knee units, prosthesis users rising with the Power Knee move with greater symmetry with hip force closer to that exhibited by able-bodied individuals.[76] To sit using a Power Knee, the user must pause to activate the default standing mode, then slowly lower the body to the chair. If the sitting motion is stopped midway, the Power Knee will support the user in a squat until the prosthesis is unweighted. Transferring the weight to the sound limb allows further knee unit bending.

Some MPKs provide special function modes that allow squatting or prolonged standing. The C-Leg, for instance, permits prosthetic weight bearing with the knee unit flexed to any angle between 7 and 70 degrees allowing maximal support for squatting or bent-knee standing. The Compact knee, designed for K2 level users, offers the same function in a 0- to 30-degree range. This mode is activated by handheld wireless remote control unit, with predetermined physical cues such as bouncing quickly on the forefoot, but also more intuitively by lowering the body to the desired degree of knee flexion and then slightly straightening the prosthetic knee to turn on the maximal knee flexion resistance needed to squat.[17] The Power Knee facilitates squatting by locking when the user stops the stand-to-sit motion at the desired degree of knee flexion.[11]

Training solutions: When sitting, the MPK user should place the hands on the armrests to enhance safety and decrease the chance that the wearer will fall backward. Using armrests, however, shifts the body weight backwards onto the heels rather than forward onto the forefeet as in able-bodied sit-to-stand transitions. For those who demonstrate the potential to stand unassisted, transferring weight forward over the forefeet can be practiced from surfaces of decreasing height as the person improves. The user's hands can be positioned anteriorly or on the thighs while arising. Placing both feet behind the knees helps advance weight over the forefeet but can be difficult due to limited prosthetic ankle dorsiflexion. Keeping the spine straight minimizes patellar compressive forces and back pain. Practicing at different speeds on different seat heights and while holding objects of different weights can prepare the user for a range of functional activities.

To develop the strength and control to squat, the user should practice single-limb squats with the sound limb. If unable, the wearer can start by performing a wall squat with a chair at hand for support. Methods to stimulate greater contribution of hip extensors on the amputated side will help in controlling the descent to the desired knee flexion angle. Squats on an unstable surface such as a cushion or tilt board performed between parallel bars and with appropriate guarding for safety can be effective. Step-ups with the prosthesis leading also help enable knee unit extension through forceful hip extensor contractions. Gluteal strengthening exercises are essential.

Fall protection: People with leg amputation have a greater risk of falling than do able-bodied individuals, with reported incidences of 20% to 32% during rehabilitation[77,78] and 52% within the community.[79] Falls occur when the wearer unexpectedly bears weight on the flexed prosthetic knee, as can happen when a user slips, stubs a toe, or steps on a rock unbalancing the prosthetic foot and causing the knee unit to bend. Stepping onto a flexed knee can also occur when the user turns, takes small sidesteps, or stops suddenly, preventing the knee unit from fully extending and activating stance phase control. When using a hydraulic non-MPK, tripping or stepping on an object leads to swing-phase knee flexion resistance and increases the risk of falls.[80] Slips may occur on heel strike onto slick surfaces such as ice. A slip causes very high demand for gluteal muscle strength that must respond rapidly to the anteromedial shear on landing.[81] The muscles of prosthetic users, including postural muscles like the erector spinae and oblique abdominal muscles, do not consistently contract when walking and respond to slips and trips slower than the muscles of sound limbs or able-bodied people.[81] The wearer may adapt to the risk of unexpected knee instability by taking shorter prosthetic steps, which results in slow, asymmetrical gait.

Prosthetic solutions: Whether a stumble or fall will result from an unexpected step onto a flexed knee depends greatly on the MPK default setting. MPKs with swing-phase knee resistance default settings require great compensatory movements; otherwise, falls occur even in younger people whose amputation etiologies were nondysvascular.[68] Knee collapse can also occur when knee unit flexion exceeds the 30- to 35-degree range programmed for stance phase resistance capacity.[68] The Power Knee and C-Leg default to stance phase knee resistance and will prevent collapse even after swing phase is interrupted.[80] In everyday situations, stance phase default C-Leg users reported significantly fewer stumbles and falls[82] and a safer experience compared with non-MPK users.[83]

Training solutions: Because stumbling is unexpected, it is difficult to prepare the new user. However, most slips result from the foot sliding on initial contact rather than in terminal stance. Thus the gluteal muscles are the most important group to strengthen and the hip flexors are a secondary concern. Consistent contraction of the core muscles throughout gait, not typically present in prosthesis users, should be developed and strengthened to allow stronger and faster response to postural disturbances.[81] Methods for strengthening gluteal muscles and integrating abdominal contractions in gait have been presented in training solutions for asymmetric steps.

Practice in functional activities encountered in real life also prepares users to respond to stumbles and falls. Obstacle courses should include different walking surfaces and stepping up, over, and onto obstacles. Carrying items and performing dual tasks can develop overall functional ability. With training, MPK users can negotiate obstacle courses quickly with fewer steps compared with those wearing non-MPK prostheses.[84] Practice on outdoor terrain can enable the wearer to participate fully in daily activities.

Other activities: The user may wish to participate in activities that require free-swinging knee function like biking or locked knee function like prolonged standing.

Prosthetic solutions: Non-MPK hydraulic or pneumatic knees sometimes have a manual switch at the back of the knee that will switch the knee to different modes of function.[11] MPKs offer various modes of function but eliminate the need to operate a switch manually. A physical cue like pushing down on the toes three times followed by unweighting the leg for 1 second switches the mode of operation from walking to free swinging for biking or maximal knee resistance for prolonged standing.[17] Regardless of whether wireless remote or leg movements are used to switch functional modes, an electronic signal, either a series of beeps or vibrations, confirms the change in setting to the user.

Training solutions: The ability to remember how to switch modes, performing the physical cue, and hearing or feeling the confirming electronic signals varies among users. As with gait training, forefoot weight-bearing practice is a fundamental skill to develop. Having the user practice initiating the cues and perceiving the signals is important to the smooth, effective use of these MPK features.

Although clinicians may focus on gait deviations that persist despite dedicated training for even the most experienced and high-level users, wearers themselves tend to focus more on their functional abilities. One study found that gait symmetry correlated with performance measures such as gait 2-minute walk test or Berg balance scale score but not with patient-reported outcomes.[85] Even active prosthesis users typically take part in bouts of activity lasting <2 minutes and averaging only 17 steps per minute. Most wearers only engage in activity lasting more than 15 continuous minutes less than once per day.[86] Functional ability and attitude toward the prosthesis are the strongest predictors of patient satisfaction.[87] Prosthetic outcomes can be maximized through a clinical approach that addresses range of motion and strength impairments while integrating functional abilities to optimize participation in the pleasures and challenges of real life.

Outcomes

Success of prosthetic fitting can be measured by objective factors, principally energy consumption, walking velocity, and step symmetry, as well as subjective responses such as falls history and quality of life questionnaires. Overall, prosthesis users perform somewhat better and report greater satisfaction when wearing MPK prostheses than with less sophisticated components. A few investigators compared the function of people wearing prostheses with various units. Even in the presence of laboratory evidence regarding the biomechanical characteristics of MPK units, clinicians' and wearers' subjective reactions remain the mainstay of formulating prosthetic prescription and thus determining prosthetic rehabilitation outcomes.[84,88]

Physical characteristics appear to outweigh the importance of a particular prosthetic component in determining the individual's performance. Review of combat-associated amputations reveals that function and amputation limb length are directly correlated, whereas energy consumption and length are inversely related.[89] People with mid-length or longer thighs, however, showed no significant kinematic or kinetic gait differences.[67]

Gait studies: Laboratory comparisons of performance with prostheses equipped with the C-Leg and the Mauch knee generally indicate that subjects walked faster with the C-Leg by as much as 21% depending on terrain.[18,82] Faster self-selected walking speed with a C-Leg did not necessarily come at higher energy costs.[90] One research team, however, reported no significant differences in free walking speed.[66] Faster gait speeds obtained with people after transfemoral amputation using the C-Leg compared with non-MPK prostheses have also been documented in a case report of one person with bilateral knee disarticulations.[91] Laboratory comparison of subjects wearing the Endolite Intelligent Prosthesis and non-MPK units reveal similar results as those involving C-Leg.[92]

A goal of prosthetic fitting is to enable the patient to walk as inconspicuously as possible. People wearing the C-Leg exhibited less step length asymmetry than when using a hydraulic non-MPK unit.[18,40,45] Kinematic analysis of subjects walking with MPK units showed less delay between late swing-phase knee extension and heel contact than with other units.[45]

Optimum rehabilitation restores the individual's ability to walk greater distances without appreciable fatigue. In one study, subjects who wore prostheses with step counters and distance monitors took similar numbers of steps and walked for equivalent durations in the home and community environments whether using the C-Leg or Mauch knee units,[86] whereas another group reported that wearing an MPK prosthesis was associated with greater physical activity in the community.[93] Overall, people using MPK prostheses had higher functional levels than those using non-MPK prostheses.[94]

A pattern of reduced energy consumption is apparent when using a unilateral MPK compared to non-MPK prostheses.[95] Although use of different MPKs produced similar levels of oxygen consumption, the energy cost for young adults with traumatic amputation using MPK was much higher than required by the able-bodied control subjects.[96]

Metabolic demand with the Rheo Knee unit was slightly less than with the C-Leg.[97] In general, any MPK reduces energy consumption modestly compared with a non-MPK, confirmed by laboratory comparison of adults walking with several types of MPKs.[68]

Performance in other ambulatory activities: Sit-to-stand transitions required less hip force for subjects wearing the Power Knee as compared with performance with the C-Leg or the Mauch knee, although all participants relied primarily on the intact limb.[76] Performance on stair and ramp descent was safest with the C-Leg, as compared with the Rheo Knee, Adaptive 2 Knee, and Hybrid Knee.[68] On hill and stair descent, MPK users exhibited smoother maneuvering over obstacles, fewer stumbles, and superior multitasking ability, allowing many to advance to a higher Medicare functional level.[71] The Rheo Knee and the C-Leg were associated with smoother gait and decreased hip power generation as compared with performance with the Mauch knee.[98] Subjects who walked on a treadmill while solving mental problems swayed less when tested with the Intelligent Prosthesis, suggesting that it was not as cognitively demanding as less sophisticated knee units.[99]

The C-Leg offers more protection against tripping as compared with non-MPK units. Three subjects participated in a randomized study in which the examiner tugged on a cord in an attempt to cause prosthetic knee flexion. Unlike other knee units, the C-Leg either produced rapid knee extension or supported the wearer on the flexed knee.[80] Improved balance and balance confidence has occurred with fewer falls after converting from non-MPK to MPK prostheses.[100] Overall, MPK use appears to have a protective impact on falls with both people after traumatic amputations and those with diabetes experiencing reduced numbers of falls with MPK use.[22,101]

Several research teams administered questionnaires to people who wore prostheses equipped with C-Legs. Respondents expressed greater confidence, gait, and maneuverability[83] as well as overall satisfaction.[22] MPK users have also reported less depressive symptoms and improved body image.[102] Scores on the Prosthesis Evaluation Questionnaire were higher.[82,84] Subjective response to the Intelligent Prosthesis was also favorable, with users preferring it to nonmicroprocessor units when walking at different speeds and greater distances with less fatigue.[99] Survey respondents commended increased quality of life when wearing MPKs.[93,94]

Although many studies of adults wearing MPKs have been published, few have addressed issues such as mechanical durability, effect of unit weight on performance, and whether the cost of the units equates to substantially greater benefit. Ideally, future research would involve larger sample sizes. Nevertheless, at the present time, one can conclude that MPK units can improve the quality of life of many people with transfemoral amputation.[94]

Prescriptive Cases

Selecting the prosthesis that matches an individual's needs requires taking into account the person's general health, level and status of the residual limb, history of prosthetic use, features and limitations of the available prosthetic components, impact level of the intended use, and the individual's functional level. Manufacturers recommend MPKs for low- to moderate-impact activities (Table 27.4) by users at the Medicare K2 to K4 functional levels (see Table 27.2), regardless of insurance company policies. After transfemoral amputation many people may not attain the functional ability to become K3 community ambulators, who often average walking speeds >0.8 m/s (1.8 mph) and negotiating steps and curbs.[103] For K2 level walkers, MPK units like the Kenevo with stance phase control only improve balance and walking on level and slopes may be sufficient.[100,104,105] Prosthesis users who walk faster, traverse daily distances of 5 km (3.1 miles) including stairs, and engage in moderate-impact activities are at the K3 to K4 functional level, thus both stance and swing-phase features are recommended. In addition to matching prosthetic components to the individual's physical and functional needs, another inescapable consideration is the cost of incorporating an MPK. Insurance will often reimburse the price of an MPK only for users at the K3 to K4 levels. The cases that follow highlight important considerations relevant to MPK prescription.

Those with hip disarticulation or higher amputations can be considered at the K2 level if walking independently, regardless of speed, although Medicare K-levels are not intended for people other than unilateral transtibial and transfemoral amputation.

Table 27.4 Impact Levels

Impact Level	Target Activity	Typical Use
Low	Walking with small cadence variations	Daily walking with low foot forces. Examples: household tasks, gardening, shopping, and occasional non-impact sports such as golf and leisure walking.
Moderate	Walking with variable cadence	Daily walking of long durations with moderate forces. Examples: aerobics, jogging, sports like tennis, and vocational activities like lifting/carrying.
High	High cadence walking	Daily activities involving vigorous and repetitive actions with fast speeds and high loading forces. Examples: distance jogging, running, jumping, sports like basketball, and vocational activities like construction work.
Sport-Extreme	High-impact sports and activities	Daily activities with high or extreme forces common in repetitive, fast, and/or sustained activities. Examples: sprinting, long-distance running, active military service.

Case Example 27.1 The Active Athlete

A 29-year-old 110-kg (245-lb) former college athlete has a transfemoral amputation resulting from a motorcycle accident 5 years ago. He has been using a non-MPK hydraulic knee prosthesis for his everyday life, which includes work as a sales representative during the week and recreational basketball and tennis on the weekends. He jogs proficiently using the skip-hop style but has become interested in more sports activities and wants to run step-over-step and potentially compete in athletic contests. He is ready for a new prosthesis that can facilitate reaching his goals.

What type of knee unit best matches his needs? His activities show K4 level functioning and would qualify him for reimbursement of an MPK prosthesis by many insurance companies. Although an MPK prosthesis would be an excellent choice for his everyday activities, they are designed for low- to moderate-impact activities and could be overloaded by the sustained and high-impact nature of his intended sports. If he is going to proceed with only one prosthesis, one with a non-MPK hydraulic knee unit such as the Mauch Knee Plus may serve him best. Such a knee could be paired with a heavy-duty energy-storing foot designed to absorb shock like the Re-Flex Shock.

Case Example 27.2 A Risk to Fall?

A 65-year-old female underwent transfemoral amputation 4 years ago resulting from a thrombosis associated with peripheral vascular and cardiovascular disease. She was active prior to amputation. Her activity has increased since the amputation and she has returned to work as a school administrator using a weight-activated friction-brake knee unit. She gardens and enjoys leisure walking in the community, although her strength and endurance limit her from walking as fast or as far as she would like. She has recently qualified for Medicare and wants a prosthesis that can help her reach her goals.

What type of knee unit best matches her needs? Her activities demonstrate K2 level prosthetic functioning with K3 level potential. Medicare and her employer-based insurance may not approve an MPK prosthesis because her functional activities do not demand a varied cadence or fast walking speed. Her age and general health status may also mitigate against her efforts to get reimbursed for the cost of an MPK prosthesis. However, community ambulating prosthesis users are at heightened fall risk.[79] Falls within her age group have annual incidence rates from 19% to 60% with 27% reporting injury at the rate of 14.1/1000 person-months.[106] Although current reimbursement practice often does not include an MPK for a K2 level patient/client, she would benefit from using an MPK prosthesis, particularly its stumble and fall protective features. Physical therapy can be used to address limited hip extension range of motion, strength, and gait speed[57,58]; use of an MPK prosthesis for a trial period has also allowed increases in walking speed of 14% to 25%.[107] Physical therapy and prosthetic intervention may help her advance to walking speeds >0.8 m/s[103] or distances >400 m[108] that may help her achieve community walking speeds and qualify for reimbursement of a K3 MPK prosthesis.

Case Example 27.3 Hemipelvectomy: Cost and Effectiveness

A 44-year-old male had a hemipelvectomy 3 months ago due to chondrosarcoma. His incision has healed and he is ready for fitting. He has never used a prosthesis but was very active until 1 year ago when he underwent tumor resection and internal hemipelvectomy and suffered a bout of depression. After the resection, he limited activity to working in an office and curtailed most sporting activities other than occasional walks in the park. Since his amputation, he has returned to work as an accountant and is adept with crutches, which he uses for light sports activities such as soccer with his children. He uses a wheelchair for traversing long distances. He complains that it is difficult to rise from a chair or hold something in his hands while using crutches. He lives with his wife and teenage sons in a suburban two-story house. He is insured through his employer and his prosthetist is confident that an MPK prosthesis will be covered by insurance. His goals are to continue work and family life with greater ease.

What type of knee unit best matches his needs? As a previously active adult who is able to walk after hemipelvectomy, he is comparable to the K2 functional level. His status has been changing and his medical and prosthetic prognoses remain unclear. He may achieve K3 level functioning. An MPK prosthesis would allow him to descend stairs and slopes with safety on two legs and walk without crutches and thus free the upper limbs for normal functions at work and social functions. However, most MPK prostheses will not provide assistance for this male in rising from a chair or ascending stairs at the same pace as his peers. Difficulty rising from a chair, walking, and negotiating stairs are complicated by fit problems common to people with hemipelvectomies who fluctuate in body weight. He may benefit from a temporary prosthesis with a non-MPK to determine his level of prosthetic use before expending the cost of an MPK prosthesis.[109]

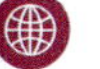

References

The complete listing of the References are available in the accompanying enhanced eBook version included with the print purchase of this textbook. Visit Elsevier eBooks+ (eBooks.Health.Elsevier.com) to access this content.

28 Athletic Options for Persons With Limb Loss*

MICHELA GOFFREDO, SANAZ POURNAJAF, MATTEO CIOETA, AND MARCO FRANCESCHINI

LEARNING OBJECTIVES

On completing the chapter, the reader will be able to do the following:

1. Discuss the relationship of physical exercise and sports to the overall health and wellness of people with limb loss.
2. Describe barriers that contribute to the lack of participation in athletics for persons with physical challenges.
3. Identify organizations that support athletic participation for persons with physical challenges, including limb loss.
4. Compare and contrast the different sports and recreational activities available for persons with limb loss.
5. Describe prosthetic components available to assist in active participation within a variety of sports.

"Games, sport, that is what we must have." Sir Ludwig Guttman,[1] Founder, Paralympic Games

Introduction

Sport for people with disabilities is an important form of expression and inclusion, providing extraordinary opportunities to overcome physical and mental challenges. Through the world of sports, these people demonstrate strength, determination, and talent, often defying stereotypes[1] Sports for people with disabilities are diverse and include swimming, athletics, tennis, basketball, soccer, etc. Each sport is tailored to the specific abilities of the athlete, allowing everyone to compete on a level playing field. Athletes with disabilities constantly demonstrate their extraordinary potential, setting records and achieving outstanding results in national and international competitions. The Paralympics, in particular, provide a global stage to celebrate the greatness and commitment of these extraordinary athletes.[2] However, sport for people with disabilities is not just about competition: participating in sporting activity offers numerous benefits, such as improving physical health, increasing self-confidence, and developing meaningful social relationships. In addition, sports help overcome mental barriers, proving that disabilities do not have to be an obstacle to achieving great feats. For this reason, sports for people with disabilities are crucial in promoting inclusion and equality.[3]

Limb amputation profoundly alters a person's life, introducing physical, emotional, and social challenges, and is a significant cause of disability in young adults.[4] The disability caused by amputation requires adjustment to the new reality: the person must learn to use a prosthesis or wheelchair, adapt to new motor skills, and face the need for constant and intensive rehabilitation. However, despite the challenges, many people with amputations develop an extraordinary determination to overcome difficulties, and over time, they learn to live fulfilling and meaningful lives. The scientific literature on prosthesis use among amputees varies in reporting the rates of successful artificial limb usage.[5] Factors influencing the level of participation for those with limb loss include the following: living independently at home,[6] with a good level of independence,[7] activities of daily living,[8] and mobility.[9] While in the subacute phase the goal of the rehabilitation process remains the restoration of an adequate level of functioning and participation in an indoor and/or outdoor activity, in the chronic phase the emergence of new needs including participation in work, social, and sports activities is evident.

As early as 2001, the World Health Organization in its International Classification of Functioning, Disability and Health introduced a revolutionary principle: disability ceases to be seen as a mere impairment of the individual and becomes a dynamic concept resulting from the continuous and changing interaction between the individual's health status and environmental and social factors.[10] Thus while limb amputation can have a negative impact on people's mobility, mental and physical well-being, and social life, sports activity in these people has beneficial physical effects on mobility.[11] The main physical benefits of sports for amputees include:[12]

- Improved cardiovascular condition: Regular physical activity, such as swimming or cycling, stimulates the cardiovascular system, increasing endurance and lung capacity.
- Increased muscle strength: The use of prostheses and involvement in sports activities require considerable muscle exertion, helping to increase the strength of the muscles involved.
- Improved coordination and balance: Sports training helps improve coordination and balance, skills that are particularly important for amputees to ensure greater safety and stability during daily activities.

*The authors would like to extend appreciation to Carol Pierce Dionne and Joshua Thomas Williams, whose work in prior editions provided the foundation for this chapter.

- Body weight maintenance: Sports help control body weight, helping to reduce pressure on joints and improve mobility.
- Reduced risk of complications: Regular physical activity can help reduce the risk of developing certain medical complications, such as cardiovascular problems, diabetes, and osteoporosis.
- Functional enhancement of prostheses: The use of prostheses during sports helps improve functional abilities by enabling amputees to refine the use of their supportive equipment.
- Increased flexibility and agility: Sports promote joint flexibility and agility, helping to maintain a wide range of motion and facilitating daily activities.

In addition to the physical benefits, sports provide an opportunity to address the psychological challenges related to amputation, enabling athletes to develop resilience, self-esteem, and a sense of belonging to a social community. In fact, sports for amputees have been shown to have numerous positive psychological effects, providing them with a significant avenue for coping with the physical and mental challenges related to disability.[13] Practicing sports after amputation can profoundly affect the emotional, social, and psychological aspects of the individual, improving quality of life and promoting a general sense of well-being.[14] The main psychological effects are as folllows:[15,16]

- Increased confidence and self-esteem: Through sports, amputees gain specific physical skills and competencies that may have been lost due to amputation. The ability to overcome challenges and achieve goals in the sports context helps develop greater confidence in their abilities and a renewed sense of self-esteem.
- Stress and anxiety reduction: Physical activity, including sports, is known for its power to reduce stress and anxiety. The production of endorphins during exercise promotes emotional well-being and may help amputees better manage the emotional trauma related to limb loss.
- Resilience development: Amputees who participate in sports develop greater adaptability and resilience in the face of adversity. Facing sporting challenges, such as learning new skills or overcoming obstacles, can result in an increased ability to cope with daily difficulties with a more positive outlook.
- Positive identity reinforcement: Playing a sport helps reinforce personal identity in a positive way. Amputees can identify themselves as athletes and as part of a sports community, moving beyond their disability status and building a sense of belonging.
- Improved social relationships: Amputee sports provide opportunities to connect with others with similar experiences. Sharing common interests and experiencing sports activity can facilitate the creation of new friendships and meaningful social relationships.
- Reducing isolation: After an amputation, many people may feel isolated or marginalized. Participation in sports can counteract this feeling by providing an inclusive environment in which amputees feel accepted and supported.
- Increased concentration and discipline: Playing sports requires concentration and discipline. Amputees who take up sports learn to focus their mental and physical energy on set goals, thereby improving their ability to concentrate and pursue goals.
- Source of fun and gratification: Sports are intrinsically linked to the experience of fun and personal gratification. Participating in a successful sporting activity or achieving set goals can increase one's sense of accomplishment and happiness.
- Improved overall mental health: Sports for amputees can help reduce the risk of depression and improve overall mental health. Regular exercise is known to promote the release of chemicals in the brain that positively affect mood and overall well-being.

Participation in sports, or more generally in physical activity, not only has physical and mental benefits, but is a significant factor in the prevention of diseases such as obesity, diabetes, hypertension, and cardiovascular disease.[17,18] Such benefits have been shown in epidemiological studies of people with disabilities by comparing them with normal subjects while performing sports activities. Moreover, that the quality of life and self-esteem of amputees who played sports were higher than those of people with limb amputation who had not participated in any physical activity. Sports and physical activity helped these individuals increase their social relationships and increase their knowledge of sports equipment and accept their disability and improve their motor skills.

Barriers and Motivation

People with limb amputation may face several barriers to sports participation.[19–22] These obstacles may vary depending on the individual's specific situation and the resources available in their community. Some of the most common obstacles include:

- Accessibility of sports facilities: Many sports facilities are not adequately equipped to accommodate people with physical disabilities, including accessible toilets, wheelchair ramps, and other necessary facilities.
- Costs of prosthetics and sports equipment: Prosthetics and adapted sports equipment can be expensive, making it difficult for some people to access the tools they need to participate in certain sports.
- Lack of information and support: People with amputation may not be aware of the sporting opportunities available to them or may not have access to adequate support to identify which sports are suitable for their abilities and interests.
- Psychological barriers: Fear of injury or not being accepted by others may discourage some people with amputation from participating in sports activities.
- Lack of inclusive programs: In some communities, there may be a lack of inclusive sports programs specifically adapted for people with limb amputation.
- Physical and functional limitations: Depending on the extent of the amputation and the level of prosthetic adaptation, some people may face specific challenges in participating in certain sports.
- Logistical concerns: Transportation to attend sporting events, especially if limited mobility situations, can be an obstacle.

- Lack of social support: Sports participation may be affected by the lack of a supportive and social environment that encourages and promotes physical activity.
- Stereotypes and negative perceptions: Some people may be discouraged from sports participation because of stereotypes and prejudices about disability.

To overcome these obstacles, it is crucial to promote greater awareness about inclusive sports participation for people with limb amputation. Creating adapted sports programs, raising disability awareness, and improving accessibility to sports facilities can help facilitate participation and ensure that everyone has the opportunity to experience the benefits of sports.

Organizational Support for Sports or Recreation Participation

Organizational support for the sports participation of people with disabilities is critical to ensuring an inclusive, rewarding, and safe experience for all athletes. Key types of organizational support include sports organizations and associations creating programs specifically designed for people with disabilities.[1] This enables athletes with disabilities to benefit from technical support and specialized coaching to improve their sports skills and competencies. These professionals are trained to work with athletes with disabilities and understand the specific challenges they may face. Of course, sports facilities must be designed and equipped to be accessible to people with disabilities, including accessible toilets, ramps, and elevators, and adequate spaces for spectators with disabilities. It is also important that sports organizations provide training and awareness raising for staff, coaches, and athletes on disability issues, including effective communication and respect for different abilities.

Sports for athletes with physical impairments are regulated by various disability sports organizations and disability-specific national governing bodies. Several organizations exist in the United States and Europe to support and develop athletes with limb loss.

ORGANIZATIONS IN THE UNITED STATES

There are several organizations and associations in the United States that promote and support sports for people with disabilities.[23–27] Here are some notable ones:

- United States Olympic & Paralympic Committee (USOPC): The USOPC is responsible for supporting and training athletes for the Paralympic Games. They provide resources and funding for Paralympic sports programs.
- Adaptive Sports USA: This organization promotes sports for individuals with physical disabilities, providing resources, events, and support to athletes and coaches.
- Disabled Sports USA: Now known as Move United, this organization offers adaptive sports programs nationwide, focusing on increasing opportunities for individuals with disabilities to participate in sports.
- National Wheelchair Basketball Association: This organization governs wheelchair basketball in the United States, supporting athletes, teams, and events at all levels.
- USA Deaf Sports Federation: Governing body for Deaf sports in the United States, promoting athletic competition and representing the United States in international Deaf sports competitions.
- Special Olympics USA: Provides year-round sports training and competition in a variety of Olympic-type sports for children and adults with intellectual disabilities.
- Wounded Warrior Project: Offers sports programs and events for wounded veterans to promote physical and mental health through sports.
- Paralyzed Veterans of America: Provides sports and recreation programs for veterans with spinal cord injuries.
- Achilles International: Focuses on providing athletic programs for people with all types of disabilities, including running, cycling, and swimming.
- Challenged Athletes Foundation: Provides grants and support to athletes with physical challenges, enabling them to participate in sports.
- National Center on Health, Physical Acivity and Disability: Provides resources and support to promote physical activity and sports among youth with disabilities.

ORGANIZATIONS IN EUROPE

There are numerous organizations and associations in Europe that promote and support sports for people with disabilities.[28–34] Some of the leading European organizations include:

- European Paralympic Committee (EPC): The EPC is the European Paralympic Committee and represents athletes with disabilities in Paralympic competitions.
- European Deaf Sports Organization (EDSO): The EDSO is a European sports federation that organizes events and promotes sports for athletes with hearing disabilities.
- Special Olympics Europe Eurasia: Special Olympics provides sports opportunities for people with intellectual disabilities in Europe and Eurasia.
- Cerebral Palsy Sport Europe: This organization promotes sport for athletes with cerebral palsy and similar motor disabilities in Europe.
- European Powerchair Football Association (EPFA): EPFA is responsible for the promotion and organization of electric wheelchair soccer in Europe.
- European Blind Union (EBU) Sports Group: The EBU Sports Group promotes sports for blind and visually impaired athletes in Europe.
- European Amputee Football Federation: This federation is responsible for the promotion and organization of soccer for athletes with amputations in Europe.

Sport Classification

In Paralympic sports, classification is a system used to ensure fair competition among athletes with different disabilities. The classification process categorizes athletes into groups based on the extent of their impairment, ensuring that they compete against others with similar functional abilities.[35] This system is essential to maintain a level playing field and ensure that success in Paralympic sports is determined by skill, training, and effort rather than the degree of impairment. The classification process varies depending on the sport, but it generally involves a thorough assessment of an athlete's impairment by qualified classifiers. Classifiers, who are often medical professionals and experts in the sport, evaluate an athlete's physical and functional abilities relevant to the specific sport's demands.

The main goals of sports classification in the Paralympics are the following:[36]

- Fair Competition: Ensuring athletes compete against others with a similar level of functional ability, providing an equitable and competitive environment.
- Integrity: Preserving the integrity of Paralympic sports by preventing athletes from gaining a competitive advantage due to their impairment.
- Inclusivity: Providing opportunities for athletes with various types and levels of impairments to participate and excel in their chosen sport.
- Skill Assessment: Evaluating an athlete's skills and abilities relative to the specific demands of the sport.
- Growth and Development: Supporting the growth and development of Paralympic sports by establishing standardized and consistent classification systems.

Athletes are assigned a sport class, typically denoted by a letter and a number, which is used to group them with others who have similar impairments. The classification system varies for each sport and is regularly reviewed and updated to ensure its effectiveness and relevance. It's important to note that sport classification is continually evolving and is subject to ongoing research and improvements. The process strives to strike a balance between ensuring fair competition and recognizing the diverse abilities of Paralympic athletes.

Summer Paralympic Sports

Summer Paralympic sports available to those with limb loss include archery, athletics (track and field), badminton, boccia, cycling, canoeing, equestrian, fencing, triathlon, powerlifting, rowing, wheelchair rugby, shooting, swimming, table tennis, tennis, sitting volleyball, taekwondo, and wheelchair basketball. Each sport has its own unique set of requirements, which may necessitate a modification of the traditional rules of the sport to allow the athlete with physical challenges to compete.

ARCHERY

Archery has been a medal sport since the first Paralympic Games in Rome in 1960.[36] Athletes with physical disabilities demonstrate their shooting precision and accuracy from either a standing or seated (wheelchair) position, in male and female categories. The paralympic competition format is identical to that of the Olympic Games. Paralympic archers shoot 72 arrows from a distance of 70 m at a target of 122 cm using a recurve bow (Fig. 28.1A) or from a distance of 50 m at a target of 80 cm using a compound bow (Fig. 28.1B). The two longest distances use a 122-cm target, while the two shorter distances use an 80-cm target. Distances are 90, 70, 50, and 30 m for males and 70, 60, 50, and 30 m for females. For competitions other than the Paralympics, athletes shoot at each of four distances, with 36 arrows shot at each distance. Depending on the athletes' classification, their level and number of amputations, and their functional ability, they may use either a recurve bow or a compound bow. Archery competition is open to male and female athletes with upper- or lower-extremity amputation/limb loss. Most athletes with limb loss will be classified into the "open" division. This classification includes athletes in wheelchairs who have relatively normal arm function and athletes who compete while standing but have impairments that affect their balance, arms, and/or trunk.[36] Specialized devices are also available to assist athletes with upper-extremity prostheses in drawing back the bow and releasing the string.

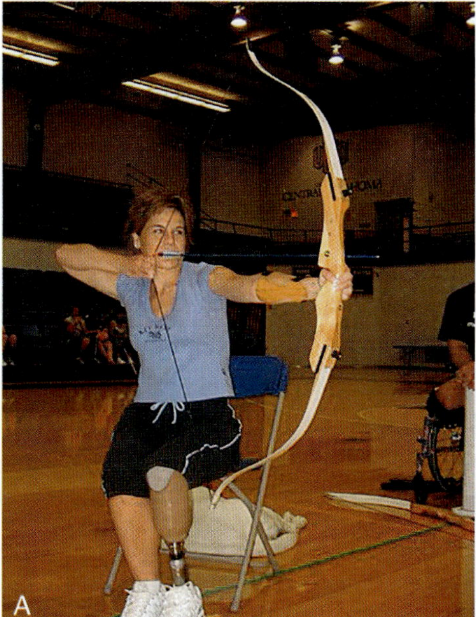

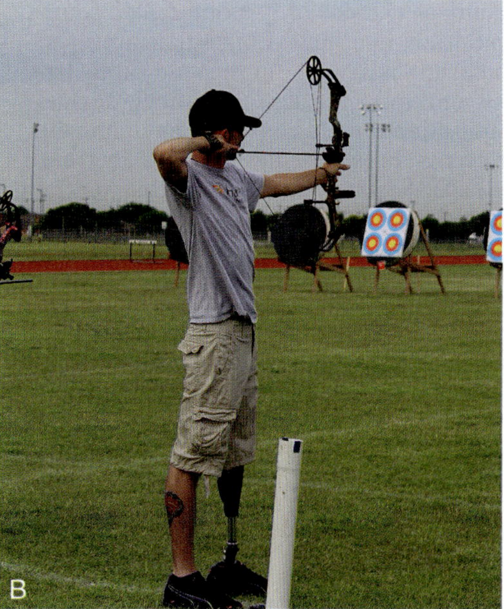

Fig. 28.1 (A) Archery recurve bow. (B) Archery compound bow. (A, Courtesy Disabled Sports USA; B, Photos taken and given with permission from Raiber O and Williams J, OUHSC.)

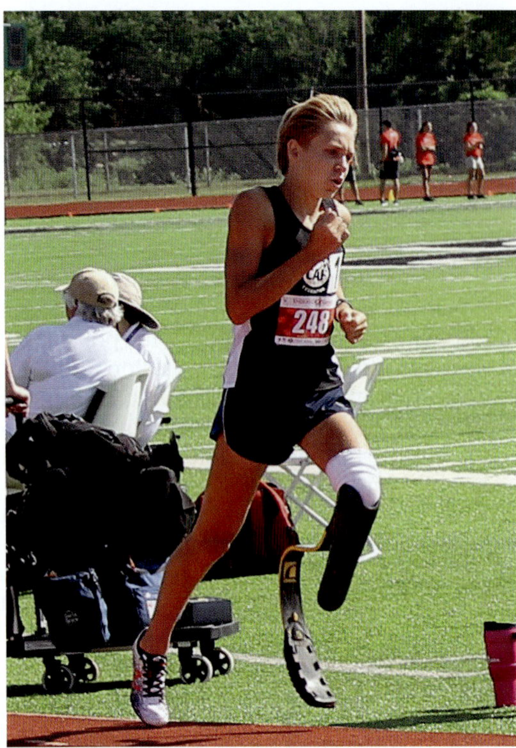

Fig. 28.2 Track and field event. (Photos taken and given with permission from Raiber O and Williams J, OUHSC.)

ATHLETICS (TRACK AND FIELD)

Athletic events are open to athletes in all disability classes and have been a part of the Paralympic program since the first Paralympic Games in Rome, Italy, in 1960.[36] Events include track (running distances from 100 m to 10,000 m and 4 × 100-m and 4 × 400-m relays); throwing (shot put, discus, and javelin); jumping (high jump, long jump, and triple jump); pentathlon (athlete competes in five events: long jump, shot put, 100-m run, discus, and 400-m run); and the marathon. The rules of the Paralympic track and field are almost identical to those of its nondisabled counterpart. Paralympic track and field competition are open to male and female athletes with upper- and/or lower-extremity single or multiple limb loss. Prosthetic devices may be used, or the athlete with limb loss may compete in the wheelchair events. Prosthetic devices used for track and field have been specifically developed to withstand the demands of sports competition (Fig. 28.2). A large variety of classifications exist for track and field. Track events and field events are classified separately. For athletes with limb loss competing with a prosthesis, there are seven different classifications (T45–T47 and T61–T64).[36] For athletes with limb loss competing in a wheelchair, four different classifications exist (T51–T54).[36] Likewise, athletes can compete in standing field events under the F42 to F46 or F61 to F64 classifications or in wheelchairs under the F51 to F57 classifications.[36]

BADMINTON

Disabled badminton is played by people with many different disabilities, including those with both upper- and lower-extremity limb loss.[36] Participants may compete either standing or in a wheelchair. The sport made its Paralympic debut at the 2021 Games in Tokyo. Badminton provides players of different disabilities and backgrounds an opportunity to participate in a common sport. Although more common in Europe, most people in the United States become involved in badminton through word of mouth and people introducing others to the sport. It is a growing sport with an increasing number of participants taking up the game either socially, competitively, or both. Both males and females in all age groups participate in badminton. For badminton, there are two classification levels for athletes who compete in wheelchairs (WH1 and WH2) and three classification levels for athletes competing while standing (SL3, SL4, and SU5) and one for short stature (SH6).[36]

BOCCIA

Boccia was practised for many years as a leisure activity before being introduced at the New York 1984 Paralympics as a competitive sport.[36] It is one of only two Paralympic sports that do not have an Olympic counterpart (goalball being the other) and is governed by the Boccia International Sports Federation (BISFed). Boccia is split into four classes, BC1–BC4, where all players compete in wheelchairs due to severe coordination impairment affecting both legs and arms. BC1 athletes have severe activity limitations affecting their legs, arms, and trunk, and are typically dependent on a powered wheelchair. BC2 players have better trunk and arm functions than those in class BC1. The abilities of their arms and hands often allow them to throw the ball overhand and underhand and with a variety of grasps. BC3 class athletes have significant limitations in arm and leg functions, and poor or no trunk control. They are unable to consistently grasp or release the ball and are unable to propel the ball consistently into the field of play and allowed to use a ramp with the help of a Sport Assistant. The BC4 class includes players with noncerebral impairments that impact their coordination.[36]

CANOEING

Canoeing made its Paralympic debut in the summer of 2016 in Rio de Janeiro.[36] The sport is identical to the competition in which able-bodied athletes compete. Males and females may compete in kayaks using a double-bladed paddle over a 200-m course. Additional competition and recreational events, including both kayaks and outrigger canoes such as va'a boats, are available at the international level, but are currently not a part of the Paralympic competition. Athletes competing in canoeing compete in one of three different classifications (KL1, KL2, or KL3).[36]

CYCLING

Cycling was first introduced as a Paralympic sport in 1984 in Mandeville, England, and involved only those athletes with cerebral palsy.[36] However, it was not until 1992 that athletes with limb loss competed at the Paralympic Games in cycling. At the 2004 Paralympic Games in Athens, handcycling (for wheelchair users) made its debut as a medal event.

Athletes compete in both track (velodrome) and road events. Track events generally consist of sprints as short as

200 m to time trials and pursuits up to 4 km. Relay races consisting of three-person teams are also contested on the track. Competition on the roads consists of time trials and road races. In time trials, athletes start individually in staggered intervals, racing mostly against themselves and the clock. Road races consist of mass starts. Distances vary based on the host country's discretion, ranging from 5 to 65 km in length. Paralympic cycling competition is open to male and female athletes with upper- and/or lower-extremity single or multiple amputation/limb loss. There are different sport classes for handcycling, H1–5, where lower numbers indicate restrictions in both upper and lower limbs, and higher numbers indicate restrictions in lower limbs only. Tricycle athletes are divided into two classes, T1 and T2, with the former being allocated to athletes with more significant coordination impairments. Athletes who are able to use a standard bicycle compete in the five sport classes C1–5, with lower numbers indicating a more severe limitation in the lower and/or upper limbs.[36]

EQUESTRIAN

Equestrian made its debut appearance at the Paralympic Games in 1996, with riders from 16 countries competing.[36] By the Paralympic Games in 2008 in Beijing, that number had grown to 73 riders from 28 countries. Riders compete in two dressage events: a championship test of set movements and a freestyle test to music. There is also a team test for three or four riders. Competitors are judged on their display of horsemanship skills demonstrated through their use of commands for walk, trot, and canter. Paralympic equestrian competition is open to male and female athletes with upper- and/or lower-extremity single or multiple limb loss who are classified into one of five groups (Ia–IV).[36]

FENCING

Fencing has been part of the Paralympic Games since 1960. Athletes compete in wheelchairs that are fixed to the floor. They rely on ducking, half-turns, and leaning to dodge their competitors' touches. However, fencers can never rise up from the seat of the wheelchair. The first fencer to score five touches is declared the winner. Athletes play the best out of three rounds and compete in single and team formats. Weapon categories for males include foil, epee, and sabre. Females compete in foil and epee. Paralympic fencing competition is open to male and female athletes with upper- and/or lower-extremity single or multiple limb loss. Most athletes with limb loss will fall into classification category A for fencing.[36]

TRIATHLON

Triathlon is an emerging sport that is quickly gaining popularity and was first included in the Summer Paralympic Games at the 2016 games in Rio de Janeiro. The sport is similar to the able-bodied version with athletes competing in the "sprint" distances of a 750-m swim, a 20-km cycling event, and a 5-km running event. The sport is governed by the International Triathlon Union, and national championships are held in more than 27 different countries. Paralympic triathlon is open to male and female athletes with upper- and/or lower-extremity single or multiple limb loss. There is a single classification category for athletes competing in wheelchairs (PT1) and three different categories for ambulatory athletes (PT2–PT4).[36]

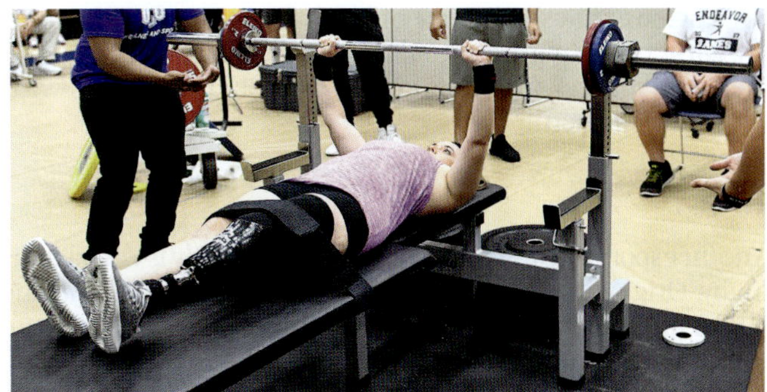

Fig. 28.3 Powerlifting. (Photos taken and given with permission from University of Central Oklahoma Endeavor Games.)

POWERLIFTING

Powerlifting is one of the fastest growing Paralympic sports. Paralympic athletes have been competing in powerlifting since 1964; however, it was initially offered only to lifters with spinal cord injuries. Currently, athletes from many different disabled sports groups participate in the sport, assimilating rules similar to those of nondisabled lifters. Athletes compete only in the bench press (Fig. 28.3), and they draw lots to determine order of weigh-in and lifts. Athletes compete lying on an official World Para Powerlifting approved bench, which is 2.1-m long. The width of the bench is 61-cm wide and narrows to 30 cm where the head is placed. The height of the bench varies between 48 and 50 cm from the ground. World Para Powerlifting approved discs must conform to several standards outlined in the sport's rules and regulations. After the athletes are categorized within the 10 different weight classes (male and female), they each lift three times (competing in their respective weight class). The heaviest "good lift" (within the weight class) is the lift used for final placing in the competition. Paralympic powerlifting competition is open to male and female athletes with upper- and/or lower-extremity single or multiple limb loss. Based on disability, there is only one classification category for powerlifting.

ROWING

Rowing is a relatively new Paralympic sport, making its first appearance in Beijing in 2008. The sport was selected for Paralympic inclusion in 2005, just 3 years after adaptive rowing made its debut on the world championship level in 2002. The rowing events include the male and female single sculls, the trunk-arms double sculls, and the legs-trunk-arms mixed four with coxswain. Paralympic rowing competition is open to male and female athletes with upper- and/or lower-extremity single or multiple limb loss. There are three sport classes: PR1 are rowers with minimal or no trunk function who primarily propel the boat through arm and shoulder function. These rowers have poor sitting balance, which requires them to be strapped to the boat/seat; PR2 are rowers that have functional use of arms and trunk but have weakness/absence of leg function to slide the seat; PR3 are rowers with residual function in the legs that allows them to slide the seat. This class also includes athletes with vision impairment.[36]

RUGBY

Another sport gaining a lot of popularity recently is wheelchair rugby. Originally called "murderball," it was developed in the 1970s and originally included only athletes with quadriplegia. However, the sport has opened up to athletes with a variety of different disabilities. Wheelchair rugby was a demonstration sport at the 1996 Paralympic Games in Atlanta and was subsequently included as a medal sport in the 2000 Sydney Games. The International Wheelchair Rugby Federation is the governing body of the sport and has developed rules that combine elements of able-bodied rugby, handball, and basketball. The sport is played on a regulation basketball court, where two teams of four athletes compete. Like wheelchair basketball, athletes are grouped by demonstrated playing ability, rather than strictly by medical classification. Wheelchair rugby is open to both males and females with upper- and/or lower-extremity single or multiple limb loss. Athletes are classified into one of four sport classes (0.5, 1.5, 2.5, or 3.5), and the total number of sports class "points" on the court at any one time may not exceed 8.[36]

SHOOTING

Shooting, divided into rifle and pistol events, air and 0.22 caliber, has been a Paralympic sport since 1976. The rules governing Paralympic competition are those used by the International Shooting Committee for the Disabled. These rules take into account the differences that exist between disabilities, allowing ambulatory and wheelchair athletes to compete shoulder-to-shoulder. Shooting matches athletes of the same gender, with similar disabilities, against each other, both individually and in teams. The competition format is very similar to that of able-bodied shooting sport—the goal of shooting is to place a series of shots inside the center ring ("bullseye") of the target. The target is comprised of 10 concentric scoring rings with a score grade of 1 to 10; the central ring gives 10 points. In many events the scoring rings are each further subdivided into an additional 10 scoring zones to give a decimal scoring system, with 10.9 being the very center of the target and the highest possible score per shot. To illustrate the level of precision required in air rifle events, athletes aim at a bullseye that is just 0.05 cm wide—about the size of a period on a printed page! Shooting competitions are divided into two disciplines: rifle and pistol, with competitions at three distances: 10 m, 25 m, and 50 m. The rules depend on the firearm (0.177 air or 0.22 smallbore caliber), the distance, the target, or the shooting position. Paralympic shooting competition is open to male and female athletes with upper- and/or lower-extremity single or multiple limb loss who may be classified into one of six different classification categories based on both the type of disability and the shooting event.[36]

SWIMMING

Swimming for males and females has been a part of the Paralympic program since the first Paralympic Games in 1960 in Rome, Italy. Races are highly competitive and among the largest and most popular events in the Paralympic Games. Paralympic swimming competitions occur in 50-m pools and, while competing, no prostheses or assistive devices may be worn. Athletes compete in the following events: 50-, 100-, and 400-m freestyle; 100-m backstroke; 100-m breaststroke; 100-m butterfly; 200-m individual medley; 4 × 100-m freestyle relay; and 4 × 100-m medley relay. Paralympic swimming competition is open to male and female athletes with upper- and/or lower-extremity single or multiple limb loss. Different classification categories exist for breaststroke compared with the other three events. There are ten different classification levels for the majority of the events, with nine different classification levels for breaststroke. A lower classification number (i.e., 1 vs. 7) indicates a more severe limitation as it relates to swimming.[36]

TABLE TENNIS

Table tennis has been a part of the Paralympic program since the inaugural Paralympic Games in 1960. Rules governing Paralympic table tennis are the same as those used by the International Table Tennis Federation, although they are slightly modified for players using wheelchairs. Athletes demonstrate the same quick technique and finesse as their counterparts without disabilities, competing in various disability groups, including male and female categories, as well as singles, doubles, and team contests. All matches are best-of-five games to 11 points. Paralympic table tennis competition is open to male and female athletes with upper- and/or lower-extremity single or multiple limb loss. There are five classification levels for those using wheelchairs to compete and five different classifications for those who stand to compete.[36]

TAEKWONDO

Taekwondo made its Summer Paralympic Games debut at the 2021 games in Tokyo. Taekwondo includes both kyorugi (sparring) and/or poomsae (forms), but only kyorugi was included in the Tokyo 2021 Games. Kyorugi consists of three 2-minute rounds with a 1-minute rest period between each round. Athletes score points similar to the able-bodied version, and the athlete with the most points at the end of three rounds is the winner. Taekwondo is open to both males and females with upper-extremity single or multiple limb loss and full use of both lower extremities. Although four different classification categories exist (K41–K44),[36] only a combined K43 to K44 category competed in the Tokyo Games.[37] In addition, athletes compete in one of three different weight classes.

WHEELCHAIR TENNIS

Wheelchair tennis first appeared at the Paralympic Games in Barcelona in 1992 and is played on a standard tennis court and follows many of the same rules as tennis. However, in wheelchair tennis, a player is allowed to let the ball bounce twice, if necessary, before hitting a return shot and the doubles court lines are used for both singles and doubles. In addition, the athlete's wheelchair is considered to be a part of the body, so rules applying to the player's body apply to the chair as well.

Paralympic wheelchair tennis competition is open to male and female athletes with upper- and/or lower-extremity single or multiple limb loss. There are three categories athletes compete in: men's, women's, and quads; each division has singles and doubles tournaments. Athletes with limb loss will compete in the "Open" classification category.[36]

SITTING VOLLEYBALL

Instituted in 1976 as a standing Paralympic sport, Paralympic volleyball has become exclusively a sitting sport. Paralympic volleyball follows the same rules as its able-bodied counterpart, with a few modifications to accommodate the various disabilities. In sitting volleyball, the net is approximately 3½ feet high and the court is 10 × 6m with a 2-m attack line. Players are allowed to block serves, but one buttock "cheek" must be in contact with the floor whenever they make contact with the ball. Paralympic volleyball competition is open to male and female athletes with upper- and/or lower-extremity single or multiple limb loss. Athletes will compete in gender-specific teams with six athletes being on the court at any one time. Being unable to stand is not a requirement for playing sitting volleyball. There are two sport classes depending on the severity and impact on the core functions in sitting volleyball: VS1 and VS2 (less impaired). Impairments can be either upper or lower limb or both. Teams can have up to two VS2 on the roster.[36]

WHEELCHAIR BASKETBALL

Basketball has been a part of the Paralympic Games since 1960 and was originally played only by males with spinal cord injuries. Currently, both male and female teams throughout the world, with a variety of disabilities, compete in the sport. Many of the same rules from its able-bodied counterpart apply in the wheelchair game. Although plays and tactics are similar, special rules, such as those to accommodate dribbling from a wheelchair, are also in place. The sport is governed by the International Wheelchair Basketball Federation. The International Wheelchair Basketball Federation governs all aspects of the game, including court size and basket height, which remain the same as in able-bodied basketball. Athletes in this event are grouped by demonstrated playing ability, rather than strictly by medical classification. Athletes are classified into one of five categories (1.0, 2.0, 3.0, 4.0, or 4.5), and a team of five players is allowed to have a total of only 14 classification points on the court at any one time.[36] Paralympic basketball competition is open to male and female athletes with upper- and/or lower-extremity single or multiple limb loss.

Winter Paralympic Sports

Just like the Summer Paralympic Games, the Winter Paralympic games are held every 4 years following the conclusion of the Winter Olympic Games in the host city of the Olympics. Paralympic athletes with limb loss compete in six winter sports: alpine skiing; biathlon; cross-country skiing; curling; snowboarding, and sled (sledge) hockey.

ALPINE SKIING

Paralympic alpine skiing competition is open to male and female athletes with amputation. There are four individual events in alpine skiing: downhill, which started as a demonstration event at the 1980 Paralympic Games in Norway; slalom; giant slalom, which was introduced as a demonstration event in 1984; and super-G. Mono-skiing was introduced in both alpine and Nordic events in 1988 at the Games in Innsbruck, Austria. Skiing equipment varies, depending on the athlete's level and number of amputations. Athletes with double-leg limb loss above the knee (transfemoral) typically use two skis with two outriggers but may also choose to

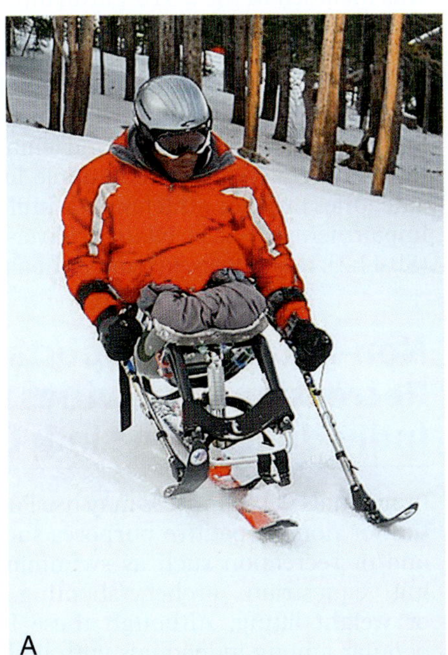

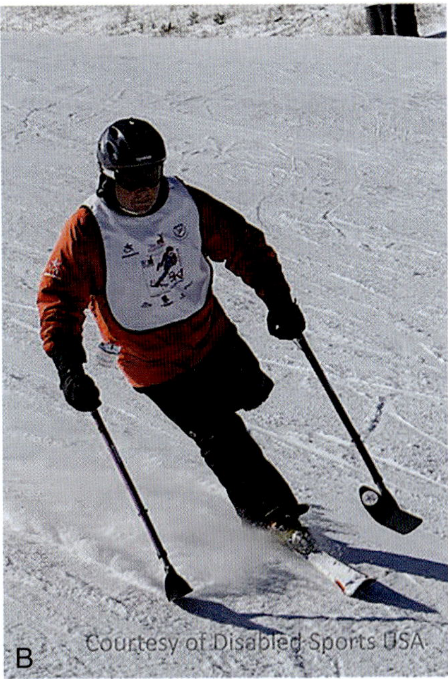

Fig. 28.4 (A and B) Alpine skiing. (Courtesy Disabled Sports USA.)

sit-ski in a mono-ski (Fig. 28.4A). Athletes with single transfemoral amputation often use one ski with two outriggers (Fig. 28.4B). Athletes with double-leg below-knee (transtibial) amputation and those with single-leg transtibial amputation may use two skis with two ski poles. Athletes with double-upper-extremity amputations, regardless of level, ski with two skis but no ski poles, whereas single-upper-extremity amputee athletes use two skis and one ski pole. If athletes have one upper-extremity and one lower-extremity amputation, they may use ski equipment that facilitates the athletes' best function. Seven different classification categories exist for standing skiers (LW1, LW2, LW3, LW4, LW5/7, LW6/8, and LW9), and three different categories exist for sit-skiers (LW10, LW11, and LW12). In October 2022 new categories were added for people with vision impairments: B1–B3. Athletes in these sport classes ski with a guide, who verbally gives directions to the athlete.[36]

NORDIC SKIING

Paralympic Nordic skiing is a Winter Paralympic sport consisting of two events: biathlon and cross-country skiing. Biathlon combines elements of cross-country skiing and target shooting. Athletes ski three 2.5-km loops (7.5 km total), stopping after the first two loops to shoot at five targets (10 targets total). One minute is added to the athlete's finishing time for each miss. Biathlon has been a part of the Paralympic Winter Games since 1992. Cross-country skiing started with the Paralympic Games in Sweden in 1976. Cross-country races range from 2.5 to 20 km depending on disability and gender. Paralympic Nordic skiing competition is open to male and female athletes with limb loss. Classification categories exist for those with lower-extremity impairments (LW2, LW3, and LW4); those with upper-extremity impairments (LW5/7, LW6, and LW8); those with both upper- and lower-extremity impairments (LW9); and sit-skiers (LW10–LW12).[36]

CURLING

Paralympic curling is a wheelchair sport that was introduced at the 2006 Paralympic Winter Games in Torino. As in able-bodied curling, teams are composed of two competitors who throw "stones" by hand or by the use of a stick towards a target at the opposite end of the ice. However, there is no sweeping and only competitors in wheelchairs are allowed to compete. The object of the game is to get a team's stones as close to the center of the target (the "house") as possible. Six ends are played, with a possible extra end if the teams are tied after six. Paralympic wheelchair curling competition is open to male and female athletes with limb loss.

SLED (SLEDGE) HOCKEY

Sled hockey is a variation of ice hockey in which the athletes compete on the ice by means of a sled. Just as in ice hockey, sled hockey is played with six players (including a goalie) at a time. Players propel themselves on their sled by use of spikes on the ends of two three-foot-long sticks, enabling players to push themselves and shoot and pass the puck. Rinks and goals are regulation Olympic size, and games consist of three 15-minute stop-time periods. Sledge

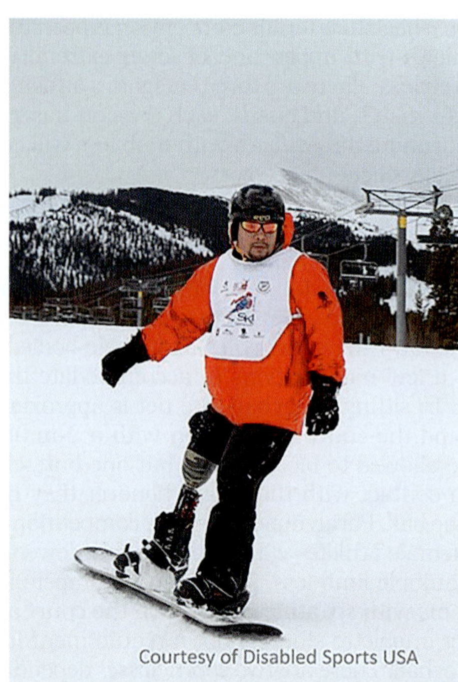

Fig. 28.5 Snowboarding. (Courtesy Disabled Sports USA.)

hockey became a medal sport in the 1994 Paralympic Games. Paralympic sled hockey competition is open to male athletes with lower-extremity limb loss, and there is only one classification category in sled hockey.[36]

SNOWBOARDING

Snowboarding debuted at the Winter Paralympic Games in 2014 in Sochi. Athletes with disability may compete in one of four different snowboarding disciplines: snowboard cross head-to-head, banked slalom, snowboard cross-time trial, and/or giant slalom. Only the snowboard cross-time trial was included in the 2014 Paralympic Winter Games; however, medals were awarded in both time trial and banked slalom at the 2018 Pyeong Chang Games. Athletes may use specialized equipment to adapt the snowboard and/or use orthopedic aids to allow them to compete (Fig. 28.5). Snowboard is open to males and females with upper- and/or lower-extremity single or multiple limb loss. Classification categories exist for athletes with unilateral lower-extremity impairment (SB-LL1); bilateral lower-extremity impairment (SB-LL2); and upper-extremity impairment (SB-UL).[36]

Non-Paralympic Sports and Recreational Activities for Individuals With Limb Loss

Individuals with limb loss may use Paralympic sports activities for noncompetitive purposes such as physical activity and/or recreation such as swimming, skiing/snowboarding, equestrian, archery/shooting, water sports, and/or weight lifting. Although these Paralympic sports are popular among individuals with limb loss, there are many other sports and recreational activities available to this population. Many of these sports require little or no adaptation for participation by those with limb loss, allowing participation and/or competition between able-bodied and individuals and those with limb loss.

FISHING

Fishing is a sport that can be enjoyed by anyone.[38] There are many different types of specialized equipment available to the disabled angler such as rods, reels, line, rod holders, and tackle, as well as easy cast and electric fishing reels for individuals who may have difficulties casting and reeling in a fish. There are also harness rod holders that can mount on a wheelchair or the side of a boat and allow an individual with limited use of their arm(s) to participate in recreational fishing. Pontoon boats can provide easy accessibility for those in wheelchairs. The Paralyzed Veterans of America sponsors a variety of fishing tournaments for people with disabilities, and there are disability fishing groups and clubs that cater to children with disabilities who enjoy fishing. They offer several bass fishing tournaments where those interested in fishing can learn new skills or improve old ones. The Paralyzed Veterans of America Bass Tour offers Team/Open Competition, pairing disabled anglers with able-bodied boat partners. Those who prefer not to fish from a boat can participate in the Bank Competition. Both novice and experienced anglers can compete for significant cash and other prizes. Fishing Has No Boundaries, Inc. is another nonprofit organization for all persons with disabilities that has grown into a national organization with 23 chapters in 11 states. Fishing Has No Boundaries enables thousands of people with disabilities to participate fully in the recreational activity of fishing.

HUNTING

As with fishing, hunting is a recreational activity that can be enjoyed by all, and any disability can be offset by adaptive hunting equipment and adaptive hunting techniques.[38] There are many different types of adaptive equipment that can be used by either gun or bow hunters with either upper- or lower-extremity limb loss. This includes hunting blinds that are more wheelchair friendly, protective clothing to make cold weather hunting more enjoyable, adaptive tree stands, tripod-mounted crossbow or gun rests, and wheelchair-based gun rests. Federal, state, and local governments are providing easier access to thousands of acres of trails, parks, and wilderness areas. There are organizations and clubs with programs for persons with disabilities who want to participate in hunting activities.

GOLF

Just about anyone, regardless of ability level, can participate in golf.[39] This makes it one of the best sports for people with disabilities, especially those with limb loss (Fig. 28.6). Anyone with limb loss can successfully play golf, including those with lower-extremity prostheses, where a torsion absorber and rotator allow them to pivot to finish their swing. Those with upper-extremity amputation may play with just one arm, or, if they play with one arm and a prosthesis, there are a number of pieces of adaptive hardware that allow them to attach their prosthetic arm to their club, allowing them to swing with both hands. If they are unable to walk a full 18-hole course, they may play golf from a seated position on a single-rider golf cart. Numerous other devices exist to help golfers with amputation tee-up and retrieve their ball, better grip the club, and aid their game.

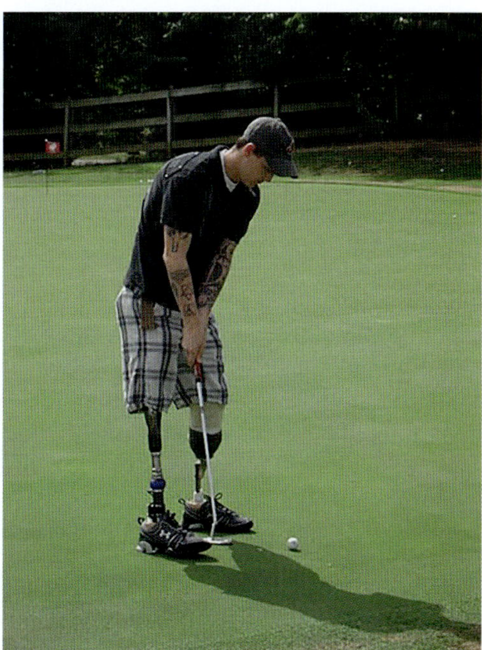

Fig. 28.6 Golfing. (Courtesy Disabled Sports USA.)

TRAIL ORIENTEERING AND CLIMBING

Conventional orienteering combines fast running with precise navigation, typically through forests or over moorland.[40] Trail orienteering is a discipline of the sport designed so that people with disabilities can have meaningful orienteering competitions. It completely eliminates the element of speed over the ground but makes the map-interpretation element more challenging. Able-bodied people can compete on equal terms with the physically challenged. Depending on the level of difficulty, up to five control markers are placed at each site, and only one will correspond exactly with the control description and control circle position. Sites are chosen so that they can be seen from a wheelchair-navigable path or area, but they may be quite a distance into the forest or over unnavigable terrain. The only special equipment needed is a compass. An escort can provide physical assistance to the competitor by pushing a wheelchair, holding and orienting the map and compass, and marking the control card (which records the competitor's progress through various checkpoints) based on the competitor's instructions. However, it is an important rule that escorts must not help in the decision-making process; they can give as much physical help as may be necessary but must not offer advice or opinions to the competitor. For serious competitions, escorts are "swapped" so they do not know the competitor they are helping.

Along with trail orienteering, other ambulatory sports/activities may be appropriate for individuals with amputation. For those who enjoy the outdoors, hiking, mountain climbing, rock climbing, and ropes courses are popular

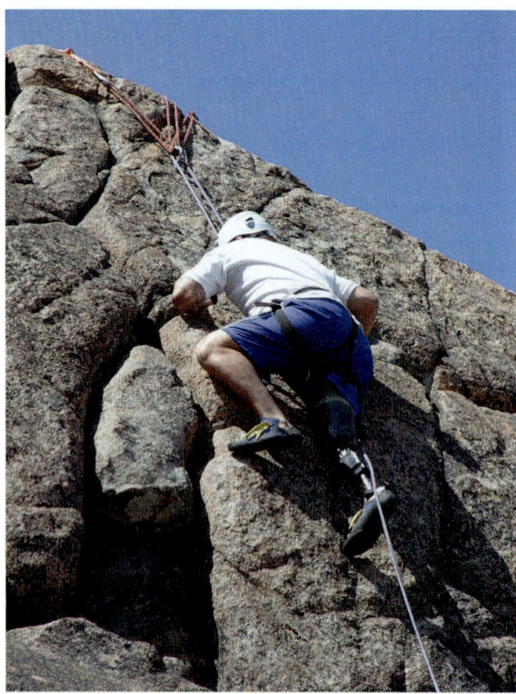

Fig. 28.7 Rock climbing. (Courtesy Disabled Sports USA.)

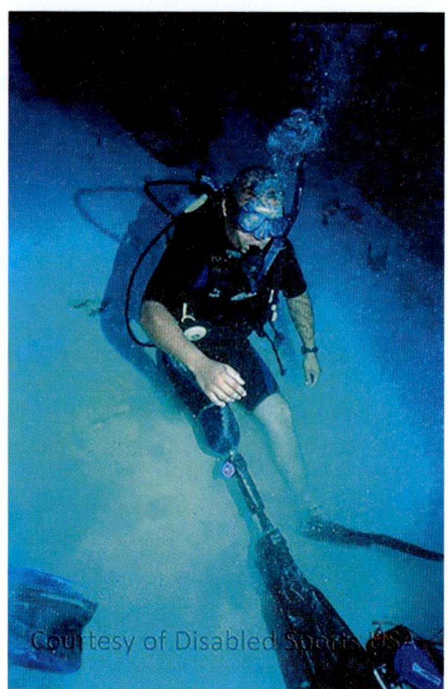

Fig. 28.8 Scuba diving. (Courtesy Disabled Sports USA.)

(Fig. 28.7).[41] These activities are easily done with able-bodied friends and can be done safely as long as normal outdoor precautions are observed. For those activities that require additional training or practice, there are many qualified instructors available at most recreational areas for lessons or instructions to increase enjoyment and reduce the likelihood of injury while participating in these sports.

SKY DIVING

Skydiving is a sport that can involve skydivers who have one or more amputated limbs.[42] Because of their prosthetic devices, amputee skydivers often have to compensate for the change in weight with the positioning of their body for both themselves and other divers in a formation. Many of these individuals begin skydiving in tandem, making jumps while attached to a certified jump instructor. However, as individuals become more experienced, many progress to solo (accelerated free fall) jumps. Modifications to prosthetic devices, particularly lower-extremity prostheses, may need to be made because of the forces incurred during landing after the jump.

Additional Water Sports and Activities

People with amputations can participate in a variety of adapted water sports, allowing them to enjoy the benefits of movement in water and participation in sports activities.[43–45] Besides swimming, there are numerous other water sports individuals with amputation may participate in such as surfing, kayaking, sailing, and scuba diving. Adapted surfing involves the use of boards and equipment adapted to the needs of people with disabilities, including people with amputations. Boards can be modified to facilitate stability and safety while surfing. Canoe and kayak can be adapted to allow amputees to participate in these sports. Boats can be modified to allow greater stability and easy access to the interior. Adapted sailing provides opportunities for people with disabilities to participate in sailing experiences and regattas. Boats can be adapted with special seating and customized controls. Adapted scuba diving is an underwater activity for people with disabilities, including amputees, using specific equipment and techniques to enable a safe and enjoyable underwater experience (Fig. 28.8). It is important to note that participation in these adapted water sports requires an individual assessment of each athlete's physical capabilities and ability. Amputees interested in participating in a water sport should consult with experts, qualified instructors, or specialized sports organizations to find the option best suited to their needs and interests.

Surfing for people with amputations can be a fun and exciting sport.[43] Individuals can begin surfing by lying down on the board, transitioning from sitting, quadruped, kneeling, and finally standing. Once standing, individuals can choose to sail with or without their prosthetic device (Fig. 28.9).

Until recently, windsurfing[45] was an inaccessible sport for people with limb loss. However, equipment modifications have made windsurfing accessible to people with all types of disabilities. Beginners can start windsurfing on a fixed or swivel seat attached to the windsurfing board. Stabilizers or flat-bottomed pontoons can be attached to the sides of the windsurfing board to provide additional stability. A vertical rail can be used on the board to allow someone to stand with an instructor for support. One or two sails can be used so that instructors can be on the windsurfing board to assist. Such adaptations open the sport to males and females with all types of disabilities, including amputation.

Water skiing[45] has been adapted so that people with physical disabilities can participate and compete. The competition is held in three events (slalom, stunt, and jump) for

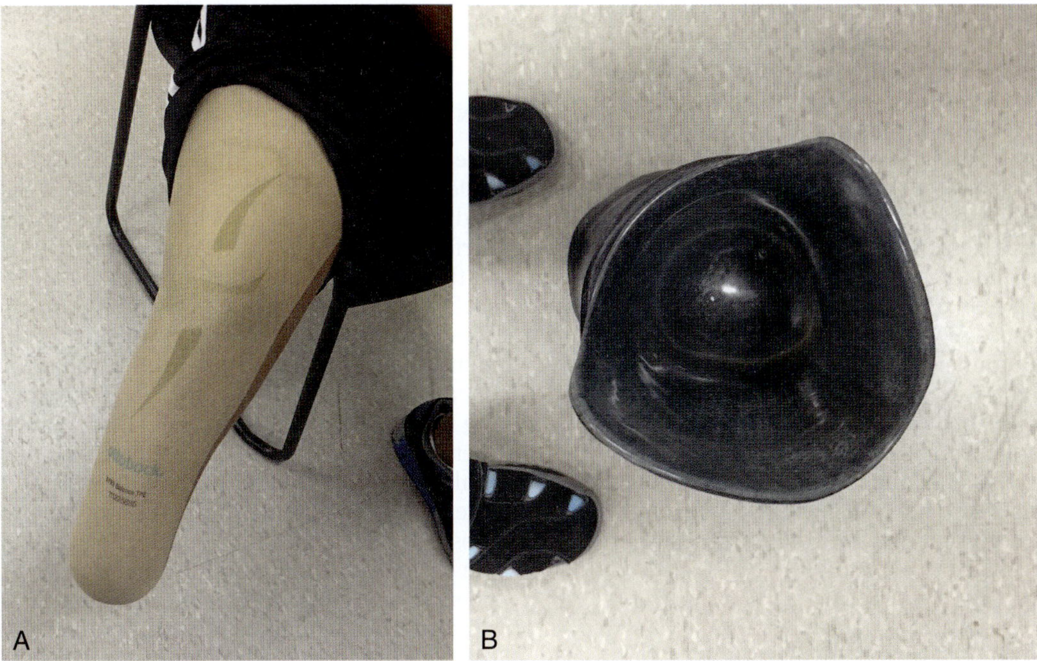

Fig. 28.9 (A) Prosthetic liner. (B) Prosthetic socket. (A and B, Photos taken and given with permission from Dionne CP, OUHSC.)

individuals with upper and lower limb loss regardless of the level of amputation. Skiers compete with the same water ski equipment used by able-bodied skiers; however, the use of a prosthetic device is optional.

Kayaking can be done alone or in tandem. To avoid entrapment, a water sports prosthesis that can be attached to the outside of the boat for easy access is recommended. For those with upper limb amputations, one-handed paddles can be used, or heavy tape or rubber rings can secure their grip on the paddle, as conventional prosthetic devices are not designed to hold paddles effectively. Rowing prostheses are also available for amputees using other types of boats. For safety reasons, wetsuits, helmets, and flotation devices are recommended for all participants.

Scuba diving can be an excellent recreational activity for people with amputations. Because of the buoyancy provided by water, mobility problems are significantly reduced, and scuba diving can be taught to swimmers with both upper and lower limb loss with virtually no modifications. For some, scuba diving represents total freedom because it provides the opportunity to move without an assistive device in an environment free of barriers and gravity. Many people choose to dive without their prostheses, but water sports prostheses are available. As with able-bodied divers, the same basic safety and equipment concerns apply.

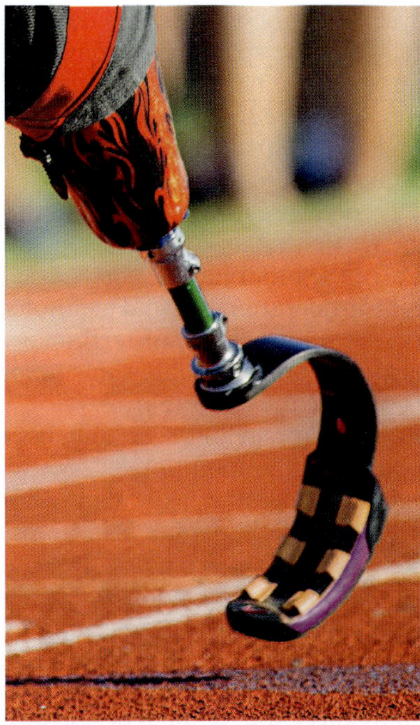

Fig. 28.10 Prosthesis without knee articulation. (Photos taken and given with permission from Raiber O and Williams J, OUHSC.)

Prosthetic Components for Athletes With Limb Loss

The substantial progress made during the past decade in disability sports cannot be discussed without mentioning the impact of Oscar Pistorius.[46] The South African athlete with a bilateral amputation below the knee, nicknamed "Blade Runner," uses carbon-fiber blade-shaped prosthetics. Although Pistorius was not the first athlete with a disability to take part in the Olympic Games, his participation has had a profound and lasting effect on the world of sports. While experts continue to debate the limits of assistive technology, athletes with disabilities push the boundaries, challenging the fundamental concepts of competition, technology, and human capability (Fig. 28.10). In fact, opportunities for people with limb loss to participate in sport and physical activity have increased over the past 20 years. An essential contributing factor to this phenomenon has been a consumer-driven demand for advances in prosthetic technology and design as well as limb loss awareness.[47] Plus, the benefits of participation in sports and activities of everyday life, now well-known, are numerous both at the individual and social levels. On the other hand, advanced tailored rehabilitation programs and sport enthusiast groups have created market demand for improvement and acceleration of modifications to everyday-use prosthetic limb and the creation of more sport-specific designs.

However, the most significant challenge in developing effective sport prostheses is achieving seamless cooperation between the user and the prosthesis in the complex context of sports. To attain a sense of complete control, the athlete must develop an "extended sensation" of the prosthetic limb and its components. The human-machine system must therefore be developed in such a way that a direct link is created between the activation of the body's own physiological systems (muscles and joints) and the movement of a prosthesis.

To succeed in this aim, each element that makes up the sports prosthesis must be made with suitable materials, such as to favor both the high level of performance and the comfort of the athlete during use.

Prosthetic Components for Athletes With Lower Limb Loss

In the field of prosthetic orthopedics, it is necessary to distinguish between prostheses used for daily life and those designed specifically for sports. Everyday prostheses have seen significant advancements, such as three-dimensional-printed prostheses to reduce costs, especially with new materials like light titanium becoming compatible with printers. Additionally, brain-computer interfaces have been developed to control prostheses through thought alone, and intelligent synthetic skin now provides tactile and sensory feedback. On the other hand, sport-specific prosthetics require careful consideration to avoid technological doping, which refers to the improper use of technology to enhance athletic performance unfairly, that is, misuse of technology to artificially enhance the performance.

Prostheses for Athletes with lower limb loss are classified according to the type of amputation

- Transfemoral (TF): prosthesis for above-the-knee amputation at the level of the femur. The necessary components for TF prosthetic fit are a prosthetic foot, the knee joint, the connecting components to the socket and, in many cases, the cuff, which connects the prosthesis to the residual limb.
- Transtibial (TT): prosthesis for below-the-knee amputation, which involves the removal of portions of the tibia and fibula. The necessary components for TT prosthetic fit are prosthetic foot and the connecting components to the socket and the cuff, which connects the prosthesis to the residual limb.

Moreover, amputation can be unilateral or bilateral: consequently, an athlete can run with one or two TF or TT prostheses.

In particular, the International Paralympic Committee classifies athletes in the following categories, in order to create homogeneous groups in the competition:

- T42–44: athletes with impairment of one or both lower limbs (use of prosthesis is not mandatory);
- T61–64: athletes with TF or TT bilateral or unilateral amputation (use of prosthesis is required).

LINER

The liner plays a very important role as a link between the residual limb and the socket. It is actually a cuff that covers and protects the residual limb, ensuring a greater contact surface with the socket. Its role is also to limit the movement of the prosthesis and the consequent friction between the socket and the stump which could damage the skin. The liner evens out the forces generated on the leg during movement, avoiding the formation of localized pressure points. It can be formed from three different materials depending on the state of the stump: silicone, polyurethane, and thermoplastic elastomers, which are mainly indicated for athletes with transtibial amputations and a medium-low level of mobility, rarely for transfemoral ones. Other added prosthetic suspensions (straps, sleeve) may be required for the prosthesis to remain intimate to the residual limb, considering expected changeable limb volume during play. The residuum skin must be protected during participation in recreational sports, as well as everyday activities.

Lower-limb prosthetics are commonly composed of a means of suspension, a prosthetic socket, joint articulation (as needed), shaft (or pylon), and foot. Prosthetics have now become modular in construction such that the athlete can still use the prosthetic socket of choice and interchange certain components to meet the demands of a specific sport.[40,42,47–49] Even recreational athletes with limb loss can enjoy sports using their usual prosthetics with additional or interchangeable modification. However, committed athletes with limb loss must consider the biomechanical demands of their sport and apply the components that allow safe and competitive participation and choose prosthetic components accordingly. For example, triathletes may choose to use a swimming prosthetic leg or opt not to use a prosthesis during the swimming portion of the competition. In addition, prosthetic design has advanced to the creation of sport-specific prosthetics, such as for swimming and track and field competition. However, affordability for these devices poses an obstacle to common accessibility.

Once the residuum has sufficiently recovered from amputation surgery and "matured" to be able to accept the shear, torsion, and load demands of a desired sport, athletes with limb loss can be fitted with prosthetics to help meet the rigors of training.[49–51] Considerations must be made for sports that demand high levels of shear, such as those that involve running or cutting. These excessive forces increase the risk of soft tissue breakdown, pain, and time out of the prosthesis and away from the sport.[49] High levels of activity also increase added perspiration within the prosthetic socket, increasing the risk of infections and related skin problems.[52] Regardless of the choice of prosthetic components, proper prosthetic management and skin care are essential in sports.

SOCKETS

The socket is certainly the most important component: it is the effective prosthesis-residual limb interface and, therefore, allows the movement and control of the prosthesis.

Total surface–bearing prosthetic sockets are in fact recommended because they are designed to disperse forces evenly over the entire surface area of the residuum-socket interface to minimize the risk for soft tissue breakdown. The design of prosthetic sockets is always customized because each individual's residual limb has a unique shape and size. For the socket surface material, rigid surface sockets are commonly made from lamination resins and polypropylene. Laminating epoxies crosslink together with a hardener at room temperature, above 25°C or hot; they are characterized by excellent mechanical and thermal resistance (over 150°C), low viscosity, excellent wettability of the fibers and resistance to yellowing as well as a high surface finish. Polypropylene (PP) is a very resistant thermoplastic polymer from a chemical point of view. Up to 120°C it maintains its characteristics of mechanical resistance and its processing is relatively simple.

In addition to rigid sockets, flexible surface sockets are modern and applicable for all types of amputation. These sockets feature thin, flexible, and transparent surfaces, combined with a rigid load-bearing frame made of laminated carbon fibers, which transfers the load effectively to the prosthetic skeleton. The socket itself is made of polyethylene, a light but very resistant material with a high resistance to chemical agents, shocks and water. Polyethylene is used widely due to its low coefficient of friction, making it ideal for application to the abutment. Additionally, it exhibits excellent resistance to fatigue, which is the tendency of a material to weaken or break under repeated stress even when the loads remain within its elastic limit. The flexible and transparent socket is inserted in the supporting structure: this can be made from carbon fibers but also from nylon, kevlar, dacron or glass fibers. Dacron is polyethylene terephthalate (PET),[51] that is, a thermoplastic resin that is transparent, flexible, and resistant to traction, tearing, and impact. It has excellent mechanical, thermal, and chemical resistance. This type of socket allows for very high comfort: during movement, muscle contractions modify the shape and geometry of the abutment. Consequently a flexible socket adapts better to these volumetric variations.

TUBULAR STRUCTURE

The tubular structure of a prosthesis consists of several structural modules that connect the socket to the knee and ankle joints. Their function is to assume the role of the femur, fibula, and/or tibia, depending on the type of amputation. The modules are made of materials that are light, rigid, and resistant to external stresses, especially compression. Therefore titanium alloys, aluminum alloys, and carbon fiber are the preferred choices for these applications. Titanium, in particular, is the best material for the tubular structure, as it is light and has good mechanical properties, although it is more expensive than the other materials. Aluminum is present in the final alloy in a concentration of more than 90%. The great advantage of this material is that it is very light, although it has lower mechanical properties.

PROSTHETIC KNEE JOINTS

Prosthetic knee joints are a crucial component of lower limb prostheses for individuals with above-knee amputations.

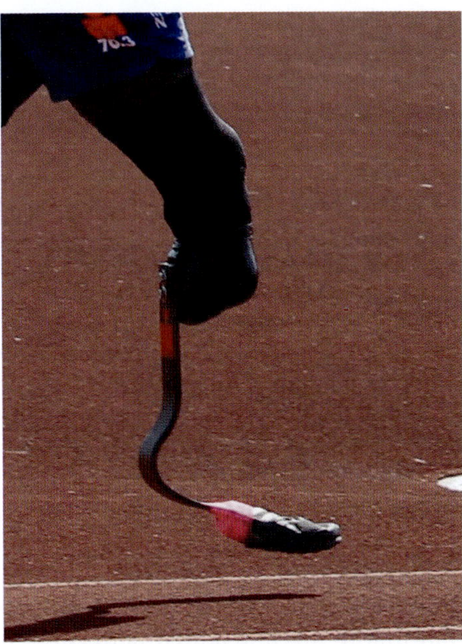

Fig. 28.11 **Carbon fiber foot.** (Photos taken and given with permission from Raiber O and Williams J, OUHSC.)

These knee joints are designed to mimic the function of a natural knee joint, providing stability, flexibility, and adaptability to support various activities and movements. There are a variety of computerized knee joints on the market that offer user-matched walking speeds. However, there is not yet a computerized knee joint designed to withstand the rigors of "stop-start" running, cutting, jumping, or swimming.[53] The athlete with transfemoral limb loss can choose to use a mechanical running limb because it is a simpler, more reliable knee joint design that can be controlled in "real time" (Fig. 28.11). However, athletes usually depend on the energy-storing running foot and the power of the hip extensors to substitute for natural knee function, or these athletes can choose to use no articulation at all, such as when competing in track and field events.[50,54] There are different types of prosthetic knee joints available, each with its own features and capabilities. Here are some common types of prosthetic knee joints:

- Single-axis knee: The single-axis knee is a simple and cost-effective design. It allows flexion and extension, making it suitable for basic walking and activities with limited demands on stability.
- Polycentric knee: Polycentric knees have multiple pivot points, which provide improved stability during walking and better control over the knee's movements. They are commonly used for everyday activities and can handle varied terrains.
- Geared polycentric knee: This type of knee joint incorporates gears or mechanical components that enhance the knee's stability and control during walking and other activities.
- Fluid or hydraulic knee: Hydraulic knee joints use fluid or oil to control the knee's movement, providing both stability and adaptability. These knees offer smoother and more natural movements during different gait phases.
- Microprocessor-controlled knee (MPK): MPKs are technologically advanced knee joints with built-in sensors

and microprocessors that continuously adjust the knee's resistance and support based on the user's movements. These knees can adapt to different walking speeds, terrains, and activities, offering enhanced stability and safety.

- Locking or stance-control Knee: Locking knees have a mechanism that locks the knee in extension during the stance phase of walking, providing added stability and reducing the risk of falls. The knee unlocks during the swing phase to allow the leg to move forward.
- Hydraulic-microprocessor-controlled knee: This is a combination of hydraulic and microprocessor-controlled technology, offering the benefits of both systems. It provides stability, smooth movement, and adaptability in various situations.

The choice of prosthetic knee joint depends on factors such as the individual's activity level, lifestyle, and functional needs. Prosthetists work closely with the user to assess their requirements and select the most appropriate knee joint to optimize mobility and overall function. Regular follow-ups and adjustments are essential to ensure that the prosthetic knee joint continues to meet the user's needs as they engage in various activities and sports.

LOWER LEG/FOOT/ANKLE COMPONENTS

Prosthetics have become modular in construction allowing the athlete to use the best-fitted socket and change the prosthetic components to minimize risk and maximize performance. Application of the appropriate prosthetic foot to maximize efficiency towards symmetric step lengths during varied walking speeds enables the recreational amputee to participate in higher levels of activity.[55] In some cases, prosthetic foot/ankle/knee components can be interchanged using a "quick-release" coupler for use in specific sport-like activities.[56]

Forces untoward residuum health must be minimized with proper selection of prosthetic components. Pylons, special-designed prosthetic ankles, and heels that absorb and dissipate energy during loading are important considerations. Athletes with either transtibial or transfemoral limb loss who are required to run or sprint typically use an energy-storing foot.[56] This specialized foot is constructed of materials that essentially "store" the energy during locomotion and transfer energy with significant efficiency to propel the athlete forward in walking or running gait. This particular prosthetic foot is posteriorly attached to the prosthetic socket. For athletes involved in running or sprinting, these high-performance carbon-fiber foot components (i.e., "blades") have become essential (Figs. 28.10 and 28.11). This design enables the athlete with bilateral or unilateral, transtibial, or transfemoral limb loss to participate and successfully compete in sports never before considered. However, there are limitations to these designs. Athletes who play sports on uneven ground and need ankle designs that simulate foot pronation and supination must depend on the older, mechanical designs to compete with less risk for injury and falls.[56]

Other Materials

In addition to the main components of modular sports prostheses, there are other materials and accessories that can help improve performance depending on the sport.

For example, in a racing prosthesis, there are other elements such as the bolts made of titanium and the insoles, which are often characterized by plastic inserts to which the nails can be attached. The insole attached to the part of the carbon blade that corresponds to a person's forefoot is designed to replicate the functionality of a cleated shoe typically used by able-bodied sprinters to provide stability and grip on the track during a race.

Athletes With Upper Limb Loss

Although there are fewer people with upper-extremity limb loss than with lower-extremity limb loss, there is a growing number of those who are competing in sports who require skilled use of the arms and hands.[57] As with lower-extremity prosthetics that incorporate advanced technologies, upper-extremity prosthetics also present significant challenges for practical use in sports. So, prosthetic designers have created human-powered prosthesis terminal devices that are used to throw and catch a ball or hold a bow and arrow.[56] The devices do not simulate human anatomy and are designed for function.

Children With Limb Loss in Sport

Prosthetic design for children with limb loss is typically simple when the child is small. However, as the child develops and grows, more complicated, adult-level components are added.[58] Current pediatric knee components usually

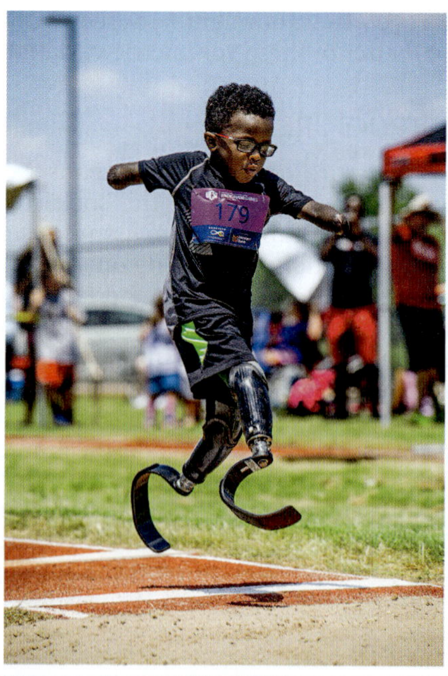

Fig. 28.12 Pediatric components. (Photos taken and given with permission from University of Central Oklahoma Endeavor Games.)

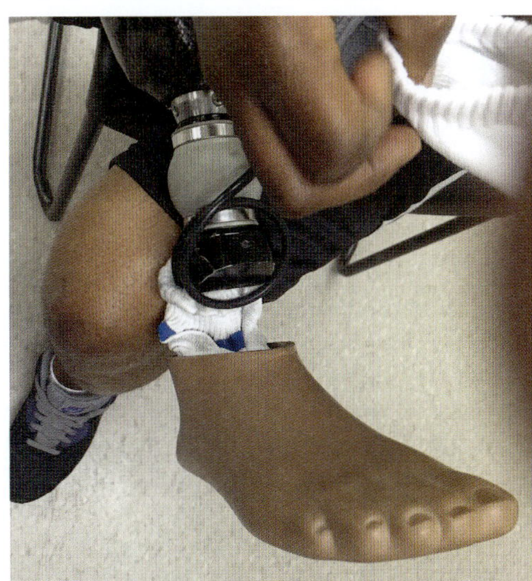

Fig. 28.13 Prosthesis with a foot. (Photos taken and given with permission from Dionne CP, OUHSC.)

provide control, shock absorption, and freedom to move like a growing child. The use of carbon-fiber, energy-storing prosthetic feet is considered the norm in these components. Components must be light, yet strong and sufficiently durable to enable young athletes to compete (Fig. 28.12). Tackling existing barriers such as prosthesis failure and high costs as well as advancements in prosthetic design and technology facilitate increasing opportunities for children with lower limb absences to participate in sport and physical activity.[22]

Prosthetics in Sports: What Is Best?

People recovering from limb amputation surgery that plan to participate in a sport should closely consult with the rehabilitation team, composed of the surgeon, physical therapist, occupational therapist, athletic trainer, and specifically the prosthetist to create a prosthesis to meet that goal.[59] Despite many advances in the design and composition of either upper- or lower-extremity prosthetic limbs, there is no tangible evidence as to which component designs are best suited for any one particular sport or consumer group. Several studies have set out to determine the effectiveness of a group of prosthetic foot-ankle or knee joint designs. However, due to the poor quality and lack of comparability of the research designs, no definitive conclusions have been drawn.[57] Regarding prostheses for athletes competing in speed events, further research on the biomechanics of running and advancements in biomaterials is needed. These studies will lead to significant improvements in the design and shape of the prostheses, making them more efficient and athlete friendly. In addition, the development and combination of new materials will result in prostheses that offer a comfortable, technical, and balanced performance. The use of increasingly advanced composite materials will allow greater joint control and offer increasingly precise correction work in the flight phase in speed competitions. With the help of additional, national-level funding of research, technology has advanced sport-specific prosthetic designs tailored to those at the most elite level of competition,[60] but these prosthetics are cost prohibitive to the everyday athlete with limb loss. Decisions regarding prosthetics for competitive athletes are currently guided by an individualized, case-by-case, expert opinions. These experts may include healthcare professionals, biomechanists, bioengineers who assess the specific needs of each athlete to optimize their performance and comfort in competitive sport (Fig. 28.13).

References

The complete listing of the References are available in the accompanying enhanced eBook version included with the print purchase of this textbook. Visit Elsevier eBooks+ (eBooks.Health.Elsevier.com) to access this content.

29 Rehabilitation for Children With Limb Deficiencies*

GIOVANNI GALEOTO AND ANNA BERARDI

LEARNING OBJECTIVES

On completion of this chapter, the reader will be able to do the following:

1. Outline the rehabilitation pathways to address physical and psychosocial concerns for infants, toddlers, school-age children, and adolescents.
2. Compare prosthweetic options for children of various ages with upper- or lower-limb deficiencies.
3. Specify the training goals for children of various ages fitted with upper- and lower-limb prostheses.
4. Design a habilitation program for an infant.
5. Use and recommend the best evaluation tool to assess the needs of children with amputation.

Introduction

CLASSIFICATION AND CAUSES OF LIMB DEFICIENCIES

Congenital limb amputations and deficiencies are missing or incomplete limbs at birth. The overall prevalence is 7.9/10,000 live births. Most are due to primary intrauterine growth inhibition or disruptions secondary to intrauterine destruction of normal embryonic tissues. The upper extremities are more commonly affected.[1,2] In Portugal, the prevalence of congenital limb malformations was 2.16 cases per 10,000 live births between 1980 and 2019.[2,3]

Congenital limb deficiencies have many causes and often occur as a component of various congenital syndromes. Teratogenic agents (e.g., thalidomide, vitamin A) are known causes of hypoplastic/absent limbs. The most common cause of congenital limb amputations is soft-tissue and/or vascular disruption defects, such as amniotic band–related limb deficiency, in which loose strands of amnion entangle or fuse with fetal tissue.

The most commonly used classification in congenital deficits is the International Society for Prosthetics and Orthosis classification, which divides these deficits into transverse and longitudinal[4] (Fig. 29.1).

The standard nomenclature divides limb deficiencies into two basic types—longitudinal and transverse. Longitudinal deficiencies involve specific maldevelopments (e.g., complete or partial absence of the radius, fibula, or tibia). Radial ray deficiency is the most common upper-limb deficiency, and hypoplasia of the fibula is the most common lower-limb deficiency. About two-thirds of cases are associated with other congenital disorders, including Adams-Oliver syndrome (aplasia cutis congenita with partial aplasia of the skull bones and terminal transverse limb malformations), Holt-Oram syndrome, thrombocytopenia-absent radius syndrome, Fanconi anemia, and VACTERL (vertebral anomalies, anal atresia, cardiac malformations, tracheoesophageal fistula, renal anomalies and radial aplasia, and limb anomalies) syndrome.

Congenital limb defects involve missing, incomplete, supernumerary, or abnormally developed limbs present at birth.

Transverse deficiencies present as limb anomalies where all elements beyond a certain level are absent, making the limb resemble an amputation stump. The most common cause of transverse deficiencies is amniotic bands, which result in varying degrees of deficiency depending on the band's location. Typically, these cases do not exhibit other defects or anomalies. However, other instances of transverse deficiencies are often associated with underlying genetic syndromes, such as Adams-Oliver syndrome, or chromosomal abnormalities.

With a transverse or longitudinal deficiency, depending on the etiology, infants may also have hypoplastic or bifid bones, synostoses, duplications, dislocations, or other bony defects; for example, in proximal femoral focal deficiency, the proximal femur and acetabulum do not develop. One or more limbs may be affected, and the defect type may differ in each limb. Central nervous system abnormalities are rare.

It is important to categorize limb reduction defects in the correct specific subtypes as these tend to differ by etiology and pathogenesis (Table 29.1).[5,6]

Precise numbers for other forms of congenital limb differences (i.e., limb length discrepancies, neuromuscular pathology leading to differences in limb) and joint deformities (i.e., contractures) are unknown.

Acquired amputations most commonly occur from trauma or disease (i.e., neoplasm or infection.) A retrospective study done in the United States determined that more than 110,000 children younger than 18 years presented to emergency rooms with traumatic amputation injuries during a 12-year period. The average age was 6.18 years, patients were predominantly males (65.5%), and finger amputations comprised 91.6% of the amputations.[7]

POSTOPERATIVE CARE

Postoperative care is simpler for young children undergoing amputation than for adolescents and adults. Ordinarily,

*The authors would like to extend appreciation to the memory of Joan Edelstein, whose work in prior editions provided the foundation for this chapter.

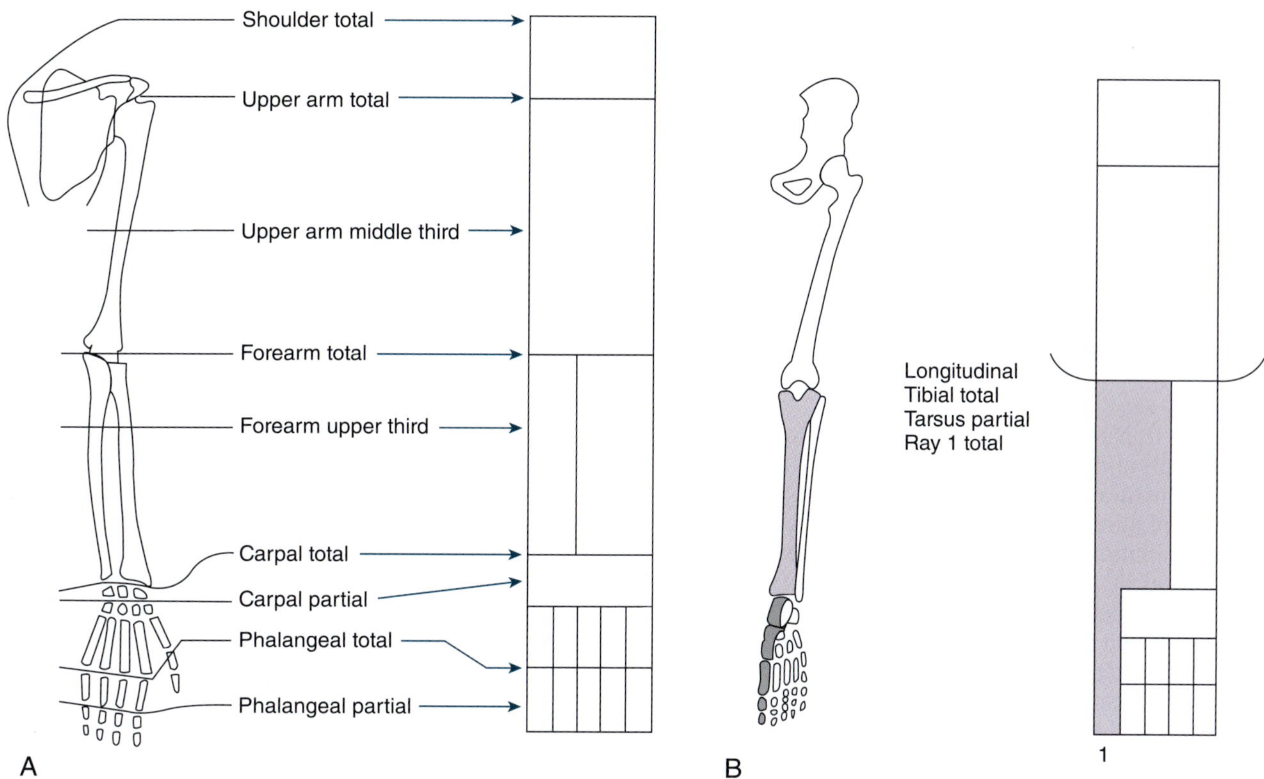

Fig. 29.1 (A) International Organization for children with Standardization/International Society for Prosthetics and Orthotics system for classifying upper-limb congenital limb deficiencies. Lower-limb transverse deficiencies are named in a similar fashion. Levels can also be described by naming the absent bone(s). (B) Lower-limb longitudinal limb deficiency. The *shaded area* represents missing segments. (Reprinted with permission from Murdoch G, Wilson AB, eds. *Amputation: Surgical Practice and Patient Management*. Butterworth Heinemann; 1996:352.)

Table 29.1 Classification of Amputation

Axis of the Limb	Segment	Involvement
Complete absence	All segments	Amelia
	Intercalary	Absence or severe hypoplasia of part of limb with normal or nearly normal terminal
		Segment, including: ■ Typical and atypical intercalary defects ■ Femoral hypoplasia
Longitudinal	Preaxial	Radial, tibial, first digit/toe (with or without the involvement of second digit/toe)
	Axial	Hand/foot only: Third ray involved (with or without second and fourth ray)
		Includes typical split-hand/foot and split-hand/foot monodactyl type
	Postaxial	Fifth digits/toes (with or without fourth digit/toe involved)
Mixed		Any other combination of two or more subtypes; e.g., femoral-fibula-ulnar complex

the residual limb presents little or no edema, and the wound heals rapidly.

Adults with amputation commonly experience phantom limb sensations. However, little literature discusses the impact of phantom limb sensations and pain on pediatric patients.[7] Phantom pain is associated with the extent of preoperative pain and is generally short lived.[8] The prevalence of phantom limb pain varies depending on the cause of amputation. In pediatric traumatic amputation, the prevalence of phantom limb pain ranges from 12% to 83%, 3.7% to 20%, and 48% to 90% for traumatic, congenital, and oncology-related amputation, respectively.[9] Symptoms are highly variable, ranging from the perceived ability to voluntarily move the phantom limb, to sharp pain, to tingling sensations. Furthermore, these symptoms typically last for minutes and can be almost constant and highly distressing. Episodes typically occur in the afternoon and evening and may be triggered by physical (e.g., bumping/injuring the amputated limb or long periods of walking or standing) and psychosocial (e.g., meeting new people or stress) triggers.[9]

Treatment for phantom limb sensations varies based on the individual's symptoms, age, and impact on their function. Desensitization techniques such as rubbing or massaging the uninvolved limb at similar points to those in which they are experiencing the phantom limb sensation of the amputated limb can be used to control symptoms.[7] A pain diary may help older children and adolescents to cope with phantom pain from traumatic amputation. Most of the research for nonpharmacologic treatments has focused on mirror therapy in pediatric cancer. Mirror therapy uses the facilitation of an illusion of the unaffected limb, thus helping to reorganize the brain's somatosensory cortex to reduce phantom limb pain/sensations.[7–10] Pharmacologic treatments are usually managed by a pain management team. Currently, no one medication is standard of practice, but several pharmacologic treatments have demonstrated effectiveness. Gabapentin, tricyclic antidepressants, and opioids effectively treat phantom limb pain. Wang and colleagues found that preoperative use of gabapentin in pediatric patients with oncology-related amputation had a beneficial impact on postoperative pain intensity and phantom limb pain prevention when compared with a placebo.[11] Other agents such as nerve blocks or epidural catheters have also been described in pediatric postoperative pain management protocols[7–10] (see Fig. 29.2).

Infants

Infants learn to trust when their basic needs are met. The baby with limb anomaly needs as much trusting, responsive care as the infant with intact limbs. Infants respond to the anxieties of parents and others who interact with them. Successful habilitation depends on the parents' replacing the expectation of a "perfect" infant with the reality of a baby with a limb deficiency. The birth of a baby with a limb deficiency can elicit intense emotion. Because such an event is rare in any hospital, medical staff may display shock and feelings of helplessness or revulsion. Some parents characterize the first few weeks after birth as a nightmare. They believe they are alone with a unique and hopeless problem when questions go unanswered or evaded. Reactions of the infant's grandparents, siblings, and other family members influence habilitation. Mourning for the loss of the ideal child is part of the coping process.[11–13] Newborns are too young for prosthetic fitting; nevertheless, early referral to a specialized clinic is highly desirable. The core team comprises a pediatrician, physical therapist, occupational therapist, and prosthetist. The team should be able to draw on the expertise of psychologists, social workers, orthopedists, and engineers, depending on the needs of the child and family.[13–15] Effective clinical team management involves the family in rehabilitation decisions and weighs management recommendations considering the immediate impact on the child's welfare and the long-term consequences on his or her appearance and function as an adult. An important resource is the Association of Children's Prosthetic-Orthotic Clinics (Rosemont, Illinois; http://www.acpoc.org). The association, founded in 1958, has held an annual interdisciplinary conference since 1972.

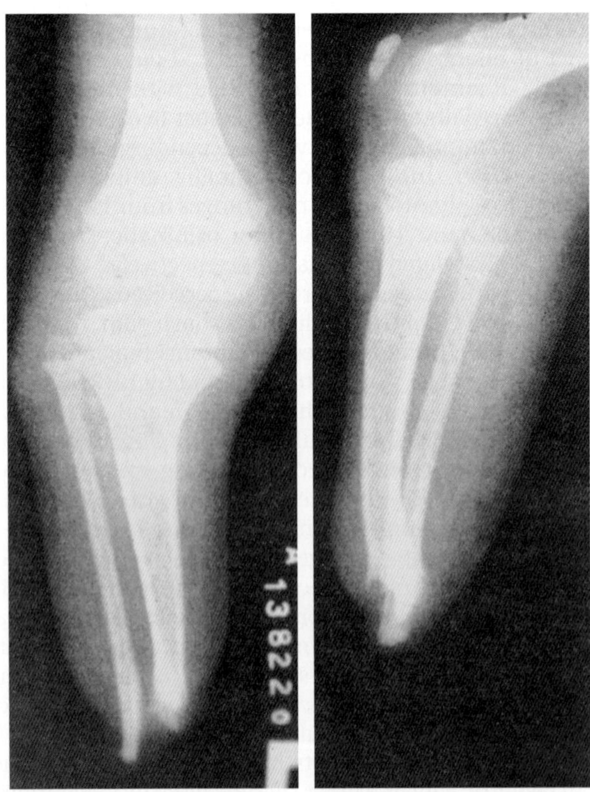

Fig. 29.2 Bony overgrowth of the fibula in the transtibial amputation limb of a 7-year-old child. In the original amputation surgery, the fibula was slightly shorter than the tibia. (Courtesy J.E. Edelstein.)

The clinical team creates an atmosphere where parents and their youngsters are welcome, encouraging conversation about feelings and obtaining answers to questions. The team's approach aims to maximize the child's function while learning the parents' style of dealing with unexpected events. Team members should empathize with parents' grief, which can bear little relation to the extent of the infant's disability. Some parents resist holding the baby, hide the deformity, avoid direct contact, or withdraw into silence. When clinicians hold the baby, parents usually realize the infant is lovable. Rather than denying any difference, the team fosters the attitude that they know the child is different but recognize and accept the infant for who the person is and what he or she can do.

Families may be interested in seeing pictures or examples of the type of prosthesis the child will probably use. However, expectations regarding the extent of prosthetic restoration may be unrealistic. Parents should understand what prosthetic and surgical possibilities exist so they can make rational decisions for their children. Infants usually receive the first prosthesis at approximately 6 to 9 months of age.[13,14] One study comparing children fitted with an upper-limb prosthesis before the age of 1 to those fitted later showed no significant difference in satisfaction or functional use of the prosthesis.[14] Some parents find it difficult to accept the prosthesis, believing it draws attention to the limb deficiency.

The team can also help parents of children who undergo amputation because of trauma or disease cope with guilt and shock. Team members assist the family in realizing that they were not negligent in protecting the child against injury or not recognizing symptoms of a disease process early enough to prevent amputation.

In addition to clinical team management, families benefit from peer support groups to share concerns, exchange information, and observe children of various ages playing with and without prostheses. Some groups publish newsletters sharing information with those far from the meeting site. The Amputee Coalition (Knoxville, Tennessee; www.amputee-coalition.org) is a peer advocacy organization that produces a magazine, monographs, and videos; has annual conferences; operates the National Limb Loss Information Center; and sponsors a youth camping program, national peer network, and limb-loss education and awareness program, among many other activities.

Parental acceptance of and active cooperation in the training program are the most important factors in its success and largely determine whether the child regards the prosthesis as a tool in daily activities.[12] Families need to learn skin care, prosthetic operation, maintenance, and the capabilities and limitations of the prosthesis. Outpatient training is preferable to avoid homesickness. The constant presence of one or both parents during therapy sessions enables the entire family to learn about prosthetic use and maintenance. Putting a prosthesis on an active child is a skill that takes time for parents to master. Scheduling appointments after naps and meals is generally more productive than attempting to coerce a tired, hungry child to participate in therapy. Clinicians should incorporate many brief activities in the treatment session, recognizing that young children have short attention spans. Therapists who treat infants must interpret nonverbal indications of comfort, discomfort, satisfaction, or dissatisfaction with the prosthesis. The infant who coos, smiles, and engages in play is probably content with the prosthesis and its function, whereas a cranky, crying person may be contending with an ill-fitting socket. As with all patients, the clinician must frequently examine the skin, particularly for persistent redness, indicating high pressure, and irritation, which may signal dermatitis.

Toddlers

Toddlers must develop self-control to acquire the autonomy necessary to cope with their environment. The interval between 1 and 3 years of age is characterized by developing language and functional communication, asserting independence, and interpersonal control. Children as young as 3 years should be informed of any impending surgery, whether to revise a congenital anomaly or treat disease or injury. Doll play can help the child to understand surgery and rehabilitation. Special dolls that depict amputations at various levels, with and without prostheses, are available from A Step Ahead Prosthetics (Hicksville, New York; www.weareastepahead.com).

Children must resolve feelings of deprivation and resentment accompanying the visible alteration of their bodies. Mobility, control, exploration, initiative, and creativity are prime emotional developmental milestones for older toddlers and young school-age children. Parents and professional staff should encourage the child's independence. Facile use of a prosthesis helps youngsters to achieve their psychological potential. Children compare themselves with others and ask, "Where is my other hand (or leg)?" Patients form two body images, one with and the other without the prosthesis. Parents should give a simple, truthful answer, clearly stating that the child will not grow another hand, saying something like "You were born this way." Similarly, toddlers who undergo amputation need a realistic answer to the question, "What happened to you?" The child may engage parents in a power struggle regarding prosthetic wearing. A firm yet gentle approach with a range of acceptable choices usually enables the youngster to incorporate autonomy needs while gaining prosthetic proficiency.

The clinical team should respect the parents' comments and involve the family in all aspects of care. The waiting room should have a variety of safe toys to make visits more pleasant. Parents should be present during the child's examination and prosthetic fitting to increase communication and thereby reduce anxiety and maximize the effectiveness of the prosthetic prescription and fitting process.

School-Age Children

School-age children need to become industrious and engaged in planning and executing tasks. The upper- or lower-limb prosthesis can be instrumental in fostering this important psychological task. The clinical team can help to prepare the child and family for encounters with teachers, scout masters, clergy, and other adults.

In group experiences, the student may have to deal with feelings of social devaluation. The teacher or other group leader can bolster the child's self-worth. The first day at school or camp can be the occasion for the child to display the prosthesis and demonstrate its function. The presentation usually dispels the mystery of the appliance and shows that a prosthesis is simply a tool that makes it easier for its wearer to engage in certain activities. The teacher should be aware of the appearance of the residual limb, the child's function with and without the prosthesis, any environmental or programmatic adaptations that may be advisable, and how to cope with prosthetic malfunction. Anticipating awkward situations helps to develop coping strategies. For example, in a circle game, classmates may be reluctant to hold hands with someone who wears an upper-limb prosthesis. If the teacher holds the child's prosthetic hook, the other students will likely realize that doing so is not scary or unacceptable. School officials may be concerned about the ability of a child with a prosthetic leg to maneuver in the classroom and playground. Classmates' natural curiosity should be dealt with through honest, simple answers. Although teasing is inevitable, the secure young student understands that taunts are merely crude expressions of interest.

Among school-age children with limb deficiencies, demographic variables (such as age, sex, socioeconomic status, and degree of limb loss) are not significant predictors of self-esteem. In contrast, social support, family functioning, self-perception, and microstressors affect the child's adaptation. Many school-age and older children respond favorably to scouting, camping, and other recreational activities. Sports programs, such as skiing, horseback riding, and track events, are fun and give children with disabilities pride in athletic achievement.

Older Children and Adolescents

Adolescents face the critical step of developing a satisfying identity within themselves and with their peers. The teenager may select times when prosthetic wear is not desirable (e.g., eschewing an upper-limb prosthesis during a football game or discarding the leg prosthesis when swimming or playing beach volleyball). Adults should nurture young adults, so they develop sufficient self-esteem to make satisfying decisions about when to use or remove the prosthesis. Teenagers with limb loss must cope with being visibly different. Young adults must adapt to a culture designed for those who do not have a disability and must evaluate whether people relate to them as individuals or as people with handicaps. Feelings such as "Why did this happen to me?" often intensify during adolescence. Adolescents constantly reexamine their body image; group showering after physical education class may be especially stressful for those with limb loss. Other developmental concerns in which limb loss plays a role are choosing a vocation, obtaining a driver's license, and engaging in sexual activity. The family and clinical team must be sensitive to privacy, confidentiality, and independence concerns.

Adolescents with bone cancer who undergo an amputation typically pass through a stage of initial impact when they learn that the treatment plan includes amputation. This news may be met with despair, discouragement, passive acceptance, or violent denial. Informing the adolescent of the rehabilitation process and the achievements of others can be helpful. The next stage is a retreat, during which the adolescent experiences acute grief. Anger may be part of the coping process. The goal of grieving is relinquishing hope of retrieving the lost object. The staff can reinforce the patient's strengths and encourage maximal independence. The third stage is acknowledgment, when the adolescent is willing to participate in rehabilitation and has incorporated the changed appearance into his or her body image. Reconstruction, the final stage, involves the return to developmentally appropriate activities, such as school, sports, and dating.

Upper-Limb Prosthesis

According to the ISO 9999 standards, a prosthesis is an orthopaedic aid that substitutes or partially substitutes a missing limb, providing both functional and aesthetic replacement. Prostheses must generally use fundamental characteristics such as functionality, pleasant esthetics, reliability, limited weight, and size. The prosthesis must become a tool that is part of the person; it must not cause discomfort or pain and must be practical.[15] Children's prosthetic needs are complex due to their small size, constant growth, and psychosocial development.[16] When dealing with the young amputee, it is necessary to simplify the prosthetic program so that it parallels motor development.[17] The rapid growth of their limbs requires the replacement of all or part of the prosthesis every year.[18] it has been demonstrated that children who start wearing prostheses before the age of 2 are less likely to abandon them[19]; therefore in the case of the pediatric age, prosthesis placement as early as possible is desirable.[15] Children who wear prostheses early, in fact, not only become able to function more successfully, but also grow up having incorporated the prosthesis into their body image. A child with a congenital condition can be fitted with a passive hand within 60 to 90 days of birth. This theoretically allows the child to acquire more normal bimanual and quadrupedal development.

The child with a traumatic or acquired amputation should ideally be mounted within 30 days to encourage prosthesis acceptance and continuation of bimanual activities.[17] In his early years, the child amputee rarely requires sophisticated equipment, often working well with very simple devices.[18] The international standard ISO 9999 identifies upper-limb prostheses in class 06 to 18 according to the level of amputation or congenital deformity in the order indicated: For the newborn and up to the age of 1½ years, we are moving towards the manufacture of passive prostheses that allow bimanual grip and therefore activities such as catching a ball and holding a bottle.

Children older than 3 years can be trained to control all available devices. Younger patients or those with congenitally deficient limbs sometimes lack sufficient neuromuscular control to operate complex devices. Passive, mechanical, and electrical elbows are all available to the child amputee.[15] The esthetic prostheses have the purpose of reconstructing the missing part allowing the restoration of the body image.[20] They move only passively. If properly positioned, elementary actions such as pressing buttons, writing, and so on, are possible for functional purposes.[21] Passive or esthetic prostheses of the traditional type have as their main function the esthetic one of resembling the natural limb; they are fixed prostheses that do not allow any type of movement other than the opposability of the thumb by means of a spring mechanism. Silicone esthetic prostheses are the most popular thanks to their versatility and compatibility for all types of amputations, high degree of customization, and complete adherence to the abutment.

The passive prostheses of the modular type are characterized by being made up of tubular and modular components capable of carrying out the load-bearing and functional function, leaving the esthetic role to a cover of spread material shaped with reference to the residual limb. What is obtained is an excellent esthetic result since the prosthesis is soft to the touch and has a high degree of customization.

This kind of prosthesis is mainly applied for transhumeral amputations and interscapular amputations. The advantages of passive prostheses appear to be lightness, reliability, resistance, and the absence of electric energy accumulators (batteries), but they have important disadvantages such as limited grip strength, numerous functional limitations mainly for important amputation levels, and more strenuous movements.[22] Functional prostheses aim at acquiring the fundamental grip and position movements compared to those of a healthy limbt.[20] It has been well established that children of all ages, including toddlers, can be trained to use externally powered prostheses.

Transradial is by far the most common and most successful level of amputation with these prostheses,[23] but they can be applied from wrist disarticulation up to shoulder disarticulation level.[22] Functional body energy prostheses (Kinematics) exploit the movement of a still active body part for the articulation of the prosthetic part of interest, using cables that are operated by harnesses. They are operated mechanically, placing cables in tension using particular movements: the abduction of the scapula by opening the hand, the elevation of the arm stump for elbow flexion, and the shoulder depression for locking and unlocking the elbow.[22] So, with this kind of prosthesis, the functions are limited to hand opening, flexion-extension, and blocking-unblocking of a possible elbow.[22]

They are generally well tolerated due to their relative lightness, reliability, robustness, and absence of electric accumulators, and allow the patient good feedback during their use; however, they are not able to develop a high gripping force and require a greater expenditure of energy than other active prostheses.

Myoelectric or electronically controlled extracorporeal energy functional prostheses use the energy supplied by accumulators to drive a direct current electric motor. The advantages of these prostheses are the high grip strength and the high degree of functionality, while the factors that may discourage the application of the above are the presence of electromyographic signals that are insufficient or cannot be controlled independently, as well as the weight which appears to be higher.[22]

Myoelectrically controlled prostheses exploit the electromyographic signals generated by the isometric contraction of the stump muscles to activate the functional elements of the prosthesis.

These signals, if of adequate intensity, varying between 40 and 100 μV, can be detected on the skin surface by specific electrodes, subsequently conveyed to an amplifier, and exploited to obtain a functional movement.

At 2 to 3 years of age, an instruction program using a myoelectric prosthesis can be undertaken.

The energy source is represented by a rechargeable accumulator at about 4.8 V in children's prostheses placed inside the socket.

A prerequisite for the application of a myoelectric prosthesis is the possibility for the patient to operate the muscle groups independently and voluntarily; for example, in the case in which the extensor muscles of the carpus are used to open the prosthetic hand and the flexors to close it.[18] Electrical games are used to train the selected muscle groups once the optimal sites have been identified.

In very young children with limb impairment, often only one muscle site is available for functional myocommand, enabling automatic hand opening and closing.[24] A myoelectric hand has a superior pinching force and is capable of controlled opening and closing throughout the full range of motion of the arm and can be operated independently of elbow function. However, it cannot be submerged in water, is heavier, and is not as adept at picking up smaller items.[18] Among the active extracorporeal energy prostheses, there are also electronically controlled prostheses that are generally used in cases of bony prominences that can activate pressure sensors, as occurs in cases of amelia or shoulder disarticulations.[15]

These devices make full use of external energy supplied by batteries. They function by pressing sensors with bony protrusions such as the acromion, using an anterior and a posterior sensor for the two components of a movement (flexion-extension), and a central button to divert energy to another area.[21] They function by pressing sensors with bony protrusions such as the acromion, using an anterior and a posterior sensor for the two components of a movement (flexion-extension), and a central button to divert energy to another area. In cases of phocomelia, the voluntary and easily controllable movement of the fingers at shoulder level can be used to activate microsensors, which then activate the various prosthetic components.[15]

Hybrid prostheses involve the use of a myoelectrically controlled hand combined with an elbow controlled by body energy. These prostheses have the advantage of having a lighter weight than the solution, which involves using an electromechanical elbow to ensure good functionality. However, they are not always applicable as the length of the transhumeral stump must generally be greater than the middle third. There must be good mobility of the shoulder to operate the braces.[22] Each prosthesis has its advantages and disadvantages and can often be combined. However, only one type of prosthesis should be used for the very young child, and as children mature, they should be given the opportunity to experiment with different ones.[18]

The worn prosthesis should not only be functional but also esthetically pleasing. The child is socially dependent.[17] The more cosmetic the prosthesis, the greater the possibility of a positive reaction by the child.[18] Electric drives and mechanical devices have been improved in recent years to meet the needs of children; however, the cost of maintenance and replacement is a barrier for many families.

Thanks to three-dimensional (3D) printing technology and open-source electronic prosthetics, it is now easier and cheaper to make a prosthetic mechanism than in the past.[16]

The use of these new production technologies has significantly lower costs; it allows the availability of sophisticated prostheses already from the first years of age, which can naturally accompany the child's growth up to adulthood.[25]

The prostheses with 3D printing, of high engineering at low costs, already from the first months or in the first years of life, are used as preparatory work for more complex devices on the bioengineering side. In fact, 3D printing allows you to set up rudimentary prostheses on the child from the first 6 months of life.

The dimensions are adapted to the progressive growth up to the definitive prosthesis. In addition to the low cost, these aids can perform small movements of opposition and grip through rudimentary electrical circuits. This functionality is sufficient to keep the plasticity of the cerebral cortex active in preparation for more sophisticated devices, such as the latest generation myoelectric prostheses.[24]

REHABILITATION OF CHILDREN WITH UPPER-LIMB AMPUTATION

Because functional use of an upper-limb prosthesis often involves control of a terminal device (substitute for the missing hand), the prosthetic design and the rehabilitation program should be appropriate for the child's motor, cognitive, and perceptual development levels.

Infants

Prosthetic fitting and training should complement an infant's development. Although a prosthesis usually is not fitted until babies are at least 6 months of age, earlier developmental accomplishment paves the way for successful prosthetic use (see Fig. 29.3).

The first prosthesis is usually passive (i.e., it does not have a cable or other operating mechanism). The terminal device may be a hook or a passive mitt. To disguise its mechanical appearance, the hook is covered with pink or brown resilient plastic. The plastic also blunts the impact of the hook as infants explore with it, swiping themselves and others in the vicinity. The hook may be a voluntary-opening design without a cable. Parents can place a rattle or other object in the hook to acquaint the baby with prehension on the deficient side. A few children start with the Child Amputee Prosthetics Project (University of California at Los Angeles, Los Angeles, California) terminal device (Fig. 29.4), which functions in the voluntary-opening mode. Some infants have a voluntary-closing hook on the first prosthesis (Fig. 29.5); without a cable, the hook holds the toy secured with tape or a rubber band. The three options offer little difference in function. A fourth terminal device option is the infant passive mitt. The mitt has a less mechanical appearance than other terminal devices but has no prehensile function; objects can be taped to it for the baby's amusement. The absence of a hooked configuration hampers the mitt use when the baby attempts to pull to standing at the side of the crib or playpen. Whatever the design, the terminal device is generally fitted into a wrist unit at the distal end of the socket.

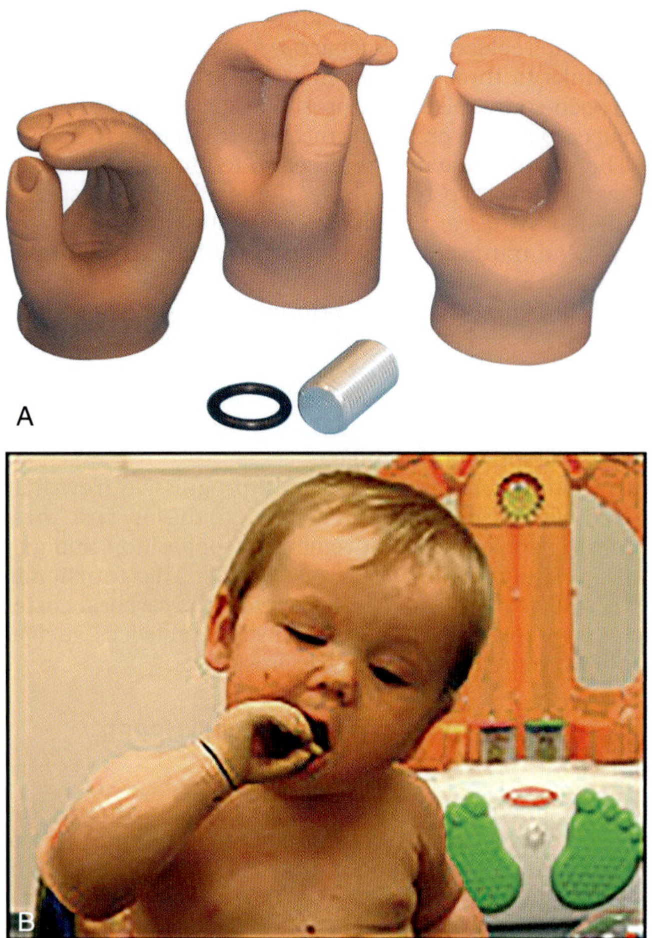

Fig. 29.3 Infant prosthetic hands. (A) Greek Series Hands are soft and flexible. (B) Infant mouthing on toy with Alpha hand. (A and B, Courtesy TRS, Inc., Boulder, Colorado.)

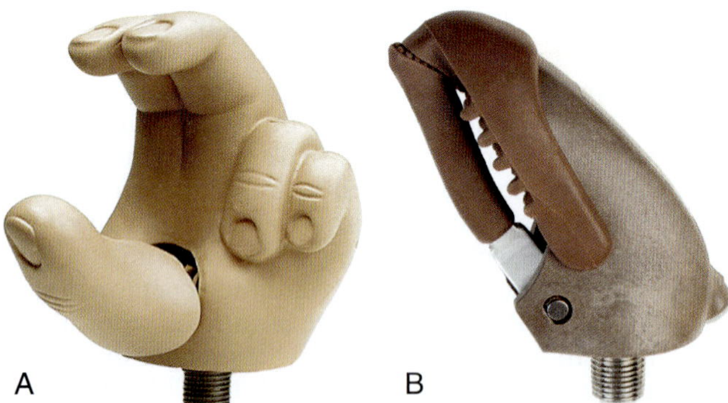

Fig. 29.4 Children's terminal devices. (A) Voluntary-closing hand. (B) CAPP (Child Amputee Prosthetics Project) voluntary-opening terminal device. (A, Courtesy TRS, Inc., Boulder, Colorado; B, Courtesy Fillauer Companies, Inc., Chattanooga, Tennessee.)

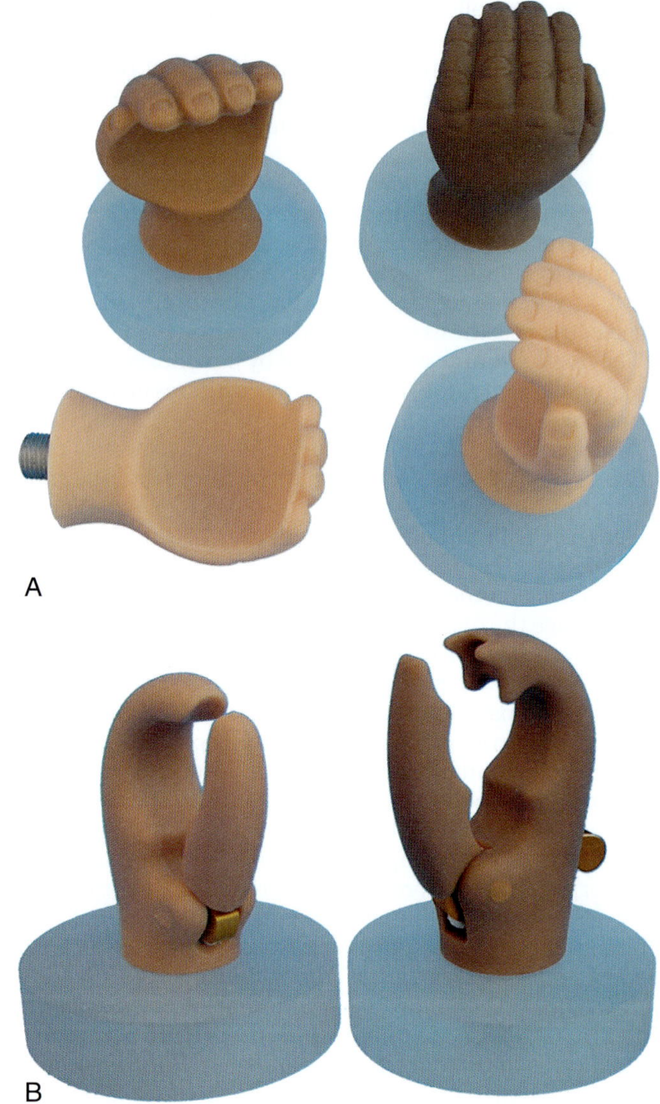

Fig. 29.5 Voluntary-closing terminal devices on prostheses. (A) Lite-Touch hand. (B) Adept hook. (Courtesy TRS, Inc., Boulder, Colorado.)

The thermoplastic socket may be custom molded to a plaster model of the child's residual limb. A fabric sock protects the skin from pressure concentration imposed by the socket. A snug fit is needed around the humeral epicondyles to stabilize the prosthesis on the child's residual limb. Changes may be needed every 2 to 4 months, depending on the growth rate. If the anomaly is higher, the first prosthesis usually does not have an elbow unit, even if the limb anomaly is comparable with transhumeral amputation.

Increasingly, prosthetic components, especially for children, are being created by 3D printing.[26] Medical application of 3D printing is additive manufacturing in which 3D objects, such as a prosthetic hand or socket, are created under computer control. The object is made by successively adding viscous plastic or other material. Alternative prosthetic fabrication is either subtractive, in which material is removed from a plaster model of the body part, or molded over a plaster model. 3D manufacturing dates from the 1980s. In most prosthetic applications, the patient's limb is scanned with a handheld device or photographed by a digital camera, thereby recording its shape and enabling the creation of a digital model. The rapidity of the 3D process is ideal for accommodating the need to create a larger socket or hand[27–30] when the patient has outgrown the previous device. The process has also been used to make a transhumeral prosthesis.[9]

Regardless of the level of limb loss, the prosthetic socket is suspended on the infant's torso by a harness, which typically has more straps than an adult harness. The toddler harness inhibits the infant's attempts to remove the prosthesis, deliberately or inadvertently, during rolling and crawling.

Clothing problems arise when a prosthesis is worn. The rigid parts of the prosthesis can cause holes in the fabric. Shirts and blouses worn over the prosthesis should be loose fitting. Raglan sleeves are roomier than sleeves set at the natural shoulder line; the latter can interfere with cable operation.

Training the infant fitted with a passive prosthesis usually begins with two sessions in 1 week and then at periodic follow-up appointments. The first meeting should be held when the baby is well rested and content. The therapist or parent puts the prosthesis on the infant, then places it on the floor with various toys. The therapist encourages the parents to play with and handle the baby while the infant wears the prosthesis. The baby may ignore the prosthesis because its socket eliminates the sense of touch and because the length of the prosthesis feels awkward. Parents should present large toys that require the use of both arms. The basic prosthesis allows the infant to cuddle a teddy bear, swat at a dangling toy, and use both upper limbs for rolling and crawling. Training involves instructing the parents, siblings, and other caregivers to gain familiarity with the prosthesis, care for the infant's skin by ensuring that the socket and harness do not exert undue pressure, and provide toys that require bimanual prehension (Box 29.1). Placing a rattle or other noise maker in the terminal device is another way to acquaint the infant with a grasp of limb deficiency. At the end of the session, the therapist and parent remove the prosthesis to inspect the child's skin for signs of irritation from the socket or harness. Parents learn how to apply the prosthesis and how to encourage full-time wear except during baths, naps, and bedtime. The youngster may be awkward when sitting and moving while adjusting to the weight of the prosthesis. Toys suitable for the child's developmental level, such as large balls, dolls, stuffed animals, balloons, xylophones, and other noisy and colorful objects, provide incentives for enjoying the prosthesis. Parents can put a mallet or other toy in the hook so the infant can enjoy using the prosthesis. Push and pull toys are appropriate when the child can stand and cruise.[31] Arranging blocks is a good activity for the new prosthesis wearer.[32]

Box 29.1 Prosthetic Training Goals for Infants

Therapy sessions are designed to increase the infant's:
- Comfort with the prosthesis
- Wearing tolerance
- Ability to clasp large objects
- Ability to use the prosthesis to aid in sitting and crawling

Parents of an infant with a prosthesis should:
- Apply and remove the prosthesis correctly
- Care for the child's skin
- Care for the prosthesis
- Recognize and report to the clinical team any problems with the prosthesis or child

Printed instructions, augmented by audiotapes or videotapes, are useful guides for the family. Instructions can address parental concerns regarding the possibility that the child may catch the prosthesis on table legs or use it to strike themselves or others; children recover balance readily, and peers can usually defend themselves.

Ideally, the therapist can assess the parents' experiences at the second training session a few days later. Donning and doffing the prosthesis should be reviewed. Initially, the child may tolerate the prosthesis only for a few minutes. It should be frequently applied during the day. Eventually, the youngster should be able to wear it most of the day, except when sleeping and bathing.

Subsequent follow-up sessions focus on the adequacy of prosthetic fit and the child's readiness for the addition of a cable to the prosthesis or substitution of a myoelectrically controlled prosthesis for a passive one, or, in the case of the child with transhumeral amputation, the addition of an elbow unit.

Toddlers

When the child is between the ages of 15 and 18 months, control cables may be added to traditional, body-operated prostheses (Fig. 29.6). Active control may not become reliable until the toddler is approximately 2.5 years of age when the understanding of cause and effect is well established. Readiness for the cable is indicated when the child wears the prosthesis full time, can follow simple instructions, has an attention span of at least 5 minutes, and will allow the therapist and prosthetist to handle him or her. A toddler who resists instruction from someone other than the parent may be too immature to learn to control the prosthesis.

If the prosthesis has a voluntary-opening hook, it should be fitted with a half- or a quarter-width rubber band to facilitate opening. The tension in the terminal device should be sufficient to let the child hold objects but not so great that

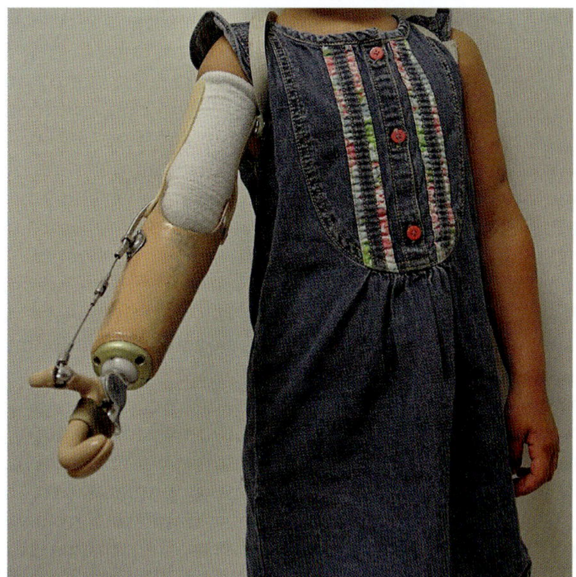

Fig. 29.6 Toddler with congenital transverse upper-limb difference using a body-powered prosthesis. (From Le JT, Scott-Wyard PR. Pediatric limb difference and amputations. *Phys Med Rehabil Clin N Am*. 2015;26(1):95–108.)

Box 29.2 Prosthetic Training Goals for Toddlers

Therapy sessions are designed to increase the toddler's:
- Control of the terminal device
- Control of the elbow unit
- Use of the prosthesis in bimanual prehension
- Use of the prosthesis in functional activities

Parents of toddlers with prostheses should:
- Provide toys that require bimanual prehension
- Encourage use of the prosthesis as an assistive device
- Inspect the skin to determine whether the prosthesis causes undue irritation

opening the hook is difficult. Young children use the voluntary-closing hook as easily as traditional voluntary-opening terminal devices. Box 29.2 summarizes the goals of prosthetic training for toddlers.

The training environment should be quiet, with a low table holding a few toys that require a bimanual grasp, such as large beads and a string with a rigid tip. For the child with unilateral amputation, the terminal device holds an object, such as a bead, while the child threads the string through the bead. The therapist is on the child's prosthetic side, holding the child's forearm at 90 degrees of elbow flexion, the optimal position for cable operation. This position also keeps the terminal device and the grasped object within the child's view. The adult moves the child's forearm forward, flexing the shoulder, tensing the cable, and causing the hook to operate. The terminal device changes position when the arm is moved back (shoulder extension). A voluntary-opening hook opens with shoulder flexion, whereas a voluntary-closing hook closes with shoulder flexion. The therapist encourages the child to help with the control motion. With either design, the initial training involves placing a toy in the hook and encouraging the child to discover how to keep it in place. With a voluntary-opening hook, the child simply relaxes to allow the rubber bands or springs to keep the hook fingers closed. The voluntary-closing hook requires the wearer to exert tension on the control cable by the harness to keep the hook closed. Children use the same control motions as adults, namely shoulder flexion or shoulder girdle protraction, for terminal device operation. The toddler may revert to the earlier practice of opening the terminal device with the sound hand; eventually, he or she will find that cable operation is more efficient, allowing more complex bimanual play maneuvers.

Reaching for objects with the sound hand is the child's initial preference. To provide the child the necessary practice with the prosthesis, the therapist or parent should offer large objects or toys that require a bimanual grasp to operate. Another technique to encourage prosthetic use is to have the child hold one object in the sound hand and another in the prosthesis. For example, two handbells are twice as tuneful as one. For some young patients, prosthetic training merely involves using the terminal device as a stabilizer rather than as a prehensile tool; for example, the child may lean the prosthesis onto a mailbox replica while placing objects in the slot with the sound hand. The prosthesis also stabilizes paper while the child draws and colors pictures.

Although children as young as 18 months have been fitted with myoelectrically controlled transradial prostheses, those who are at least 3 years of age have an easier time learning to contract the appropriate flexors and extensors to close and open the hand (see Fig. 29.6). The prosthesis is heavier, more fragile, and needs more maintenance than does a cable-operated device. Weight should be gradually added to the passive prosthesis to prepare the child for a myoelectric prosthesis. Rudimentary training begins with practice with the prosthesis of the arm. At first, the therapist may place an electrode on the sound forearm and ask the child to flex and extend the wrist to close and open the fingers of the prosthetic hand. The therapist then places an electrode on the forearm on the amputated side and encourages the child to discover that contraction of the forearm musculature on that side achieves the same results. Motorized toys can be used to help the child practice deliberate contraction of flexors and extensors to cause an electric train, for example, to go backward and forward, depending on which electrode is stimulated. The prosthetic socket can be made with electrodes when the child gains reasonable proficiency. Care must be taken to achieve and maintain a snug fit so that the electrodes are in constant contact with the skin. Empirical evidence regarding functional differences between cable- and myoelectrically operated prostheses for children is lacking.[33]

Fitting a myoelectrically controlled transradial prosthesis before the patient is 2 years old has been associated with greater long-term acceptance.[34–36]

Whether the prosthesis is cable or myoelectrically controlled, practice to gain prosthetic proficiency is the same. The beginner experiences many instances of dropping objects while learning the muscle contraction or cable tension needed to maintain suitable terminal device closure. The ability to close the terminal device around an object develops before active release. Grasping an object from the tabletop is difficult. Children attempting to put objects into their mouths discover that the change in shoulder position alters the tension on the control cable. Similarly, children who drop toys and try to retrieve them from the floor discover how to hold their shoulders to maintain adequate cable tension. Those wearing myoelectrically controlled prostheses also notice that the prosthesis is easier to operate in some forearm positions than in others.

Moving pegs on a board affords the child practice in opening and closing the terminal device. Tossing a beanbag or playing card games are useful for teaching terminal device opening and closing. Cutting paper is another satisfying activity. The child holds the paper in the terminal device and uses the scissors in the sound hand. Prosthetic training should acquaint the child with objects of various textures, sizes, and shapes. Resilient foam toys are easier to grasp than those made of rigid material. Playing with sewing cards, nested barrels, and snap-apart beads; removing objects from a drawstring bag; opening a zipper; removing loose clothing; opening small boxes of raisins; opening and closing felt-tipped pens; and playing the xylophone entice the child to attempt grasping, holding, and releasing motions with the terminal device. Moving checkers or other markers from one location to another on a game board is a good drill. The prosthesis is helpful when swinging and climbing on the playground, rolling a wheelbarrow or doll carriage, jumping rope, and riding a tricycle. Children with unilateral amputation usually regard the intact limb as the dominant one. Many children with unilateral amputation refer to the prosthesis as the helper, which correctly identifies its role as a device that assists the intact hand.

Functional training depends on the child's ability to reach the mouth, waist, hips, feet, and perineum. Feeding, dressing, writing, and personal hygiene are incorporated at the appropriate times. Thirty-month-old children can throw and catch a ball, start uncomplicated dressing, and eat with a spoon with minor spillage. Children play in sand, earth, and water and engage in rough-and-tumble activities, which can damage the prosthesis and the skin. Daily inspection and attention to minor problems help to avoid major prosthetic repairs and skin disorders.

A 2-year-old with transhumeral amputation may have a prosthesis with an elbow unit, although mastery of the elbow-locking cable is unlikely to occur before the third birthday. Strategies to self-manage donning and doffing the prosthesis can be introduced to children as young as 3. Most find removing the prosthesis easier than donning it.

At 3 years of age, the child may begin to be curious about the rotational possibilities of the wrist unit. Objects of various shapes within reach oblige the child to turn the terminal device in the wrist unit to the suitable position. Most objects can be manipulated with the terminal device in the pronated position; however, paper and other thin items are more easily managed with the terminal device in mid-position, and small balls are best cradled in the terminal device when rotated to the supinated position. Holding the handlebars of a tricycle or manipulating hand controls in other wheeled toys helps the child to learn how to use terminal device rotation in the wrist unit. Prosthetic activities for the toddler should include eating, drinking, dressing, and managing crayons and other writing implements. Three-year olds blow soap bubbles, pull up pants, pull a belt through loops in pants, and fill a cup with water from a spigot.

Throughout the toddler phase, work periods should alternate with free play that may or may not involve the prosthesis. Weekly training sessions are effective. Parents should inspect the axilla; persistent redness indicates the harness is applying undue pressure. The home program should include written suggestions regarding activities to promote bimanual prehension, instructions concerning the care of the prosthesis and the care of the child's skin, terminology pertaining to parts of the prosthesis, and ideas regarding clothing that will not impede prosthetic function.

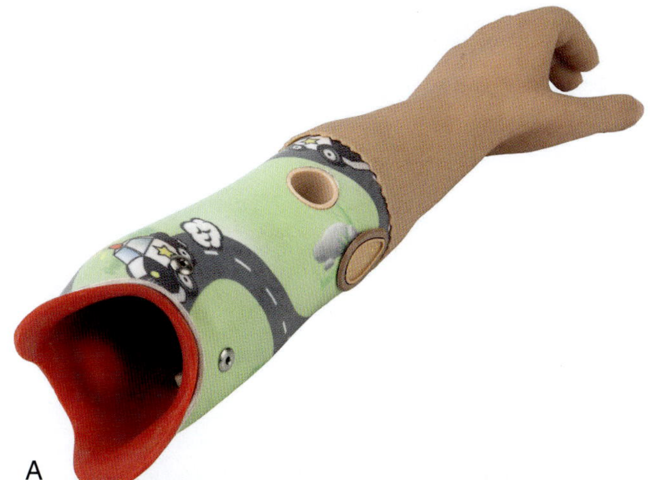

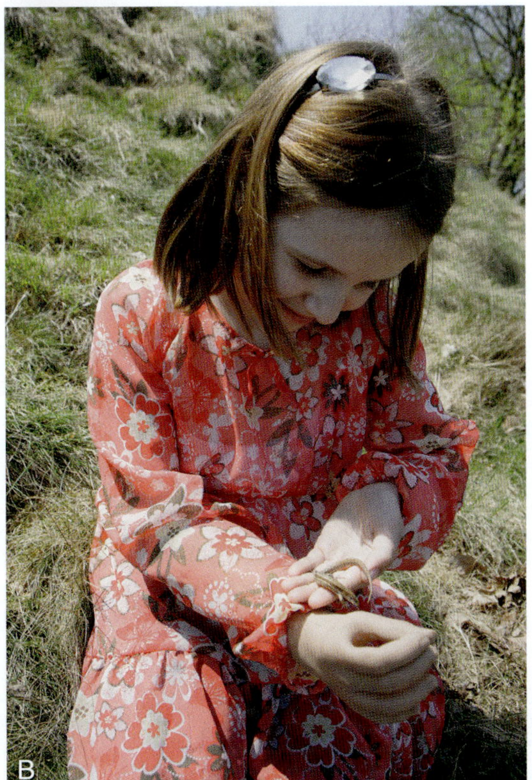

Fig. 29.7 (A) Myoelectric prosthesis. (B) Girl contracting forearm muscles to operate a myoelectrically controlled terminal device. (Courtesy Ottobock Orthopedic Industry, Inc., Minneapolis, Minnesota.)

School-Age Children

An important consideration for the growing child is a large socket for a comfortable fit and adequate prosthetic control.

The 4-year-old child is usually coordinated enough to grasp fragile objects without breaking or crushing them. With a voluntary-opening hook, the child must maintain tension on the control cable to prevent the hook fingers from snapping shut. A voluntary-closing terminal device necessitates the application of gentle tension on the cable rather than forceful shoulder motion. With a myoelectrically controlled hand, the child must contract flexors minimally so that the fingers close on the object without undue pressure (Fig. 29.7). Four-year-olds can pour from containers, peel a banana, sharpen a pencil with a handheld sharpener, sew, hammer nails, and apply adhesive bandages (Fig. 29.8). The average 5-year-old can open a milk container and sweep with a brush and dustpan. Box 29.3 summarizes the goals of prosthetic training for school-age children. Performing an activity with the sound hand may facilitate accomplishing the same task with the prosthesis.[37]

Assessing the ability of a child to grasp various objects may include stringing four large beads, opening four 35-mm film cans, separating three nested screw-top barrels, assembling 10 interlocking beads, and separating a five-piece notched plastic block. More challenging activities are using a sewing card, stringing small beads, sticking an adhesive bandage to the table, cutting a paper circle

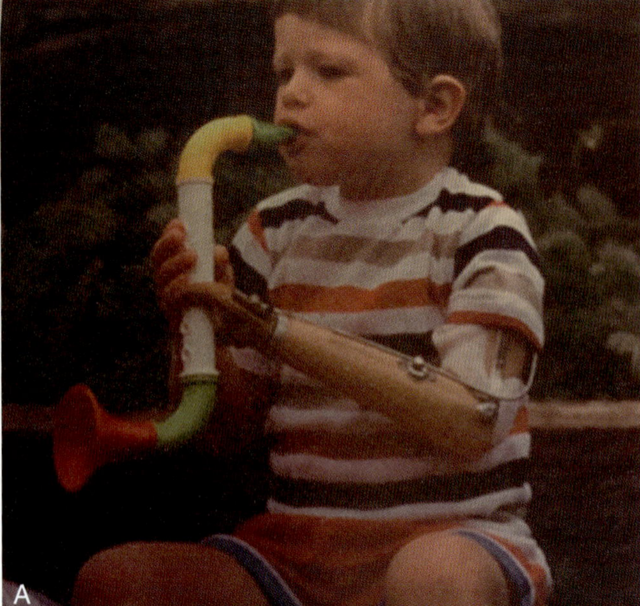

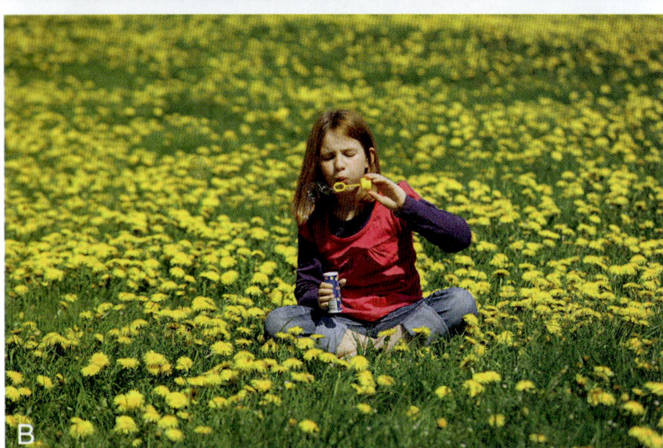

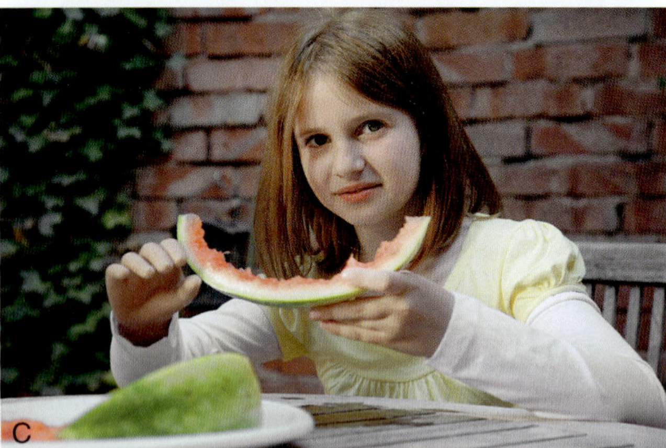

Fig. 29.8 Bimanual activities. (A) Playing a toy saxophone. (B) Blowing bubbles. (C) Girl wearing right prosthesis while eating watermelon. (A, Courtesy TRS, Inc., Boulder, Colorado; B and C, Courtesy Ottobock Orthopedic Industry, Inc., Minneapolis, Minnesota.)

and gluing it to another paper, and opening a small package of facial tissues. The most demanding tasks include cutting modeling plastic with a knife and fork, discarding five playing cards from a hand of 10 cards, lacing a shoe and making a bow, and wrapping a book.

Box 29.3 Prosthetic Training Goals for School-Age Children

Therapy sessions assist the school-age child to:
- Maintain proper prosthetic fit
- Grasp firm and fragile objects without dropping or crushing them
- Open and close the terminal device reliably
- Don and doff the prosthesis independently
- Dress independently
- Recognize when the prosthesis needs repair or alteration

Parents of school-aged children with prostheses should:
- Ensure their child is independent in daily activities and play

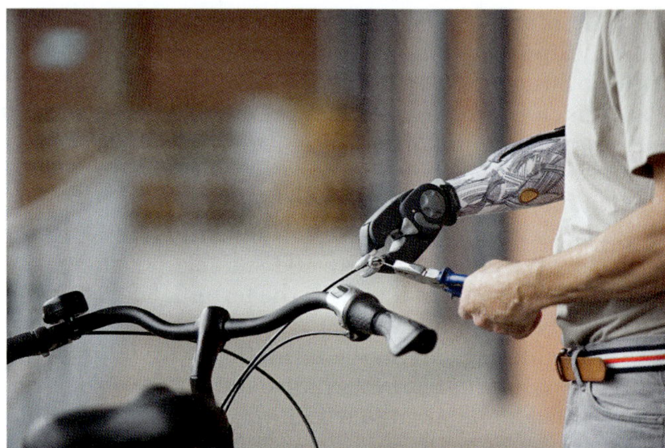

Fig. 29.9 Myoelectric Greifer terminal device on right transradial prosthesis. (Courtesy Ottobock Orthopedic Industry, Inc., Minneapolis, Minnesota.)

Card games often fascinate children in elementary school. Maintaining several cards in the terminal device and then releasing the desired card involves a gradation of tension on the control cable for prostheses equipped with a voluntary-opening or -closing terminal device. Card playing is more difficult with a myoelectrically controlled prosthesis because the child must contract the forearm flexors and extensors with the correct amount of force at the appropriate time. The 5-year-old should dress independently, except for small buttons, shoelaces, pullover shirts, and sweaters. The child must also learn how to care for the prosthesis, keep it clean, and ask for help when parts malfunction. Skin inspection is an essential part of training.

Older Children and Adolescents

Many children and adolescents can incorporate prostheses into school activities. A myoelectric hook terminal device (Fig. 29.9) may be practical for teenagers interested in repairing bicycles and cars. Sports prostheses, such as those with a terminal device designed to hold a basketball, give wearers more opportunities to participate in group activities (Fig. 29.10).[38] Teenagers may find that playing a musical instrument is pleasurable. Simple adaptations, such as fingering a trumpet with the sound hand and supporting it with the prosthesis, can open a world of enjoyment to the

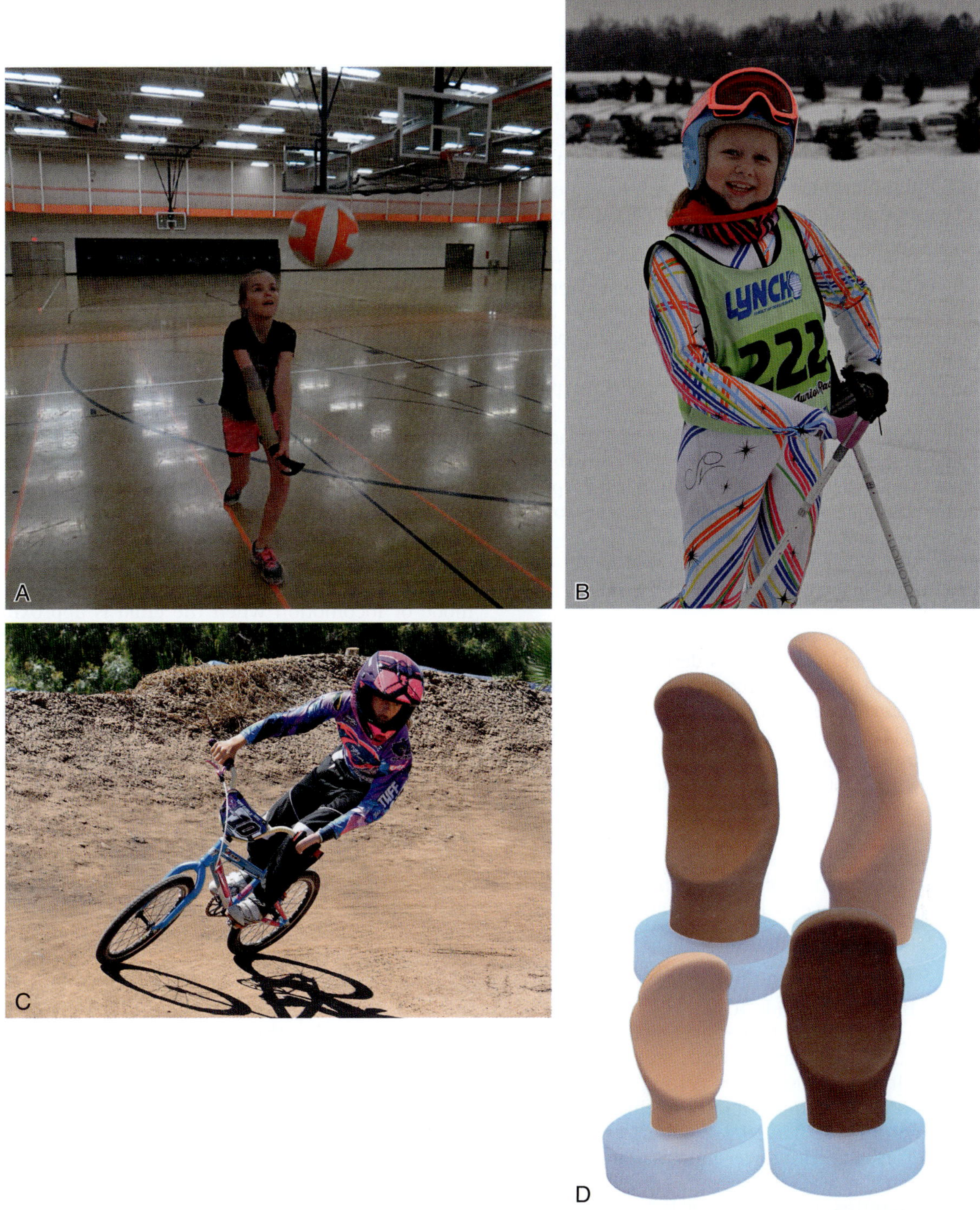

Fig. 29.10 Activity-specific terminal devices. (A) Girl playing volleyball with Barrage terminal device. (B) Girl downhill skiing with right Downhill Racer Ski terminal device. (C) Girl mountain biking wearing a transradial prosthesis with Swinger terminal device. (D) SuperSport terminal device. (C, Courtesy M.A. Sweezy and TRS, Inc., Boulder, Colorado.)

musician. Older adolescents should have vocational exploration, vocational assessment, and, when indicated, job training. Obtaining a driver's license is a meaningful event for most teenagers. Using a prosthesis does not influence the capacity to drive; however, those with upper-limb deficiency are more likely to use adaptive devices when driving than those with lower-limb deficiency.[39,40]

Some adolescents with unilateral limb deficiency seek escape from parental control by abandoning their prostheses, preferring to manage with the intact limb. Peer acceptance and social integration appear to be more important for adolescents than the functional benefits that may be achieved with prosthetic use.[41] Certain activities are more easily accomplished without the prosthesis or cannot be done with a prosthesis. For example, prostheses are not worn when showering. Individuals with transradial amputation may prefer to use elbow flexion to stabilize objects in the antecubital fossa rather than use a prosthetic terminal device. Simple equipment adaptation can facilitate one-handed performance, such as using a book holder, guitar pick band, or camera grip. Some individuals become facile with the remaining upper limb, learning to hit a baseball and folding laundry with one hand. Most people develop strategies that enable them to perform all desired activities.[42]

The function of children fitted with unilateral upper prostheses can be measured by the Prosthetic Upper Extremity Functional Index administered to parents and older children[43] or the similar University of New Brunswick Test of Prosthetic Function (UNB).[44] Results from formal testing compare favorably with questionnaires regarding prosthetic use.[45]

Older children report quality of life about the same for those who do and do not wear prostheses,[46] with prostheses used for specific activities.[47] Overall, children with upper-limb deficiency are as socially competent as able-bodied peers.[48]

REHABILITATION OF CHILDREN WITH LOWER-LIMB LOSS

Children with lower-limb deficiencies deserve clinic team management similar to that described for those with upper-limb deficiencies. Early referral to a clinical team is equally important for the family with a child who has a lower-limb amputation or limb deficiency. Peer support is also invaluable for parents who must share concerns, suggestions, and camaraderie with others coping with a similar situation. Treatment should suit the patient's developmental stage so that prosthetic use fosters the achievement of key milestones.[49] Parents serve as the primary instructors of their children, with the guidance of the physical therapist and other members of the clinical team.

Infants

Sitting balance is a major guide to lower-limb prosthetic fitting. The average age when babies accomplish independent sitting is 6 months. Sitting depends on postural control and antigravity muscle strength. Sitting balance and trunk stabilization are also important for freeing the hands to explore the environment. Box 29.4 summarizes the rehabilitation goals of infants with lower-limb malformation or amputation.

Infants 5 to 7 months of age discover the mobility possibilities of crawling and creeping, moving from supine to four-point and sitting positions, and moving to the hands and knees from the sitting position. Crawling involves the alternate action of the opposite arms and legs as in walking. Hip extensors strengthen during crawling and kneeling. Rocking on four points before crawling is another important precursor to walking.

Most babies can overcome gravity to pull up to a standing position and rise from kneeling to standing at approximately 8 months. When pulling to a standing position, the baby expends great energy bouncing and actively disturbing balance. Bouncing gradually gives way to shifting weight from side to side. The initial standing posture is wide based, with the hips abducted, flexed, and externally rotated. The base accommodates the child's new center of gravity position, which is higher than when crawling. Maintaining an upright posture depends on sufficient maturity of the visual, proprioceptive, and vestibular systems.

Box 29.4 Prosthetic Training Goals for Infants With Lower-Limb Deficiency

Therapy sessions are designed to facilitate the infant's:

- Comfort with the prosthesis
- Wearing tolerance
- Ability to stand by leaning against a table
- Ability to cruise around furniture
- Ability to walk with and without support from a doll carriage or other supporting toy

Parents of infants with lower-limb prostheses should:

- Apply and remove the prosthesis correctly
- Care for the child's skin
- Care for the prosthesis
- Recognize and report any problems with the prosthesis

Stepping movements are common among 7-month-olds who are supported. Cruising along furniture is a preferred mode of locomotion when the child is approximately 10 months old. Cruising strengthens the hip abductors. The typical nondisabled child stands alone at approximately 11 months and walks alone at 12 months.[16] The urge to walk is the culmination of the endless pulling and standing activity that has occupied the baby for several preceding months.

Some infants undergo surgery either to transform a congenitally anomalous limb into one that is more suitable for a prosthesis or as part of the treatment of a limb that has been involved in trauma or in the presence of a tumor. In these instances, skin grafting does not result in adverse functional outcomes.[50] Another intervention applicable to a few children is limb lengthening using an Ilizarov apparatus.[51,52] For children born with proximal focal femoral deficiency, where there is a shortening of the thigh with an intact foot, a knee rotationplasty is often performed. This involves sectioning the limb and rotating the distal portion posteriorly; the foot thus serves as a partial leg, enabling fitting with a transtibial prosthesis (Fig. 29.11).[53,54] Very few children with myelodysplasia undergo amputation of lower limbs that have severe contractures or have intractable ulcers.[55]

Regardless of the etiology of limb deficiency, prosthetic fitting aims to facilitate the child's attainment of motor milestones. The infant who is missing a lower limb should have prosthetic restoration at approximately 6 months when the baby has enough trunk control for sitting and is ready to pull to a standing position. A simple prosthesis fosters symmetric sitting balance and aids the baby's attempts to pull to standing. In addition, the prosthesis equalizes leg length, adds weight to the anomalous side, and obviates the tendency to compensate with a one-legged standing pattern. Reducing the weight asymmetry inherent in limb deficiency facilitates rotational control of the trunk. The prosthesis enables standing and walking. Otherwise, the world is circumscribed by the confines of the stroller or playpen, and the deficiency becomes a source of shame. Fitting before

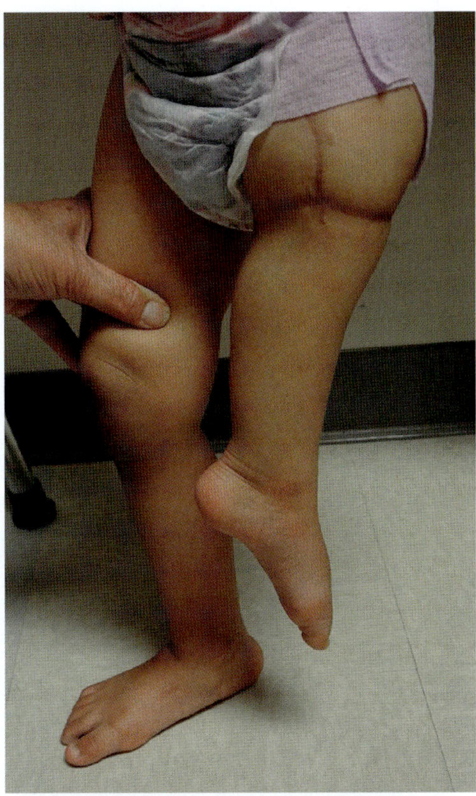

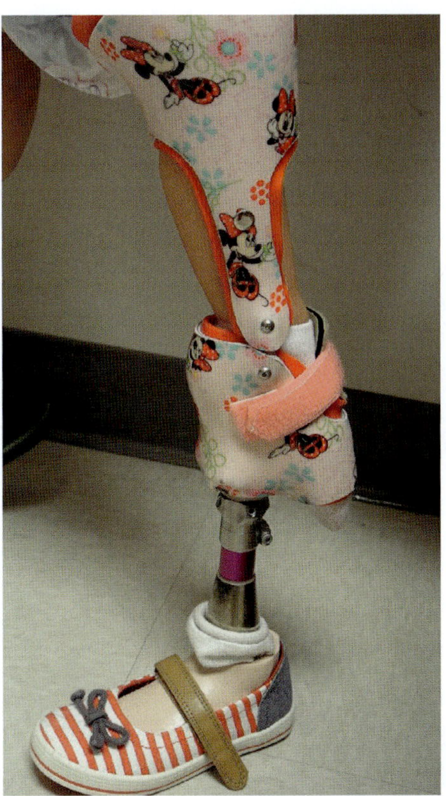

Fig. 29.11 (A) A child with proximal focal femoral deficiency after rotationplasty (B). Same child from (A), now wearing prosthesis. The presence of ankle function offers superior control and function over a mechanical prosthetic knee. (From Le JT, Scott-Wyard PR. Pediatric limb difference and amputations. *Phys Med Rehabil Clin N Am*. 2015;26(1):95–108.)

6 months might hinder the baby's efforts to turn from prone to a supine position and back again.

The first prosthesis includes a solid-ankle, cushion-heel foot, the smallest foot manufactured (Fig. 29.12). Rubber-soled shoes give the infant more traction and are therefore preferable to leather-soled shoes. The prosthesis must be comfortable when the baby stands, sits, squats, crawls, and climbs. A silicone socket liner (Fig. 29.13) is desirable to protect sensitive skin from chafing in the socket. The toddler with transfemoral amputation may start with a prosthesis having a locked knee (Fig. 29.14).[56,57] Another type of knee joint available to the pediatric population is a polycentric knee (Fig. 29.15). A four-bar linkage system allows the axis of motion to be posterior during stance, allowing greater stability, and anterior during swing to assist in clearance. Polycentric knee units are incorporated into prostheses for young toddlers and often into the child's first prosthesis. Teenagers are often fitted with hydraulic-, pneumatic-, or microprocessor-controlled knees that allow for greater variability of movement and physical activities. The drawbacks to hydraulic and pneumatic knees are added weight, cost, and intricacy of adjustments, so they are typically reserved for the adolescent population.

During the first training session, the therapist and parent confirm that the prosthesis fits comfortably, without redness of the residual limb. Most of the handling of the child should be done by the parent rather than the therapist, so that the family gains confidence in managing the child at home. Useful equipment includes a play table, an elevated sandbox, a floor mat, a rolling stool, a full-length mirror, steps, and a ramp. The parent should encourage the child to stand on both feet by supporting the trunk and gradually reducing the support. The young child gains prosthetic tolerance and standing balance by being near the table. Initially, the child may lean the torso against the table while manipulating toys that require both hands. Toys should be moved to places on the table where the child must reach in different directions, shifting weight. Eventually, the child will move along the table's periphery to place objects in the desired location. When first learning to walk with a prosthesis, the child moves cautiously. Initially, the child takes small steps and has a wide base, keeping the trunk upright and arms abducted. The new prosthesis wearer resembles normal peers who begin walking with increased hip and knee flexion, full-foot initial contact, short stride, increased cadence, and relative foot drop on the sound side in the swing phase.[14–16]

At home, a sturdy table chest high for the child encourages standing balance and cruising during play with toys on the table. Raised sandboxes, blocks, finger paints, and pans of water with floating toys all promote standing balance. A playpen is a good environment for the baby to pull to standing, cruise the perimeter, and sit when the baby wishes. Balls are useful in prosthetic training. Kicking a ball requires balance on one leg and flexion of the other leg. The baby starts by holding on to a stable object with both hands, then with one, and eventually letting go. Throwing a ball requires good balance and usually sustains the infant's interest. Wheeled toys, such as a doll carriage, enable the child to walk with a modicum of support. Placing toys

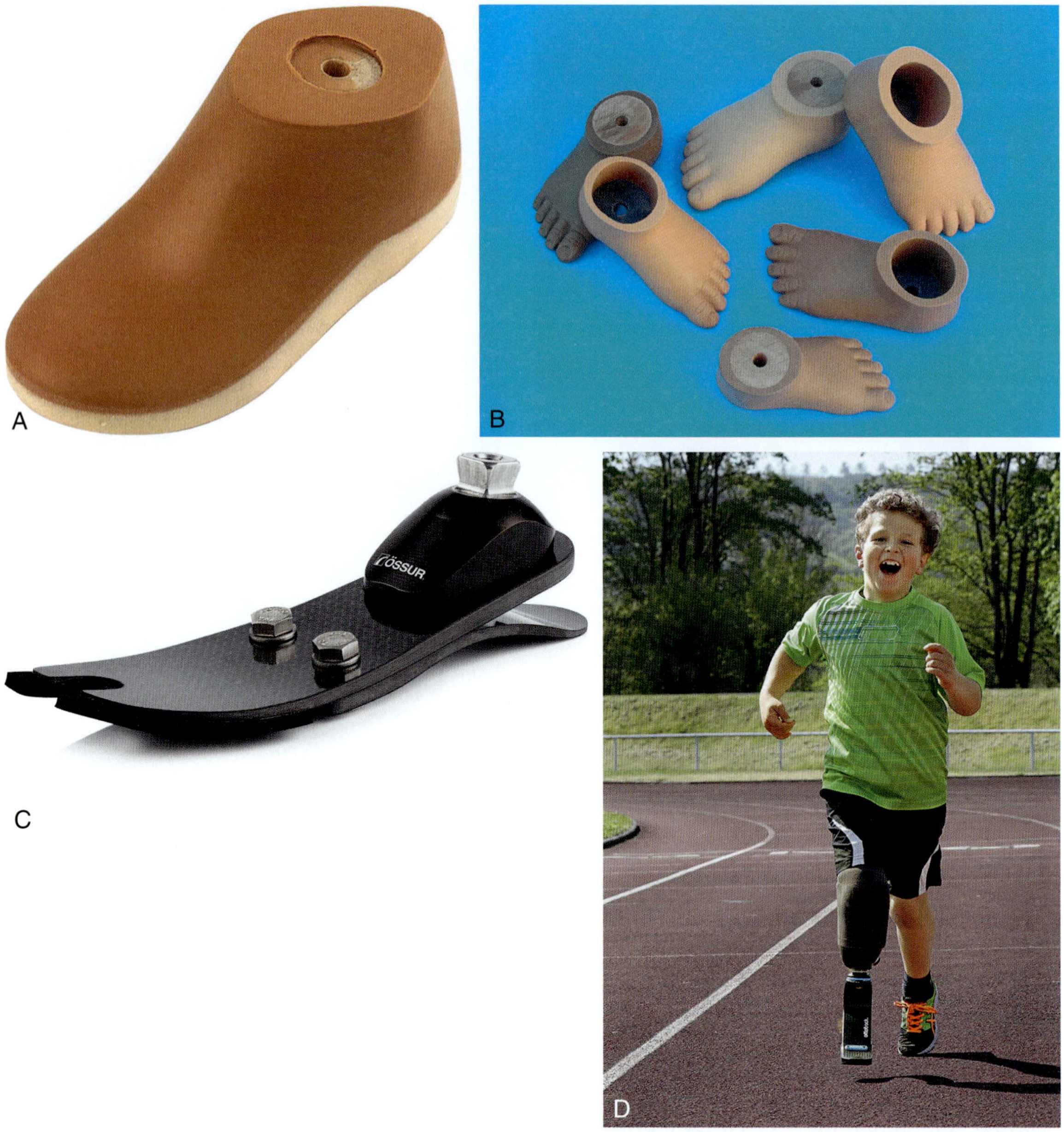

A

B

C

D

Fig. 29.12 Children's prosthetic feet. (A) Solid-ankle, cushion-heel (SACH) foot. (B) SACH feet adaptable for crawling and walking. (C) Flex Foot Junior. (D) Boy running while wearing transtibial prostheses with Runner Junior feet. (A and D, Courtesy Ottobock Orthopedic Industry, Inc., Minneapolis, Minnesota; B, Courtesy TRS, Inc., Boulder, Colorado; C, © Össur.)

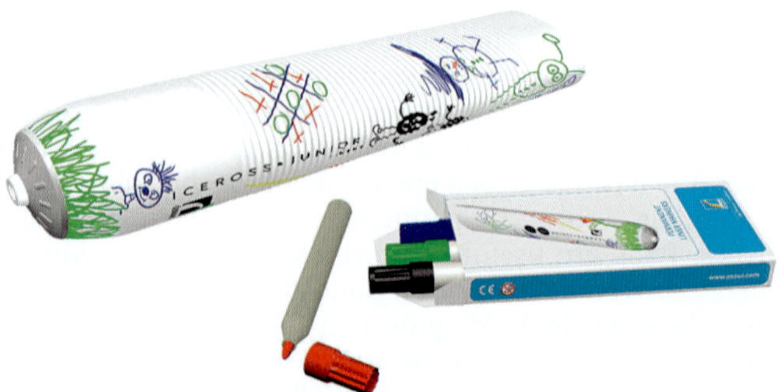

Fig. 29.13 Silicone socket liner suspension system. Uses a pin-locking mechanism to attach to the distal end of the socket. (© Össur.)

where the child must take a few steps to reach them fosters independent walking.

Young children frequently revert to crawling and sitting on the floor as they grow accustomed to the prosthesis. Falling is seldom a problem since the child generally lands on the buttocks as a nondisabled child would. When the child falls or tries to retrieve a toy on the floor, the parents and therapist should let the young person explore the movement and not be overly protective. Just as other children learn to walk by supporting themselves on furniture, the child who wears a prosthesis should have the same experience to develop confidence. Parallel bars, walkers, and harnesses are seldom advisable for children with unilateral or bilateral transtibial amputation.

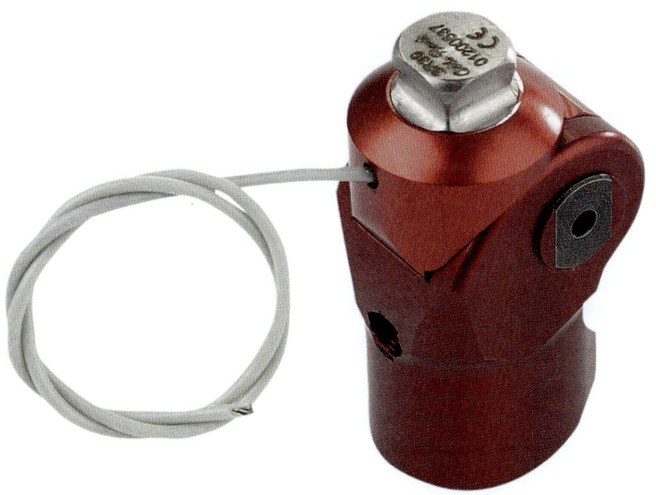

Fig. 29.14 Single-axis knee units with manual lock. (Courtesy Ottobock Orthopedic Industry, Inc., Minneapolis, Minnesota.)

A prosthesis imposes weight-bearing loads on portions of the leg not ordinarily used for this purpose. Consequently, building tolerance to prosthetic wear is important so that skin overweight-bearing areas can adjust to the pressure. During the first week, most infants tolerate 1 hour of wear, after which the prosthesis should be removed, and the skin examined. The prosthesis can be reapplied for another hour after a 10- to 15-minute rest period. Signs of fatigue, limping, and the avoidance of standing on the prosthesis indicate that the prosthesis is irritating and should be removed. The infant with a transfemoral prosthesis should be checked to determine whether skin near the proximal part of the prosthesis is irritated by urine or feces, which may leak from the diaper.

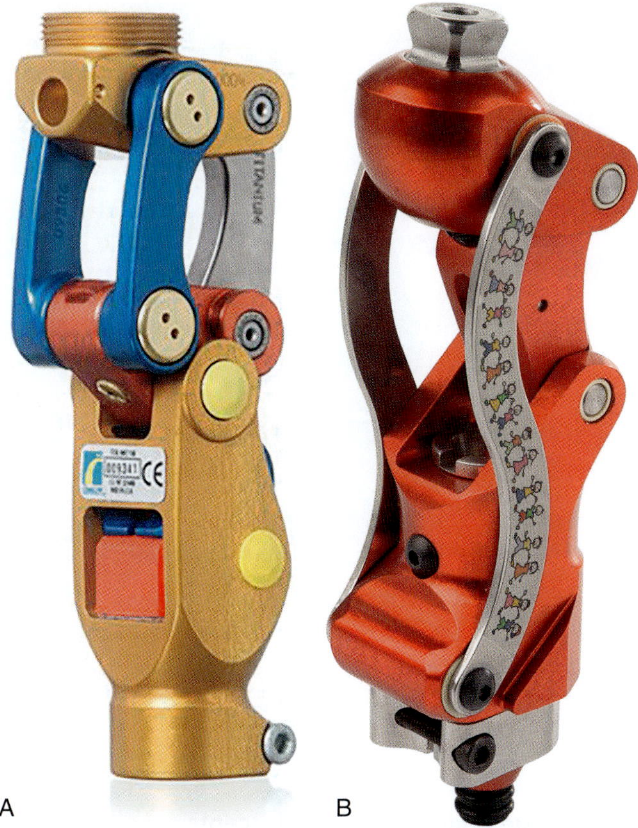

Fig. 29.15 Polycentric knee units used to provide stability and aid in initiation of smooth gait pattern. (A) Total Knee Junior. (B) 3R66 Knee Joint for Children. (A, © Össur; B, Courtesy Ottobock Orthopedic Industry, Inc., Minneapolis, Minnesota.)

Toddlers

By 15 months, toddlers are upright and mobile. The heel-toe sequence replaces flat-foot contact during the second year. Neurologic maturation, changes in physique, and improved strength are evident as the child's base of support narrows. Muscular activity has matured into the adult pattern. Goals for rehabilitation (Box 29.5) reflect the developmental activities of a preschool-age child. Young children with transfemoral amputation who were fitted with a prosthesis having an articulated knee used the prosthesis successfully.[58]

Another milestone expected of all children, including those with a prosthesis, is running, which begins between 2 and 4 years of age. The flight phase (double float), when both feet are off the ground, occurs by strong application of propulsive force during a late stance. The prosthetic foot offers much less energy storage and release than the gastrocnemius. Consequently, the child with a prosthesis adopts an asymmetric running gait that emphasizes propulsion on the sound side. Two-year-olds can kick a ball accurately, steer a push toy, and jump. As with running, jumping with a prosthesis is primarily an action of the sound side. Games of throwing and catching a ball or beanbag and tossing darts help the toddler to refine balance with the prosthesis.

The 3-year-old will probably leap, jump, gallop, climb stairs step over step, and ride a tricycle. The tricycle pedal may have a strap to secure the prosthetic foot. Jumping from a step and hopping are other toddler stunts. Playground equipment, such as a jungle gym, slide, swing, seesaw, sandbox, and tunnels, is enticing. Children with unilateral transtibial amputation achieve an almost normal gait and have no difficulty climbing inclines and stairs. Opportunities for kneeling, managing various types of chairs, and getting to and from the floor are additional elements in rehabilitation. The child will need help in removing and donning the prosthesis.

Box 29.5 Prosthetic Training Goals for Toddlers With Lower-Limb Deficiency

Goals of rehabilitation for toddlers with lower-limb deficiency include:

- Full-time wear of the prosthesis, except for bathing and sleeping
- Use of the prosthesis in age-appropriate ambulatory activities

Parents of toddlers with lower-limb prostheses should:

- Encourage use of the prosthesis
- Provide toys and equipment that require age-appropriate activities
- Inspect the skin to determine whether the prosthesis causes undue irritation

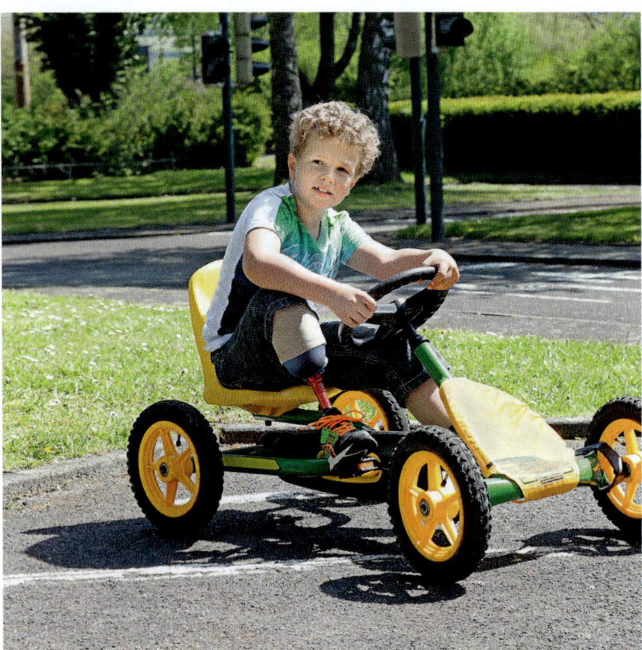

Fig. 29.16 **Boy wearing transtibial prosthesis pedaling an adaptive bike.** (Courtesy Ottobock Orthopedic Industry, Inc., Minneapolis, Minnesota.)

School-Age Children and Adolescents

By 4 years of age, most children can descend stairs step over step, ride a bicycle, and roller skate (Fig. 29.16). Five-year-olds skip rope and play dodgeball. Accurate kicking demonstrates balance on one foot while transferring force to the ball. By 6 years of age, most children can don and doff the prosthesis independently. They can start, stop, and change direction easily, and skip and hop for long distances. The child also moves toward independence in prosthetic management, taking more responsibility for donning and doffing, skin inspection, and prosthesis maintenance (Box 29.6). A minimal difference exists between the gait performance of children wearing Syme prostheses and those with transtibial prostheses.[59,60]

Children who undergo lower-limb amputation after 5 years may respond favorably to balance and gait training similar to that appropriate for adults.[61] Video games that involve weight shifting, such as bowling and tennis, improve balance engagingly.[62] Physical therapy emphasizes dynamic stability, weight shifting, and control of the prosthetic foot and the knee unit in the case of the child with transfemoral amputation (Fig. 29.17). The C-leg can be fitted to adolescents who are tall enough to accommodate the size of the microprocessor-controlled knee unit.[63]

Sports are particularly useful for developing self-esteem, strength, and coordination. Most children with amputations take part in physical education classes at school, sometimes with modified activity. Carbon acrylic or graphite reinforcements enable the prosthesis to withstand high stresses. The child should understand that shoes must always be worn; the plantar surface of most prosthetic feet is not durable enough to withstand abrasion by a sidewalk, and the alignment of the foot is intended for a shoe.

Box 29.6 Goals for School-Age Children and Adolescents With Lower-Limb Deficiency

In later childhood and adolescence, rehabilitation includes:

- Monitoring and maintaining proper prosthetic fit
- Inspecting the skin
- Donning and doffing the prosthesis independently
- Dressing independently
- Engaging in the full range of ambulatory activities with the prosthesis
- Recognizing when the prosthesis needs repair or alteration

Parents of school-age children and adolescents with lower-limb prostheses should:

- Encourage the young person's independence
- Provide opportunities for sports participation

Teenagers who sustained amputation in an earthquake displayed similar quality of life, although those with transtibial amputation achieved higher activity levels than those with transfemoral amputation.[64]

Some activities are more easily performed without a prosthesis or do not require a prosthesis. Children should learn how to use crutches as an alternate mode of locomotion when the prosthesis is being repaired. Bathing is facilitated by sitting on the shower floor or using a sturdy bath seat. Most people prefer to swim and scuba dive without a prosthesis. They hop or use crutches from the dressing room to the water's edge. Sports prostheses can be constructed, such as a swimming prosthesis with a fin in place of the foot. Bicycling, skiing, and mountain climbing are other sports that can be enjoyed with or without a prosthesis.

REHABILITATION OF CHILDREN WITH MULTIPLE LIMB AMPUTATION

Babies with lower-limb deficiency and anomalies of one or both upper limbs generally do best by being fitted first with simple lower-limb prostheses to foster sitting balance. The introduction of upper- and lower-limb prostheses simultaneously is apt to overwhelm the infant and family.

A simple bilateral fitting counteracts the tendency toward developing positional scoliosis when both upper limbs are anomalous. The baby with bilateral upper-limb deficiency should receive prostheses after independent walking is established; otherwise, prostheses make it more difficult to crawl, move on the floor, and pull to standing with the chin for support. Those with bilateral upper-limb deficiency become quite skillful with foot prehension. The extent to which foot use should be encouraged is controversial. Foot prehension is so rarely observed in public that the child using the feet may experience unwanted stares. Nevertheless, feet have the tactile sensation and considerable dexterity that prostheses lack. Children with bilateral longitudinal deficiencies have partial or complete hands; they would be encumbered by wearing prostheses. Functional activities with and without prostheses should be introduced according to the physical and emotional maturity of the child. Adaptive aids may be required for some functions, such as personal hygiene.

Infants with trimembral or quadrimembral limb deficiency move about by rolling along the floor.

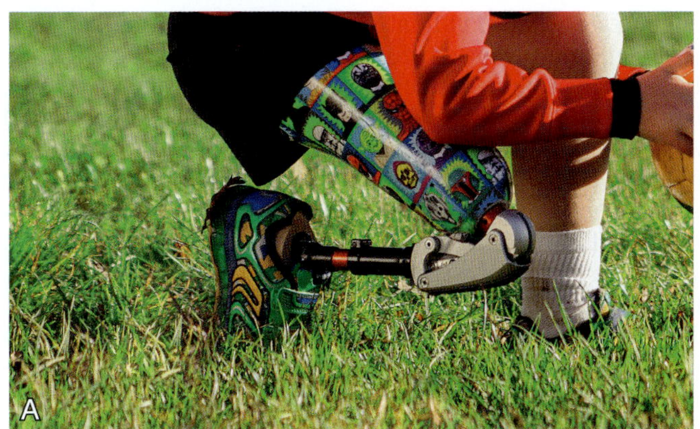

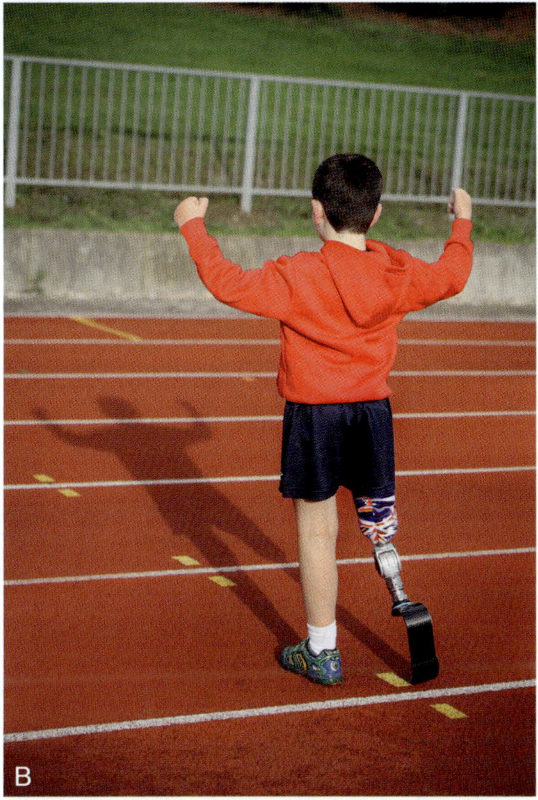

Fig. 29.17 (A) Boy wearing transfemoral prosthesis with hydraulic knee kneeling to pick up a ball. (B) Same child wearing a prosthesis fitted with a modular hydraulic sports knee. (Courtesy Ottobock Orthopedic Industry, Inc., Minneapolis, Minnesota.)

Occupational Therapy for Children With Upper-Limb Loss

The occupational therapy intervention for children promotes engagement and participation in children's daily life roles. Children's roles include developing personal independence, becoming productive and participating. The practices of pediatric occupational therapists have evolved and changed based on research and theory, such as family-centered care and the World Health Organization's International Classification of Functioning, Disability, and Health.[65] Whether they wear a prosthesis or not, most children with upper-limb loss have the potential to live full, productive lives.[68] The child may face varying degrees of difficulty due to limb reduction. These challenges depend on the extent and location of the reduction. Some limitations could include delays in the normal development of motor skills, limitations in performing activities of daily living (ADLs), and possible impact on emotional social well-being due to their appearance.[66] The inability to participate in play or recreational activities can cause marginalization, social isolation, and lowered self-esteem. The occupational therapist will have to identify the individual needs of the person and structure a rehabilitation program that helps the individual to achieve autonomy in carrying out significant occupations.[65] In collaboration with the parents, the therapist must select and tailor intervention choices to match the child's goals, preferences, and potential for improvement.[65] Occupational therapists select interventions for children based on an analysis of the child's performance in daily living roles, how their performance is affected by their disability, and how their environment supports or limits their performance. Based on the Person Environment Occupation model, it considers the three elements that compose it, while also taking into account the complexity of the situation and the interaction of all aspects involved. The therapist then also performs an environmental intervention by introducing aids or evaluating the possibility of using electronic and automatic devices that can help precarious or impossible movements and reevaluate the arrangement of tools, materials, and furniture; for this reason, it is important that they also go to his home. This specific competence of being able to intervene directly on environmental factors, on the person or through the provision and instruction in the use of aids, allows the therapist to be able to identify the barriers and facilitators relating to the patient's environments of interest, in order to implement changes that allow them to achieve the highest possible degree of autonomy, satisfaction, participation, and social inclusion.[65] In the preprosthetic phase, the occupational therapist should undertake targeted treatment concerning wound healing, active mobilization of the residual upper extremity and the sound limb, and reduction of edema and pain.[67] The stump, understood as a "segment of a limb between the section surface and the immediately proximal joint," must use specific characteristics and qualities to be evaluated as a functional basis for accommodating the prosthesis. In the following phases, the patient will be informed about the different possibilities of prostheses and their relative advantages and disadvantages. The prosthesis should be evaluated when delivered to the patient to ensure it complies with the prescription and clinic standards. The rehabilitative period is structured with a training program aimed at strengthening the muscles necessary for movement, the one for specific movements that are directly connected to the action of the prosthesis, and with a prosthesis exercise program based on the level of amputation and its characteristics.[65] The occupational therapist is responsible for providing both new strategies and support, as well as telling parents how to correctly fit and remove the prosthesis and maintain the prosthesis in good hygienic condition. The fit, comfort, and function of the prosthesis in normal use, along with the stability of the grip and the sling, are observed. The occupational therapist teaches the child to open the terminal device. Two to three short training sessions per week for 2 to 3 months are reasonable to reinforce prosthesis movement control learning and to provide a successful experience for the child.[68] The occupational therapist teaches the child to open the terminal device. Two to three short training sessions per week for 2 to 3 months are reasonable to reinforce prosthesis movement control learning and to provide a successful experience for the child.[68] In this phase, the therapist will work on targeted gestures, progressively dosed, coarse and fine and right-left motor coordination (bimanual), increasing unilateral skills and providing suitable auxiliary means.[67] Once the patient has mastered the movements, perfecting the movement is addressed. Although some children become more spontaneous than others, practice and repetition are an important part of building a habit pattern.[69] The occupational therapist encourages the child to use the prosthesis in normal play activities and helps the child to participate in ADLs (eating, dressing, washing, writing, etc.), demonstrating adapted techniques and experimenting with adapted equipment. The limb-deficient child can do part or the whole task quite easily. Because dressing and toileting skills require considerable practice, coordination, and effort, the individual may not achieve independence until adolescence. For some activities, assistance may always be required.

The concept of adapted performance, such as "encouraging the patient to approach and solve tasks adaptively using the whole body and to look beyond the conventional methods of using the arms and hands to stabilize, grasp and move objects in space," is essential for the child with severe upper-limb loss, as prostheses never provide total independence.[68] To allow the child to interact with the environment, the therapist will propose activities that allow functional activities to be kept intact and/or new ones to be stimulated: ludic-recreational activities, coordination, balance, attention and concentration activities, activities for school reintegration, recreational and social activities, and sports support activities.[70]

Outcome measure for children with prothesis

Most current prostheses require frequent visits to healthcare professionals for adjustments or replacements, which can lead to abandonment.[70] The assessment of prosthetic use in children is limited by a lack of adequate outcome measures, particularly in areas such as device acceptance or rejection, long-term use and abandonment, cost-effectiveness, and the functional and psychosocial outcomes associated with prosthetic use.

It is believed that there is a positive relationship between early fitting and increased prosthetic ability associated with child growth, that wearing a prosthesis encourages the use of the affected limb, thereby promoting symmetrical functional development, and that a natural-looking prosthesis helps improve self-image and self-esteem, but these clinical observations have not been tested. Observational assessments of an individual's abilities may not reflect specific performance in various real-life activities.[71] The ongoing controversy over the cost-effectiveness of providing upper extremity prostheses to children has spurred considerable interest and research into evaluating prosthetic use.[72] In the last decade, several prosthetic outcome measures have been designed and validated for children and adolescents: Assessment of Capacity for Myoelectric Control (ACMC),[81] Prosthetic Upper Extremity Functional Index (PUFI), Unilateral Below Elbow Test (UBET), UNB, and the Child Amputee Prosthetics Project-Functional Status Inventory (CAPP-FSI).[71] The ACMC is a rating scale of myoelectric control ability, an observational assessment of the performance of 30 bimanual movements during a chosen ADL, with a myoelectric prosthesis. Elements include gripping, holding, releasing, and coordinating objects in the hands. The score reflects the quality of movement control on a 4-point scale ranging from "not capable" to "spontaneously capable."[73] The UBET is developed for children ages 2 to 21 with transverse reduction deficiencies wearing a prosthetic device. The test consists of nine bimanual activities selected from the UNB test. It takes approximately 15 to 20 minutes to complete the test under each condition (i.e., with and without a prosthetic device). Task completion is rated on a five-point scale (4 = no difficulty, 3 = minimal difficulty, 2 = moderate difficulty, 1 = maximum difficulty, 0 = unable to complete the task). The method of use is a nominal scale that describes the grasping and stabilization methods for both prosthesis wearers and nonresidents: A for active use of the extremity device (recipients) or residual extremity manipulation (nonresident), P for passive use of the resuscitator device (recipients) or forearm stabilization (nonresident), E for elbow or trunk grasping, and N for no use of the affected limb.[74]

The PUFI assesses how frequently a child uses the prosthesis for daily activities. It evaluates the "ease of performing tasks" with and without the prosthesis, the "method of execution," and the "perceived utility of the prosthesis."[75] Includes 38 items for 7- to 18-year-olds and 26 items for 3- to 6-year-olds. Considers various activities: toilet, dressing, housework, games, schoolwork.[71]

The UNB is an assessment tool for children ages 2 to 13 with unilateral upper extremity amputations who wear powered or conventional prostheses. The test provides 10 bimanual activities for four age levels (i.e., 2–4, 5–7, 8–10, and 11–13 year olds) and has three versions. It has a dual rating scale, one for ability and one for spontaneity of prosthetic function, both rated on a five-point scale. Skill scores range from 4 (active use of the terminal device is quick, dexterous and fluid, grip is always maintained) to 0 (prosthesis not used). Spontaneity scores range from 4 (immediate, automatic, and consistent use of the terminal device for active grasping) to 0 (prosthesis not used or used only on request).[74]

Parent- or child-reported functional status questionnaires to measure the effective functional benefit of upper-limb prosthetic devices were developed by Pruitt: the CAPP-FSI for children aged 8 to 17 years (1996), the CAPP-FSI version for preschool children (1998), and the CAPP-FSIT for toddlers (1999). These inventories include a list of common ADLs (dressing, eating, drawing, playing, and recreational activities), evaluating the prostheses functionally only, and the respondent is asked to indicate (1) whether the individual performed the activity and (2) whether the prosthesis was used.[76]

The Child Amputee Prosthetics Project-Prosthesis Satisfaction Inventory (CAPP-PSI) questionnaire is a new outcome measure to evaluate satisfaction of the

Table 29.2 Assessment Tools for Children With Amputation

Scale	First Author	Year	Language	Sample	Mean Age/SD	Amputation Level	Indication for Amputation	Gender (M/F)	Administration	Cronbach's Alpha
Child Amputee Prosthetics Project-Functional Status Inventory for Preschool children (CAPP-FSIP)	Pruitt S.D.	1998	English	41	4.9 ± 1.2 (range 4–7)	Lower limb 21; upper limb 20	Congenital limb 84%; acquired 16%	Boys 54%	Parent report	Does the activity α = 0.97; "Uses a Prosthesis" α = 0.94
Child Amputee Prosthetics Project-Prosthesis Satisfaction Inventory (CAPP-PSI)	Pruitt S.D.	1997	English	97	8.1 ± 4.5 (range 1–17)	Upper limb 41%; lower limb 59%	Congenital 78%; acquired 22%	Boys 49%; girls 51%	Parent report	parent satisfaction with prosthesis α = 0.80; (parent rated) child satisfaction with prosthesis α = 0.87; parent satisfaction with service α = 0.90
Child Amputee Prosthetics Project-Functional Status Inventory (CAPP-FSY)	Pruitt S.D.	1996	English	65	11.7 ± 2.6 (range 8–17)	Lower-limb deficiency 43; upper-limb deficiency 22	Congenital limb deficiency 75%; acquired limb impairments 25%	Boys 51%; Girls 49%	Parent report	α= 0.96
Child Amputee Prosthetics Project-Functional Status Inventory for Toddlers (CAPP-FSIT)	Pruitt S.D.	1999	English	20	2.41 ± 0.73 (range 1–4)	Upper limb 13 (1 had bilateral impairment); lower limb 7 (2 had bilateral impairment)	Congenital 19; acquired 1	Boys 12; girls 8	Parent report	Upper extremity items on the "Does the Activity" α= 0.95; lower extremity items on the "Does the Activity" α = 0.83; upper extremity items on the "Uses a Prosthesis" α = 0.96; lower extremity items on the "Uses a Prosthesis" α = 0.94

F, female; *M*, male; *SD*, standard deviation.

prosthetic component prescribed for children with limb deficiency. The satisfaction scale was developed by Pruitt in 1997 and is in addition to the outcome measures available for children with amputations. There are no other validations than the original version (1). The CAPP-PSI is widely used in several countries, such as the Netherlands[75], China[76], France[77], Canada[78], Turkey[79], and Sweden.[80] It can be used in both etiologies (congenital and acquired), single and double and at all prosthetic levels.

It has also been used to examine the use of 3D printing for the development of prostheses for patients with upper or lower-limb amputees in low- and middle-income countries.[76] The questionnaire is aimed at children with an amputation aged between 1 and 17 years. It is compiled by parents reporting their and their children's satisfaction with the prescribed prosthetic device concerning function, fit, appearance, and service. The elements of the CAPP-PSI were generated from a literature review on pediatric limb impairment and solicitation from experienced clinicians (physicians, physical and occupational therapists, and psychologists).

The questionnaire is made up of 14 elements, divided into three subscales:

1. Child's satisfaction with the prosthesis (reported by the parent).
2. Parental satisfaction with the prosthesis.
3. Parental satisfaction with the service: delivery times, instructions provided, repair times, child rehabilitation, follow-up.

Here's the proofread version of the sentence: Parents select one answer for each question using the following categories, which have scores from 0 to 4: "not at all" = 0, "a little" = 1, "somewhat" = 2, "very" = 3, or "extremely" = 4.

Each CAPP-PSI scale is scored by summing the scores for each item within the scale. The CAPP-PSI produces a total summary score: a sum of the scores on each scale.

Higher scores reflect greater satisfaction with the prosthesis (Table 29.2).

Summary

Habilitation or rehabilitation of children with limb deficiencies can be most gratifying. The physical therapist and all members of the clinical team should design the program to assist the child in achieving developmental milestones associated with maturing upper- and lower-limb function. Psychosocial factors govern the behavior of all children, although it appears that those with limb deficiency behave comparably manner to nondisabled peers. Peer support is very helpful for children and parents. Clinic team members need to recognize the basis for parental distress while fostering realistic expectations for the child's function by demonstrating that the child is lovable regardless of the condition of the limbs.

References

The complete listing of the References are available in the accompanying enhanced eBook version included with the print purchase of this textbook. Visit Elsevier eBooks+ (eBooks.Health.Elsevier.com) to access this content.

30 Prosthetic Options for Persons With Upper Extremity Amputation*

INGA WANG

LEARNING OBJECTIVES

On completion of this chapter, the reader will be able to do the following:

1. Identify the factors that influence the choice of prosthetic devices for individuals with upper extremity amputation.
2. Describe the functional goals and outcomes associated with different types of upper extremity prostheses.
3. Discuss the role of medical professionals and prosthetists in the assessment, fitting, and training of individuals with upper extremity prostheses.
4. Identify the psychological, social, and emotional factors that may influence the acceptance and use of upper extremity prosthetic devices.
5. Compare and contrast the features and functionality of myoelectric, body-powered, and hybrid prosthetic devices.
6. Explain the benefits and limitations of various upper extremity prosthetic options.
7. Analyze the impact of advances in prosthetic technology on the design and functionality of upper extremity prosthetic devices.
8. Discuss emerging trends and future directions in upper extremity prosthetic technology and design.

Overview

While orthotics are designed to assist an existing body part, prostheses, or prosthetic devices, are artificial replacements for missing body parts, typically limbs (arms or legs), but can also include other body parts such as fingers, hands, feet, or facial structures. Prosthetics is the field of healthcare concerned with the design, fabrication, and fitting of prostheses. Devices are custom made to suit the individual's needs and are designed to restore function, mobility, and esthetics to those who have experienced limb loss or congenital limb deficiencies, and to provide amputees with a renewed opportunity to perform various functions despite limb loss.

The prosthetic management of individuals with upper extremity amputations presents a unique set of challenges for healthcare professionals, including prosthetists and therapists. In addition to the initial assessment, device selection, and fitting, prosthetic management involves training individuals with a suitable prosthetic device to help them regain as much function and independence as possible. This is an ongoing process, and periodic adjustments, repairs, or replacements of the prosthetic device may be necessary over time. For the prosthetic device to be effective, its design must meet the user's expectations, and its operations must address their needs. In addition to functionality, other aspects such as reliability, appearance, comfort, usability, and affordability are crucial factors that determine the device's clinical utility and help prevent device disuse and abandonment.[1]

*The author extends appreciation to Susan Spaulding and Tzurei Chen, whose work in the prior edition provided substantial foundation for this chapter.

Individuals facing upper extremity limb loss encounter unique challenges compared to those with lower extremity prostheses. Unlike lower extremity prostheses, which can be concealed by pants, socks, and shoes, the terminal device (TD) of an upper extremity prosthesis is often left uncovered. This lack of concealment presents additional obstacles for individuals in terms of physical appearance. Those with upper extremity limb loss experience the loss of some of the most complex movement patterns and functional activities of the human body. Additionally, upper extremity limb loss deprives the patient of an extensive and valuable system of tactile and proprioceptive inputs that previously offered feedback to guide and refine functional movement.[2,3] Even the simplest tasks related to grasp and release become challenging. The positioning of prosthetic limb segments in space and the maintenance of advantageous postures necessary for manipulating objects pose continuous challenges for the medical community, urging improvements in both functional and esthetic outcomes for patients in this population.[4–6]

As the prosthetic technology continues to advance, many design challenges have been addressed through the integration of new and emerging technologies. These innovations have made it possible, in some circumstances, to successfully "fit" a patient with high-level amputation who previously would have little or no reasonable expectation to succeed with traditional technology and fitting techniques.[7,8] Advanced socket interface designs and material science now empower prosthetists to provide stronger and more stable platforms for all levels of amputation, often with substantial weight savings. Moreover, innovative suspension strategies and interface materials have expanded the functional ranges of motion that patients can comfortably achieve.[9] Recenly, the advent of bionic limb technoloty[10–29] and the utilization of three-dimensional (3D) printing[30–39] has revolutionalize the prosthetic world, offering users alternative option and the freedom to choose different designs, forms, sizes and colors of their prostheses. These advancements have profoundly and positively impacted the comfort, function, and compliance of both body-powered and externally powered prostheses at all levels of amputation. The significant progress in externally powered prosthetics has been largely driven by these breakthroughs and technological advancements.

This chapter presents a comprehensive examination of upper extremity amputation, encompassing aspects such as prevalence, etiology, and preprosthetic care. Additionally, we will delve into the essential components of upper limb prosthetic prescription, explore various upper limb prosthetic options including none, passive, body-powered, hybrid, externally powered, and activity-specific devices. Furthermore, we will briefly touch upon the advancements in bionic arm technology and the emergence of 3D-printed prosthetics.

Prevalence of Upper Extremity Amputation

Determining the prevalence of major amputation poses challenges as many countries lack records documenting the number of individuals with limb amputation.[40–42] In 2017 it was estimated that around 57.7 million individuals worldwide were living with limb amputation due to traumatic causes.[41] According to the Amputee Coalition,[43] the United States currently has a population of nearly 2.1 million individuals living with limb loss. Vital and Health Statistics indicate that approximately 185,000 individuals undergo limb amputations annually in the United States,[44] with lower limb amputations accounting for 159,000 of these cases.[44] Projections indicate that the number of individuals living with limb loss will surpass 3.6 million by the year 2050.[40]

Etiology of Upper Extremity Amputation

Amputation is frequently linked to various underlying conditions, including trauma (e.g., motor vehicle collisions, machinery accidents), dysvascular disease, complications related to diabetes, cancer-related factors, infection, and congenital limb deficiencies.[45–49] Traumatism stands as the primary cause of upper limb amputation, followed by neoplasia, vascular or infectious diseases.[50]

Beyond the aforementioned causes, war and conflict are also significant contributors to the sporadic occurrence of limb amputations in both military veterans and civilian populations. Among soldiers in the US Army wounded in action during World War II, about 15,000 (2.5%) required major amputations.[51,52] Since 2001, more than 1500 US service members have lost a limb as a result of explosive devices during the conflicts in Iraq and Afghanistan.[53,54]

Length of the Residual Limb

Amputations to the upper extremity can be classified or named by the limb segments affected (Fig. 30.1). Levels of

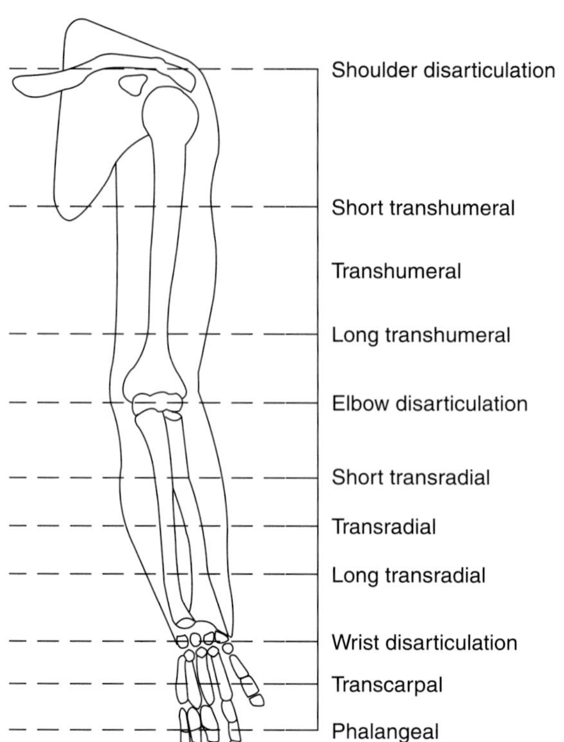

Fig. 30.1 Classification of upper extremity amputation and residual limbs. (From Murdoch G, Wilson AB. *Amputation: Surgical Practice and Patient Management*. Butterworth; 1996:308.)

upper extremity amputations include: Fingers or partial-hand (transcarpal), at the wrist (wrist disarticulation), below the elbow (transradial), at the elbow (elbow disarticulation), above the elbow (transhumeral), at the shoulder (shoulder disarticulation), and above the shoulder (forequarter).

The most distal are at the finger, partial-hand, or transcarpal levels. Amputations that separate the carpal bones from the radius and ulna are referred to as wrist disarticulations. Amputations that occur within the substance of the radius and ulna are classified as transradial amputations. When the humerus is preserved but the radius and ulna are removed, the amputation is referred to as an elbow disarticulation. Those that leave more than 30% of humeral length are designated as transhumeral amputations. Residual limb length less than 30% of the proximal humerus is treated like shoulder disarticulation because of the lack of humeral lever arm. More proximal amputations that invade the central body cavity, resecting the clavicle and leading to derangement of the scapula, are described as interscapulothoracic (forequarter) amputations.

For those with transverse amputations of the forearm, the length of the residual limb affects the amount of functional elbow flexion and functional forearm pronation and supination that will be retained independent of prosthetic intervention.[2] Articulations between the radius and the ulna along the entire forearm are necessary to provide for natural anatomic movements in supination and pronation; as the level of amputation moves proximally from the styloid process of the radius toward the elbow, the ability to perform and to use pronation and supination during functional activities is progressively lost (Fig. 30.2). In addition,

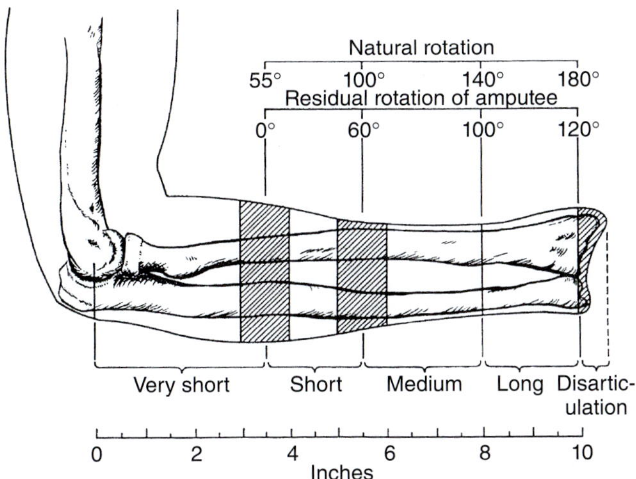

Fig. 30.2 **Potential for pronation and supination of transradial residual limbs of differing lengths.** (From Taylor CI. The biomechanics of control in upper extremity prosthetics. *Orthot Prosthet.* 1981;35:20.)

not all available transverse motion can be fully captured in the prosthetic socket. When the residual forearm is extremely short, all transverse motion is essentially lost, and it is difficult to gain any active functional forearm rotation for prosthetic use.

Amputations at the level of the elbow (elbow disarticulation) derive little functional benefit from the added length because the length of the limb limits options for cosmetic and functional placement of elbow units within the prosthesis without substantially improving functional leverage.

Although the primary concern of surgeons who perform an upper extremity amputation is adequate closure of the wound, they must also consider the potential advantages of a fairly long lever arm, balanced by an understanding of the space requirements for prosthetic components. Provided that adequate skin and tissue viability are not compromised, consideration should be given to adequate room for a full array of prosthetic componentry.

Preprosthetic Care

All patients experiencing upper extremity amputation, regardless of cause, require some level of prosthetic management. Early postoperative care goals encompass strengthening of the joints proximal to the residual limb, core strengthening, psychosocial support, and care of the residual limb including edema control, wound healing, pain management, and desensitization.[55] Shrinkers, immediate postoperative prostheses, and preparatory prostheses play a crucial role in achieving these goals. Effective care is best achieved through coordination within a multidisciplinary team, involving the surgeon, physiatrist, prosthetist, nurses, physical and occupational therapists, counselors, and other necessary professionals.[56]

The timeliness of patient evaluation, prosthesis fitting, and training significantly influences the likelihood of a positive rehabilitation outcome.

Malone and colleagues[57] highlighted the advantages of early postoperative fitting, including reduced edema, decreased postoperative and phantom pain, accelerated wound healing, improved rehabilitation, shorter hospital stays (potentially reducing costs), increased prosthetic use, maintenance of continuous proprioceptive input through the residual limb, and enhanced psychological adaptation to amputation. Malone et al.[57] found a difference in rehabilitation success between patients fitted within 30 days of surgery and those fitted more than 30 days after surgery. Specifically, all 13 patients fitted within 30 days of surgery, who had job-related injuries, returned to work, whereas only 15% (3 out of 20) of those fitted more than 30 days after surgery returned to work.[57]

Most professionals concur that there exists a relatively brief window of opportunity during which the chances for successful rehabilitation are at their peak, although there is some disagreement regarding the duration of this "optimal rehabilitation" period. Initially, most patients are primarily concerned with restoring their body image[58] and achieving independent bimanual function. Brenner proposes an ideal timetable for prosthesis fitting after wrist disarticulation or transradial amputation (Table 30.1).[59] The timing and type of prosthesis are contingent on factors such as the level of residual limb healing, comorbidities, and patient-centered considerations (Fig. 30.3).

Irrespective of the intervention type, rehabilitation should center on the patient and their preferences. Postoperative rehabilitation goals aim to improve upper extremity strengthening, facilitate residual limb healing,

Table 30.1 Timelines for Prosthetic Fitting After Amputation

Type of Prosthesis	Postoperative Application
Immediate or early postoperative prosthesis	24 hours to 14 days
Preparatory/training body-powered prosthesis	2–4 weeks
Definitive body-powered prosthesis	6–12 weeks
Preparatory/training electronic prosthesis	2–12 weeks
Definitive electronic prosthesis	4–6 months

Reprint with permission from Krajbich JI, Pinzur MS, Potter BK, Stevens PM. *Atlas of Amputations and Limb Deficiencies.* Fourth ed. American Academy of Orthopaedic Surgeons; 2018.

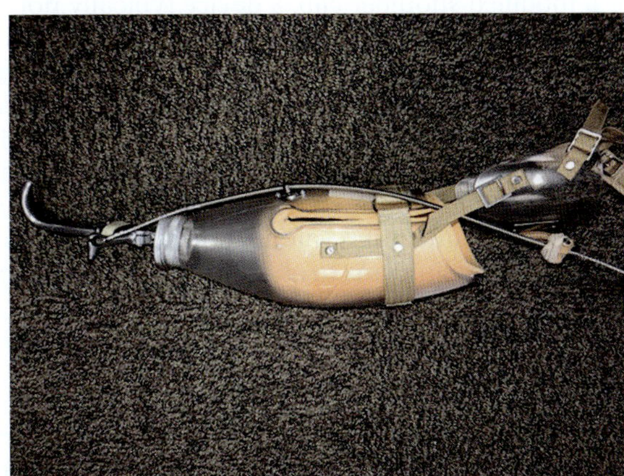

Fig. 30.3 The postoperative upper extremity prosthesis can help to improve edema control, wound healing, pain control, desensitization, proximal joint and core strengthening, and psychosocial adaptation. (Courtesy Hanger Clinic, Austin, Texas.)

provide psychosocial support, restore body image and independent bimanual function, and enable a return to the patient's desired lifestyle. Once the wound site is adequately protected and bandaged, compressive wraps or shrinkers should be employed when an early postoperative or preparatory prosthesis is deemed inappropriate. In most cases, multidirectional shrinker garments prove more effective in controlling volume and shaping the residual limb compared to other methods, such as elastic bandages.[60]

When properly worn, shrinkers are less prone to migrating or shifting position on the residual limb, making them more effective at creating a consistent distal-to-proximal pressure gradient. Ideally, the compressive garment should terminate proximal to the joint above the amputation site. For transhumeral amputations, this necessitates the inclusion of a modified shoulder cap, a device typically not commercially available and usually requiring custom fabrication. Diligence is crucial to ensuring the achievement and maintenance of appropriate tension and compression gradients.

Any volume management protocol inherently initiates limb maturation and desensitization concurrently. Moreover, effective and timely volume management influences not only residual limb volume and shape but has also been employed by clinicians to assist in managing phantom pain.[61]

Prosthetic Options

Upper extremity prosthetics provide a range of options to meet the diverse needs of individuals with upper limb amputations or limb differences. Common types of upper extremity prosthetics include: cosmetic or passive prosthetics, body-powered prosthetics, myoelectric prosthetics, hybrid prosthetics, cosmetic or passive prosthetics, activity-specific prosthetics, bionic arms and hands, and customized 3D-printed prosthetics (Fig. 30.4). Depending on the patient's lifestyle and physical condition, the prosthetic team can make a number of recommendations. The physician, prosthetist, therapist and patient must consider the benefits and limitations of the various prosthetic options to best meet patients' needs.[62]

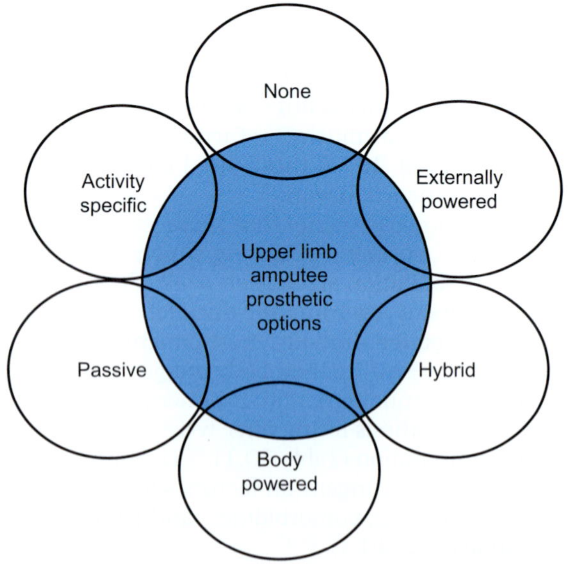

Fig. 30.4 Upper limb prosthetic options. (From Melton DH. Physiatrist perspective on upper limb prosthetic options: using practice guidelines to promote patient education in the selection and the prescription process. *J Prosthet Orthot*. 2017;29:40–44.)

There are various reasons why individuals with upper extremity amputations might choose not to regularly use a prosthesis. Some may find the prosthesis uncomfortable or unwieldy, leading them to prioritize greater comfort without the device. If the prosthesis fails to deliver the necessary functionality or meet the user's specific needs, they may opt not to use it. In certain activities or tasks, individuals may deem the use of a prosthesis impractical or unnecessary. Others might prioritize their appearance or prefer the natural look of their residual limb, leading them to forgo a prosthesis for cosmetic reasons.

The learning curve associated with using a prosthesis can be steep, and some individuals may encounter challenges in adapting to the device. This could result from poorly implemented prosthetic care or a lack of adequate training.[63,64] Prosthetic devices can be costly, limiting accessibility for some individuals who may not have access to affordable or comprehensive prosthetic care. Additionally, certain medical conditions or complications may render the use of a prosthesis unfeasible. Individuals with skin sensitivity, pain, or unresolved medical issues may opt not to use a prosthetic device.

Advanced materials have enabled prosthetists to create lighter, stronger, and more comfortable systems,[65,66] as well as extremely cosmetic restorations.[67] Consideration of adaptive tools and resources such as "One-Handed in a Two-Handed World" and the Amputee Coalition should be discussed to address each patient's needs.[68,69] Ultimately, the decision to use or not use a prosthesis is highly individualized. It involves a careful consideration of various factors, and individuals may reassess their preferences and needs over time based on changes in their circumstances and the availability of new prosthetic technologies.

PROSTHETIC PRESCRIPTION

Assessment of individuals with upper extremity amputations should include complete evaluation of the level of amputation, residual limb condition, upper extremity musculoskeletal condition, cognitive ability, and presence of degenerative conditions or comorbidities.[70] Practitioners must identify the patient's perspectives and priorities about their own needs for control, durability (maintenance), function (speed, work capability, type of grip, ruggedness, high grip force, visibility), comfort (harness, weight, effort), cosmesis (appearance), and reliability.[71] When asked, "what is the goal of the upper limb prosthesis?," the answer always depends on the goals of the wearer.[72] Satisfaction with a prosthesis is associated with clear clinician-patient communication,[73–75] the relationship with their prosthetist, and focused attention to patient preferences.[76,77] Recognizing patient priorities helps strike a balance between the benefits and limitations of various prosthetic options. Prosthetists and patients often compromise between form and function when selecting components, design features,[71,78,79] and surgical procedures.[80]

The prosthetic prescription (Box 30.1) includes a base code and add-on codes. Prosthetic and orthotic L-codes within the Healthcare Common Procedural Coding System (HCPCS) allow for patient specificity in which the team may select various combinations of codes to address patient-specific needs. HCPCS L-code base codes imply the design (e.g., preparatory or definitive), the control, and often basic elements of the prosthesis. For example, the myoelectric prosthesis base code (Table 30.2) includes the electrodes, cables, two batteries, and a charger. L-codes also include (1) the initial patient evaluation; (2) consultation with the physician or nurse practitioner; (3) measurements, casting, and scanning; (4) parts cost; (5) shipping, receiving, and restocking charges; (6) fabrication; (7) fitting trial appointments; and (8) follow-up appointments or adjustments for 90 days after the patient goes home with the completed prosthesis.[81] The add-on codes state specific elements of the prosthesis such as the type of socket interface (e.g., socks, foam insert, gel insert), suspension mechanism (e.g., harness, suction, roll-on liner, and pin), TD, wrist unit (if applicable), elbow unit (if applicable), and shoulder unit (if applicable).[79] Tables 30.2 and 30.3 provide examples of two prostheses with different components and types of control. However, some design elements may be similar between them: both include test sockets, frame type socket design, and acrylic laminations.

If the rehabilitation goal requires the prosthesis to be as lightweight as possible, the team may select an endoskeletal design (Fig. 30.5). Using endoskeletal components and/or lightweight materials requires less suspension and less harnessing and may enhance comfort for the user. Endoskeletal prostheses have a tubular structure connecting the socket

Box 30.1 Elements of the Upper Limb Prosthetic Prescription

- Socket type
- Test sockets
- Interface (e.g., liner, socks, sheaths, foam insert, roll-on liner)
- Control system (passive functional, body powered, externally powered, hybrid, or activity specific)
- Suspension mechanism (e.g., harness, anatomic, suction, lanyard, or pin)
- Components: terminal device, glove, wrist, elbow (if applicable) and shoulder (if applicable)

Table 30.2 Example of a Prescription for an Upper Extremity Externally Powered Prosthesis

Base Code and Description	Add-on Codes and Descriptions
L6935: Below elbow, external power, self-suspended inner socket, removable forearm shell, Ottobock or equal electrodes, cables, two batteries and one charger, myoelectronic control of terminal device	L6680: Upper extremity addition, test socket, wrist disarticulation or below elbow
	L6687: Upper extremity addition, frame type socket, below elbow or wrist disarticulation
	L7403: Addition to upper extremity prosthesis, below elbow/wrist disarticulation, acrylic material
	L7007: Electric hand, switch or myoelectric controlled, adult
	L6881: Automatic grasp feature, addition to upper limb electric prosthetic terminal device
	L6882: Microprocessor control feature, addition to upper limb prosthetic terminal device
	L6629: Upper extremity addition, quick-disconnect lamination collar with coupling piece, Ottobock or equal
	L6890: Addition to upper extremity prosthesis, glove for terminal device, any material, prefabricated, includes fitting and adjustment
	L7499: Upper extremity prosthesis, not otherwise specified

Table 30.3 Example of a Prescription for an Upper Extremity Body-Powered Prosthesis

Base Code	Add-on Codes
L6110: Below elbow, molded socket, (muenster or northwestern suspension types)	L6680: Upper extremity addition, test socket, wrist disarticulation or below elbow
	L6687: Upper extremity addition, frame type socket, below elbow or wrist disarticulation
	L7403: Addition to upper extremity prosthesis, below elbow/wrist disarticulation, acrylic material
	L6706: Terminal device, hook, mechanical, voluntary opening, any material, any size, lined or unlined
	L6704: Terminal device, sport/recreational/work attachment, any material, any size
	L 6615: Upper extremity addition, disconnect locking wrist unit
	L6616: Upper extremity addition, additional disconnect insert for locking wrist unit, each
	L6675: Upper extremity addition, harness, (e.g., figure-of-eight type), single cable design
	L6655: Upper extremity addition, standard control cable, extra

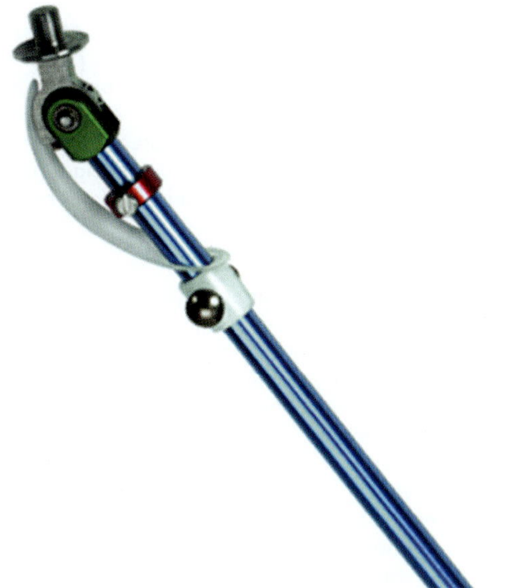

Fig. 30.5 Example of a lightweight endoskeletal prosthesis. (Courtesy Steeper Group.)

to the components, which is covered by a protective foam, whereas exoskeletal prostheses have a rigid outer shell that provides structure and shape.[82] Although endoskeletal prostheses are lighter in weight, currently available upper limb componentry is limited and not as durable as lower limb endoskeletal componentry. Therefore most upper limb prostheses are exoskeletal. Both endoskeletal and exoskeletal components may be operated passively or through cable and harnessing (body powered).

An interdisciplinary approach is necessary due to the specialization and complexity of the necessary skills and knowledge when working with this small population of individuals with upper limb loss. The rehabilitation team (e.g., physician, nurse, psychologist, prosthetist, physical therapist, occupational therapist, social worker, and pharmacist) has shared treatment goals toward improving the patients' quality of life. This interdisciplinary rehabilitation team approach is well recognized in upper extremity rehabilitation.[4,83–86] Clear chart note documentation from all team members is necessary to enhance interdisciplinary communication/collaboration and best meet the rehabilitation goals. Box 30.2 lists information that must be documented in the patients' charts.[79]

Prosthetic Socket

Upper extremity prosthetic sockets secure the prosthesis onto the residual limb, extending control functions (movement and direction) to distal components (e.g., wrist, TD). Depending on the control system, sockets facilitate force transmission for body-powered TD operation or stabilize skin electrodes for myoelectric control.

Design considerations include skin condition, soft tissue volume, residual limb characteristics, and patient-specific functional needs. Key elements for effective designs involve comfort, cosmesis, stabilization, suspension, anatomic contouring, contralateral/ipsilateral involvement, range of motion (ROM), and vocational/personal needs.[87] Balancing these elements is crucial, acknowledging their interconnected and sometimes inversely related nature.

Socket fit refers to the stability of the socket on the residual limb and the comfort from the patient's perspective. Patient comfort with the socket interface plays a major deciding role in whether a patient will use their prosthesis.[88] Strategically placed socket pressures reduce residual limb movement inside the socket,[89] consequently improving rehabilitation outcomes.[90]

Socket pressures are evaluated using the Tekscan pressure measuring system.[91,92] Daly et al.[91] found that pressure measurements did not strongly correlate with socket discomfort scores. This suggests that while pressure data is valuable, it may not fully capture the subjective experience of discomfort reported by the prosthesis user. Schofield et al.[92] identified unique pressure distribution patterns among transhumeral participants. This emphasizes the variability in how individuals experience pressure within the socket, reinforcing the need for personalized evaluations. Prosthetists need to strike a balance between a patient's ability to tolerate pressure and the stability the socket provides.

Limb volume refers to the amount or size of space occupied by the residual limb or the remaining part of a limb after amputation. Reducing residual limb volume during

Box 30.2 Supporting Documentation for an Upper Limb Prosthesis and Prosthetic Training

Physician or Nurse Practitioner Documentation

- The cause, date, level of limb loss, include right or left or bilateral.
- The patient's preamputation level of independence and function, as well as the potential to return or increase in function when successfully using a prosthesis.
- Comorbidities that could interfere with function of the prosthesis.
- Pain interference of function (including residual pain).
- Adequate neurologic and cognitive ability to operate the prosthesis effectively.
- The type of prosthesis being prescribed (preparatory or definitive).
- Rehabilitation treatment plan describing the long-term and short-term goals and the anticipated timeline for recovery.

Prosthetist Documentation

- The individual's perspectives about their
  - Vocational and avocational needs including information about the specific activity or activities that the prosthesis will be used for
  - Motivation to use the prosthesis
  - Lifestyle: habits, interests, opinions
  - Social network support
  - Use environment
  - Hand dominance
  - Perspectives and priorities with respect to function, cosmesis, reliability, comfort, and cost.
- Functional assessment of the need for function, cosmesis, durability, protection, support, control, and perceived ability to learn and use a prosthesis.
- Myotesting results: minimum microvolt threshold and whether this would allow operation of a myoelectric prosthesis.
- Prosthetic treatment plan describing the long-term and short-term goals, barriers and facilitators of desired outcomes, and interdisciplinary communication.
- Patient-specific justification for each element of the prosthesis.

Therapist Documentation

- Occupational/functional evaluation of activities of daily living, instrumental activities of daily living, and vocational and avocational needs.
- The individual's perspectives about their
  - Motivation to use the prosthesis
  - Lifestyle: habits, interests, opinions
  - Social network support
  - Use environment.
- Occupational/functional assessment of the client's need for function, cosmesis, durability, protection, support, control, and perceived ability to learn and use a prosthesis.
- Myotesting results: minimum microvolt threshold and whether this would allow operation of a myoelectric prosthesis.
- Therapy treatment plan describing the short-term and long-term goals, type, amount, intensity, duration and frequency of therapy visits, complicating factors, and interdisciplinary communication.

the early postoperative and preprosthetic care phases is essential because variations in residual limb volume affect stabilization, anatomic contouring, and suspension which then affect comfort and function of the prosthesis for the patient. Limbs with large longitudinal contours or bulbous distal contours are least desirable because these adversely influence the ability to capture the skeletal structures. In these cases, surgical reconstruction may be necessary to remove the redundant tissues.[93]

Upper extremity sockets often provide suspension to avoid use of harnessing. Suspension may be provided through anatomic shape, suction, harness, or roll-on liner and pin. Selection of suspension method is determined by the residual limb condition and the functional needs of the individual, such as ease of donning and the weight of objects being manipulated.

Influences on the advancement of socket designs can be attributed to advances in material science and upper extremity prosthetic specialists.[65] Most contemporary upper extremity prosthetic socket designs use some type of flexible interface with a rigid frame exterior. The interface material is often composed of a high–silicone content conformable elastomer. These elastomers have dramatically improved patients' perceptions of fit and function with regard to comfort.[66,94]

In summary, the socket secures the prosthesis to the patient's body. The prosthetist needs to ensure that the socket (a) matches the patient's anatomy; (b) is comfortable and stable; (c) provides suspension and ROM; (d) is easy to don/doff; and (e) supports the patient's vocational, avocational, and personal needs. Alignment between the socket and the distal components needs to be considered to reduce compensations at the proximal joints. Socket fit is an ongoing dynamic process. The prosthetist makes changes to the socket over a patient's lifespan as the patient's body condition changes (e.g., weight, atrophy).

Passive-Functional Prostheses

Passive functional prostheses refer to a category of prosthetic devices that do not have active components or mechanisms, such as motors or electronics, but are designed to provide functional benefits to the user through their passive features. This category of prostheses consists of systems that do not have the ability to actively position a mechanical elbow in space or actively provide grasp and release. Some advantages of passive-functional prostheses include simplicity and durability, lightweight design, natural appearance, lower cost, reduced learning curve, and lower maintenance. These systems most frequently have a self-suspending design and use a realistic-appearing hand as a TD. Suspension may be achieved with specific socket interface geometry, suction, roll-on liner, and pin/lanyard. These devices are extremely functional in terms of supporting objects or stabilizing items during bimanual tasks and activities.[95] They appear to be important for social integration[96] and psychosocial well-being.[97] Low body image is associated with depression and general anxiety in individuals with upper extremity amputation.[98]

The finish of these devices varies widely. Production polyvinyl chloride (PVC) cosmetic gloves provide a cost-effective short-term outcome for patients; short term because PVC readily stains and deteriorates in ultraviolet light. Silicone gloves provide an added benefit of longevity, because they can be cleaned with soap and water. In general, the additional cost of silicone is mitigated by its superior cosmesis, durability, and increased coefficient of friction.

Many individuals seek out esthetic, or transparent, restorations (Fig. 30.6). These restorations require greater investments in time and financial resources. Options to enhance the esthetic appearance may include enhanced or acrylic nails, skin shading, and the addition of hair. Laser scanning and computer modeling may create near perfect "mirror" images of high-level amputations, such as shoulder disarticulations and scapulothoracic amputations. This investment is most often rewarded with an esthetic, natural, and transparent-appearing body image.

The appearance of a prosthesis can be described from three perspectives: the *passive cosmesis* based on the static visual appearance, the *cosmesis of wearing* based on the esthetics while wearing the prosthesis such as while walking, and the *cosmesis of use* based on the appearance during activity performance.[58] Although patients may not

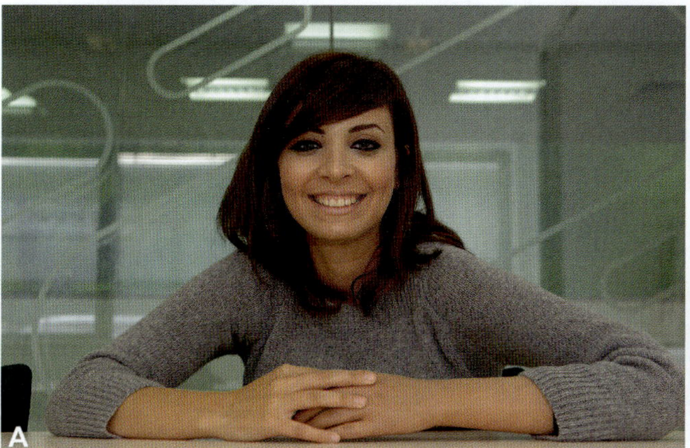

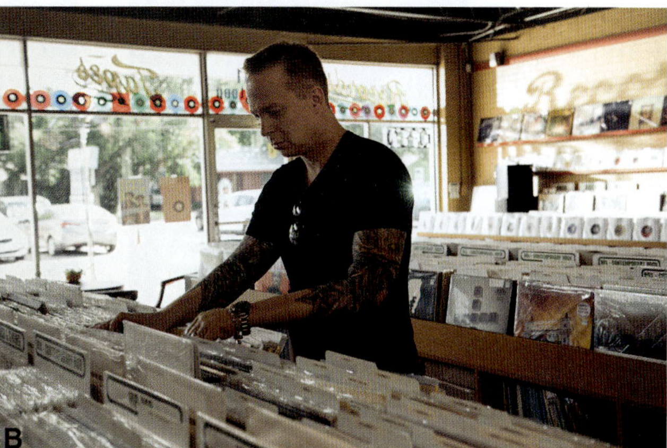

Fig. 30.6 Esthetic restorations address the psychosocial needs of individuals by reducing social stigma and enhancing community participation to optimize healthcare outcomes. (A) A female working in customer service. (B) Skin restoration with tattoos. (A, © Össur; B, Courtesy Ottobock Health Care, www.ottobockus.com.)

voice their insecurities about the cosmesis (transparency) of wearing or using a prosthesis, they often avoid activities that require unnatural movements. During training, the patient needs instruction about how to move in a natural way with and without their prosthesis.[58]

Partial-Hand Prostheses

Partial-hand prostheses are devices designed to replace a part of the hand that has been amputated or is congenitally missing. Unlike full-hand prostheses, which replace the entire hand, partial-hand prostheses focus on specific segments or digits of the hand, such as fingers or portions of fingers. By restoring hand function, partial-hand prostheses empower individuals to regain independence in daily living.[99]

Individuals who undergo partial-hand amputation face challenges in returning to their previous jobs, even with prosthetic restoration. Berger et al. found that less than half of individuals who underwent partial-hand amputation returned to their same job, with particular difficulties observed in cases involving thumb or multiple finger amputations ($n = 48$).[100,101]

The partial-hand amputation presents design challenges for the prosthetist because of its long residual limb length. Longer residual limb length reduces the amount of space to place components, sometimes resulting in a bulky and less esthetically appearing prosthesis. In addition, the prosthetist aims to preserve open sensate areas to allow sensation (and sometimes mobility) while finding enough area to distribute socket pressures to achieve a secure "fit" between the limb and the prosthesis. Because of these challenges, surgical reconstruction may be preferred.[95] Preoperative consideration of the sensation and mobility of remaining functional digits should not be understated. If functional range and sensation are inadequate, the surgeon may consider a more proximal level of amputation. The patient, surgeon, prosthetist, and therapist should discuss the prosthetic design challenges, surgical interventions, and hand function in advance to avoid unrealistic expectations and to achieve optimal outcomes.[102]

Partial-hand prostheses may be categorized as passive (static or adjustable) or active.[103] Passive partial-hand prostheses are nonelectronic, nonmotorized devices that do not have any movable parts. Active partial-hand prostheses are electronic and may include motors, sensors, and other components to enable movement and control. Among passive types, static (passive) partial-hand prostheses are nonarticulating devices that do not incorporate movable components or joints. They maintain a fixed position and lack the ability to mimic natural finger movements. Adjustable (passive) partial-hand prostheses incorporate movable components or joints that allow for adjustment and manipulation of the device. These prostheses aim to enhance functionality by providing limited articulation, enabling users to perform basic hand movements.

Passive-static tools (oppositional posts) are most useful when either the thumb is remaining and fingers are missing or when fingers are missing and thumb is remaining.[104] They allow the patient to regain grasp and release capability of the affected limb and can be fabricated for heavy-duty activities, depending on the condition of the residual limb. Passive-static hands (esthetic or transparent) are shaped to appear as a "typical" hand and allow for reduced social stigmatism, as described earlier. Users of prosthetic hands consider appearance and function a priority.[103] When designed to match the individual's specific needs, passive prostheses enhance activity performance.

Active partial-hand prostheses include both body-powered and externally powered partial-hand prosthetic options. Body-powered partial-hand prostheses allow independent and immediate operation of each finger such as playing the piano (Fig. 30.7A) and performance of heavy-duty activities in dusty environments (see Fig. 30.7B). Externally powered advancements of small electric componentry permits electric control despite lack of clearance with long residual limbs (Fig. 30.8).

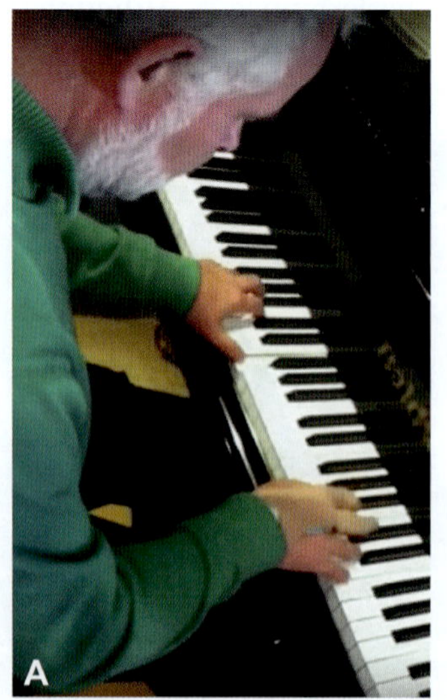

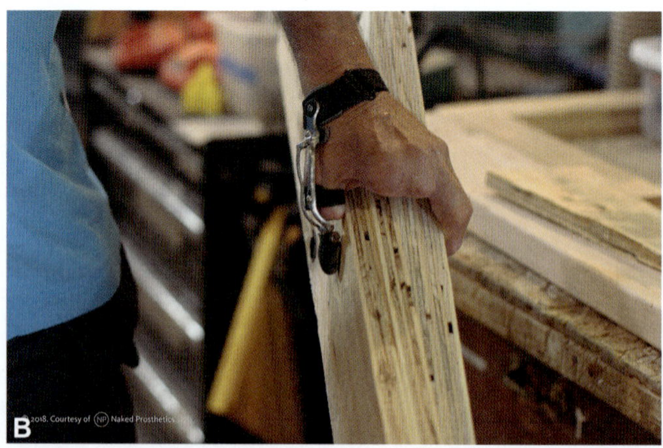

Fig. 30.7 Body-powered active partial-hand prostheses operate with immediate response and require no battery power. (A) Professional piano player who had lost his fingers in an accident. He had not sat down at a piano since his accident, 2 years prior. (B) Demonstrating the ability to hold heavy and bulky loads in dusty environments. (A, Courtesy Didrick Medical; B, Courtesy Naked Prosthetics.)

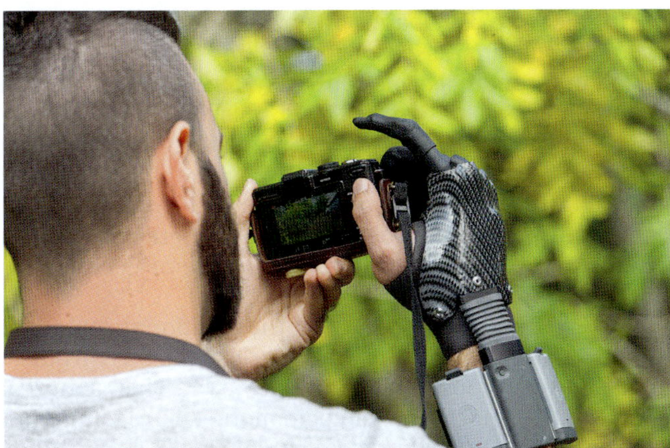

Fig. 30.8 Externally powered active partial-hand prostheses are designed based on the remaining digits and the functional needs of the individual. The multiarticulating iLimb allows for single-digit operation. (© Össur.)

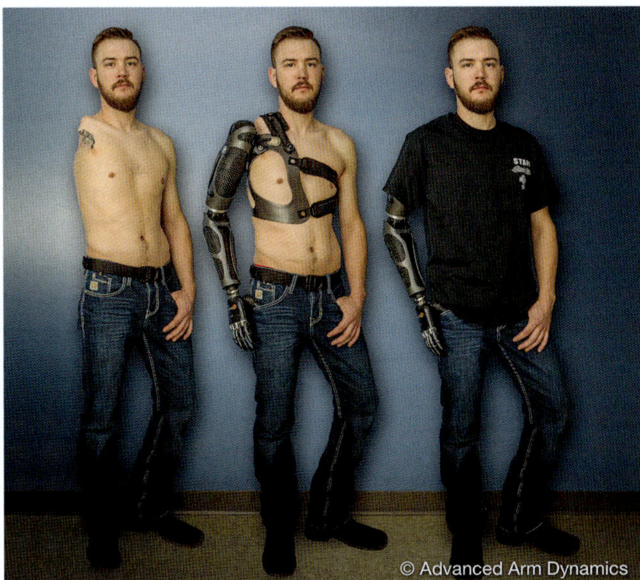

Fig. 30.9 Prosthetic care of individuals with shoulder disarticulation presents complex functional and esthetic needs. (Courtesy Advanced Arm Dynamics.)

Disarticulation Considerations

Disarticulation amputation refers to the surgical removal of a limb or body part at a joint, allowing for the separation of bones without cutting through them. In this type of amputation, disarticulation amputations provide a long lever. Their anatomy allows for suspension and preserves rotational control for functional performance. However, the disadvantages of disarticulations for prosthesis use include reduced clearance between the end of the socket and the prosthetic componentry. Reduced clearance means that there is limited space for batteries and fewer component options. For wrist disarticulation, the reduced clearance may lead to a difference in arm length with the wrist and prosthetic hand unit secured, which negatively affects functional performance. For elbow disarticulation, the reduced clearance requires the use of body-powered external locking elbow hinges. The finished prosthesis with outside-locking hinge technology is less ideal for a few reasons: they are bulky, making it difficult to fit into shirt sleeves; they lack durability; and they do not include options for flexion assist or externally powered options. At the shoulder disarticulation level, the clinical team needs to consider many more variables. Here, the rehabilitation goals not only include grasp and stabilization of objects for bimanual function but also body image and postural symmetry (Fig. 30.9).

If the surgeon removes the bony anatomy (styloids or condyles) or leaves hypersensitive distal tissues,[59] the benefits (self-suspension and rotation control) of disarticulation are lost. Therefore additional bony length should be removed to improve functional performance when using a prosthesis. The ideal residual limb length is the compromise between form and function—the benefits of having a longer limb with costs of reduced cosmesis and loss of functional control.

Transradial and Transhumeral Considerations

In a transhumeral amputation, the amputated limb includes the entire hand, wrist, forearm, and a portion of the upper arm. The amputation occurs above the elbow joint, which is no longer present. In a transradial amputation, the amputated limb includes the hand, wrist, and a portion of the forearm. The elbow joint is preserved.

Componentry for transradial and transhumeral prostheses is selected based on functional needs, patient's habitus, and level of amputation. For transradial level limb loss, the lateral epicondyle is typically the bony landmark used for reference length measurements. On the contralateral side, the measurement is taken from the lateral epicondyle to the radial styloid. On the affected side, the measurement is taken from the lateral epicondyle to the distal end of the residual limb. To accommodate the length of a quick-disconnect unit, a difference of at least 5.7 cm is needed, whereas 8.9 cm or more of difference is sufficient to allow for an electric wrist rotator (Lang M, personal communication, February 2, 2018).

At the transhumeral level, the acromium is typically the bony landmark used for reference length measurements. The measurement is taken from the acromium to the distal aspect of the olecranon on the contralateral side and from the acromium to the distal end of the residual limb on the affected side. To accommodate all potential internal-locking elbow units, 14 cm of space must be present beyond the distal residual limb. Certain elbow units are more compact and will fit within 10.2 cm while maintaining symmetry. Additional skeletal length significantly enhances suspension and force distribution, especially at the transhumeral level. Therefore Lang recommends that the length of amputation should not be dictated solely by the availability of components.

For individuals with a short residual humerus, a body-powered prosthetic system may not be realistic, and even an externally powered prosthesis may be difficult or problematic to fit, suspend, and control. When the residual humerus is very short (<4 cm), it may be necessary to treat a transhumeral limb loss functionally as a shoulder disarticulation level to capture stability.

Body-Powered Components

Body-powered components in prosthetics refer to mechanisms and devices that are activated and controlled by the movement of the user's body. Some key components associated with body-powered prosthetics include control cables, TD (hooks, grippers), harnessing systems, locks and brakes, and wrist units.[105]

TERMINAL DEVICES FOR BODY-POWERED PROSTHESES

The TDs most often used for body-powered prostheses are either hook prostheses or hands and grippers. Both are available as a voluntary opening system (closed at rest, opened by means of the cable) or as a voluntary closing system (opened at rest, closed by means of the cable). Each configuration has its own inherent strengths and weaknesses.

Voluntary opening devices enable the wearer to apply volitional force and excursion of the cable (using shoulder flexion or protraction/biscapular abduction) to open the TD (Fig. 30.10). Once tension is released from the cable, the object being grasped is "trapped" in the device, allowing the wearer to position the object in space as the task demands. The individual does not need to generate force or excursion to maintain grasp. The prehensile force (grip strength) is determined by some external closing mechanism, most frequently springs or elastic bands. Significant prehensile forces can be generated by using multiple layers of elastic bands or multiple springs but must match the wearer's ability to create and sustain cable excursion when less than maximum grip force is desired. Because grip force with a voluntary opening terminal device (VO TD) is determined by the number of elastic bands or springs used, the maximum force cannot be increased when handling heavy objects. The friction inherent in a cable control system slightly increases the force necessary to open the TD above the closing force achieved by the elastic bands or spring systems. Finding the right prehensile force to perform the variety of activities one performs throughout the day can be challenging. Several manufacturers market voluntary opening prehensors with settings the wearer can adjust to increase or decrease the prehensile force (Fig. 30.11).[106]

With voluntary closing TDs, the volitional force and excursion supplied by the wearer closes the TD from its normally open position (Fig. 30.12).[107] This action is similar to the natural physiologic motion of reaching and grasping. The key advantage of a voluntary closing TD is the possibility of significantly higher forces that can be applied through the cabling system as compared with the VO TD. In fact, with most voluntarily closing TDs, voluntary prehensile force is limited only by the strength available from the wearer or by discomfort from the harness or the residual limb. When using a voluntary closing TD, the individual must maintain both excursion and power so as to retain the object in the TD grasp, unless using a cleat or cable lock and retainer system. The sustained force allows for the ability to volitionally grade prehensile force, adapting it to the characteristics of the object to be held.[108] In addition, graded prehension allows for activities requiring fine motor control.

Voluntary closing devices are selected less often for individuals with transhumeral amputations using a body-powered prosthesis with a dual-control cable system. This is because the dual-control cable system operates both the elbow and TD, thus requiring more excursion. Functionally, much of the cable excursion would be used to close the TD, leaving less available to position the forearm. Although

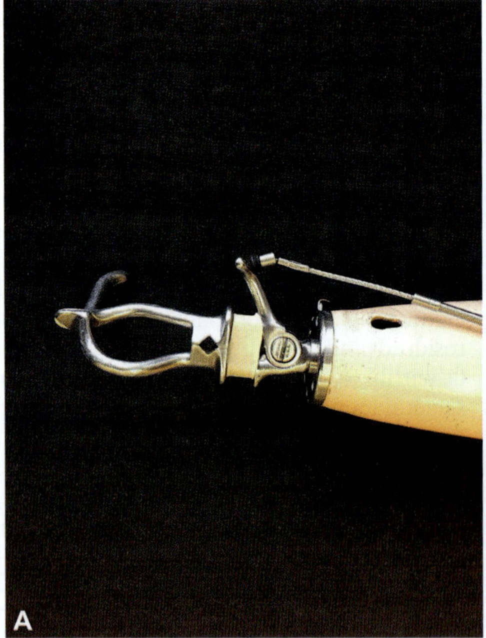

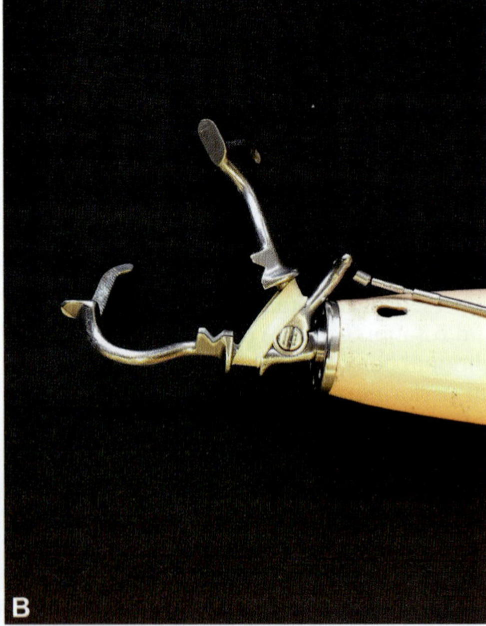

Fig. 30.10 The voluntary opening terminal device grip force is dependent by the number of elastic bands or springs. The individual must introduce force and excursion to open the hook. (A) Voluntary opening hook without tension on the cable. (B) Voluntary opening hook with full tension on the cable.

those with transhumeral amputation frequently have adequate strength and motor control to position the forearm in space, many are quite challenged to produce enough excursion to effectively operate the elbow throughout full ROM while maintaining a graded prehension of the TD. These actions become even more challenging when the residual transhumeral limb is relatively short. In addition, because cable excursion is typically limited for those with bilateral amputations, VO TDs are also the TDs of choice if bilateral body prostheses are recommended. Consequently, the passive closure (i.e., elastic bands or spring) of VO TDs tends to be more functional for individuals with limited excursion capacity (Fig. 30.13).

Several groups have attempted to design body-powered TDs that can be switched between voluntary open and voluntary close mode because each mechanism has its own advantage and disadvantage.[109,110] The challenges to design a voluntary open and voluntary close TD include higher cost, increased weight, and variable need for cable excursion.

WRIST UNITS FOR BODY-POWERED PROSTHESES

A wrist unit is used to attach and preposition the TD for activities. Several wrist types exist to accommodate different functional needs.[111] *Friction Wrists* are simple wrist

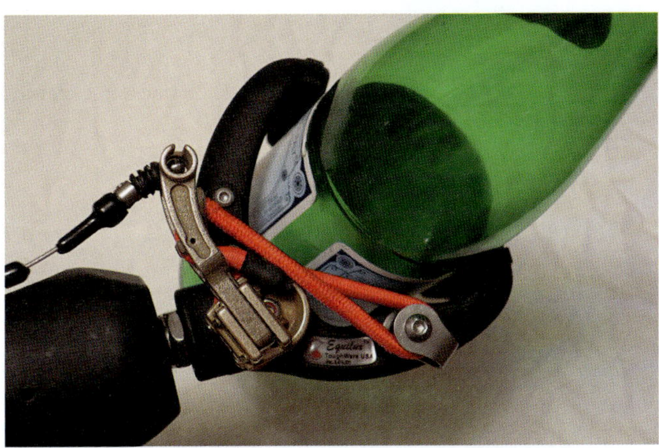

Fig. 30.11 The V2P terminal device has a variable grip closure mechanism that allows the individual to grasp objects with more or less grip force. The lever is currently positioned for maximum grip force. The individual rotates the lever to reduce grip force. (Courtesy ToughWare Prosthetics.)

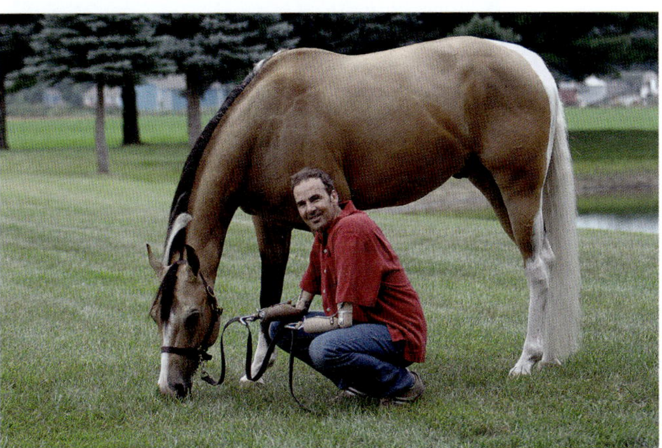

Fig. 30.13 Individuals with bilateral transhumeral limb loss may participate in activities that require dexterity in wet and dirty environments. This individual is using internal-locking elbows with voluntary opening terminal devices. (Courtesy Fillauer.)

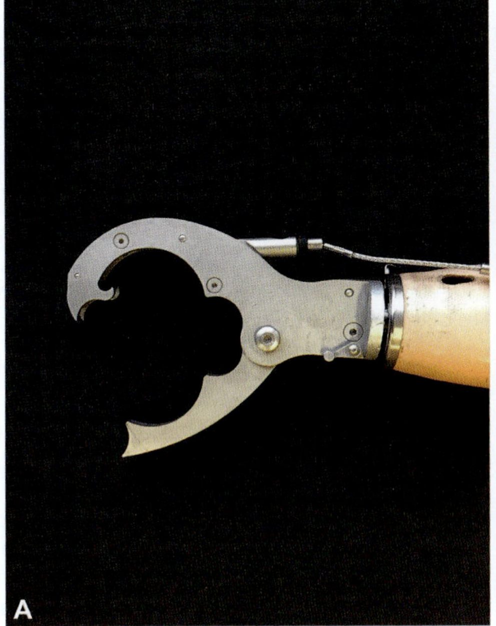

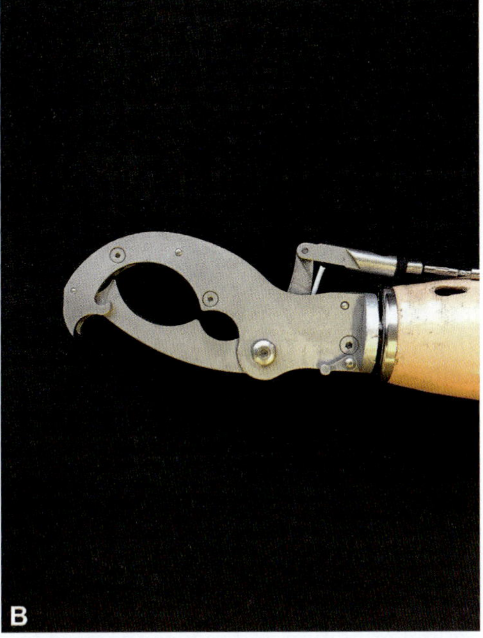

Fig. 30.12 The voluntary closing terminal device grip force is dependent only on the individual's strength and excursion capacity. The individual must introduce force and excursion to close the hook. (A) Voluntary closing hook without tension on the cable. (B) Voluntary closing hook with tension on the cable.

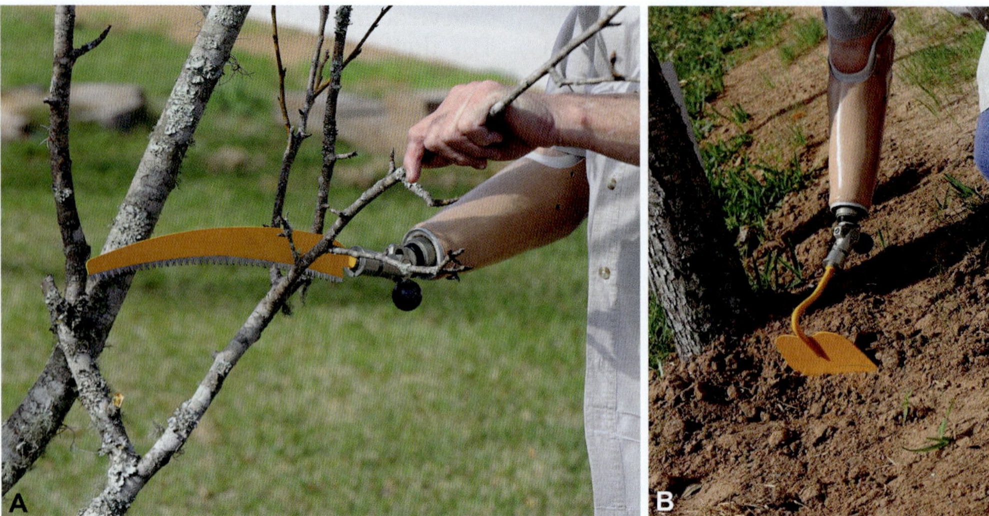

Fig. 30.14 Quick-disconnect wrist joints allow the individual to switch out terminal devices (TDs) for various work activities. (A) Cutting a tree branch with a pruning saw TD. (B) Gardening with a hand hoe TD. (A, Courtesy Texas Assistive Devices; B, Courtesy Texas Assistive Devices.)

units that use friction to control the TD positions. These wrists can be prepositioned by the other hand. Individuals with bilateral limb loss may preposition the wrist by pushing the TD against a stable object or securing the TD between the thighs and then rotating the socket and forearm. *Locking Wrists* can lock the wrist in various fixed positions to facilitate grasping and lifting heavy objects and stop transverse rotation of the TD. *Quick-Disconnect Wrists* allow quick swapping of different TDs. In addition, some quick-disconnect models are designed to allow precise locking position of pronation and supination (Fig. 30.14). *Flexion Wrists* provide wrist flexion, which is essential to perform several functional activities at midline of the body, such as feeding, dressing, and personal hygiene, especially for individuals with bilateral upper limb loss. *Multifunction Wrists* combine multiple degrees of freedom (DOF), enhance ergonomic postures, and reduce compensatory movements (Fig. 30.15).

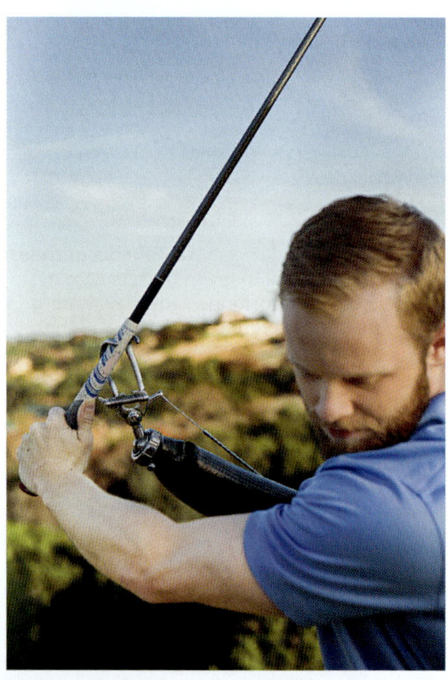

Fig. 30.15 Mobility of the wrist joint reduces compensatory motions in the proximal joints, permitting movement that is more natural and ergonomic. The position on the terminal device with the Robo wrist is adjusted by rotating the base of the wrist unit. (Courtesy Ottobock Health Care, www.ottobockus.com.)

ELBOW UNITS FOR BODY-POWERED PROSTHESES

A mechanical elbow unit is necessary for elbow disarticulation, transhumeral prostheses, and above to allow control of elbow flexion, extension, and transverse rotation. Two types of elbow locking system are used: *Outside-Locking Hinges* (Fig. 30.16) and *Internal-Locking Elbows*. *Outside-Locking Hinges* are used for long transhumeral residual limb and elbow disarticulation that do not have sufficient space for an elbow unit. However, they lack durability and are more bulky as compared with internal-locking elbows. *Internal-Locking Elbows* have the advantage of allowing manual transverse rotation of the forearm to compensate for the loss of humeral internal and external rotation.

For transradial prostheses, elbow hinges aid in suspension of the socket. *Flexible Elbow Hinges* allow natural residual limb supination and pronation and reduce the need to manually preposition the TD. *Rigid Elbow Hinges* restrict residual limb supination and pronation but provide transverse rotational stability between the limb and the socket. The full humeral cuff may be used with the rigid hinges to relieve loads from the residual limb by distributing pressure to the humerus. Rigid elbow hinges may be selected for individuals who perform work with heavier objects or for individuals with a short residual limb when voluntary supination and pronation are absent and transverse rotational stability is needed.

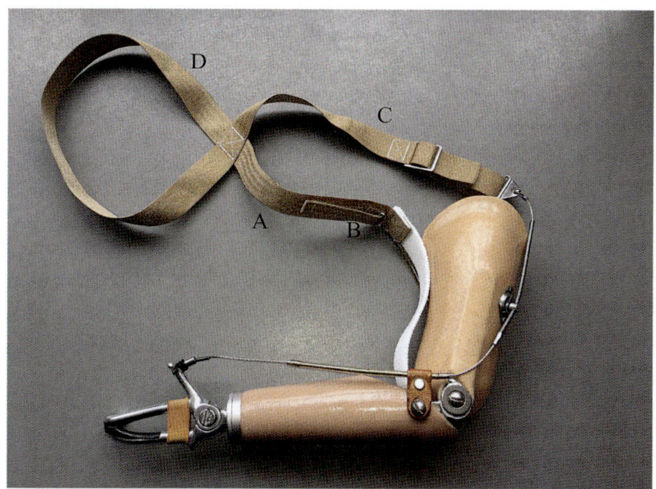

Fig. 30.16 This elbow disarticulation prosthesis uses outside-locking hinges with a figure-of-eight harness and dual-control cable. The harness includes *(A)* an anterior suspension strap, *(B)* an elbow lock control strap to control the locking and unlocking of the elbow, *(C)* a control attachment strap, and *(D)* a contralateral axilla loop. The lateral suspensor, the main suspensor for the transhumeral prosthesis, is missing from this harness. It originates at the posterior upper portion of the axilla loop and extends horizontally over the anterior support strap and over the acromion to the lateral proximal aspect of the socket.

Body-Powered Control

Body-powered control in prosthetics refers to a control system where the movement and positioning of the prosthetic device are achieved through the use of the user's own body movements. In a body-powered prosthetic system, control cables are connected to specific points on the user's body, typically the remaining limb or other body parts, to transmit mechanical forces.

Both force and excursion are necessary to operate body-powered components. Excursion can be defined as the length that the cable needs to be pulled to operate the components, measured in inches or centimeters. Compared with externally powered prostheses, body-powered prostheses are more durable, are easier to maintain, require shorter training time and fewer adjustments, and provide more sensory feedback.[4] However, several areas of improvements in body-powered prosthetic operation have been identified by its users, such as wrist movement and control, task completion time, coordination, and sensory feedback.[4] The individual must use specific strategies to effectively create enough excursion in the cable to operate the TD or preposition the forearm in space. In most instances, glenohumeral flexion contributes the largest amount of excursion in body-powered prosthesis control. Additional excursion can be achieved through scapular and biscapular abduction (scapular protraction). These secondary movements allow a well-trained and skilled prosthesis wearer to increase their functional work envelope, the space in which the wearer can effectively control the TD.

For most body-powered upper extremity prostheses, the functional envelope is limited to a relatively small area below the shoulders, above the waist, and not far outward past shoulder width. Many individuals have significant difficulty with tasks that involve grasp-and-release tasks above the head or down near their feet. Because the control strategy involves generating cable excursion through flexion or protraction, or both, tasks and activities occurring behind the back are not possible. Despite these functional limitations, body-powered prostheses have provided many individuals with reliable and durable prosthetic systems.

FIGURE-OF-EIGHT HARNESS FOR SUSPENSION AND CONTROL

A figure-of-eight harness in prosthetics refers to a specific type of harnessing system used in the context of body-powered prosthetic devices. The harness is shaped like the figure-eight, with two loops that encircle different parts of the user's body. One loop encircles the contralateral (non-amputated) shoulder, while the other loop goes around the ipsilateral (amputated) shoulder. The loops cross over the user's back, creating an "X" shape in the mid-back region (see Fig. 30.16). The crosspoint (center of the figure-of-eight) can be positioned just below the seventh cervical vertebra and slightly toward the contralateral side to increase cable excursion. The axillary loop can be adjusted through its attachment to a circular ring or fixed with a sewn crosspoint. The use of a center ring often makes the donning process less difficult and appears to provide the most satisfactory ROM. The size of the axillary loop determines the location of the crosspoint and determines the relation of comfort versus excursion capability. A larger and looser axillary loop is more comfortable but limits the individual's ability to capture excursion due to the slack in the material and the relative location of the control attachment strap across the back. To capture as much excursion as possible, the control attachment strap should be taut and positioned over the lower third of the scapula. Harnessing materials are most frequently fabricated with medium-weight Dacron webbing with both leather and plastic integrated components.

Individuals with transradial amputations control the TD by means of a single-control (Bowden) cable.[112] In most instances a triceps cuff is used to secure the cable housing in an optimal position, as well as provide an integral link to the forearm section (Fig. 30.17). Metal flexible hinges can be substituted for the Dacron flexible hinges in circumstances in which extremely heavy axial loads can be expected (i.e., if a wearer must carry or move heavy objects at work).

Individuals with transhumeral amputations need a dual-cable harness with an anterior single-control cable that controls the locking and unlocking of the elbow unit and a dual-control cable that controls the TD (if the elbow is locked) or moves the prosthetic forearm (if the elbow is unlocked). This second (longer) dual-control cable that attaches to the TD requires a split-cable (fairlead) housing system (Fig. 30.18). The proximal portion of the housing is attached to the humeral section, while the distal portion is attached just distal and anterior to the elbow center.

Most elbow units have multiple locking positions at equally spaced intervals moving from full extension to

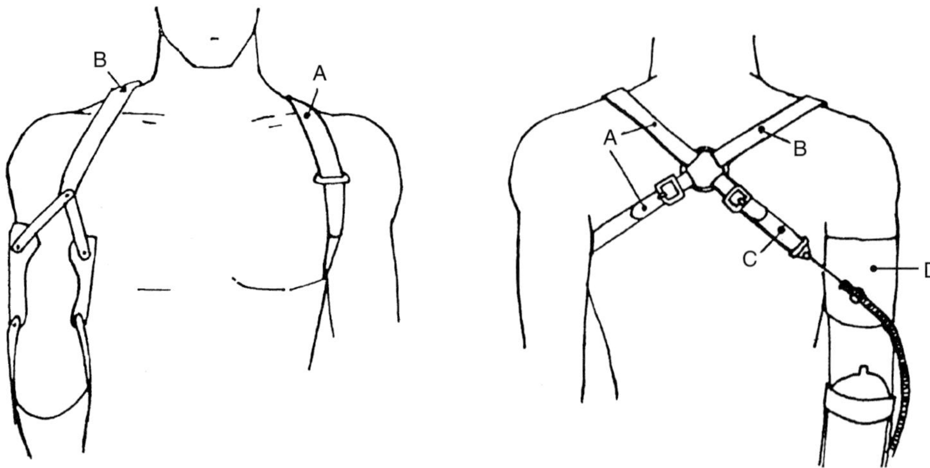

Fig. 30.17 Anterior and posterior view of a figure-of-eight harness system for a transradial prosthesis, with *(A)* the axillary loop, *(B)* the anterior support strap that provides stability during a downward pull, *(C)* the attachment strap for cable control of the terminal device, and *(D)* the triceps pad that anchors the control cable in the most effective position. (Modified from the Northwestern University Printing and Duplicating Department, Evanston, Illinois, 1987.)

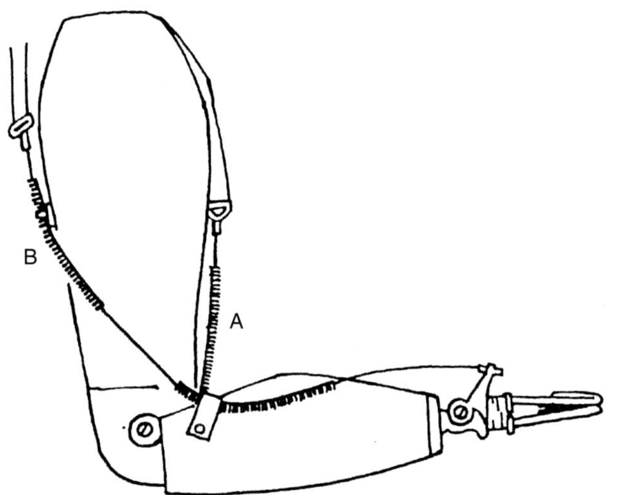

Fig. 30.18 Dual control cable and forearm lift tab of a body-powered transhumeral prosthesis with *(A)* an elbow lock cable and *(B)* a dual-control cable. (Modified from Northwestern University Printing and Duplicating Department, Evanston, Illinois, 1987.)

flexion. The locking mechanism is most frequently activated using a rapid and forceful shoulder extension and abduction. When the elbow unit is "locked" in any given position, this quick and forceful ipsilateral shoulder depression and extension pulls the elbow lock cable that releases the lock; subsequent shoulder flexion or scapular abduction (protraction) affecting the dual-control cable repositions the prosthetic forearm in space. This happens because the dual-control cable running to the TD is aligned anterior to the axis of rotation of the elbow unit; when the elbow is unlocked, tension through this dual-control cable causes the forearm to rise in flexion. When the forearm reaches the desired inclination for the task at hand, another quick down-and-back motion will reengage the lock. Once the elbow unit is locked, cable control is transferred to the TD, and subsequent shoulder flexion or protraction operates the prosthetic hook or hand. To achieve live lift with the dual-control cable, the amount of force required to open the VO TD needs to be greater than that needed to flex the forearm. If the force to open the VO TD is less than the force needed to flex the forearm, then the TD will open before the forearm lifts. Live lift is the ability to flex the forearm while holding something in the TD. Because this control strategy with the dual-control cable is always sequential in nature, careful consideration and assessment must be given to the force-excursion ratio. Failure to maximize these criteria results in incomplete elbow flexion or incomplete TD control. Challenges in operation of the dual-control cable can be addressed with the triple-control harness; however, care must be taken to avoid crossover contamination between control motions.

CONTROL AND SUSPENSION FOR BILATERAL PROSTHESES

For individuals with amputation of both upper extremities, careful clinical consideration must be given to ease donning and control. Instead of using a traditional figure-of-eight harness with a contralateral axillary loop for each prosthesis, the two anterior suspension components can be linked. In this arrangement, the bilateral prosthetic system is effectively stabilized by the equal counteracting forces from each prosthesis. On the basis of an individual's functional needs, the prosthetist may use either a single-ring, dual-ring, or biomechanically aligned harness anchor ring system to maximize the efficiency of the body-powered prostheses.

Some individuals with bilateral amputations opt to use separate and completely independent harness systems for their prostheses, especially if they are a new prosthesis user, or sometimes wear only one prosthesis, or if their prostheses are dissimilar. For example, an individual with bilateral transradial amputations might elect to use a body-powered system on their nondominant side and a self-suspending externally powered prosthesis on their dominant residual limb.

Electric Components

Electric components in prosthetics refer to the electrical elements integrated into certain types of prosthetic devices, particularly those classified as externally powered or myoelectric prosthetics. These includes (1) electric component(s) that are (2) activated by the electronics to acquire and process the input signal(s), (3) directed by the controller, and (4) powered by the battery such as myoelectric sensors, microprocessors, motors/actuators, batteries, wiring and connectors, control interface, bluetooth and wireless technology, and sensors for feedback (Fig. 30.19).

ELECTRIC TERMINAL DEVICES

Electric terminal devices are components of externally powered or myoelectric prosthetic systems that serve as the functional end or hand of the prosthesis. Common categories for electric terminal devices include grippers, multiaxis hands, prehensors, artificial hands with individual finger movement, externally powered hands, and customized terminal devices. With advancements in technology, some currently available electric systems are quite robust (Fig. 30.20).

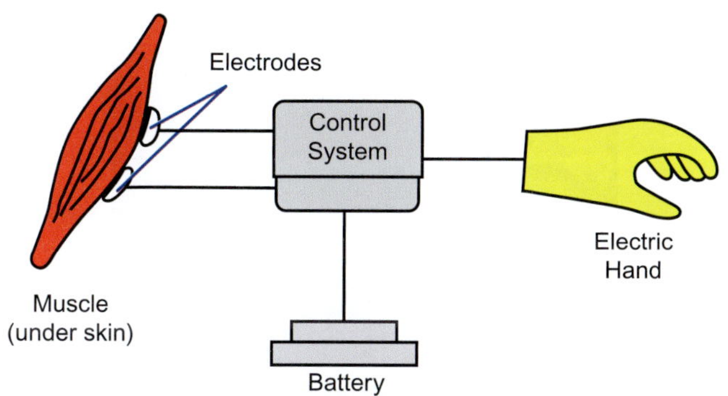

Fig. 30.19 Basic concept of myoelectric control: myoelectrodes, controller, battery, and electric component. (From Muzumdar A. *Powered Upper Limb Prostheses*. Springer; 2004:36.)

Selection of the TDs depends on the type of activity, the environment and the shape, size, and weight of the objects being manipulated, and the specific characteristics of the TD. Hands are available in "single degree-of-freedom" (single-DOF) designs allowing combined movement between the thumb and fingers and "multiple degree-of-freedom" (multi-DOF or multi-articulating) designs allowing independent movement of each digit, including the proximal interphalangeal and distal interphalangeal joints. All hands are capable of a "three-jaw chuck" and palmar pinch grasp pattern between the thumb and first two digits, which is ideal for grasping cylindrical objects such as cups, steering wheels, and hand rails (Fig. 30.21A).

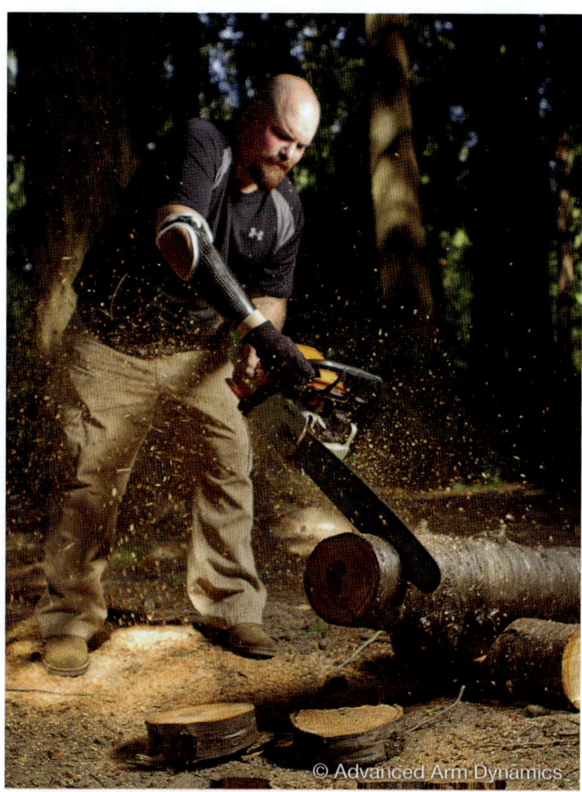

Fig. 30.20 Performing heavy-duty activities with self-suspension and an externally powered prosthesis. (Courtesy Advanced Arm Dynamics.)

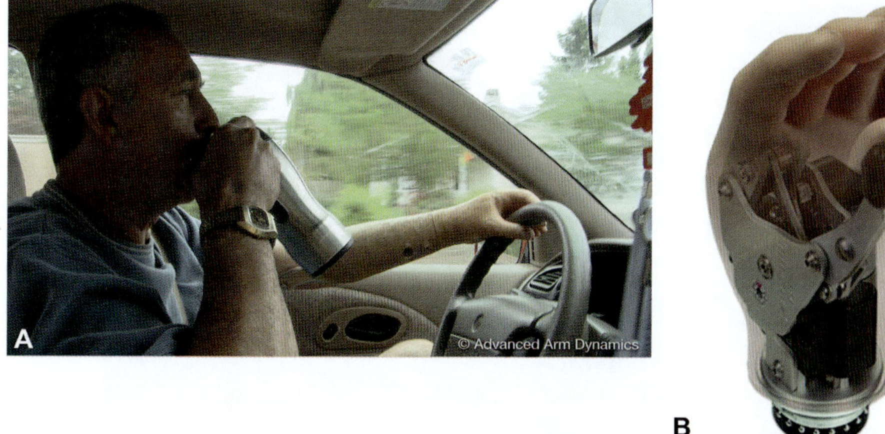

Fig. 30.21 Single degree-of-freedom hand. (A) Three-jaw chuck grasp of steering wheel enhances driving performance. (B) The internal mechanism of the three-jaw chuck hand is visible through the outer structure. The motor controls movement of the index and middle fingers, while the fourth and fifth digits follow. (A, Courtesy Advanced Arm Dynamics; B, Courtesy Steeper Group.)

Single-DOF hands are limited to simple opening and closing of the thumb and the digits; most often the first two digits move toward the thumb while the remaining fingers (digits four and five) follow passively (see Fig. 30.21B). Some hands include sensors in the digits to provide slip control. This allows objects to be retained in the grasp without conscious control from patient input (Fig. 30.22).

Significant grasp forces can be achieved with single-DOF electric hands; in fact, pressures can be so significant that individuals must be cautioned during early training about the amount of force production. With proportional control, maximum grip strength is achieved with corresponding maximum input signal generated by forceful muscle contraction. The maximum grip force of a multiarticulating hand is somewhat lower than the single-DOF (noncompliant) hand. However, the amount of grasp necessary to stabilize an object is dependent on the type of grasp, number of contact points and friction between the fingers and object, and the weight and geometry of the object.[27] The reduced grip force of multiarticulating hands as compared with single-DOF hands is offset by the additional surface area and contour of multiple fingers around an object (Fig. 30.23).

Multiarticulating hands permit many activities that were previously impossible to perform with single-DOF hands because of the variety of grasp patterns. For example, single-DOF hands do not have the capability of fully opening or allowing for single-digit movement. Multiarticulating hands allow for variation in individual preferences and manipulation strategies (Figs. 30.8 and 30.24). For those who had the option of six grasp patterns for use in their home environment (power, tool, chuck, fine pinch open, fine pinch close, and lateral pinch), lateral grip followed by chuck then pinch closed were most often selected by the individual.[113] Substantial variation of grasp pattern use exists between professions (housekeeper vs. machinist), as

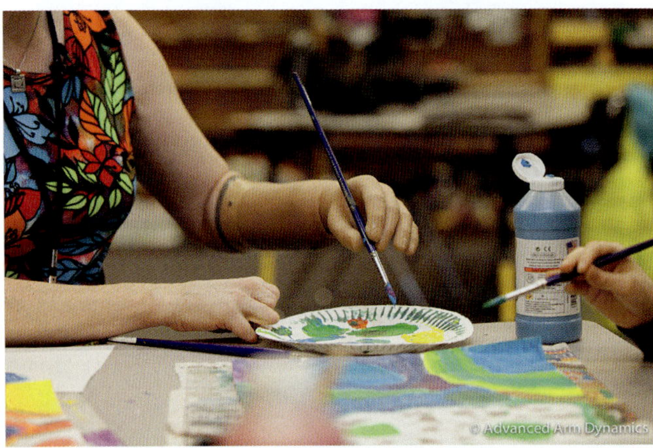

Fig. 30.22 The individual can concentrate on the activity rather than on the operation of the terminal device with the Sensor Hand Speed. (Courtesy Advanced Arm Dynamics.)

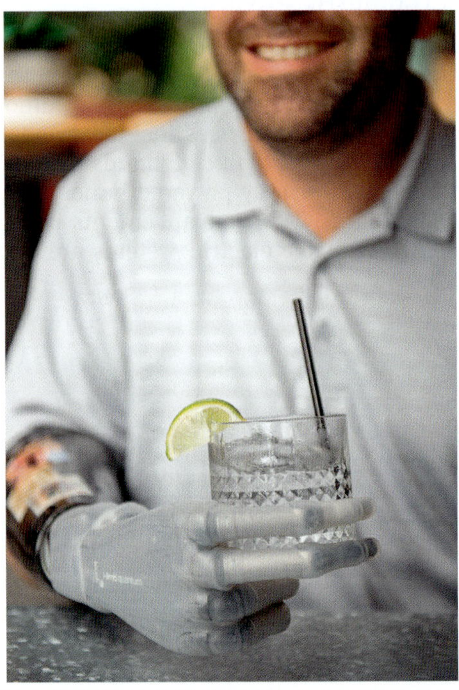

Fig. 30.23 Multiarticulating hands are also called "compliant hands" because they comply to the shape of the object being grasped. Grasping the object with greater surface area provides a secure hold on the object. (© Össur.)

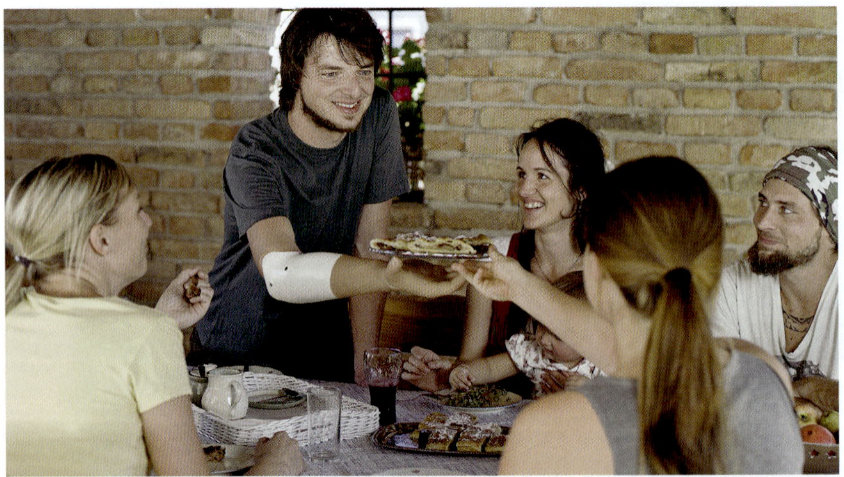

Fig. 30.24 Variable grip patterns allow the individual to hold, stabilize, and grasp objects of various sizes and shapes. Stabilizing a plate with a Michelangelo Hand. (Courtesy Ottobock Health Care, www.ottobockus.com.)

well as between individuals within those professions when performing different activities.[113,114] Because increasing DOF is associated with enhanced activity performance, powered opposition of the thumb that allows active movement from lateral prehension to palmar prehension is a prosthetic hand design recommendation.[27] This ability to move between palmar prehension (Fig. 30.25A) and lateral prehension (see Fig. 30.25B) reduces compensatory motions at the proximal joints.

Because most prostheses include a quick-disconnect option for the TD, prosthetic wearers can easily change TDs to suit their functional demands. Nonanthropomorphic (hook-style or utility) electric prehensors range from tools that closely resemble portable vices (Fig. 30.26A) to terminal hardware that closely mimics the functional characteristics of an electric hook (see Fig. 30.26B). Many of the nonanthropomorphic prehensors can generate even greater forces than the corresponding hands. The geometries of the opening mechanism allow these alternative tools to easily grasp larger, cylindrical, and irregularly shaped objects. The smaller tips of some of these prehensors allow individuals to grasp smaller and flatter objects and have less obstruction of the visual field. To date, no one TD is commercially available that satisfactorily replicates the lost proprioception and sensation or combines the function, durability, and cosmesis of the anatomic hand.

ELECTRIC WRISTS

Wrist units are necessary to connect the TD to the prosthesis and substitute for lost pronation and supination and sometimes for radial-ulnar deviation and flexion-extension motions. These movements may require prepositioning by the contralateral extremity unless using an electric rotator. Loss of wrist motion leads to compensatory motions.[115,116] Use of electric wrists with active DOF often requires more clearance and adds weight to the distal end of the prosthesis, thus requiring clinical decisions about the cost and benefits. Although two DOF electric wrist units exist, the additional weight and clearance requirements limit their clinical use.[117] Some TDs incorporate wrist flexion/extension or ulnar/radial deviation within the TD components, which provide the individual with advantageous approaches for improved grasp (Fig. 30.27).

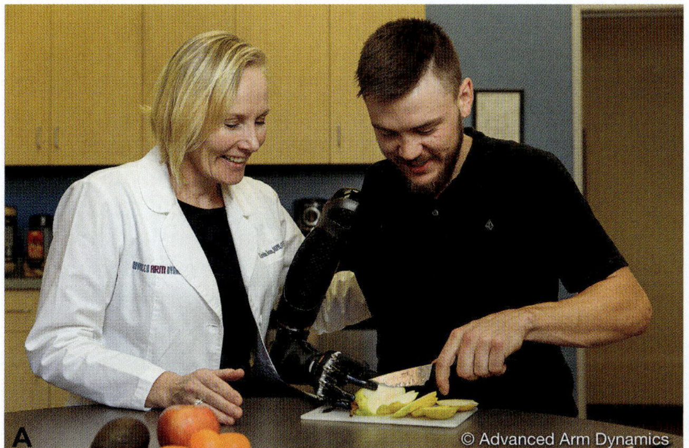

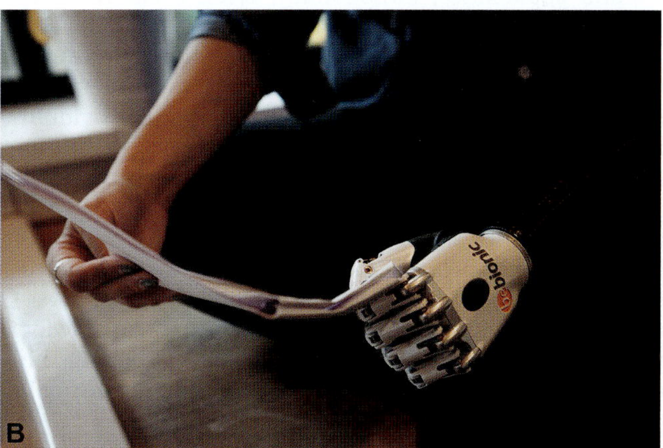

Fig. 30.25 Powered adduction of the thumb allows for both palmar and lateral prehension grasp patterns. (A) Palmar prehension allows for grasp of round or cylindrical objects. (B) Lateral prehension is one of the most common grasp patterns used during daily activities. (A, Courtesy Advanced Arm Dynamics; B, Courtesy Ottobock Health Care, **www.ottobockus.com**.)

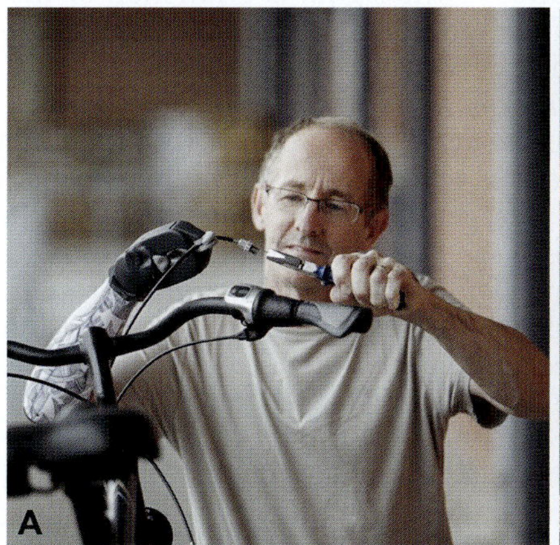

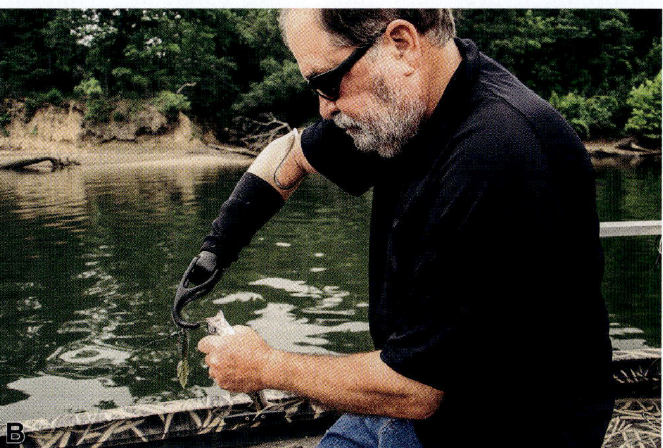

Fig. 30.26 Nonanthropomorphic terminal devices for externally powered prostheses. (A) The Griefer opens with a parallel grasp and can provide the extremely strong grasp forces. (B) The electric terminal device opens with a nonparallel grasp and allows for activities in wet environments. (A, Courtesy Ottobock Health Care, **www.ottobockus.com**; B, Courtesy Fillauer.)

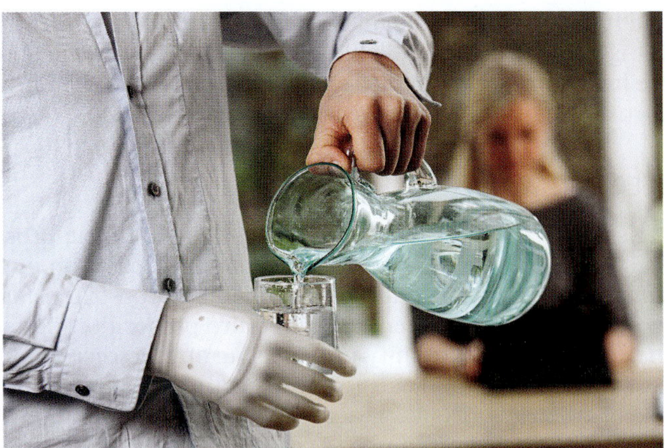

Fig. 30.27 The Michelangelo hand incorporates a wrist that allows ulnar deviation for ergonomically correct positions. (Courtesy Ottobock Health Care, www.ottobockus.com.)

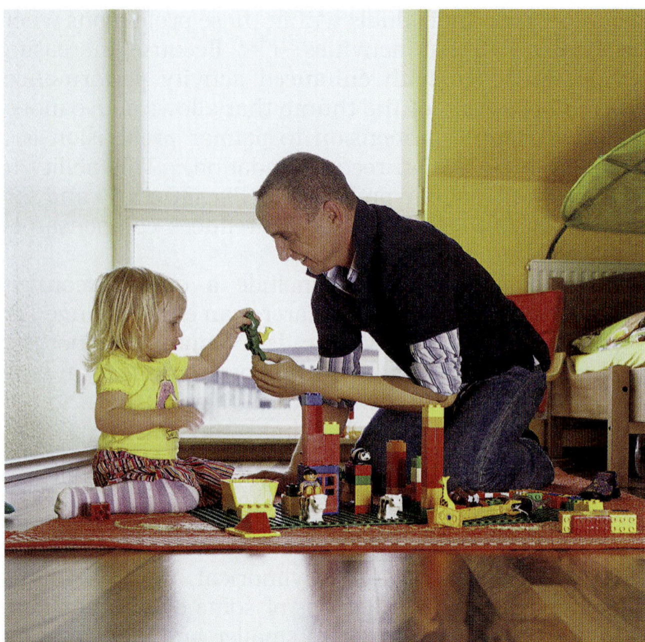

Fig. 30.28 The electric elbow provides elbow flexion, whereas the electric wrist rotator pronates the hand after the hand grasps the object from the floor. (Courtesy Ottobock Health Care, www.ottobockus.com.)

ELECTRIC ELBOWS

A number of electric elbow components are commercially available. Each electric elbow uses proprietary signal processing and drive mechanisms to achieve design-specific functional capabilities. Functionally, electric elbow units provide powered flexion and extension at the elbow joint (Fig. 30.28). Substitution for internal and external rotation of the shoulder is more difficult. Most systems integrate a passive friction humeral rotator that allows the individual to reposition the forearm and TD in the desired amount of internal or external shoulder rotation though powered rotation is commercially available.[105] For individuals with exceptionally short transhumeral limbs and shoulder disarticulation, most prostheses use a mechanical device to replace the shoulder joint that can be passively repositioned, although electrically actuated locks are available for clinical use and provide an effective means of locking the position of the humerus relative to the midline of the body for individuals with high-level amputations.

Externally Powered Control

Externally powered control in prosthetics refers to the method of controlling a prosthetic limb using external power sources, typically electric motors or actuators. For the externally powered prosthesis, the control system includes the input devices and the controller. The electronics to acquire the input signal(s) are called input devices. Examples of input devices include myoelectrode assemblies, switches, linear transducers (servos), and force-sensing resistors (touch pads); these are discussed in the myoelectric and alternative control system sections later in this chapter. The controller translates the signal from the input device to the correct command then transmits the commands to the motor in the electric component.[118,119]

MYOELECTRIC CONTROL SYSTEMS

Myoelectric control relies on the detection of electrical signals (myoelectric signals [MESs]) generated by the user's residual muscles.[120] Electrodes placed on the skin surface or implanted within muscles capture muscle contractions, and the signals are processed by a microprocessor. Among the advantages of myoelectric control are cosmesis,[4] increased prosthesis use in activities of daily living,[64] psychosocial adaptation,[121] reduced cortical reorganization and reduction of phantom limb pain intensity,[4] strengthening of muscle tone, and comfort. For an individual with a transradial amputation, the greatest advantage of myoelectric prostheses is the elimination of the harness. The harness is the most common source of prosthesis discomfort;[63] with the harness eliminated, the prosthesis is easier to don and doff, even when the person is fully dressed.[122]

The MES is the small electrical activity generated by the ionic activity of the contracting muscles and detected by surface electrodes. Modern circuitry and sophisticated filters allow most individuals, even those with small signals, the potential for reasonable control. "The amplitude and appearance of the signal is a function of many variables: *depth* of the muscle, *size* of the muscle, *strength* of the contraction, overlying *tissue*, as well as the *type, location, and orientation* of electrodes."[119]

Specific to myoelectric control, the practitioner must evaluate the MES to determine the minimum microvolt threshold and whether this would allow operation of a myoelectric prosthesis, the number of muscle sites or switches that can be independently controlled, signal separation, and the cognitive ability of the user (Box 30.3). These attributes are analyzed in consideration of the number of components and the DOFs needed for control.

Before the MES is sent to the controller, it is processed through a differential amplifier and filtered (dual-site control also requires that the MES be rectified and smoothed). Some software programs (Motion Control and Touch Bionics) allow prosthetists the ability to alter the smoothing algorithm. The MES inherently carries noise from a variety

Box 30.3 Myoelectric Input Signal Evaluation

- Myoelectric signal minimum microvolt threshold
- Cognitive ability of the user
- Specific to direct control
  - Number of muscle sites or switches that can be independently controlled
  - Signal separation

of sources, which is a problem because the noise may be confused with the true intended MES. Noise is reduced through a variety of mechanisms (Table 30.4). Common mode voltage is the noise from the environment that appears as an offset on both electrodes; the signal is literally common (belonging equally to both) electrodes. Devices that plug into outlets in the United States use a 60-Hz frequency, whereas in most other countries it is 50 Hz. The differential amplifier and notch filters reduce this common mode voltage.

Motion artifact occurs with vertical and horizontal movement of the electrode over the surface of the skin. It may be problematic during dynamic contractions, vigorous activities, or when lifting heavy loads.[119] Skin motion artifact is avoided by a snug and well-fitting socket. This means that the socket fit and the control system have been evaluated as the individual performs activities in various positions within their work space.

For dual-site myoelectric control, it is critical to identify isolated signals during myotesting and myotraining because signals from neighboring muscles can distort the amplitude and timing of the desired signal. To avoid crosstalk contamination, the gain is reduced or a location identified with less interference from the undesired MES. Physiologic noise can be reduced only by repositioning the electrode further away from the source of the tissues that generate the interfering electrical signals.

After processing the signal (filtering out the noise, amplification, rectification, and smoothing), the MES can be thought of conceptually as a command that triggers the motor. When the MES is greater than the threshold, the controller sends a signal to the motor to be active. The clinician can alter the threshold or the gain setting to adjust the sensitivity of activation.

If the MES does not provide a varying voltage, the controller sends a fixed speed command to the motor. This digital speed control is in contrast to proportional control in which the MES provides a varying voltage that can control the speed, force, and position of the component(s). In other words, the speed and force of the electric component are proportional to the contraction level and intensity of the MES. This graded control enables individuals to develop extremely precise speed and grip strength function. Because of its superior function, most systems use proportional control. Clinicians need to adjust the gain setting so that the MES lies within the control range when using proportional control. Setting the amplification of the signal too high (i.e., gain setting) may result in loss of control-efficiency as strong MES may exceed the control range. Depending on the strength and isolation of the signals, the prosthetist selects the appropriate control scheme such as dual-site control or pattern recognition control and sequential control or simultaneous control.

Table 30.4 Various Sources of Signal Noise

Signal Noise Source	Resolution
Common mode signal	Differential amplifier
	Notch filter
Motion artifact	Well-fitting socket
Crosstalk contamination[a]	Reduce the gain or reposition the sensor to reduce the signal level
Physiologic noise	Locate sensor further away from the source

[a]Crosstalk contamination is not permitted in pattern recognition control.

EMG
Differential amplification
Rectification smoothing
Controller maps one-site (signal) to one-function

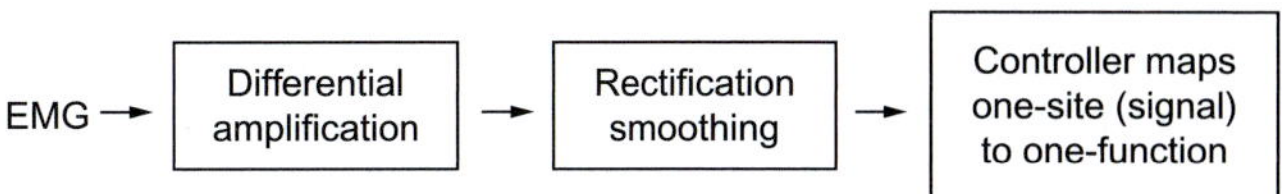

Fig. 30.29 Basic illustration of the stages of electromyography (EMG) myoelectric signal processing with single-site and dual-site myoelectric control.

Sequential and simultaneous control refers to the operation of one or more components. Sequential control means that each component's motion is operated one at a time from the same input. For example, the controller sends a signal to the elbow to operate, then the controller switches modes from the elbow to the wrist for wrist operation. With simultaneous control, the same two MESs at the biceps and triceps can be used to control movement of elbow and wrist at the same time. Individuals use their biceps to simultaneously close the TD and pronate the prosthetic forearm or use their triceps to simultaneously open the TD and supinate the prosthetic forearm. For example, the person could grasp something off the floor with a pronated wrist and then flex their elbow while simultaneously positioning the wrist in neutral (see Fig. 30.28). Although simultaneous control is more challenging to operate, it allows for more seamless and efficient movement patterns. For a beginning prosthesis user, sequential control is recommended.

Dual-Site Control

Single-site and dual-site controls refer to the number of myoelectrode sites: one site and two sites, respectively (Fig. 30.29). In other words, dual-site control involves using two distinct muscle sites for control, often in close proximity to each other. Ideally, the prosthetist tries to identify two independent MESs in a set of physiologically paired (agonist and antagonist) muscles. The advantage is the reduction of the risk of crosstalk between muscle signals, enhancing control accuracy, allowing for more nuanced control and versatility.

For those with transradial limb loss, electrodes are typically positioned over flexor muscle residuum in the forearm to control grasp (closing of the TD) and the extensor muscle residuum to control release (opening of the TD). Many individuals who, with sufficient training, master independent contraction of these muscle groups are candidates for even more sophisticated control. The traditional dual-site sequential control scheme for an individual using an externally powered transhumeral prosthesis might include one myoelectrode to capture MES of the biceps and a second myoelectrode over the triceps. Assuming both MESs are of satisfactory amplitude and differentiation, successful myoelectric control of two devices—an electrically powered elbow and an electrically powered TD—can be successfully achieved. To extend the elbow, the individual purposefully contracts the triceps. The MES is provided continuously until the forearm and elbow reach the desired position in space. The elbow locks in this position by holding the elbow steady (no longer flexing or extending) through a predetermined and programed time interval. The controller then cycles to TD (hand) control, using the same two electromyography (EMG) inputs. To grasp an object, the individual purposefully contracts the biceps. The most commonly used sequential control scheme is contraction of the triceps to open the hand or extend the elbow and contraction of the biceps to close the hand or flex the elbow. Again, the beginning user might initially use this sequential control scheme. As they progress, some microprocessors can be adjusted to allow simultaneous control during therapy sessions until they are ready for it full time.

A prosthetic control scheme with sequential control of two or more components or components with multiple DOFs (i.e., multiarticulating hands) requires a method for mode selection. Various selection methods, ways to use an MES trigger to switch modes or hand positions, exist. MES selection methods include a cocontraction, quick-slow contraction, impulse contraction (single, double, or triple), or a sustained hold-open contraction.

Many individuals wearing transradial myoelectric prostheses can use a quick cocontraction of forearm flexors and extensors to switch control between operation of the hand and the wrist unit, whereas those with transhumeral prostheses use a quick cocontraction of biceps and triceps to switch between control of the electric elbow, wrist, and hand. Cocontraction mode selection is based on the simultaneous timing of contraction of two muscles (usually antagonistic muscles). Effective mode selection with cocontraction requires an individual to fire antagonistic muscles above a predetermined threshold at nearly the same instant, which presents a training challenge for the therapist. Early in training, many new myoelectric prosthesis users focus on forcefulness of contraction in an effort to increase amplitude of the signal, rather than on producing the desired quick cocontraction. If an individual struggles or is unable to master cocontraction, the clinician can program a different MES trigger.

If an individual struggles or is unable to master mode selection with MES triggers, alternative control strategies are available. Non-MES inputs such as a button, Bluetooth beacons, radio-frequency identification tags, or movement of the device (gesture control) may be integrated to select a component or specific hand position. In addition, many systems allow the user a default mode (usually to the TD) to which the mode selector reverts after a predetermined time interval.

Pattern Recognition Control

Pattern recognition control involves using advanced algorithms to recognize complex patterns in myoelectric signals associated with specific movements. Pattern recognition control for multifunctional control has been discussed since the early 1970s[123] and has demonstrated improving accuracy and timely performance.[124] Individuals report that pattern recognition is closer to true intuitive control and more consistency of performance as compared with dual-site control.[124] When using pattern recognition, individuals contract their muscles as if they are opening/closing their hand, rotating their wrist, or flexing/extending their elbow commonly while imagining they are performing these motions with their phantom limb. The MES signals are sent to the controller for processing, which involves feature extraction from all MES signals. These features are then classified to determine the motion (or no motion) that is most likely intended by the prosthesis wearer. The controller then sends a motion command, which includes the relative speed, to actuate the prosthesis (Fig. 30.30).[125,126]

Pattern recognition control reduces some of the challenges of dual-site myoelectric control, such as muscle coactivation and EMG crosstalk contamination. Most importantly, it eliminates the need for mode selection. For example, if an individual using a prosthetic hand and a wrist rotator would like to grasp an object, he or she would send an intuitive MES that means "pronate wrist" then a signal that means "open hand" followed by a signal that means "close hand" (Fig. 30.31). There is no need for the user to send a separate MES to switch control between the wrist and hand components because the intuitive signals

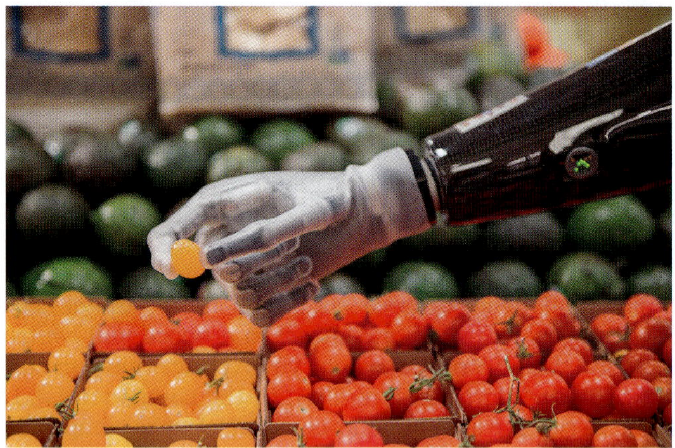

Fig. 30.31 With pattern recognition, the individual's intuitive motor patterns are used to select the desired grasp position and to select operation of the desired component. Here the individual produces a distinct motor pattern to grasp the tomato with index and thumb and a separate motor pattern to rotate the wrist. (© Össur.)

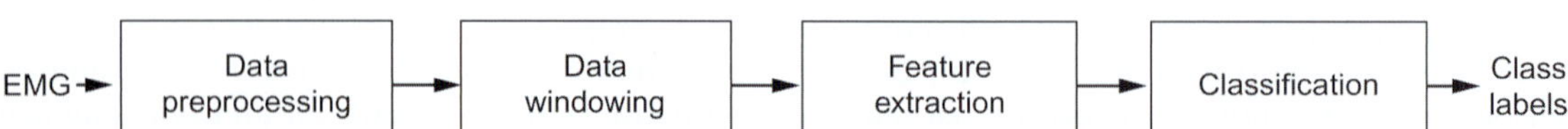

Fig. 30.30 Basic illustration of the stages of electromyography (EMG) myoelectric signal processing with pattern recognition myoelectric control. (From Scheme E, Englehart K. Electromyogram pattern recognition for control of powered upper limb prostheses: state of the art and challenges for clinical use. *J Rehabil Res Dev*. 2011;48(6):643–659.)

are directly mapped to those motions. In addition, pattern recognition allows the individual to easily select a hand position of choice, such as three-jaw chuck, finger point for computer use, or lateral grip when using a multiarticulating hand (see Fig. 30.31).

The key for optimal user control is consistency and distinguishability of the MES patterns. Nonstationarities (i.e., variation) in MES patterns may be related to fatigue, sweat, changes in tissue location in the socket with donning, and surface motion of the electrodes such as during dynamic contractions, unusual static postures, vigorous activities, or lifting heavy loads. Variation in the MES patterns is well recognized by engineers who have designed the controller to select some MES features to account for the variation, as well as systems to allow the user to recalibrate the control system. The therapist's greatest challenge when training an individual to use a prosthesis with pattern recognition control is related to training muscle relaxation, as well as training how to generate a repeatable and distinct MES pattern.

ALTERNATIVE CONTROL SYSTEMS

If effective myoelectric control is too difficult to master for an individual immediately after amputation surgery, the prosthetist may opt to use an alternative means to operate the electric prosthetic components. Alternative control systems may include switch control, linear potentiometers, force transducers, and force-sensing resistors.

Switch control does not require myoelectric sensors against the skin. Simple switch control systems require extremely small movement to trigger—typically an excursion in millimeters and a force in fractions of pounds. This reduced excursion reduces the force required for control as compared with body-powered components that required larger cable excursions to operate the TD or lock or unlock the prosthetic elbow. The ease of operation of grasp and release can be mastered fairly readily by most new prosthesis users and the reduced forces for excursion limit exposure to stresses on the recently amputated residual limb. In addition to being used in early postoperative fittings, switches can be used in definitive prostheses because the small excursion and light force required to operate switch control makes prosthesis use feasible for individuals with limited ROM or strength. Although most switches are activated by pulling a cable or strap, other applications are activated by depressing a lever or button. Some switches are complex in nature because they have numerous functions that are dictated by the position of the switch. When switches are used to trigger electric prosthetic components, proportional control (graded action where the action of the device is proportional to the effort made to trigger its operation) is not possible. Unfortunately, this absence of proportional control is a limiting factor in many switch control applications.

Proportional control of all externally powered devices (especially of elbows and the TDs) enables individuals to achieve fine control of speed and force with less effort as compared with digital control.[127] Technology has enabled proportional control to further expand the functional range of the prosthesis, with higher-speed drive motors and clutches that allow extremely responsive and rapid control. When proportional control is coupled with circuitry designed to create and maintain stable prehensile patterns within the electric components, wearers can achieve increasingly complex and sophisticated tasking patterns.

To achieve true proportionality, a servo-resistor or other sensing resistor is necessary. Transducers detect biomechanical signals (force or excursion) and turn them into electrical signals.[118] These devices may (1) interpret the travel (excursion transducers or linear potentiometers) applied to the system and translate this input quantitatively with predetermined electrical outputs, or they may (2) translate force (force transducers or servos) simultaneously or independently of excursion to create a proportional output. Force transducers, as compared with linear potentiometers, are more challenging for the user to control because their activation requirements are minimal; thus a sleep mode is necessary to prevent inadvertent activation.

Force-sensitive resistors (FSRs, also called touch pads) have found utility as a possible control driver in instances when MESs are not readily available. FSRs are designed to interpret surface pressure on the pad and supply a resultant proportional output. Because these devices are extremely flat and small in diameter, they are well suited for applications such as residual limb buds in children with congenital limb deficiencies or in partial-hand prostheses. However, special consideration must be given to the location and preparation of sites in which an FSR is to be used. These devices can become problematic if the base on which they are placed is not perfectly flat. Even a small radius can cause the conductive gel inside the sensor to fail. The location must be placed strategically to allow any perspiration to settle away from the sensor. In addition, FSRs can be challenging to operate for the prosthesis user. Because minimal movement is required to activate the sensor, they may detect inadvertent pressures from positioning the limb and/or the prosthesis in space. This makes it is difficult to determine how much force is being volitionally applied and thus sent to the controller.[72]

Engineers continue to develop alternative methods to produce control signals and create more intuitive control schemes.[128,129] However, despite the technologic advancements in externally powered prosthetics, lack of relevant sensory feedback of touch and proprioception within the system confines the intuitive nature of movement and requires visual and cognitive input for control of the components.[72,118] When considering the prosthesis design, the rehabilitation team (including the patient) needs to recognize this functional limitation when considering the desired functional performance outcomes.

Hybrid Prostheses

Some prosthetics combine both body-powered and myoelectric components, providing users with the benefits of both systems. Prosthetic systems can be configured to use an electric elbow with a body-powered mechanical prehensor or an electric prehensor with a body-powered elbow. Hybrid control refers to prostheses that combine body-powered control with externally powered control.[122] Compelling arguments can be made for various control systems; the ultimate decisions for components and control systems are based on an individual's ability to capture the necessary excursion and use proprioceptive feedback from the cable system, as well as the available inputs for the electric components.

Frequently, hybrid systems are sought due to insufficient range or strength available to provide complete functional control at the elbow joint and prehensor with body-powered systems. This may be the result of a frozen shoulder, an unstable joint that is vulnerable to frequent subluxation, or shoulder disarticulation. If the residual limb muscles can generate satisfactory MESs, despite the more proximal shoulder involvement, then myoelectric control of the prehensor can be achieved. Placement of the forearm in space can then be assisted using a large variety of spring-assisted or forearm-balancing mechanical devices. Advantages of hybrid designs include the potential for simultaneous control of elbow and prehensor, reduced overall weight of the prosthesis, and a wider selection of prosthetic components. The prosthetist must consider the compatibility of the components, whereas the therapist considers the specific training strategies with the control scheme.

Activity-Specific Prostheses

Most of this chapter's discussions have revolved around functions that relate to ADLs and vocational pursuits. Most individuals with upper extremity amputations want to be involved in various pursuits beyond ADLs and vocational activities, just as they were before their amputations. However, few individuals with limb loss participate in exercise and sports. Participation following amputation is lower than preamputation level.[130] A number of unique prosthetic interventions, as well as adaptations and assistive tools for an existing prosthesis, can effectively address the recreational and avocational desires of individuals.[131] Although conventional wisdom suggests that these pursuits not proceed until complete maximal rehabilitation has occurred with the primary prosthetic device, this is not always the case; being able to return to an important avocational activity might be a major motivating factor in rehabilitation. However, few individuals have the financial resources for specialized prostheses for vocational and avocational activities. Most prosthetists make every attempt to implement activity-specific devices within the primary prosthetic design. Because the array of activities in which individuals participate is limitless, so too is the creation of specific tools and adaptations to accommodate these needs. Quick-disconnect wrists allow for a myriad of options in place of the existing TD. Commercial application of TDs can include nearly any imaginable adaptation for sport and recreational pursuits (Fig. 30.32). Specific challenges such as exposure to the elements, vibration, and impact may require more significant modification to ensure acceptable durability of the device.

Bionic Arms and Hands

Bionics, or biologically inspired engineering, involves using biological mechanisms from nature to study and design engineering systems and modern technology. In the context of bionics, a bionic arm captures electric signals from muscles and/or nerves above the amputation level, translating them into intuitive movements of the bionic hand. Surgery is often required, with correct interfacing of residual nerves being critical. Additional sensors may be implanted and integrated with the neural system.

Various types of bionic arm interfaces have been proposed.[10–28] A commonly used surgical procedure used in the context of prosthetics is targeted muscular reinnervation (TMR).[132,133] The goal of TMR is to enhance the control of prosthetic devices by rerouting nerves from the amputated limb to specific target muscles. The procedure involves connecting the remaining nerves of the amputated limb to nearby, available muscles. These reinnervated muscles then act as biological amplifiers for the signals generated by the nerves, providing a more intuitive and precise control interface for prosthetic devices. For example, in the case of an upper limb amputation, nerves from the residual limb can be surgically connected to muscles in the chest. The ulnar nerve may be connected to the medial third of the clavicular head of the pectoralis major, while the median nerve is surgically attached to the sternal head of the pectoralis major. The musculocutaneous nerve can be reinnervated laterally on the pectoralis major muscle. Additionally, half of the radial nerve can be reinnervated into the serratus muscle, while the other half is innervated into the remaining tricep muscle. When the individual thinks about moving their missing hand, the reinnervated chest muscles generate electrical signals that can be detected and used to control the movements of a prosthetic arm. This allows for a more natural and coordinated control of the prosthetic limb, improving the user's ability to perform various tasks.

TMR is one of several surgical techniques aimed at improving the functionality and user experience of prosthetic devices, enhancing the integration of the artificial limb with the user's remaining anatomy and neural control systems. For instance, In some cases, transversal intrafascicular multichannel electrodes (TIMEs)[134] can be implanted within the nerves. These specialized electrodes are designed to penetrate the epineurium and reside within the nerve, serving as a corrective neural prosthetic interface for recording and stimulating the peripheral nerve. An array of surface electromyogram (EMG) electrodes is placed on the surface of the reinnervated muscles that can be utilized to receive EMG singals to control a motorized prosthetic arm.

Beyond the motor signals, medical professionals and surgeons may connect existing sensory nerves in the chest to reinnervated nerves to enhance sensory feedback. For instance, the intercostobrachial nerve, originating from the skin, can be deinnervated and subsequently reinnervated by the median nerve, while the supraclavicular nerve can be reinnervated by the ulnar nerve. This process is known as target sensory reinnervation. To facilitate sensory perception, tactile, position, or force sensors can be integrated into the bionic hand. During grasping or manipulation, these sensors transmit signals that stimulate the reinnervated skin, eliciting a "false" but realistic sensory feedback sensation to the user's brain.

As the signals originate from the individual's residual nerves, the stimulation of reinnervated chest muscles occurs when the user envisions moving their absent hand in the brain. Subsequently, these signals are captured through recording electrodes and utilized to control the movements

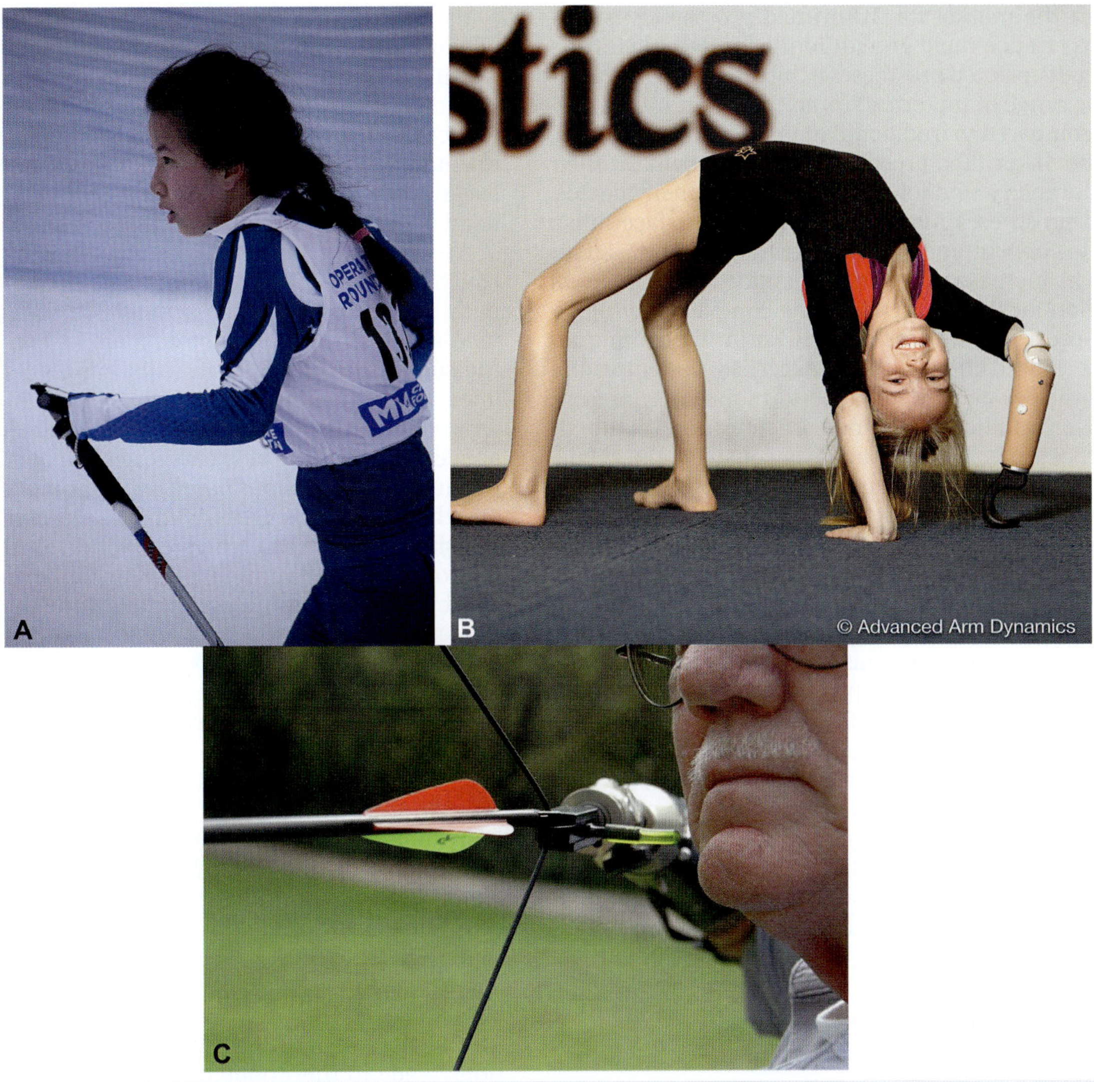

Fig. 30.32 Activity-specific prostheses allow for participation in various recreational activities across the lifespan. (A) Winter sports, (B) gymnastics, and (C) archery. (A, Courtesy TRS Prosthetics; B, Courtesy Advanced Arm Dynamics; C, Courtesy Texas Assistive Devices.)

of the robotic arm. Bionic limbs offer several advantages, including enhanced sensation, improved reintegration and embodiment of the artificial limb, and enhanced controllability. However, the direct surgical implantation of electrodes for nerve stimulation presents certain drawbacks, including the high cost associated with the surgery, potential pain during the recovery period, risk of nerve damage, possibility of infection, and potential scarring. These factors could ultimately impede the effective stimulation of the nerve.

3D-Printed Prostheses

Utilizing 3D printing technology allows for the creation of customized and cost-effective prosthetic devices tailored to an individual's unique anatomy. The 3D printing technology[30–39] gives prosthetic users an alternative option and the freedom to choose different designs, forms, sizes and colors of their prostheses. These advancements have had a profound and positive effect on the comfort, function, and compliance of both body-powered and externally powered prostheses at all levels of amputation. There are many advantages of 3D-printed prostheses, including customization, affordability, rapid prototyping, lightweight and comfort, and personalization. 3D printing enables the creation of prostheses that are tailored to the individual's unique anatomy and specific needs. This customization ensures a better fit and improved functionality compared to traditional mass-produced prostheses. 3D printing technology has the potential to reduce the cost of prosthetic devices by eliminating the need for expensive molds or specialized equipment. Combing with 3D scanning, 3D printing allows for quick iteration and modifications during the design process. Prototypes can be produced and tested in a shorter timeframe, accelerating the development and refinement of prosthetic devices. 3D-printed prostheses can be designed with lightweight materials, which could reduce fatigue and strain on the residual limb. 3D printing enables the incorporation of personalized designs, colors, and patterns into prosthetic devices. This allows users to express their individuality and enhance their self-confidence.

Although the market for 3D-printed prosthetics is projected to experience rapid growth in the foreseeable future, the existing 3D-printed prostheses exhibit a number of limitations. The range of materials suitable for 3D printing may be limited compared to traditional manufacturing methods. Many of the 3D-printed prosthetics are unknown for their strength, durability, and longevity of the prosthetic device. 3D-printed prostheses may have a rougher surface finish compared to conventionally manufactured prostheses. This can result in increased friction, discomfort, and potential skin irritation for the user. Developing complex and highly functional prosthetic devices using 3D printing techniques requires specialized knowledge and expertise. Designing and optimizing the device for optimal performance may present challenges for traditionally trained practitioners. As the 3D printing process involves layer-by-layer construction, ensuring consistent quality and structural integrity of the prosthetic device is crucial. Any defects or inconsistencies in the printing process could impact the overall performance and reliability of the prosthesis. The regulatory landscape for 3D-printed prostheses is still evolving. Ensuring compliance with safety and quality standards, as well as addressing any legal and ethical considerations, can pose challenges for manufacturers and healthcare providers.

As part of the NIH 3D, e-NABLE (https://3d.nih.gov/collections/prosthetics) is an online global community of "digital humanitarian" volunteers from all over the world who are using their 3D printers to make free and low-cost prosthetic upper limb devices for children and adults in need. The goal of this collection is to provide a central repository for all open-source assistive technology designs. With the continual advancements in 3D printing technology, it is anticipated that 3D printing will have a transformative impact on the production and accessibility of prosthetic devices.

Summary

Prosthetic rehabilitation of persons with upper limb loss is both challenging and rewarding. In addition to understanding the individual's needs, consideration of the needs and expectations of spouse, children, and extended family is important. Once functional, psychosocial, and other healthcare needs are completely understood, the team develops careful and thoughtful rehabilitation treatment plans. The rehabilitation team (including the physician, nurse, prosthetist, therapist, psychologist, and the individual) needs to explicitly define the patient-specific rehabilitation goals.

Upper extremity prosthetic technology has made rapid advancements, especially over the past decade. With engineering advancements in osseointegration[135] and osseoperception[136] and other technologies,[137] further progress is expected. Upper extremity prosthetic care requires attention to detail. Because of the rapid advancement, unique problem-solving, and the infrequent patient population, referral to an upper extremity prosthetic specialist is recommended.

An effective prosthetic prescription will specify (1) the control system (passive-functional, body-powered, externally powered, hybrid, or activity specific); (2) the socket type and interface (e.g., socks, foam insert, gel insert); (3) the suspension mechanism (e.g., harness, suction, roll-on liner, and pin); and (4) the appropriate TD components, wrist unit, elbow unit (if applicable), and shoulder unit (if applicable). Each of these categories can be subdivided, with the number of divisions based on the complexity of the case and the clinical resources available. A prescription for therapy should accompany the prescription for the prosthesis.

Prosthetic intervention plays an important role in the rehabilitation of the individual. Although each clinician has a specific focus, maximizing functional potential for community reintegration is the overarching rehabilitation goal. Clear communication and coordination are critical to enhance treatment outcomes. Rehabilitation success may be determined when the needs of the individual are met; when the technology is intuitive, functional, and comfortable from the individual's perspective; and when the individual is able to resume their participation in society at the same or higher level than before their amputation. Follow-up and continued care throughout the lifespan are critical to ensure a healthy lifestyle.

ACKNOWLEDGMENTS

The authors wish to express their gratitude for the contributions made to this chapter by Susan Spaulding and Tzurei Chen. Their prior work and expertise have been instrumental in shaping the content and expanding the body of knowledge presented in this updated edition.

References

The complete listing of the References are available in the accompanying enhanced eBook version included with the print purchase of this textbook. Visit Elsevier eBooks+ (eBooks.Health.Elsevier.com) to access this content.

31 Rehabilitation for Persons With Upper Limb Amputation*

MARIKA DEMERS

LEARNING OBJECTIVES

On completion of this chapter, the reader will be able to do the following:

1. Identify the key components of a comprehensive evaluation for clients with upper limb amputation.
2. Develop an appropriate plan of care for clients with upper limb amputation in each of the phases of rehabilitation.
3. Recognize the key characteristics of therapeutic interventions in the preprosthetic and prosthetic training phases of rehabilitation for body-powered and myoelectric prosthetic devices.
4. Describe evidence-based therapeutic activities and interventions to facilitate functional independence in activities of daily living with and without a prosthesis.
5. Identify the current research and advancements in prosthetic technologies for upper limb amputation and analyze how these may have future implications on functional outcomes for clients.

Rehabilitation After Upper Limb Amputation

Upper limbs have important contributions to everyday activities. Specifically, human hands are complex sensory and motor organs capable of interpreting and interacting with the environment. The fine manipulative skills and intricate grasp patterns of the hand cannot be duplicated. When a hand is lost, the ability to perform normal daily activities is greatly disrupted, which consequently impacts quality of life and social participation.[1] Although a prosthesis does not duplicate hand function, it can help to provide for basic grasp in the performance of normal daily activities and help to maintain bilateral hand function.

This chapter discusses the rehabilitation of adults with upper limb amputation including the assessment and treatment of people with upper limb amputation at each stage of the rehabilitation process. The rehabilitation of adults with amputation requires an interdisciplinary team approach. The client is at the center of the interdisciplinary team and has an active role in their rehabilitation plan of care. The therapist must facilitate the individual's return to maximum performance of daily occupations and roles that contribute to living a meaningful life.[2]

Incidence and Causes of Upper Limb Amputation

The primary cause of acquired upper limb amputations is trauma, with approximately 80% of upper limb amputations being traumatic.[3,4] The most common causes of traumatic injury are work-related accidents such as crush injuries or electrical burns, gunshot wounds, and, in times of active warfare, traumatic injuries sustained in combat. Congenital anomalies, infections, and tumors are examples of nontraumatic causes of amputation. Approximately 34.5% of limb amputations in the United States are in the upper limb.[5] Because upper limb amputations are typically work-related, they primarily occur in young or middle-aged adults, and the ratio of males to females is about 3:1.[6] This contrasts with lower limb amputations, which occurs more predominantly in older adults with end-stage diabetes or peripheral vascular disease.[5]

Classification and Functional Implications

There are various terminologies used to describe levels of upper limb amputation. In this chapter, we will use the International Standards Amputation terminology,[7] since it is a common terminology used in research and practice. The classifications for levels of upper limb amputation are described anatomically. Amputation of the upper limb can also be described as either major or minor. The term disarticulation describes an amputation through the joint. From proximal to distal, the term intrascapulothoracic disarticulation forequarter describes an amputation of the upper limb at the scapulothoracic and the sternoclavicular joints. Transhumeral describes an amputation of the upper limb between the shoulder joint and the elbow joint, whereas transradial describes an amputation between the elbow joint and the wrist joint.

Since upper limb amputation occurs in younger individuals, it can result in significant disability and substantial psychosocial and vocational consequences.[4,8] In a retrospective study of limb amputations in the United States, people with upper limb amputation had a significantly greater combined disability rating than those with lower limb amputations (82.9% vs. 62.3%).[8] Functionally speaking, with more proximal levels of amputation, fewer joints and muscles are available to control the prosthetic device. Although a longer residual limb provides better mechanical advantage for prosthetic use, limb length does not always correspond to

*The author extends appreciation to Margaret Wise and Annemarie E. Orr, whose work in prior editions provided the foundation for this chapter.

an increase in prosthetic function. For example, the length of the residual limb in an elbow disarticulation or long transhumeral amputation limits the space available for an elbow unit and affects both cosmesis and function of the prosthesis.

Stages of Rehabilitation

The rehabilitation of individuals with upper limb amputation can be divided into four phases: (1) perioperative, (2) preprosthetic, (3) prosthetic training, and (4) lifelong care. Although certain goals and activities are unique to each phase, there is overlap between each phase, which allows for bidirectional movement and flexibility based on the client's progression, tolerance, goals, wound healing, and psychological readiness. Phases 2 to 4 may be repeated with each prosthetic device the client receives.

ASSESSMENT AND ANALYSIS

Regardless of the stage of rehabilitation, rehabilitation should include a comprehensive interdisciplinary assessment to obtain baseline information about the client's past medical history and current functional status (medical, functional, and psychological; see Table 31.1 for an overview of the elements of a comprehensive evaluation). The interdisciplinary assessment establishes a baseline level of function to prepare the ensuing rehabilitation plan.[9] A comprehensive assessment begins with conducting a thorough history and gathering preliminary or background data, including: (1) the cause and date of amputation, (2) any associated injuries that might influence the rehabilitation process, (3) hand dominance, (4) all medications the client is currently taking, and (5) modifiable/controllable health risk factors. The rehabilitation assessment also includes identification of occupational roles, home and work environments, and leisure interests. The therapist assesses the client's upper limb range of motion (ROM), strength, sensation, wound and skin healing, limb volume, pain, activities of daily living (ADL) performance, and psychological adjustment postamputation.

The examination continues with an assessment of the psychosocial environment as a resource for rehabilitation and discharge planning. The therapist assesses the following client characteristics:

- The availability of family and other support systems
- Living situation
- Level of education
- Prior occupation and leisure interests

The therapist then considers the condition of the residual limb, documenting the following:

- The presence and description of any phantom limb sensation
- The presence and description of any pain the client is experiencing
- The length of the residual limb
- The presence of edema, measured by limb circumference
- Skin condition, wound healing, and the presence of scar tissue or soft tissue adhesion
- ROM of the residual limb to identify any contractures or tightness that may be present
- Bilateral upper limb strength
- Possible sites for placement of electrodes for myoelectric control

Multiple outcome measures can be used to assess upper limb impairments and activity limitations. Outcome measures can be divided into performance-based and self-reported measures. In a recent systematic review, the performance-based measure with the highest psychometric properties were Activities Measure for Upper Limb Amputees, University of New Brunswick Test of Prosthetic Function (UNB) skill subscale, UNB spontaneity subscale, Box and Block Test, and heavy cans and light cans subtests of the modified Jebsen-Taylor Test of Hand Function. Similarly, the highest rated self-reported measures were Disabilities of the Arm, Shoulder and Hand (DASH), Patient Rated Wrist Evaluation overall score and functional recovery subscale, QuickDASH, Hand Assessment Tool, and International Osteoporosis Foundation Quality of Life Questionnaire.[10]

The comprehensive examination concludes with a consideration of mobility and functional status, including the following:

- Posture and skeletal alignment because of the missing limb
- Pertinent limitations of the lower limb
- Postural control (static, anticipatory, and reactionary balance)

Table 31.1 Clinical Assessment Using the International Classification Of Functioning, Disability, and Health Framework

Body Function and Structure	Activity and Participation	Contextual Factors
Physical:	*Activities of daily living:*	*Environmental:*
Endurance	Arm and hand use	Health services, system, and policies
Motor function	Feeding	Living situation
Edema	Mobility	Support and relationships
Pain and sensation	Self-care	
Posture and body alignment		
Range of motion		
Skin integrity		
Strength		
Sensation:	*Instrumental activities of daily living:*	*Personal factors:*
Pain	Housekeeping	Age
Sensory disturbance	Laundry	Comorbidities
	Manage finances	Coping mechanisms
	Meal preparation	Modifiable risk factors
	Shopping	Motivation
	Take medication	
	Use of transport	
Affective:	*Leisure and productivity:*	
Body image	Recreation activities	
Psychological adjustment	Work or volunteering	

- Current and potential abilities to perform activities of special interest to the individual (e.g., self-care, work, leisure activities)

If the client previously used a prosthesis, a prosthetic history is taken that includes the type of prosthesis used, how long the prosthesis was worn each day, and how the prosthesis was used in basic and instrumental ADLs. The findings from the initial comprehensive evaluation will guide the rehabilitation plan of care to assist the client in meeting their functional goals. Reevaluation should also be performed routinely to determine the effectiveness of rehabilitation intervention and adjust the treatment plan.

PERIOPERATIVE

The perioperative phase of rehabilitation starts after the upper limb amputation, or the decision has been made that amputation is necessary. The initial goals of rehabilitation during this phase must be modified according to the client's medical status. Goals of the perioperative phase of rehabilitation are as follows:

- To perform a comprehensive evaluation of the client
- To manage pain
- To promote wound healing
- To establish a strategy for effective edema control
- To preserve ROM, flexibility, and body symmetry
- To provide psychological support

In the perioperative phase of rehabilitation, clear communication is crucial to ensure coordinate care. Multiple rehabilitation interventions can be initiated during this phase to manage pain, promote wound healing, control edema, maintain ranges of motion, retrain ADLs, and provide support to help the client adjust to their loss.

Pain Management

Pain from various etiologies is frequent after an upper limb amputation. It is important for the therapist to understand how each type of pain is distinct and its effect on a client's prosthetic rehabilitation. Common pain types may include overuse syndrome, phantom pain, hyperesthesia, neuromas, or heterotopic ossification. Overuse syndrome is common after upper limb amputations. To compensate for lost motion in the upper limb, people with upper limb amputation tend to adopt compensatory movements, such as excessive motion in other articulations, or repetitive use of the nonaffected limb. The changed kinematics and repetitive use of the nonaffected limb can lead to persistent/recurrent musculoskeletal pain and deteriorated musculoskeletal function of the nonaffected upper limb.[11–13] Prevention and education about the likelihood of overuse and repercussions are the most effective approaches for overuse injuries.[11] Residual limb hyperesthesia, or an overly sensitive residual limb, is also common after amputation. Reduction of hypersensitivities through desensitization techniques improves the client's tolerance to wearing a prosthesis. Desensitization techniques including tapping and vibration and introduction of various textures to the skin are performed after wound closure.[14,15]

Phantom limb sensation is a normal phenomenon experienced by most clients with upper limb amputation. It is a painless sensation of the limb that is no longer there. Phantom limb sensation can be divided into three categories: kinetic sensations, kinesthetic components, and exteroceptive perceptions.[16] Clients typically report that they feel all or part of their amputated limb. Some describe a pulling, tingling, or burning sensation in the missing limb, and the distal aspect of the limb is most frequently felt. Phantom limb pain is highly prevalent, with up to 80% of individuals with amputation experiencing phantom limb pain.[17] Clients often describe the pain as stabbing, burning, or throbbing. Pain frequently decreases in intensity and duration in the first 6 months after amputation, but some clients may experience residual pain throughout their life.[18,19] Phantom pain management is complex and should involve an interdisciplinary team.[17] Treatment methods include active participation in functional tasks, desensitization techniques, analgesics, mirror therapy, biofeedback, transcutaneous electrical nerve stimulation, prosthetic wear, and surgical revision.[20–22] Unfortunately, there is currently limited evidence to support pharmacological and nonpharmacological approaches to prevent or treat phantom limb.[17,23] Evidence from systematic reviews and clinical practice guidelines recommend the use of mirror therapy to reduce short-term phantom limb pain.[9,24] However, high-quality, large randomized control trials have not yet been conducted.

Wound Healing

Various procedures are used to promote wound healing depending on the type and size of the wound. During therapy sessions, wound dressings can be removed to assess the incision and the skin. A thorough wound assessment should include the anatomic location; measurements (length, width, and depth in centimeters); color and quality of the wound (i.e., closed incision); type and color of exudate; odor; pain; and a description of the peri wound skin.[25] Additional assessment data may be required depending on the type and character of the wound, and treatment protocols may vary according to physician or facility preference. Therapists should feel comfortable cleansing the wound and reapplying new dressings. Wound debridement is occasionally required, and the therapist may collaborate with the physician, the nurse, or the wound specialist to determine appropriate debridement practices during dressing changes. In general, closed incisions should be treated with nonadherent dressings or they may be left open to air after 1 to 3 days postoperatively. If they are located directly under a prosthesis or other device, they may require additional protection. Skin grafts need to remain covered with nonadherent dressings for several weeks postoperatively, and measures should be taken to avoid shearing forces along the site of the graft.

Edema Control

Immediately following surgery and limb closure, edema control is initiated. Limb wrapping is used to decrease edema and promote optimal shaping of the residual limb. The residual limb is wrapped with an elastic bandage in a figure-of-eight configuration for distal to proximal compression. Education should be provided to the client and family members about edema control to avoid restricting circulation by wrapping the limb in a circular fashion. Once clearance is obtained from a physician, the client can be fit with an elastic shrinker or compression garment. The client is educated to always wear the shrinker for edema control and perform skin checks two to three times daily. Ideally, the bandage should continue up and over one joint proximal to the amputation (e.g., above the elbow in transradial amputation; Figs. 31.1 and 31.2). Active exercises and elevation can also be used as modalities for edema control.

Range of Motion, Flexibility, and Body Symmetry

Implementation of a comprehensive exercise program is of utmost importance in the weeks following upper limb amputation. To avoid the development of soft tissue contractures, early active movement of all proximal joints should be initiated the first day after amputation. Once medical clearance has been given, the rehabilitation team will engage the client in exercises to maintain and increase proximal joint ROM and strength. Early ROM exercises are used to gently elongate tissues of joints most at risk of contracture formation. Reduced passive ROM at the shoulder is associated with reduced shoulder and elbow weakness, decreased activity performance, and lower satisfaction with prothesis.[26] It is therefore imperative to maintain ROM, strength, and flexibility of the joints in the remaining upper limb. Exercises should be progressed to active-assistive ROM in all planes of motion for residual and contralateral limb.[9] Therapeutic activities can be performed in front of a mirror to provide visual feedback and promote body awareness. Maintenance of body symmetry and proper trunk alignment following upper limb amputation can decrease the risk of overuse injuries of the upper limb, neck, or back.[27]

Basic Training in Activities of Daily Living

Following amputation, one of the main goals for rehabilitation is to achieve independence in basic self-care activities. It is important for the client to begin to feel a sense of independence and gain control over their environment. Once a client is medically stable, basic training in ADLs can be initiated. The ADL training should include compensatory strategies to perform basic self-care activities (e.g., self-feeding, toileting, and oral hygiene).[15] Therapists can provide education on one-handed techniques, adaptive equipment and environmental modifications that will set the client up for success with basic self-care activities. Adaptive equipment such as universal cuffs, bidets, adapted clothing, and wall-mounted scrub brushes can provide initial independence for the client. When the dominant upper limb is amputated, dominance retraining can be initiated for activities such as writing and eating. Clients learn to adapt and compensate quickly and often initiate ADL performance with their non-dominant hand. Although independence in self-care with and without a prosthesis is encouraged, it is important to facilitate opportunities for bimanual use of the upper limbs

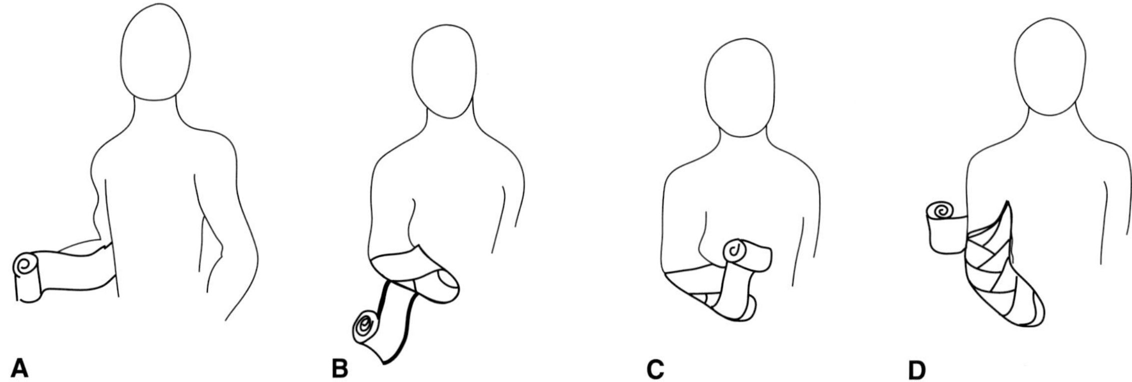

Fig. 31.1 (A) To apply a compressive wrap to a transradial residual limb, the client anchors the elastic bandage between the elbow and trunk and wraps it around the distal end of the limb. Next, a series of overlapping figure-of-eight layers of the wrap (B and C) are applied, creating a distal-toward-proximal pressure gradient. The wrap should continue proximally for several inches above the elbow joint (D).

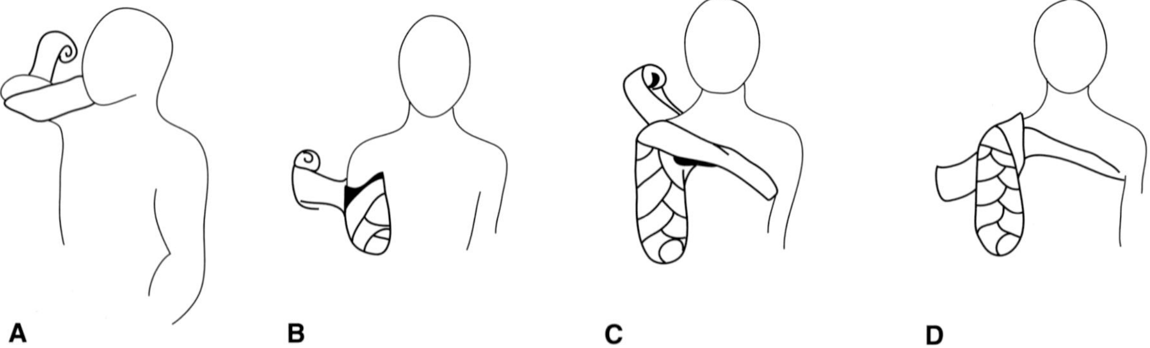

Fig. 31.2 (A) To apply a compressive wrap to a transhumeral residual limb, the client anchors the elastic bandage between the chin and clavicle and wraps it over and behind the distal end of the residual limb. (B) Once the initial figure-of-eight layer is applied to anchor the end of the bandage, the client continues to apply overlapping layers, creating a distal-toward-proximal pressure gradient. The wrap continues up and over the shoulder (C), over the anterior chest wall under the contralateral axilla, and then around the back, over the residual shoulder, and under the axilla before being secured in place (D).

for ease of performance and to minimize risk of overuse syndrome of the remaining limb.

Psychological Support

Psychological adjustment following amputation is multifactorial. The client's personality, quality of social support, and sociocultural response to amputation all contribute to the individual's process of adjustment following limb loss.[28] Initially, the client may experience shock, dismay, and anger, typical initial emotional reactions, following a traumatic amputation.[29] Depression and posttraumatic stress disorders are also frequent in people receiving rehabilitation services following upper limb amputation.[28] Clinical practice guidelines recommend that clients be screened for cognition, mental health conditions such as posttraumatic stress disorder and depression, and pain during the initial evaluation and across the continuum of care.[9] Psychological support should be addressed throughout each phase of the rehabilitation process, from initial amputation through reintegration into the community. It is the responsibility of the therapist to build a relationship of trust with the client. This rapport encourages an open discussion about the individual's psychological adjustment to loss of their limb. An individual's response to amputation is complex and individualized. Concerted work by an interdisciplinary team, including mental health services, should be offered to support individuals with amputation and their social support systems and minimize psychological distress. Mental health professionals may play an important role in normalizing patients' emotions and experiences and in promoting psychological adaptation.[30] Peer-support and self-management programs could be explored as strategies to help adjust to upper limb loss.[9,28]

The perioperative phase ends when the incisions on the residual limb are closed and free of infection, the medical condition is stable, and basic ADLs using alternative strategies are progressing.[9]

PREPROSTHETIC

The primary goal of this phase is to prepare the client and their residual limb to be fit with a prosthetic device. The preprosthetic training phase begins after wound closure and ends with the client being fit with a preparatory prosthesis. Time spent in this phase of rehabilitation depends largely on the client's limb volume, ROM, pain and hypersensitivity, and psychological status. Many of the interventions from the perioperative care phase carry over and advance in the preprosthetic training phase. Therapists play an important role in the preparation of the client for prosthesis fitting and optimal use.[31] Intervention priorities for the preprosthetic training phase include the following:

- Psychological support
- Edema control and limb shaping for optimal fit of a prosthesis
- Enhancing ROM and strengthening
- Myosite testing and training
- Training in ADLs

Considerations for Prothesis Prescription

Input from all the members of the team, including the client, is vital for the initial prothesis prescription. Based on the 2022 Veterans Affairs/Department of Defense clinical

Case Example 31.1 A Client With Bilateral Traumatic Amputation of the Forearm

T.M. is a 17-year-old high school soccer player who underwent traumatic amputation of his right and left forearms when the sleeves of his winter jacket became caught in the blades of a running snow blower that had jammed, then suddenly released, as he was trying to clear the mechanism. T.M. was home alone when the accident occurred and had significant blood loss before he was able to reach a neighbor's home for assistance. At the local hospital, tourniquets were placed to control blood loss, wounds were flushed and cleaned, intravenous fluids with antibiotics and packed red blood cells were begun, and morphine was administered. T.M. was prepared for emergency transfer to the nearest trauma center.

On arrival at the trauma center, he was immediately taken to surgery for débridement and closure of his wounds. His parents arrived at the trauma center while he was in surgery. The right transradial residual limb had 7 cm of radius and ulna preserved and required a split-thickness skin graft to close (the donor site was the anterior right thigh). The left transradial residual limb had 18 cm of radius and ulna preserved and was closed without skin graft.

Two days have passed since T.M.'s surgery, and he is recovering in the surgical intensive care unit. His white blood cell count and temperature are moderately elevated. His residual limbs are in bulky dressings with elastic compressive wraps, with significant serosanguineous drainage noted at dressing changes. A morphine pump is being used for pain management. T.M. is currently receiving supplemental oxygen by nasal cannula and is sleeping fitfully. On questioning, he is semialert, oriented to family members and place, but not to others or time.

QUESTIONS TO CONSIDER

- What questions and assessments are most appropriate to include in the evaluation at this point in the postoperative phase of T.M.'s care? How will the information collected guide the development of a plan of care for this young man?
- What specific intervention strategies should the rehabilitation team use to address issues of pain control, limb volume and edema, and wound healing in the next 2 to 5 days? How should client and family education be best integrated with these strategies?
- What specific ROM is most important to target for T.M. with a short transradial residual limb on the right and a long transradial residual limb on the left, anticipating the need for bilateral prostheses in his future? Which upper limb joints are most at risk of contracture formation and why? What specific intervention strategies should the therapists initiate to preserve as much functional ROM as possible? How might pain, medications, and level of consciousness influence the potential development of soft tissue contractures?
- In what ways can the team help to establish an effective relationship with T.M. and his parents in these early days of care? What information is most important to help the family cope with adjustment to this situation and prepare for the days ahead? How will the rehabilitation team assess the family's understanding of the situation and need for emotional support?

practice guidelines,[9] essential elements to be included in an upper limb prosthesis prescription are as follows:

- Design (e.g., preparatory vs. definitive)
- Control strategy (e.g., passive, externally powered, body powered, hybrid, activity specific)
- The anatomical side and amputation level of the prosthesis
- Type of socket interface (e.g., soft insert, elastomer liner, flexible thermoplastic)
- Type of socket frame (e.g., thermoplastic or laminated)
- Suspension mechanism (e.g., harness, suction, anatomical)
- Terminal device (TD)

If applicable, wrist, elbow, and shoulder unit should also be considered. Elements of prothesis prescription and prosthesis options are discussed in more detail in Chapter 30. Factors such as the client's strength, ROM, handedness, cognition, vocational pursuits, significant daily activities, and long-term goals are important determinants of an individual prosthetic plan. Information about the prothesis should be provided to the client. A meta-analysis of the qualitative literature identified six main themes that could affect prosthetic choice: (1) physical (i.e., a person's body), (2) activities and participation, (3) mental thinking and feelings, (4) social relations and functioning in society, (5) rehabilitation, cost, and prosthetist services, and (6) prosthesis-related factors.[32] The prosthetist and therapist begin by educating the client on the advantages and disadvantages of the various upper limb prosthetic systems available, with the goal of selecting the control strategy and system that will allow the client the most function. The prosthetist provides education on the specific prosthetic options and componentry selection whereas the occupational therapist informs the client regarding how the prosthesis relates to occupational performance. Thorough discussions between the client and the interdisciplinary team will help to guide decision-making.

Psychological Support

Psychological support is an integral part of the early rehabilitation program and should be made available for the family and client.[28] Psychological support encompasses education throughout the recovery process, self-management, and the therapeutic use of self.[14] In the preprosthetic training phase, psychological support is continued and modified to appropriately respond to the rapidly changing needs of the client.[14] Similarly to the perioperative phase, clients may benefit from peer support in the form of meeting with a peer mentor or with individuals who have experienced similar amputations. Discussion with peers may help to facilitate understanding of the rehabilitation process and can assist in setting expectations for the client to return to their life roles.

Residual Limb Management

In the preprosthetic training phase, the client must continue to use compression to control the edema and shape the limb for prothesis fitting. Frequent changing of compression dressing is essential to maintain adequate pressure around the residual limb and to reduce edema.[33] As limb volume decreases, the shrinker or tubular elastic bandaging should be adjusted to continue to provide compression on the residual limb. In addition to compressive dressings, edema can further be reduced through soft tissue mobilization, retrograde massage, and elevation.[33,34] However, while widely used in clinical practice, the evidence to support retrograde massage to control hand edema is limited.[35] Active participation in self-care and use of the arm to assist during functional bimanual activities is encouraged for edema control. Once the wound is closed, scar massage can be useful to prevent skin adhesion.[33] Stump massage can also train the client to tolerate the pressure associated with contact between the stump and socket of the prothesis in the later stage of recovery.[22]

Daily ROM exercises are important to prepare the client for use of a prosthetic device. Having as close to full upper limb ROM as possible allows the client to use the prosthesis to its full capability. Physical therapy interventions such as heat modalities, soft tissue mobilization, gentle stretching, and active ROM exercises can often improve motion in clients with recently developed tissue tightness and ROM restriction. Stretching of residual musculature should be continued in all the subsequent stages to prevent the impact of compensatory movements, loss of weight of the limb, and less use of the distal extremity.[9]

According to the level of upper limb amputation, a graded exercise program will be provided to maximize ROM and strength. As a strengthening exercise, the therapist will position the residual limb in the desired posture and ask the client to hold the appropriate muscles in place. Isometric exercises allow the client to participate in an exercise program without equipment. As the client progresses, equipment such as elastic bands, strap-on weights, and adaptive cuffs with D-rings can be incorporated. For control and operation of a body-powered prosthesis or a hybrid prosthesis, clients must strengthen the muscles that control shoulder flexion, scapular protraction, retraction, and depression. It is the responsibility of the therapist to guide the client through a home exercise program for self-stretching and upper limb strengthening in preparation for use of a prosthesis.

Myosite Testing and Training

For clients who choose an externally powered or myoelectric prosthesis, myosite testing should be carried out to identify the optimum control site locations. Specifically, externally powered or myoelectric prosthesis use electromyographic (EMG) signals to control the prosthetic device. When a muscle contracts, it generates an EMG signal. The EMG signals produced by an activated muscle or muscle group in the residual limb are detected by surface electrodes placed in the socket of the prosthesis and are used to control operations of the prosthesis. Selection of optimal muscle sites is based on what is most intuitive to the client.[14] In their most basic form, myoelectric devices rely on agonist-antagonist pairs to operate the prosthesis.[36] With new advances in pattern recognition technology, specific EMG patterns from several synergistic muscles can be used to provide more intuitive control and natural transitions between movements (see section on "*Current Research and Advancements in Technologies*")."[37] Externally powered devices can also be controlled using control inputs, such as force sensitive resistors, linear transducers, toggle and rocker switches, and inertial measurement units.[9] This stresses the importance of a close collaboration between the client, the therapist, and the prosthetist to inform the control strategy.

Myosite testing can be initiated once the limb volume is stable (i.e., when the edema is controlled). It consists of the identification of precise electrode placement to optimize the control of a myoelectric prosthesis. The therapist or the prosthetist can complete myosite testing with the client. Generally, distal myosites are preferable to allow adequate space within the prosthetic socket for electrode placement and good suspension. Myosite testing is performed with a biofeedback system or myotester to measure the strength of EMG signal produced by the residual muscle or muscle group. A surface electrode is placed over the myosite and connected to biofeedback equipment, such as a Myolab II (Motion Control, Salt Lake City, Utah) or the MyoBoy with the Prosthetist's Assistant for Upper Limb Architecture (PAULA) (Otto Bock HealthCare, Vienna, Austria) (Fig. 31.3). The strength of the EMG signal is read from the meter, and precise electrode placement is adjusted as necessary. The therapist and prosthetist will identify the minimum signal necessary to operate the myoelectric system.

Once the best electrode sites have been located, the client will begin myosite training with the therapist. The goals of myosite training are to teach the client to use specific residual limb musculature independently and efficiently to activate and perform basic myoelectric prosthesis functions. This will ensure the client will be able to immediately operate the myoelectric prosthesis at the first fitting.[14] For effective use of a myoelectric prosthesis, good muscle control is more important than overall strength of contractions. During control site training, the client typically will learn to

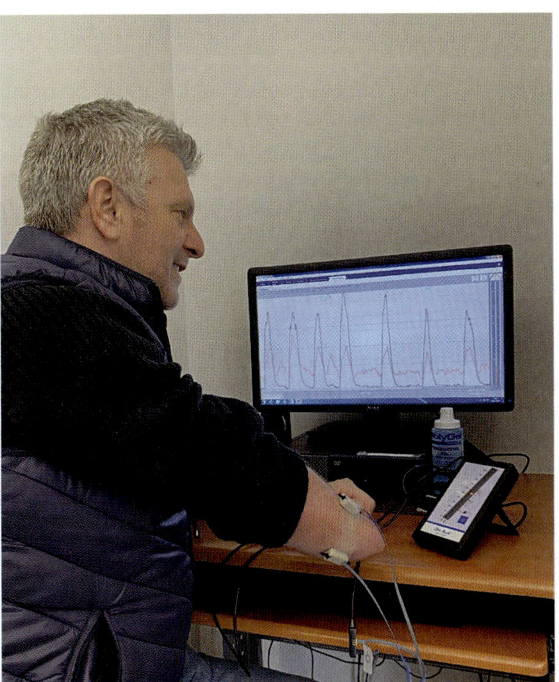

Fig. 31.3 A Myoboy system with surface electrodes is used to locate potential myosites and provide biofeedback to help clients master the types of contractions necessary to control actions of a myoelectric prosthesis.

consciously control the muscle contraction, level of activation, and isolation through repetitive exercises. An example of pattern of muscle activation is:

1. To contract one muscle (muscle A, agonist) to a specific level, while leaving the other (muscle B, antagonist) at rest or in a quiet state.
2. To contract muscle B to a specific level while leaving muscle A at rest or in a quiet state.
3. To perform quick and equal cocontractions of muscles A and B.

Myosite training will aim to increase endurance of the targeted muscles. Biofeedback equipment, or muscle trainers, can be used to master effective, efficient muscle control. In recent years, a mobile, game-based approach to myoelectric prosthesis training has also emerged to improve rehabilitation success rates and provide myosite training outside of the clinical environment.[38]

Training in Activities of Daily Living and Instrumental Activities of Daily Living

During the preprosthetic phase, training in ADLs should be continued. Adaptative techniques for dressing, bathing, grooming, and toileting without a prosthesis, such as one-handed techniques, should be taught and instrumental ADL training can be initiated. An assessment for personal equipment and assistive devices to perform ADLs can be initiated, along with training to use equipment or assistive devices. As the client continues to progress, independence in more complex ADLs can be targeted.[9] As appropriate, change of dominance training is continued.

Education

Therapists play an important role in providing education to their client. Depending on individual needs, education can be provided on the following topics:

- Stump care
- Positioning
- Energy conservation
- Pain management
- Edema management
- Limb protection
- Prosthetic timeline
- Equipment needs
- Life with an amputation
- Coping methods

BASIC PROSTHETIC TRAINING

For clients deemed candidates to proceed to prosthetic fitting, the prosthetic training phase marks a turning point in rehabilitation.[9] This phase starts when the client receives their prosthesis and continues until the client demonstrates desired functional outcomes with proper prosthetic use during meaningful daily activities. Training in the use of the prothesis is essential to promote the seamless integration of the prothesis in ADLs and ensure best outcomes. In a recent qualitative study on the perspectives of people with upper limb amputation, early experiences with learning to live with an amputation were formative milestones that shaped perceptions of ability and prosthesis use.[39]

Case Example 31.2 A Client With Transhumeral Amputation

R.O. is a 37-year-old automobile mechanic who underwent a traumatic transhumeral amputation of the right upper limb 3 weeks ago after he sustained a crush injury when a car fell off the jack during a tire change. He struggled to get out from under the vehicle and seriously strained his right rotator cuff. At this point, all surgical drains and sutures have been removed, and the wound has closed except for a ¼-inch area on the medial distal humerus that continues to leave slight signs of clear drainage on the nonadherent dressing. R.O. is currently using a double layer of elasticized Tubigrip (Mölnlycke HealthCare, Gothenburg, Sweden) for limb volume control and shaping. He reports a sensation of a tight constrictive cuff around his "missing" right elbow and a somewhat unpredictable shooting "electric" sensation into his missing forearm and hand. He tends to hold his residual limb in a flexion pattern across his lower chest. R.O. experiences pain in his right shoulder with movement in all planes.

Active ROM at the shoulder is currently 0 to 90 degrees of flexion, 0 to 70 degrees of abduction, 0 degrees of internal rotation, and 0 to 25 degrees of external rotation. His shoulder and residual limb can be passively moved into 115 degrees of flexion, 90 degrees of abduction, 10 degrees of internal rotation, and 40 degrees of external rotation.

As a husband and father of two preschool-age children, R.O. is having a difficult time imagining how he will be able to return to work to support his family. He is discouraged and impatient with his postoperative pain and phantom sensation. He is reluctant to allow his residual limb to be moved, passively or with active assistance, toward any end ROM at the shoulder because of impingement pain. He does not incorporate his paretic limb in daily activities. He is discouraged with the skill level he has reached in self-care with his nondominant left upper limb.

QUESTIONS TO CONSIDER

- What are R.O.'s most immediate educational and support needs now that he has begun the preprosthetic training phase of care? What strategies would help to strengthen rapport with R.O., help him to understand the next steps in the process, and enhance his outlook and motivation?
- Given the length of his residual limb and the status of his incision line, what specific strategies for volume control, edema, and limb shaping should be recommend at this time? What are the indicators of readiness for prosthetic fitting?
- Given his current level of discomfort and the concurrent rotator cuff dysfunction, what contractures are most likely to develop at R.O.'s shoulder? Considering his hopes to return to work as an auto mechanic, what shoulder motions would be most important to preserve and enhance in preparation for prosthetic training? What specific strategies should be used to accomplish this?
- What impact might a rotator cuff injury have on R.O.'s potential to use a prosthesis successfully? How should the severity of his rotator cuff impairment be assessed? What strategies could be used to improve the function of his shoulder, given the acuity of his rotator cuff injury?
- What types of muscle performance are most important to address at this point? What muscles could be used for myosite training for R.O. specific to his level of amputation? What strategies should be used to address strength, power, and control of the various types of muscle contractions R.O. will need to use his prosthesis effectively?
- What basic ADL skills should be priorities for training at this point? What strategies should be used to enhance motor learning of skilled activity with his left (nondominant) hand? How might his residual limb be incorporated during these functional activities? What types of adaptive equipment may be beneficial to R.O. for performance of basic self-care activities without a prosthesis?

Many interventions initiated in the previous two phases are continued, including physical interventions (i.e., pain management, ROM, strengthening), education, and psychological support. Moreover, needs should be reassessed (e.g., driving evaluation and training, use of prosthesis in daily and recreational activities, pain management, vocational rehabilitation), and discharge planning should be adjusted as appropriate. Potential complications that can occur during prosthesis use (i.e., redness, irritation, skin breakdown, pain, discomfort, contractures) should also be carefully monitored.

Residual Limb Hygiene and Care of the Prosthesis

Education on residual limb hygiene is provided to the client and family members early in the prosthetic training phase. Perspiration is common with prosthetic use and can cause irritation or maceration of the skin. The client is instructed to perform skin inspections of the residual limb each time the prosthesis is removed, to look for redness or irritation. Regardless of the control system being used, the residual limb and axilla must be washed daily with mild soap and water, and the socket of the prosthesis must be wiped clean with a damp cloth. The harness should be removed and cleaned as needed. Clients using a body-powered prosthesis often wear prosthetic socks as an interface between the skin and socket surface. A fresh, clean sock should be used each day; in hot weather, the sock may need to be changed several times per day. Prosthetic components should be maintained according to the manufacturer's guidelines. The therapist and prosthetist should guide the client through basic maintenance of their prosthetic device to include socket cleaning, componentry maintenance, harness adjustment, cable system modifications, and battery-charging procedures.[14]

Wearing Schedule

On initial fitting of a prosthesis, the wearing schedule is established to increase the client's tolerance to the device over time and to decrease the risk of skin breakdown. Initially, the prosthetic wearing period is short (e.g., 10–30 minutes). After each wearing period, the prosthesis is removed, and skin condition carefully examined. Areas of redness (reactive hyperemia) that persist for more than 10 minutes after the residual limb is out of the socket may indicate areas of high pressure. If no skin issues develop, wearing time and frequency is gradually increased according to the client's tolerance, skin condition, and need for prosthesis use. Ultimately, the goal will be to tolerate the prothesis approximately 8 hours per day.[14] The client is advised to consult with their prosthetist, therapist, or physician if the following occur:

- Ongoing pain in the residual limb or associated with the prosthetic harness
- Skin breakdown
- Change in limb volume (weight gain or loss)
- Change in the ability to don and doff the prosthesis
- Change in pattern of usage[9]

Donning and Doffing the Prosthesis

Independence in donning and doffing the full prosthetic system is one of the most important goals for prosthetic training and should be addressed during the initial treatment sessions. Training in how to independently don/doff the residual limb sock, the prosthetic socket, and/or the harness is provided during therapy sessions. Depending on the harness and the type of prosthesis, different methods to don/doff the prosthesis should be explored with the client to identify the method of choice for each client, using a collaborative approach. The client may also develop their own technique. For individuals with high levels of amputation or bilateral amputations, special equipment such as a dressing tree or wall-mounted hooks may be used to allow for independent donning and doffing of prosthetic devices.

Controls Training and Functional Use Training

There are two phases of prosthetic training: prosthetic controls training and functional use training. The goal of controls training is to achieve smooth, consistent movement of each operation of the prosthesis with minimal awkward movement or delay. Functional use training translates the skills in controls training to task performance and functional application of the prosthetic device. Initially, each component of the prosthesis is trained on individually, prior to combining movements into functional performance. Progression of controls training for body-powered prostheses and myoelectric prostheses begins with education on operation of each component of the prosthetic device. Once the client has demonstrated continuous, smooth control of each component in a natural sequence, clients progress to performing grasp and release in different body positions (e.g., seated and standing). This will encourage prepositioning of the shoulder, elbow, and TD for optimal use. Training progression includes the use objects of various size, shape, and densities, placed at various heights and distance from the body. Initially, rote tasks are practiced, but eventually, more complex and functional tasks are integrated in the treatment program. Clients are trained to manipulate objects with proportional control to increase proprioceptive awareness of their prosthesis and minimize the potential for crushing items, such as a Styrofoam cup. Once the client has demonstrated how to operate and control each prosthetic component, they can transition to functional use training. Functional use training minimizes awkward and compensatory movements by emphasizing prepositioning of each prosthetic joint, increasing prosthetic tolerance and muscle endurance, and promoting incorporation of the prosthetic device into task performance. During training, clients should be encouraged to avoid maladaptive compensatory movements, such as shoulder hiking, extreme shoulder flexion, trunk displacement for objects within reach, elbow abduction, or excessive internal humeral rotation.[40,41] The use of external feedback may be used to minimize compensatory movements (e.g., verbal cues, mirrors, video feedback). The role of the therapist is to guide each individual to identify appropriate challenges and have realistic expectations in task performance, as the ability to accurately control a prosthesis may vary between individuals and prosthesis type.[9]

Control and Functional Use of Body-Powered Prostheses

In a body-powered prosthesis, forces generated by gross body motions are translated through the harness and cable system to activate each prosthetic component (Fig. 31.4). Depending on the level of amputation, the control of movements used to operate the TD will differ. For example, for a transradial prosthesis, the TD is operated through scapula abduction and glenohumeral flexion. In contrast, transhumeral prosthetic devices may use a dual-control cable system, requiring scapular depression and shoulder extension and abduction. Shoulder disarticulation prostheses may use a manually operated, friction-held shoulder unit, whereas clients with high levels of amputation or those with nerve involvement may also need to use chest expansion to operate the prosthesis.

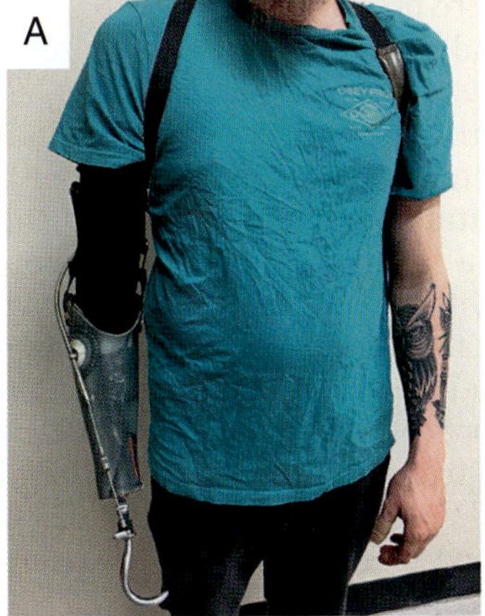

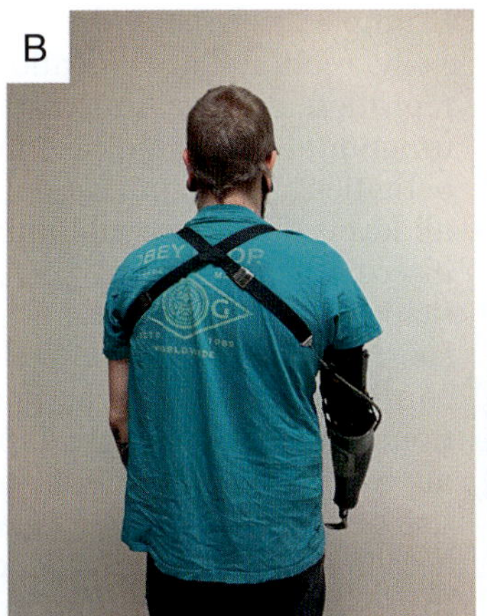

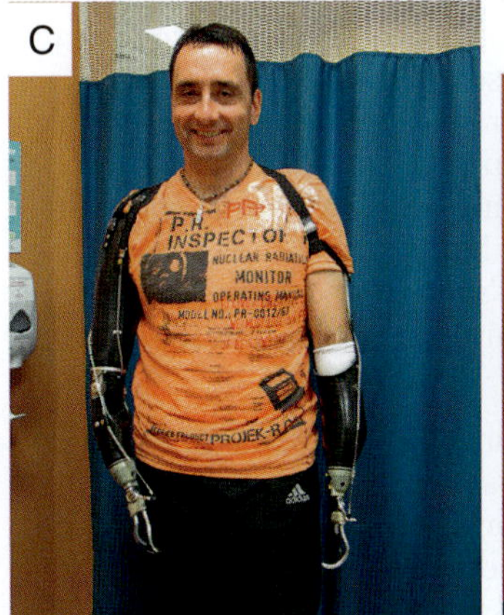

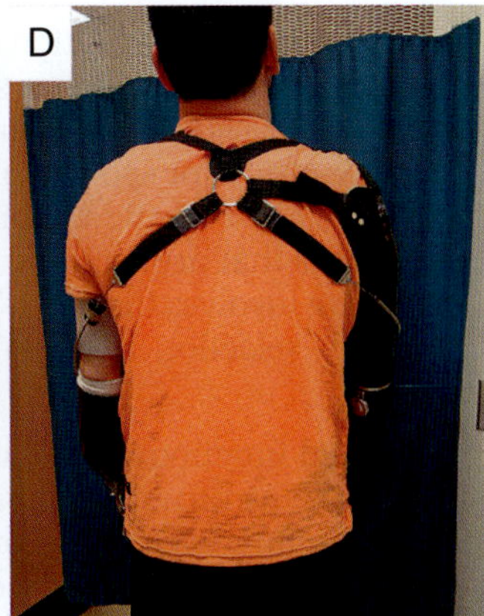

Fig. 31.4 Body-powered prothesis with a figure-eight harness for a unilateral amputation (A and B) or a bilateral transradial and transhumeral amputations, and (C and D). Front view (A and C), back view (B and D).

Control and Functional Use of the Myoelectric Prosthesis

Myoelectric prostheses have various control schemes based on the client's prosthetic system componentry and the individual's musculoskeletal integrity. Typically, a two-site control system is used. When using two-site control the individual with a transradial amputation must switch from hand (or other TD) mode to wrist mode. Several options exist for control of the wrist. The wrist unit can be passively positioned, or the wrist rotator can be electrically controlled. Clients are trained to contract their muscles to produce a signal that corresponds to that prosthetic control. For example, the wrist extensors typically control hand open. A controlled contraction of those muscles will open the hand proportionally to the strength and speed of the muscle signal provided. To supinate the wrist unit, the same wrist extensors are used, but the client will give a quick muscle contraction and hold it to activate that motion. Control schemes are dependent on the componentry and programming can be done by the prosthetist to maximize the client's control of the prosthesis.

Clients with transhumeral myoelectric prostheses must manage the additional complexity of controlling the TD, wrist, and elbow units. Typically, transhumeral control schemes use the biceps and triceps to operate the prosthetic device. Biceps contractions operate elbow flexion and hand close, whereas triceps contractions operate elbow extension and hand open. Control training is performed to practice smooth transitions from elbow to TD mode.

Controls training for myoelectric prostheses begin with open/close of the TD in various positions to ensure the electrodes are maintaining good contact with the skin in each position. The client will be trained in proportional control to include opening the TD through one-third, one-half, and three-fourths range. Practice drills will be performed for each prosthetic joint to maximize functional use and minimize extraneous movement and energy.

LIFELONG CARE

After learning to control and use the prosthesis, the client is ready to begin incorporating prosthetic use in activities. There are five characteristics of advanced functional skills training that can assist in guiding the treatment plan:[14]

1. The client's rehabilitation plan is individualized, and each person has their own set of goals.
2. The client uses tools or interacts with an object such as a writing utensil or sports equipment.
3. Advanced prosthetic training involves complex, multistep tasks that are typically bimanual.
4. Training involves the client's prosthetic device of choice.
5. Activity selection and training is meaningful to the client.

Advanced functional use training will focus on incorporation of the prosthesis into basic and instrumental ADLs. There are many ways to accomplish most tasks; therefore the therapist will guide the client through use of the prosthesis in an efficient way that is practical and allows them to meet their goals. Different TDs can also be used to facilitate ADL and instrumental ADL performance (see Fig. 31.5 for an example of customized TD for bathing). Clients are also taught to analyze each activity and its relation to the environment. Often the environment in which the activity is performed can be modified or used to assist the client in activity performance. When possible, the therapist should bring clients into the actual environment in which the activity is performed to promote realistic training and allow the client to use their prosthesis in a meaningful way. In general, individuals with unilateral upper limb amputation can learn quickly how to adapt and perform activities with one hand. Education can be provided on different strategies to incorporate the prosthesis into bimanual activities for stabilization or support. Clients with unilateral or bilateral upper limb amputations often incorporate adaptive equipment into their daily life to achieve maximal independence. Adaptive equipment may include items such as a rocker knife for cutting, suction cup brushes for bathing, zipper pulls on jackets to increase ease of dressing, and a bidet for toileting. Examples of assistive devices are provided in Fig. 31.6.

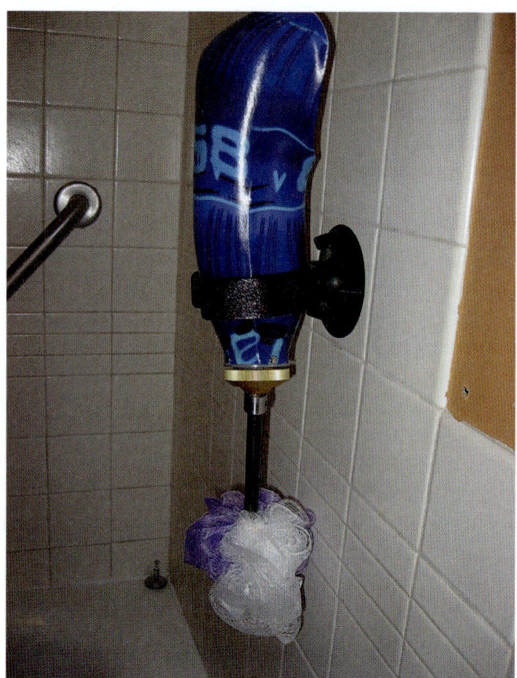

Fig. 31.5 Customized prothesis for bathing.

Recreational and vocational activities, community reintegration, driving, and adaptive sports are part of advanced functional skills training. There are a variety of recreational activities and adaptive sports available for individuals with all levels of upper limb amputations. Each member of the interdisciplinary team plays a key role in promoting participation in meaningful activities, recreation and adaptive sports as part of the rehabilitation program. Modifications can be made to prosthetic devices to allow for participation in ADLs and adaptive sports programs (Fig. 31.7). This allows for the opportunity to train in advanced functional use of the client's prosthetic system of choice or of their activity-specific prosthetic device. Participation in adaptive sports and recreation not only promotes advanced use of the prosthesis but also promotes social and psychological health that assists individuals with limb loss to focus on their abilities rather than their limitations.[42] After the end of the rehabilitation, people with upper limb amputation will continue to learn and develop their own strategies to accomplish their goals with support networks and resources from the broader community.[39]

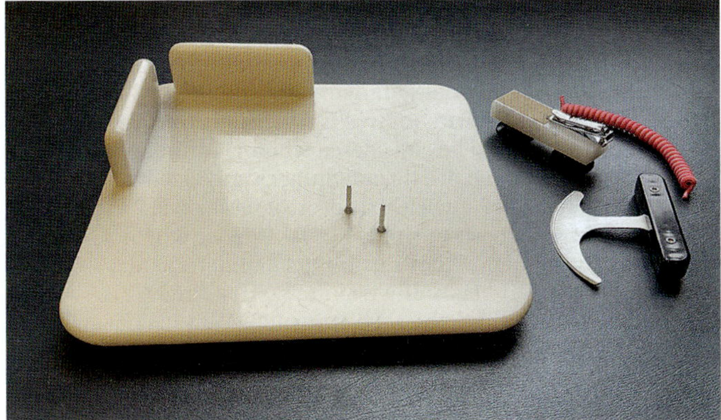

Fig. 31.6 Assistive devices to facilitate activities of daily living with one hand. Left: adaptative cutting board, top middle: nail clipper with suction cup base, top right: no tie elastic shoelace, and bottom right: rocker knife.

After the end of the rehabilitation, people with upper limb amputation should be followed at least every year to assess any changes in medical or functional status and ensure the prothesis still fits and functions properly. Social support systems should also be evaluated. As indicated, the client should be referred to specialists. Strategies about secondary complication prevention can be useful to continue during annual follow-up visits.[9]

Prosthesis Abandonment

Despite rehabilitation efforts and improvement in technology, dissatisfaction with the available technology and prothesis abandonment remains high among people with upper limb amputations.[3,31,43,44] In adults with upper limb amputations, a literature review identified mean rejection rates of 26% for body-powered protheses and 23% for myoelectric prostheses.[44] The decision to wear or not protheses is influenced by predisposing factors, including origin of limb amputation, gender, bilateral amputation, and, most importantly, level of limb amputation.[44] Another significant factor influencing acceptance of the prosthetic device is early fitting.[31,44] When medically able, early fittings have been shown to increase the client's incorporation of the prosthesis into daily activities and increase functional use

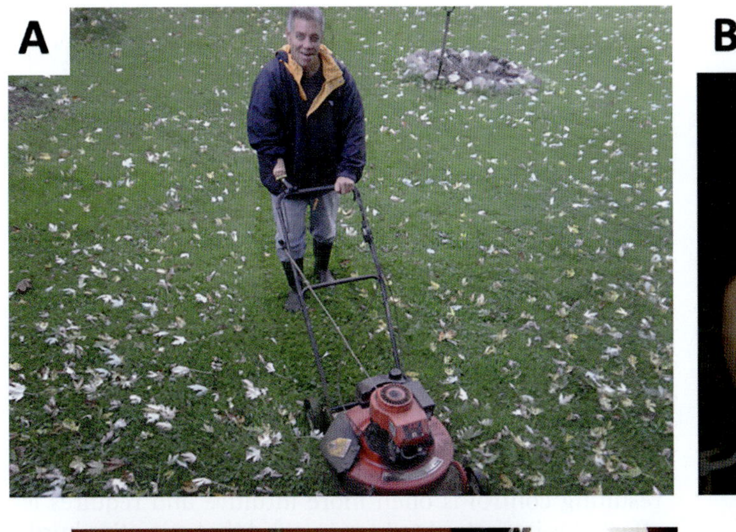

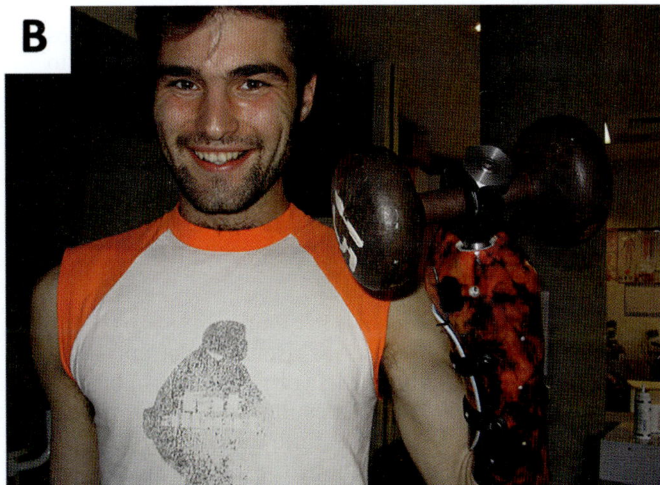

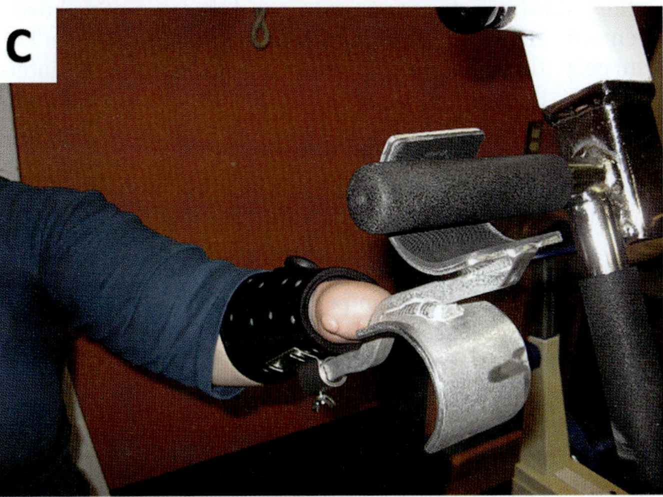

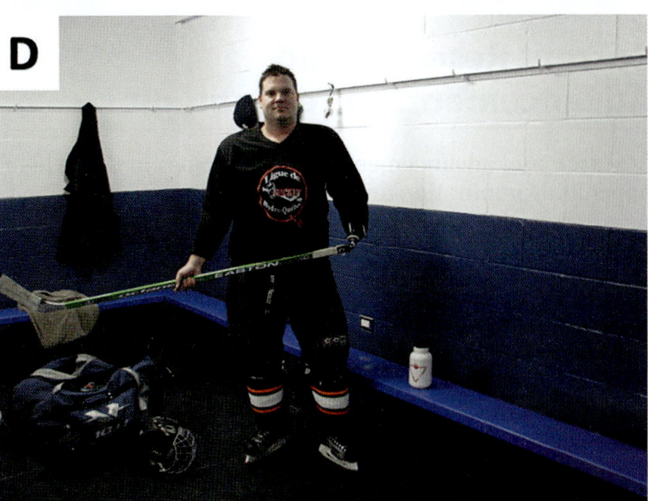

Fig. 31.7 Custom modifications to upper limb prosthetic devices allow instrumental activities of daily living, leisure, or sports: (A) mow the lawn or use a bicycle, (B) lift weights, (C) train at the gym, and (D) play hockey.

Case Example 31.3 A Client With Bilateral Upper Limb Amputation After Electrocution

E.H. is a 19-year-old college freshman studying to become a marine biologist. Six months ago, he participated in a school project on a boat with an instructor and other students to measure lake depth and take samples of underwater plants. The day before, the local power company had begun stringing power lines that extended over the edge of the lake and inadvertently left these wires lower than intended. E.H. was using an aluminum pole to measure water depth and accidentally touched these live wires with the pole. He was immediately electrocuted, rendered unconscious, and fell into the water. The other students pulled him from the lake and resuscitated him. He was medically evacuated to the trauma center, where he was found to have burns on both hands and forearms. The entrance wound, where the electrical current entered his body, was in his right (dominant) hand. The exit wounds were in his left forearm and thigh. As a result of the burns and subsequent tissue damage, amputation was necessary on the right side at the midtransradial level and on the left at midhumeral level; he received a skin graft on his left thigh and left arm.

E.H. was hospitalized for 2 months near his home and then discharged to live with his family (parents and brother) and receive outpatient therapy. At the time of discharge, in addition to bilateral upper limb ROM limitations, E.H. had severe balance deficits and limited lower limb strength and flexibility bilaterally. He was completely dependent in ADLs.

Three months later, he was referred to an outpatient prosthetic center for prosthetic fitting and therapy. The goal is to train him to use his prostheses to become as independent as possible, including returning to school to pursue his career in marine biology. E.H.'s wounds are well healed. His arms are well contoured, show minimal edema, and have few adhesions and full ROM. Hip flexion is limited to 85 degrees, extension to neutral. He is able to stand on the right foot for 20 seconds and the left for 5 seconds. Because of inactivity, E.H. is 40 lb overweight. E.H. received his prostheses 3 weeks after beginning prosthetic rehabilitation.

QUESTIONS TO CONSIDER

- What tests and measures are currently appropriate? What are the most important goals in his current rehabilitation phase? How will his goals change as prosthetic rehabilitation progresses? How many weeks will likely be required?
- What factors should be considered when planning prosthetic options? What are the advantages and disadvantages of body-powered or myoelectric prostheses for E.H.? Will one type of prosthesis meet his needs? Why or why not?
- Should his initial prosthetic training be unilateral or bilateral? Why? If beginning training with a single prosthesis, which side should be targeted? Why? What basic components should be recommended for each of his prostheses?
- How can the team assist E.H. in learning to use his myoelectric devices? What control motions are needed for the right (transradial) side? What motions are needed for the left (transhumeral) side? How might E.H. progress from simple activity to more complex and functional activities with his TDs to facilitate learning while minimizing frustration?
- What effect does elbow function have on hand positioning? How will elbow function affect the use of his transradial prosthesis? What is the sequence that E.H. needs to master to control elbow function of his transhumeral prosthesis? What kinds of activities would help him to master elbow control in both single-limb and bimanual tasks? How would training tasks be graded to ensure success?
- What vocational and recreational activities can be integrated into E.H.'s rehabilitation plan to assist him in meeting his goals?

for bimanual tasks.[31,44] Perceived usefulness of one's prosthesis also contributes to actual use of prostheses in basic and instrumental ADLs.[39,45] These results stress the importance of providing people with upper limb amputation with individualized and targeted prosthetic training to increase optimal, active prosthesis use in ADLs.[45]

Current Research and Advancements in Technologies

Research and advancements in technologies in the field of upper limb amputation and prosthetics continue to expand. As a result of the collaboration between various medical, engineering, government, academic, and research institutions, advancements are being made in upper limb prosthetic socket design, signal control schemes, prosthetic componentry, and surgical techniques. The next section will describe four new advancements in technologies: Targeted muscle reinnervation, sensory feedback, pattern recognition, and osteointegration.

Targeted muscle reinnervation (TMR) is a surgical technique used to increase the number of myosites available in the residual limb to enhance prosthetic control.[46] This surgical procedure takes residual nerves in the arm and transfers them to surgically denervated areas of unused musculature in the residual limb or chest.[47] The EMG signals of the target muscle now correspond to the motor commands of the limb. The resulting myosites, when successful, correspond physiologically to the prosthetic control functions. While resulting control is often more intuitive and requires less effort, it is important to keep in mind that cognitive burden remains high. In a transhumeral amputation with TMR surgery, the distal radial nerve will innervate the lateral head of the triceps for hand open and the median nerve will innervate the short head of the biceps for hand close.[47] The structured rehabilitation protocol developed in a recent Delphi study by Sturma et al.[48] can be used to guide rehabilitation for people undergoing high upper limb TMR surgery. TMR has also been shown to elicit a targeted sensory reinnervation in which sensory nerves in the residual limb can be redirected, resulting in perceived touch of the phantom limb. Targeted sensory reinnervation is being researched to provide sensory feedback within a prosthetic device.[49]

One key area of research is exploring ways to provide precise control and sensory feedback to upper limb prosthetic devices.[50] The Hand Proprioception and Touch Interfaces (HAPTIX) program is part of the Defense Advanced Research Project Agency. HAPTIX technologies are being designed to use sensory and motor signals in the residual limb to allow the individual to control their prosthetic device with the same neural signaling used for their intact limbs.[50] The goal is to provide intuitive control of multiple degrees of freedom of the hand while providing sensory feedback to improve grip force, precision, and proprioception with a prosthesis.

Pattern recognition is a type of myoelectric control that uses multiple surface electrodes versus the typical two-site control scheme to recognize the pattern that is generated by the muscle contractions in the residual limb.[37] Pattern recognition does not require isolated myosites for control; instead, it allows the individual to control the various movements of the prosthetic device by reproducing the natural motions of the amputated limb and translating that pattern into prosthetic control. To be effective, pattern recognition requires additional muscle signal input. In more proximal amputation levels, such as shoulder disarticulation and transhumeral amputations, the use of TMR enhances the myoelectric signals available for control. Pattern recognition paired with TMR surgery optimizes those myoelectric signals in the residual limb to create more natural, intuitive prosthetic control for the myoelectric prosthesis.[51,52]

Osseointegration (OI) is a surgical procedure that provides direct skeletal attachment of a prosthetic device to the residual limb.[53] An implant is surgically fixed into the bone of the residual limb, with a skin-penetrating abutment for skeletal attachment of the prosthesis. This procedure eliminates the need for a prosthetic socket or suspension system.[54] OI was developed as an alternative for individuals with upper and lower limb amputation who have difficulty using a conventional prosthetic system because of issues such as skin breakdown, residual limb length, or shape and have significant limitations in function.

Summary

This chapter presents rehabilitation techniques and interventions for adults with upper limb amputation, including perioperative care, preprosthetic training, basic prosthetic training, and lifelong care. Expertise on the part of the interdisciplinary team is essential in the rehabilitation of upper limb amputations, with the client having an active and central role in this team. Comprehensive evaluation and a client-centered approach to therapeutic intervention, combined with effective communication with the interdisciplinary team, can make the rehabilitation process rewarding while ensuring the best functional outcomes for clients with upper limb loss are achieved.

Acknowledgments

I would like to acknowledge the contributions of Marie-Hélène Forest, occupational therapist, and Josée Dubois, certified prosthetist from the Centre intégré universitaire de santé et de services sociaux du Centre-Sud-de-l'île-de-Montréal, Institut de réadaptation Gingras-Lindsay de-Montréal, for their valuable clinical expertise.

References

The complete listing of the References are available in the accompanying enhanced eBook version included with the print purchase of this textbook. Visit Elsevier eBooks+ (eBooks.Health.Elsevier.com) to access this content.

Index

Note: Page numbers followed by *f* indicate figures, *t* indicate tables, and *b* indicate boxes.

J

K

L

M

T

V

W

Y

Z